Pediatric Skills

for Occupational Therapy Assistants

Pediatric Skills
for Occupational Therapy Assistants

4TH EDITION

JEAN WELCH SOLOMON, MHS, OTR/L, FAOTA

Occupational Therapist
Berkeley County School District
Moncks Corner, South Carolina

JANE CLIFFORD O'BRIEN, PhD, MS, EdL, OTR/L, FAOTA

Professor
Department of Occupational Therapy
University of New England
Portland, Maine

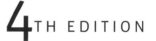

ELSEVIER

3251 Riverport Lane
St. Louis, Missouri 63043

Content Strategy Director: Penny Rudolph
Content Development Manager: Ellen Wurm-Cutter
Associate *Content Development Specialist:* Katie Gutierrez
Publishing Services Manager: Jeff Patterson
Senior Project Manager: Jodi M. Willard
Design Direction: Ryan Cook

Printed in United States of America

Last digit is the print number: 9 8 7 6 5 4 3 2 1

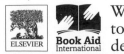

We dedicate this edition to OTA and OT students, COTAs, and OTRs who use the knowledge gained from reading this textbook to provide the best evidence-based occupational therapy services to children and adolescents and their families, teachers, and others actively engaged in their lives.

Contributors

Patricia Bowyer, EdD, MS, OTR, FAOTA
Associate Director/Professor
School of Occupational Therapy—
    Houston
Institute of Health Sciences
Texas Medical Center
Texas Woman's University
Houston, Texas
Applying the Model of Human Occupation
    to Pediatric Practice

Gilson J. Capilouto, PhD, CCC-SLP, FASHA
Professor and Director of Undergraduate
    Research
College of Health Sciences
University of Kentucky
Lexington, Kentucky
Assistive Technology

Ricardo C. Carrasco, PhD, OTR/L, FAOTA
Professor and Founding Chair
Entry Level Doctor of Occupational
    Therapy (OTD) Program
Department of Occupational Therapy
College of Health Care Sciences
Nova Southeastern University—Tampa
Tampa, Florida
Sensory Processing /Integration and
    Occupation

Nancy Carson, PhD, MHS, OTR/L
Associate Dean for Academic and
    Faculty Affairs
Associate Professor, Occupational
    Therapy Division
Medical University of South Carolina
Charleston, South Carolina
Community Systems

Judith Clifford Cohn, MS, SpEd
Certified Elementary School Teacher
Certified Therapist in Pet-Assisted
    Therapy
Barrington, Rhode Island
Animal-Assisted Activities and Therapy

Patty C. Coker-Bolt, PhD, OTR/L, FAOTA
Associate Professor
Department of Health Professions
Medical University of South Carolina
Charleston, South Carolina
Cerebral Palsy
Positioning and Handling: A
    Neurodevelopmental Approach

Elizabeth W. Crampsey, MS, OTR/L, BCPR
Assistant Clinical Professor
Department of Occupational Therapy
University of New England
Portland, Maine
Play and Playfulness
Motor Control and Motor Learning

Michelle Desjardins, MS, OTR/L, CBIS
Adjunct Clinical Professor
Department of Occupational Therapy
University of New Hampshire
Durham, New Hampshire
Activities of Daily Living and Sleep/Rest

Nadine K. Hanner, MSOT, OTR/L
Faculty, Academic Fieldwork
    Coordinator
OTA Program
Trident Technical College
North Charleston, South Carolina
Therapeutic Media: Activity with Purpose

Karen S. Howell, PhD, OTR/L, FAOTA
Chair, Institute of Occupational Therapy
Department of Occupational Therapy
University of St. Augustine
St. Augustine, Florida
Neurosciences for the Pediatric Practitioner

Caryn Husman, MS, OTR/L
Assistant Professor
Health, Wellness, and Occupational
    Studies
University of New England
Biddeford, Maine
Instrumental Activities of Daily Living

Jane Kleinert, PhD, CCC-SLP
Associate Professor
Division of Communication Sciences and
    Disorders
University of Kentucky
Lexington, Kentucky
Assistive Technology

Jessica M. Kramer, PhD, OTR/L
Assistant Professor
Department of Occupational Therapy and
    PhD Program in Rehabilitation Sciences
Boston University
Boston, Massachusetts
Applying the Model of Human Occupation
    to Pediatric Practice

Melissa E. Kronberger, BA, COTA/L
Academic Fieldwork Coordinator
Occupational Therapy Assistant Program
American Career College
Anaheim, California;
Former Faculty Member
Stanbridge College
Irvine, California
Medical Systems

Dianne Koontz Lowman, EdD
Director of Counseling and Advocacy
Safe Harbor
Richmond, Virginia
Principles of Normal Development
Development of Performance Skills
Development of Occupations

Angela Chinners Marsh, AHS, COTA/L
Occupational Therapy Assistant
Department of Exceptional Children's
Services
Charleston County School District
Charleston, South Carolina
Therapeutic Media: Activity with Purpose

Margaret Q. Miller, MS, OTR/L, C/NDT
Clinical Specialist
Department of Occupational Therapy
St. Luke's Rehabilitation Institute;
Adjunct Faculty Member
Occupational Therapy Assistant Program
Spokane Falls Community College
Spokane, Washington
Pediatric Health Conditions

Erin Naber, BS, DPT
Senior Physical Therapist
Fairmount Rehabilitation Programs
Institution Kennedy Krieger Institute
Baltimore, Maryland
Cerebral Palsy

Randi Carlson Neideffer, AA, AHS(OT), MSOT, OTR/L
Department of Exceptional Children
Services
Charleston Country School District
Charleston, South Carolina
Therapeutic Media: Activity with Purpose

Jane Clifford O'Brien, PhD, MS, EdL, OTR/L, FAOTA
Professor
Department of Occupational Therapy
University of New England
Portland, Maine
Scope of Practice
Development of Performance Skills
The Occupational Therapy Process
Childhood and Adolescent Psychosocial and
*   Mental Health Disorders*
Play and Playfulness

Mashelle K. Painter, MEd, COTA/L
Faculty, Distance Education
    Coordinator
Occupational Therapy Assistant
    Program
Linn-Benton Community College
Lebanon, Oregon
Educational Systems
Animal-Assisted Activities and Therapy

Mary Elizabeth Patnaude, MS, OTR/L
Assistant Clinical Professor
Department of Occupational
    Therapy
University of New England
Portland, Maine
Motor Control and Motor Learning

Teressa Garcia Reidy, MS, OTR/L
Senior Occupational Therapist
Fairmount Rehabilitation Programs
Constraint Induced and Bimanual
    Intensive Programs
Kennedy Krieger Institute
Baltimore, Maryland
Cerebral Palsy

Deborah A. Schwartz, OTD, OTR/L, CHT
Product and Educational Specialist
Department of Physical
    Rehabilitation
Orfit Industries America
Leonia, New Jersey
Orthoses, Orthotic Fabrication, and Elastic
*   Therapeutic Taping for the Pediatric*
*   Practitioner*

Jean Welch Solomon, MHS, OTR/L, FAOTA
Occupational Therapist
Berkeley County School District
Moncks Corner, South Carolina
Scope of Practice
Educational System
Principles of Normal Development
The Occupational Therapy Process
Anatomy and Physiology for the Pediatric
*   Practitioner*
Childhood and Adolescent Psychosocial and
*   Mental Health Disorders*
Intellectual Disabilities
Functional Task at School: Handwriting

Susan A. Stallings-Sahler, PhD, OTR/L, C/SI, C/NDT, FAOTA
Professor
School of Occupational Therapy
Brenau University—North Atlanta
    Campus
Norcross, Georgia;
Executive Director
Sensational Kids Pediatric
    Rehabilitation, Inc.
Augusta, Georgia
Sensory Processing/Integration and
*   Occupation*

Barbara J. Steva, MS, OTR/L
Independent Contractor
Saco, Maine
Instrumental Activities of Daily Living

Kerryellen G. Vroman, PhD
Associate Professor, Department Chair
Department of Occupational Therapy
University of New Hampshire
Durham, New Hampshire
Adolescent Development: Becoming an
*   Adult*
Childhood and Adolescent Psychosocial and
*   Mental Health Disorders*
Childhood and Adolescent Obesity

Pamela J. Winton, BA, MA, PhD
Senior Scientist and Outreach Director
Frank Porter Graham Child
    Development Institute
University of North Carolina at Chapel
    Hill
Chapel Hill, North Carolina
Family Systems

Robert E. Winton, MD
Psychiatrist, Private Practice
Duke University Psychiatry Department,
    Retired
Durham, North Carolina
Family Systems

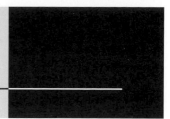

Preface

This book has been written for the occupational therapy assistant (OTA) student and the certified occupational therapy assistant (COTA) working in the pediatric practice setting. The language is consistent with the *Occupational Therapy Practice Framework* (3rd edition).[1] Each chapter emphasizes practical information that may readily be used by students, certified occupational therapy assistants (COTA), and entry-level registered occupational therapists (OTR) who work with children and adolescents. Theories, frames of reference, and practice models are introduced and integrated into the content so they can be easily applied. When possible, the text differentiates between the roles of the COTA and OTR. The term *occupational therapy practitioner* refers to OTRs and COTAs and is used during discussions of procedures that can be performed by either.

All of the chapters contain the following elements: outline, key terms, objectives, summary, review questions, and suggested activities to help readers understand material and apply concepts in practice. Each chapter begins with an outline that identifies the main topics included in each chapter. Key terms are listed in the order they appear in the text and are bolded within the text. The chapter objectives concisely outline the material readers will learn from studying the chapter. A summary at the end of each chapter reemphasizes the key points of the chapter. Review questions help readers synthesize the information presented. Suggested activities are designed to reinforce information in interesting ways. These activities can be completed individually or in small groups.

Boxes, case studies, tables, and figures are used throughout the chapters to reiterate, exemplify, or illustrate specific points. Interspersed throughout each chapter are "Clinical Pearls"—words of wisdom based on the authors' clinical expertise. The clinical pearls contain helpful hints or reminders that have been consistently useful for OT practitioners working with children and youth. Several chapters include additional appendixes useful in clinical practice.

The first five chapters present an overall framework of occupational therapy practice with children and youth and the settings in which practitioners work. Chapter 1, *Scope of Practice*, provides an overview of occupational therapy practice with children and youth, including a discussion of recommended pediatric curriculum content, selected practice models, COTA supervision, establishment of service competency, and a review of the OT Code of Ethics. The next four chapters—*Family*

Systems (Chapter 2), *Medical Systems* (Chapter 3), *Educational Systems* (Chapter 4), and *Community Systems* (Chapter 5)—delineate the variety of settings in which practitioners who work with children and families practice and describe contexts, team members, intervention approaches, and laws governing occupational therapy services.

The next group of chapters provides readers with an overview of typical development that serves as a foundation for clinical practice. *Principles of Normal Development* (Chapter 6) offers an overview of the periods and principles of normal development. Using the *Occupational Therapy Practice Framework*[1] as a guide, *Development of Performance Skills* (Chapter 7) explains the development of performance skills from infancy to adolescence. *Development of Occupations* (Chapter 8) presents information about the typical sequence of development of areas of occupation (e.g., education, feeding, dressing, bathing, toileting, play, rest, and sleep). *Adolescent Development: Becoming an Adult* (Chapter 9) portrays the uniqueness of adolescence and the journey into adulthood.

The Occupational Therapy Process (Chapter 10) addresses the manner in which OT practitioners evaluate, intervene, and measure outcomes of intervention. The authors provide an overview of documentation, practice models (frames of reference), and measurements using a variety of case examples. An explanation of anatomy, physiology, and neuroscience structures, functions, and terminology for practice with children and youth are covered in Chapter 11 (*Anatomy and Physiology for the Pediatric Practitioner*) and Chapter 12 (*Neuroscience for the Pediatric Practitioner*).

A variety of chapters explain the etiology, signs, and symptoms of pediatric conditions/disorders that an OT practitioner may encounter and include current intervention models and strategies. Chapter 13 (*Pediatric Health Conditions*) describes a variety of medical conditions, and Chapter 14 (*Childhood and Adolescent Psychosocial and Mental Health Disorders*) reviews disorders affecting psychosocial functioning. Chapter 15, *Childhood and Adolescent Obesity*, explores issues surrounding the health and wellness of children and includes information on intervention planning specific to this population. Two common conditions are examined in Chapter 16 (*Intellectual Disabilities*) and Chapter 17 (*Cerebral Palsy*). Specific intervention strategies for children with cerebral palsy are outlined in Chapter 18 (*Positioning and Handling: A Neurodevelopmental Approach*) using case studies to illustrate its application to practice.

Chapters 19 through 22 examine areas of intervention of primary importance to OT practitioners and include specific strategies for intervention related to occupations, specifically, *Activities of Daily Living and Sleep/Rest* (Chapter 19), *Instrumental Activities of Daily Living* (Chapter 20), *Play and Playfulness* (Chapter 21) and *Functional Task at School: Handwriting* (Chapter 22). Each chapter elaborates on intervention techniques, strategies, and outcomes using case studies to illustrate key concepts and principles.

OT practitioners often use media to assist children in achieving their therapeutic goals. Chapter 23 (*Therapeutic Media: Activity with Purpose*) provides sample activities, describes grading and adapting activities, and outlines the process for matching activities to children's therapeutic goals. Chapter 24 (*Motor Control and Motor Learning*) describes principles that practitioners may use to teach motor skills. The authors provide an overview of research evidence while outlining strategies that can easily be implemented in practice with a variety of children and adolescents.

The remaining chapters explore specialized areas of practice. *Sensory Processing/Integration and Occupation* (Chapter 25) defines sensory processing and integration, describes intervention strategies, and discusses the underlying theory and principles of a sensory integrative approach. *Applying the Model of Human Occupation to Pediatric Practice* (Chapter 26) defines the components of this model and describes how it can be applied to design and conduct effective intervention for children and youth. *Assistive Technology* (Chapter 27) explains the process of selecting assistive technology and gives examples of types of assistive technology. *Orthoses, Orthotic Fabrication, and Elastic Therapeutic Taping for the Pediatric Population* (Chapter 28) reviews types of orthoses, describes principles and reasoning related to orthotic fabrication, and summarizes strategies and principles regarding elastic therapeutic taping (e.g., kinesio taping). The final chapter, *Animal-Assisted Activities and Therapy* (Chapter 29), presents readers with innovative ideas for incorporating animals in occupational therapy practice with children and youth. The authors provide examples of pet-assisted therapy projects.

This book has evolved from many years of teaching pediatric skills to students and is intended to present readers with theoretical and practical knowledge required for occupational therapy practice with children and youth. All chapters have been revised and updated to reflect current professional philosophy, research, and practice. A new chapter has been added on neuroscience to better prepare practitioners for practice. Case examples are embedded throughout to illustrate concepts more clearly. Each chapter offers numerous clinical pearls based on the expertise of the author. Readers are urged to examine the tables, boxes, and figures that clarify topics. This fourth edition includes additional content throughout to assist readers in applying concepts to occupational therapy intervention for children and youth. Chapters are written in clear and concise language, with numerous examples to help readers understand and use concepts to design and implement interventions. In addition to the textbook, the Evolve Learning Site has been updated and revised to better meet the reader's needs.

The Evolve Learning Site includes new material (e.g., video clips, student multiple-choice questions, and Web resources) to help readers comprehend information and apply it in practice. A variety of video clips are available to illustrate key concepts from specific chapters. For example, video clips illustrate the use of therapeutic media, hand skill intervention, play, dressing, and feeding. Additional video clips display typical and atypical development, family-centered care, and community and rehabilitation intervention. To develop increased observational skills, questions are supplied for readers to consider while viewing video clips. Student multiple-choice questions (with rationales) assist in focusing student reading and are designed to cue students toward important content. Students are urged to examine the questions and review content in the textbook to reinforce learning. The Evolve Learning Site also includes a compilation of websites that provide resources useful in practice. For example, websites regarding orthotic material, assistive technology, therapeutic media ideas, and creative intervention plans are provided.

The fourth edition of *Pediatric Skills for Occupational Therapy Assistants* represents the expertise of an impressive group of contributing authors who have developed up-to-date, practical, and innovative material. The authors represent expertise in a variety of areas. We are grateful to the authors, reviewers, and contributors for their wisdom and skill. We hope you will enjoy reading and using all the learning materials provided in the textbook and Evolve Learning Site.

Jean Welch Solomon

Jane Clifford O'Brien

1. American Occupational Therapy Association. (2014). Occupational therapy practice framework: domain and process (3rd ed.). *Am J Occup Ther*, 68(Suppl. 1), S1–S48.

Acknowledgments

On this fourth edition, we had the opportunity to work with many talented and dedicated professionals who are passionate about the care of children and youth who have special needs. The authors come from various areas of the country, represent a wide range of practice areas, and have extensive clinical experience and knowledge that they share with the readers. It was fun and exciting reconnecting with colleagues and friends who participated in this project, and we are thankful for their work. We thank Morgan Midgett Taylor for transforming our words into pictures/illustrations and for having such patience for requested detailed changes. Jordan Hennsley (Berkeley County School District, Moncks Corner, South Carolina) provided many photographs of children who attend St. Stephen Elementary School. MaryBeth Patnaude, Barbara Price, Scott McNeil, Judy Cohn, Caitlin Cassis, Keeley Heidtman, and numerous contributing authors also provided photographs to illustrate concepts.

We acknowledge the following people for their work providing quality video for the Evolve materials: Dr. Elaine Norton; Kayla Drake, COTA/L; and children Liahna, Nicholas, Gabby, Jacob, and Annslee. Furthermore, we are appreciative of the children and families and team members with whom we work and who have inspired much of the writing throughout this textbook. We also acknowledge Henry Powell (Class of 2016); Scott O'Brien, Brendan Salvas, and Kelly Dolyak (Class of 2017); and Kelcey Briggs (Class of 2017) who were all so positive and helped on short notice with the Evolve materials and glossary.

We appreciate the hard work of the Elsevier editorial and production staff—Penny Rudolph, Jolynn Gower, Katie Gutierrez, Jodi Willard, and Ryan Cook. It has been such a pleasure working with everyone on this textbook.

Contents

JEAN WELCH SOLOMON
JANE CLIFFORD O'BRIEN

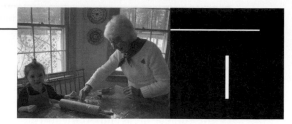

Scope of Practice

CHAPTER *Objectives*

After studying this chapter, the reader will be able to accomplish the following:

- Describe the centennial vision of the American Occupational Therapy Association (AOTA).
- Describe the basics of the *Occupational Therapy Practice Framework: Domain and Process,* 3rd edition, and its relationship to clinical practice.
- Identify eight subject areas in which entry-level certified occupational therapy assistants need to have general knowledge.
- Describe the four levels at which registered occupational therapists supervise occupational therapy assistants.
- Define service competency and give examples of ways it may be obtained.
- Outline AOTA's Code of Ethics and apply the code to pediatric practice.
- Define and give examples of the different types of scholarship in which practitioners may engage.

CHAPTER *Outline*

This chapter provides an overview of occupational therapy (OT) practice with children and adolescents. The chapter begins with a discussion of the subject areas important in pediatric OT curriculum followed by a description of the centennial vision of the American Occupational Therapy Association (AOTA), with respect to issues of children and youth. To understand the OT process, a review of the Occupational Therapy Practice Framework: Domain and Process (OTPF) is provided. Using case examples, the authors provide descriptions of levels of supervision and service competency requirements. The scope of OT practice with children and adolescents would not be complete without an understanding of the AOTA Code of Ethics. Lastly, the authors emphasize lifelong learning scholarship to enhance practice.

During the past 20 years, significant changes have occurred in the provision of pediatric OT services.[2,3,8] Numerous federal laws that expand the services available to infants, children, and adolescents who have special needs or disabilities have been implemented. Approximately 20% of all occupational therapy assistants (OTAs) work in pediatric settings.[11] OT practitioners provide pediatric services in medical settings such as outpatient clinics and hospitals, as well as in community settings such as schools, homes, and daycare centers.[11] Because numerous practitioners work with infants, children, and adolescents, it is important that both entry-level occupational therapists and OTAs have a solid foundation in pediatrics.

The AOTA has identified eight subject areas to be included in any pediatric curriculum.[4,8] An entry-level OT practitioner must have knowledge in the following areas:

Normal development: OT practitioners working with children who have special needs or atypical development patterns must have a firm knowledge of normal development and the expected range of performance to understand children and design effective interventions. (See Chapters 6 to 9.)

Importance of families in the OT process: Families are the most consistent participants on the pediatric team and are central to the child's well-being. Understanding the needs of families and children is essential to the therapeutic process. (See Chapter 2.)

Specific pediatric diagnoses: Pediatric OT practitioners use knowledge of specific pediatric diagnoses as a guideline for determining which assessments, strategies, and methods are the most appropriate for the child or youth. OT practitioners use knowledge of the diagnosis to understand factors such as prognosis, precautions, medical interventions, and guidelines that are considered in practice decisions. (See Chapters 3, 13, 14, 15, 16, 17.)

OT practice models (i.e., frames of reference): Understanding models of practice and frames of reference are necessary for organizing and developing interventions based on evidence from the profession. Knowledge of the principles and techniques allows OT practitioners to develop interventions for children with a variety of diagnoses and conditions. Understanding the theory and principles for intervention allows practitioners to develop intervention plans for children with a variety of conditions interfering with occupational performance. (See Chapters 10, 18, 22, 23, 24, 25, 26, 27, 28.)

Assessments appropriate for a child with a specific disability or diagnosis: OT practitioners work with children and youth who have a variety of conditions and diagnoses that interfere with occupational performance. Therefore OT practitioners must have knowledge of a variety of assessments as well as the ability to use clinical reasoning to choose, interpret results of, develop, and carry out intervention plans. Practitioners also use data from assessments to measure outcomes of interventions. (Interspersed throughout chapters).

Age-appropriate activities: OT practitioners working with children need to adjust therapy activities to suit the age, developmental needs, and intervention goals of each individual child. Knowledge of a range of age-appropriate activities and the ability to carefully analyze the client factors required for performance is essential to practice. OT practitioners use creative activities to address occupational performance goals. (See Chapters 6, 7, 8, 9, 20, 21, 29.)

Differences among systems in which OT services are provided: OT services are provided in a variety of settings. These settings exist within systems that have different missions. OT practitioners work within these settings and design interventions to meet the needs of their clients as well as those of the system. For example, children receiving services in a public school system require educationally relevant therapy goals and objectives, whereas children receiving services in a hospital require medically necessary goals and objectives that allow them to engage in a variety of occupations. (See Chapters 1, 2, 3, 4, 5.)

Assistive technology: OT practitioners who work with infants, children, and adolescents with disabilities or special needs must have knowledge of the range of assistive technologies that promote safe and independent living and allow children to engage in a variety of occupations. (See Chapter 27.)

CENTENNIAL VISION

In 2017, the OT profession will be 100 years old. AOTA developed a **centennial vision** that recognizes occupational therapy as a science-driven and evidence-based profession that continues to meet the occupational needs of clients, communities, and populations.[1] To reach this vision, AOTA is actively promoting that OT practitioners assume leadership roles and contribute to outcome databases that support evidence-based practice.[1]

The centennial vision specifically addresses areas of pediatric practice, including the health and wellness of children and youth (e.g., programs to prevent childhood obesity), and the psychosocial needs of this population.[7] AOTA, through its vision, suggests that practitioners continue to provide evidence of the importance of occupation and intervention.[1] The centennial vision advocates that practitioners working with children and youth develop programs for children with autism, target the mental health issues of children and youth, use standardized assessments to measure outcomes, and disseminate intervention results. The vision encourages practitioners to become leaders in the profession and to support the profession through participation in AOTA, scholarship (at many different levels), and clinical practice.[1]

OCCUPATIONAL THERAPY PRACTICE FRAMEWORK

The **Occupational Therapy Practice Framework: Domain and Process, 3rd edition** (the Framework) defines both the process and domain of occupational therapy.[6] (Subsequent chapters in this text discuss the Framework in detail and apply the concepts to practice.) The Framework was developed to assist practitioners in defining the process and domains of occupational therapy.[6] It is designed for use by occupational therapists, certified occupational therapists, consumers, and health care providers. Figure 1-1 identifies the domains of occupational therapy as areas of occupations, client factors,

performance skills, performance patterns, contexts and environments, and activity demands. Occupations include activities of daily living (ADLs), instrumental activities of daily living (IADLs), rest and sleep, education, work, play, leisure, and social participation.[6] OT practitioners examine client factors to determine how they are influencing occupations. Client factors include specific capacities and characteristics of beliefs that reside within the person and influence how they perform.[6] Client factors include values, beliefs and spirituality, body functions, and body structures.[6] For example, a child may have cerebral palsy, resulting in muscle tone that interferes with his ability to use his hand effectively (e.g., body function), influencing his ability to feed himself (area of occupation). His body functions (muscle tone) influence his occupations. Practitioners examine performance skills (sensory, motor, process, social, cognitive, and emotional skills) and patterns (habits, routines, roles, and rituals) associated with occupations. OT practitioners may design interventions to address all domains. Equally important is an examination of the contexts and environments in which an occupation occurs. According to the Framework, these contexts and environments are cultural, personal, physical, social, temporal, and virtual (Table 1-1). Contexts influence how an occupation is viewed, performed, and evaluated. For example, when considering the temporal context, practitioners expect differences in social behavior between a 2-year-old toddler and 6-year-old child. The practitioner evaluates the activity demands (objects, properties, social, space, actions, and body functions needed) as part of the occupational therapy process.

The Framework defines occupational therapy as a dynamic ongoing process that includes evaluation, intervention, and outcomes. Figure 1-2 presents a definition of each process of service delivery. *Evaluation* provides an understanding of the clients' problems, occupational

AREAS OF OCCUPATION	CLIENT FACTORS	PERFORMANCE SKILLS	PERFORMANCE PATTERNS	CONTEXT AND ENVIRONMENT	ACTIVITY DEMANDS
Activities of Daily Living (ADL)*	Values, Beliefs, and Spirituality	Sensory Perceptual Skills	Habits	Cultural	Objects Used and Their Properties
Instrumental Activities of Daily Living (IADL)	Body Functions	Motor and Praxis Skills	Routines	Personal	Space Demands
Rest and Sleep	Body Structures	Emotional Regulation Skills	Roles	Physical	Social Demands
Education		Cognitive Skills	Rituals	Social	Sequencing and Timing
Work		Communication and Social Skills		Temporal	Required Actions
Play				Virtual	Required Body Functions
Leisure					Required Body Structures
Social Participation					
*Also referred to as *basic activities of daily living (BADL)* or *personal activities of daily living (PADL)*.					

FIGURE 1-1 Aspects of occupational therapy's domain. All aspects of the domain transact to support engagement, participation, and health. This figure does not imply a hierarchy. (From the American Occupational Therapy Association. (2014). Occupational therapy practice framework: domain and process (3rd ed.). *Am J Occup Ther,* 68(Suppl. 1), S4.)

TABLE 1-1

*Definitions of Contexts**

CONTEXT	DEFINITION	EXAMPLE
Cultural	Customs, beliefs, activity patterns, behavior standards, and expectations accepted by the society of which the individual is a member. Includes political aspects, such as laws that affect access to resources and affirm personal rights. Also includes opportunities for education, employment, and economic support.	Family believes that mothers should stay home and care for children, while fathers work. The child is the youngest of three children. They live in a rural community where resources for children are limited. Considers factors such as ethnicity, family attitude, beliefs, values.
Personal	"[F]eatures of the individual that are not part of a health condition or health status."[1] Personal context includes age, gender, socioeconomic status, and educational status.	5-year-old boy who attends first grade classroom.
Physical	Nonhuman aspects of contexts. Includes accessibility to and performance within environments having natural terrain, plants, animals, buildings, furniture, objects, tools, or devices.	Child lives in a city with public transportation, park nearby, and many accessible buildings.
Social	Availability and expectations of significant individuals, such as spouse, friends, and caregivers. Also includes larger social groups that are influential in establishing norms, role expectations, and social routines.	Child engages in play with friends at school. She joined a dance class after school and enjoys going to school events with her two best friends. Relationships with individuals, groups, or organizations; relationships with systems (political, economic, institutional).
Temporal	"Location of occupational performance in time."[2]	Young child who is learning to separate from parents and develop friendships at school. Refers to stages of life, time of day, time of year, duration.
Virtual	Environment in which communication occurs by means of airways or computers and an absence of physical contact.	Adolescent who communicates with peers via Snapchat. Refers to situations such as those online that provide realistic simulation of an environment.

Adapted from the American Occupational Therapy Association (2014). Occupational therapy practice framework: domain and process (3rd ed.). *Am J Occup Ther, 68*(Suppl. I), S1–S48. http://dx.doi.org/10.5014/ajot.2014.682006
*Context refers to a variety of interrelated conditions within and surrounding the client that influence performance.
[1]World Health Organization (2001). *International classification of functioning, disability and health* (ICF). Geneva, Switzerland: WHO.
[2]Crepeau, E., Cohn, E., & Boyt-Schell, B. (2009). *Willard and Spackman's occupational therapy (11th ed.)*. Philadelphia: Lippincott Williams & Wilkins.

history, patterns, and assets.[6] *Intervention* includes the plan (based on selected theories, models of practice, frames of reference, and evidence), implementation, and review. *Outcome* refers to how well the goals are achieved. The practitioner and client collaborate throughout. The practitioner completes an occupational profile that informs the intervention plan, implementation, and review. However, a practitioner may also revisit the occupational profile during intervention as new information emerges. At the same time, the practitioner measures outcomes throughout the intervention. The context and environment may influence all stages of the process.

The Framework advocates that practitioners focus on occupations instead of its components. The goal of OT services is to enable children and youth to engage in daily occupations within their own environments

(Figure 1-3). For example, a practitioner may identify that poor hand skill is interfering with a child's ability to write in the classroom. Intervention may be targeted to improve hand skills. However, the practitioner who targets the occupation of success in the academic setting may provide the child with an alternative method (such as iPad access) to communicate in class and work on writing outside of class time. The goal is to enable the child's success in the occupation of academics (i.e., school).

THE OCCUPATIONAL THERAPY PROCESS

The OT practitioner uses a model of practice to organize his or her thinking and chooses a frame of reference to design interventions based on the child's and

---

EVALUATION

Occupational profile—The initial step in the evaluation process that provides an understanding of the client's occupational history and experiences, patterns of daily living, interests, values, and needs. The client's problems and concerns about performing occupations and daily life activities are identified, and the client's priorities are determined.

Analysis of occupational performance—The step in the evaluation process during which the client's assets, problems, or potential problems are more specifically identified. Actual performance is often observed in context to identify what supports performance and what hinders performance. Performance skills, performance patterns, context or contexts, activity demands, and client factors are all considered, but only selected aspects may be specifically assessed. Targeted outcomes are identified.

INTERVENTION

Intervention plan—A plan that will guide actions taken and that is developed in collaboration with the client. It is based on selected theories, frames of reference, and evidence. Outcomes to be targeted are confirmed.

Intervention implementation—Ongoing actions taken to influence and support improved client performance. Interventions are directed at identified outcomes. Client's response is monitored and documented.

Intervention review—A review of the implementation plan and process as well as its progress toward targeted outcomes.

OUTCOMES (Supporting Health and Participation in Life Through Engagement in Occupation)

Outcomes—Determination of success in reaching desired targeted outcomes. Outcome assessment information is used to plan future actions with the client and to evaluate the service program (i.e., program evaluation).

FIGURE 1-2 Process of service delivery. The process of service delivery is applied within the profession's domain to support the client's health and participation. (From the American Occupational Therapy Association (2014). Occupational therapy practice framework: domain and process (3rd ed.). *Am J Occup Ther, 68*(Suppl. 1), S10)

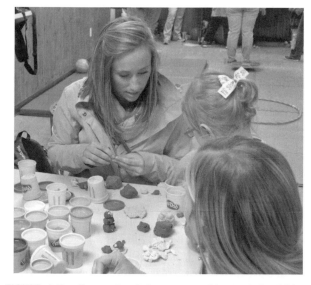

FIGURE 1-3 Occupational therapy practitioners help children engage in occupations such as play.

the family's needs (see Chapter 10 for specifics on model of practices and frames of reference). The frame of reference helps the practitioner decide what to do during therapy sessions. The OT process begins when a parent, physician, teacher, or other concerned professional requests a referral for occupational therapy. The OT decides whether the referred client should be screened to help determine whether the client will benefit from OT services.[3,8,9] If the screening shows that the child is likely to benefit from OT services, an evaluation is performed. The occupational therapist determines the areas to be evaluated and may assign portions of

the evaluation to an OTA. The evaluation process helps the occupational therapist identify the child's strengths and weaknesses. Long-term goals and short-term objectives are established on the basis of the occupational therapist's interpretation of the assessment. In collaboration with the OTA, the occupational therapist develops an intervention plan based on these goals and objectives[2] (Figure 1-4). Depending on the client's progress and periodic reassessments, the plan is implemented and modified. The intervention is designed to address the goals and objectives based on a selected frame of reference. When deciding on a frame of reference, clinicians consider the diagnosis, client's age and stage in life (e.g., toddler, adolescent, adult), setting, their own clinical expertise, and current evidence-based research, as well as the client's goals. Clinicians must stay informed about current research and intervention strategies to develop effective interventions for the children they serve. The client is discharged when all of the goals and objectives have been met or if the occupational therapist decides that services should be discontinued. (For a more detailed discussion of the OT process, see Chapter 10).

ROLES OF THE OCCUPATIONAL THERAPIST AND OCCUPATIONAL THERAPY ASSISTANT

The occupational therapist is responsible for all aspects of the OT process and supervises the OTA. The extent to which the OTA supervises the occupational therapist depends on a variety of factors, including the OTA's knowledge, skill, and experience. In any case,

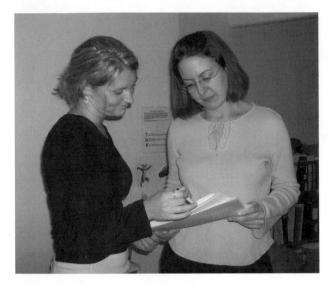

FIGURE 1-4 The occupational therapist and occupational therapy assistant collaborate on goals and an intervention plan.

TABLE 1-2

Supervision of Occupational Therapy Assistants

LEVEL OF SUPERVISION	TYPE OF SUPERVISION
Close	Direct and daily contact; on-site supervision.
Routine	Direct and regularly scheduled contact; on-site supervision.
General	Indirect supervision as needed and direct contact once a month or as mandated by state regulatory board.
Minimum	Direct and indirect supervision as needed or as mandated by state regulatory board.

occupational therapists and OTAs are both considered OT practitioners, and therefore they share the responsibility of communicating with each other about their clients.[3,9]

QUALIFICATIONS, SUPERVISION, AND SERVICE COMPETENCY

Entry-level OTAs must meet basic qualifications to practice in the field of occupational therapy. As they gain experience by working with occupational therapists, OTAs require less supervision and gradually become more competent at providing occupational therapy services.[3]

Qualifications

Entry-level OTAs must meet specific qualifications, which include successful completion of course work in an accredited OTA program and passing the certification examination administered by the National Board for Certification in Occupational Therapy.[3] In addition, OTAs must meet specific requirements established by OT regulatory boards in their respective states and obtain a license if required by state law.

Supervision

Four **levels of supervision** have been delineated by AOTA: close, routine, general, and minimal. *Close* supervision is direct, daily contact between the OTA and the occupational therapist at the work site. *Routine* supervision is direct contact between the OTA and the occupational therapist at the work site at least every 2 weeks and interim contact through other means, such as telephone conversations or e-mail messages. *General* supervision is

minimum direct contact of 1 day per month and interim supervision as needed. *Minimum* supervision is that provided on an "as-needed" basis. It is important to note that individual state OT regulatory agencies may require stricter guidelines than those established by AOTA. Stricter state guidelines supersede those of AOTA.[2,3,8,9]

The level of supervision that OTAs require varies with their level of expertise. AOTA defines three levels of expertise: entry, intermediate, and advanced.[3] OTAs progress from one level to another based on their acquisition of skills, knowledge, and proficiency and not on their years of experience. Entry-level OTAs are typically new graduates or those entering a new practice setting who have general knowledge of the population or setting but limited experience. Intermediate-level OTAs have acquired a higher level of skill through experience, continuing education, and involvement in professional activities. Advanced-level OTAs have specialized skills and may be recognized as experts in particular areas of practice. Although the extent to which a particular OTA is supervised varies according to the individual, the level of supervision generally falls into one defined by AOTA based on the OTA's expertise. An entry-level OTA requires close supervision, an intermediate-level OTA requires routine or general supervision, and an advanced-level OTA requires minimum supervision (Table 1-2).[3]

Service Competency

Levels of supervision are closely related to establishing service competency. AOTA defines **service competency** as "the determination, made by various methods, that two people performing the same or equivalent procedures will obtain the same or equivalent results."[2,3,8,9] Service competency is a means of ensuring that two individual

OT practitioners will have the same results when administering a specific assessment, observing a specific performance area or component, or providing intervention. Communication between the OTA and the occupational therapist is an essential part of the entire OT process but is especially important when establishing service competency. Occupational therapists must be sure that they and the OTAs are performing assessments and intervention procedures in the same way. Once an occupational therapist has determined that an OTA has established service competency in a certain area, the OTA may perform an assessment or intervention procedure (within the parameters of that particular area) without close supervision by the occupational therapist. Ensuring service competency is an ongoing mutual learning experience.[3]

AOTA has specific guidelines for establishing service competency. For standardized assessments and intervention procedures that require no specific training to administer, the occupational therapist and OTA both perform the procedure. If they obtain equivalent results, the OTA may be allowed to administer subsequent procedures independently. For assessments and intervention procedures requiring subjective interpretations, direct observation and videotaping are valuable tools that can be used to establish service competency. These tools allow practitioners to observe a client performing a particular task and compare their individual interpretations of the performance. Likewise, an occupational therapist can tape a client, have an OTA watch the tape, and compare and contrast the observations that have been made. If the occupational therapist and the OTA consistently have similar interpretations, the OTA has established competency in observing and interpreting the particular area of performance.[2,3,8,9] Specific examples of establishing service competency are provided here.

Videotaping

Teresa, an OTA, used the biomechanical approach to intervention when providing care for Abigail, a 10-month-old who experienced a brachial plexus injury at birth. Before working with Abigail, Teresa reviewed a videotape of her supervising occupational therapist treating another child with the same injury. Teresa's discussion of the tape with the occupational therapist revealed that she understood the intervention procedures used. Abigail's next therapy session, which was led by Teresa, was videotaped. The occupational therapist watched the tape and observed that Teresa carefully positioned the child and successfully carried out the intervention plan. The occupational therapist determined that Teresa established the service competency needed to treat Abigail. The occupational therapist and Teresa agreed that as part of the ongoing learning process, each month they would videotape and subsequently discuss one of Abigail's intervention sessions.

Co-Treatment

Raja, a 4-year-old boy diagnosed with cerebral palsy recently received a nerve block to decrease flexor tone in his right arm. Since then, Alejandro, the occupational therapist, was treating him. Alejandro asked Richard, an OTA, to assist him in treating Raja. Richard prepared for the co-treatment by reading about nerve blocks and carefully observing Alejandro's one-on-one intervention session with Raja. Richard asked pertinent questions and expressed a keen interest in working with Raja. After several successful co-treatment sessions during which Alejandro and Richard obtained equivalent outcomes from the procedures used, Alejandro assigned Raja's case to Richard. Richard then received only general supervision from Alejandro because he demonstrated service competency when working with Raja.

Observation

Missy, an OTA, used the rehabilitative approach to treat Dewayne, a 6-year-old who obtained an amputation below the elbow. Before becoming an OTA, Missy volunteered regularly at Shriner's Hospital (on the unit that specialized in trauma and burn cases) and she observed many clients being fitted with prostheses; she frequently assisted the therapists. After graduating as an OTA, she was hired to work in the OT Department at Shriner's Hospital. As an OTA, she worked closely with an occupational therapist, who developed intervention plans for clients with injuries similar to Dewayne's. Missy also observed and assisted in administering the department's prosthetic checklist, which was designed to assess the care, application, and use of prostheses. Missy began working with Dewayne when he was fitted for his first prosthesis at the age of 3. The occupational therapist observed Missy administering the procedures on the prosthetic checklist; their findings were equivalent. When Dewayne was fitted with a new prosthesis, the occupational therapist was confident that Missy could independently and accurately complete the checklist procedures. Missy demonstrated service competency in administering the assessment.

AOTA CODE OF ETHICS

The Representative Assembly of AOTA approved the updated Occupational Therapy **Code of Ethics** in 2010.[5] This new code was tailored to better address the ethical concerns of the profession. This is a public statement of the principles used to promote and maintain high standards of conduct by all OT personnel. The Code of Ethics is based on seven principles:

- Beneficence
- Nonmaleficence
- Autonomy and confidentiality
- Social justice

- Procedural justice
- Veracity
- Fidelity

Beneficence refers to the benefit of services to consumers, which may include clients, families, and community. For example, if a child is not progressing or benefiting from OT services, then discontinuation of services would be considered an ethical decision. *Nonmaleficence* refers to the principle of not inflicting or imposing harm on clients. The OT practitioner avoids activities or interventions that may hurt the child or adolescent. For example, the practitioner carefully observes the child's response to multisensory inputs and is alert to prevent sensory overload. The principles of *autonomy* and *confidentiality* relate to the rights and privacy of clients. OT practitioners actively involve children and families in the intervention process and respect and uphold their rights to privacy and confidentiality. The OT practitioner is careful not to speak in public places about children or tell others about the child's services. The principle of *social justice* refers to providing fair and equitable OT services for all clients.[5] Thus, OT practitioners must make sure that all clients receive the same level of services despite such things as ability level, socioeconomic status, or culture. For example, the OT practitioner does not schedule more sessions just because the parent's insurance will cover the cost, rather sessions are scheduled based on the child's needs. The principle of *procedural justice* necessitates that OT practitioners comply with state and federal laws and AOTA policies. Furthermore, this principle ensures that practitioners provide OT services in accordance with established policies and procedures. In terms of the relationship between the occupational therapist and the OTA, procedural justice ensures that supervision is provided within the required guidelines established in state laws. *Veracity* means honesty in all professional matters. Practitioners adhering to the principle of veracity accurately document services provided, including the child's progress. Veracity also includes being honest about one's professional qualifications and level of competency. *Fidelity* refers to respect, fairness, discretion, and integrity. In practice, practitioners are following the principle of fidelity when they provide the same quality of care to all clients, regardless of payment schedules, culture, or disability. OT practitioners are expected to adhere to the profession's code of ethics at all times.[5]

SCHOLARSHIP

Occupational therapy practitioners must be lifelong learners to be competent in the provision of services. **Scholarship** is a form of leadership and enables practitioners to expand their knowledge base and to maintain competence. Scholarship involves the dissemination of findings, either formally or informally. OT practitioners may choose a variety of options for disseminating their findings, including in-service training, conference presentations, poster sessions, publications, journal club discussions, and informal networking. Practitioners may choose to network with others by using *social media*, such as blogging. Scholarship may involve formal learning, such as enrolling in a course. Some practitioners may wish to demonstrate knowledge through practical application.

Boyer defined four types of scholarship: discovery, integration, application, and teaching.[10] *Discovery* scholarship includes work that contributes to the body of knowledge of a profession, thus increasing evidence-based practice options. For example, searching the literature to review various intervention methods is a form of discovery scholarship.

Integration scholarship involves interpreting and synthesizing research findings to identify linkages across disciplines. Exploring interventions used in physical therapy, speech therapy, or education and relating those findings to occupational therapy is a form of integration scholarship.

Frequently, OT practitioners are interested in applying professional knowledge to solve clinical problems and to assess outcomes. This type of scholarship is called *application* scholarship.

OT practitioners frequently educate other practitioners and clients' family members on intervention techniques and, as such, are interested in examining their teaching effectiveness. *Teaching* scholarship is used to determine how the client best learns. It is also used when OT faculty and practitioners examine how the OTA student learns in the classroom and when on fieldwork.

OT practitioners are encouraged to actively engage in scholarly activities at various levels on a regular basis. For instance, participation in a journal club to discuss a particular client group, laws, or systems in one's state can benefit the practitioner and client. Presenting new interventions or interesting findings at state conferences or through in-service training often is helpful in refining or further developing ideas. Engaging in a variety of scholarship activities benefits practitioners, clients, and the OT profession.

SUMMARY

This chapter presented an overview of pediatric OT practice beginning with an overview of the AOTA centennial vision and how it relates to OT practice with children. An overview of the OTPF was followed by a discussion of the OT process. The role of the occupational therapist and the OTA were defined throughout the chapter, with an emphasis on the qualifications, supervision, and service competency requirements for the entry-level OTA.

Examples throughout the chapter illustrated how levels of supervision and service competency are used in delivery of OT services within the realm of the OTPF. A discussion of the AOTA Code of Ethics was presented, using pediatric examples to reinforce key concepts. Finally, the authors defined scholarship, providing examples to illustrate how OTAs can contribute to the professions' work in pediatrics.

References

1. American Occupational Therapy Association. (2014). AOTA *centennial vision priorities: FY 2015.* http://www.aota.org/aboutaota/get-involved/bod/news/2014/fy15-cv-prioritites.aspx.
2. American Occupational Therapy Association. (2013). Guidelines for documentation of occupational therapy. *Am J Occup Ther,* 67(Suppl.), S32–S38.
3. American Occupational Therapy Association. (2009). Guidelines for supervision, roles, and responsibilities during the delivery of occupational therapy services. *Am J Occup Ther,* 63(6), 707–803.
4. American Occupational Therapy Association. (September 30, 2008). *Occupational therapy assistant model curriculum,* https://www.aota.org/-/media/Corporate/Files/Education Careers/Educators/Model%20OTA%20Curriculum%20-%20October%202008.pdf.
5. American Occupational Therapy Association. (2010). Occupational therapy code of ethics and ethics standards. *Am J Occup Ther,* 64(Suppl. 6), S17–S26.
6. American Occupational Therapy Association. (2014). Occupational therapy practice framework: domain and process (3rd ed.). *Am J Occup Ther,* 68(Suppl. 1), S1–S48.
7. American Occupational Therapy Association. (2004). Psychosocial aspects of occupational therapy. *Am J Occup Ther,* 58, 669–672.
8. American Occupational Therapy Association. (2010). Scope of practice. *Am J Occup Ther,* 64(Supp.), S70–S77.
9. American Occupational Therapy Association. (2005). Standards of practice for occupational therapy. *Am J Occup Ther,* 59, 663–665.
10. Boyer, E. L. (1997). *Scholarship reconsidered: priorities of the profession.* San Francisco, CA: Jossey-Bass.
11. American Occupational Therapy Association. (2006). Occupational therapy salaries and job opportunities continue to improve: 2006 AOTA workforce and compensation survey. *OT Practice.*

Recommended Reading

Boyt-Schell, B., Gillen, G., Scaffa, M., & Cohn, E. (Eds.). (2014). *Willard and Spackman's occupational therapy* (12th ed.). Philadelphia: Lippincott Williams & Wilkins.

O'Brien, J., & Hussey, S. (2010). *Introduction to occupational therapy* (4th ed.). St. Louis: Mosby.

Jacobs, K., MacRae, N., & Sladyk, K. (2014). *Occupational therapy essentials for clinical competence* (2nd ed.). Thorofare, NJ: Slack, Inc.

REVIEW *Questions*

1. List and describe five content areas in which a pediatric OT practitioner needs to have knowledge while working with children and adolescents.
2. Provide an overview regarding the domain and process of occupational therapy as described in the OTPF. Use a pediatric example to illustrate this.
3. What is service competency? How is it established?
4. How would each type of scholarship (as defined by Boyer) enhance OT practice for children and youth?
5. Define the seven ethical principles, and provide a clinical example of each.

SUGGESTED *Activities*

1. Interview an OTA or an occupational therapist who works in pediatrics. The focus of the interview should be supervision and service competency. Questions might include the following:
   (a) Which courses in school have proved to be the most useful to you as a pediatric OT practitioner?
   (b) How many years of clinical experience do you have?
   (c) What is the level of supervision that you receive (OTA) or give (occupational therapist)? What are the means by which this occurs?
   (d) How is service competency established between the occupational therapist and the OTA in your workplace?

2. Observe an OT practitioner and describe the OT domain and process as outlined in the OTPF.
   (a) List and describe the domains that the practitioner addressed.
   (b) What aspects of the process did the practitioner use?
   (c) Describe the dynamic nature of the OT process by using the example of what you saw.
3. Choose an article that addresses OT practice with children and youth. Summarize the findings and describe how this would inform practice. Identify which type of scholarship is represented in the article and describe your rationale for this response.
4. Provide an example illustrating how a practitioner follows the Code of Ethics in practice.
   (a) Review occupational therapy ethical violations and describe the ethical principle(s) violated. (Some states record these decisions.)
   (b) Describe all the various forms of plagiarism. Discuss which code of ethic principle covers plagiarism. How does your school handle plagiarism?

PAMELA J. WINTON
ROBERT E. WINTON

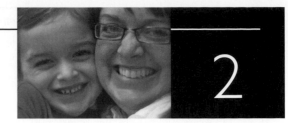

Family Systems

2

KEY TERMS

Domain
Client-Centered
Prescriptive
Consultative
Morphostatic Principle
Morphogenetic Principle
Equifinality
Life Cycle
Normative Life-Cycle
   Events
Nonnormative Life-Cycle
   Events
Adaptation
Resources
Perceptual Coping
   Strategies
Acknowledgment

CHAPTER *Objectives*

After studying this chapter, the reader will be able to accomplish the following:

- Describe why it is important for an occupational therapy practitioner to have knowledge of and skills related to working with families.
- Describe the differences between prescriptive and consultative professional roles.
- Understand the way a therapy program for a child always has an effect on the family unit.
- Describe the key concepts of family systems and life-cycle theories and the roles of these concepts in interventions for children.
- Recognize and appreciate that all families have unique ways of adapting and coping with life events and that effective therapy builds on these existing coping strategies.
- Describe several communication strategies that an occupational therapy practitioner can use to promote familial–professional partnerships.

CHAPTER *Outline*

The Importance of Families

Current Issues Affecting Occupational Therapy Practitioners and Families
CHANGES IN POLICIES AND SERVICE DELIVERY MODELS
EXPANSION OF PRACTITIONERS' ROLES
DEMOGRAPHIC CHANGES IN THE U.S. POPULATION
IMPLICATIONS FOR PRACTICE

Family Systems Theory
DESCRIPTION
GENERAL SYSTEMS THEORY CONCEPTS
IMPLICATIONS FOR PRACTICE

Family Life Cycle
DESCRIPTION
IMPLICATIONS FOR PRACTICE

Family Adaptation
DESCRIPTION
IMPLICATIONS FOR PRACTICE

Essential Skills for Successful Intervention with Families

Summary

CASE *Study*

Margarita Sanchez, 3 years old, has been diagnosed with pervasive developmental delays and mild to moderate cerebral palsy. She lives in a small apartment with her paternal grandmother, great aunt, parents, and three siblings who are 11 months, 5 years, and 6 years of age. When Heather McFall, the occupational therapy (OT) practitioner, arrives for a routine visit, she learns that Margarita's mother has not been working with Margarita on the toilet training program that was discussed during the last visit. Heather recommended that they start the program because she thought it was important that Margarita be toilet trained in time to begin a public school prekindergarten program in the fall. After some discussion, it becomes apparent that in the winter Mrs. Sanchez is unable to deal with the wet, soiled clothes that invariably accompany a toilet training program. After further discussion, Heather and Mrs. Sanchez agree to wait until the weather gets warmer to begin toilet training. During their conversation, Heather also realizes that she needs to plan a time for the Sanchez family to visit the prekindergarten class and see what they think of the program. Although Heather is enthusiastic about the academic and social experiences that Margarita would have in the class, Mrs. Sanchez seems hesitant and uncharacteristically quiet when they talk about the program. Heather has learned that Mrs. Sanchez tends to become quiet when she has reservations about an idea.

As Heather leaves the apartment, she thinks about her relationship with the family and how it has developed during the 2 years she has been working with Margarita. At the beginning of the relationship, Heather was often frustrated by Mrs. Sanchez's seeming disinterest in, or inability to follow through with, some of the home program ideas that Heather introduced. She fretted and fumed but tried to help Mrs. Sanchez see the importance of taking Margarita's needs seriously and devoting the necessary time to therapy. It was only after discussing the case with a colleague that Heather realized she had departed from the guidelines of the 2014 Occupational Therapy Practice Framework (OTPF).[1] She got caught up in her own expertise in the **domain** of occupational therapy and had strayed from a **client-centered*** consultative process.

As Heather recalls this, she laughs to herself as she recognizes that she has "done it again" with regard to the toilet training directive. She is also happy that she recovered her client-centered role and helped Mrs. Sanchez develop a plan that incorporates some of her ideas into the family routines. Mrs. Sanchez's silent response also has clued her in to the fact that she departed from the client-centered

consultative role related to the preschool issue. She resolves that on the next visit she will attempt to remain client centered as she revisits the idea of preschool.

THE IMPORTANCE OF FAMILIES

The vignette of Margarita and her family underscores the reason it is important for OT practitioners to understand family systems. Box 2-1 contains the key reasons for using a family-centered approach in early intervention when working with young children who have disabilities.

Families have the most significant environmental influence on a young child's life and development. As evident in this case, the majority of Margarita's time is spent with her family. If the family members are not convinced of the benefits of therapy or are unable to find time to carry out the intervention plan, optimal improvement in Margarita's case is unlikely to occur. As interventionists, OT practitioners enter children's lives for relatively brief periods. Family members are the "constants" in most children's lives.

The OT practitioner may function in two distinct roles in his or her involvement with a family—**prescriptive** and **consultative**. When working directly with the child, the OT practitioner functions primarily in the prescriptive and directive role; when working with the family, he or she functions primarily in the consultative role. Consulting with the family on the possibility of achieving the desired goals for the child and for the family builds collaboration and trust, which are key ingredients for intervention success with families.

CLINICAL *Pearl*

Developing a trusting and collaborative relationship with families is a key ingredient for intervention success.

BOX 2-1

Reasons Families Are Important

- A family has a significant environmental influence on a young child's life and development.
- Interventions with children inevitably affect the family.
- Laws and current service delivery models promote a family-centered approach.
- Professional organizations, including the American Occupational Therapy Association, have identified the areas of competency and created recommended guidelines for working with families.

---

*The OTPF[1] defines the term *client* as the individual or the individual within the context of a group (i.e., a family). The terms *client-centered* and *family-centered* are used interchangeably in this chapter.

Interventions with children have an inevitable effect on the life of the family; therefore, interventions are most effective when the family is consulted and invests in the development of the intervention plan. Margarita's story reveals the importance of considering the whole family with regard to the intervention plan. It also illustrates the advantages of the OT practitioner functioning in a family-centered, consultative role, one that acknowledges and supports a family's central function in the design and implementation of intervention plans. Margarita's therapist learned the importance of this concept when she recalled her initial failed attempt to help the family institute a toilet training program and again when introducing the idea of preschool for Margarita.

The family-centered approach is also the focus of many current laws and health care delivery models. Public Law 99-457, which was passed in 1986 (IDEA, Part C), is considered revolutionary because of its emphasis on the central role a family plays in interventions with young children.[7] This law and its subsequent interpretations have altered the way in which services for young children are planned and delivered. Some of the highlights of the early intervention component of the law include the following:

1. Families are mandated co-leaders on state-level advisory boards that make recommendations about the way in which service systems are designed.
2. Family concerns, resources, and priorities guide the development of individual intervention plans.
3. Families play an important role in children's assessments and evaluations.
4. Families have certain rights to confidentiality, record keeping, notification, and other procedures related to the programs and agencies that serve their children.[7]

The law ushered in additional changes that ultimately benefit families, such as promoting interdisciplinary and interagency collaboration. The importance of collaboration among families and professionals from different agencies and disciplines became apparent when numerous stories surfaced about the challenges for families when professionals did not collaborate with each other.[5]

Professional organizations, including the American Occupational Therapy Association (AOTA) and the Division for Early Childhood of the Council for Exceptional Children (DEC/CEC), identified particular areas of competency and certain guidelines to emphasize the importance of practitioners having the skills and knowledge necessary to work effectively with families.[3] The dramatic changes in the relationship between families and professionals, which were catalyzed by Public Law 99-457, as well as the increased focus on the importance of families in all human service organizations, did not develop overnight. The existing workforce had to develop new collaboration and communication skills.

University and community college training programs had to retrain faculty and upgrade curricula to prepare students adequately for the newly defined pediatric roles (Box 2-2).[3] Professional organizations have supported the changes by creating recommended practice guidelines and areas of competency.

CURRENT ISSUES AFFECTING OCCUPATIONAL THERAPY PRACTITIONERS AND FAMILIES

Changes in Policies and Service Delivery Models

As mentioned previously, policies and legislation passed in the past decades affected service delivery models and recommended OT practices. The resulting changes include emphasis on the following approaches to service delivery:

- Interdisciplinary and family-centered approaches are used when planning and implementing interventions.
- Children with disabilities are included in regular educational settings.
- Therapists act as consultants, providing pediatric treatment that is integrated into the children's regular routines and natural environments instead of using "pull-out therapy"* (Figure 2-1).

Expansion of Practitioners' Roles

Recent changes in service delivery and implementation resulted in an expansion of the role of OT practitioners. Their duties now also include the following:

- Assessing family interests, priorities, and concerns;
- Observing and gathering information about the daily routines of children and families in their homes and in the classrooms;
- Gathering and sharing information with families about development and intervention strategies; and
- Implementing therapy in collaboration with parents, caregivers, and general educators.

Demographic Changes in the U.S. Population

In addition to changes in laws, policies, and recommended practices, the demographic makeup of the children being served has also changed. Nearly half (49.9%) of the children in the United States under the age of 5 years are racial or ethnic minorities.[6] In contrast, although the U.S. population is becoming more diverse, the members of health-assessing and treating professionals (i.e., nurses, therapists, dietitians, pharmacists) are predominantly (83%) white.[2]

Pull-out therapy is therapy that is not provided in the context of a child's daily routine.

BOX 2-2

DEC-Recommended Practices in Early Intervention/Early Childhood Special Education

FAMILY PRACTICES

Family practices refer to ongoing activities that (a) promote the active participation of families in decision making related to their child (e.g., assessment, planning, intervention); (b) lead to the development of a service plan (e.g., of a set of goals for the family and child and the services and supports to achieve those goals); or (c) support families in achieving the goals they hold for their child and the other family members.

Family practices encompass three themes:

1. *Family-centered practices*: Practices that treat families with dignity and respect; are individualized, flexible, and responsive to each family's unique circumstances; provide family members complete and unbiased information to make informed decisions; and involve family members in acting on choices to strengthen child, parent, and family functioning.

2. *Family capacity-building practices*: Practices that include the participatory opportunities and experiences afforded to families to strengthen existing parenting knowledge and skills and promote the development of new parenting abilities that enhance parenting self-efficacy beliefs and practices.

3. *Family and professional collaboration*: Practices that build relationships between families and professionals who work together to achieve mutually decided outcomes and goals that promote family competencies and support the development of the child.

We recommend the following family practices for practitioners:

F1. Practitioners build trusting and respectful partnerships with the family through interactions that are sensitive and responsive to cultural, linguistic, and socioeconomic diversity.

F2. Practitioners provide the family with up-to-date, comprehensive, and unbiased information in a way that the family can understand and use to make informed choices and decisions.

F3. Practitioners are responsive to the family's concerns, priorities, and changing life circumstances.

F4. Practitioners and the family work together to create outcomes or goals, develop individualized plans, and implement practices that address the family's priorities and concerns and the child's strengths and needs

F5. Practitioners support family functioning, promote family confidence and competence, and strengthen family–child relationships by acting in ways that recognize and build on family strengths and capacities.

F6. Practitioners engage the family in opportunities that support and strengthen parenting knowledge and skills and parenting competence and confidence in ways that are flexible, individualized, and tailored to the family's preferences.

F7. Practitioners work with the family to identify, access, and use formal and informal resources and supports to achieve family-identified outcomes or goals.

F8. Practitioners provide the family of a young child who has or is at risk for developmental delay/disability, and who is a dual-language learner, with information about the benefits of learning in multiple languages for the child's growth and development.

F9. Practitioners help families know and understand their rights.

F10. Practitioners inform families about leadership and advocacy skill-building opportunities and encourage those who are interested to participate.

Source: Division for Early Childhood. (2014). DEC recommended practices in early intervention/early childhood special education. Retrieved from http://www.dec-sped.org/recommendedpractices

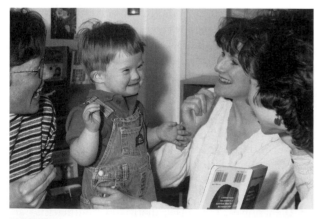

FIGURE 2-1 Therapist working with the mother, child, and early childhood teacher at a child-care center. This is an example of interdisciplinary collaboration and embedding therapy into the daily routine. (Courtesy Don Trull, FPG Child Development Institute, University of North Carolina—Chapel Hill, Chapel Hill, NC.)

Implications for Practice

The myriad changes taking place in the OT environment affect service delivery and implementation in numerous ways, including the following:

- OT practitioners are more likely than ever to be working with children and families whose cultural backgrounds and native languages are different from their own. They may need to use translators or interpreters. They must develop the ability to appreciate and respect cultural differences, which may mean developing an awareness of their own cultural identities, the acknowledgment of inherent biases and values, and knowledge of other cultures.

- Young children with disabilities are more likely than ever to be in regular early childhood and educational programs. OT practitioners must be able to embed therapy into the daily routines of home,

BOX 2-3

Family Systems Theory Concepts

MORPHOSTATIC PRINCIPLE

Like all systems, family systems are organized with recognizable feedback loops and "rules." These rules may be consciously recognized and spoken by family members; however, most are nonverbal and shared assumptions of family functioning. An example of a spoken "rule" is: "In our family, parents always inquire about his or her child's day and the child always responds." An example of a nonverbal "rule" is a parent expressing anger at a child and the child withdrawing to avoid conflict. Deviation from either pattern by the parent or the child would be met with corrective (morphostatic) action. Failure of the parent to inquire or the child to respond in the first instance would draw the immediate attention of the other, leaving him or her to wonder if there was a problem. In the second example, an arguing response could be met with increasing anger from the parent until the child finally withdraws; if the parent fails to respond angrily to an "infraction," the child might escalate the misbehavior until the angry response occurs.

MORPHOGENETIC PRINCIPLE

Families do evolve; that is, they change. Just as a child grows and develops, families do, too. In the examples given here, the parent who usually asks how his or her child's day was might get caught up in work or in taking care of a younger sibling and not be available when the now older and more independent child arrives home. The child might start

volunteering information about his or her activities without being asked. In the latter example, the child, as he or she grows older and gains experience outside the family, may see this as undesirable and no longer be willing to continue the sequence. Either the parent or the child will initiate a conversation that leads to an agreement to make changes in the sequence.

EQUIFINALITY

This concept is, in many ways, a subset of the morphogenetic principle. Simply stated, it says that any system can change in an infinite number of ways. If we again take the second example, a positive change was described. Another version might be that the now 16-year-old boy becomes increasingly belligerent, gets into a physical fight with his father, and either runs away or is kicked out of the house. Even in this extreme example, it is important to recognize that the "family" continues and the notion of equifinality still applies. The child could become addicted to drugs, with the parents forever grieving, or he could eventually get into the military, receive the GI bill, do well in college for a couple of years, and be reunited with his family, who then support him through graduate school and he subsequently wins the Nobel prize. Equifinality does not imply an end point but, rather, a series of way stations in the life of a family. For the OT practitioner, it is the most important idea, one of hope and optimism.

child-care, and regular educational settings and must develop expertise in consulting with early childhood teachers, families, and other specialists. OT practitioners need the knowledge and skill to work as members of interdisciplinary teams, which requires interpersonal, communicative, and collaborative skills.

• OT practitioners must obtain information on a wide range of community-based programs and services, both specialized and generic, to meet the individual needs of the various families and children with whom they work.

FAMILY SYSTEMS THEORY
Description

Family systems theory is a core framework for guiding interactions with families.* It is a group of ideas that describe the many ways that individuals in families are connected across time and space, and its implications for

*The definition of family in this chapter is inclusive: "…two or more people who regard themselves as a family and who perform some of the functions that families typically perform. These people may or may not be related by blood or marriage and may or may not usually live together."

the families with whom practitioners work are far reaching. Developing and increasing an understanding of the family as a system significantly affects the way practitioners working with families perceive their own roles, determine which potential outcomes are positive, and understand family changes. The core concepts of family systems theory are provided in Box 2-3.

General Systems Theory Concepts

Each living system (including family), to be recognizable as such, must have some order, no matter how undesirable or chaotic it appears to an outside observer. The maintenance of this order has been termed the **morphostatic** (form maintenance) **principle**. Examples for families include daily family rhythms such as meals, bedtime, expectations for bathing, greetings or departures, and affectionate naming. At the same time, these systems have a capacity for change, which has been named the **morphogenetic** (form-evolving) **principle**. Examples for families include gaining or losing a member through marriage, divorce, birth and death, and the shifting roles of members through marriage, school progression, or aging. Change is possible only through the introduction and assimilation of new information into the system, such as gaining or losing members.

A feature of the form-evolving (morphogenetic) aspect of living systems is their capacity to evolve along different paths and yet arrive at a given "destination." It implies that no single past event predicts a system's current form, nor does any specific current event specifically predict a future form. This has been named **equifinality**. The practitioner will see families that are similar in many ways but whose lives have been affected in dramatically different ways by the introduction of a child with special needs. A clear example is one in which the family seems to have been drawn closer together, in contrast with that in which the family has become emotionally disconnected.

Implications for Practice

The OT practitioner is an agent for bringing new information into the system. In addition to the core knowledge (the domain of the profession) the practitioner brings, he or she must develop communication skills to help the family assimilate this new information. To do so, the OT practitioner is guided by these basic ideas: (a) "I must acknowledge and accept current family form and function" (support the current form); and (b) "I must ally myself with the system's capacity for change" (support the assimilation of the new knowledge I bring). These ideas form the basis for the consultative role.

The OT practitioner leverages his or her ability to support change by eliciting from the family its desired outcomes and integrating his or her ideas into a collaborative plan aimed first and foremost at achieving the family's goals. Figure 2-2 shows collaboration between family and practitioner. This is truly a family-centered practice, with the family being the client and the OT practitioner being a consultant rather than a prescriptive interventionist.

A major goal when working with families is to establish a trusting relationship, particularly with key members. One of the first steps to establishing trust is to identify the outcomes that family members desire. Given that different family members have different priorities, helping them find verbal expression for outcomes that everyone can endorse builds that trust in a powerful way. Sometimes families simply have the basic desire to help their children grow and develop. Regardless of whether a family's goals are vague, it is important to acknowledge the ways they perceive the current situation and priorities while helping them agree on goals.

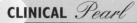

CLINICAL *Pearl*

The first step in a successful intervention is identifying what the family hopes to accomplish.

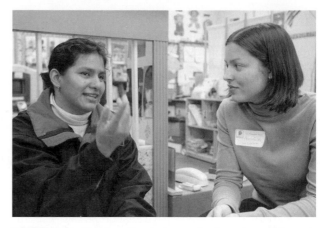

FIGURE 2-2   Collaboration between family and practitioner is essential for achieving goals that enable children to participate in meaningful occupations. (Courtesy Don Trull, FPG Child Development Institute, University of North Carolina—Chapel Hill, Chapel Hill, NC.)

CLINICAL *Pearl*

Intervention efforts should begin with a clarification and acknowledgment of the way in which family members perceive their situation and define their priorities, however unfocused their goals may seem.

The second step in building a trusting relationship is developing strategies for accomplishing the family's goals. The strategies should be developed in collaboration with the family to ensure adherence to its beliefs and daily living patterns. In the case of Margarita, Heather began the intervention process by working with the mother, which, given her key role, was the appropriate way to begin establishing a trusting relationship. However, even if Heather successfully consulted with the mother at the previous visit to determine that toilet training was a desirable goal for the family, she departed from the consultative role when she decided on the time line for Margarita's toilet training. Instead, once the family endorsed the idea, Heather should have consulted with Mrs. Sanchez about the practical realities and timing of implementing the training. To implement the toilet training even more powerfully, she should have included the father, grandmother, and aunt in developing strategies once they endorsed these ideas as desired goals. This would have avoided some of the constraints created by Mrs. Sanchez's already complex life. Because Heather failed to include the other family members in the planning process, she missed some opportunities to support the intervention/change process. Fortunately, Heather was able to shift out of the prescriptive and directive role, which previously led to frustration.

Margarita's story illustrates a common occurrence—the professional role of the OT practitioner as the prescriber of intervention clashing with existing family functioning. This can significantly reduce the efficiency and effectiveness of any intervention. The paradox is that families desire professional expertise and assistance and it is hard for practitioners to resist the temptation to take a directive role. At the same time, families do not like being told what exactly to do by someone else, especially as interventions may disrupt family routines and behaviors. Some families can be creative and take a prescribed intervention and weave it into existing family routines, beliefs, and daily living patterns, but many will do less well or discard the intervention altogether. Staying in a consultative role is key to intervention success. The OT practitioner helps families integrate the interventions that move them toward the goals on which they agreed and into their daily living patterns as well as they can. As the consultant, the OT practitioner not only helps families integrate new intervention strategies but also helps them troubleshoot those aspects of the plan that they were unable to actually accomplish. "Trying harder" rarely works. Changing the process, the goals, and the time line, however, are all reasonable adaptations to current family functioning. Figure 2-3 shows an interventionist modeling an intervention strategy in a home setting.

With this approach, families are more likely to take full advantage of the practitioner's expertise. OT practitioners who are able to relinquish their felt power as experts and provide consultation in a truly family-centered fashion often are able to make the most of their professional skills and expertise.

CLINICAL *Pearl*

The likelihood of families following through with intervention plans depends on the extent to which those plans are constructed to fit within families' existing routines, beliefs, and patterns of family life.

OT practitioners also should be aware that success with a family is an evolving process. As in the case of Heather, the only real mistake is the one that is not recognized. An easy way to enhance the family's trust is to consult with them on intervention plans gone awry. Being truly curious to learn about the family and collaborating with the family to add or change elements in a plan not only improve the odds of success but also further the family's acceptance of the therapist. Developing a trusting relationship with families takes time. Differences in cultural and linguistic backgrounds and heritages also influence how quickly and easily relationships are formed, but adhering to the consultative role does accelerate the process.

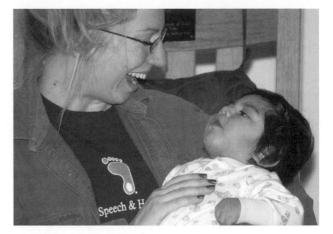

FIGURE 2-3 Modeling intervention strategies in a home setting allows family members to participate in the process that supports follow-through and the achievement of goals. (Courtesy Don Trull, FPG Child Development Institute, University of North Carolina—Chapel Hill, Chapel Hill, NC.)

FAMILY LIFE CYCLE
Description

Another concept important to consider is the family **life cycle**. Like individuals, families also go through normal or typical developmental phases. No consensus exists on the number of phases that should be considered, which is not surprising considering that family development is a fluid process and not a discontinuous series of steps. Critical stages of the family life cycle are those involving life transitions: birth, marriage, leaving home, and death.

Perhaps one of the most important points about the phases of the life cycle is the fact that moving from one phase to another causes stress and requires the family to adapt. Stress is completely normal and necessary for the evolution (morphogenesis) of the family system. Life-cycle changes bring about changes in the needs, interests, roles, and responsibilities of each family member. For instance, becoming a parent entails learning a whole new set of skills and alters the relationships between parents and among parents and their extended family and friends. Families often can benefit from the extra support of friends, neighbors, or extended family members during life-cycle transitions.

Children with disabilities have special needs and undergo numerous stressful life-cycle events. These events may include unexpected hospitalization for a lengthy period, unusual and sometimes painful treatments, and participation in special education and early intervention programs. These events often involve new relationships with numerous different professionals. Forming new relationships, especially when individual choice does not exist (as when a practitioner is assigned a case), can be stressful. In the case of Margarita, the arrival of an OT practitioner in the Sanchez household created a certain degree of stress. As Heather, the therapist, shifted into a more consultative role, the stress of intervention was no longer dealt with by dropping the prescribed intervention and changing nothing (morphostatic principle); rather, the intervention (toilet training) was integrated into a family plan for change that was endorsed, at least in its timing, by Mrs. Sanchez and was therefore more likely to succeed (adhering to the morphogenetic principle).

Watching a child miss typical milestones can create stress for a family. For example, the realization that a child has not started walking or talking by the appropriate age can be very stressful. In Margarita's case, the fact that her younger 11-month-old sister had begun to walk whereas the 3-year-old Margarita had not, clearly highlighted the ongoing and unexpected stress caused by Margarita's extended dependency for basic functions such as feeding and toileting.

Because certain events—for example, frequent hospitalizations, participating in OT interventions, or not reaching important milestones—are not **normative life-cycle events** (i.e., the usual or expected transitional events), families experiencing these events have fewer people with whom to share their experiences. For instance, parents of adolescents often find it helpful to share "war stories" with other parents about transitional events (e.g., teaching the adolescent to drive). The majority of parents of adolescents can relate to the challenges and triumphs associated with this event. Research has shown that sharing experiences and getting support from family, friends, and neighbors are effective strategies for dealing with stress.[4] However, few parents can relate to **nonnormative life-cycle events** (not the usual or expected transitional events), such as the experience of raising a child who will never be able to walk.

Implications for Practice

The life events that have been described are somewhat arbitrary and obviously overlap, so they are grossly inadequate representations of the wide range of family experiences that exist. Cultural factors also can affect how these events and life stages are perceived and experienced. For example, is it acceptable for an adult child to be living with his or her parents? In the case of many white families, this situation would be perceived as a failure on the part of the child, whereas this may be normal in many Hispanic families. Practitioners tend to attach meanings, usually rooted in their own backgrounds, beliefs, and experiences, to the phases of the family life cycle. This tendency can potentially put practitioners at odds with certain families. This is illustrated in the case study about Margarita. Heather, with her Anglo-Saxon values, recommended that Margarita attend the prekindergarten program in a public school because she thought it would enhance the child's social and cognitive development. Mrs. Sanchez became

quiet when Heather made that suggestion, an action that Heather came to recognize as a sign of disagreement. Perhaps the Sanchez family considered it unusual for children to attend any school at such a young age, or they may have preferred a neighborhood parochial school with several bilingual nuns on staff.

Being sensitive to family transitional events (normative and nonnormative) also is important. Events such as the death of a parent, an adult child leaving home, or a job transition can take the time and attention of the family away from intervention efforts. Consider the big picture when working with a family. Family-centered consultation is clearly preferred under such circumstances.

During nonnormative transitional events, the families of children who have disabilities sometimes find it extremely helpful to be connected with each other. They can share information, similar experiences, and methods of coping. Parent-to-parent programs exist in many communities, and research has demonstrated their helpfulness.[4,5]

FAMILY ADAPTATION
Description

In what ways do families adapt to unexpected events such as the birth of a child who has developmental delays? Crises, which are brought on by overwhelming stress, are not always negative. Families are living systems that evolve in response to internal events (e.g., illness, death, birth, emancipation) and external events (e.g., the loss of a job, a move to another city, the involvement of the OT practitioner). Like all living things, families are generally adaptive (the morphogenetic principle) by nature. Although serious crises can precipitate alcoholism, separation or divorce, or family violence, in some cases they can enable rapid positive changes, such as recommitment to a marriage or resolution of a long-standing conflict. For many years, research on the families of children with disabilities was focused on family dysfunction, stress, and pathology. However, in recent years research has revealed what some families had been saying for years: Despite the stress caused by their child's disability, dealing with the disability strengthened the family or changed it in some positive way.[4]

Families react and adapt to crises in individualized and unique ways. Family **adaptation** is affected by the interaction of family **resources** (e.g., time, money, and friends) and perceptions (the way events are defined). Social support plays an extremely important role in family and individual well-being. For the families of children with disabilities, the informal support of extended family, friends, and neighbors appears to be more important than the formal support received from professionals and institutions. Of course, an important factor is the way families define their resources. In the Sanchez family, the

BOX 2-4

Perceptual Coping Strategies

PASSIVE APPRAISAL
Ignoring a problem and hoping it will go away

REFRAMING
Redefining a situation in ways that make it more manageable

DOWNWARD COMPARISON
Identifying a situation that is worse than your own

USE OF SPIRITUAL BELIEFS
Using philosophic or spiritual beliefs to make sense of and find meaning in a situation

extended family is a source of positive support for Margarita's parents, whereas in other families, a mother-in-law or an aunt living in the home could be a source of additional stress.

In addition, the way families define and understand a particular event, such as the birth of a child with a disability, is an important component of family adaptation. Specific **perceptual coping strategies** are listed in Box 2-4.

At times practitioners get impatient with families who seem to ignore or minimize problems. Although it may be tempting to be judgmental in these situations, it is important to recognize that these families are using their own coping strategies. Families adapt as a whole, and this adaptive capacity should be supported. OT practitioners should not assess a given situation and assign direct responsibility to any specific factor. For example, a practitioner cannot accurately assume that George, a 6-year-old who cannot tie his shoes, would be able to if he had started occupational therapy at age 3. Too many other variables are relevant. For example, family financial demands, time constraints, and emotional strain may have been significant factors when George was 3. Beginning occupational therapy at that age could have forced George's father, who had just overcome his drinking and spousal abuse problems, to regress. In turn, this could have caused George to regress and lose his toileting skills. No individual, not even an OT practitioner, can conceive of all the potential positive outcomes and all the ways to achieve those outcomes (equifinality). Families and OT practitioners have attitudes and biases about the causes of problems and the possibilities of overcoming them. Nevertheless, the adaptive potential of a family as a whole is unlimited, and remembering this can help families as well as OT practitioners achieve the best possible outcomes.

Implications for Practice

When meeting a family for the first time, it is important to be interested in learning about the unique ways in which the parents adapt to their child's disability—the ingenious ways that they cope in their daily lives. In Margarita case, Heather regained this curiosity and interest when she recognized Mrs. Sanchez's indirect feedback, that is, her quietness. This indicated that Heather shifted away from the consultative role.

CLINICAL *Pearl*

When meeting a family for the first time, it is important to express curiosity and interest in the unique ways in which they are adapting to their child's disability without judging and evaluating.

It also is important to use and support existing resources in families' lives. OT practitioners sometimes get so excited about specialized support services that they forget about generic support services such as churches, neighborhood playgrounds, and community recreation centers that are closer to home. If OT practitioners are not careful, their clients may suddenly realize that they have lost touch with neighbors and friends because of the time spent taking their children to specialized programs far from home. They could end up in a specialized world inhabited mainly by professionals.

Families must carry out daily tasks to perform their basic functions.[1] Family functions include activities related to education, recreation, daily care, affection, economics, and self-identity.[4] Family routines must be considered when home therapy programs are developed; otherwise, time-consuming programs that simply cannot be done within the parameters of the daily household routines and time schedule may be prescribed.

ESSENTIAL SKILLS FOR SUCCESSFUL INTERVENTION WITH FAMILIES

For OT practitioners, having good communication skills is just as important as having the proper knowledge to treat a client. Some essential communication skills include the following:

- *Solution-focused curiosity and interest:* People generally have an extremely positive response to practitioners who are nonjudgmentally interested in them and their situations. The focus should be on strengths, achievements, and desires rather than on the traditional problems and deficits. This "solution focus" allows the practitioner to support the adaptive (morphogenetic) potential of the family while not challenging or criticizing its current status. In the example of the Sanchez family, it would have been better for Heather to have asked Mrs. Sanchez, "What have you found that works best for feeding Margarita?" rather than "What problems do you encounter when feeding Margarita?"

- *Collaborative goal setting:* A family that has requested or been referred for OT services has some goals, even if only vague ones, that they hope the services will help achieve. The practitioner may have a very different idea of what the goals should be. Collaborating with the family to clarify and develop a common set of goals helps practitioners efficiently and effectively manage the intervention planning process. Staying close to the plan that was agreed on while being willing to change the plan as family needs evolve builds trust, and family members perceive the therapist as being interested in helping them achieve their goals. For example, after introducing herself, Heather should have asked Mrs. Sanchez about Margarita and what she hoped to accomplish by getting involved in the early intervention program. Asking "What are Margarita's biggest problems?" is a deficit-oriented approach. Stating, "I think we should work on Margarita's toilet training so that she is ready for kindergarten" could slow the development of a relationship between Heather and the Sanchez family. Carefully eliciting and acknowledging the family's wishes would create a solid basis for working with them. Starting with the family's hopes, dreams, and moments of pride reinforces the capabilities and competence of its members. After listening carefully to Mrs. Sanchez's expressed wishes for Margarita, Heather could say something like "So, you aren't sure about what you want to accomplish, but no matter what we do, Mrs. Sanchez, you want Margarita to feel like she is a part of the whole family." If Mrs. Sanchez nods and smiles, Heather would know that she identified a primary goal of the Sanchez family. She should keep that as a major feature of the intervention planning process.

CLINICAL *Pearl*

Build on family strengths, dreams, and hopes. When talking with families, ask "how" rather than "why" questions. Ask them to describe rather than explain situations. Instead of trying to establish some sort of linear cause-and-effect relationship among different factors, try to simply understand the relationships among events, people, and situations.[5]

- *Acknowledgment:* "Solution-focused curiosity and interest" and "collaborative goal setting" are skills that are grounded in the central communicative tool

known as **acknowledgment**, which practitioners can use to assure their clients that what they are saying is being heard and understood. OT practitioners can acknowledge the clients with whom they are speaking by providing appropriate feedback. This feedback can be in the form of verbal repetition or confirmation of the clients' statements (e.g., "So you have lived here for 5 years" or "I see"), nonverbal body movements (e.g., nodding the head, sitting forward with an interested expression), or paraverbal cues (e.g., "uh-huh" or "mm-hmm").

- *Continuity:* The OT practitioner's arrival and departure are the most important moments of contact with a family. At both times, the practitioner should be solution focused or future oriented. When arriving at the home, the practitioner is attempting to establish or reestablish positive rapport with the family. After discussing any relevant events that have taken place since the previous visit, the practitioner elicits from the family a desired outcome for that visit or restates an agreed-upon goal to guide activities during the current visit. When departing from the home, the practitioner and family identify events that will or may take place before the next visit as well as discuss a potential goal for the next visit. It can be difficult and frustrating for a practitioner to leave after a visit in which little progress has been made. In such cases, it is often helpful to leave the family with some "homework" related to their goal—to look for and note circumstances that relate to it—so that the practitioner can use the information as a stepping-stone for the next session. For example, imagine that the parents want their daughter to be able to dress independently and have identified their daughter using the zipper of a dress as their goal; however, the goal seems unreachable, and little progress is being made. The OT practitioner could ask them to pay attention to the circumstances under which their daughter attempts to touch or play with the zipper. The visit can then end on a more positive note, with the family having to focus on a smaller goal.

SUMMARY

Family systems theory provides a useful framework for thinking about families and the ways in which they operate. The challenges and triumphs of parenting a child who has a disability are similar to others that families without children with disabilities face. An important factor in determining whether families can successfully adapt to these challenges is the strength and support of their relationships with other key individuals. An OT practitioner is one of these key players—a person who has the opportunity to make a difference in the life of a family through a sensitive, individualized intervention approach.

References

1. American Occupational Therapy Association. (2014). *Occupational therapy practice framework: domain and process* (3rd ed.). Bethesda, MD: Author.
2. Chou, C.-F., & Johnson, P. J. (2008). Health disparities among America's health care providers: Evidence from the integrated health interview series, 1982 to 2004. *J Occup Environ Med, 50,* 696–704.
3. Division for Early Childhood. (2014). DEC recommended practices in early intervention/early childhood special education. Retrieved from http://www.dec-sped.org/recommendedpractices.
4. Turnbull, A., Turnbull, R., Erwin, E. J., Soodak, L. C., & Shogren, K. A. (2010). *Families, professionals, and exceptionality: positive outcomes through partnerships and trust* (6th ed.). New York, NY: Pearson.
5. Turnbull, A., Winton, P., Rous, B., & Buysse, V. (2010). *CONNECT module 4: family-professional partnerships.* Chapel Hill: University of North Carolina, FPG Child Development Institute, CONNECT: The Center to Mobilize Early Childhood Knowledge.
6. U.S. Census Bureau. Retrieved from http://www.census.gov/acs/www/about_the_survey/american_community_survey/.
7. U.S. Department of Education. (n.d.). Individuals with Disabilities Act Part C Regulations, 34 CFR Part 303. http://idea.ed.gov/part-c/regulations/1.

Recommended Reading

Turnbull, A., Winton, P., Rous, B., & Buysse, V. (2010). *CONNECT module 4: family-professional partnerships.* Chapel Hill: University of North Carolina, FPG Child Development Institute, CONNECT: The Center to Mobilize Early Childhood Knowledge.

Turnbull, A., Turnbull, R., Erwin, E. J., Soodak, L. C., & Shogren, K. A. (2010). *Families, professionals, and exceptionality: positive outcomes through partnerships and trust* (6th ed.). New York, NY: Pearson.

Winton, P. J., Brotherson, M. J., & Summers, J. A. (2008). Learning from the field of early intervention about partnering with families. In M. Cornish (Ed.), *Promising practices for partnering with families in the early years* (pp. 21–40). Greenwich, CT: Information Age.

Winton, P., Buysse, V., Turnbull, A., & Rous, B. (2010). *CONNECT module 3: communication for collaboration.* Chapel Hill: University of North Carolina, FPG Child Development Institute, CONNECT: The Center to Mobilize Early Childhood Knowledge.

REVIEW *Questions*

1. What are the differences between prescriptive and consultative professional roles?
2. How does a therapy program affect a family unit?
3. Describe three key concepts related to family systems theory and the implications of these concepts for OT practitioners.
4. Explain why nonnormative transitional events may be more stressful than normative transitional events.
5. With the information provided on family systems and family adaptation, explain why it is important to individualize therapy programs for children and families.
6. What are four communication strategies that could be used during the initial home visit with a family?

SUGGESTED *Activities*

1. Spend time with a child with special needs in his or her natural environment (e.g., home, neighborhood). Observe the various activities taking place. Keep a list of the ways different therapy activities could be embedded in these routines. Imagine the way therapy concepts could be introduced to the parents and then implemented. Write these ideas down.
2. Talk with the families of children with disabilities and with OT practitioners. Ask each group to describe the characteristics of an OT practitioner that they think are important. Take notes, and summarize the comments. Compare the comments of the two groups. Create a personal list of the skills and competencies of an effective OT practitioner.
3. Go online to CONNECT Module 4 on Family-Professional Partnerships. Review the videos demonstrating effective communication practices with families and participate in the suggested activities associated with the videos. http://community.fpg.unc.edu/connect-modules/learners/module-4.

MELISSA E. KRONBERGER*

Medical Systems

KEY TERMS

Pediatric medical care
  system
Primary care
Secondary care
Tertiary care
Quaternary care
Neonatal intensive care
  unit (NICU)
Acute
Pediatric intensive care
  unit (PICU)
Medical/surgical/general
  care unit
Hematology/oncology
  unit
Subacute unit
Pediatric acute
  rehabilitation
Outpatient services
Long-term care
Assistive technology
  services
Screening
Evaluation
Interprofessional
  collaboration
SOAP note
Universal precautions

CHAPTER *Objectives*

After studying this chapter, the reader will be able to accomplish the following:

- Describe occupational therapy practice in a medical system.
- Identify the key members of a pediatric medical system.
- Differentiate among pediatric acute care, pediatric acute rehabilitation, subacute care, long-term care, outpatient services and specialty clinics, and home care medical settings.
- List commonly assessed areas of function in a pediatric medically based occupational therapy evaluation.
- Discuss the roles of the occupational therapist and the occupational therapy assistant during the process of intervention and documentation in a pediatric medical system.
- Identify equipment commonly found in hospital settings.
- Identify challenges faced by occupational therapist practitioners working in a pediatric medical practice setting.
- Describe infection control procedures for occupational therapy practitioners.

CHAPTER *Outline*

Medical Care Settings
LEVELS OF MEDICAL CARE
NEONATAL INTENSIVE CARE UNIT
PEDIATRIC INTENSIVE CARE UNIT
MEDICAL/SURGICAL/GENERAL CARE UNIT
SPECIALTY SERVICES
SUBACUTE SETTING
PEDIATRIC ACUTE REHABILITATION PROGRAMS
HOME CARE
OUTPATIENT SERVICES AND SPECIALTY CLINICS

Moving Through the Medical System Continuum

Role of Occupational Therapy in the Pediatric Medical System
ROLE OF THE OCCUPATIONAL THERAPY PRACTITIONER
PHYSIOLOGIC PARAMETERS

MEDICAL EQUIPMENT
NUTRITION

Interprofessional Collaboration

Documentation

Modalities

Reimbursement

Challenges for OT Practitioners Working in the Medical System
INFECTION CONTROL
CHARACTERISTICS OF A SUCCESSFUL HEALTH CARE
  PROVIDER
LEGAL AND ETHICAL CONSIDERATIONS IN A MEDICAL
  CARE SYSTEM

Summary

*We acknowledge the review by and contributions from Margaret Miller during the preparation of the fourth edition.

The medical system represents a significant sector of care in the United States. Medical systems continuously change and access to care continuously evolves. Legal, legislative, societal, ethical, and financial factors influence health care delivery. The role of the occupational therapy (OT) practitioner in the medical setting is to facilitate the ability of the infant, child, or adolescent to engage in everyday occupations while supporting medical stability for discharge. The OT practitioner facilitates community reentry by providing outpatient services and recommending community resources. Understanding the types of settings and the role of OT practitioners among teams is essential to providing quality services to children and youth.

MEDICAL CARE SETTINGS

A medical system includes many team members, including children, families, specialists, generalists, nurses, physicians, physical therapists, physical therapy (PT) assistants, child life or therapeutic activity specialists, speech and language pathologists, occupational therapists, and certified occupational therapy assistants (COTAs). A **pediatric medical care system** comprises a group of individuals who form a complex and unified whole dedicated to caring for children who are ill (Box 3-1).[9] A variety of personnel work as part of the team, including medical laboratory technicians, audiologists, pharmacists, dietitians, orthotists, social workers, case managers, psychologists, and recreational therapists. Support personnel may include phlebotomists who draw blood, radiology technicians who take x-rays, cardiac technicians who do studies of the heart (including electrocardiograms), and electroencephalogram technicians. A medical-based OT practitioner has to become familiar with the roles and responsibilities of other disciplines. This knowledge facilitates team collaboration and benefits children and their families.

CLINICAL *Pearl*

The number of specialties included in the pediatric medical care system may be challenging for the new OT practitioner to remember. Learn the names of the medical team members and their specialties. Carry contact information when working on the unit to facilitate ease of communication and consulting.

Levels of Medical Care

OT practitioners need to be aware of the level of medical care under which services are being provided to children. The increased number of uninsured or underinsured children and families has resulted in expansion of medical care practice outside of the more traditional arena (i.e., inpatient, center-based care, in-home services).

Primary care is considered the "first level" of medical care and includes visits to one's primary physician.[4]

Pediatric primary care is strongly grounded in the understanding that caregivers must receive assistance to recognize the need for routine and follow-up medical care. Practices such as immunizations, vaccinations, regularly scheduled checkups, and ongoing monitoring of chronic conditions are all examples of strategies that are used under the primary care model to promote and support health in children. All medical personnel who provide services under this model of care are responsible for participating in educating family members, caregivers, and significant others.

Second-level **(secondary)** medical **care** involves follow-up that occurs once a child has become ill. In secondary care, a primary care physician refers a child to a specialist for complex medical or developmental concerns. This level of medical care involves caregiver education, focusing on caregiver recognition of the importance of adherence to guidelines regarding care, sanitation, dispensing medication, and observation for signs of improvement or worsening of a condition.[4] This level of care is more intense than in the primary care model. The increased level of medical care is provided to prevent the necessity of tertiary medical care.

Third-level **(tertiary)** medical **care** involves the need for hospitalization.[4] At this point in the medical care continuum, serious concerns have arisen regarding involvement of the child's body system(s) and that additional body systems will be affected by primary or secondary causes associated with the child's illness. As in all other levels of medical care, caregiver education is provided. However, a greater level of responsibility for the child's recuperation is dependent on interventions provided by medical personnel.

Quaternary care is an extension of tertiary care and is less common, highly specialized, and provided in circumstances such as severe trauma, significant burns, heart transplants, and experimental services.[4] These medical interventions are not found in every hospital.

CLINICAL *Pearl*

The occupational therapy assistant (OTA) will typically work in primary, secondary, and tertiary care.

Comprehensive pediatric medical care occurs over a continuum of various settings, including neonatal intensive care unit (NICU), step-down nursery or pediatric intensive care unit (PICU), medical/surgical/general care unit, acute rehabilitation unit, subacute setting, the home, or a residential (long-term care) facility.

The role of the OT and the COTA and types of occupational therapy services delivered in each unit of care varies. However, the core of service delivery remains the same: evaluation, intervention, and outcome review. Medical care centers require that all inpatient

BOX 3-1

Medical and Allied Health Team in the Medical Setting

PHYSICIAN SPECIALISTS

- *Hospitalist:* A physician in charge of medical care during hospitalization (e.g., emergency, critical care, medical units).
- *Neonatologist:* A physician who specializes in the study, care, and treatment of neonates. The team leader of the neonatal ICU.
- *Pediatric intensivist:* A pediatrician who specializes in the care of infants and children who are in the ICU because of severe illnesses.
- *Pediatric medical subspecialists:* Physicians specializing in specific diagnostic areas in the care of children.
- *Anesthesiologist:* A physician specializing in in the branch of medicine that understands the autonomic, neuromuscular, cardiac, and respiratory physiology; the relationship with the control of acute and chronic pain and use of sedative, analgesic, hypnotic, antiemetic, respiratory, and cardiovascular drugs. The anesthesiologist is involved with preoperative, intraoperative, and postoperative care.
- *Cardiac surgeon:* A surgeon specializing in performing surgery on clients with cardiac disorders.
- *Cardiologist:* A physician specializing in the treatment of heart disease (i.e., congenital heart defects)
- *Developmental optometrist:* An eye doctor with postgraduate training in the eye health and efficient vision for functioning in daily occupations; a specialist in children's vision.
- *Gastroenterologist:* A physician specializing in the anatomy, physiology, and treatment of disorders related to the digestive organs (i.e., digestive disorders, difficulty absorbing certain nutrients, reflux, failure to thrive, malabsorption, motility disorders).
- *Geneticist:* A specialist in genetic disorders.
- *Genetic counselor:* A health care professional who specializes in the education and support of patients, families, or prospective parents about inherited diseases that they or their offspring may be susceptible.
- *Head and neck surgeon (HNS; formerly called ENT):* A specialist in the science of the ear, nose, and the throat, and their functions and diseases (i.e., hearing impairment, craniofacial anomalies, cleft lip/palate, problems with airway, tracheostomies)
- *Hematologist:* A physician who specializes in the diagnosis and treatment of blood disorders and blood-forming tissues.
- *Nephrologist:* A physician who specializes in the structure and function of the kidney and related diseases.
- *Neurologist:* A specialist in the study and treatment of diseases of the nervous system; involved in identification and diagnosis of neurologic problems (i.e., seizure disorders, cerebral palsy, transverse myelitis, Guillain-Barré, brain tumors).
- *Nurse practitioner:* A licensed registered nurse who has obtained advanced preparation for practice in the diagnosis and treatment of illness. The nurse practitioner may diagnose medical problems, order treatments, and make referrals. The practitioner may work collaboratively with physicians or independently in private practice or nursing clinics. In some states, the nurse practitioner is able to prescribe medications.
- *Oncologist:* A physician who specializes in the diagnosis and treatment of tumors and cancer-related disorders.
- *Ophthalmologist:* A physician who specializes in the treatment of disorders of the eye.
- *Orthopedist:* A specialist in the branch of medical science that deals with the prevention or correction of disorders involving the skeleton, joints, muscles, fascia, ligaments, and cartilage.
- *Physiatrist:* A physician who specializes in physical rehabilitation and medicine. The physiatrist is the medical team leader of the acute rehabilitation unit and provides service for children requiring inpatient or outpatient rehabilitation.
- *Physician assistant:* A specially trained and licensed individual who performs tasks usually done by physicians and works under the direction of the supervising physician.
- *Pulmonologist:* A physician trained and certified to treat pulmonary diseases (e.g., chronic lung disease, cystic fibrosis)
- *Surgeon:* A medical practitioner who specializes in surgery. For children, the surgeon may place feeding tubes (e.g., gastrostomy or jejunostomy) or help stabilize children who have had a trauma (e.g., injury to abdomen from car accident)

ALLIED HEALTH PROFESSIONALS

- *Art therapist:* A professional holding a master's degree in art therapy who uses the creative process, art media, and the resulting artwork to explore feelings, reconcile emotions, foster self-awareness, manage behavior, and develop skills to improve or restore a client's sense of well-being. Art therapists are trained in art and human development, psychology and counseling.
- *Audiologist:* A specialist who can identify and evaluate hearing loss, and can rehabilitate those with hearing loss, especially those whose loss cannot be improved by surgical or medical means.
- *Case manager:* An individual who coordinates the interprofessional medical care for a patient to improve quality and continuity of care and to decrease hospital costs. The case manager coordinates the individualized medical plan for children with complex needs or chronic medical problems, and acts as a liaison between family and team members for optimal communication before discharge.
- *Child life specialist:* A professional with expertise in helping children and their families overcome challenging life events, particularly those related to health care and hospitalization, via play, preparation, and self-expression.
- *Clinical neuropsychologist:* A professional with specialized knowledge and training in the applied science of brain behavior relationships including assessment, diagnosis, treatment and rehabilitation of clients across the life span who have neurologic, medical, developmental,

BOX 3-1

Medical and Allied Health Team in the Medical Setting—cont'd

or psychiatric conditions. The pediatric clinical neuropsychologist provides service on the medical and acute rehabilitation units of the children's hospital.

- *Clinical nurse specialist:* A nurse who holds a master's degree with competence in a specific area such as intensive care, cardiology, oncology, obstetrics, or psychiatry. The pediatric clinical nurse specialist provides care to infants and children.
- *Dietitian (RD):* An individual trained in the area of nutrition who evaluates and provides intervention regarding the dietary needs of the healthy and the sick. Registered dieticians are certified with the American Dietetic Association.
- *Hospital school teacher:* A certificated teacher responsible for the education of children who are hospitalized.
- *Music therapist:* A professional trained to assess the strengths and needs of a patient and use music within a therapeutic relationship to address physical, psychological, cognitive, and social needs of the individual.
- *Occupational therapist (OTR):* A professional who provides assessment and intervention for occupational performance. Occupational therapists help clients engage in everyday activities (occupations) that provide clients with a sense of meaning and identity.
- *Certified occupational therapy assistant (COTA):* The COTA provides intervention to enable clients to engage in meaningful activities and occupations that provide them a sense of identity and purpose. COTAs work under the supervision of an OT.
- *Orthotist:* A professional who designs, constructs, and adjusts orthotics, orthopedic braces, and other structures that support the body or its parts.
- *Pharmacist:* A professional licensed to prepare and dispense drugs. A pharmacist may advise on the selection, dosages, interactions, and side effects of medications.

- *Physical therapist:* A licensed individual trained in the management of the client's movement system who provides examination and intervention to alleviate disability, impairments, and functional limitations.
- *Physical therapist assistant:* A trained paraprofessional who provides selected interventions for clients under the supervision of a physical therapist.
- *Prosthetist:* A specialist in the branch of surgery or physiatry dealing with the construction, replacement, and adaption of missing or damaged limbs.
- *Registered nurse (RN):* A nurse licensed to work in a specific state. The pediatric RN is prepared to care of infants and children. RNs work closely with team members and administer medication, provide medical care, and assist families with psychological issues.
- *Respiratory therapist:* A person skilled in managing the techniques and equipment used in treating clients with acute and chronic respiratory diseases.
- *Social worker:* Pediatric social workers provide supportive services to neonatal, pediatric, and adolescent clients and their families. Assistance includes adjustment to disability, illness, grief or loss, and addressing personal, financial, legal and environmental difficulties for solving and coping with everyday problems.
- *Speech-language pathologist:* A health care professional trained to evaluate and treat people who have voice, speech, language, swallowing or hearing disorders, especially those that affect their ability to communicate or consume food.
- *Therapeutic recreation specialist:* An individual who specializes in planning and directing recreational activities for patients recovering from physical or mental illness or who are attempting to cope with a permanent disability.

Adapted from Venes, D. (2009). *Taber's cyclopedic medical dictionary* (21st ed.). Philadelphia: FA Davis.

occupational therapy evaluations be completed within 48 hours of the client's admission.

Neonatal Intensive Care Unit

Infants who have experienced complications with birth may be placed in the **neonatal intensive care unit (NICU).** The goal of the NICU team is to address the **acute** or extremely severe symptoms or conditions of infants so that they can become physiologically stable (i.e., maintain a stable body temperature, heart rate, and respiratory rate).

The medical team closely monitors the medical status of NICU infants. A neonatologist serves as the leader of the NICU team (Figure 3-1). In addition to conducting a neonatal assessment, the neonatologist consults with

other professionals on the medical team about the specific needs of the infant. Infants with the following conditions may be admitted to the NICU:

- Cyanosis: the infant turns blue because of insufficient oxygen
- Bradycardia: the infant has a heart rate of less than 100 beats per minute (bpm)
- Low birth weight (LBW): the infant weighs less than 2500 grams
- Very low birth weight (VLBW): the infant weighs less than 1500 grams
- Extremely low birth weight (ELBW): the infant weighs less than 750 grams
- Premature birth (less than 37 weeks gestational age)

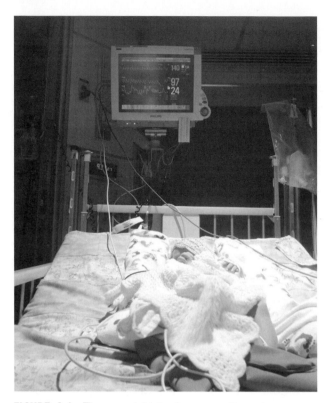

FIGURE 3-1 The neonatal intensive care unit can be an overwhelming environment. (From Parham, L. D., & Fazio, L.S. (2009). *Play in occupational therapy for children* (2nd ed.). St. Louis: Mosby.)

- Respiratory difficulties
- Presence of congenital anomalies
- Neurologic injury or abnormality
- Infants requiring surgery

When presented with an infant who has one or more of these conditions, additional medical team members take part in consultations and interventions. Pulmonologists (lung specialists), cardiologists (heart specialists), gastroenterologists (digestive specialists), neurologists (brain specialists), social workers, and respiratory therapists may be needed to address the needs of infants in the NICU. OT practitioners may address positioning for function, range of motion, and age-related motor and sensory development. In certain states, the occupational therapist addresses feeding and swallowing concerns of the critical care infant and provides lactation consultation.

CLINICAL *Pearl*

Families with children experiencing life-threatening illnesses may express various types of emotions at any given time. The skilled OT practitioner incorporates characteristics of therapeutic use of self while interacting with the individual coping with a loved one's illness.

Only highly qualified allied health professionals perform NICU-based intervention. Therapists who work in the NICU are required to have advanced education and certification in NICU-based intervention. For example, therapists in the NICU must have a thorough knowledge of life signs, which are key indicators of the infant's status (e.g., color, respiration rate, body temperature, extremity movement). Changes in these indicators are noted by the therapist through sight, hearing, and touch. A role for the OTA in the provision of NICU services has not been identified.[1] OT practitioners who want to work with this special client population should obtain the necessary education and certification required to ensure that intervention is provided safely and appropriately.

Pediatric Intensive Care Unit

The **pediatric intensive care unit (PICU)** is a specialized unit that addresses the critical medical needs of the infant, child, or adolescent from birth to 21 years. The pediatric intensivist, also referred to as the pediatric critical care medicine specialist, is the medical team leader of the PICU. The pediatric intensivist directs the care of the infant, child, or young adult by administering direct care or consulting with a variety of experts to determine the best course of intervention for these medically fragile, high-risk children.[4] For example, the pediatric intensivist may consult with the pediatric infectious disease physician regarding a child with a rare or infectious disease. The following conditions may indicate the need for admission to the PICU:

- Open heart surgery
- Brain injury (e.g., trauma from accident, near drowning, aneurysm)
- Brain surgery (e.g., posterior fossa syndrome)
- Significant life-threatening illness (e.g., transverse myelitis)
- Respiratory complications resulting from diagnoses (e.g., Guillain-Barré, multiple sclerosis)
- Nonaccidental trauma (e.g., shaken baby syndrome)
- Transfer from the NICU

CLINICAL *Pearl*

When working with medically fragile infants and children, check with nursing regarding timing of intervention. Therapy times may require scheduling around medical procedures or naps.

In the PICU, the OT practitioner encounters patients with a wide variety of medical diagnoses and ages. The occupational therapist and the COTA closely monitor the medical condition of the patient while providing evaluation and intervention for basic self-care, transfer training, postural control, range of motion, orthotics and splinting, contracture prevention, and sensory stimulation. They also may provide interventions to target

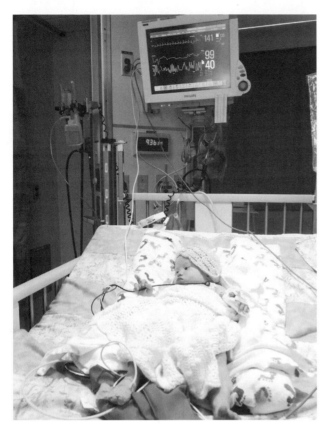

FIGURE 3-2 Infants are transferred to a step-down nursery or pediatric intensive care unit when they have the ability to maintain satisfactory physiologic functioning. (Courtesy Dawn B. Oakley and Kathleen Logan-Bauer, Bayside, NY.)

instrumental activities of daily living (IADL), sleep and rest, feeding and swallowing concerns, as well as lactation consultations. The frequency and duration of OT service varies from two to five times per week for 30 to 60 minutes, depending on the patient's condition.

Providing intervention in a step-down nursery or PICU also requires related experience to ensure the provision of the most appropriate treatment. However, unlike the situation in the NICU, OTAs who have received service competency training can assume a role in providing medical services in the step-down nursery and PICU.[1] OTAs working in the step-down nursery or PICU benefit from obtaining continuing education units and on-the-job training (Figure 3-2).

Medical/Surgical/General Care Unit

Children receiving care on a **medical/surgical/general care unit** require 24-hour medical attention. Diagnoses may include orthopedic conditions, trauma, drowning, falls, sports-related injuries, pneumonia, flu, severe asthma attacks, and cardiac conditions. A variety of specialty physicians and team members serve on these units, including OT practitioners. The OT practitioner

monitors medical status related to function while providing interventions to address areas of occupation (e.g., ADLs, IADLs, sleep and rest, play and leisure, education). Practitioners may recommend adaptive equipment. The OT practitioner documents and relays medical status and progress during unit rounds or team conferences. The frequency and duration of OT intervention varies from two to five times per week for 30 to 60 minutes.

> **CLINICAL** *Pearl*
>
> To improve time-management skills, quickly learn where ADL items and clean linen are stored on each unit/floor. Take the stairs going down, not up, if time is short.

> **CLINICAL** *Pearl*
>
> The child admitted to an in-patient medical unit may experience feelings of isolation and depression due to acute medical need. It is important for the OT practitioner to coordinate with nursing and child life services for engagement in intervention sessions and for play and leisure participation.

Specialty Services

Large children's hospitals may designate beds in a unit to provide care for particular procedures in a specific specialty. For example, a unit may provide care for those children having cardiac surgery or otolaryngology (i.e., ear, nose, throat) procedures. This means that instead of the child or young adult recovering on a general medical unit, 24-hour direct patient care is provided by nursing staff specifically trained for addressing needs that typically follow the specific procedures. They may request that OT practitioners provide services on these units as medically necessary for ADL and IADL tasks.

Hematology/Oncology Unit

An occupational therapist or OTA can be assigned to a specialty unit such as the **hematology/oncology unit.** The OT practitioner evaluates and develops intervention to address basic ADLs, IADLs, sleep and rest, play and leisure, and education. Helping clients engage in daily meaningful activities can add to their quality of life. Practitioners may evaluate client factors interfering with engagement in one's occupation such as range of motion, strength, endurance, posture, visual perception, and fine and gross motor skills. Practitioners evaluate and recommend adaptive equipment to allow children to engage in activities. OT practitioners use knowledge that engaging in activities to help children and youth maintain their identity while experiencing illness. The intervention plan and schedule may follow medical protocol/guidelines and consider the child's chemotherapy and/or radiation schedule. Intervention typically varies between 30 and 60 minutes, one to five times a week.

Palliative Care

Palliative care services are provided in large children's hospitals on all medical units. Palliative care provides comfort care for the dying infant, child, adolescent or young adult by providing medical interventions and sensory interventions to calm and decrease anxiety. This care also provides comfort to family members. The palliative care nurse consults with team members, including OT practitioners and medical social workers.

Many children's hospitals have child life services that provide social and leisure activities for children and youth facing procedures that cause pain, depression, and anxiety. They may provide individual or group activities to help children and youth focus on play and leisure. This may help children coping with illness or disability. OT practitioners and child life specialists share information on the client's performance skills and psychosocial status to better address the client's needs.

Subacute Setting

Subacute units serve infants and children up to age 21 who are not ready to return home. These infants, children, and young adults may exhibit generalized weakness, respiratory deficits, cardiac conditions, neuromuscular deficits, and other limitations that interfere with age-appropriate function and engagement in daily occupations. They may require medical interventions not available in outpatient clinics or at home.

Clients in these subacute settings are typically more medically stable than those in the NICU, step-down nursery, or PICU. However, OTAs working in these settings must be familiar with the signs of physiologic distress and be prepared to respond properly as in the other medically based practice settings.

Box 3-2 provides two examples of the types of children who may receive care in a subacute setting.

Pediatric Acute Rehabilitation Programs

Pediatric acute rehabilitation programs are a specialty service that may be found in the children's hospital or a rehabilitation hospital. Acute rehabilitation programs are directed by a pediatric physiatrist and provide occupational therapy, speech therapy (ST), and physical therapy (PT) services five to six times a week for 3 hours per day. The practitioners work with children who have sustained a serious injury or illness to maximize their independence in meaningful daily activities.

OT practitioners provide interventions to enable children and youth to participate in daily occupations

---

BOX 3-2

Examples of Children Receiving Care in Subacute Setting

1. The infant is improving and no longer requires the level of care provided in the PICU but cannot be discharged home because the family lives too far from a medical facility. The infant still requires frequent monitoring of blood pressure and heart rate. The infant is beginning to show adequate suck-swallow-breathe but is not yet consistent. This child is transferred to the subacute setting where intervention goals reflect the medical needs of the infant and the desires of the infant's caregivers. The OT practitioner encourages a suck-swallow-breathe pattern and provides consultation to the parents on infant development expectations as related to their infant's condition. The practitioner reviews soothing techniques and positioning suggestions as part of the plan. Finally, the practitioner provides community resources for additional support upon discharge and listens to the parents as they describe fears. The practitioner provides psychosocial support and develops a therapeutic relationship through listening.

2. An adolescent is recovering from new onset of Guillain-Barré syndrome. This patient easily and quickly fatigues, sometimes requires respiratory interventions, and is dependent in basic self-care. The OT practitioner provides evaluation and intervention for basic ADLs (feeding, dressing, bathing, toileting). The practitioner addresses swallowing and evaluates client factors that interfere with occupational performance. Specifically, the practitioner works with the client to facilitate range of motion, endurance, breathing techniques, and daily routine planning. As the adolescent gains endurance, the practitioner explores energy conservation techniques and the use of adaptive equipment. Furthermore, the OT practitioner provides psychosocial support by listening to the adolescent, encouraging, and educating the adolescent on the rehabilitative process.

(e.g., ADL, IDAL, sleep and rest, education, play and leisure, and social participation). They develop group and individual intervention sessions to develop cognitive, motor, and psychosocial performance skills. For example, OT practitioners may develop intervention to enhance self-care skills, cooking abilities, school reentry, community participation, and leisure. They may emphasize gross and fine motor skills, visual motor and visual perceptual training, cognitive, or feeding and swallowing skills. In some settings, weekly team conferences are provided for families to prepare for discharge. The length of stay can be from 1 week to 3 or more months.

Home Care

The medical team and caregivers formulate discharge plans as the client's status improves. The goal for pediatric patients is to return home. OT practitioners develop discharge plans to promote the continued acquisition of age-appropriate skills, engagement in social and play activities and return to school. Often with young children, an agency (such as early intervention [EI] state agency) coordinates the child's medical needs and home-based therapeutic services. Typically children over 3 years old are served in outpatient clinics, community-based EI, or Early Head Start programs

States provide community support services for children and families, such as Miracle League, Autism Speaks, and Special Olympics. The knowledgeable clinician seeks out resources and networks within the community to help children and families participate in their community.

> ### CLINICAL *Pearl*
>
> Practitioners must respect the families' values, beliefs, and customs while providing home-based occupational therapy services for children.

Once at home, there are multiple physical and psychosocial occupational therapy goals. These goals may include facilitating caregiver and infant bonding, promoting the continued acquisition of age-appropriate developmental skills, engagement in social and play activities, and return to school. OT practitioners working in home environments, outpatient clinics, or community-based settings evaluate and implement individual intervention. The practitioner working in these settings considers the family's communication styles, values, customs, time commitments, and environment when developing and implementing the intervention plan. The frequency and duration of occupational therapy services varies, depending on the child's diagnosis, current level of function, and the accessibility of service to the child and family.

Outpatient Services and Specialty Clinics

A variety of **outpatient** occupational therapy **services** are available to children with specific medical diagnoses who are in need. OT practitioners working in an outpatient setting provide evaluation, intervention, and consultation to allow the child to engage in meaningful daily activities (i.e., ADL, IADL, sleep and rest, play and leisure, social participation, education). They educate family members and provide community resources, including support systems and assistive technology supports.

Traditional medically based pediatric outpatient occupational therapy services are provided at rehabilitation, children's, and community hospitals. OT service delivery consists of evaluation, intervention, and outcome review for areas of occupation as well as a review of client factors that may be typically associated with a given condition. For example, children with neurologic deficits may benefit from a thorough assessment of muscle tone and how it influences voluntary movement for home, school, and community activities. The practitioner may reevaluate adaptive seating options and consult with the school teacher on positioning for academics in the classroom. Some specialty clinics may specialize in hand therapy, whereas others may focus on feeding and swallowing, vision rehabilitation, or sensory integration. The OTA can provide service delivery in these settings once they have established service competency. Specialty clinics may include the following:

- Patients who have had an acute rehabilitation inpatient stay;
- NICU baby follow-up clinic/high-risk infant clinic;
- Hypertonicity clinic;
- Spinal bifida clinic;
- Rheumatology clinic;
- Cystic fibrosis clinic;
- Neuro-oncology clinic; and
- Cleft palate clinic.

Each specialty clinic is structured to monitor the medical needs of the infant, child, or adolescent and their family. A child may receive intervention (e.g., Botox injections for hypertonicity; gastroenterology procedures to prevent oral aversion) or consultation from professionals (e.g., occupational therapy consult regarding new wheelchair or adaptive equipment). Children attending clinics may also be referred to other health care professionals.

The OT practitioner contributes to the child's evaluation. The practitioner may recommend occupational therapy services, consult with practitioners in the community, or provide strategies to child and families at the clinic session. See Box 3-3 for examples of occupational therapy participation in specialty clinics.

It is important to note that the OTA does not provide direct service in a specialty clinic. The OTA may provide service to the child in the community or school.

> ### CLINICAL *Pearl*
>
> The OTA working in the medical setting needs to be resourceful to children and families by having awareness of local support groups and community programs.

BOX 3-3

Examples of Role of OT Practitioner in Specialty Clinics

The following examples illustrate the role of the occupational therapy practitioner in a specialty clinic.

Rehabilitation clinic: Child receives an appointment to attend the rehabilitation clinic within 6 weeks of leaving the hospital inpatient stay. The occupational therapy completes an evaluation (or quick screening) for ADLs using the WeeFIM and also completes range of motion evaluation, manual muscle test, visual screening, feeding/swallowing assessment, and evaluation of orthotic needs. The therapist interviews the parent to determine how the child is functioning at home, at school, and in the community. Based on the information gathered, the therapist makes changes to the positioning equipment, updates the child's orthoses, and refers the parent to a local clinician who specializes in feeding. The occupational therapist remains concerned that the child is not achieving in school. The therapist collaborates with the neuropsychologist, social worker, and school occupational therapist to make sure the adaptive equipment recommendations for school are provided and monitored. The OTA at the school discusses the progress and they collaborate to find a solution for the child.

Hypertonicity clinic: Children who exhibit muscle tone deficits may benefit from attending this clinic. Children who sustained a serious brain injury, have developmental delays (e.g., cerebral palsy or spinal bifida), or those with neurologic disorders may exhibit hypertonicity. Occupational therapy practitioners working in this clinic frequently monitor muscle tone and its influence on ADL, IADL, play and leisure, social participation, and education. They may evaluate upper extremity function (using the Ashworth Scale) and make recommendations for serial casting, orthotics or custom splinting. The practitioner develops a home program and consults with the OT assistant regarding follow-up at school.

Long-Term Care

During discharge planning, parents, families, or primary caregivers may decide that they are unable to handle the child's specific medical needs. Some children may require **long-term care** (residential) to meet their specific medical needs. This is a difficult decision, commonly seen when the child has complex medical problems that require significant medical intervention (e.g., feeding tubes, oxygen, specialized positioning, ventilator support). In these cases, medical team members consult and research available residential (long-term care) facility options.

The team presents the options to caregivers for the final placement decision. The goals of long-term care are to provide appropriate medical care and therapy services. OT practitioners working in long-term care facilities provide services to help children and adolescents engage in daily occupations. They provide interventions to prevent or minimize losses in range of motion, prevent contractures, optimize positioning, encourage interaction, stimulate sensorimotor activity, develop oral motor skills, promote participation in ADLs, and provide adaptive equipment and assistive technology. Occupational therapy interventions in long-term care focus on performance skills and client factors with the goal of enhanced occupational performance.

Parent and Child Support Groups and Community Programs

Community support groups may address a variety of important issues such as grieving, coping, or bullying; support groups may focus on topics related to specific conditions such as spinal cord injury, juvenile arthritis, or cerebral palsy. The OT practitioner may lead the group or provide consulting services and/or guest lectures. Practitioners may provide insight regarding the engagement of child in occupations, experience in the medical setting, understanding of the continuum of medical care and related community reentry needs. Some clinics provide individual or group OT interventions and "camps" addressing the needs of children who have specific diagnoses or needs (e.g., constraint-induced movement therapy, cancer, spinal cord injury).

Organizations such as Autism Speaks or Special Olympics support children's and adolescent's participation. The knowledgeable clinician seeks out support networks and may even start a network within the practice setting to maximize the child's return to participation in daily activities.

Assistive Technology in the Outpatient Setting

Assistive technology refers to devices and services for the disabled. **Assistive technology services** may be located at hospitals, universities, community organizations, or schools. OT practitioners may obtain special certification through the American Occupational Therapy Association (AOTA) in environmental modification or obtain continuing education before they can provide service delivery in the area of assistive technology. See Chapter 27 for details on assistive technology.

MOVING THROUGH THE MEDICAL SYSTEM CONTINUUM

The extent to which a child is involved in the medical system continuum changes as the child's circumstances change. For example, a child may be admitted to an acute care facility because of an acute illness. The child may be subsequently discharged and return home but then be admitted to a long-term care facility because of extenuating circumstances at home. This is just one example of the way a child's involvement in the pediatric medical care system can change. The case study presented here follows the progression of one child through pediatric medical care settings.

CASE *Study*

Justine was born at 34 weeks' gestation after a difficult pregnancy to a 19-year-old single mother who already had a 2-year-old. Ultrasound at 23 weeks' gestation revealed that Justine had multiple anomalies including cleft lip and palate, shortened limbs, small corpus callosum, and enlarged ventricles and duodenal atresia.

Justine was born by cesarean delivery and was apneic at birth. She was resuscitated and needed ventilator support for 2 days. She transitioned to continuous positive airway pressure (CPAP) and then to oxygen per cannula. Her birth weight was 1830 grams (4 pounds, 1.5 ounces).

A number of medical specialists were involved in her care including a neonatologist, a head and neck surgeon (ENT), a plastic surgeon for management of cleft palate, and a general surgeon who surgically repaired her duodenal atresia. A pediatric neurologist and pediatrician also were part of the team of medical specialists.

Justine received surgery for duodenal atresia on day of life 6 followed by briefly requiring ventilator support. She received intravenous (IV) nutrition for 14 days until feeds into her stomach could be initiated. She was able to suck on a pacifier. The team expressed significant concerns regarding feeding and swallowing in view of prematurity and cleft lip and palate. She was able to nipple a small volume of fluid/formula but was not efficient with oral feeding. A nasogastric tube was placed. The tube provided the majority of her nutrition. Oral feeds were trialed for 10 days followed by surgery for a gastrostomy tube (g-tube) when she was term age. Justine failed her hearing screen and further testing showed she had abnormally formed ear structures. Her head circumference was closely monitored for risk for developing hydrocephalus.

Justine was readmitted to the hospital eight times during her first year of life for various reasons: three times for surgical repair of the cleft palate, once for an infection in her gastrointestinal system, once for respiratory syncytial virus, once for the surgical revision of the g-tube and twice for breathing difficulties. She was in the PICU when she had breathing problems and for the first 2 days following each surgery. After one admission, she was discharged to a subacute setting for a month near the hospital because of ongoing medical needs. She was fitted for hearing aids at 2 months.

Occupational, physical, and speech therapies were involved with Justine throughout her NICU stay, focusing on positioning, range of motion, and oral skills (nippling) during therapy sessions with Justine and her mother. Justine's mother received education on Justine's level of arousal and her sensory development. The OT practitioners taught the mother how to recognize and help Justine organize her alertness with strategies for calming and console herself. The practitioners educated the mother on social interaction strategies to engage Justine in meaningful ways.

OT services were provided to Justine at the hospital, subacute setting, and at the home. Although she continued to demonstrate delays in skills, Justine made developmental gains at her pace. She learned to calm with support of her mother and caregivers with slow gentle movement. Justine was visually attentive, held her head up by 4 months, and sat unsupported at 8½ months. She had difficulty with prone positioning, also known as "tummy time," which is common for children with g-tube placement. She was hypersensitive to touch and movement, and especially avoided touch near her mouth.

Pediatric medical care often is required to treat complications resulting from genetic defects. Children may need medical care for accidental injuries, neurologic and musculoskeletal traumas, and birth-related trauma. Occupational therapy services were provided during Justine's time in the NICU, step-down nursery, transition home, and subsequent hospitalizations during her first year including the 1-month interval at a subacute facility. OT services supported age-related development and ongoing caregiver education and support. Each level of care addressed Justine's changing needs, progress, and family concerns (see Chapter 2 for additional information on working with families). Hospital-based OT services and in-home services focused on helping Justin develop ADLs (e.g., feeding, bathing, toileting, grooming, dressing), play and leisure, and sleep and rest. Intervention activities included but were not limited to activities targeting: range of motion, positioning, oral motor development, sensory development, gross and fine motor skill development, visual development, parent education and role modeling, and adaptive equipment to enhance Justine's participation in daily life. The OTA and occupational therapist monitored Justine's ability to eat by mouth and taught the mother strategies to decrease oral hypersensitivity for feeding. Justine was reevaluated in NICU follow-up clinic every 3 months; she attended the cleft palate clinic for additional support and monitoring.

CLINICAL *Pearl*

State regulations may determine the role and the responsibilities of the OT practitioner related to feeding and swallowing services.

ROLE OF OCCUPATIONAL THERAPY IN THE PEDIATRIC MEDICAL SYSTEM

CLINICAL *Pearl*

Childhood is filled with many typical developmental stages and events. Normal developmental progression can be negatively affected by atypical experiences and events, such as prolonged hospitalization.

Prolonged hospitalization of an infant or child is not a normal event. A hospitalization of more than a few days puts a typical child at risk for some degree of developmental delay. For example, to develop meaningful social and emotional bonds, infants and children need to be comforted and held by other human beings. Children and infants who are hospitalized typically are not held as often as those who are not in a hospital. These children and infants may have difficulty developing the social and emotional skills needed for successful interactions with members of their families and their peers. The OT practitioner trains parents and caregivers by role modeling and providing strategies to assist the child to develop social interaction skills, learn to receive comfort, and develop emotional regulation skills and self-soothing strategies.

The knowledge necessary to work in the NICU is made up of three components:

1. An understanding of the equipment;
2. An understanding of the standards of care that govern operations in these settings; and
3. An understanding of medical status signs that will guide the provision of therapeutic services.

The level of care required by the children admitted to one of these settings is high, and the status of these children is monitored regularly. Children may also need scheduled medication(s). The equipment found in these settings varies depending on the population of children being served. Some examples of the equipment found in these settings are shown in Box 3-4.

Some examples of standards of care include adherence to treatment guidelines (where and when treatment can occur), sign-out practices (children's locations must be recorded at all times), medical supervision (treatment must be provided in accordance with medical orders), and caregiver/parental expectations (guardian expectations and goals are included in the development of a comprehensive plan of care). OTAs providing services in these settings must accommodate all of these factors.

In addition to the equipment that monitors the children's status, the OT practitioner needs to perform ongoing monitoring to assess their readiness to receive

---

BOX 3-4

Equipment Examples

APNEA MONITORS
Monitor respiration

IV LINES/TUBES
Pass through the skin and into the veins

PULSE OXIMETER
Measures pulse and oxygen saturation levels (i.e., amount of oxygen found in the blood)

FEEDING TUBES
Oral tubes can be placed in the mouth and empty into the stomach; nasal tubes can be placed in the nose and empty into the stomach; and gastrostomy tubes can be placed in the abdomen and empty into the stomach.

ULTRAVIOLET LIGHTS
Light ray frequencies used to treat illness

WARMING BLANKETS/LIGHTS
Temperature control coverings (may be placed directly over a protective covering on the body or above a bed) used to assist in the maintenance of body temperature

Adapted from Venes, D. (2009). *Taber's cyclopedic medical dictionary* (21st ed.). Philadelphia: FA Davis.

therapy services or their ability to tolerate specific therapeutic interventions. Once the clinician has the opportunity to develop a level of comfort for service provision in the medical setting, he or she will develop a site-specific medical status checklist. Box 3-5 shows a medical status checklist for an entry-level OTA working with a child.

The checklist serves only as a general guideline. The clinician and child share the ultimate responsibility of determining whether a therapeutic intervention is successful. Because it is not uncommon for medically fragile children to experience distress when they are moved or touched, clinicians need to develop monitoring ranges that are acceptable for intervention.

Role of the Occupational Therapy Practitioner

The fundamental principle of occupational therapy is to promote optimal performance in each of the areas of occupation: play/leisure, ADLs, IADLs, social participation, sleep and rest, and education. OT practitioners working with children and youth use play activities to facilitate the acquisition of age-appropriate developmental skills (e.g., gross motor, fine motor, cognitive, social, oral-motor).

BOX 3-5

Medical Status Checklist

HEALTH STATUS
Client well enough to receive therapy services
- Alert
- Awake
- Blood pressure and heart rate remain within guidelines.

HEART RATE
Established guidelines maintained during activity.

OXYGEN SATURATION
Levels
Child-specific, established guidelines

Color
Typical shading, as demonstrated by the child when not in distress.
Color remains consistent during activity.
Examine fingernails and lips.

SKIN TEMPERATURE
Warm to the touch (unless child presents with a condition that affects internal temperature regulation).
Child is not overly sweating.
Responds to changes in external temperature.

BREATHING PATTERN
Should be typical of the child when not in distress (e.g., based on either age-appropriate or diagnosis-related breathing patterns)
Regular, rhythmic breathing.
Chest does not indicate labored breathing.
Child/infant able to participate in activity.

AFFECT
Presenting behavior is typical of a child.
Child is ready to engage in activity.
Calm and engaging.
Appears to feel safe.

SLEEP–WAKE CYCLE
Existing patterns have not been interrupted.
Child is rested.
Activity is presented at time when child is ready to engage.

MOVEMENT PATTERNS
Developmental levels (gross motor, fine motor, oral motor, socioemotional, cognitive, self-care, play)
Muscle tone
Range of motion
Strength
Voluntary
Symmetric movements
Coordinated
Able to move in a variety of ways
Posture/balance allows for movement

ORAL MOTOR/FEEDING
Status of feeding
Liquid intake
Food consistency
Suck-swallow-breathe
Nutritive and nonnutritive sucking
Oral motor control

Occupational therapists working in medical settings are responsible for conducting screenings and evaluations, formulating and carrying out daily intervention plans, documentation, and supervision of OTAs. The OTA's responsibilities include formulating (with the occupational therapist) and carrying out daily intervention plans and documentation. Based on the OTA's service competency, he or she also assists with or conducts portions of the screening and contributes to the evaluation and discharge planning.

After receiving a referral from a physician, pediatric screening and evaluation are completed by the occupational therapist within 24 hours and 48 hours, respectively. The **screening** and **evaluation** are conducted through formal and informal measurement tools, clinical observations, and interview. Throughout the assessment process, the OT practitioner considers that certain factors, such as time, severity of illness, and stress associated with being in a hospital environment, may mask a child's true abilities in a given performance area.

The occupational therapist interprets the findings and develops an intervention plan (consulting with the OTA). The plan includes long-term goals and short-term objectives that are meaningful to the child and family. Once the child is medically stable, the OT practitioner initiates intervention. The goals of the intervention plan are gradually integrated into the child's environment.

The responsibilities of OTAs may be dictated by the facility in which the services are being provided. The OTA may conduct parts of the initial developmental screening, collaborate on the evaluation, provide interventions, update goals, and collaborate with team members on the discharge plan.

The plan of care developed for a child admitted to a medical setting incorporates information reflecting the child's preadmission status as well as his or her current status. This information, along with the child's medical diagnosis and medical course, is used to develop goals that will lead to discharge. The OT practitioner may gather information on the following areas to understand client factors that may interfere with occupational performance:

- Cognitive: level of alertness, orientation, behavior, moods, activity level, memory, attention to task;
- Sensory: visual, auditory, oral, tactile, vestibular, gustatory, pain;
- Neuromuscular system: extremity movements and limitations, strengths, weaknesses, prior injuries/surgeries, presence or absence of age-appropriate reflexes;
- Cardiovascular and respiratory systems: blood pressure, breathing patterns, prior activity and fatigue levels;
- Voice/speech/respiration: verbal or nonverbal communication, quality of voice, ability to sustain conversation;
- Digestive/metabolic: eating, absorption, energy return on caloric intake
- Skin: intact, abrasions, cuts, wounds, injection or access sites;
- Sleep and rest functions; and
- Elimination function: output schedule, level of independence.[3]

Experienced practitioners evaluate children on a daily basis to record their progress and address their changing needs. The OTA's knowledge of body systems and how strengths or deficits in one system affect the performance of another system facilitates the development of an appropriate plan of care (inclusive of objectives and goals that maximize a child's optimal level of occupational performance).[3]

Physiologic Parameters

The OT practitioner working in a medical setting needs knowledge of physiologic parameters of infants and children. The status of fragile infants and children can change quickly. As infants and children grow, heart rate (HR) and respiratory rate (RR) slows, blood pressure increases, and oxygen saturation remains steady. Refer to Table 3-1 for ranges of normal physiologic measures. The practitioner communicates changes in physiologic

measures to the health care team (e.g., nursing, occupational therapists, doctor, respiratory therapist). Children in the hospital are typically placed on monitors to measure HR, RR, and oxygen saturation.

Physiologic data provided by monitors and clinical observations provides an accurate clinical picture. Along with RR, practitioners note "work of breathing" by observing the ease of breathing and how the child breathes. Practitioners observe the use of accessory muscles (e.g., shoulder girdle elevation) with breathing. The presence of "retractions" that are observed as "indentations" between the ribs (intercostal retraction) or below the ribcage (subcostal retractions) may indicate stress. "Pursed lip" breathing may be indicative of increased respiratory effort. Practitioners observing signs of labored breathing modify the activity. If there is decline in oxygen saturations greater than 5%, therapy should be significantly modified or discontinued.

Additionally, the OT practitioner must be aware of IV lines and be careful not to dislodge them or the monitor leads. The OT practitioner needs to be mindful of the tubing from the medicine bags to the IV lines. For example, when transferring a child, practitioners place IV tubing so the child can be moved easily without getting tangled in the tubing. See Table 3-2 or types of IVs and associated precautions.

Medical Equipment

Infants and children in the hospital may need additional interventions and medical equipment of which the practitioner needs to be aware. These include respiratory support ranging from oxygen per nasal cannula to ventilator support. When children receive oxygen per nasal cannula, they receive oxygen through tubing placed in the nose. The tubing needs to remain connected to the oxygen source and not be stretched during therapy.

When children are very ill, they may need ventilator support. The OT practitioner may need to provide positioning supports and gentle range of motion exercises. It is imperative to keep the endotracheal tube (ETT) in

TABLE 3-1

Physiologic Parameters

AGE	RESPIRATORY RATE (BREATHS/MIN)	HEART RATE
Infant (< 1 year)	30–60	100–160
Toddler (1–3 years)	24–40	90–150
Preschooler (4–5 years)	22–34	80–140
School age (6–12 years)	18–30	70–120
Adolescent (13–18)	12–16	60–100

From Marx, J., et al. (2014). *Rosen's Emergency Medicine: Concepts and Clinical Practice.* (8th ed). Philadelphia: Saunders.

place. The OT practitioner can ask the nurse to remain at bedside during interventions to ensure the ETT remains secure.

Nutrition

Children may need a range of nutrition supports. Infants and children may require additional calories mixed in the formula or drink. If the infant or child is unable to take in enough nutrition, the child may need supplemental nutrition by nasogastric tube (into the stomach) or nasoduodenal tube (into the duodenal section of the small intestine). The OT practitioner needs to mindful of tube placement during handling to prevent dislodging the tube. Infants and children may need a gastrostomy or jejunostomy tube, which is surgically inserted into the stomach to allow longer-term nutrition support. During occupational therapy, the practitioner needs ensure the tube remains in the proper place and avoid any unnecessary pull on the tube.

Some children with certain medical conditions and those with swallowing disorders may not be able to eat by mouth. This should be noted in the chart as well as posted in the room. NPO means nothing per oral (not by mouth). The OT practitioner needs to be aware of this, particularly when the child is completing oral motor tasks, including toothbrushing.

CLINICAL *Pearl*

Infants with gastrostomies require time in the prone position, also referred to as "Tummy Time." Tummy Time can be adapted by placing an infant over forearm to provide sensory experience of being prone without putting pressure on the g-tube site. The OT practitioner can also adapt Tummy Time by placing soft blanket rolls around g-tube in prone to decrease pressure on the tube site. Remember, when using soft rolls with infants, they need to be supervised at all times.

INTERPROFESSIONAL COLLABORATION

Interprofessional collaboration is important in any medical setting. Collaboration with professionals plays a particularly essential and integral part of medical and therapeutic intervention in pediatric care. Before the initiation of a therapeutic intervention, OT practitioners consult with the physicians and nurses assigned to the client's care and obtain updates on the status of their clients. Areas of particular importance include medications, physiologic stability, nutritional status, and sleep patterns. OT practitioners may obtain this information from written reports and during rounds and medical team meetings.

The medical team members meet daily, weekly, or biweekly to discuss patient care and plan. Frequency is based on medical necessity and pending discharge date. Meeting time varies from 15 minutes to 2 hours and family/caregivers may or may not be present. The OT practitioner present updates the team on the occupational therapy plan and patient's progress and provides information relevant to discharge planning that may include adaptive equipment and follow-up services.

CLINICAL *Pearl*

For an interprofessional team to be effective, the team members must trust and respect each other so that they are comfortable with role release (i.e., relinquishing certain professional duties to other team members).

DOCUMENTATION

The OT practitioner's ability to clearly document the events that occur in a pediatric medical setting is crucially important. Documentation is used for many purposes, including updating others on client status, justifying the necessity for OT services, and explaining

TABLE 3-2

Types of Intravenous (IV) Lines and Precautions

NAME OF IV LINE	PURPOSE	PRECAUTIONS
PIV (peripheral IV)	Provides fluids and medicines for several days or a week	Some immobilization at insertion site. Note if joint movement is limited by the IV board.
PICC (peripherally inserted cardiac catheters)	Catheter goes through vein into the heart. Provides long-term IV access for children needing medications and IV fluids for an extended time. Can be in place for up to 30 days.	Needs to have sterile occlusive dressing. Be careful of the tape around IV.
Arterial line (art line)	Used in intensive care setting when child needs careful monitor of blood pressure and frequent checks of oxygen levels in blood (blood gases). Often placed in wrist or in the femoral artery in the groin area.	Do not move the arterial line. Nurse able to adjust the arterial line if necessary to move the extremity with the arterial line.

requests for supplies and reimbursements.[6] Documentation also serves as a legal record of services.

OT practitioners working in a medical setting complete a screening or initial assessment of the infant or child.[10] A screening determines whether a comprehensive evaluation is needed. Screenings and evaluations include medical history, general observations, gross and fine motor functions, visual and perceptual function, cognitive function, sensory function (when applicable), ADL function, summary, recommendations, frequency, and long- and short-term goals. Box 3-6 contains an example of a medical evaluation. The information is used to establish baseline functioning and provides the basis for the intervention plan.

Accrediting and licensing agencies require documentation. If the occupational therapy process is not documented, then occupational therapy services did not occur. Consequently, entries in a medical record should be concise, clear, accurate, complete, and chronologically ordered. The Health Information Portability and Accountability Act protects a client's medical information, otherwise known as patient health information.[7]

CLINICAL *Pearl*

The WeeFIM (UB Foundation Activities, Inc., Queens, NY) is a functional assessment used to describe a child's performance during essential activities.[11] It measures those activities that children can actually carry out and not what they may merely be capable of doing. The assessment can be used to clarify a child's functional status, provide information for team conferences, facilitate goal planning, and provide information on burden-of-care issues, that is, those issues related to the person who is meeting the child's basic needs (i.e., eating, bathing, dressing, grooming, transferring, moving, and toileting).[10,11]

The WeeFIM provides a uniform language for practitioners to use when measuring and documenting the severity of disabilities and outcomes of pediatric rehabilitation. It allows practitioners to measure disability types as well as determine the amount of help a child needs to perform basic activities. The assessment is conducted by direct observations or through interviews with the caregiver and can be used in inpatient and outpatient settings. However, it is not meant to be the *only* diagnostic tool. Before using

---

BOX 3-6

Medically Based Occupational Therapy Education

ST. MARY'S HOSPITAL FOR CHILDREN INITIAL OCCUPATIONAL THERAPY EVALUATION

Name: Kevin   *Unit:* CUW
DOB: 7/13/02   *Sex:* Male
Medical Record #: 12345
Diagnosis: Duchenne muscular dystrophy
2/28/10: Doctor's orders received. Full evaluation with recommendations to follow.

MEDICAL HISTORY

Kevin, 7 years and 8 months old, has Duchenne muscle dystrophy. On 3/21/2006, he underwent a spinal fusion and multiple tendon releases. He was subsequently placed in two long-leg casts with bars. Kevin was born at 36 weeks' gestation and weighed 5 lb 5 oz. Kevin was a healthy child until he was diagnosed with Duchenne muscular dystrophy at age 5.

GENERAL OBSERVATIONS

Kevin is a thin, frail boy, who has an overall decreased affect. He has a scar from spinal surgery that extends from approximately T1/T2 to his coccyx. He is able to verbalize his needs by speaking in a soft, high-pitched voice. Kevin is able to visually track objects in all planes. He is seated in a reclined wheelchair with his lower extremities elevated and in a spica cast.

GROSS MOTOR FUNCTION

Kevin has hypotonicity throughout his trunk and upper extremities. He is able to transition from the prone position to the supine position, and vice versa. Kevin requires significant assistance to maintain the sitting posture. He exhibits pectus excavation, bilateral scapular winging, a kyphotic posture, and bilateral rib flaring.

UPPER EXTREMITY FUNCTION

Passive range of motion (PROM) is within normal limits (WNL). Goniometric active range of motion (AROM) measurements are as follows:

	RIGHT	LEFT
Shoulder flexion	No ROM at either shoulder; uses compensatory techniques (e.g., climb arms on cest)	
Elbow flexion	Flexes both elbows in a gravity-eliminated plane	
Wrist extension	0–30 degrees	0–25 degrees
Wrist flexion	0–60 degrees	0–55 degrees
Ulnar deviation	0–30 degrees	WNL
Radial deviation	0–20 degrees	WNL
Supination	WNL	WNL
Pronation	WNL	WNL

Courtesy Kathleen Logan-Baucer, Bayside, NY.

the WeeFIM assessment, both OTRs and COTAs are required to be certified with the UB Foundation.

After the initial screening or assessment has been completed, the OT practitioner notes the child's progress and changes in the status over time. The progress is recorded in the form of a daily note, weekly progress note, or monthly progress note in a narrative or **SOAP-note** format (see Chapter 10). SOAP stands for Subjective information (general statements concerning the child by the caregiver or child), Objective information (what is observed), Assessment (interpretation of findings), and Plan (what will be done).[6] An example discharge note based on the SOAP format might be as follows:

S Nursing reports that child is in a "great mood" today and drank 8 oz of formula this morning.
O Patient is a 14-month-old male who presents with a diagnosis of prematurity, bronchopulmonary dysplasia, and a gastrointestinal tube (GT) placement. He receives OT, PT, and ST services twice weekly for 30 minutes each. He is medically stable and receives his nutrition by way of a combination of oral and overnight GT feedings.

   At present, patient is alert and oriented to person and place. He is able to cruise with contact guard. He demonstrates right and left unilateral hand skills (active grasp and release in response to verbal prompts). Child is able to attend to light-up/auditory toys for approximately 45 seconds with moderate cueing. He tolerates hand-over-hand assistance to participate in cause-and-effect activities in approximately 75% of the trials.
A Patient presents with developmental delays in the areas of postural control, bilateral hand function, eye-hand coordination, and attention to a task, which interfere with his ability to engage in self-care, social participation, and play. Patient would benefit from home-based or community based OT services to promote his continued improvement in the areas of independent mobility/transition, in-hand manipulation, visual perception, and sustained attention skills needed for engagement in self-care, play, and social participation.
P Discharge home with referral to the early intervention (EI program) for continued occupational therapy services.

Progress notes are important for justifying interventions, continuing services, and planning discharge. OT practitioners record clearly and concisely therapeutic interventions, the child's responses to them, and the justification for specialized equipment. Insurance sources may approve or deny a request based on an OT practitioner's ability to justify the necessity for the requested item. OT practitioners justify the necessity for equipment by identifying the ways in which equipment will benefit the child's level of function. For example, OT practitioners may discuss how the equipment will improve respiratory, cardiac, musculoskeletal, esophageal, and gastrointestinal functions. OT practitioners emphasize how the equipment helps the child in terms of safety as well. See Box 3-7 for an example of a letter of justification. The letter includes information regarding the way the requested equipment will

---

BOX 3-7

Letter of Equipment Justification

RE: Frankie
Diagnosis: Severe tracheomalacia, gastroesophageal reflux, and supraventricular tachycardia
Medicaid #: GF12345U
DOB: 7/12/2009

TO WHOM IT MAY CONCERN
Frankie is a 10-month-old male who had severe tracheomalacia, gastroesophageal reflux, and supraventricular tachycardia at birth. He has decreased head and postural control as well as tracheotomy.

   Current equipment: Currently Frankie does not have any equipment.

   Equipment ordered: One Panda stroller with swivel-front wheels, a combined sun/rain hood, and foot straps.

   Justification: Frankie is an active, alert, and oriented 10-month-old male with decreased head and trunk control, which affects his ability to assume and maintain independent, upright postural sets. Frankie's inability to maintain an upright and erect posture places him at risk for occluding his tracheostomy and limits his ability to achieve his full respiratory capacity. These limitations affect his endurance and gas exchange.

   A Panda stroller will assist Frankie with maintaining a neutral posture, which will facilitate his mechanical efficiency and therefore, improve his endurance for maintaining an upright position. Improvement in his endurance will increase his upper extremity use, which will foster the acquisition of age-appropriate fine motor skills. The stroller will help prevent bony deformities and joint contractures, thereby preventing the need for future surgeries. Frankie's ability to swallow and digest will also be improved if he can maintain a neutral position. A neutral position allows Frankie to use gravity to help him carry out the previously stated functions.

   Thank you in advance for your assistance with this matter.

   Therapist's signature_____
   Physiatrist's signature_____

Courtesy: Nechama Karman, Dawn B. Oakley, Queens, NY, 1996.

improve the child's ability to function in the areas of respiration, trunk control (musculoskeletal), endurance (cardiac and respiratory), and swallowing and digestion (physiologic).

CLINICAL *Pearl*

Always remember a child and his or her diagnosis are not one and the same (examples: **Yes:** Jack is a child, who presents with autism. **No:** Jack is an autistic child).

MODALITIES

OT practitioners working with children and youth in medical settings may use a variety of modalities to help children improve performance skills. These modalities include thermotherapy, cryotherapy, paraffin wax, fluidotherapy, neuromuscular electrical stimulation (NMES), functional electrical stimulation (FES), VitalStim, and serial casting. Ultrasound is not recommended for children under the age of 21 due to contraindications related to bone growth.

Occupational therapists are specially trained in the use of these techniques. In certain states, advanced practice licensing is required to administer these modalities. The OTA must be deemed service competent in various aspects of each technique before administering it. In certain states, the OTA must work directly under the occupational therapist with the advanced practice licensing. This means, if the certified OTA is deemed service competent and the primary OTR on the case does not have the advanced practice licensing, the OTA may not administer the adjunctive method to the particular child.

NMES and VitalStim therapy involve the administration of small, electrical impulses to the muscles of the arm (NMES) or swallowing muscles in the throat (VitalStim) through electrodes attached to the skin overlaying the musculature. The therapist determines which musculature would benefit from this facilitation through a patient evaluation. Once the electrodes are placed and current intensity set to a satisfactory level, the therapist either engages the patient in oral exercises with the patient (VitalStim) or allows the patient to comfortably receive impulses (NMES). The goal of these interventions is to stimulate muscle fibers and reinervate the muscle that has lost nerve function.

FES is designed to provide electrical impulses concurrent with a functional activity for improved performance while reaching and grasping during play or self-care tasks. The FES device is for use on muscles that have active nerve function. The goal of FES is to increase muscle strength, range of motion, and motor control.

CLINICAL *Pearl*

The entry-level COTA is exposed to the variety of physical agent modalities and adjunctive methods available in clinical practice. Advanced education and service competency is required before a COTA may use the physical agent modality or specific method during intervention sessions.

Serial casting is a weekly program designed to gradually increase range of motion of a specific joint to improve function, joint alignment, reduce spasticity, and prevent contractures. Serial casting involves the use of plaster and/or fiberglass casts to restore or improve range of motion, reduce muscle contracture, and improve movement and alignment of joints in the arms (see Chapter 28). Constraint-induced movement therapy attempts to promote hand function by using intensive practice with the affected hand while restraining the less-affected hand (see Chapter 17).

REIMBURSEMENT

Reimbursement for medical services constantly changes. As of 2014, each state monitors medical insurance by requiring citizens to register. Due to ongoing decision making regarding reimbursement, it is important for the OT practitioner to be actively aware of the federal and state requirements for specific documentation to justify the services rendered for each payor source. For example, health maintenance and preferred provider organizations (HMOs and PPOs) require frequent documentation to justify the initiation and continuation of services. In certain instances, specific clinics and vendors must be used. A hospital social worker or case manager is the best source of information regarding insurance requirements and coverage.

Charitable organizations are another reimbursement source. They are usually nonprofit companies or organizations that raise funds to be given to other nonprofit organizations. A charitable organization makes a donation to a pediatric institution or agency, which, in turn, deposits the donation into an appropriate general fund. The agency then determines the way to distribute these funds to pay for the specific expenses of individuals.

CHALLENGES FOR OT PRACTITIONERS WORKING IN THE MEDICAL SYSTEM

In addition to rehabilitative services (e.g., OT, PT, ST), a variety of specialized service personnel constitute the medical system, including radiology technicians, medical laboratory technicians, audiologists, pharmacists, dietitians, orthotists, social workers, case managers, psychologists, and recreational therapists. A medical OT practitioner has to become familiar with other pediatric disciplines and their roles in the medical institution. This knowledge facilitates team collaboration.

OT practitioners must have extensive knowledge of medical diagnoses and terminology when working in medical settings. The study of the basic word roots used in pediatric medical practice helps practitioners develop this much-needed knowledge base. A thorough understanding of diagnoses, including etiology, progression, signs, symptoms, and interventions is required when working in medical settings.

Children with certain conditions such as pneumonia, asthma, diabetes, and cerebral palsy may be admitted to hospitals frequently.[10] These children may develop episodes of acute illness or the need for corrective surgery. Children who are frequently hospitalized require unique approaches to intervention to maintain a sense of continuity with aspects of their lives outside the hospital. The OT practitioner draws upon models of practice, such as the Model of Human Occupation (MOHO), Canadian Occupational Performance Measure (COPM), or Person, Environment, Occupational Performance (PEOP) to develop comprehensive intervention plans that integrate the children's preadmission habits, routines, and roles with their current levels of performance.

Practitioners working in medical care systems may have to address issues related to palliative care. Children who have been diagnosed with terminal illnesses may be treated in a medical care setting or home setting and may require OT services. The focus of OT intervention services for children diagnosed with terminal illnesses varies depending on their medical and current functional status. Initially, the OT practitioner may focus on the restoration or maintenance of function related to the ability of the child or caregiver to carry out performance skills. As the child's status declines, the focus of therapy services may shift to the maintenance and integration of energy-conservation techniques that assist in easing the performance of independent or assisted performance skills. The clinician also may integrate the use of intervention modalities that allow the caregiver's and child's memories to be recorded in a permanent manner as a source of future comfort for the family after the child dies. As a child enters the final stage of life, the OT practitioner may focus on ensuring that the child is comfortable and work closely with the caregiver to provide the child opportunities for meaningful occupations and interactions.

Infection Control

Infection control is the responsibility of every OT practitioner, who must follow **universal precautions** when working with any client. These precautions are expressed as a set of rules instituted by the Centers for Disease Control and Prevention. When health care workers face the risk for being exposed to blood, certain other body fluids,

or any other fluid visibly contaminated by blood, they must assume that all individuals with whom they come in contact may be infected with HIV or HBV and therefore follow these precautions at all times.

All professionals working within medical care settings must adhere to infection control practices. One of the first lines of defense against the spread of infection is proper hand washing. Medical care settings provide detailed orientation sessions to educate employees on practices to prevent the spread of infection. Some medical facilities employ a nurse who is responsible for overseeing infection control. This nurse monitors the status of communicable infections; assists in the quarantine of an infected child, caregiver, or medical personnel; and works to prevent the spread of contagious infections to other medically compromised children. Health care professionals use personal protective equipment (e.g., masks, eye shields, gloves, and gowns) to prevent the spread of infection. Policies and procedures for the appropriate disposal of waste materials (e.g., diapers, soiled linens, blood, or other body fluid spills) must be followed to prevent further infection.

Hand Washing

Proper hand washing is the single most important component of infection control and one of the first lines of defense against the spread of infection. Hands should be washed before and immediately after working with a client or whenever an individual comes into contact with any type of body fluid. Proper hand washing requires washing for 20 seconds with warm water and soap. Hands should be washed after removing gloves. Many hospitals also provide hand sanitizer, located in the patient room and hallways. The hand sanitizer is sufficient for nonblood or nonfluid hand cleaning. However, it is important to note that hand sanitizers are not effective after the fourth consecutive use and are not sufficient for cleansing after exposure to a certain virus or bacteria.

> **CLINICAL** *Pearl*
>
> Wash your hands before and after working with a child. Hand sanitizer can be used up to four consecutive times before hand washing is necessary.

Use of Gloves

OT practitioners wear gloves when there is a possibility of coming into contact with infected material or exposure to body fluids (e.g., during oral motor intervention, which requires the OT practitioner to place fingers in a child's oral cavity, or when changing diapers). Gloves should also be worn by OT practitioners who have scratches on or breaks in their skin.

Types of Precautions

Children who have communicable diseases may be isolated from others. The conditions requiring isolation usually involve gastrointestinal illnesses or respiratory illnesses such as RSV, tuberculosis, or measles. The OT practitioner recognizes and respects specific isolation precautions. The child is placed in a private room with the door closed with an isolation sign on the door. The signage provides guidelines for anyone entering the room. Types of precaution signs are as follows:

- **Contact precautions:** Wash hands when entering and leaving the room. Wear gown and gloves.
- **Droplet precautions:** Wash hands when entering and leaving the room. Wear gown, gloves, and mask.
- **Airborne precautions:** Wash hands when entering and leaving room. Wear gown and gloves. Wear fit-tested N-95 or higher disposable respirator mask or special protective mask.

Hepatitis B Vaccination

The Occupational Safety and Health Administration (OSHA) standard regarding bloodborne pathogens requires employers to offer a free three-injection hepatitis B vaccination series to employees who are exposed to blood or any other potentially infectious material during their routine duties. This policy includes OT practitioners and other health care workers. Vaccinations must be offered within 10 days of initial assignment to a job in which exposure to blood or other potentially infectious materials can be "reasonably anticipated."[12]

Cleaning of Equipment and Toys

OT practitioners need to maintain equipment and toys in good, clean working order. Although equipment and toys are not sterilized after children use them, all of these items should be properly sanitized. OT practitioners can also require that families provide the children's favorite toys for use during therapy. They can educate the families about the safest and most effective methods of cleaning their children's toys.

According to OSHA, facilities and agencies must provide workers with policies and procedures for cleaning and disinfecting.[12] These procedures are beyond the scope of this chapter. It is the responsibility of practitioners to become familiar with their facilities' policies and procedures for disinfecting.

Characteristics of a Successful Health Care Provider

OT practitioners working in medical settings must understand the concept of therapeutic use of self. This includes professional behaviors, interpersonal skills, compassion, empathy, honesty, active listening, and effective business and professional communication with clients and team members. This concept incorporates nonverbal communication skills and effective use of humor.

> **CLINICAL *Pearl***
>
> The most important tool a clinician brings to the therapy session is therapeutic use of self. The most important skill a clinician brings to a team meeting is active listening.

The pace of a medical care setting is fast. OT practitioners who exhibit high energy level, actively pursue new knowledge, and feel confident in expressing their findings to other team members will find success in this setting. Articulating sound clinical reasoning skills and being willing to listen to others' ideas is beneficial to all team members, family and support systems.[7]

Expert OT practitioners in medical care settings exhibit advanced technical skills, knowledge of current intervention strategies, assessments, and documentation guidelines. As in all specialty areas of occupational therapy, skilled practitioners respect other team members' time, opinions, and professional expertise. They are able to advocate for clients and families in multiple contexts.

Legal and Ethical Considerations in a Medical Care System

Each health care profession has a national organization that has adopted a code of ethics to govern the behavior of its members and establish standards of care for the profession. All OT practitioners are expected to abide by the AOTA's Code of Ethics (see Chapter 1 for an overview of the code of ethics). In general, the AOTA Code of Ethics provides guidelines for ethical practice that include the following:[2]

1. Beneficence
2. Nonmaleficence
3. Autonomy and confidentiality
4. Social justice
5. Procedural justice
6. Veracity
7. Fidelity

These seven principles provide the standards of practice related to competence (therapy skills and abilities), honesty (as related to the provision of care and interactions with others), and clear communication (as related to services provided and interactions with peers, patients, and caregivers).[2] For example, the principle of autonomy and confidentiality suggest that it is every OT practitioner's responsibility to ensure confidentiality for each patient and to allow patients to make decisions about their intervention plans.

SUMMARY

The pediatric medical care system is composed of individuals dedicated to caring for children with various illnesses. The six major settings in the pediatric medical care system include:

1. NICU;
2. Step-down nursery or the PICU;
3. Acute care;
4. Subacute;
5. Residential or long-term care; and
6. Home care.

The complex nature of the pediatric medical care system poses a unique challenge for OT practitioners working in medical systems. OT practitioners are required to possess not only basic OT skills but a working knowledge of the pediatric medical specialties, the ability to use and interpret pediatric medical terminology, and information about the frequent changes in the pediatric health care environment. OT practitioners working with children and youth in medical settings are responsible for understanding medical terminology, equipment, and changes in the health care system. They work closely with a variety of interprofessional team members and advocate for services for children and their families within the systems in which they work. This requires knowledge of documentation, billing, reimbursement, and resources. OT practitioners develop a sound understanding of conditions that children may experience in medical settings so they can help children and youth engage in occupations of childhood.

References

1. American Occupational Therapy Association. (2009). Guidelines for supervision, roles, and responsibilities during the delivery of occupational therapy services. *Am J Occup Ther, 63*, 797–803.
2. American Occupational Therapy Association. (2010). Occupational therapy code of ethics and ethical standards. *Am J Occup Ther, 64*(Suppl. 1), S17–S26.
3. American Occupational Therapy Association. (2014). Occupational therapy practice framework: Domain and process (3rd ed.). *Am J Occup Ther, 68*(Suppl. 1), S1–S48.
4. Anderson, K. N. (2005). *Mosby's medical, nursing, and allied health dictionary* (7th ed.). St. Louis, MO: Mosby.
5. Dudgeon, B. J., Crooks, L., & Chapelle, E. (2014). Hospital and pediatric rehabilitation services. In J. Case-Smith, & J. O'Brien (Eds.), *Occupational therapy for children and adolescents* (7th ed.). (pp. 704–726). St. Louis, MO: Mosby.
6. Morreale, M. J., & Borcherding, S. (2013). *The COTA's guide to documentation: writing SOAP notes* (3rd ed.). Thorofare, NJ: Slack Inc.
7. Judson, K., & Harrison, C. (2012). *Law and ethics for health professions* (6th ed.). New York: McGraw-Hill.
8. Oakley, D., & Bauer-Logan, K. (1996). *Traumatic brain lecture series*. Queens, NY: St. Mary's Hospital for Children.
9. Slee, V., & Slee, D. (2001). *Slee's health care terms* (4th ed.). St. Paul, MN: Tringa Press.
10. Venes, D. (2009). *Taber's cyclopedic medical dictionary* (21st ed.). Philadelphia: FA Davis.
11. Uniform Data System for Medical Rehabilitation. (2014). *WeeFIM system workshop*. Queens, NY: UB Foundation Activities.
12. U.S. Department of Labor, Occupational Safety and Health Administration. (2011). *Bloodborne pathogens—hepatitis B vaccination protection fact sheet*. Washington, DC: Author.

REVIEW *Questions*

1. When might a child be transferred from one medical setting to another?
2. Which functional areas are assessed in a pediatric medically based occupational therapy evaluation?
3. In what ways could a medical practitioner's documentation have an effect on the intervention and equipment needs of a child?
4. Describe the various levels of medical care and the role of the OT practitioner.
5. Who are the various team members within a medical system?
6. What equipment might an OT practitioner find in a medical setting?
7. What challenges do OT practitioners face in medical settings?
8. What types of precautions are considered in medical settings?
9. Describe the role of the OT practitioner in speciality units.
10. How do OT practitioners help children and youth who are in medical settings engage in occupations?

SUGGESTED *Activities*

1. Create three examples of a narrative or SOAP note based on three observations of children in a natural setting (e.g., schoolyard, playground).
2. Purchase and review flash cards of common roots of medical terms.
3. Visit children in a hospital. Ask them about the things they like to do when they are at home or play a game with them. What did you learn from them?
4. Research a pediatric health condition that an occupational therapy practitioner may find in a medical setting. What occupations may be affected by the condition/disease? Write three potential long-term goals the OT practitioner may consider addressing during the child's in-patient hospital stay. Where else may the practitioner work with the child? Describe the various medical settings.
5. Interview a health care professional who works in a medical setting. Describe the professional's roles, duties, and scope of practice. How does this professional work with the OT practitioner?
6. Examine the roles and duties of multiple interprofessional team members who work in medical settings. Describe how these professionals help children and their families.

MASHELLE K. PAINTER
JEAN WELCH SOLOMON

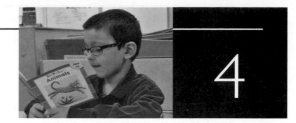

4

Educational Systems

CHAPTER *Objectives*

After studying this chapter, the reader will be able to accomplish the following:
- Identify the federal laws that govern the provision of educational services to children with disabilities.
- Explain the formation and function of an Individualized Educational Program team.
- Explain the process involved in an Individualized Educational Program.
- Compare and contrast the roles of the occupational therapist and the occupational therapy assistant in the school setting.
- Distinguish between the clinical and educational models for occupational therapy service delivery.
- Describe the techniques for working with teachers and parents in schools.
- Differentiate between direct, monitoring, and consultation types of occupational therapy service delivery.

CHAPTER *Outline*

One fourth (25%) of occupational therapists and 21.6% of occupational therapy assistants (OTAs) report that they work with children and adolescents in public school systems.[13] Despite these statistics, occupational therapy (OT) practitioners in public schools often find that they work alone, with a limited support network. This is especially true in rural areas, where one practitioner may provide therapy services to several small school districts or a cooperative educational service area. Being a member of an educational team requires that practitioners broaden their focus on the ways children function in their families, communities, and schools. This mode of thinking contrasts with the traditional medical model of "evaluate and treat," with its focus on the disabilities or limitations of children. As part of a multidisciplinary educational team, OT practitioners working in school systems interact with a variety of people. They must therefore possess specialized technical skills and have knowledge of the educational system, current special education laws, and regulations.[3,7,9]

OT practitioners working in educational settings apply their knowledge and intervention skills in the context of a school setting while communicating effectively with parents* and educators.

OT practitioners working in the public school setting collaborate with regular education and special education teachers, psychologists, speech therapists, physical therapists, and other team members based on the student's individual educational needs. They work with the student in the classroom whenever possible. Sometimes taking the student to a separate room might be the optimal learning situation for the student (Figure 4-1). OT practitioners develop strategies to facilitate educational goals. Strategies and suggestions may be provided to the teacher to better enhance the student's learning.

CLINICAL MODELS VERSUS EDUCATIONAL MODELS

Providing OT services in an educational setting requires a shift in thinking and a change in philosophy from the clinical (medical) setting (Table 4-1). OT practitioners traditionally trained under a medical model view services for children based on dysfunction and its underlying components. In this model, therapists evaluate and treat physical problems and environmental factors that can support or hinder a child's performance. The focus of a medical model is the remediation of the underlying components of dysfunction and the removal of pathologic processes so that development can continue.

In the school system, the practitioner evaluates the student's performance in the classroom to determine whether physical, emotional, or behavioral aspects interfere with the student's ability to perform classroom tasks. The student's abilities are described in functional terms (rather than in terms of disability or diagnosis) and the capacity to meet classroom demands.[2,3]

Federal, state, and local educational agency regulations established guidelines for the provision of OT services in the school system.[2,10-12] Practitioners working in schools may serve more children by working with them in groups. This provides peer support and is a natural part of school. Consulting with the teacher and classroom staff helps resolve many problems and may have an effect on many children. The OT practitioner may become more directly involved if a student's skills deteriorate or the OT practitioner thinks that a short period of direct service will help the student become more independent. Appendix 4-A provides some commonly used acronyms used in school settings.

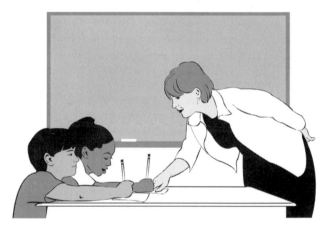

FIGURE 4-1   Working with a child in a separate room may help facilitate educational goals.

TABLE 4-1

Comparison Between Clinical and Educational Settings

CLINICAL SETTING	EDUCATIONAL SETTING
Patient goals are primary	Educational goals are primary
Treat acute conditions or conduct short-term intense intervention for chronic conditions	Reduce the effects of chronic or newly diagnosed conditions so child can benefit from the educational program
Focus is on addressing developmental issues and components of movement within functional skills	Focus is on addressing functional skills and providing adaptations that promote the attainment of educational objectives

---

*In the chapter the term *parents* is used in the general sense and refers to the legal guardian who is the child's primary caregiver and is responsible for the child's well-being. For example, the parent may be a grandparent, aunt, uncle, or even a friend of the family.

CLINICAL *Pearl*

Goal writing is much easier if the practitioner takes the time to ask the teacher, parent, or child what they hope to get out of the occupational therapy sessions. Start out with very broad questions (e.g., "What would you like to do better?" "What is causing you trouble in school?" "What is interfering with the child's ability to learn?"), and then ask specific questions (e.g., "What aspects of reading are causing you trouble?" "What about your writing: Is it a problem?" "Do you tire easily?" "Is it messy?" "Do you have trouble holding the pencil?" "What does the child do in class that interrupts others?"). Continue until you have a clear visual picture of what the child hopes to accomplish. The OT practitioner works collaboratively with the student's case manager (typically the special education teacher) to establish annual goals and objectives.

Students who are eligible for special education services may also qualify to receive related services such as occupational or physical therapy at no cost to the student or the family. However, OT practitioners working in schools can bill Medicaid for educationally related services. Medicaid was created to provide medical and health-related services for financially needy children. It pays for health services for those who are eligible and is not dependent on where the services are provided. When therapy is provided in the school, it decreases the student's absence from school and is thus an effective way to provide medical care related to the education of children.

Although children with medical conditions or diagnoses may benefit from occupational therapy in the school setting, the emphasis is to help children function in the classroom, gym, cafeteria, and playground. Providing services in the least restrictive environment (LRE) often means working in the classroom. OT practitioners provide educationally relevant services, which makes the practitioners part of the educational team. In recent years, educational agencies and third-party payors have increased their requests for OT practitioners to use outcome-based practices in pediatric settings. Practitioners identify and treat problem areas, quantify functional performance, and consider multiple factors including neuromuscular and psychosocial processes, the student's potential for improvement, social skills, environmental demands, and family priorities.[1]

CLINICAL *Pearl*

OT services are most integrated when provided in the classroom. An informal exchange of ideas and effective intervention strategies naturally evolve among team members when the OT practitioner works with children in their classrooms. This allows for the carryover of strategies and changes that allow children to be successful in school.

FEDERAL LAWS

In an educational system setting, occupational therapy services are mandated by federal laws.[4,10-12] Box 4-1 summarizes the laws that have an effect on OT services in public school systems. Education is an important occupation of children (Figure 4-2). As such, OT practitioners working in school systems have the opportunity to directly affect the child's occupation. They are afforded the luxury of seeing the results of their interventions daily within the context for which it is intended. Their role is to improve the child's ability to function within the school environment; they must become skillful in advocating for the needs of the children within the contexts of this setting and the laws.

BOX 4-1

Summary of Federal Laws That Affect Occupational Therapy in Educational Settings

1973
PUBLIC LAW 93–112, SECTION 504 OF THE REHABILITATION ACT
- Discrimination against people with disabilities when offering services is prohibited.

1975
PUBLIC LAW 94–142: EDUCATION FOR ALL HANDICAPPED CHILDREN ACT (RENAMED EDUCATION OF THE HANDICAPPED ACT [EHA])
- All children have the right to free and appropriate public education.

1986
PUBLIC LAW 99–457, PART H (ADDED TO EHA)
- Birth-to-3 services should be equal in all states and counties.

1990
AMERICANS WITH DISABILITIES EDUCATION ACT
- In areas of public services, discriminatory practices against individuals with disabilities by employers are prohibited.
- EHA is renamed Individuals with Disabilities Education Act (IDEA).

1997
- IDEA is revised (IDEA-R).
- Part H of IDEA-R is renamed Part C.

2001
- No Child Left Behind stresses the use of scientifically based or evidence-based programs and practices.

2004
- IDEA-R reauthorized

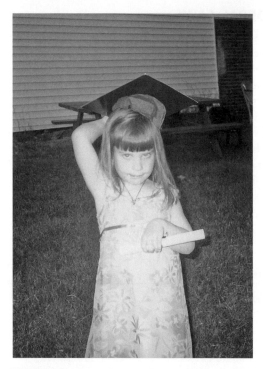

FIGURE 4-2   Education is an important occupation.

Education of the Handicapped Act (Public Law 94-142)

In 1975, the U.S. Congress passed the Education of the Handicapped Act (EHA; Public Law 94-142) requiring schools to provide **free appropriate public education** to all children from ages 5 to 21 years.[2,3]

Children with special needs have the right to have their educational programs geared toward their unique needs, regardless of the nature, extent, or severity of their disabilities. In 1986 the law was amended so that public schools could be responsible for providing educational services to children at age 3 years.

Provisions under this law guarantee children the right to be educated in the **least restrictive environment** (LRE) and to receive other services that may be required for them to benefit from their educational program. The law also outlines the rights and the legal course of action for parents and children. Parents have the right to **due process**—that is, voluntary mediation and impartial hearing—to resolve differences with the school that cannot be resolved informally.

Least Restrictive Environment

The right to be educated in the LRE allows a student who has special needs to be educated in a regular classroom whenever possible.[10] He or she is entitled to interact with peers who do not have disabilities. Before this law was enacted, students with disabilities were placed in special schools with other students who had disabilities, or they were placed in self-contained classrooms in a separate school building with no opportunity to interact with typically developing peers. The LRE guidelines provided the impetus for the development of mainstreaming and **inclusion models** (i.e., models in which children with disabilities are able to spend time in general education classrooms). School personnel determine whether a student who has a disability can receive an appropriate education in a general education classroom with the aid of support services and necessary modifications. The team considers whether the student may benefit from any time in a general education classroom. The spirit of the EHA requires that schools provide an entire continuum of services to those students with special needs.[2,4,10] For some students this may mean placement in a general education classroom that has been modified to meet their needs (e.g., one that has been equipped with positioning devices). For other students it may mean placement in a general education classroom that allows them to go to a resource room for assistance from a special education teacher. Some students need individualized instruction from a special education teacher, allowing students to spend most of the day in the self-contained classroom as well as participate in certain classes or activities in the general education classroom. This individualized instruction is known as **specially designed instruction** (SDI). SDI is instruction that has been modified or adapted to meet the specific learning needs of a student with a disability. Some of the modifications may include changes to the amount of class work the student is expected to complete, the way the instruction is presented, the amount of assistance provided in class, and so on. Students who are identified as needing SDI are placed on an **Individualized Education Program** (IEP), which outlines the way in which the instruction will be provided for the student and the process for specifically addressing the student's needs though goals and objectives. The IEP will also describe any related services that the student may need. Students who have difficulty transitioning from one area to another can benefit from reverse mainstreaming, where the general education students come into the special education classroom during certain courses.

Related Services

According to the EHA, schools are required to provide **related services** as necessary for the student to benefit from the educational program. These services include transportation, physical therapy, occupational therapy, speech therapy (ST), assistive technology services, psychological services, school health services, social work services, and parent counseling and training.[9,10] Except for ST, these services are available only to a student classified as a special education student. ST is the only therapy service that may be either a related service or a "stand-alone" service. In some cases, a student's only need for specially designed instruction is ST.

Rehabilitation Act and Americans with Disabilities Act

The educational rights of children with disabilities are protected by two additional federal laws: Section 504 of the Rehabilitation Act (1973) and the Americans With Disabilities Act (ADA; 1990).[3,7] Section 504 of the Rehabilitation Act stipulates that any recipient of federal aid (including a school) cannot discriminate when offering services to people with disabilities. The ADA prohibits discriminatory practices in areas related to employment, transportation, accessibility, and telecommunications. A student with a disability who is not eligible for special education services but requires reasonable accommodation in his or her regular educational program may be eligible to receive related services under these laws. To be eligible, the student must have a condition that "substantially limits one or more major life activities," with learning being a major life activity (Figure 4-3).[7,10]

CASE *Study*

Jack is a 5-year-old boy with spina bifida. He attends a regular kindergarten class and is able to perform academic activities in a manner equal to his peers. Jack comprehends the information provided, but due to the diminished strength and endurance caused by his disability, he is slower than others in completing his work. Jack needs to be catheterized twice a day by the nurse. Jack qualifies for related services under Section 504 of the Rehabilitation Act. Specifically, the following accommodations will allow Jack to use educational services:

1. He must complete 50% of his work in class; other work will be sent home.
2. He will have extra class time to complete work whenever possible.
3. Classroom supplies will be readily available and placed in front of him before a task begins.
4. OT services will be provided to increase strength and endurance for academic functions.
5. A peer or an adult will accompany him when he leaves the classroom.
6. He will use his iPad for classroom assignments.

Public Law 99-457

Public Law 99-457, which was passed in 1986, added Part H (which is now known as Part C) to the EHA. This law mandates services for preschoolers with disabilities and provided the impetus for the development of early intervention services for infants and toddlers from birth to 3 years of age.

Although the specific policies, procedures, and time lines for birth-to-3 programs vary from those of the public

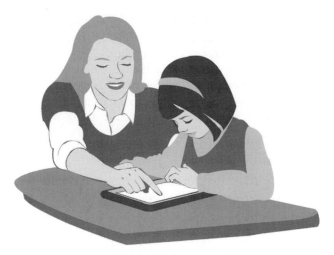

FIGURE 4-3   Child working on handwriting for school.

school setting, both systems follow a similar framework that includes identification and referral, evaluation, determination of eligibility, development of the Individualized Educational Program (IEP) or Individualized Family Service Plan (IFSP), and transitions.

Individuals with Disabilities Education Act

The EHA was renamed the **Individuals with Disabilities Education Act** (IDEA) in 1990; it was revised in 1997 and is now known as IDEA-R. This Act encourages OT practitioners to work with children in their classroom environment (inclusion) and provide support to the general education teacher (integration). It also encourages schools to allow students with disabilities to work toward meeting the same educational standards as their peers. IDEA-R changed the process for the identification, evaluation, and implementation of IEPs.[8] Under IDEA the role of the OT practitioner includes determining the need for assistive technology that allows the child to remain in a regular classroom. The practitioner may consult with others on positioning, train team members, and consult with others on strategies to increase the likelihood of success in the classroom. The role of the occupational therapist under IDEA-R is to assist children with special needs so that they can participate in educational activities. In 2004 IDEA-R was replaced with the Individual's with Disabilities Education Improvement Act and renamed IDEA. IDEA mandates that related service support access to and progress in the general education curriculum or natural environments.[10] This mandate has significantly affected the location and delivery of occupational therapy services.

No Child Left Behind Act

The **No Child Left Behind Act** (NCLB) was enacted in 2001 to improve teaching standards and students' learning results. NCLB supports the use of scientifically based practices by professionals working in the educational setting. Therefore educators and OT practitioners are required to consider research when selecting instructional or interventional practices. Schools must report adequate yearly progress through a single accountability system that applies the same standards to all students. These standards are based on each state's academic achievement standards. Teacher quality and paraprofessional competencies are also parts of this Act, yet it does not specifically address the competencies of related services such as occupational therapy.[12] OT practitioners need to collaborate and consult with the team to prioritize the student's needs. Therapy is integrated into the classroom and provides consistent follow-through. Student-centered IEP goals and objectives enhance success in the educational environment.[8]

RIGHTS OF PARENTS AND CHILDREN

The IDEA-R outlines several procedural safeguards for children with disabilities and for their parents. These procedures are detailed in the U.S. Code of Federal Regulations, Title 34, Subtitle B, Chapter III, Part 300.[11] To summarize, the safeguards include notifying parents in writing of all proposed actions (prior written notice), obtaining written consent to evaluate/reevaluate and allowing parents to attend IEP team meetings. Additional procedural safeguards include the right to request an independent evaluation and the right to appeal school decisions through mediation. Mediation is a voluntary process in which an impartial officer helps schools and families reach an agreement without going through a due process hearing. The IDEA-R requires that school districts inform parents of their rights in a written format. [11]

IDENTIFICATION AND REFERRAL

Physicians and health care professionals frequently refer children to special programs. Screening clinics offered by agencies, schools, and early intervention programs aid in identifying children who need special education services. Referrals are made to the appropriate agency (e.g., Child Find, early intervention clinic, or public school system). Once a referral is made, the responsible agency determines whether screening or an evaluation is needed.

Once children enter the school system, teachers often identify those who experience difficulty meeting educational expectations. Children receiving special education services may be referred to occupational therapy, or may qualify for services under Section 504. The **Individualized Education Program team** (e.g., parent, teacher, special educator, OT therapist) determines a student's need for services (including occupational therapy). For example, children needing assistance with fine motor

skills typically require evaluation by an occupational therapist. Likewise, students showing cognitive skill deficits require evaluation by a special educator; those with speech and language issues are referred to a speech therapist. The professional members are responsible for evaluating these children and determining whether they would benefit from related services. The interdisciplinary team collaborates and reviews the needs of students to determine their eligibility for related services.

EVALUATION

After a referral for OT services is received and parental consent is obtained, an evaluation can be initiated. (Some state and Medicaid conditions require a physician's order as a prerequisite to initiating these services.) Evaluations measure the student's abilities at that particular time. Therefore it is important to consider the viewpoint of everyone involved with the student, including teachers and parents. Knowledge of the student's strengths and needs may be gained from consultation with the teacher, parent, child, and staff. Standardized tests and clinical observations provide important information. State, local, and school policies may dictate what type of assessment will be used. However, practitioners must consider the child's needs in choosing assessment tools. See Chapter 10 for extensive list of assessments used when evaluating a student who may benefit from occupational therapy at school. Occupational therapy practitioners use a combination of both standardized assessments and observations of functional performance in determining the need for occupational therapy services. Observation of the child in the classroom, cafeteria, playground, and bathroom provides information about his or her functional skills.[1] Many children are able to perform certain activities in a quiet one-on-one situation but have difficulty generalizing or modulating them in a busy classroom. Students may also perform better when they are not aware that someone is watching or observing. Consultation with the teacher is key in identifying the specific problems and needs of the student. A questionnaire or referral form completed by the teacher is helpful to the team. The occupational therapist is responsible for completing the evaluation (with input from the OTA), interpreting the information, and presenting the report to the IEP team. The skills of the student should be reassessed before different goals are formulated. Students are reevaluated as needed or if requested by parents, teachers, or team members. The federal laws mandate that the student be reevaluated at least every 3 years.

ELIGIBILITY

The IEP team determines the student's eligibility once all evaluations are completed. Eligibility for services in

BOX 4-2

Determining the Need for Occupational Therapy in the School

- Does the child have an EEN? Because occupational therapy is a related service, the child must have an EEN or qualify under Section 504 of the Rehabilitation Act to be eligible to receive OT services provided by the school system.
- Does the evaluation indicate the need for OT services? The evaluation may consist of standardized tests, portfolio reviews, classroom and school environment observations, and consultations with parents and teachers.
- Does the child demonstrate a significant delay in motor, sensory or perceptual, psychosocial, or self-help skills compared with the established norms of other children of the same age? A significant delay is one that is more than 1 SD below the norm and affects school performance.
- Is occupational therapy a related service that may be required for the child to benefit from and participate in an educational program? Factors that affect the answer to this question include the child's program, other related services received, and the demands of the classroom, the child's level of function, and the potential for improvement or skill development.
- Does the child require the specialized skills of an OT practitioner, or can other personnel carry out tasks and interventions? For example, a teacher may be able to help a child learn eating skills by using adaptive equipment provided by an OT practitioner.

conducted an IEP team evaluation and meeting to determine whether she was eligible for OT services. The team members' evaluation revealed that Mary had age-appropriate learning and thinking skills (cognition) and communication skills, although she sometimes drooled and spoke unclearly. Mary walked independently, moved around the building, and independently performed classroom tasks (e.g., printing, managing materials such as books and paper/pencil). Observations from team members led to the conclusion that she interacted well with her teachers and classmates and was an active participant in the classroom. The OT practitioner reported that Mary had mild spasticity in her left upper extremity, decreased control (isolation and precision) of her left upper extremity, and difficulty with bilateral tasks but that she successfully compensated for these factors and could participate in all classroom activities. She played with other children on the playground and handled self-feeding well. Mary participated in regular gym classes. She was independent in toileting.

The IEP team determined that although Mary had a documented disability (cerebral palsy), it did not interfere with her ability to receive an appropriate education. Therefore an EEN did not exist and special education and OT services were not required for Mary to participate in and benefit from her educational program. If Mary's family thought that she would benefit from OT services to resolve issues related to her muscle tone, range of motion, fine motor skills, and bilateral coordination skills, the family could seek and secure OT services in a clinic on an outpatient basis. For a child to be eligible to receive OT services in the public school setting, the services and goals must be educationally relevant.

public schools is based on **exceptional educational need (EEN)**. Box 4-2 contains questions to assist practitioners in determining whether a student needs OT services and which level of service is recommended. The IEP team must consider all of the information obtained through the evaluations to determine whether the disability or condition interferes with the student's ability to participate in an educational program and whether the student needs related services to benefit from an educational program.[2,3] The presence of a disability does not necessarily mean that a student cannot participate in the regular educational program, nor does it mean that the student has an EEN as illustrated in the following case.

CASE *Study*

Mary, an 8-year-old girl in second grade, is diagnosed with cerebral palsy (left hemiplegia). Her parents requested an evaluation through the school district, which, in turn,

INDIVIDUAL EDUCATIONAL PROGRAM

For school-age children (3–21 years of age) who receive special education services, an IEP is developed to outline present levels of academic and functional skills, service delivery model and amount of time as well as the goals and objectives for the academic year. It is a written plan as well as a process. The IEP team consists of the student's parent(s) or guardian, general education teacher, special education teacher or provider, representative of the school district who is knowledgeable about the general curriculum, an individual who can interpret the instructional implications of evaluation results (i.e., the way certain factors may affect the student's ability to learn), and related services personnel. The representative of the school district, frequently given the title of local education agency (LEA) representative, may be the principal. The LEA representative is responsible for making sure that the programs outlined on the IEP are followed in the educational environment. The person who interprets the evaluation results is often the school psychologist or a clinical psychologist. The student may be present at the meetings. The parents may invite anyone they wish to be present, such as a private therapist or parent advocate. If the family brings a lawyer to the IEP meeting to assist with the process, then the school district may also bring a legal representative.

When developing the IEP, the team considers all evaluation results and the extent of the student's educational needs.[4] Goals, objectives, and methodologies (service and frequency) are developed at the meeting. The IEP is reviewed at least annually or sometimes more frequently if requested or necessary. The format of the IEP varies by state and school district. Box 4-3 contains information that must be included in an IEP.

Sometimes when a child enters school at 3 years of age, he or she already has a written **Individualized Family Service Plan** (IFSP). Box 4-4 lists components included in the IFSP. This document is the result of the collaboration between the parents and the birth-to-3 program professionals and is reviewed every 6 months. IFSPs emphasize the family's goals for the child, whereas an IEP focuses on educational goals that the student works on in school and is reviewed annually. Both documents require the parents to accept all or a portion of the recommended services. The parents or the school district have the option of going to due process if the team is unable to agree on the program or services recommended for the child. Children receiving special services are given progress notes with each report card.

Data collection sheets detail the child's objectives, frequency of performance in selected tasks, and success to date. This information is used to document the child's progress in quarterly reports. Performance is measured in a variety of contexts, with the goal being integration. Progress notes include information from the data sheets and rely on consultation and collaboration with teachers and staff to ensure that the performance represents actual achievement in the occupation (e.g., education).

BOX 4-3

Components of an Individual Educational Plan

- Statement of a child's present level of educational performance, including the way the child's disability affects his or her involvement in the general curriculum or age-appropriate activities
- Statement of measurable annual goals, including short-term objectives related to increased involvement and progress in the general curriculum and other (non)educational needs, such as those involving social and extracurricular activities
- Description of special education and related services and supplementary aids and services
- Description of program modifications or support to be used by school personnel to enable the child to attain goals; involvement and progress in general curricular, extracurricular, and nonacademic activities; and education and participation in activities with other children, both with and without disabilities
- Explanation of the extent to which the child will not participate in the regular classroom and IEP activities with children who do not have disabilities
- Statement of any individual modifications needed for the child to participate in formal assessments of student achievement (e.g., state- or district-wide tests)
- Projected date for beginning services and educational modifications; anticipated frequency, location, and duration of services
- Transition services, including linkage with other agencies
- Statement of the way that progress toward annual goals is measured
- Descriptions of methods to regularly inform parents of their child's progress (at least as often as the parents of children without disabilities are informed)

CLINICAL *Pearl*

Occupational therapy objectives are embedded in the special education teacher's goals and other team members reinforce objectives. As a result, everyone on the team is responsible for the goals and objectives of the IEP.

TRANSITIONS

Children undergo various transitions from infancy to 21 years of age. Students' services and programs change as they enter and leave the birth-to-3 program and the public school system. A transition plan includes steps that should be taken to support students and their families as they go through these changes so that the transitions

---

BOX 4-4

Components of an Individual Family Service Plan

The format of the written plan may differ from program to program, but an IFSP must contain the following information:

- Child's current level of development
- Summaries of evaluation reports
- Family's concerns
- Desired outcomes (goals)
- Early intervention services and support necessary to achieve outcomes
- Frequency of, method for providing, and location of services
- Payment arrangements (if any)
- Transition plan

can be smooth and successful. **Transition planning** informs families about the different services and agencies available.

When a student reaches age 14, transition services such as vocational education and job coaches are discussed with the student and the family to help in identifying his or her interests and preferences. Students nearing the age of majority (sometimes at age 17) are informed of their rights under the IDEA-R. The family is notified that all rights accorded to parents transfer to the student but that they will continue to receive required parental notices. For the parents to retain their rights, they must be recognized as the student's legal guardians by the courts.

ROLES OF THE OCCUPATIONAL THERAPIST AND THE OCCUPATIONAL THERAPY ASSISTANT

Occupational therapists and OTAs have related but distinct roles in the educational setting. A successful partnership between the two ensures effective and efficient use of education and training, encourages creativity, and promotes professional growth and respect.[2,3] All OT services provided in the educational setting must comply with federal and state regulations. Additionally, professional standards of practice help occupational therapists and OTAs with **role delineation** in the educational setting. OT practitioners work together to provide the best possible service to the child.

OT practitioners may be employed directly by the local educational agency (school district) or contracted through a local hospital, health care agency, or private practice. Those employed by the local educational agency must comply with the supervision and employment practices of the school district's structure. If the OT services are contracted through another agency (e.g., a hospital or health care agency), the practitioners are considered employees of that agency and may be supervised by one of its employees. Supervision guidelines and expectations should be closely coordinated between the employer and the local educational agency. In either situation, all licensing and state regulations regarding caseload and supervision standards must be followed.[3,5]

> ### CLINICAL *Pearl*
>
> In 48 states teachers are held accountable for meeting the **Common Core State Standards (CCSS).** Therefore the OT practitioner must be familiar with specific common core state standards. Box 4-5 provides more information regarding CCSS.

The occupational therapist is legally responsible for all aspects of the OT process. The OTA is responsible for providing services within his or her established level of competence. Professional supervision is a partnership that requires communication and mutual responsibility to clarify competencies and responsibilities. The practice standards established by the American Occupational Therapy Association delineate levels of supervision (see Chapter 1). The required level of supervision depends on many factors such as the OTA's level of experience and service competency, the complexity of the evaluation and therapy methods used, and the current practice guidelines and regulations of the state or local educational agency. Supervision in a school district often can be challenging because of the large number of schools and the geographic distance. Having the occupational therapist and OTA work together in the same school at the same time allows ongoing supervision of and communication with the OTA. Occupational therapists are ultimately responsible for service performance.[2,3] If an occupational therapist is not comfortable with an OTA's performance of a particular task, it should no longer be delegated to the OTA. Likewise, an OTA who is not comfortable performing a certain task is responsible for communicating this concern to the supervising occupational therapist.

Each of the practitioners has a role in screening and evaluation, IEP formation, treatment planning, and intervention. During the evaluation, occupational therapists determine which data are collected and which tools and methods to be used. OTAs can assist with data collection by making clinical observations and administering and scoring tests within their service competency level. Occupational therapists are responsible for analyzing,

---

BOX 4-5

Common Core State Standards

- Definition: The CCSS are educational expected outcomes applicable to all students receiving public education. State chief school officers and governors in collaboration with educators, administrators, and other experts, developed these standards.
- Purpose: The CCSS provide a consistent and clear understanding of what students are to learn.
- Instructional areas: The CCSS provide a high-quality framework for grade-level instruction in English/language arts/literacy and mathematics. Expected outcome: The focus of the students' education should be relevant to the real world and ensure that graduates have the knowledge and skills necessary for success in college, careers and life no matter where you live in the United States.

interpreting, and reporting information verbally and in writing. During the IEP formation, OTAs assist with developing goals and may attend the IEP meeting (under the direction of an occupational therapist) to report the findings and recommendations. Although OTAs do not interpret the findings or negotiate changes in levels of service or goals, they may suggest changes or reevaluation. OTAs are responsible for communicating observations, ideas, interpretations, and suggestions.

For the intervention phase, OTAs must first demonstrate service competency to the occupational therapist. Then they are responsible for developing intervention activities related to the goals and objectives (after initial direction from an occupational therapist). OTAs provide intervention aimed at improving children's occupations ranging from printing, cutting with scissors, using a keyboard, and performing lunchroom activities to managing clothing for toileting or recess. The OTA also collaborates and works with the teacher and other school personnel on appropriate positioning of the student and determining which materials or methods can be used in the classroom to increase the student's ability to participate successfully. The OTA is responsible for informing the occupational therapist of changes in the student's environment and providing current data regarding his or her performance.[2,3]

OTAs may be responsible for collecting data to establish evidence-based intervention. Because the domain of OT is occupation, the collected data must address occupation. Although goals and objectives must be measurable, practitioners must ensure that they are also meaningful to children, families, and educators. Table 4-2 provides a sample of school-based goals and intervention activities. By collecting data on activities that are valued by educators, families, and children, practitioners support the importance of the profession. Goals and objectives that are too far removed from the actual occupation may be measurable, but if they are not meaningful much time is wasted. For example, consider the following goal: Marcie will cross the street with 75% accuracy. Although this goal is measurable, it is not meaningful and is, in fact, dangerous. Marcie's mother's comment is: "What about the 25% of the time that she does not meet this goal?" Another commonly written goal states the following: "Mike will bring a spoon halfway to his mouth." As this goal is written, Mike does not even get any food during mealtime. A better goal would be as follows: "Mike will bring a spoon to his mouth; the first half of the distance will be hand over hand, and he will complete the second half of the distance 7 out of 10 spoonfuls." OTAs can assist the occupational therapist in developing measurable and meaningful goals by describing the behaviors in the context of the classroom. Once the goals are established, the OTA may be responsible for collecting and recording the data on a regular basis.

TABLE 4-2

Sample School-Based Goals and Intervention Activities

GOAL	ACTIVITY
Sam will write four sentences with 80% accuracy (spelling, legibility).	Hand strengthening, warm-up exercises Compensatory techniques, including laptop, frequency words available, Benbow Hand program, adaptive writing tool
Sam will write all his assignments in his daily planner, with verbal reminders from the teacher for 10 school days.	Teacher and parent will begin by reminding him (and fade cueing). Clinician adds a fun game to the assignment; if Sam remembers it, he gets a reward (i.e., bring in a picture of you and your pet).
Sam will participate in 45 minutes of regular gym class, with physical modifications made as needed.	Clinician will consult with gym teacher to provide modifications as necessary. OT clinician will consult with gym teacher about games and activities that the whole class may benefit from (e.g., parachute games, relay races, "Simon Says," dancing, etc.)

TYPES OF SERVICE

OT services can be delivered through direct service, monitoring, or consultation. The members of the IEP team decide which service delivery level is appropriate for each child. Therapy emphasizes the child's ability to perform in the school environment rather than in the therapy room.[7,13] IDEA mandates that the child participate in the regular curriculum to the maximum extent possible, so therapy in the classroom is recommended whenever possible. Occupational therapy plays a supportive role in helping the student participate and benefit from the special education program. This requires continuous collaboration between the teacher or other school staff member and the therapist.

In the classroom, paraprofessionals (such as teacher aides) benefit from training on and explanations of ways to work with children with special needs. For example, the OTA can teach and model how to perform proper body mechanics while lifting and handling a child with a severe disability. In addition, explaining to the staff how to feed, dress, and position children with various diagnoses is essential to carrying out integrated services and creating a safe educational environment.

Direct Services

With direct services, the OT practitioner works with the student so that he or she can acquire a skill. Direct therapy may be conducted one on one with the child or in a group setting; the time and frequency depend on the needs of the child.

For example, an OT practitioner working with several students in a regular grade 2 class could treat the children in the classroom during the regularly scheduled handwriting time. The OTA would be present for the handwriting session and work directly with the children designated in the IEP. Before the handwriting session, the OTA may encourage warm-up exercises. The entire class may do these exercises, but the OTA pays particular attention to the children under the IEP. As the students work on assignments, the OTA may review posture, provide cues for beginning the assignment, help with pencil grip, and provide verbal or tactile feedback, among other strategies. Direct service requires collaboration with the parent or teacher for follow through and optimal learning. Practitioners who partner with teachers show the most success in this type of approach.

Monitoring Services

OT practitioners following monitoring services create programs for the child that the teacher, other staff member, or family can follow. The practitioner contacts them frequently so that the program can be updated or altered as necessary. The personnel who follow the program are well trained and need to have a clear understanding of its goals. Billing procedures or state regulations may not acknowledge the monitoring service. Under this service, the practitioner is responsible for ensuring that the child's goals are met.

Consultation Services

Consultation services are provided when the occupational therapist's expertise is used to help other personnel achieve the child's objectives. OT practitioners may contact others only once or on an as-needed basis as set up by the team. Ongoing contact with the teacher or caregiver may be necessary. Consultation services are useful for adapting task materials or the environment, designing strategies to improve posture and positioning, or demonstrating how to handle a situation.

For example, an OT practitioner may consult with the teacher about a sensory diet for a student who needs help organizing sensory input. The practitioner would work with the teacher to create sensory suggestions for the child in the classroom. Equipment such as a weighted vest, trampoline, vibrator, and weighted lap pad would be purchased or made for use by the student and staff as necessary. Sensory suggestions could be outlined for the staff to use with the student on a daily basis. Table 4-3 is an

TABLE 4-3

Sensory Strategies

WHAT IT LOOKS LIKE FOR THE BRAIN	SENSORY DIET
TACTILE SENSE	
Seeks touch and deep pressure	Provide deep pressure
	Provide weighted items
	Provide resistive finger/hand fidgets
Seeks touch by touching objects and people around him	Provide weighted vest or weighted lap pad
Seeks soft, silky material	Provide silk-like sheets or clothing
	Place a piece of silk on his seat
	Provide a piece of silk to calm
VESTIBULAR SENSE	
Seems to seek vestibular movement by spinning or rocking	Provide swings, rocking chairs, balls or ball chairs
	Activity suggestions: "Sit and move" chair cushion
Gets overstimulated by activities in the environment	Encourage student to go to the quiet area in the corner of the room
	Have student rock in the rocking chair
PROPRIOCEPTIVE SENSE	
Seeks high impact by touching other people	Provide weights, joint compression, vibration toys
Pushes himself against other people	Provide weighted vest, joint compression, and vibration
AUDITORY SENSE	
Very sensitive to noise	Work in noiseless environment
	Try mufflers or headset to decrease noise
	Play quiet ocean sounds in the background
	Try rhythmic sounds, like a metronome
Easily distracted by sound	Keep verbal cues to a minimum and avoid extraneous noise
VISUAL SENSE	
Easily distracted by objects	Decrease visual distractions
Gets easily over stimulated by too much visual stimulation	Remove visual distractions from the wall; work in a cubicle

example of an outline with sensory strategies that could be provided to the teacher. The practitioner would then consult with the staff to set up a daily schedule of sensory needs, which could be adjusted as necessary.

DISCONTINUING THERAPY SERVICES

Dismissing a child from OT services can be difficult because of the rapport that has been established among the child, family, and practitioner. Children may be dismissed from occupational therapy when all of the intervention goals and objectives have been accomplished or therapy is not resulting in the desired changes. In cases of plateauing (i.e., the child does not make any progress toward the goal), the child may benefit from working with another therapist or an alternative approach. If possible, practitioners should avoid discharging a child from therapy when he or she is undergoing a transition, such as changing schools. Frequently, a child is eased out of therapy by decreasing the quantity and going from direct therapy to consultation service to dismissal.[7] Children may require consultation on positioning when undergoing physical changes. Any change in service (including frequency) is discussed with the IEP team (including parents). For example, students entering middle school may not have had refined fine motor and self-care skills addressed. Service delivery is a dynamic process that requires flexibility and adaptability to the changing needs of the school and the child. Consultation with the teacher will help serve the child's needs in an effective manner. If this type of delivery does not work, the practitioner may decide to provide direct service. It is helpful to explain to parents the dynamic nature of OT services and the IEP process.

> **CLINICAL** *Pearl*
>
> Remember that the teacher is the manager of the classroom. The OT practitioner is a guest, and his or her presence should not disrupt the routine.

> **CLINICAL** *Pearl*
>
> Adolescents may need OT consultation to discuss their strengths and weaknesses for vocational activities. Children entering high school may benefit from consultation with an OT practitioner about study habits, strategies to succeed, and issues surrounding physical changes.

CASE *Study*

Tamara, an OTA, intended to work with Jovan in his first-grade classroom during art class. The objective for the session was for Jovan to hold a crayon with a static tripod grasp and imitate a circle. However, when Tamara entered the classroom, the teacher informed her that the art class had been canceled; they were now involved in playing "Simon Says" and other inside games because it was raining and the kids were all "wound up." Instead of insisting that Jovan participate in the scheduled art activity, Tamara decided to incorporate Jovan's second goal of improving postural control for writing activities. She quickly changed her intervention to facilitate the trunk and upper arm strengthening required for writing. Tamara asked the teacher if she could be the leader of the game. The teacher appreciated the break after a hectic rainy morning. Tamara led the activities for the entire class and provided hands-on help to Jovan as needed. The children performed arm pushups, wheelbarrow walks, crab walks, and sit-ups, among other physical activities. Jovan was proud of himself because he knew how to do the crab walk and got to show the others. Tamara ended the session by asking the children ("Simon says") to sit in their seats, put their heads down, count quietly to 20, and then look up. This helped quiet the children. The teacher enjoyed seeing the variation of "Simon Says" activities. Tamara explained that these were great prehandwriting activities and that all the children could benefit from them. Tamara agreed to write them down for the teacher.

TIPS FOR WORKING WITH PARENTS AND TEACHERS

Parents and teachers are key players on any team involving children in school systems.[5,6] Children and families benefit by OT practitioners who establish therapeutic relationships early. Since parents may not regularly attend school, OT practitioners are responsible for setting up systems to communicate clearly and often with parents regarding the child's progress and goals. Working with teachers also requires negotiation and strategies to be successful. The following tips and strategies may prove useful when working with parents and teachers.

Tips for Working with Parents*

1. Parents know their child! Listen to what they have to say, and try to address their concerns. They may not know why their child is behaving in a particular manner (professionals may help with this), but they are aware of the behaviors.
2. Parents and caregivers may not understand the language that professionals use in meetings. Present information in layman's terms so that explanations are not needed. For example, say, "John has trouble

---

*Tips provided by Judy Cohn, MS, ED, and Jane O'Brien, PhD, OTR/L, FAOTA

getting around without tripping or bumping into things" instead of "John has dyspraxia."

3. Parents attending IEP meetings may be nervous and may feel uncomfortable. Put them at ease by beginning the meeting asking them what they hope to achieve from the meeting or what they see as their child's strengths.

4. IEP team meetings frequently highlight the child's weaknesses and present only briefly the child's strengths. Begin your report with the child's strengths; follow it by describing problem areas, with a plan for how to address these concerns.

5. When discussing the child's performance, be clear about what has been tried in the classroom and how it has or has not worked. This gives the team information on future goals, objectives, and intervention strategies.

6. Parents may become frustrated with a long list of problems. Order the list of problem areas in such a way that the most important issues may be targeted immediately for intervention. You can always address other problems later.

7. Ask the parents what works or does not work at home. You may be able to provide them with strategies to help their child, or they may be able to help you with strategies. Children benefit when both the parents and professionals are working on the same page.

8. Provide suggestions and/or strategies for helping the child function within the classroom. Using a previously developed list is acceptable, but make sure you have individualized it to the child. Use his or her name. Remember that any written information sent to others is a reflection of you. You do not want to give the parents the impression that you are too busy to work with their child.

9. Follow up with the parents. Sending letters home with the child, e-mail messages, or brief phone calls let the parents know that you are working with them to help their child. Keep information confidential and protected. For example, there are some things you do not want to e-mail, but letting the parents know that "John had a great day in occupational therapy" is always welcomed.

Tips for Working with Teachers*

1. Most importantly, remember that the job of an OT practitioner in a school setting is to help the child function within the classroom. The teacher is in charge of the classroom. Therefore you must observe the teacher's style, rules, and classroom expectations before designing the intervention for a specific child.

2. Spend time in the classroom without making suggestions or judging the teacher.

3. Ask the teacher what he or she sees as the problem areas for the child. Ask the teacher how you could help the child function better within the classroom.

4. Prioritize strategies for the teacher. He or she must work with the entire class, so providing them with one or two effective strategies for a child is sufficient. You can always add more later.

5. Provide the teacher with short written strategies, and follow up as necessary.

6. Respect the teacher's time. Teachers get very few breaks during the day. Discussing a child over lunch may seem like a good solution to you but may add stress to the teacher's day and not allow for a much-needed break. Another solution may be to ask to lead a 30-minute "handwriting" seminar for the entire class every Friday morning. You can work with the entire class, targeting the needs of a small group at the same time. This helps build rapport with the teacher, fosters carryover in the classroom, and benefits the entire class.

7. E-mails and short notes are effective means of communication with teachers.

8. Help determine good child–teacher fits. Once you understand the style and expectations of a classroom you can assist in the placement of children with special needs. For example, some teachers are extremely organized and may work best with children who have difficulty with organization. Other children require flexibility and accommodation.

9. Present yourself to teachers as a resource. For example, it may be helpful to provide them with writing kits full of activities to enhance writing skills, fine motor games, visual motor games, or crafts that may be easily implemented into the classroom. You may want to lead morning exercises or warm-ups to address the sensory needs of the students while modeling activities for teachers.

10. Help teachers out by using OT resources. Establish a relationship between the nearby occupational therapy educational program. College students are frequently looking for projects that may help teachers and schools. Box 4-6 lists some examples of projects that may assist teachers and OT students.

11. Provide solutions to teachers concerning children with special needs. Gain their trust through collaboration, which works best by listening, discussing, and following through. Team members must be able to critically analyze their work and look for alternative solutions.

12. Use layman's terms when speaking with teachers. It is best to describe the observed student's behavior in simple language rather than by using medical or psychological terms to describe behaviors. Speaking

*Tips provided by Judy Cohn, MS, ED, and Jane O'Brien, PhD, OTR/L, FAOTA

BOX 4-6

Projects That May Assist Teachers and Students in Programs for the Occupational Therapy and the Occupational Therapy Assistant

- Design a fine motor kit for classrooms.
- Develop games associated with the seasons.
- Provide the regular education teacher with a handwriting kit with a variety of pencil grips, pencils (size, color, type) and paper (e.g. highlighted lines, raised edged).
- Provide the teacher with finger fidgets to be available for the students in regular education classrooms.
- Provide the teacher with scents for calming or alerting behaviors.
- Make pieces of equipment, toys, or other items needed for the classroom (positioning equipment must be checked out by the practitioner).
- Design and implement a finger puppet show (to improve finger individuation) based on a book (to encourage reading).
- Participate in a health fair at a local school.
- Volunteer for story time; find a book about children with special needs.
- Volunteer for a field trip or evening workshop.
- Develop teacher/parent handouts with strategies for children with organizational problems.
- Organize a teacher appreciation day.

about what one observes limits misunderstanding. For example, instead of saying, "John is tactually defensive, which is why he has trouble modulating his behavior," say, "John does not like to be touched by other children unexpectedly; he finds this type of contact annoying, which is why he may hit other children." Then you can provide a solution (e.g., allow John to be in the back of the line. Sometimes he will also want to be in the front of the line. When John is the "line leader," observe carefully and ask him to lead the way from the front. You do not want John to feel left out and never be allowed to be the line leader).

Tips for Providing Intervention in the Classroom*

1. Develop a collaborative relationship with the teacher before providing intervention in the classroom. Be aware of the teacher's style, rules, routine, and classroom expectations.

* Tips provided by Judy Cohn, MS, ED, and Jane O'Brien, PhD, OTR/L, FAOTA.

2. Discuss with the teacher what you would like to do. Decide on a time that this fits in with other classroom activities. Be open to adjusting your schedule to fit in with the teacher's agenda.
3. Working in small groups makes the intervention less obvious and intrusive.
4. Keeping a regular schedule allows the class to feel comfortable with you.
5. Walk into the classroom at a nondisruptive time (e.g., after the bell rings, when the children are settling down). It is not helpful if you interrupt quiet reading or testing to work with a child.
6. Provide intervention as the child participates in the activities. For example, a child with poor handwriting may complete a worksheet by repeating correct strokes during writing practice. You may help a child with hand movements to a song while standing by and providing trunk stabilization so that the child can move his or her arms.
7. Providing intervention in the classroom requires the OT practitioner to adjust the intervention so that the child can be successful at the activities. For example the teacher may choose the activities while you adapt and grade the activities. This requires you to be flexible and "think on your feet." It is important that you have the child's goals and objectives firmly in mind.
8. Flexibility is easily achieved when you are aware of the child's goals and objectives. If the classroom activity changes, you may select a different goal for the session. Once you are clear about the desired objective, you may adapt and modify the activity to address it.
9. Be responsible for developing a weekly activity plan for the entire class. Attend the class at the same time (for consistency) and complement the teacher's lesson plan. For example, if the first-grade class is learning about animals, you could design an entire session on animals. Students could make animal noises and walk like an animal (gross motor), match animal cards of mothers and babies (visual perceptual), pick out animal textures (fur for a bear, slippery snakeskin) or plastic shapes (stereognosis), and make an animal craft (cutting, drawing, coloring) (fine motor).
10. Communicate clearly with the teacher. You could e-mail the teacher to let her know the plan for the following week. It is important to be respectful of the teacher by being well prepared for the class and letting her know in advance if you are unable to attend a class. It would be very helpful to the teacher if you have all the materials prepared (along with the lesson plan) in case you are unable to attend.
11. Ask for and accept feedback. Set up a system whereby the teacher can give you feedback. Make

changes based on the feedback, and follow up with suggestions of your own. Teachers are more likely to listen to you if they feel you are listening to them. Be sure to ask how the children responded to your sessions. Some of these sessions may make the children more attentive for the rest of the day, whereas others may cause the children to become restless.

SUMMARY

OT practitioners must possess technical knowledge and skills as well understand child development, family systems, learning theory, community resources, and current federal and state regulations. Although there are federal regulations that dictate broad policies, OT practitioners must keep abreast of state regulations and local educational agency procedures to ensure compliance in all areas.

Communicating and working as a team is key to school-based practice. Practitioners must be prepared to discuss OT knowledge in a language that educators and families understand. Successfully functioning as part of a team requires the members to value the educational philosophy and listen carefully to parents and teachers. Practitioners working in schools have the unique opportunity to help children function in the place where they work (school). Incorporating therapy into classroom activities takes skill and negotiation. Practitioners may need to "think outside the box" and provide therapeutic activities in a busy, crowded classroom. OT practitioners are responsible for modeling and teaching skills to others so that the educational staff can provide services to children on a daily basis. Practitioners working in educational settings analyze children in terms of their ability to perform occupations in the school, family, and community rather than in terms of their deficits in performance components. By working with a team of dedicated professionals, clinicians may improve a child's ability to learn, socialize, and function in school.

References

1. American Occupational Therapy Association. (2014). Occupational therapy practice framework: domain and process (3rd ed.). *Am J Occup Ther*, 68(Suppl. 1), S1–S48.
2. American Occupational Therapy Association. (2007). *Occupational therapy services for Children and youth under IDEA*. Rockville, MD: Author.
3. American Occupational Therapy Association. (2011). *Occupation therapy services in early childhood and school-based settings*. Rockville MD: Author.
4. American Occupational Therapy Association. (2006). *Transforming caseload to workload in school-based early intervention occupational therapy services*. Bethesda, MD: Author.
5. Barnes, K. J., & Turner, K. D. (2001). Team collaboration between teachers and occupational therapists. *Am J Occup Ther*, 55, 83–89.
6. Bose, P., & Hinojosa, J. (2008). Reported experiences from occupational therapists interacting with teachers in inclusive early childhood classrooms. *Am J Occup Ther*, 62, 289–297.
7. Carrasco, R. C., Skees-Hermes, S., Frolek-Clark, G., et al. (2007). Occupational therapy service delivery to support child and family participation in context. In L. L. Jackson (Ed.), *Occupational therapy services for children and youth under IDEA* (3rd ed.). Bethesda, MD: AOTA.
8. Council for Exceptional Children. (1999). *IEP team guide*. Arlington, VA: Author.
9. Hanft, B. E., & Shepherd, J. (2008). *Collaborating for student success: a guide for school-based occupational therapy*. Bethesda, MD: AOTA.
10. Individuals with Disabilities Education Act, IDEA 2004, *Final Regulations* 300.34 (2006). National Governors Association Center for Best Practices (NGA), Council of Chief State School Officers (CCSSO). (2010). Common Core standards state initiative. Washington, DC: NGA: CCSSO.
11. Opp, A. (2007). Reauthorizing no child left behind: opportunities for OTs. *OT Practice*, 12, 9–13.
12. Senior, R. (2012, March 12). *The 2012 ADVANCE Salary Survey*. http://occupational-therapy.advanceweb.com/Archives/Article-Archives/The-2012-ADVANCE-Salary-Survey.aspx.
13. Swinth, Y., & Handley-More, D. (2003). Update on school-based practice. *OT Practice*, 8, 22–24.

REVIEW *Questions*

1. What are some of the federal laws that have an effect on the provision of OT services in the public school system?
2. Which factors determine whether a child is eligible to receive OT services in a school setting?
3. In what ways do therapy services provided according to an educational model differ from those provided according to a medical model?
4. How do the roles of an occupational therapist and an OTA differ in a school setting?
5. What are the components of the IEP?
6. What are some tips for working with teachers and parents?
7. What are some tips for providing intervention in the classroom?

SUGGESTED *Activities*

1. Visit or volunteer in a public school, and observe the various programs and environments that have been developed for students with special needs, such as a learning disabilities resource room and a self-contained classroom.
2. Be politically aware and active. Keep abreast of changes in local, state, and federal laws. Participate in public hearings, and contact legislators when laws affecting the provision of OT services are being debated.
3. Volunteer with an occupational therapist or an OTA in the public school system to understand ways to integrate therapy services in the regular classroom.
4. Make a list of the various assessment tools used by an OT practitioner working in an educational system. Describe the assessments and ask practitioners to explain why they selected the assessment. Describe what the assessment measures, how it is administered, and the age range of the children it is intended. Review the manual and develop questions.
5. Develop a notebook with resources for children, teachers and parents that may help children receiving occupational therapy services in educational settings.
6. Develop an intervention plan to address a variety of educationally relevant goals.

Acronyms Frequently Used in the Educational System

GENERAL TERMS

AT: Assistive technology
ABA: Applied behavioral analysis
BIP: Behavior intervention plan
CCSS: Common Core State Standards
DD: Developmental delay
EEN: Exceptional educational need
EOY: End of school year
ESY: Extended school year
Gen.Ed.: General education
ID: intellectual disability
IEP: Individualized Education Plan
IFSP: Individualized Family Service Plan
LEA: Local educational agency
LRE: Least restrictive environment
NCLB: No Child Left Behind
OHI: Other health impairment
O&M: Orientation and mobility
PSC: Preschool self-contained classroom
PT: Physical therapist
RtI: Response to intervention
SC: Self-contained classroom
SLP: Speech and language pathologist
SPED: Special education
SS: Standard or scaled score
ST: Speech therapist and/or speech therapy
SY: School year
UDL: Universal design for learning

INTERVENTION AND REPORTING TERMS

ASD: Autism spectrum disorder
BD: Behavior disorder
CA: Chronologic age
CWS: Correct word sequences
DOB: Date of birth
DOE/DOA: Date of evaluation/assessment
ED: Emotional disorder
ELA: English language arts
FM: Fine motor
GM: Gross motor
IQ: Intellectual quotient
LD: Learning disability
LPM: Letters per minute
ODD: Oppositional defiant disorder
PBSI: Positive behavior support intervention(s)
PI: Push in
PO: Pull out
POC: Plan of care
PSI: Preschool itinerate teacher
SD: Standard deviation
TWW: Total words written
VI: Vision itinerant teacher
VP: Visual perception
VMI: Visual motor integration
WPM: Words per minute
%: percentile ranking compared with same-aged peers

SCHOOL-SPECIFIC EXAMPLES

WES: Whitesville Elementary School
BES: Berkeley Elementary School
BIS: Berkeley Intermediate School
BMS: Berkeley Middle School
BHS: Berkeley High School
THS: Timberland High School

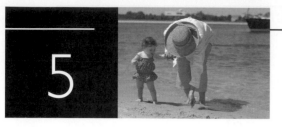

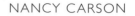

Community Systems

KEY TERMS

Community
Community-based
  practice
Community-built
  practice
Health
Clients
Therapeutic use of self
Therapeutic relationship
Public health
Precede-Proceed Model
  (PPM)
Community Mental
  Health Center Act
  of 1963
Cultural competence

CHAPTER *Objectives*

After studying this chapter, the reader will be able to accomplish the following:
- Understand the difference between community-based practice and community-built practice.
- Understand the importance of therapeutic use of self in providing services in the community and in building community partnerships.
- Identify the different service delivery methods occupational therapists may utilize in community settings.
- Identify the different community systems in which occupational therapists work.
- Understand the influence of public health on community interventions.
- Identify the challenges to providing services in the community.

CHAPTER *Outline*

Community-Based and Community-
  Built Practice

Therapeutic Use of Self

Public Health Influence

Community Mental Health
  Movement

Community Occupational Therapy
  Interventions

Challenges in Practice in Community
  Systems

Summary

The delivery of occupational therapy (OT) services has expanded far beyond the traditional medical model that served the majority of clients in the past. As health care expands to meet the unique needs of an increasingly diverse society, the intervention setting has changed so the needs of the clients can more efficiently be addressed. This requires occupational therapy services to be provided in a community setting in which the child lives, learns, plays, or is otherwise occupationally engaged. It should be a setting that is accessible and appropriate for the child or youth and which allows for successful intervention to occur.

There are many community systems or community-oriented service delivery models in which occupational therapists and occupational therapy assistants (OTAs) can provide services to children. Community systems can include schools, preschools, afterschool programs, day cares, faith-based programs, community recreational programs, community mental health centers, community health clinics, camps, group homes, residential care facilities, homeless shelters, and home health agencies. Any type of facility, outside of the traditional medical model presented in a hospital or clinic setting, that provides health-related programs or services to individuals in the community can be considered a community system. Any organization that offers programs or services in the context of one or more community settings also can be thought of as a community system. There also are a variety of service delivery models that may exist within each of these community systems (Figure 5-1). Service delivery models may include approaches such as individual therapy, group therapy, skill-building, coaching, mentoring, family education and training, teacher or caretaker education and training, and program consultation.

COMMUNITY-BASED AND COMMUNITY-BUILT PRACTICE

In order to understand how therapists practice in these settings and how this may differ from traditional hospital-based practice, it is necessary to define a **community**. Understandably, *community* is a broad term and many definitions of a community exist. One definition for community is that it is a "person's natural environment, that is, where the person works, plays and performs other daily activities."[21, p. 2] Another definition for community is "an area with geographic and often political boundaries demarcated as a district, county, metropolitan area, city, township, or neighborhood ... a place where members have a sense of identity and belonging, shared values, norms, communication, and helping patterns."[9, p. 256] To further understand the practice of occupational therapy in community systems two definitions are provided to articulate service delivery models. **Community-based practice** is defined as "skilled services delivered by health practitioners using an interactive model with clients" and **community-built practice** is defined as when "skilled services are delivered by health practitioners using a collaborative and interactive model with clients."[21]

Community-based practice is usually initiated by the medical model and results from referrals from other health care workers. Community-built practice is presented from a public health perspective focusing on health promotion and education. Treatment involves defining the community and working with the community in a variety of ways to support the client and enhance occupational functioning (Figure 5-2). Although both types of community practice emphasize an interactive model, it is the community-built practice that involves collaboration and a strong emphasis on empowerment and wellness.[21]

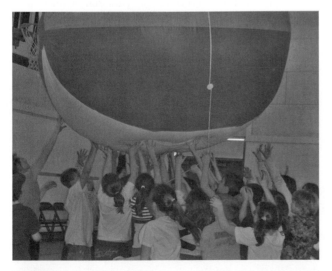

FIGURE 5-1 Wellness in the community: OT students promote physical activity and give back to the community by organizing fun games for children.

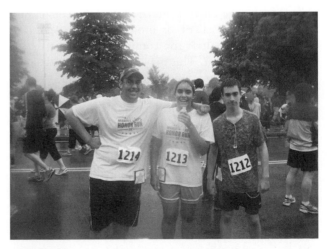

FIGURE 5-2 High school students give back to the community by running a race in honor of those who serve.

It is imperative that the OT practitioner be aware of the community systems in which the client is engaged. Even if services are not provided in the context of a community agency, the environmental implications of the communities in which the child interacts on a daily basis must be considered to allow for optimal occupational functioning and health. The definition of **health** provided by the World Health Organization[22] states that "health is a state of complete physical, mental and social well-being and not merely the absence of disease or infirmity." To support optimal health for the child, the OT practitioner must understand the community in which the child functions and how community systems and community resources can support successful occupational functioning.

The Occupational Therapy Practice Framework: Domain and Process (3rd ed.)[1] defines **clients** as persons, groups, and populations within a community being classified as a group. When the client is a child referred for intervention, treatment may focus primarily on the child, the caregiver, or teacher. The context and environment must be considered as part of the domain of occupational therapy. Specifically, the social environment includes the community groups they are part of and that affect the child's occupational performance. The context in which the child interacts with these community groups must be considered for effective intervention to take place.[1]

Herzberg[10] emphasizes the declining trend of health care being provided in traditional in- and outpatient medical model settings and the increasingly predominant trend of health care services being offered in a community environment or through a community agency. A variety of perspectives on community interventions are presented and the need for OT practitioners to develop the skills for working in communities to enhance full inclusion and social participation for the individual is discussed. Skills for the OT practitioner may include consultation, policymaking, and program development. Defining who the client is may result in the community agency being the client or broadening the definition of the client to include the community at large that is supporting the client. This may be necessary so that the most effective occupational therapy is provided to the individual client. The distinction between community-based and community-built practices is discussed in the context of how the role of the OT practitioner differs depending on the focus of the community organization. Here, the focus of community-based practice is discussed as the delivery of skilled services and addressing the client's deficits by direct intervention in a community setting. Likewise, community-built practice involves the delivery of skilled services along with collaboration with and support from the appropriate community resources and building a sense of client empowerment to resolve client-defined issues. The need for both types of community practice is strongly emphasized and the two approaches are viewed as existing on a continuum.

OT practitioners are encouraged to expand their services to include roles on this continuum and roles that are focused in community environments.[10]

THERAPEUTIC USE OF SELF

Although the move toward a greater awareness and involvement in community systems is generally perceived as a positive trend in health care, the practitioner should be mindful of the possible negative perceptions of the recipients of these types of services. Silverstein, Lamberto, DePeau, and Grossman[15] unexpectedly found that low-income parents of children receiving multiple community and social services had negative experiences and perceptions of the community resources they used. Qualitative analysis of 41 interviews revealed parental perceptions of having to make important decisions based on choices that were often less than satisfactory. A lack of control was experienced as a result of accepting community services that were sometimes seen as being ineffective due to lack of individualization.[15] Employees of community agencies were sometimes perceived as being judgmental or too personal and the need to compromise value systems was sometimes perceived by these parents.

It is essential for occupational therapists and OTAs to practice effective **therapeutic use of self** when engaging with clients, their families, and individuals within the client's community health care system. Therapeutic use of self has been described as the therapist's "planned use of his or her personality, insights, perceptions, and judgments as part of the therapeutic process"[14 p. 285] and conscious use of self in therapy as "the use of oneself in such a way that one becomes an effective tool in the evaluation and intervention process."[13, p. 199] Effective therapeutic use of self requires the therapist to have a thorough self-understanding of personal values and expectations as well as an understanding of the client's values and cultural needs. Understanding how to negotiate a relationship most effectively by using personal skills to an advantage, while respecting the client's values and beliefs, is a skill that one must learn to be an effective therapist. When working with children, the relationship between the practitioner and the child's caretaker(s) also must be considered. When providing services in community settings there also may be other individuals such as teachers or community resource providers involved in the child's care. It therefore becomes a multilayer network of relationships that must be nurtured and developed to ensure the best outcomes for the child. The relationship between the OT practitioner and these individuals needs to be considered to ensure effective treatment for the child. Figure 5-3 shows a practitioner using therapeutic use of self while engaging a child in a cooking activity. Therefore practitioners working with children in community settings need to have excellent communication and negotiation skills as well as an acute ability to

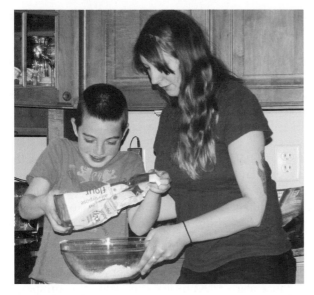

FIGURE 5-3 The practitioner uses therapeutic use of self (collaboration) when working towards a child's goals.

The Intentional Relationship Model's Therapeutic Modes as Defined by Taylor

MODE	DEFINITION
Advocating	Ensure that the client's rights are enforced and resources are secured.
Collaborating	Expect the client to be an active and equal participant in therapy and ensure choice, freedom and autonomy where possible.
Empathizing	Continually strive to understand the client's thoughts, feelings, and behaviors while suspending judgment.
Encouraging	Instill hope and celebrate a client's thinking or behavior through positive reinforcement.
Instructing	Structure therapy activities and be explicit about the plan, sequence, and events of therapy.
Problem solving	Facilitate pragmatic thinking and solving dilemmas by outlining choices, posing strategic questions and providing opportunities for analytic thinking.

Data from Taylor, R. R. (2008). *The intentional relationship: occupational therapy and use of self*. Philadelphia: F. A. Davis.

network with others to establish effective resources for each child. Furthermore, all of this requires a thorough understanding of the mission of the community system in which the child is engaged and how this mission relates to the services being provided by occupational therapy.

The **therapeutic relationship** has been defined as a "trusting connection and rapport established between practitioner and client through collaboration, communication, therapist empathy and mutual respect."[8, p. 49] The *intentional relationship model* is a conceptual practice model that thoroughly explains the relationship between the OT practitioner and the client.[17] This model is specific to the field of occupational therapy and explores in detail how therapeutic use of self promotes occupational engagement facilitating a positive therapeutic relationship that allows for successful therapy outcomes. One aspect of the model is an understanding of one's therapeutic modes. In all, there are six therapeutic modes that a therapist might use. A therapeutic mode is defined as an interacting style that a therapist employs when interacting with a client. A therapist may employ more than one mode and the use of these modes is a function of the individual's innate personality traits and natural communication style. The modes identified in this model include advocating, collaborating, empathizing, encouraging, instructing, and problem solving. Box 5-1 provides definitions of the modes. Ideally, a therapist strives toward being able to use all of the modes and develops the ability to recognize which mode is most appropriate to use in any given situation.[17]

Effective therapeutic use of self allows for the development of a therapeutic relationship. As defined, the therapeutic relationship embodies collaboration. It is through this collaboration that client empowerment evolves. When working with children, it is necessary to establish a therapeutic relationship with the child, the caretaker(s), and appropriate individuals within the community system(s) involved in the child's health care. This requires the therapist to be acutely aware of the many different relationships that must be nurtured and maintained to promote the most successful outcomes for the child. Not only must the child be empowered but the significant figures in the child's live must be empowered as well. This requires the therapist to strive to maintain multiple therapeutic relationships and this may require different approaches and strategies with the different individuals involved in the child's care. This may be in contrast to a traditional medical model where the therapist may be minimally involved and only in contact with the person transporting the child to therapy.

CLINICAL *Pearl*

Therapeutic use of self is a very important tool for the OT practitioner when working with the child as well as when communicating with the individuals within the community setting. OT practitioners should constantly engage in self-evaluation of communication and interpersonal skills and strive to increase their ability to work well with others. The OT practitioner must be able to communicate, empower, and motivate the child and those involved with achieving the child's therapy goals. Treating the child alone is not enough for successful outcomes; it takes the whole community working together.

PUBLIC HEALTH INFLUENCE

The influence of **public health** on community practice for many health care disciplines cannot be underestimated. In considering community systems from a very broad perspective, the field of public health employs community-based and community-built approaches for many of its initiatives. Most of the interventions implemented by public health educators are done within community settings and organizations.[12]

Understandably, a larger number of people can receive intervention when it is provided to groups of people versus individuals or is provided through organizations that include people with similar needs. Traditionally, many occupational therapy services have been provided individually and this is necessary for specific types of treatment. However, as medical costs rise and health care services continue to move more to community settings, the need and opportunity to broaden the service delivery of occupational therapy is expanding.

Developing an appreciation for public health approaches is useful for understanding community-based and community-built services for occupational therapists. For both types of service delivery models, thorough knowledge and awareness of the community is needed to provide effective treatment. Community-based services may be individual services provided in a community setting but still functioning like the medical model, whereas community-built services can be considered individual or group approaches that embrace and empower the client and the community service providers and may be provided in community settings or through community organizations. The approach used will depend on the needs of the individual or group of clients being served.

Many of the initiatives addressed by the public health discipline are addressed in the *Healthy People 2020* objectives.[20] Traditionally, health care in the United States has not been focused on preventive care. In recent years this trend has changed. *Healthy People* originated in 1979 through the Centers for Disease Control and Prevention as a mechanism of identifying objectives and strategies for the prevention of illness and premature death. Every 10 years, national health priorities are identified and objectives for prevention are established. *Healthy People 2020* is the fourth revision of

this initiative and provides a framework for prevention for the people of the United States. The four overarching goals of *Healthy People 2020* are to increase healthy years of life for all individuals, achieve health equity and end health disparities, create healthy social and physical environments, and promote healthy behavior and quality of life.[20]

Healthy People 2020 consists of 26 leading health indicators, 42 topic areas, and more than 1200 objectives. The leading health indicators are a smaller subset of the objectives and are used to measure the health of the citizens of the United States. Many of the topic areas and corresponding objectives identified in *Healthy People 2020* are areas of interest to occupational therapy. The relevant topic areas include educational and community-based programs, mental health and mental disorders, nutrition and weight status, physical activity, and substance abuse.[20] As health care delivery continues to evolve and health care practitioners are challenged to provide services in a variety of settings, the opportunities for occupational therapists are numerous. By being aware of the objectives set forth in the *Healthy People 2020* initiative, OT practitioners can partner with other health care providers in the community to meet the health needs and improve the quality of life of clients (Figure 5-4).

Childhood obesity is an example of a public health concern that occupational therapists can be effective in addressing. Childhood overweight and obesity is a growing concern; in 2011 to 2012 approximately 17% of children and youth ages 2 to 19 years were obese. Broken down by age, 8.4% of children 2 to 5 years of age, 17.7% of children 6 to 11 years of age, and 20.5% of adolescents 12 to 19 years of age were obese.[6] Over the past 20 years, the number of adults considered obese has also grown significantly; in 2009 to 2010 more than one-third of U.S. adults (35.7%) were obese.[7]

Campbell and Crawford[4] present a review of data that suggests that eating behaviors are likely to be established early in life and may be maintained into adulthood. Steinbeck[16] suggests focusing more on intervention and prevention in children to establish lifelong healthy eating patterns and regular engagement in physical activity because it has been documented that treating established adult obesity and overweight is difficult and has poor outcomes overall. Community interventions designed to address physical activity and nutrition in children are an excellent opportunity for occupational therapists. Programs can be designed for schools, day-care centers, or afterschool settings. Programs should address a variety of influences that affect the child's weight. Collaboration with caregivers and teachers is essential for effective outcomes. OT practitioners have the necessary skills to provide this type of program and because of the public recognition of

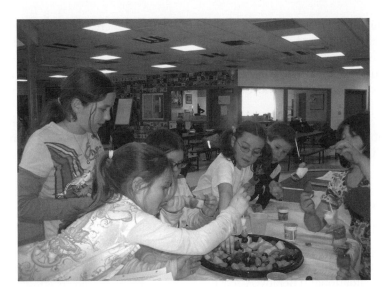

FIGURE 5-4 OT students provide an afterschool program to children to promote health nutritional habits and reduce childhood obesity.

childhood obesity as a national concern, the need for such programs is substantial. Chapter 15 of this text presents more information on childhood obesity.

In planning a community intervention it is necessary to have a well-devised model to follow. A widely used model for planning, implementing, and evaluating community interventions in public health is the **Precede-Proceed Model** (PPM).[9] PPM consists of eight phases that provide a framework for intervention. It is an educational and ecological model that incorporates planning for evidence-based best practices, intervention, and integration of evaluation methods for quality improvement. PPM involves careful and thorough assessments of the community systems and the influences on the health behavior being addressed. PPM provides one example of an appropriate framework to use; however, the practitioner should make sure to develop a complete understanding on the use of the model in planning and implementing community interventions.

COMMUNITY MENTAL HEALTH MOVEMENT

Possibly the most significant example of the move from hospital-based care to community care has occurred in the mental health system. During the 1960s there were many changes in American society. Political, social, and cultural changes resulted from the Civil Rights Movement and activities of the time. Prolonged institutionalization of individuals with disabilities was viewed negatively and political support for deinstitutionalization increased. As a result, the **Community Mental Health Center Act of 1963** was signed by President John F. Kennedy and funds were approved to build comprehensive community mental health centers that would provide a range of mental health services.[3]

In some states, occupational therapists were integrated into the community mental health services and in some states their roles were replaced by other health care providers. This occurred for a variety of reasons including lack of awareness of occupational therapy, unavailability of therapists interested in mental health treatment, higher cost to include occupational therapy on staff, and other health care professionals providing services deemed to be similar to occupational therapy. For those practitioners wanting to work in mental health, the need to advocate for the profession and the ability to demonstrate the benefit of occupational therapy to the mental health director and administrators is necessary to create a role in the community mental health setting. Thinking outside of the box and looking at a variety of settings in which to provide services can open up new opportunities. With increased emphasis on the mental well-being of children, there are opportunities to provide community-built occupational therapy services to children with mental illness.

In a review of community-based mental health occupational therapy interventions, Ikiugu[11] presents a model for the design and implementation of community programs. The steps in the model include:

1. "Educating clients, case managers, other professionals, and the public at large regarding the role and scope of occupational therapy in community mental health
2. Establishing a client referral system
3. Identifying appropriate assessment instruments and completing client evaluation
4. Integrating family caregivers and other key persons controlling community resources in the therapeutic process

5. Implementing individualized interventions as much as possible within the client's natural environment
6. Supporting the client as he or she attempts to reintegrate into the community, for instance by introducing him or her to key individuals within the community."[11, p. 371]

This model provides another effective framework for approaching occupational therapy intervention in the community.

COMMUNITY OCCUPATIONAL THERAPY INTERVENTIONS

The school system is the largest community system that employs occupational therapists and OTAs. According to the 2010 American Occupational Therapy Association Workforce Study, 21.6% of OT practitioners work in school systems.[2] In many schools, OT practitioners primarily address handwriting skills, fine motor skills, attention to task, and sensory integration. However, the school system provides the opportunity for OT practitioners to address a variety of other health care concerns such as mental health issues, social skills, overweight and obesity, and physical activity. With so many OT practitioners working in the school systems, this is an opportunity to embrace the school as a community system and provide services beyond the individualized one-on-one treatment in which the occupational therapist may only be interacting with the child's classroom teacher. The opportunity to address a health concern shared by a large group of students and the opportunity to work within a community system to create effective outcomes is possible in the school community. However, it requires the OT practitioner to use an effective model or framework for implementing a health intervention program that is occupationally based and addresses the social, political, and environmental demands of the community system. The OT practitioner also must be willing and able to communicate effectively with administrators, teachers, parents, and children. Excellent communication and negotiation skills are needed. A variety of service delivery methods may be employed too, such as mentoring, training, educating, and consultation. The OT practitioner may initiate the idea for a service or program that benefits the school system and serve as an organizer or leader in its initiation but not the implementation. Preschools, afterschool programs, and day-care centers can provide these same types of opportunities.

There are other community systems as well that can offer the opportunity for OT practitioners to provide services that are community-built interventions. These may include faith-based programs, community recreational programs, community health clinics, camps, group homes and residential care facilities, and homeless shelters.

With the increase in medical diagnoses such as autism, attention deficit disorder, and a variety of developmental disorders, and the increase in health concerns such as obesity, school violence, and behavioral problems, the need for pediatric services is constantly expanding. Treatment and interventions to address these medical issues and concerns must be provided in community settings as most require long-term attention.

CLINICAL *Pearl*

Volunteering is a good way to introduce yourself to a community setting that does not currently employ OT practitioners. Providing in-services regarding the potential role of occupational therapy in the community setting can increase awareness and facilitate productive relationships with other team members.

CHALLENGES IN PRACTICE IN COMMUNITY SYSTEMS

There are a variety of challenges that exist when working within a community system. The biggest challenge facing occupational therapists may be funding. Although occupational therapy services are required under the Individual with Disabilities Education Act[19] for defined disabilities, these services may not be comprehensive in scope to meet the child's needs or the child may have health-related concerns that do not meet the defined disabilities. OT practitioners wishing to expand services in the school system may face funding and time constraints. OT practitioners working with children in settings other than the school systems may be challenged to receive reimbursement for services from insurance or self-pay mechanisms. Grants and donations may be one source or partnering with community organizations that can absorb the costs of the intervention and provide compensation for therapist time may be a possibility. These options require an investment of time and energy upfront to network and establish working relationships with the community organizations. The ability to define the need for occupational therapy to provide the services and to establish positive working relationships is needed. The use of evidence-based practices and the ability to articulate this to the appropriate individuals within the community systems as well as to the consumer is also needed to work effectively in a variety of community systems and with a variety of community organizations.

Another challenge to working within community systems is the ability to maintain good communication between the practitioner and the child's guardians, caretakers, teachers, other health care providers, and administrative or other support persons within the community system. With multiple people involved in the system at different levels, it can be difficult to maintain effective lines of communication regarding the child's care. Support is generally needed to follow through on the child's plan of care or to reinforce certain behaviors and skills. Without a plan for establishing and maintaining open lines of communication it can be difficult to achieve effective outcomes. Fragmentation of community services can affect communication and outcomes as well by making it more difficult to interact with individuals involved in the child's care.

The **cultural competence** of the therapist may also be a challenge when working within a community system. As we look toward the future, the U.S. Census Bureau[18] projects that by 2043 no single racial group will represent a majority of the population, the United States will become a majority-minority nation with the non-Hispanic white population remaining the largest single race. Minority populations will continue to increase in the United States resulting in an increasing need for culturally competent health care practitioners. One definition of cultural competence comes from the nursing literature and defines cultural competence as a process that requires the health care professional to address five constructs:

1. Cultural awareness: Being respectful and sensitive to the values and beliefs of a client's culture and requires one to be aware of personal prejudices and biases about other cultures.
2. Cultural knowledge: Involves understanding the client's worldview.
3. Cultural encounters: The experience of interacting with clients from culturally diverse backgrounds.
4. Cultural skill: The ability to identify significant cultural data relevant to the client's health status and therapy goals.
5. Cultural desire:[9] The health care practitioner's motivation to be culturally competent and motivated to work through the process.[5] Therapists who are not culturally competent and those who are unwilling to work through the process to develop cultural competence will be challenged to provide effective community services as most communities are culturally diverse.

SUMMARY

The future of occupational therapy is exciting as health care continues to evolve into more diverse settings within the community. OT practitioners are well suited for community practice. Occupational therapy's focus on treating the whole person by addressing the occupational needs of the child as well as consideration of the environmental influences that affect the child's functioning provides for the ability to practice in a variety of settings. OT practitioners have the skills to address the physical,

sensory, behavioral, and psychosocial concerns of the child in the community as health care moves more into this context of service provision.

The need to carefully evaluate the community systems in which the child lives, goes to school, and plays, as well as community systems providing other services or care to the child, continues to be of upmost importance. Community systems and services are constantly changing and there continue to be increasing opportunities for health care services to be provided in different types of community settings. These settings may include schools, preschools, afterschool programs, day-care centers, faith-based programs, community recreational programs, community mental health centers, community health clinics, camps, group homes, residential care facilities, homeless shelters, and home health agencies.

The need for the OT practitioner to continually evaluate and refine interpersonal skills, therapeutic use of self, cultural competence, and other abilities such as program development and consultation is important for successful community practice. The challenges of community practice include funding and reimbursement issues, the challenge of interacting with multiple individuals involved with the child's care, awareness of the different community systems affecting the child's treatment, and addressing cultural influences. As health care opportunities continue to increase in the community environment and more emphasis is placed on evidence-based outcomes and preventive care, occupational therapy will continue to be a vital service for children. Therapists need to be aware of developing opportunities and be on the forefront of providing services to children in a multitude of community settings.

CASE *Study*

Mary is an OTA working in a school system. She is primarily interested in working with children with psychiatric diagnoses. A K-12 school in the district provides services for 125 children with psychiatric and emotional disorders and works with the community mental health center to address these problems. The community mental health center provides psychiatric evaluations and therapy but does not employ an occupational therapist. Currently these students are not receiving occupational therapy. Mary discusses with her supervisor her interest in working with children in this community school setting. At first her supervisor does not support Mary based on her current full-time schedule at other schools within the district. Mary does, however, receive support to meet with the school principal, teachers, and mental health counselors to discuss the possible need for occupational therapy services. Mary reviews data on the student population including diagnoses, academic performance, socioeconomic status, family situation, home environment, and current mental health services provided to these students. She also conducts a literature review of services currently provided in other school districts and networks with other therapists who work with this population to provide current and evidenced-based data regarding the role and efficacy of occupational therapy in this setting. She develops a plan for integrating occupational therapy services into the school setting by offering individualized occupation-based intervention following assessment by one of the district occupational therapists. She requests input from the staff for referrals and screens these children. The school is supportive of occupational therapy involvement and requests services. Mary negotiates with her supervisor to begin with one student at the school and to expand services if successful. Her supervisor agrees with the plan based on the support and request from the school. To expand services within the school district, Mary has successfully promoted occupational therapy and built relationships within the community of the school system in which she is employed.

References

1. American Occupational Therapy Association. (2014). Occupational therapy practice framework: domain and process (3rd ed.). *Am J Occup Ther*, 68(Suppl. 1), S1–S51.
2. American Occupational Therapy Association. (2010). *Your career in occupational therapy: workforce trends in occupational therapy*. http://www.aota.org/-/media/Corporate/Files/EducationCareers/Prospective/Workforce-trends-in-OT.PDF. 2014.08.30.
3. Bruce, B. A., & Borg, B. (2002). *Psychosocial frames of reference: core of occupation-based practice* (3rd ed.). Thorofare, NJ: Slack, Inc.
4. Campbell, K., & Crawford, D. (2001). Family food environments as determinants of preschool-aged children's eating behaviors: implications for obesity prevention policy: a review. *Aust J Nutr Diet*, 58(1), 19–25.
5. Campinha-Bacote, J. (2001). A model of practice to address cultural competence in rehabilitation nursing. *Rehabil Nurs*, 26(1), 8–11.
6. Centers for Disease Control and Prevention. (2014a). *Childhood obesity facts*. http://www.cdc.gov/obesity/data/childhood.html. 2014.08.30.
7. Centers for Disease Control and Prevention. (2014a). *Adult overweight and obesity*. http://www.cdc.gov/obesity/adult/index.html. 2014.08.30.
8. Cole, M. B., & Mclean, V. (2003). Therapeutic relationships re-defined. *Occup Ther Ment Health*, 19(2), 33–56.
9. Green, L. W., & Kreuter, M. W. (2005). *Health program planning: an educational and ecological approach*. New York: McGraw-Hill.
10. Herzberg, G. L. (2004, March). Preparing ourselves for working with communities. *HCHSIS*, 11, 2–4.
11. Ikiugu, M. N. (2007). *Psychosocial conceptual practice models in occupational therapy: building adaptive capability*. St. Louis, MO: Mosby, Inc.
12. McKenzie, J. F., Neiger, B. L., & Smeltzer, J. L. (2005). *Planning, implementing, and evaluating health promotion program: a primer* (4th ed.). San Francisco: Benjamin Cummings.
13. Mosey, A. C. (1996). *Psychosocial components of occupational therapy*. New York: Lippincott, Williams, & Wilkins.
14. Punwar, J., & Peloquin, M. (2000). *Occupational therapy: principles and practice*. Philadelphia: Lippincott.
15. Silverstein, M., Lamberto, J., DePeau, K., & Grossman, D. C. (2008). "You get what you get": Unexpected findings about low-income parents' negative experiences with community resources. *Pediatrics*, 122(6), 1141–1147.
16. Steinbeck, K. S. (2001). The importance of physical activity in the prevention of overweight and obesity in childhood: a review and an opinion. *Obes Rev*, 2, 117–130.
17. Taylor, R. R. (2008). *The intentional relationship: occupational therapy and use of self*. Philadelphia: F. A. Davis.
18. U. S. Census Bureau. (December 12, 2012). *U.S. Census Bureau projections show a slower growing, older, more diverse nation a half century from now*. https://www.census.gov/newsroom/releases/archives/population/cb12-243.html. 2014.08.30.
19. U. S. Department of Education. (n. d.). *Building the legacy: IDEA 2004*. http://idea.ed.gov/. 2014.08.30.
20. U. S. Department of Health and Human Services. (n.d.). *Healthy People 2020*. http://www.healthypeople.gov/2020/about/default.aspx. 2014.08.30.
21. Wittman, P. P., & Velde, B. P. (2001). Occupational therapy in the community: what, why, and how. *Occup Ther Health Care*, 13(3-4), 1–5.
22. World Health Organization. (1948). Preamble to the Constitution of the World Health Organization as adopted by the International Health Conference, New York, 19-22 June, 1946, signed on 22 July 1946 by the representatives of 61 States and entered into force on 7 April 1948. *Official Records of the World Health Organization*, 2, 100.

REVIEW *Questions*

1. What is the difference between a community-based and a community-built practice?
2. Why is it important to understand the community in relation to occupational therapy services for the child?
3. How can adopting a public health approach support OT practitioners in community practice?
4. What are some of the different service delivery methods OT practitioners employ in community settings?
5. What are some of the challenges to providing services in the community?

SUGGESTED *Activities*

1. Interview an OT practitioner working with children in a community setting to understand the effect of the community on the occupational therapy intervention. Identify three examples of how the OT practitioner's understanding of the community supports effective treatment.

2. Conduct a review of pediatric occupational therapy interventions in the occupational therapy literature for the past 5 years and identify the number of interventions that occur in a community setting versus hospital-/clinic-based setting. Identify the types of setting and the service delivery methods used.

3. Identify a community-built approach to addressing a public health need of children that you may treat. Describe where this approach would be implemented, the type of treatment activities involved, and the treatment goals that would be addressed. How would you gain the support of the community in implementing this intervention?

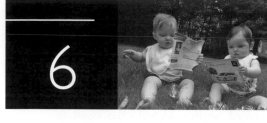

DIANNE KOONTZ LOWMAN
JEAN WELCH SOLOMON

Principles of Normal Development

6

KEY TERMS

Principles of
    development
Context
Normal
Typical
Development
Growth
Periods of development

CHAPTER *Objectives*

After studying this chapter, the reader will be able to accomplish the following:

- Explain the importance of knowing and understanding the characteristics of typical development while working with children and youth.
- Discuss the relationship among typical development, areas of performance, and contexts.
- Define and briefly describe the periods of development.
- Describe the general principles of development.
- Apply the general principles of development to develop intervention for skills acquisition in areas of occupational performance.

CHAPTER *Outline*

General Considerations
  DEFINITIONS OF TERMS
  PREDICTABLE SEQUENCE OF SKILL ACQUISITION
  RELATIONSHIP BETWEEN TYPICAL DEVELOPMENT AND
    CONTEXT

Periods of Development
  GESTATION AND BIRTH
  INFANCY

EARLY CHILDHOOD
MIDDLE CHILDHOOD
ADOLESCENCE

Principles of Normal Development

Summary

Sally is an occupational therapy assistant (OTA) who is employed by the local public school system. She is assigned a new client, a 3-year-old girl named Amy. The supervising occupational therapist began the occupational therapy (OT) evaluation and requested that Sally schedule a visit to assess the child's self-care and play skills to determine whether Amy is functioning at the appropriate age level in these areas. Sally realizes that to accurately assess Amy's skills relative to her chronologic age, she needs to review normal development definitions and principles.

The OT practitioner must understand development and the process of typical development. The sequence of acquisition in relation to occupational performance skills and areas is the foundation for OT assessment of and intervention with children who have special needs. The sequence of skill acquisition is predictable in the typically developing child.[1] The OT practitioner's knowledge of normal development guides the order of expectations and choice of activities for children who are not developing typically. In atypical development, delays in performance skills may make it difficult or impossible for a child to perform activities of daily living (ADLs), engage successfully in play activities, or acquire functional work and productive skills. The OT practitioner identifies the occupational performance skills deficits (e.g., motor and process skills) that interfere with the child's occupational performance. The practitioner relies on knowledge of typical development to assist the child in developing useful, functional skills.

GENERAL CONSIDERATIONS

An OT practitioner who is attempting to grasp the basics of normal development considers general pediatric terms, the predictable sequence of skill acquisition in normal development, the **principles of development,** and the relationship between development and **context**. An understanding of the general terms used by pediatric therapists is necessary for effective communication. The OT practitioner must understand the relationship between typical development and the occupational performance contexts as delineated in the American Occupational Therapy Association's Occupational Therapy Practice Framework: Domain and Process (3rd ed.).[3]

Definitions of Terms

A basic understanding of the terms used by pediatric OT practitioners helps practitioners and other individuals working in the area of pediatrics to communicate effectively. **Normal** is defined as that which

---

> **BOX 6-1**
>
> ## *Definition of Typical Development*
>
> *Typical development* is defined as the natural process of acquiring skills ranging from simple to complex.

occurs habitually or naturally.[2] In this chapter, *normal* is used interchangeably with **typical** in the discussions on development. **Development** is the act or process of maturing or acquiring skills ranging from simple to more complex.[2] **Growth** is the maturation of a person.[2] Because the concepts of development and growth are analogous, these terms are used interchangeably in this chapter (Box 6-1).

Predictable Sequence of Skill Acquisition

The normal development of skills in terms of performance and areas of occupation occurs in a predictable sequence.[1,4,5,7] The OT practitioner uses knowledge of typical development while working with children who have special needs as a way to identify the areas in which there are deficits and to develop a plan to improve their ADLs, play, and academic skills. Although developmental checklists and other tools may help a practitioner identify the presence or absence of certain skills, understanding the process of how and why children are able to develop these skills is more useful in the clinical setting. For example, an OT practitioner may use an observational checklist to determine whether a child can independently finger feed him or herself. A practitioner who has knowledge of normal development and its predictable sequence of events understands that children usually learn to eat with their fingers before learning to eat with a spoon. Therefore, if a child has not begun finger feeding, the practitioner would not introduce spoon feeding (depending on the circumstances). Knowledge and understanding of normal development guide the OT practitioner in the intervention planning process.

Relationship Between Typical Development and Context

OT practitioners need to understand the relationship between typical development and context. Because the events of normal development are sequential and predictable, the chronologic age of the child (i.e., how old the child is) has an effect on the child's level of skill development in performance and areas of occupation.[1,4,5,7] Although practitioners obviously cannot change the age of a child, they can offer age-appropriate

BOX 6-2

Contexts

CULTURAL CONTEXT
Customs, beliefs/values, standards, and expectations

PERSONAL CONTEXT
Features of the person such as age, gender, socioeconomic status, and level of education

PHYSICAL CONTEXT
Nonhuman aspects of the environment

SOCIAL CONTEXT
Significant others and the larger social group

TEMPORAL CONTEXT
Stage of life, time of day, and time of year

VIRTUAL CONTEXT
Computer or airways, simulators, chatrooms, and radio

Adapted from the American Occupational Therapy Association (2014). Occupational therapy practice framework: domain and process (3rd ed.), *Am J Occup Ther,* 68, S1–S50.

activities during intervention sessions. Being familiar with age-appropriate activities helps OT practitioners choose tasks for therapy sessions with children. For example, a practitioner may use colored blocks when performing fine motor and sorting activities with a 3-year-old, but the use of blocks would not be suitable in a session with a 14-year-old. It would be more appropriate to have the adolescent use objects like coins for fine motor and sorting activities.

Although normal development is predictable and sequential, the rate of skill acquisition varies among children. This variability greatly depends on the context and environment (Box 6-2). These contexts include cultural, personal, physical, social, temporal, and virtual aspects.[3]

The cultural environment, which comprises customs, beliefs, activity patterns, and behavior standards, also influences the rate of skill development and performance in areas of occupation.[3] Anticipation of behaviors refers to an individual's expectation of repetition of a daily schedule (e.g., waking up, eating, bathing, and dressing—in that order) or consistency of cause and effect behaviors (e.g., washing the dishes and cleaning the room, which cause the mother to be pleased with the child). An adolescent whose parents believe that only adults should be employed may develop work skills later in life than one whose parents believe that summer and afterschool jobs are appropriate and should be encouraged. In certain cultures,

using eating utensils is not the adult norm. Children in this cultural environment may never learn to use a fork or spoon.

The personal context includes the child's age, gender, socioeconomic status, and educational level.[3] For example, a 2-year-old boy from a rural community will have different goals and enjoy different activities than would a 10-year-old girl from an inner city.

The physical, or nonhuman, aspects of the environment have an effect on the rate of skill acquisition in both performance and areas of occupation.[3] For example, if a child lives in a climate that requires warm clothing, he or she will learn to don and doff a sweater or a coat more quickly than one who lives in a temperate climate. A child who lives in a two-story house will more likely learn to ascend and descend stairs before one who lives in a single-story house.

The social context refers to the availability and anticipation of behaviors by significant others, which influences the rate of skill acquisition in occupations.[3] An infant who is breastfed will not acquire the ability to drink from a bottle or cup as quickly as one who is bottle fed. An infant who is carried frequently may not develop gross motor and mobility skills as quickly as one who is allowed to move around on the floor or in a playpen.

It is important for OT practitioners working with children to understand the temporal context, which refers to the stage of life, time of year, and length of occupation.[3] Adolescents and toddlers have very different goals and experiences. Toddlers experience the "terrible 2s" for a short period (it varies for each child). However, a 5-year-old child should be well past this phase, so the observation of this behavior past the expected duration indicates a cause for concern.

The virtual context includes communication by means of computers and airways.[3] Children use computers, cell phones, and other electronic means to communicate. These virtual environments provide opportunities for children but also must be monitored.

Studying the process of typical development allows practitioners to learn about its predictable sequences and contextual variability. Although this knowledge is important, having the skills to solve problems related to the developmental process is more useful than memorizing the sequences of skill acquisition in performance and areas of occupation. Carefully studying this chapter as well as the next two and participating in the suggested activities will give OT practitioners an excellent basis for using the problem-solving approach in the developmental process. One framework to use when studying development is based on the generally accepted periods of development. Another framework involves understanding the general principles of development. Each will be described in the following sections.

CLINICAL *Pearl*

It is widely accepted in the field of child development that environmental factors may have a significant effect on the development of the baby, toddler, and child.[10] The child who has all his or her needs met in a safe and secure environment is free to actively explore surroundings and learn from these explorations. However, there are environmental factors that may have a potentially adverse effect on the child's development. Potential environmental risk factors may include low socioeconomic status, inadequate parental caregiving, abuse or neglect, poor nutrition, and so on.[10] It is important to note that not all children living in poverty have developmental delays. The presence of protective factors helps families deal adaptively and ward off the possible negative impact; examples of protective factors include social supports and connections to extended supportive family networks. [11]

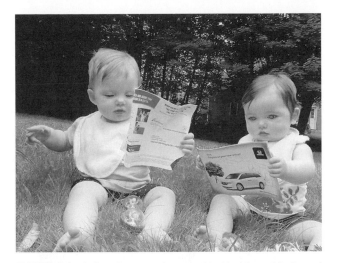

FIGURE 6-1 Infants learn to sit up and hold objects. Madie and Sadie enjoy a day at the park.

BOX 6-3

Periods of Development

GESTATION AND BIRTH
From conception to the moment at which the neonate can survive on its own without placental nutrients

INFANCY
From birth through 18 months of age

EARLY CHILDHOOD
From 18 months through 5 years of age

MIDDLE CHILDHOOD
From 6 years of age until the onset of puberty (12 years of age for girls and 14 years of age for boys)

ADOLESCENCE
From puberty until the onset of adulthood (usually 21 years of age)

PERIODS OF DEVELOPMENT

Periods of development are intervals of time during which a child increases in size and acquires specific skills.[2] Pediatric OT practitioners work with children of varying chronologic ages. The following normal developmental periods are used as the basis for comparison in subsequent chapters dealing with normal development (Box 6-3).

Gestation and Birth

Gestation refers to the developmental period of the fetus, or unborn child, in the mother's uterus. This period begins with conception and ends with birth.[2] The gestational period is also referred to as the prenatal (before birth) period.[2] Gestation typically lasts 40 weeks.[2] The birthing process is also known as the perinatal (around birth) period. This period varies greatly in duration for a variety of reasons, the discussion of which is beyond the scope of this book. The perinatal period ends when the infant is able to independently sustain life without placental nutrients from the mother. The postnatal (after birth) period is the immediate interval of time after birth. During the postnatal period, the infant is known as a neonate, or new baby.[2]

Infancy

Infancy is the period from birth through approximately 18 months of age.[9] It is characterized by significant physical and emotional growth.[9] Typically developing infants grow considerably in height and weight during the first 18 months of life.[9] They develop sensory and motor skills, and by 18 months of age they are walking, talking, and performing simple self-care tasks such as eating with a spoon, drinking from a cup, and undressing (Figure 6-1).

Early Childhood

Toddlers and preschool children represent the period of early childhood, which begins at 18 months of age and lasts through age 5 years.[2,9] During the early childhood period, children become increasingly independent and establish more of a sense of individuality (Figure 6-2).

Middle Childhood

Middle childhood begins at 6 years of age and lasts until puberty, which begins at approximately 12 years

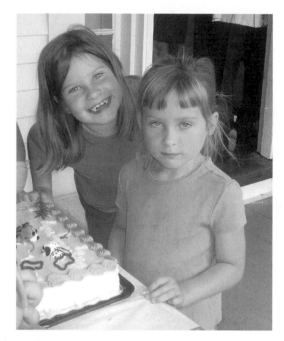

FIGURE 6-2   Children in early childhood establish a sense of individuality. Molly enjoys her birthday cake with friends.

of age in girls and 14 years of age in boys.[9] Children in this developmental period spend the majority of their time in educational settings; therefore, the major influence on the child shifts from parents to peers (Figures 6-3).

Adolescence

Adolescence is the period of physical and psychological development that accompanies the onset of puberty. Puberty is a stage of maturation in which a person becomes physiologically capable of reproduction. This period is marked by hormonal changes and their resulting challenges.[2] Adolescence ends with the onset of adulthood (usually 21 years of age), when individuals begin to function independent of their parents.[2]

OT practitioners use the periods of development as reference points when working with children who have special needs. Knowledge of the sequence of development within each period is used as a guide for the OT process. Practitioners need to know the general principles of development to understand the reasons children gain skills predictably and sequentially (Figure 6-4).

PRINCIPLES OF NORMAL DEVELOPMENT

The general principles of development are widely accepted in the various pediatric disciplines (Box 6-4). The following principles are tools used by OT practitioners to solve problems related to the acquisition of skills.

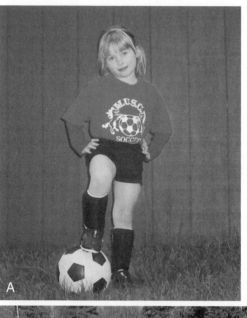

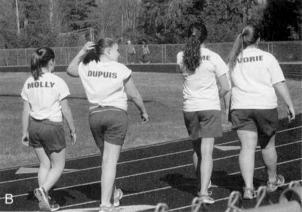

FIGURE 6-3   Middle childhood refers to ages 6 to 12 years. **A.** Children refine motor skills (such as those needed for soccer) during middle childhood. **B.** Children participate in team activities involving rules and competition.

- Normal development is sequential and predictable. The rate (speed) and direction (vertical or horizontal) of development vary among children, but the sequence remains the same.[1,4,5,7,8] For example, infants who are typically developing acquire head before trunk control (an example of vertical development). Head and trunk control are necessary for them to sit independently. Infants learn to roll, then sit, then creep, and finally walk. Although most developmental theorists agree that the sequence is the same for all children, recent research in motor control theory demonstrates that motor development does not always follow a set sequence.[1] In either case, each child acquires these skills at a unique rate.
- Maturation and experience affect a child's development.[4-8] Maturation and experience influence the rate and direction of normal development.

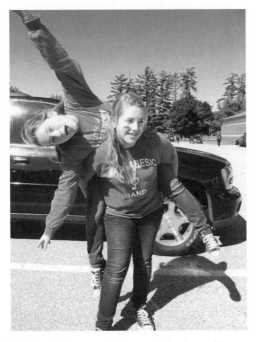

FIGURE 6-4 Adolescents enjoy socialization with peers and function independently from their parents. Teens frequently act silly with each other and dress alike.

BOX 6-4

General Principles of Development

- Development is sequential and predictable.
- Maturation and experience affect development.
- Development involves changes in the biologic, psychological, and social systems.
- Development occurs in two directions: horizontal and vertical.
- Development progresses in order in three basic sequences.
  1. Cephalad to caudal
  2. Proximal to distal
  3. Gross to fine

Maturation is the innate (natural) process of growth and development, and experience is the result of interactions with the environment.[2] In addition, current research on motor control introduces the concepts of arousal states and motivation as additional factors that have an effect on motor learning. The child must be aroused in order to be motivated to move and interact with the environment.[1] Although most developmental theorists agree that maturation, experience, arousal state, and motivation have an effect on a child's development, their opinions vary about which one is the more significant.

- Throughout the course of normal development, changes occur in the biologic, psychological, and social systems.[5] Therefore, development is a dynamic and continuously changing process. Changes in the biologic system include those related to the functions and processes of internal structures.[6,9] Changes in the psychological system affect the emotional and behavioral characteristics of the individual.[9] Changes in the social system include those that affect individuals in their immediate environment and society as a whole.[5,6,9] These changes occur in all three systems throughout the course of typical development. A change in one system influences the other two.

- Development progresses in two directions: vertical and horizontal.[5,8] As children progress through the various developmental levels related to the specific performance skills or areas of occupation, they are progressing vertically. For example, in the occupational area of ADLs, children learn to eat with their fingers before they learn to eat with a spoon. As children learn to roll, then crawl, and finally walk, they are progressing vertically in gross motor performance skills. In both examples, development is occurring in a vertical direction within a specific performance skill or area of occupation. Development that involves different performance skills and areas of occupation indicates horizontal progression. A child who is simultaneously learning to finger feed, use a pincer grasp, and creep is progressing horizontally because several different performance skills and areas (i.e., ADLs, fine motor skills, and gross motor skills) are involved.

Motor development follows three basic rules:

1. Development progresses cephalad to caudal, or head to tail.[5] For example, a baby is first able to control head and neck movements (beginning at around 2 months), then the arms and hands (grasping begins at about 3 months), then the trunk (most babies sit well by 8 months), and finally the legs and feet (most children walk by 14–15 months).

2. Development progresses in a proximal to distal direction, which means that children develop control of structures close to their body (such as the shoulder) before they develop those farther away from their body (such as the hand).[4] For example, a baby can swat at an object by 3 to 4 months but cannot reach straight ahead and grasp an object in the fingers until around 8 months.

3. Development progresses from gross control to fine control, which means that children gain control of large body movements before they can perform more refined movements.[4] For example, children are able to catch a large ball using both arms and the body before they learn to catch a tennis ball with one hand. They use the larger arm muscles to catch a large 8-inch ball

and the smaller wrist and hand muscles to catch a tennis ball.

These general principles of development provide a framework for OT practitioners to use when solving developmental problems. The principles can be used to guide the intervention planning process when working with children who have special needs.

SUMMARY

Normal development is sequential and predictable. OT practitioners rely on their knowledge and understanding of typical development when working with children with special needs. Practitioners also must consider the relationship between normal development and contexts.

The periods and general principles of development help provide a framework for organizing and understanding information related to typical development. The periods include gestation and birth, infancy, early childhood, middle childhood, and adolescence. The general principles of development are widely used in the various pediatric disciplines and help OT practitioners plan evaluations and interventions when working with children who have special needs.

References

1. Alexander, R., Boehme, R., & Cupps, B. (1993). *Normal development of functional motor skills.* Tucson, AZ: Therapy Skill Builders.
2. *American heritage dictionary of the English language* (5th ed.) (2011). Boston, MA: Houghton Mifflin.
3. American Occupational Therapy Association. (2014). Occupational therapy practice framework: domain and process (3rd ed.). *Am J Occup Ther*, 68(Suppl. 1), S1–S48.
4. Boehme, R. (1988). *Improving upper body control: an approach to assessment and treatment of tonal dysfunction.* Tucson, AZ: Therapy Skill Builders.
5. Case-Smith, J., & O'Brien, J. (2015). *Occupational therapy for children* (7th ed.). St. Louis, MO: Elsevier.
6. Kielhofner, G. (2009). *Conceptual foundations of occupational therapy* (4th ed.). Philadelphia, PA: FA Davis.
7. Kramer, P., & Hinojosa, J. (2009). *Frames of reference for pediatric occupational therapy* (3rd ed.). Philadelphia, PA: Lippincott Williams & Wilkins.
8. Llorens, L. A. (1976). *Application of a developmental theory for health and rehabilitation.* Rockville, MD: American Occupational Therapy Association.
9. Meyer, W. J. (1997). *Infancy, Microsoft Encarta 98 encyclopedia.* Redmond, WA: Microsoft.
10. Shonkoff, J. P., & Phillips, D. P. (2000). *From neurons to neighborhoods: the science of early childhood development.* Washington, DC: National Academy Press.
11. Epps, S., & Jackson, B. J. (2000). *Empowered families, successful children: early intervention programs that work.* Washington, DC: American Psychological Association.

REVIEW *Questions*

1. Explain the following terms: *normal, typical, development,* and *growth*.
2. List and describe the periods of development.
3. List and describe the general principles of development.
4. Define *context*.
5. Describe how contexts have an effect on intervention.
6. How would you use the principles of development to intervene?

SUGGESTED *Activities*

1. Visit a day-care center or playground to observe children playing. Note the variety of approaches that are used by different children to accomplish the same task.
2. In small study groups, discuss the general principles of development, and then describe these principles in your own words. Give examples of these principles in relation to your own development.
3. In small study groups, describe your cultural background and how it influences your goals and the occupations that you perform. How would it influence the intervention of a child?
4. Provide examples of how contexts (cultural, personal, physical, social, temporal, and virtual) influence development. Discuss the techniques practitioners could use to address each context.
5. Describe the main milestones for each period of development.

DIANNE KOONTZ LOWMAN
JANE CLIFFORD O'BRIEN

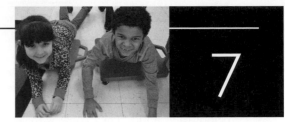

Development of Performance Skills

CHAPTER *Objectives*

After studying this chapter, the reader will be able to accomplish the following:

- Define performance skills.
- Provide examples of the specific performance skills required for a variety of childhood occupations.
- Describe significant physiologic changes that occur at each stage of development.
- Identify the sequences of motor skill development (gross and fine motor).
- Outline the stages of process development (cognitive) as defined by Piaget's theory.
- Describe the developmental changes for each phase of social interaction skills (psychosocial development) using the theories of Erikson and Greenspan.
- Analyze the performance skills children and youth use to engage in their desired occupations.

CHAPTER *Outline*

Children's development progresses in a predictable pattern, with easier skills developing before complex skills. For example, children sit up before they stand. They chew with whole wide movements before chewing using rotational patterns. They use one-word sentences before making up stories. The rate of development varies, but understanding the overall progression of performance skills allows practitioners to anticipate the next steps in an intervention plan. OT practitioners use knowledge of development to create goals and objectives that are attainable, logical, and within the child's reach. Goals are created from a careful analysis of performance skills.

According to AOTA practice framework, **performance skills** refer to **motor skills (gross** and **fine motor skills)**, **process skills** (cognition), and **social interaction skills** (communication and psychosocial) (Box 7-1).[2] Performance skills are "goal-directed actions that are observable as small units of engagement in daily life occupations." [2, p. S7] Deficits in any of these skills may interfere with the child's performance in the areas of self-care, play, education, and social participation. For example, a child must *stabilize* and *align* his or her body to engage in feeding. Stabilizing and aligning the body are motor performance skills. The child assigns taste to the food and decides food preferences, which is an example of process skills. Finally, the child may request additional food, express pleasure, or engage in light conversation while eating, all examples of social interaction skills. Occupations are made up of a variety of performance skills that interact with each other. OT practitioners often target performance skills as a way to enable children to engage in occupations.

A definition and review of performance skills are provided. The authors describe typical developmental sequences to assist occupational therapy (OT) practitioners in identifying potential deficits or delays in performance skills. Case examples are provided throughout to illustrate the concepts for practice.

PERFORMANCE SKILLS

As children and youth complete daily occupations, they perform motor skills (such as gripping, moving, lifting); they choose between objects, initiate activity, and sequence (process skills); and they interact with others, communicate, and respond in a timely manner (social interaction skills). OT practitioners examine performance skills required to complete occupations and develop interventions to enable performance. Performance skills are observable actions.[2] Because they are observable actions and many performance skills are required to complete an occupation, the OT practitioner may target performance skills during intervention. Performance skills are categorized into motor, process, and social interaction skills.

Motor Skills

Motor skills are observable actions observed as the child interacts and moves objects and self in the environment.[2] Motor skills involve gross and fine motor actions, including the following: aligns, stabilizes, positions, reaches, bends, grips, manipulates, coordinates, moves, lifts, walks, transports, calibrates, flows (uses smooth and coordinated movements), endures, and paces.[2] This list is not all inclusive. OT practitioners prioritize key performance skills to address during intervention.

For example, a child playing on the playground may use the following motor performance skills:

- *Stabilizes* his body to move.
- *Walks* toward a variety of equipment, or *runs* to play a game.
- *Endures* 1 hour of physical activity outside.
- *Coordinates* both sides of his body to pump swing.
- *Grips* the ropes on the swing.
- *Bends* to tie his shoes.

Along with motor skills, the child makes decisions and plans movement, referred to as process skills.

BOX 7-1

Performance Skills

MOTOR SKILLS

Motor skills are those involved in moving and interacting with objects or the environment and include posture, mobility, coordination, strength, effort, and energy. Examples of motor skills include stabilizing the body and manipulating objects.

PROCESS SKILLS (COGNITION)

Process skills are those used in completing daily tasks and include energy, knowledge, temporal organization, organizing space and objects, and adaptation. Examples of process skills include maintaining attention to a task, choosing appropriate tools and materials for the task, and accommodating the method of task completion in response to a problem.

SOCIAL INTERACTION SKILLS

Social interaction skills refer to those needed to interact with other people and include physicality, information exchange, and relations. Examples of communication and interaction skills include gesturing to indicate intention, expressing affect, and relating in a manner that establishes rapport with others.

Adapted from the American Occupational Therapy Association (2014). Occupational therapy practice framework: Domain and process (3rd. ed.). *Am J Occup Ther, 68*(Suppl.1), S1–S48.

Process Skills

Children plan, make decisions, and problem solve during everyday occupations. They use these cognitive process skills to adjust and adapt to changes in the environment, physical self, or social situations while engaging in ADLs, IADLs, play (leisure), education, or work. The observable actions that constitute process skills include the following: paces, attends, heeds, chooses, uses, handles, inquires, initiates, continues, sequences, terminates, searches/locates, gathers, organizes, restores, navigates, notices/responds, adjusts, accommodates, and benefits.[2]

For example, a child on the playground playing a game of tag engages in the following process skills:

- *Paces* himself so he can complete the entire game.
- *Chooses* who he wants to run after to tag.
- *Initiates* play with his peers.
- *Continues* to run when not tagged.
- *Terminates* the activity (running) when he is tagged.
- *Searches* for other friends in the game.
- *Adjusts* his activity by going to a new location.
- *Navigates* his body around obstacles and peers.
- *Benefits* (prevents problems) by slowing down to get tagged.

While the child is clearly engaged in a motor skill, he is also processing a variety of information from the environment and making decisions to continue in the play. These process skills provide the foundation for many occupations. For example, brushing one's teeth requires a child determine how to use a tool (toothbrush) correctly, initiate the movement, sequence (add toothpaste, run water, brush), gather materials, and terminate the actions once completed. Social interactions add to the complexity of performing motor or process skills. For example, a child who is playing catch outside with his brother must adjust his body in terms of the speed and distance of the ball and position himself to catch it. The processing, motor, and social interaction skills become more complex if the child is engaging in a game of baseball on the playground at school.

Social Interaction Skills

Social interaction skills refer to those actions involved with engaging in activities with another person. Communication and language skills are considered part of social interaction skills. Social interaction skills include the following observable actions: approaches/starts, concludes/disengages, produces speech, gesticulates (uses socially appropriate gestures), speaks fluently, turns toward, looks, places self, touches, regulates, questions, replies, discloses, expresses emotion, disagrees, thanks, transitions, times response, times duration, matches language, clarifies, acknowledges and encourages, empathizes, heeds, accommodates, and benefits.[2]

Children develop and use social interaction skills to engage in a variety of occupations. For example, a child in the classroom may use social interaction skills in the following ways:

- *Approaches* the teacher in the morning to say hello.
- *Concludes* discussion with peer when class starts.
- *Produces speech* to answer a question in front of class.
- *Turns* to the child speaking when he hears his name.
- *Looks* at classmate (social partner) when engaged in conversation.
- *Regulates* responses to teacher's questions.
- *Disagrees* with classmate in appropriate manner.
- *Clarifies* homework assignment.
- *Thanks* teacher for helping him.
- *Transitions* to and from recess without becoming upset.

Children who have difficulty with social interaction skills may not read others' cues, leading to difficulties in social settings. They may perform better in smaller groups or with familiar people. Understanding the behavioral rules may help. OT practitioners may engage children in role-playing activities to help children develop social interaction skills.

Understanding the developmental progression of performance skills provides OT practitioners with a foundation to analyze occupations and design interventions. Practitioners use knowledge of developmental progression of skills as a guideline to determine the "next steps" while acknowledging that children may progress at different rates and that some variability exists in sequences.

INFANCY

Phillip is an active and happy 1-year-old. It is his first birthday party, and he is busy experimenting with and figuring out his new toys (process skills). As family and friends watch, he sits on his push toy and makes it move across the kitchen floor, propelling with his feet and steering with his hands (motor skills). When his older siblings offer help, he pushes them away and says, "No, mine" (social interaction skills). It is not uncommon for children this age to prefer to play alone.

When examining performance skills required for occupations, OT practitioners consider the child's developmental age. The following sections describe characteristics of each stage of development.

Physiologic Development

The average birth weight of an infant is 7 pounds, 2 ounces; the average length is between 19 and 22 inches. The newborn appearance is characterized by a covering comprising a layer of fluid called *vernix caseosa*; a large, bumpy head; a flat, "board" nose; reddish skin; puffy eyes; external breasts; and fine hair called *lanugo* covering the body.[10] At 1 minute after birth, the newborn's physiologic status is tested using the **Apgar scoring** system, which rates each of the following five areas on a scale of 0 to 2: color, heart rate, reflex irritability, muscle tone, and respiratory effort. The scores are computed at 1 and 5 minutes after birth. The closer the total score (sum of scores for the five areas) is to 10, the better is the condition of the newborn; scores of 6 or less indicate the need for intervention.[9]

The infant's first 3 months of life are characterized by constant physiologic adaptations. Structural changes in the newborn's cardiopulmonary system include the expansion of the lungs and increased efficiency of blood flow to the heart. The developing central nervous system (CNS) participates in the body's regulation of sleep, digestion, and temperature.[8]

Physical growth is dramatic—from birth to 6 months of age, infants experience a more rapid rate of growth than at any other time, except during gestation.[15] During the first year, infants triple their body weight, and their height increases by 10 to 12 inches. Their body shape changes, and by 4 months the size of their heads and bodies are more proportionate. By 12 months, average infants weigh 21 to 22 pounds and are 29 to 30 inches tall. During the second year of life, physical growth slows. By 24 months, an average toddler weighs about 27 pounds and is 34 inches tall. The posture of toddlers is characterized by *lordosis* (forward curvature of the spine) and a protruding abdomen, which toddlers retain well into the third year.[29]

Sleep Patterns

Six behavioral states can be observed in the newborn: deep sleep; light sleep; drowsy or semi-dozing; alert, actively awake; fussy; and crying.[7] At 4 months, sleep patterns begin to be regulated, and some infants may sleep through the night. By 8 months, the average infant sleeps 12 to 13 hours per day, but the range can vary from 9 to 18 hours per day. Toddlers typically nap during the day (up to 2 to 4 hours). Toddlers and young children require 10 to 12 hours of sleep per night, whereas adolescents require 8 to 10 hours.

Motor Skills

Motor skills develop as infants experience the environment and explore. Exploration begins as the sensory systems develop. For example, an infant moves her hand and processes this sensation. Practicing this skill and sensation leads to further movement and additional exploration. Infants and toddlers repeat movements as they develop new skills; this is often referred to as mastery.

As they gain skill, earlier movements become automatic, and they are able to refine their skills. Refining skills allows them to perform in a variety of conditions and to make subtle adjustments, which improves the quality of movement. This stage is referred to as achievement.

Sensory Skills

Newborns have vision at birth and can see objects best from about 8 inches away, which is the typical distance between the caregiver's face and the infant's.[25] By the first month of life, an infant shows a preference for patterns and can distinguish between colors. By 3 months, visual acuity develops enough to allow distinction between a picture of a face and a real face.[8] By 12 months, the infant's visual acuity is about 20/100 to 20/50.[20]

Hearing is well developed in newborns and continues to improve as they grow. They tend to respond strongly to the mother's voice.[21] During the first 2 months, infants respond to sound with random body movements. At 3 months, they move their eyes in the direction of sound.[8] At 6 months, they localize sounds to the left and right.[6]

At birth, newborns are able to taste sweet, sour, and bitter substances. Between birth and 3 months, infants are able to differentiate between pleasant and noxious odors. They are very sensitive to touch, cold and heat, pain, and pressure; one of the most important stimuli for infants from birth to 3 months is skin contact and warmth.[23] Holding and swaddling the infant provides skin contact and maintains the infant's body temperature.[10]

Gross Motor Skills

The newborn's body is characterized by physiologic flexion, a position of extremity and trunk flexion.[6] Flexion keeps the infant in a compact position and provides a base of stability for random movements to occur. These movements are characterized by a motion called *random burst*, in which everything moves as a unit.[1] The newborn has numerous **primitive reflexes,** which are genetically transmitted survival mechanisms. These automatic responses to stimuli help the newborn adapt to the environment. Lower levels of the CNS control primitive reflexes. As higher levels of the CNS mature, higher systems inhibit the expression of primitive reflexes. As infants learn about the environment, primitive reflexes are integrated into their overall postural mechanism, with the more mature righting and equilibrium responses that dominate their movements.[30] Under stress, these reflexes may be partially present, but they are never obligatory in normal development. Some primitive reflexes are present at birth, whereas others emerge later in the infant's development (Table 7-1).

As shown in Table 7-2, infants' gross motor skills become gradually more complex as they develop.[1,6,10] Infants begin to combine basic reflexive movements with higher cognitive and physiologic functioning to control

TABLE 7-1

Reflexes and Reactions

REFLEX OR REACTION	POSITION (P) / STIMULUS (S)	POSITIVE RESPONSE	AGE SPAN: AGE OF ONSET OR INTEGRATION	LACK OF INTEGRATION OR ONSET
Rooting	P: Supine S: Light touch on side of face near mouth	Opens mouth and turns head in direction of touch	Birth to 3 mo	Interferes with exploration of objects and head control
Sucking/swallowing	P: Supine S: Light touch on oral cavity	Closes mouth, sucks, and swallows	Birth to 2-5 mo	Interferes with development of coordination of sucking, swallowing, and breathing
Moro's	P: Supine, head at midline S: Dropping head, more than 30 degrees extended	Arms extend and hands open; then arms flex and hands close; infant usually cries	Birth to 4-6 mo	Interferes with head control, sitting equilibrium, and protective reactions
Palmar grasp	P: Supine S: Pressure on ulnar surface of palm	Fingers flex	Birth to 4-6 mo	Interferes with releasing objects
Plantar grasp	P: Supine S: Firm pressure on ball of foot	Toes grasp (flexion)	Birth to 4-9 mo	Interferes with putting on shoes because of toe clawing, gait, and standing and walking problems (e.g., walking on toes)
Neonatal positive support—primary standing	P: Upright S: Being bounced several times on soles of feet (proprioceptive stimulus)	LE extensor tone increases, and plantar flexion is present Some hip and knee flexion or genu recurvatum (hyperextension of the knee) may occur	Birth to 1-2 mo	Interferes with walking patterns and leads to walking on toes
ATNR	P: Supine, arms and legs extended, head in midposition S: Head turned to one side	Arm and leg on face side extend; arm and leg on skull side flex (or experience increased flexor tone)	Birth to 4-6 mo	Interferes with reaching and grasping, bilateral hand use, and rolling
STNR	P: Quadruped position or over tester's knees S: 1. Flexed head 2. Extended head	1. Arms flex and legs extend (tone increases) 2. Arms extend and legs flex (tone increases)	Birth to 4-6 mo	Interferes with reciprocal crawling (children "bunny hop" or move arms and then legs in quadruped position) and walking
TLR	P: 1. Supine, head in midposition, arms and legs extended 2. Prone S: Position (laying on floor); being moved into flexion or extension	1. Extensor tone of neck UE, and LE increases when moved into flexion 2. Flexor tone of neck UE, and LE increases when moved into extension	Birth to 4-6 mo	Interferes with turning on side, rolling over, going from lying to sitting position, and crawling; in older children, interferes with ability to "hold in supine flexion" or assume a pivot prone position
Landau	P: Prone, held in space (suspension) supporting thorax S: Suspension (usually), also active or passive dorsiflexion of head	Hips and legs extend; UE extends and abducts. Elbows can flex (typically used to determine overall development)	3-4 mo to 12-24 mo	Slows development of prone extension, sitting, and standing Early onset (1 mo); may indicate excessive tone or spasticity

Continued

TABLE 7-1

Reflexes and Reactions—cont'd

REFLEX OR REACTION	POSITION (P) STIMULUS (S)	POSITIVE RESPONSE	AGE SPAN: AGE OF ONSET OR INTEGRATION	LACK OF INTEGRATION OR ONSET
Protective extension UE—Parachute, downward forward, sideways, backward	P: Prone, head in midposition, arms extend above S: Suspension by ankles and pelvis and sudden movement of head toward floor P: Seated S: Child pushed: 1. Forward 2. Left, right 3. Backward	Shoulders flex and elbow and wrist extend (arms extend forward) to protect head; infant catches self in directions pushed: 1. Shoulder flexes and abducts; elbow and wrist extend (arms extend forward) 2. Shoulder abducts, elbow and wrist extend (arms extend to side) 3. Shoulders, elbows, and wrists extend (arms extend backward) to protect head	6-9 mo continues through life	Interferes with head protection when center of gravity displaced
Stagger LE—Forward, backward, sideways	P: Standing upright S: Displacement of body by pushing on shoulders and upper trunk: 1. Forward 2. Backward 3. Sideways	Infant takes ≥1 steps in direction of displacement. UEs often also have a protective reaction, with elbow, wrist, and fingers extending: 1. Shoulder flexes 2. Shoulder abducts and extends 3. Shoulder abducts	15-18 mo, continues throughout life	Interferes with ability to catch self when center of gravity displaced, causes trips and falls
Equilibrium—sitting	P: Seated, extremities relaxed S: Hand pulled to one side or shoulder pushed	*Head righting: non–weight-bearing side*—trunk flexes; UE and LE abduct and internally rotate; and elbow, wrist, and fingers extend *Head righting: weight-bearing side*—trunk elongates; UE and LE externally rotate; and elbow, wrist, and fingers abduct and extend.	7-8 mo, continues throughout life	Interferes with ability to sit or maintain balance when reaching for objects or displacing center of gravity
Standing	P: Standing upright, extremities relaxed S: Body displaced by holding UE and pulling to side	*Head righting: non–weight-bearing side*—trunk flexes; UE and LE abduct and internally rotate; and elbow, wrist, and fingers extend. *Head righting: weight-bearing side*—trunk elongates; UE and LE externally rotate; and elbow, wrist, and fingers extend and abduct	12-21 mo, continues throughout life	Interferes with ability to stand and walk and make transitional movements
Equilibrium or tilting—prone, supine	P: Prone or supine on a tilt board, extremities extended S: Board tilted to left or right	*Head righting: non–weight-bearing side*—trunk flexes; UE and LE abduct; and elbow, wrist, hip, and knee externally rotate and extend *Head righting: weight-bearing side*—UE and LE internally rotate and abduct and elbow, wrist, fingers, knee, and hip extend	5-6 mo, continues throughout life	Interferes with ability to make transitional movements, sit, and creep

Adapted from Alexander, R., Boehme, R., & Cupps B. (1993). *Normal development of functional motor skills.* Tucson, AZ: Therapy Skill Builders; Bly L. (1994). *Motor skills acquisition in the first year: an illustrated guide to normal development.* Tucson, AZ: Therapy Skill Builders; Fiorentino M.R. (1981). *Reflex testing methods for evaluating CNS development* (2nd ed.), Springfield, IL: Charles C Thomas Publisher, Ltd.
ATNR, Asymmetric tonic neck reflex; LE, lower extremity; STNR, symmetric tonic neck reflex; TLR, tonic labyrinthine reflex; UE, upper extremity

TABLE 7-2

Normal Development of Sensorimotor Skills

AGE	GROSS MOTOR COORDINATION	FINE MOTOR COORDINATION
Birth or 37-40 wk of gestation	Is dominated by physiologic flexion Moves entire body into extension Turns head side to side (protective response) Keeps head mostly to side while in supine position	Visually regards objects and people Tends to fist and flex hands across chest during feeding Displays strong grasp reflex but has no voluntary grasping abilities Has no voluntary release abilities
1-2 mo	Appears hypertonic as physiologic flexion Practices extension and flexion Continues to gain control of head Moves elbows forward toward shoulders while in prone position Has ATNR with head to side while in supine position When held in standing position, bears some weight on legs	Displays diminishing grasp reflex Involuntarily releases after holding them briefly has no voluntary release abilities
3-5 mo	Experiences fading of ATNR and grasp reflex Has more balance between extension and flexion positions Has good head control (centered and upright) Supports self on extended arms while in prone position props self on forearms Brings hand to feet and feet to mouth while in supine position Props on arms with little support while seated Rolls from supine to prone position Bears some weight on legs when held proximally	Constantly brings hands to mouth Develops tactile awareness in hands Reaches more accurately usually with both hands Palmar grasp Begins transferring objects from hand to hand Does not have control of releasing objects may use mouth to assist
6 mo	Has complete head control Possesses equilibrium reactions Begins assuming quadruped position Rolls from prone to supine position Bounces while standing	Transfers objects from hand to hand while in supine position Shifts weight and reaches with one hand while in prone position Reaches with one hand and supports self with other while seated Reaches to be picked up Uses radial palmar grasp; begins to use thumb while grasping Shows visual interest in small objects rakes small objects Begins to hold objects in one hand
7-9 mo	Shifts weight and reaches while in quadruped position Creeps Develops extension, flexion, and rotation movements, and increases number of activities that can be accomplished while seated May pull to standing position while holding on to support	Reaches with supination Uses index finger to poke objects Uses inferior scissors grasp to pick up small objects Use radial digital grasp to pick up cube Displays voluntary releases abilities
10-12 mo	Displays good coordination while creeping Pulls to standing position using legs only Cruises holding on to support with one hand Stands independently Begins to walk independently Displays equilibrium reactions while standing	Uses superior pincer grasp with fingertip and thumb Uses 3-jaw chuck grasp Displays controlled release into large containers
13-18 mo	Walks alone Seldom falls Begins to go up and down stairs	Displays more precise grasping abilities Precisely releases objects into small containers

Continued

TABLE 7-2

Normal Development of Sensorimotor Skills—cont'd

AGE	GROSS MOTOR COORDINATION	FINE MOTOR COORDINATION
19-24 mo	Displays equilibrium reactions while walking Runs using a more narrow base support	Uses finger to palm translation of small objects
24-36 mo	Jumps in place*	Uses palm to finger and finger to palm translation of small objects Displays complex rotation of small objects Shifts small objects using palmar stabilization Scribbles Snips with scissors

Adapted from Alexander, R., Boehme, R., & Cupps B. (1993). *Normal development of functional motor skills.* Tucson, AZ: Therapy Skill Builders; Clark GF. (1993). Oral-motor and feeding issues. In C.B. Royeen (Ed.), *AOTA self-study series: classroom applications for school-based practice.* Rockville, MD: American Occupational Therapy Association; Erhardt R.P. (1994). *Developmental hand dysfunction: theory, assessment, and treatment* (2nd ed.). Tucson, AZ: Therapy Skill Builders.
ATNR, Asymmetric tonic neck reflex
*From this point on, skills learned during the first 24 months are further refined.

BOX 7-2

Development of Coordinated Movement in Infancy

EXTENSION → FLEXION → LATERAL FLEXION → ROTATION

PRIMITIVE REFLEXES

Primitive reflexes are automatic movements that are usually stimulated by sensory factors and performed without conscious volition. Primitive reflexes cause the first involuntary movements to occur and allow for extension movements to emerge. Primitive reflexes are controlled at the lower levels of the central nervous system. As the higher levels (cerebral hemispheres) mature, the expression of primitive reflexes is inhibited by these higher levels (i.e., they seem to disappear).

RIGHTING REACTIONS

Righting reactions are postural responses to changes of head and body positions. Righting reactions bring the head and trunk back into an upright position. These reactions involve movements called *extension, flexion, abduction, adduction,* and *lateral flexion.*

EQUILIBRIUM REACTIONS

Equilibrium reactions are automatic, compensatory movements of the body parts that are used to maintain the center of gravity over the base of support when either the center of gravity or the supporting surface is displaced. These complex postural responses combine righting reactions with movements known as rotational and diagonal patterns. Essential for volitional movement and mobility, the use of righting reactions begins at 6 months and continues throughout life.

PROTECTIVE EXTENSION RESPONSES

Protective extension responses are postural reactions that are used to stop a fall or to prevent injury when equilibrium reactions fail to do so. These responses involve straightening of the arms or legs toward a supporting surface. Essential for mobility, the use of protective extension reactions begins between 6 and 9 months and continues throughout life.

Adapted from Alexander, R., Boehme, R., & Cupps B. (1993). *Normal development of functional motor skills.* Tucson, AZ: Therapy Skill Builders; Bly L. (1994). *Motor skills acquisition in the first year: an illustrated guide to normal development.* Tucson, AZ: Therapy Skill Builders.

these movements in the environment (Box 7-2). Between birth and 2 months, infants can turn their heads from side to side while in prone and supine positions. As physiologic flexion diminishes, they appear more hypotonic (have less muscular and postural tone), and the movements of each side of their body appear asymmetric. The asymmetric tonic neck reflex holds infants' heads to one side. By 4 months, they can raise and rotate their heads to look at their surroundings. In the supine position (on the back), 4-month-old infants begin to bring their hands to their knees and can deliberately roll from the supine position to the side. The increased head and trunk control observed

at this age is the result of emerging **righting reactions** and better postural control (see Box 7-2). At 5 months, when pulled to a sitting position, infants can bring their heads forward without lagging. By 6 months, they can shift their weight to free extremities to reach for objects while in the prone position (on the stomach). In the supine position, 6-month-old infants can bring their feet to their mouths and are able to sit by themselves for short periods. At 7 to 8 months, they are able to push themselves from the prone position to the sitting position, roll over at will, and crawl on their stomachs. Between 6 and 9 months, infants develop upper extremity **protective extension** reactions

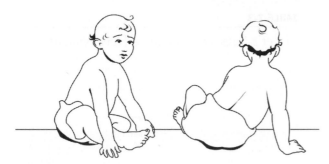

FIGURE 7-1 Equilibrium reactions allow infants to protect themselves by automatically moving forward and sideways after losing balance in the sitting position or when moving from one position to another.

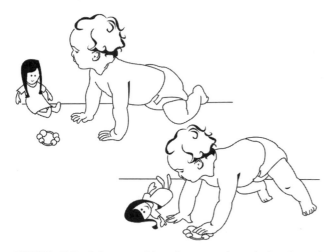

FIGURE 7-2 Infant transition from quadruped (hands and knees) position to vaulting position.

that allow them to catch themselves when pushed off balance (Figure 7-1). From 7 to 21 months, they develop **equilibrium reactions** that allow them to maintain their center of gravity over their base of support; these reactions are critical for transitional movement patterns (i.e., movements from one position to another) and ambulation (see Box 7-2 and Figure 7-2). At 10 to 11 months, infants practice and enjoy creeping. By 12 months, they learn to shift their weight and step to one side by cruising around furniture. At 13 or 14 months most infants take their first steps, and between 12 and 18 months they spend much of their time practicing motor skills by walking, jumping, running, and kicking. Mobility changes infants' perceptions of their environment. A chair is a one-dimensional object in the eyes of a 6-month-old; it is only when the toddler can climb over, under, and around the chair that he or she discovers that a chair is a three-dimensional object.[20]

Fine Motor Skills
Between birth and 3 months, infants interact with the environment through visual inspection. The grasp reflex allows the infant to have contact with objects placed in the hand.

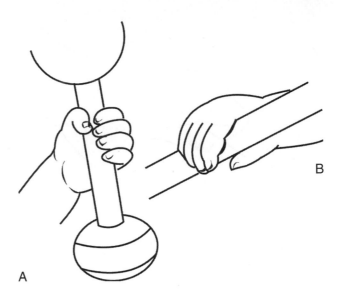

FIGURE 7-3 **A,** When using the ulnar palmar grasp, the infant places his or her fingers on the top surface of the object, pressing it into the center of the palm toward the little finger. **B,** When using the radial palmar grasp, the infant holds the object between the thumb and the radial side of the palm.

At 4 months, the infant demonstrates visually directed reaching skills. At 5 months, the infant uses an ulnar-palmar grasp. The child's fingers are placed on the top surface of an object. The fingers then press the object into the center of the palm toward the little finger (Figure 7-3, A).

At 5 to 6 months, transferring objects from one hand to another is a two-step process (the taking hand grabs the objects deposited by the releasing hand before the releasing hand lets go). By 6 months, the infant is coordinated enough to reach for an object while in the sitting or prone position. A 6-month-old infant uses a radial palmar grasp (in which the object is held between the thumb and the radial side of the palm; Figure 7-3, B) to transfer objects from hand to hand in a one-stage process (with the taking hand and releasing hand executing the transfer simultaneously).

Grasping skills change significantly between 7 and 12 months. At 7 months, the infant uses a radial digital grasp (in which objects are held between the thumb and fingertips), and the ability to voluntarily release an object begins to emerge. At about 9 months, the infant learns to use an inferior pincer grasp (the pad of the thumb is pressed to the pad of the index finger) to pick up a small object. By 10 months, the infant can release an object into a container. By 12 months, the infant uses a superior pincer grasp (the tip of the thumb is pressed to the tip of the index finger; Figure 7-4) and consistently puts objects into containers. By 12 months, fine motor skills are developed enough to allow the infant to combine objects and explore their functional uses. These fine motor skills facilitate the development of functional and symbolic play skills.[10,13]

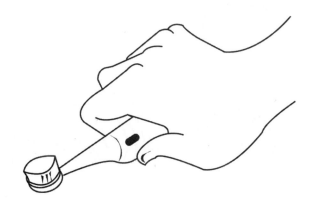

FIGURE 7-4 When using the superior pincer grasp, the infant holds a small object between the tips of the index finger and thumb. The wrist is slightly extended, with the ring and little fingers curled into the palm.

Interrelatedness of Development Skills

It is important to note how the interrelatedness of skills affects development. When the newborn is placed in the prone position during periods of alertness, the position of physiologic flexion raises the pelvis off the surface, transferring much of the infant's weight to the head and shoulders. In addition, this position places the hands beside the cheeks. As the infant turns, the head, the mouth, and cheeks rub against the surface, providing the sensory input necessary to elicit the rooting reflex. When the infant turns the head and opens the mouth to root, he or she is able to suck on the hands.[1] This input to the cheeks also helps develop oral motor skills, such as sucking and chewing. As the infant grows, time in the prone position (or "tummy time") affords the opportunity to raise the head and provides deep-pressure input to the ulnar side and the palm of the hands. This input to the hands facilitates the separation of the radial and ulnar portions of the hand in preparation for radially oriented precision and ulnar-oriented strength. By 6 months, as the infant shifts weight in the prone position, this position provides deep-pressure input to the radial side of the hand, facilitating the radial digital grasp. It is important for the OT practitioner to emphasize the importance of "tummy time" to facilitate the development of oral motor and fine motor skills.

Process Skills

The infant's cognitive development can be described using Piaget's theory, which states that individuals pass through a series of stages of thought as they progress from infancy to adolescence. These stages are a result of the biologic pressure to adapt to the changing environment and organize structures of thinking. According to Piaget, cognitive development is divided into four stages: sensorimotor, preoperational, concrete operational, and formal operations. See Table 7-3 for a

TABLE 7-3

Piaget's Stages of Cognitive Development

STAGE	DESCRIPTION
Sensorimotor (birth to 2 years)	Knows about environment through movement and sensations.
Preoperational (2 to 7 years)	Begins to think symbolically and uses words or pictures to represent objects. Tends to be egocentric.
Concrete operational (7 to 11 years)	Begins to think logically about concrete events and problems.
Formal operations (11+ years)	Begins to think abstractly. Reasons about hypothetical problems.

Adapted from Cherry, K. (n.d.). Piaget's stages of cognitive development: Background and key concepts of Piaget's theory. Retrieved June from www.psychology.about.com/od/piagetstheory/a/keyconcepts.htm.

description of each stage. During the sensorimotor stage, the infant develops the ability to organize and coordinate sensations with physical movements and actions. As shown in Table 7-4, the **sensorimotor period** has six substages.[15,23,26]

During the first stage, known as *reflexive schemes*, behavior is dominated by reflexes such as sucking and the palmar grasp. A rattle placed in an infant's hand is retained by the grasp reflex. Random motor movement causes the infant to accidentally shake the rattle.

In the second stage, referred to as *primary circular reactions*, the infant repeats the reflexive movements and patterns simply for pleasure. During this stage, he or she may accidentally get the fingers to the mouth and begin to suck on them. The infant then searches for the fingers again but has trouble getting them to the mouth because the coordination to do so has not been mastered yet. The infant repeats this action until the fingers get to the mouth.

The third stage is referred to as *secondary circular reactions*, and it is characterized by the infant beginning to use voluntary movements to repeat actions that accidentally produced a desirable result. At this age, an infant who accidentally hits a rattle with the foot while kicking would repeat the same kicking movement to reproduce the sound, thus creating a learned scheme, or mental plan, that can be used to reproduce the sound.

During the fourth stage, *coordination of secondary circular reactions*, several significant changes take place. The infant readily combines previously learned schemes and generalizes them for use in new situations. For example, the infant may visually inspect and touch a

TABLE 7-4

Piaget's Sensorimotor Substages of Cognitive Development

SUBSTAGE	OBSERVABLE BEHAVIORS
Reflexive schemes (0-1 month)	Uses newborn reflexes Uses entire body during vocalizations Slowly follows moving objects visually (tracks)
Primary circular reactions (1-4 months)	Uses simple, whole-body motor responses Uses smoother visual tracking Stops activity while focusing on object or person Begins to pat bottle with hand while being fed Puts own hands in mouth Produces increased variety of sounds
Secondary circular reactions (4-8 mo)	Imitates familiar behaviors Increasingly dissociates sounds from movement Understands concept of cause and effect Repeats patterns of actions involving objects or people that create pleasurable sensations Calls out to get attention
Coordination of secondary circular reactions (8-12 months)	Uses goal-directed behavior Uses intentional movements Is able to find hidden object (object permanence) Imitates behaviors that are slightly different Has increased ability to anticipate events Follows simple directions
Tertiary circular reactions (12-18 months)	Imitates novel behaviors Solves problems by trial and error Uses speech to name, refuse, call, greet, protest, and express feelings Searches for hidden objects in several locations Uses objects in novel ways (e.g., uses spoon to feed mom instead of self)
Mental representation (18 to 24 months)	Labels and symbolically uses mental schemes to present concepts Solves problems by self Uses make-believe play Uses speech as a significant means of communication

Adapted from McLeod, S. (2015). Sensorimotor Stage. Retrieved from www.simplypsychology.org/sensorimotor.html.

toy simultaneously. The major advancement during this period is the emergence of object permanence. The infant searches for an object that seems to have disappeared. In addition, he or she uses existing schemes to obtain a desired object. For example, the infant may pull a string to get an attached toy or object.

During the stage called *tertiary circular reactions*, he or she repeatedly attempts a task and modifies the behavior to achieve the desired consequences. The repetition helps the infant understand the concept of cause-effect relationships. Another important hallmark of this stage is the use of tools, such as using a cup to drink something.

The last stage of the sensorimotor period, known as *mental representation*, is characterized as the toddler begins using trial and error to solve problems. For example, he or she learns that pulling on a tablecloth will bring down a plate of cookies to the floor. During the last stage, the child also uses "pretend" play to create new roles for various objects. For example, stuffed animals that were previously used while teething or to hit other objects are now considered playmates.[15,23,26]

Social Interaction Skills

Language Development

The development of language is closely related to both cognitive and **psychosocial development**.[10] Undifferentiated crying characterizes the newborns' "language." By 3 months, their vocalizations are called *cooing* and usually consist of pleasant vowel sounds. Around 4 months, they begin to *babble*, or repeat a string of vowel and consonant sounds. From birth to 4 months, infants are "universal linguists"—they are capable of distinguishing among the 150 sounds that constitute all human speech. By 6 months, they recognize only the speech sounds of their native language.[19] By the age of 8 months, infants develop a sense of the existence of others, recognizing and imitating the actions of caregivers. By 12 months, infants know between two and eight words and babble short sentences. Their vocabulary increases significantly during the second year. By 24 months, toddlers may have 50 to 200 words in their spoken vocabulary.[10]

Social Interaction Development

The psychosocial development of newborns begins with the earliest emotional connections and interactions with their caregivers. The development of this emotional connection, or feeling of love, between newborns and their caregivers was first examined in the context of attachment, or the development of affectionate ties to the mother by the infant. Ainsworth outlined four stages in the development of infants' attachment to their caregivers.[3]

1. *Initial attachment:* At 2 to 3 months, infants exhibit nondiscriminating social responses.
2. *Attachment in the making:* By 4 to 6 months, infants begin to distinguish between familiar and unfamiliar persons.
3. *Clear-cut, or active, attachment:* By 6 to 7 months, infants become more attached to one primary caregiver, seeking proximity to and contact with that person.
4. *Multiple attachments:* After 12 months, infants become attached to persons other than their primary caregivers.

Another facet of the infant-caregiver relationship is called *bonding,* which is characterized by behaviors such as stroking, kissing, cuddling, and prolonged gazing. These behaviors serve two functions: expressing affection and sustaining an interaction between caregivers and infants. By the time infants are 1 month of age, most parents are able to read and interpret their cries to meet the infant's needs. Caregivers also begin to recognize the early indicators of changes in their infants' temperaments and know ways to calm them or prevent overstimulation.[3,7,23]

Two theories of psychosocial and emotional development in infancy are highlighted in Table 7-5. According to Greenspan, the first stage is called *self-regulation and interest in the world.*[18] During the first few months after birth, the infant is focused on organizing the internal and external worlds, and the job of the primary caregiver(s) is to help him or her regulate these influences. Around month 2 or 3, the infant moves into the *falling-in-love* stage, in which he or she forms strong attachment to the primary caregiver(s). The infant responds to the facial expressions and vocalizations of the caregivers with smiles and coos. From 3 to 10 months, the infant begins to learn the art of *purposeful communication.* At this stage, smiling is purposeful; he or she has learned that smiling causes adults to smile back. Around 9 or 10 months, the infant develops an organized *sense of self* and begins to realize how behaviors can be used to get different reactions from others.[18]

EARLY CHILDHOOD

Four-year-old Phillip spends time practicing his fine motor skills. He enjoys drawing pictures and telling long, sometimes exaggerated stories to go with his pictures. When playing with other children in the neighborhood, Phillip tends to play with boys. The boys tend to play rougher games than the girls.

Physiologic Development

The beginning of the early childhood period is marked by the development of autonomy, the beginning of expressive language, and sphincter control.[10] The rapid growth of infancy slows as children enter their second and third years. Their limbs begin to grow faster than do their heads, making their bodies seem less top-heavy. By 6 years, the legs make up almost 45% of the body length, and children are about seven times their birth weight. The brain of a 5-year-old child is 75% of its adult weight.[11,29,30] Changes in physiologic pathways give children the sphincter control necessary for toilet training.

The physiologic differences between children in the early childhood stage and adults are significant. The eustachian tube is shorter and positioned more horizontally than that of adults, making children more susceptible to middle ear infections. The digestive tract is not fully mature, and the shape of the stomach is straight, resulting in frequent upset stomachs. Because of the immaturity of the retina, young children are farsighted.[10]

Motor Skills

All of the basic components of motor development such as vision, touch, and gross and fine motor skills exist physiologically during the second and third years. These components are developed as skills and refined through interactions with the environment. Balance and strength increase during the early childhood period. At 2 years of age, toddlers walk with an increased stride length, and by 4 years, their walking pattern closely resembles that of an adult. The ability to run develops around 3 to 4 years; by 5 or 6 years, a mature running pattern develops. Two-year-old children can climb stairs without holding on to a support; by 3.5 years, children are able to walk up and down the stairs independently and with alternating feet.

Like gross motor skills, the coordination and precision of hand and finger movements are refined with maturation and practice, especially when children enter preschool and school. At 2 years of age, children learn to draw. The first type of grasp they learn is the palmar grasp; during the second year, they develop the ability to hold a pencil with their fingers and thumb (rather than in the fist). As thumb, finger, and hand precision improves enough to allow children to use the tripod grasp, their drawings progress from scribbles to deliberate lines and shapes. Mature, dynamic tripod grasp develops by 5 years (Figure 7-5). While 3-year-old children are able to snip paper with scissors, mature scissor skills develop around 5 to 6 years.[10]

Process Skills

Piaget's second phase of development, the **preoperational period**, occurs between the ages of 2 and 7 years. The beginning of symbolic thought and strong egocentrism and the emergence of animism characterize this substage. The ability to use symbolism means that the child is able to mentally consider objects that are not present around

TABLE 7-5

Psychosocial and Emotional Development

PERIOD	AGE (Y)	ERIKSON	GREENSPAN	TYPICAL BEHAVIORS
Infancy	0-1	TRUST VS MISTRUST Has needs gratified Gives to others in return Develops drive and hope	SELF-REGULATION (0-3 mo) Calms self Regulates sleep Notices sights and sounds Enjoys touch and movement FALLING IN LOVE (2-7 mo) Is wooed by significant others Responds to facial expressions and vocalizations Attachment PURPOSEFUL COMMUNICATION (3-10 mo) Displays reciprocal interactions when initiated by adult Initiates interactions	Has fussy periods to relieve stress Smiles Imitates gestures Uses special smiles for different people and events May experience joy and anger Fears strangers (8 mo) Gives affection Learns about cause and effect Understands concept of object permanence
Early childhood	1-3	AUTONOMY VS SHAME AND DOUBT Considers self separate from parents Develops self-control and willpower Struggles with a conflict between holding on and letting go	EMERGENCE OF ORGANIZED SENSE OF SELF (9-18 mo) Knows ways to get different types of reactions Is focused and organized when playing Initiates complex behaviors Is capable of feeling embarrassment, pride, shame, joy, empathy, anger CREATING EMOTIONAL IDEAS (18-36 mo) Uses words and gestures Participates in pretend play with others Learns to recover from anger or temper tantrums Starts associating particular functions with certain people	**Early:** Attaches to transitional object (such as blanket) Imitates others Understands function of objects and means of behaviors May experience joy and anger **Late:** Is egocentric Experiences separation anxiety (2 y) Loves an audience and attention Often says phrases like "me do it" and "no" Has difficulty sharing Begins to become independent and spends time alone
	4-6	INITIATIVE AND IMAGINATION VS GUILT Displays purpose in actions Has a lively imagination Tests reality Imitates parental actions and roles Seeks new experiences that if successful lead to sense of initiative, needs balance between initiative and responsibility for own actions Accepts consequences of actions Makes choices and plans	EMOTIONAL THINKING (30-48 mo) Differentiates between real and unreal Follows rules Understands relationships among behaviors, feelings, and consequences (is capable of feeling guilty) Interacts in socially appropriate ways with adults and peers	Seems optimistic and confident Asks why Is spontaneous Seeks other playmates Fears monsters, spiders, etc., has bad dreams (4-5 y) Plays with imaginary playmates Tells exaggerated stories

Continued

TABLE 7-5

Psychosocial and Emotional Development—cont'd

PERIOD	AGE (Y)	ERIKSON	GREENSPAN	TYPICAL BEHAVIORS
Middle childhood	5-11	**INDUSTRY VS INFERIORITY** Sees work as pleasurable Develops sense of responsibility and competence Learns work habits Learns to use tools Likes recognition for accomplishments Is sensitive to performance in comparison with others Tries new activities Becomes scholastically and socially competent	**THE WORLD IS MY OYSTER (5-7 y)** Carries out self-care and self-regulatory functions with minimum assistance Enjoys relationship with parents Takes simultaneous interest in wants and needs of parents, peers, and "me first" Forms relationships with peers Struggles to assert own will with peers Can better handle not getting own way Can better understand reasons for reality limits **THE WORLD IS OTHER KIDS (8-10 y)** Cares about role in peer group Has best friends and regular friends Maintains nurturing relationship with parents Continues to enjoy fantasy Follows rules Orders emotions and groups them into categories Experiences competition without becoming aggressive or compliant	**Early (5-7 y):** Acts assertive and bossy; acts like a "know-it-all" Is critical of self Experiences night terrors Shares and takes turns May experience joy and anger **Late (9-11 y):** Desires privacy Acts with impulsivity and more control Looks up to and focuses on being like a certain person a "hero" ("hero worship") Becomes more competitive Expects perfection from others (11 y)
Adolescence	10-19	**SELF-IDENTITY VS ROLE CONFUSION** Has a temporal perspective Experiments with roles (parents, friends, various groups) Enters sexual relationship Shares self with others Develops ideological commitments	**THE WORLD IS INSIDE ME (11-12 y)** Has a developing internal sense of right and wrong Enjoys one or a few intimate friends Takes interest in adults as role models Uses rules flexibly by understanding context Takes interest in opposite sex Has feelings of privacy about own body Has concerns about body and personality related to puberty	Acts as if *right now* is most important thing in life Accepts and adjusts to changing body Plays to imaginary audience Believes in personal fable (of infallibility) and characterized by the phrase "It won't happen to me" Begins working Achieves emotional independence

Courtesy Jayne Shepherd. Adapted from Erikson E.H. (1963). *Childhood and society* (2nd ed.). New York: WW Norton; Greenspan S.I. (1993). *Playground politics: understanding the emotional life of your school-aged child*. Reading, MA: Addison-Wesley; Greenspan S. & Greenspan, N. (1985) *First feelings: milestones in the emotional development of your baby and child*. New York: Viking Penguin.

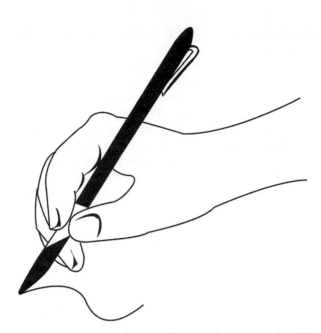

FIGURE 7-5 When using the dynamic tripod grasp, the child holds a pencil with the thumb and index and middle fingers. The fingers move, while other joints of the arm remain stable.

him or her. *Egocentrism* is the inability of individuals to realize that others have thoughts and feelings that may not be the same as their own. *Animism* is the mental act of giving inanimate objects lifelike qualities; this characteristic develops around age 3.[30] Children between the ages of 5 and 7 years are in a substage of preoperational thought called *intuitive thought*.

Social Interaction Skills

Language Development

During this phase, cognitive and language development is characterized by the use of symbolism. At this time, children begin to engage in symbolic, or pretend, play and tend to think more logically. They are able to use words and gestures to represent real objects or events.[10] Their vocabulary expands rapidly, increasing from a repertoire of 200 words at 2 years to 1500 words at 3 years. Two-year-old children label items and ask simple questions, whereas 3-year-old children can express their thoughts and feelings in simple sentences. By age 4, children can narrate long stories, which are sometimes exaggerated. At 5 or 6 years old, they are able to enunciate clearly and use their advanced language skills as a tool for learning. For example, they commonly ask questions such as "What is this for?" "How does this work?" and "What does it mean?"

Psychosocial Development

According to Erikson, the 2- to 4-year-old period of early childhood is referred to as the *stage of autonomy versus shame and doubt*. During this stage, children experience a need to be autonomous; they are determined to make their own decisions and to be independent. Central to this stage is the period known as the *terrible twos*, in which 2-year-olds try to establish their independence. According to Erikson's theories, children begin to doubt themselves and feel ashamed if they are not given adequate opportunities for self-regulation.[8,14]

Children between the ages of 4 and 6 years are in the stage Erikson calls *initiative and imagination versus guilt*.[14] On the one hand, children show initiative in activities in which their behavior produces successful, effective results and meets with parental approval. On the other hand, guilt results when children assume a sense of responsibility for their own behavior. By imitating others, they learn to take responsibility for their own actions and develop a sense of purpose. Gender role development also occurs during this stage.[32]

Greenspan identified two stages as occurring in early childhood: *creating emotional ideas* and *emotional thinking*.[18] In the creating emotional ideas stage, 2-year-olds express themselves by using words and gestures, engaging in pretend play, and starting to associate certain functions with certain people. In the emotional thinking stage, 3- and 4-year-olds are able to differentiate between what is real and what is not, follow rules, and understand the relationship between behaviors and feelings.[18]

MIDDLE CHILDHOOD

Ten-year-old Phillip is very concerned about being accepted by his peer group. He insists on wearing the same tennis shoes as the other boys. He and his friends spend hours playing seemingly endless baseball games. They follow the rules but do not really keep scores.

Physiologic Development

Between early childhood and adolescence, the growth rate slows down. Although wide variations in growth occur in both sexes during middle childhood, girls and boys typically grow an average of 2 to 3 inches per year, with their legs becoming longer and trunks slimmer.[30] Girls typically grow taller than boys during this period. Facial features become more distinct and unique, partly because baby teeth have been replaced by permanent teeth. The digestive system matures, so children retain food in the digestive system longer; they eat less frequently but have increased appetites and eat greater quantities.[10] By the age of 10, head and brain growth is 95% complete. Hearing acuity increases, and changes in the position of the eustachian tube decrease the risk for middle ear infections.[9,30]

Motor Skills

Because the rate of physical development slows down during middle childhood, children have the opportunity to refine their gross motor skills and become more adept at handling their bodies. Children in middle childhood focus on the refinement of previously learned skills. Hours of repetition leads to mastery of these skills, which creates higher self-esteem and greater acceptance from peers.[5]

Increased muscle strength and endurance allow children to become more physical; their favorite activities often include running, climbing, throwing, riding a bicycle, swimming, and skating.[30] Refined fine motor skills allow children to improve their performance of tasks such as sewing, using garden tools, and writing. The task of writing is a combination of refined grasping skills and coordinated movements that result in smooth writing strokes and smaller letters. By the age of 10 years, most children have converted from writing in printed letters to writing in cursive letters.[10]

Process Skills

The middle childhood years, ages 7 to 11, include Piaget's stage of **concrete operations**. This stage marks the beginning of the ability to think abstractly, or to mentally manipulate actions. For example, children are able to envision what might happen if they threw a rock across the room, without actually throwing a rock. Other characteristics of the concrete operational period include the following[30]:

- Being less self-centered
- Being able to recognize that others may have viewpoints that differ from their own
- Being able to identify similarities and differences among objects
- Being able to use simple logic to arrive at a conclusion
- Being able to simultaneously consider many aspects of a situation rather than just one
- Realizing that a substance's quantity does not change when its form does
- Being able to order objects by size, indicating an understanding of the relationships among objects
- Being able to imagine objects or pieces as parts of a whole

Moral Development

Kohlberg formulated schemes of moral development. He termed the early elementary years (between the ages of 4 and 10 years), the *preconventional level of moral development*.[27] At this stage children make moral judgments solely on the basis of anticipated punishment or reward (i.e., a "right" or "good" action is one that feels good and is rewarded, and a "wrong" or "bad" action is one that results in punishment).[27]

Between 10 and 13 years, children enter a stage called the *morality of conventional role conformity*. They are eager to please others and therefore tend to internalize rules (by applying them to themselves) and judge their actions according to set standards. Ten- and 11-year-olds are concerned about meeting the expectations and following the rules of their peer group. This stage is characterized by conforming, following the "Golden Rule" ("Do unto others as you would have them do unto you"), and showing respect for authority and rules.[27]

Social Interaction Skills

Language Development

During middle childhood, the vocabulary of children expands, partly as a result of their focus on reading. Puns and figures of speech become meaningful, and children's jokes are based on the dual meaning of words, slang, curse words, colloquialisms, and secret languages.[15] Communication among children during the middle childhood years has been described as *socialized communication*—conversations center around school activities, personal experiences, families and pets, sports, clothes, movies, television, comics, and "taboo" subjects such as sex, cursing, and drinking.[27]

Psychosocial Development

When children begin attending elementary school, their families are no longer the sole source of security and relationships. During this period, significant social relationships are developed outside the family in the neighborhood and school. In middle childhood, the feeling of belonging is very important to children, so they become increasingly concerned about their status among peers. They seem to have their own personal societies, separate from the adult world, that include rituals, heroes, and peer groups.[5,10,27] Peer groups usually comprise children of the same sex. Girls and boys tend to engage in their own activities, with little communication between the two groups. During this period, children experience more pressure to conform than during any other period of development. Children struggle to simultaneously participate in group activities while balancing the group's identity with their own and establishing their roles within the group.[15]

The middle childhood years include the stage Erikson named *industry versus inferiority*.[14] He believed that children must learn new skills to survive in their culture; if unsuccessful, they develop a sense of inferiority.[15] During this stage, the source of children's feelings of security switches from family to peer group as they try to master the activities of their friends.

Greenspan described the 8- to 10-year-old developmental stage as *the world is other kids*.[17] Children develop a mental picture of themselves that is based on interactions with friends, family members, and teachers. The stage called *the world inside me* is representative of an 11-year-old's definition of self, which is based on personal characteristics rather than the peer group's perceptions. At this age, children are able to empathize and understand the feelings of others. They realize that relationships require constant mutual adjustments, so they are able to disagree with a friend but still maintain the friendship.[17]

ADOLESCENCE

Fifteen-year-old Phillip wants to get a job in the music store at the mall. He thinks he would be good at the job because of his extensive knowledge of popular bands and musicians. An additional benefit is that all his friends hang out at the mall.

Physiologic Development

Adolescence is a period characterized by many dramatic physiologic changes, some of which are related to the adolescent growth spurt and some to the onset of puberty (see Chapter 9). Preadolescence, characterized by little physical growth, is followed by a period of rapid growth, indicating the onset of puberty.[35] The growth spurt is triggered by neural and hormonal signals to the hypothalamus, resulting in the increased production of and sensitivity to certain hormones. The onset of puberty in boys occurs between 10½ and 16 years, with the average age being 12½ years. The onset in girls occurs between 9½ and 15 years, with the average age being 10½ years. Although boys begin their growth spurt later than do girls, their growth spurt tends to be greater, with height increasing by 8.3 inches, compared with girls' height increasing by 7.7 inches.[12,22,35]

The onset of puberty is usually associated with the first signs of sexual development. The first visible sign of puberty in girls is breast growth, which begins around 10½ years. The average age of menarche is 12.8 years.[29] The onset of puberty in boys is signified by enlargement of the testes, which occurs between the ages of 10 and 13½ years.[12] As the age of the onset of puberty is quite variable, only a range of ages is given here.

Boys who mature earlier than others are described more positively by peers, teachers, and themselves. They tend to be the most popular, are better at sports, and begin dating with more ease than those who mature later. Boys who mature later are described as less attractive, more childish, and less masculine.[12,28,33] In the case of girls, the scenario is reversed. Those who mature the earliest sometimes have a poor body image and low self-esteem.

They tend to confide in and share their experiences with older adolescents. Girls who mature later develop at the same age as do their male peers and are likely to develop a better self-concept than do those who mature earlier.[12,28,33] These differences in the rates of development greatly affect adolescents' self-concept and self-esteem. To help ease the transition, adults can educate adolescents about the following:

- Health and preparation for puberty
- Nutrition
- Issues such as smoking prevention, automobile safety, and contraception
- Developing autonomy and independence[33]

Motor Skills

The development of gross motor skills in adolescents is directly related to the physical changes that are occurring. Increased muscle mass provides increased dynamic strength, as evidenced by better running, jumping, and throwing skills.[4] Because boys have a greater percentage of muscle mass than do girls, their strength is greater.[5] Fine motor abilities tend to differ between the sexes. Girls show greater rates of improvement in hand-eye coordination, but overall they still do not perform as well as boys do when it comes to motor skills.[5,32,35]

Process Skills

The development of **formal operational thought** is the hallmark of adolescence.[5] Adolescents have the ability to think about possibilities as well as realities. They can formulate hypotheses about the outcome of a certain situation, and after imagining all the possible results, they can test each hypothesis to determine which one is true.[12] This process is called *hypothetical deductive reasoning*.

Adolescents develop their moral thought in the period known as the *conventional level* of Kohlberg's stages. During this stage, adolescents approach moral problems in a social context; they want to please others by being good members of society. Adolescents follow the standards of others, conform to social conventions, support the status quo, and generally try to please others and obey the law.[28]

Social Interaction Skills
Language Development

In high school, adolescents manipulate language; for example, they use codes, slang, and sarcasm. The use of slang during adolescence is important for establishing group membership and being accepted by peers. They also have the cognitive ability to use language for more than simple communication. For example, they can participate in debates or class discussions and argue against a position that they do not agree with; children at younger ages do not understand this abstract use of language.[5]

Egocentrism

Adolescents tend to believe that if something is of great concern to them, then it is also of great concern to others. Because they believe that others have thoughts similar to their own, they tend to be self-conscious, or *egocentric*. This egocentrism manifests itself in adolescents as having an imaginary audience, or a perception that everyone is watching them. Another way egocentrism manifests itself is through the *personal fable*, or the idea that they are special, have completely unique experiences, and are not subject to the natural rules governing the rest of the world. Egocentrism is the cause of much of the self-destructive behavior of many adolescents who think that they are magically protected from all harm.[28]

Identity

Erikson referred to the adolescent stage of development as *identity versus identity confusion*.[14] During this stage, the main goal for adolescents is to find or understand their identities. They work to form a new sense of self by combining past experiences with future expectations. This process allows adolescents to understand themselves in terms of who they have been and who they hope to become.[14]

The establishment of an occupational identity is one part of the establishment of ego identity. A number of theories about occupational development exist. Ginzberg outlined three periods that apply to this stage: a fantasy period, a tentative period, and a realistic period.[16] Adolescents explore various occupations, identify with workers in a specific occupation, discover which occupations they enjoy, and develop basic habits of work and an identity as a worker.[34]

Peers

Peer groups support adolescents as they experience the transition from childhood to adulthood.[22] Involvement in peer groups provides opportunities to accomplish the following:

- Sharing responsibilities for their own affairs
- Experimenting with new ways of handling new situations
- Learning from each other's mistakes
- Trying out new roles[22]

Early adolescence (ages 12-14 years) is the time when children are most concerned about conforming to the values and practices of their peer groups. Older adolescents are less likely to conform to a group and more likely to rely on their own independent thinking and judgment.[22]

Parents

Although adolescents spend more time with friends, parents still have a considerable effect on them. Although adolescents seek the advice of peers on matters such as social activities, dress, and hobbies, they seek the advice of their parents on issues such as occupation, college, and money.[31]

SUMMARY

Infants and children progress through a series of stages of development that are predictable and sequential. The rate of development may vary. Contexts (personal, social, cultural) influence development. Understanding the sequences of development allow OT practitioners to analyze the performance skill requirements and develop interventions. This chapter provides an overview of developmental progression and an analysis of performance skills. Because performance skills are observable actions (motor, process and social interaction skills), they provide the basis for many intervention plans.

References

1. Alexander, R., Boehme, R., & Cupps, B. (1993). *Normal development of functional motor skills*. Tucson, AZ: Therapy Skill Builders.
2. American Occupational Therapy Association. (2014). Occupational therapy practice framework: domain and process (3rd ed.). *Am J Occup Ther*, 68(Suppl. 1), S1–S48.
3. Ainsworth, M. (1982). Attachment retrospect and prospect. In C. M. Parkes, & M. Stevenson-Hind (Eds.), *The place of attachment in human behavior*. New York: Basic Books.
4. Ausubel, D. P. (2002). *Theories and problems of adolescent development* (3rd ed.). Bloomington, IN: Writers Club Press. iUniverse, Inc.
5. Berger, K. S. (2011). *The developing person through childhood and adolescence* (9th ed.). New York: Worth Publishers.
6. Bly, L. (1998). *Motor skills acquisition in the first year: an illustrated guide to normal development*. Tucson, AZ: Therapy Skill Builders.
7. Brazelton, T. B., & Nugent, J. K. (2011). *Neonatal behavioral assessment scale* (4th ed.). London, UK: Mac Keith Press.
8. Caplan, T., & Caplan, F. (1995). *The first twelve months of life*. New York: Bantam Books.
9. Bazyk, S., & Case-Smith, J. (2015). School-based occupational therapy. In J. Case-Smith, & J. O'Brien (Eds.), *Occupational therapy for children and adolescents* (7th ed.). St. Louis, MO: Mosby.
10. Case-Smith, J. (2015). Development of childhood occupations. In J. Case-Smith, & J. O'Brien (Eds.), *Occupational therapy for children and adolescents* (7th ed.). St. Louis, MO: Mosby.

11. Dacey, J. S., & Travers, J. F. (2008). *Human development across the lifespan* (7th ed.). New York: McGraw-Hill.
12. Dusek, J. B. (1995). *Adolescent development and behavior* (3rd ed.). Englewood Cliffs, NJ: Prentice Hall.
13. Erhardt, R. P. (1999). *Developmental hand dysfunction: theory, assessment, and treatment* (2nd ed.). Tucson, AZ: Therapy Skill Builders.
14. Erikson, E. H. (1963). *Childhood and society* (2nd ed.). New York: WW Norton.
15. Freiberg, K. (1999). *Human development*. 99/00. Guilford, CT: McGraw-Hill/Dushin.
16. Ginzberg, E. (1972). Toward a theory of occupational choice: a restatement. *Voc Guide Quart, 20,* 169.
17. Greenspan, S. (1994). *Playground politics: understanding the emotional life of your school-aged child*. Reading, MA: Addison-Wesley.
18. Greenspan, S., & Greenspan, N. (1994). *First feelings: milestones in the emotional development of your baby and child*. New York: Viking Penguin.
19. Grunwald, L. (1995). The amazing minds of infants. In E. N. Junn, & C. J. Boyatzis (Eds.), *Annual editions: child growth and development*. Guilford, CT: Dushkin.
20. Haywood, K. M., & Getchell, N. (2008). *Life span motor development* (5th ed.). Champaign, IL: Human Kinetics.
21. Hetherington, E. M., et al. (2005). *Child psychology: a contemporary viewpoint* (6th ed.). New York: McGraw-Hill.
22. Kimmel, D. C., & Weiner, I. B. (1995). *Adolescence: a developmental transition* (2nd ed.). New York: John Wiley & Sons.
23. Lamb, M. E., & Bornstein, M. (2002). *Development in infancy: an introduction* (4th ed.). Mahwah, NJ: Lawrence Erlbaum Associates.
24. Leach, P. (2010). *Your baby and child: from birth to age five*. New York: Knopf.
25. Lief, N. R., Fahs, M. E., & Thomas, R. M. (1997). *The first three years of life*. New York: Smithmark.
26. McLeod, S. (2015). *Sensorimotor Stage*. www.simplypsychology.org/sensorimotor.html.
27. Minuchin, P. (1977). *The middle years of childhood*. Pacific Grove, CA: Brooks/Cole.
28. Papaplia, D. E., Olds, S. W., & Feldman, R. (2008). *Human development* (11th ed.). New York: McGraw-Hill.
29. Payne, V. G., & Isaacs, L. D. (2011). *Human motor development: a lifespan approach* (8th ed.). New York: McGraw-Hill.
30. Santrock, J. W. (2012). *Life span development* (14th ed.). New York: McGraw-Hill Humanities.
31. Sigelman, C. K., & Rider, E. A. (2011). *Life span human development* (7th ed.). Independence, KY: Cengage Learning.
32. Simon, C. J., & Daub, M. M. (2008). Human development across the life span. In E. B. Crepeau, E. S. Cohn, & B. A. Boyt-Schell (Eds.), *Willard and Spackman's occupational therapy* (11th ed.). Philadelphia: Lippincott.
33. Steinberg, L. (2013). *Adolescence* (10th ed.). New York: McGraw-Hill.
34. Super, D. E. (1957). *The psychology of careers*. New York: Harper & Row.
35. Watson, R. I., & Lindgren, H. C. (1979). *Psychology of the child and the adolescent* (4th ed.). New York: Macmillan.
36. Fine, C. (2011). *Delusions of gender: how our minds, society, and neurosexism create difference*. New York: WW Norton & Company.

REVIEW *Questions*

1. What are primitive reflexes, righting reactions, equilibrium reactions, and protective extension?
2. What activities might you use to promote the development of infants, toddlers, and adolescents?
3. Briefly describe the gross and fine motor skills of children at the following ages: 1 month, 6 months, 12 months, and 18 months.
4. What are four sequences of Piaget's stages of cognitive development? Give an example of a behavior that might be observed during each stage of cognitive development.
5. Why is Greenspan's stage for 2- to 7-month-olds called falling in love? Why is Greenspan's stage for 5- to 7-year-olds called the world is my oyster?
6. What are Erikson's five stages of development? Briefly describe each.
7. What are motor, process, and social interaction performance skills?

SUGGESTED *Activities*

1. Visit a nursery or a child-care center that serves infants and toddlers. What postural reactions do you observe? Which ones can you elicit while playing with the infants?
2. Go to a nearby playground and watch normally developing children at play. Using the American Occupational Therapy Association's Occupational Therapy Practice Framework (2014) as a guide,

record your observations. Develop a chart like the one that follows to summarize development throughout childhood.

PERFORMANCE SKILLS	NEWBORN	1 YEAR	4 YEARS	10 YEARS	15 YEARS
Physiologic development					
Motor skills: gross					
Motor skills: fine					
Process					
Social interaction/ psychosocial development					

3. Interview a parent (caregiver) of an infant, toddler, or adolescent and document the social interaction phases in which the child is currently engaging. Discuss how the child's motor and process skill development may influence his or her social interaction skills.

4. Observe a child engaged in an area of performance. List the performance skills observed by recording all observable actions.

DIANNE KOONTZ LOWMAN

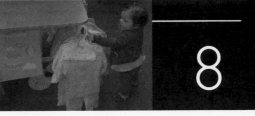

Development of Occupations

CHAPTER *Objectives*

After studying this chapter, the reader will be able to accomplish the following:

- Describe the development of specific occupations addressed with children and youth.
- Identify the sequences of activities of daily living for the categories of feeding and eating, dressing and undressing, and grooming and hygiene development.
- Describe the developmental sequence of oral motor control.
- Identify the types of food and utensils that are appropriate for infants and young children of different ages.
- Describe the progression of the instrumental activities of daily living for the categories of home management, care of others, and community mobility, including the factors that influence performance.
- Identify readiness skills required for work or productive activities.
- Explain the difference between formal and informal educational activities.
- Explain the relevance of play to occupational therapy practice.
- Describe rest and sleep patterns in infants and children.
- Describe the development of social participation.

CHAPTER *Outline*

Occupational therapy (OT) practitioners focus on improving a child's ability to perform a variety of occupations which fall into categories of activities of daily living (ADLs), instrumental activities of daily living (IADLs), rest and sleep, education, work, play and leisure, and social participation.[2] These activities occur in cultural, physical, social, personal, temporal, and virtual contexts. The OT practitioner evaluates a child's ability to perform occupations by examining the performance skills (motor, process, social interaction) and client factors. Knowledge of each **occupation** is therefore important to pediatric OT practice. This chapter provides a description of each occupation within the framework of normal development.

ACTIVITIES OF DAILY LIVING

Activities of daily living constitute one of the occupations described in the American Occupational Therapy Association's (AOTA's) Occupational Therapy Practice Framework.[2] The ADLs listed in Box 8-1 are the most basic tasks that children learn as they grow and mature.[2,3] Basic self-care skills include feeding and eating, dressing and undressing, bathing and showering, toileting and toileting hygiene, and grooming and hygiene.[2] Other ADLs include functional mobility, personal device care, and sexual activity.[2]

Feeding and Eating Skills

Because eating is a critical daily living skill essential to the child's survival, growth, health, and well-being, it falls within the OT practitioner's domain of concern.[2,3] A child with sufficient eating skills is able to actively bring food to the mouth without assistance. A child who requires feeding must receive assistance in the activity of eating.[3] *Oral motor control* relates to the child's ability to use the lips, cheeks, jaw, tongue, and palate.[28]

BOX 8-1

Activities of Daily Living

- Bathing and showering
- Bowel and bladder management
- Toilet hygiene
- Dressing
- Eating
- Feeding
- Functional mobility
- Personal device care
- Personal hygiene and grooming
- Sexual activity

From American Occupational Therapy Association. (2014). Occupational therapy practice framework: domain and process (3rd ed.). *Am J Occup Ther, 68*(Suppl. 1), S1–S48.

Oral motor development refers to feeding, sound play, and oral exploration.[19] Feeding is an oral motor skill, but some oral motor skills, such as oral motor awareness and exploration, do not involve food at all.[9]

The normal development of oral motor skills related to eating and feeding involves sucking from a nipple, coordinating the suck–swallow–breathe sequence, drinking from a cup, and munching and chewing solid foods.[13,17,18] The maturation of these skills is closely tied to the physical maturation of the infant.

Oral Motor Development

The infant's oral mechanisms differ anatomically from those of the adult; the infant's oral cavity appears to be filled by the tongue. The small oral cavity, coupled with sucking fat pads that stabilize the infant's cheeks, allows the infant to compress and suck on a nipple placed in the mouth. The limited mobility of the tongue results in the back and forth movement of the tongue known as suckling.[17,19,20] As the size ratios in the mouth change with the infant's growth, a more mature oral motor pattern emerges. By 4 to 6 months of age, the area inside the infant's mouth increases as the jaw grows and the sucking fat pads decrease. These changes allow increased movement of the infant's cheeks and lips. A "true sucking" pattern develops, as the infant's tongue can move up and down as well as forward and backward. Increased control of the jaw, lips, cheeks, and tongue allows the infant to move food and liquid toward the back of the mouth and prepares the infant to accept and control strained baby food.[19,21]

Full-term infants are born with reflexes that allow them to locate the source of food, suck, and then swallow. These reflexes are described in relation to oral motor development:[21]

- *Rooting reflex:* When the infant's cheeks or lips are stroked, he or she turns toward the stimulus. This reflex, which allows the infant to search for food, is maintained for a longer period in breast-fed infants.
- *Suck–swallow reflex:* When the infant's lips are touched, the mouth opens, and sucking movements begin.
- *Gag reflex:* The gag reflex protects the infant from swallowing anything that may block the airway.[19] At birth, the gag reflex is highly sensitive and elicited by stimulation to the back three-fourths of the tongue. This reflex gradually moves to the back one-fourth of the tongue as the infant matures and engages in oral play.
- *Phasic bite–release reflex:* When the infant's gums are stimulated, he or she responds with a rhythmic up-and-down movement of the jaw. This reflex forms the basis for munching and chewing.

- *Grasp reflex:* When a finger is pressed into the infant's palm, he or she grasps the finger. As the infant sucks, the grasp tightens, indicating a connection between sucking and the grasp reflex. Most of these early reflexive patterns begin to change or disappear between 4 and 6 months of age, when the cortex develops.[19,21]

Infancy

Oral skills develop concurrently and are closely related to the overall development of sensorimotor skills. Table 8-1 presents a brief overview of the development of normal sensorimotor, oral motor, and feeding skills during the first 3 years of life. Feeding initially requires that the adult provide head support and head–trunk alignment to enable the infant to coordinate the suck–swallow–breathe sequence. The infant's first suckling pattern predominates for the first 3 to 4 months of life.[13] Beginning at 4 months, a "true sucking" pattern—an up-and-down tongue movement—develops as head and jaw stability appears.

At 6 months, the infant has complete head control and more jaw stability, allowing for better control of tongue movements. This stability allows the infant to effectively suck from a bottle and take in soft food from

TABLE 8-1

Normal Development of Sensorimotor, Oral Motor, and Feeding Skills

AGE	SENSORIMOTOR SKILLS	ORAL MOTOR SKILLS	FEEDING SKILLS
Birth/37–40 wk gestation	Is dominated by physiologic flexion Moves total body into extension or flexion Turns head side to side in prone position (a protective response) Keeps head mostly on side in supine position Tends to keep hands fisted and flexed across chest during feeding Has strong grasp reflex	Possesses strong gag reflex Possesses rooting reflex Possesses autonomic phasic bite–release pattern Sucks and suckles when hand or object comes into contact with mouth Shows minimal drooling in supine position and increased drooling in other positions	Begins bottle- or breast-feeding with total sucking pattern Uses mixture of suckling and sucking on bottle (dependent on head position) Possesses incomplete lip closure Is unable to release nipple
1–2 mo	Appears hypotonic as physiologic flexion diminishes Practices extension and flexion Continues to gain control of head Moves elbows forward toward shoulders in prone position Possesses ATNR, with head to side in supine position Experiences weakening grasp reflex Does not possess voluntary release skills	Continues to show strong gag reflex Continues to show rooting reflex Continues to show automatic phasic bite–release pattern Continues to suck and suckle when hand or object comes in contact with mouth Drools more as jaw and tongue move in wider excursions	May lose coordination of sucking–swallowing–breathing pattern with increased head movements Opens mouth and waits for food Has better lip closure Uses active lip movement when sucking
3–5 mo	Experiences diminishing ATNR and grasp reflex Possesses more balance between extension and flexion Has good head control (centered and upright) Brings hands to mouth constantly Supports on extended arms and props on forearms in prone position Brings hand to feet and feet to mouth in supine position Props on arms, with little support in sitting position Develops tactile awareness in hands Reaches more accurately, usually with both hands Begins transfer of objects from hand to hand Does not possess controlled release skills; may use mouth to assist	Experiences diminished rooting reflex and autonomic phasic bite–release pattern Experiences diminished strong gag reflex at 5 mo Drools less in positions with greater postural stability Uses mouth to explore objects Begins to show new oral movements in association with increased head and body control	Anticipates feeding; recognizes bottle and readies mouth for nipple Demonstrates voluntary control of mouth during bottle-feeding or breast-feeding Loses liquid from lip corners Is able to receive solid food from a spoon at 5 months Uses suckling during spoon feeding; gags on new textures Shows tongue reversal after spoon is removed; ejects food involuntarily

Continued

TABLE 8-1

Normal Development of Sensorimotor, Oral Motor, and Feeding Skills—cont'd

AGE	SENSORIMOTOR SKILLS	ORAL MOTOR SKILLS	FEEDING SKILLS
6 mo	Has total head control Shifts weight and reaches with one hand in prone position Begins shifting weight in quadruped position Transfers objects from hand to hand in supine position Reaches with one hand while supporting with other in sitting position Reaches to be picked up Begins to use thumb in grasp Begins to hold objects in one hand Shows visual interest in small things	No longer has rooting reflex or autonomic phasic bite–release pattern Experiences decrease in strength of gag reflex Maintains lip closure longer in supine, prone, and sitting positions Drools when babbling, reaching, and teething; drools less during feeding	Sucks from bottle or breast with no liquid loss and long sequences of coordinated sucking–swallowing–breathing Suckles liquid from a cup with liquid loss Coughs and chokes when drinking too much liquid from cup Moves upper lip down to scrape food from spoon and uses suckling with some sucking to move food back Gags on new textures Opens mouth when spoon approaches Uses phasic up-and-down jaw movements, suckling, or sucking when presented with solids Moves tongue laterally when solids placed on side biting surfaces Begins finger feeding Plays with spoon
7–9 mo	Shifts weight and reaches in quadruped position Creeps Develops extension, flexion, and rotation; expands movement options in sitting position May pull to stand and hold on to support Reaches with supination Uses index finger to poke Develops voluntary release skills	Experiences diminishing gag reflex; becomes more similar to an adult protective gag reflex Uses facial expressions to convey likes and dislikes Uses mouth in combination with visual examination and hand manipulation to investigate new objects Bites on fingers and objects to reduce teething discomfort Produces more coordinated jaw, tongue, and lip movements in supine, prone, sitting, and standing positions; rarely drools except when teething	Suckles liquid in cup; loses liquid when cup is removed Takes fewer sucks and suckles before pulling away from cup to breathe Independently holds bottle Feeds self cracker using fingers Holds jaw closed on soft solids to break off pieces Uses variable up-and-down movement while chewing; moves tongue laterally and jaw diagonally when solids placed on biting surfaces Assists with cup and spoon feeding
10–12 mo	Creeps with good coordination Cruises holding on to support with one hand Stands independently Learns to walk independently Uses superior pincer grasp with finger tip and thumb Smoothly releases large objects	Produces more coordinated jaw, tongue, and lip movements when sitting, standing, and creeping on hands and knees; rarely drools except when teething	Easily closes lips on spoon; uses upper and lower lips to remove food from spoon Uses controlled, sustained biting motion on soft cookies or crackers Chews with mixture of up-and-down and diagonal rotary movements Feeds self independently using fingers Likes to feed self but needs assistance with using spoon; inverts spoon before putting in mouth

TABLE 8-1

Normal Development of Sensorimotor, Oral Motor, and Feeding Skills—cont'd

AGE	SENSORIMOTOR SKILLS	ORAL MOTOR SKILLS	FEEDING SKILLS
13–18 mo	Walks alone Learns to go up and down stairs Has more precise grasp and release	Moves upper and lower lips By 15–18 months, has excellent coordination of sucking, swallowing, and breathing	Uses an up-and-down sucking pattern to obtain liquid from a cup Shows well-coordinated rotary chewing movements by 18 months Has well controlled and sustained biting movements Practices self-feeding; becomes neater Holds cup and puts cup down without spilling liquid
19–24 mo	Demonstrates equilibrium reactions while standing and walking Runs with more narrow base of support	Uses up-and-down tongue movements and tip elevation Develops internal jaw stabilization Swallows with easy lip closure	Efficiently drinks from cup Has well graded and sustained bite
24–36 mo	Jumps in place* Pedals tricycle* Scribbles* Snips with scissors*	Uses tongue humping rather than tongue protrusion to initiate swallow	Possesses circular rotary jaw movements* Closes lips while chewing* Holds cup in one hand* Handles spoon more accurately* Uses fingers to fill spoon* Begins to drink from straws*

Adapted from: Alexander, R., Boehme, R., & Cupps B. (1993). *Normal development of functional motor skills.* Tucson, AZ: Therapy Skill Builders; Bly, L. (1994). *Motor skills acquisition in the first year: an illustrated guide to normal development.* Tucson, AZ: Therapy Skill Builders; Glass, R.P., Wolf, L.S. (1999). In D.K. Lowman, & S.M. Murphy (Eds.), *The educator's guide to feeding children with disabilities.* Baltimore, MD: Paul H. Brookes; Korth, K., & Rendell, L. (2015). Feeding and oral motor skills. In J. Case-Smith, & J. O'Brien (Eds.), *Occupational therapy for children and adolescents* (7th ed.). St. Louis, MO: Mosby; Lowman, D.K., & Lane S.J. (1999). Children with feeding and nutritional problems. In S. Porr, & E.B. Rainville (Eds.), *Pediatric therapy: a systems approach.* Philadelphia: FA Davis; Morris, S.E., & Klein, M.D. (1987) *Pre-feeding skills: a comprehensive resource for feeding development.* Tucson, AZ: Therapy Skill Builders.
ATNR, asymmetric tonic neck reflex.
*From this point on, skills learned during the first 24 months are further refined.

a spoon.[17] At 4 to 5 months, the infant demonstrates a reflexive phasic bite–release pattern when given a soft cracker. With practice, the rhythm progresses into a munching pattern, which involves an up-and-down jaw movement. The munching pattern is effective for eating baby food or other dissolvable foods.[13,17] By 7 to 8 months, some diagonal jaw movements are added to the munching pattern. Infants use their fingers to eat soft crackers and cookies.[13,17]

Around 12 months, infants enjoy and prefer eating with their fingers. Rotary chewing movements and a well-graded bite are observed. At this time, many infants transition from drinking from a bottle to drinking from a cup. While learning to drink from a cup, the infant's jaw initially continues to move in the up-and-down sucking pattern. In addition, the infant bites the rim of the cup to stabilize the jaw. By 15 months, the infant demonstrates some diagonal rotary movements of the tongue and jaw while chewing food. Between 15 and 18 months, the infant begins to independently eat with a spoon.[13]

Early Childhood

By 24 months of age, the foundation has been established for all adult eating patterns. At age 2, children eat independently, consuming most meats and raw vegetables (Figure 8-1). Circular rotary chewing develops between the second and third year of life and allows toddlers to eat almost all adult foods.[17,21]

By 24 months, children can hold a spoon and bring it to the mouth with the wrist supinated into the palm-up position.[19] At 30 to 36 months, children experiment with forks to stab at food. A variety of spoons are available for children learning to use utensils.[12] The size of the spoon's bowl should match the size of the child's mouth. Children learning to use spoons typically use ones with shallow bowls; they have to work harder to eat food from spoons with deeper bowls. Child-size spoons and forks are easier for children to hold and manipulate, and bowls and plates with raised edges also make it easier for children to scoop the food.[12,19]

By 24 months, toddlers can also efficiently drink from cups. Children may begin drinking through straws between 2 and 3 years of age, especially if they have been exposed early to the use of straws. Given the variety of playful long, short, and decorated straws that are available on the market, children are happy to independently use their own

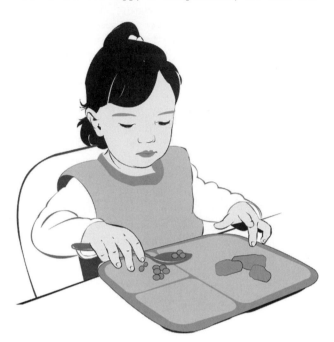

FIGURE 8-1 At age 2, children are able to sit up at the table, feed themselves, and eat almost all adult foods.

straws.[12] By 30 to 36 months, children try to serve themselves liquids and family-style servings of food.[19]

Dressing

Dressing and undressing are also essential, basic self-care skills learned in infancy and early childhood.[2] Dressing includes selecting clothing and accessories appropriate for the weather and occasion, putting clothes on sequentially, and fastening and adjusting clothing and shoes.[2] Young children develop independent dressing skills at various ages according to the family's cultural expectations for self-dressing and the types of clothing worn, opportunities for practice, and the child's motivation for independence.[8] Dressing skills require coordinated movements of almost every body part.[22] The development of independent dressing skills typically occurs at age 4 to 5 years.[8,10,27] Table 8-2 lists the general sequence of dressing and undressing skills.

Infancy

During the first year of development, the infant establishes the daily routine and begins to cooperate in dressing activities. He or she learns to remove loose-fitting clothing such as hats, mittens, and socks. By age 1, most infants have achieved many of the motor skills needed for the development of dressing skills. They can separate movements so that the arms or legs can move separate from the trunk, have begun to stabilize with one hand

TABLE 8-2

Developmental Sequence for Self-Care Skills

AGE (y)	DRESSING AND UNDRESSING SKILLS	GROOMING AND HYGIENE
1	Cooperates in dressing (e.g., holds foot up for shoe or sock, holds arm out for sleeve) Pushes arms through sleeves and legs through pants	Cooperates during hand washing and drying Has regular bowel movements
1½	Takes off loose clothing (such as mittens, hat, socks, and shoes) Partially pulls shirt over head Unties shoes or takes off hat as an act of undressing Unfastens clothing zippers with large pull tabs Puts on hat	Allows teeth to be brushed Pays attention to acts of eliminating Indicates discomfort from soiled points Begins to sit on potty when placed there and supervised (for a short time)
2	Removes unfastened coat Purposefully removes shoes (if laces are untied) Helps pull down pants Finds armholes in over-the-head shirt	Attempts to brush teeth in imitation of adults Washes own hands with assistance Shows interest in washing self in bathtub Urinates regularly
2½	Removes pull-down pants or shorts with elastic waist Removes simple clothing (such as open shirt or jacket) Assists in putting on socks Puts on front-button-type coat or shirt Unbuttons large buttons	Dries hands Wipes nose if given a tissue and prompted to do so Has daytime control of bowel and bladder; experiences occasional accidents Usually indicates need to go to toilet; rarely has bowel accidents

TABLE 8-2

Developmental Sequence for Self-Care Skills—cont'd

AGE (y)	DRESSING AND UNDRESSING SKILLS	GROOMING AND HYGIENE
3	Puts on over-the-head shirt with some assistance Puts on shoes without fastening (may be on wrong feet) Puts on socks with some difficulty positioning heel Independently pulls down pants or shorts Zips and unzips coat zipper without separating or inserting zipper Needs assistance to remove over-the-head shirt Buttons large front buttons	Washes own hands Uses toothbrush with assistance Gets drink from fountain or faucet with no assistance Uses toilet independently but needs help wiping after bowel movements
3½	Usually finds front of clothing Snaps or hooks clothing in front Unzips front zipper on coat or jacket, separating zipper Puts on mittens Buttons series of three or four buttons Unbuckles belt or shoe Puts on boots Dresses with supervision (needs help with front and back)	Pours well from small pitcher Spreads soft butter with knife Seldom has toileting accidents; may need help with difficult clothing
4	Removes pullover garment independently Buckles belt or shoe Zips coat zipper, inserting zipper Puts on pull-down pants or shorts Puts on socks with appropriate heel placement Puts on shoes with assistance in tying laces Consistently knows front and back of clothing	Washes and dries hands and face without assistance Brushes teeth with supervision Washes and dries self after bath with supervision Cares for self at toilet (may need help with wiping after bowel movement)
4½	Puts belt in loops	Runs brush or comb through hair Tears toilet tissue and flushes toilet after use
5	Puts on pullover shirt correctly each time Ties and unties knots Laces shoes Dresses unsupervised	Scrubs fingernails with brush with coaching Brushes and combs hair with supervision Cuts soft foods with knife Blows nose independently when prompted Wipes self after bowel movements
5½	Closes back zipper	Performs toileting activities, including flushing toilet, independently
6	Ties bow knot Ties hood strings Buttons back buttons Snaps back snaps Selects clothing that is appropriate for weather conditions and specific activities	Brushes and rinses teeth independently

Adapted from Case-Smith, J. (1994). Self-care strategies for children with developmental deficits. In C. Christiansen (Ed.), *Ways of living: self-care strategies for special needs.* Bethesda, MD: AOTA; Johnson-Martin, N.M. (2004). *The Carolina curriculum for preschoolers with special needs* (3rd ed.). Baltimore, MD: Paul H. Brookes; Klein, M D. (1983). *Pre-dressing skills: skill starters for self-help development* Tucson, AZ: Communication Skill Builders; Shepherd, J. (2015). Activities of daily living and sleep and rest. In J. Case-Smith, & J. O'Brien (Eds.), *Occupational therapy for children and adolescents* (7th ed.). St. Louis: Mosby.

the action of the other, and can adjust their posture during reaching.[11] Infants have the necessary control to push arms and legs through sleeves and pants or play at pulling off a hat.[11]

Early Childhood

By age 2, refined balance and equilibrium reactions provide children with the necessary motor skills to raise their arms to pull shirts over their heads. They can move their hands behind them to attempt to put their arms into the sleeves of a button-front shirt. By 3 years, children are more aware of details and can find arm and leg holes easily. By 4 years, they recognize correct and incorrect sides; as fine motor skills progress, they can also use buckles, zippers, and laces. By 5 years, all skills of balance, equilibrium, and fine motor coordination are refined enough to allow children to dress themselves unsupervised.[11] Figure 8-2 shows a child putting on her boots before going outdoors.

Personal Hygiene and Grooming

Grooming and hygiene are important self-care skills that tend to develop after the development of eating and dressing skills. (Table 8-2 shows the general sequence of personal hygiene and grooming.) The cultural expectations and social routines of the family determine when independence in grooming and hygiene is achieved.[27] Face washing, hand washing, and hair care are typical **personal hygiene and grooming** skills learned in early childhood. The infant cooperates in hand washing. By age 2, children can wash their hands but need assistance turning on water and getting soap. By age 4, children can perform hand and face washing unsupervised. With supervision and coaching, 5-year-olds can scrub fingernails with a brush and comb hair.

In early childhood, **oral hygiene** involves brushing teeth.[2] Before age 2, infants allow their parents to brush their teeth. Two-year-olds imitate parents brushing their teeth. Children continue to brush their own teeth with supervision until the age of 5 or 6 years.[27] At that time, refinement of skill in the use of tools enables children to independently complete all steps of dental care, including making the necessary preparations and then brushing the teeth and rinsing the mouth.[13]

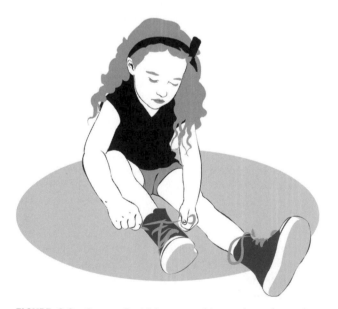

FIGURE 8-2 By age 5, children are able to dress themselves without adult supervision. They show adequate strength, balance, equilibrium, and fine motor coordination.

Bathing and Showering

Bathing and showering involve soaping, rinsing, and drying the body. Around age 2, children begin to show interest in bathing by assisting in washing while in the bathtub. Because bathing is a pleasurable activity for most children and parents, learning to wash oneself begins in the context of play.[13] Typically most children are able to wash and dry themselves with supervision by age 4. It is not until age 8 that most children can independently prepare the bath or shower water, wash, and dry themselves.[27]

Toilet Hygiene

Toilet hygiene involves clothing management, maintaining toileting position, transferring to and from toileting, and cleaning the body. Physiologically, voluntary control of urination does not usually occur until between 2 and 3 years of age. Independent toileting is a developmental milestone, which varies widely among children. During infancy, regularity in bowel movement and urination develops gradually. The infant may also indicate when diapers are wet or soiled and even sit on the toilet when placed there. Toilet training is not typically introduced until the child remains dry for 1 or more hours at a time, shows signs of a full bladder or the need to toilet, and is at least 2½ years old.[14] Daytime bowel and bladder control is usually attained between 2½ and 3 years of age, although the child may still need assistance with difficult clothing or fasteners. Nighttime bladder control may not be attained until age 5 or 6. During the day, 5-year-olds can anticipate immediate toilet needs and completely care for themselves while toileting, including wiping themselves and flushing the toilet.

Personal Device Care

Children may have **personal devices** (e.g., glasses, walker, wheelchair, technology, hearing aids, medical equipment) that help them engage in a variety of occupations. OT practitioners provide information on the care of devices and help children establish roles and routines for the maintenance of the equipment. Children may be responsible for placing devices in a safe container when not in use, cleaning devices, handling devices with care and asking for assistance as needed. The OT practitioner considers the child's age and abilities when developing a personal device plan.

Functional Mobility

The OT practitioner facilitates functional mobility in a variety of ways. The practitioner may address physical barriers in the home and community that prevent children from accessing the environment. For example, OT practitioners may assess the home and recommend modifications. They may help children gain performance skills such as postural control and endurance for mobility. Often the OT practitioner works as part of the team to recommend wheelchair or mobility technology. Helping children and youth gain movement through the environment has implications on learning and social interactions. OT practitioners strive to help children become mobile early so they can discover their environment.

Sexual Activity

As children mature, they may have many questions regarding sexual activity. OT practitioners may be asked to help children with disabilities understand how to express themselves. Allowing children to speak about these issues and helping them understand what this means for them is within the OT practitioner's realm. As the child matures, the OT practitioner may serve as a resource to parents and children. (Chapter 18 provides further description of ADL interventions.)

INSTRUMENTAL ACTIVITIES OF DAILY LIVING

Instrumental activities of daily living are complex activities of daily living that are necessary to function independently in the home, school, or community.[2] Box 8-2 lists all the categories included in IADLs and these are described in Chapter 20. During childhood,

---

BOX 8-2

Instrumental Activities of Daily Living (IADL)

- Care of others
- Care of pets
- Child rearing
- Communication management
- Community mobility
- Financial management
- Health management and maintenance
- Home establishment and management
- Meal preparation and cleanup
- Religious observance
- Safety and emergency maintenance
- Shopping

From American Occupational Therapy Association. (2014). Occupational therapy practice framework: domain and process (3rd ed.). *Am J Occup Ther, 68*(Suppl. 1), S1–S48.

---

children learn home management tasks that help them participate in family routines and community mobility skills that help them to be active outside the home. As they get older, they are given the responsibility of caring for others.[27]

Readiness Skills

Readiness skills are necessary for successful participation in home management, community mobility, and care of others' activities. Specific readiness skills are related to particular tasks. Activity analysis (dividing activity into steps) can determine the readiness skills needed to perform a specific task. For example, making a bed requires the coordination of both sides of the body, sequencing skills, and a pad-to-pad pinch. Setting the dinner table requires sequencing, balance, and dexterity while carrying and placing plates and silverware. The different readiness skills necessary to care for others can be illustrated by comparing the requirements for caring for a pet with those for babysitting a sibling. These two tasks obviously require different abilities. The contexts and environments in which they engage on a daily basis determine readiness skills acquired by children and adolescents.

Home Management

Home management activities are tasks necessary to obtain and maintain one's personal and household possessions.[2] The context significantly influences a child's or adolescent's participation in home management tasks. Children's ages and their physical, social, and cultural environments determine their roles in this domain. Children and adolescents may have chores that they are expected to complete on a regular schedule. Examples of chores include making the bed, setting the dinner table, and cutting the grass. Some children and adolescents have the incentive of a monetary allowance to complete the assigned chores, whereas others do not have a monetary incentive but are still expected to assist in the maintenance of their households.

Community Mobility

Mobility in the community outside the home is critical to the child's development. During the preschool years, **community mobility** may mean accompanying parents; during adolescence, it may be driving to run errands. Environmental factors that have an impact on mobility might be crowds, street crossings, public transportation, and architectural barriers.[27] Family and cultural expectations also determine the age and independence of community mobility skills.

Care of Others

Care of others refers to the physical upkeep and nurturing of pets or other human beings.[2] As with household management, the care of others is also significantly influenced by performance contexts. In large families, older siblings may be required to assist their parents in the care of younger siblings. A child living on a farm may assist with feeding and caring for the farm animals. A child living in an urban area may walk the family dog several times a day in the park or around the neighborhood.

REST AND SLEEP

A newborn will sleep as much as 16 to 17 hours a day, often in stretches of 3 to 4 hours. From 2 weeks of age until 3 to 4 months, it is common for babies to have a fussy period at the end of the day.[26] The infant wears out over the course of the day, becoming increasingly unable to modulate his or her response to environmental stressors. By 3 to 4 months, the baby begins to adapt to the parents' sleep–wake cycle (and the stomach is growing and holding more milk), and may sleep up to 7 or 8 hours at a time.[26] Babies of 4 to 7 months of age will sleep anywhere from 9 to 18 hours per day (the average number is 13 hours per day). Some babies may only nap 20 minutes and others, a few hours. Most babies this age nap once in the morning and again after lunch.[14]

Preschoolers sleep an average of 10 to 12 hours a night.[14] At this age, many children move into a "big boy bed." Making the bed as appealing as possible and providing fun pajamas for the child to wear creates an inviting environment. Helping the child create a place they can call their own will help them develop a sense of ownership and feelings of privacy. Going to sleep can be hard especially if the child is very tired or if older siblings are still up. The best way to prepare is to establish a bedtime routine. This routine might include turning off all electronic devices 1 hour before bedtime, playing quietly in the room, choosing one book to read, and when that book is finished, turning out the lights and going to sleep. Some 4 year olds have dreams and nightmares and will need to be reassured that these images are not real. Many 5-year-old children still need a nap as they tire while playing. A short play nap may involve falling asleep, looking at a book, talking to themselves, or listening to quiet music. Most 5 year olds begin to show less reluctance to going to sleep at bedtime. School-aged children typically need 10 to 12 hours of sleep per night.[14] Adolescents, who need about 8½ to 9½ hours of sleep per night, experience a change in their sleep patterns; their bodies want to stay up late and wake up later. Because this is not possible during the school week, teens might try to catch up on sleep over the weekend.

These inconsistent sleep patterns can actually make getting to sleep at a reasonable hour during the week even harder.[14]

CLINICAL *Pearl*

The American Academy of Pediatrics (http://www.healthychildren.org/English/ages-stages/baby/sleep/Pages/Sleep-Position-Why-Back-is-Best.aspx) recommends that healthy infants be placed on their backs to sleep, not on their stomachs or sides. When told to place the baby on his back to sleep, young parents sometimes hear "never place the baby on his stomach." The result is that some infants never get the chance to experience "tummy time." It is important for all infants to engage in tummy time when they are awake and alert, and the caregiver is present to observe and interact with the infant. Consider how physiologic flexion places the infant in the position to receive deep pressure input to the cheeks and facilitates sucking on the hand. This input to the cheeks helps develop oral-motor skills and facilitate sucking and chewing. As the infant grows, time on his tummy will give him the opportunity to raise his head and provide deep pressure input to the sides and palms of the hands. This input to the hands helps develop a voluntary grasp. As the infant begins to move, tummy time is a precursor to the infant getting up on hands and knees and crawling. In addition to the benefits to development, a certain amount of tummy time will help prevent flat spots on the infant's head.

EDUCATION

Educational activities are the opportunities that facilitate learning for children and adolescents.[27] These activities can be formal or informal. Formal educational activities are structured and may be mandated by public law for specific age groups. These activities are provided in settings such as preschool programs, day-care centers, public schools, and Sunday school classes. Informal educational activities are less structured and occur in a variety of settings. Examples of activities in which younger children engage include playing school with an older sibling and playing a shopping game with peers. Figure 8-3 shows children engaged in "playing school," a typical informal educational activity. Adolescents frequently study together, creating opportunities for informal learning.

Readiness Skills

Readiness skills are those performance abilities that are necessary to effectively engage in educational and vocational activities. Readiness is a stage of preparedness for "what comes next."[27] Different readiness skills are necessary for different tasks. Readiness skills must

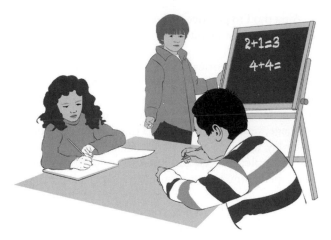

FIGURE 8-3 Children enjoy "playing school," a typical informal educational activity. Note the students attending to the "teacher."

be considered within the temporal and environmental contexts. The chronologic age of the child or adolescent is directly related to the necessary readiness skills. For example, readiness skills expected of a kindergarten student are different from those expected of a high school student. Social, cultural, and physical environments also influence expectations of readiness. This section discusses educational readiness skills for children enrolled in preschool programs, kindergarten, and elementary school.

Preschool Readiness Skills

Children entering preschool programs need certain readiness skills, which include independence in toileting with a minimum of assistance for handling fasteners, independence in self-feeding, and cooperative play behavior. Children attending a preschool program are also expected to understand rules and schedules. They need to exhibit the beginning of behavioral and emotional maturity (i.e., controlling tempers and mood swings).

Kindergarten Readiness Skills

The child attending kindergarten is expected to have the readiness skills of a typical preschooler with additional preacademic and academic skills. He or she must be able to sit quietly while listening to a story and should have adequate fine motor skills for coloring and for manipulating small objects.[4] The child must possess gross motor skills such as running, hopping, and jumping and is expected to recognize letters and numbers.

Elementary School Readiness Skills

Children attending elementary school are expected to have greater independence and skill in occupations than younger children. Independence in the bathroom and cafeteria is necessary. In addition to independence in eating, children in elementary school are expected to carry their lunch trays and assist in cleaning the table at the end of a meal. They must remain in their classroom chairs

for extended periods. The ability to remain "on task" and attend to work while seated is termed *in-seat behavior*.

Expectations of reading, writing, spelling, and math skills increase with grade level. The child attending elementary school should have adequate perceptual and motor skills to participate in games and organized sports.

Middle Childhood and Adolescent Readiness Skills

Educational readiness skills for middle childhood and adolescence build on the competencies gained during the preceding periods. Appropriate social skills and manners are expected, and increased skill in creative thinking, problem solving, and the development of ideas is required. Children learn expressive writing during this period and must be ready to perform cognitively and motorically. During middle childhood, children and adolescents also begin to seek independence. They question authority figures but must learn to work with them effectively in educational settings.

WORK/VOCATIONAL ACTIVITIES

In preparation for entering the world of **work** as adults, adolescents engage in a variety of **vocational activities**. These activities are work related and typically have a monetary incentive or salary.[1] Like educational activities, vocational activities can be formal or informal. An example of a formal vocational activity is having a job. Public laws determine the age at which a person may hold a job. Informal vocational activities include neighborhood lemonade stands and cutting a neighbor's grass for a fee. Figure 8-4 shows a child "selling" cookies to a friend. Like home management and the care of others, vocational activities in which a child or adolescent might participate are significantly influenced by performance contexts for that individual.

Readiness skills for formal and informal vocational activities are varied. To successfully engage in formal vocational activities, skills such as promptness, appropriate dressing, and effective communication with peers and supervisors are important. Activity analysis is beneficial when considering appropriate formal and informal vocational activities.

PLAY/LEISURE ACTIVITIES

Play is the occupation of childhood. Through play, children learn cognitive, socioemotional, motor, and language skills.[23,25] In adulthood play often takes the form of **leisure** activities, which are not associated with time-consuming duties and responsibilities.[2] During play and leisure activities children, adolescents, and adults refine skills, relax, reflect, and engage in creativity. Children develop problem-solving skills and flexibility as well as motor skills during play. Importantly, children need a variety of skills to engage in play, such as motor skills (e.g., coordination, strength, balance, timing, sequencing), social (e.g., sharing, negotiating, communicating), and cognitive skills (e.g., problem solving, creativity, planning). OT practitioners evaluate the play of children to determine ways to facilitate play and enable children to play at their highest potential. In this way, OT practitioners assist children in gaining skills for adulthood.

Definition of Play

Scholars have struggled for centuries to define play.[5-7,10,23-25] Play has been viewed as:

1. A method to release surplus energy
2. A link in the evolutionary change from animal to human being (recapitulation theory),

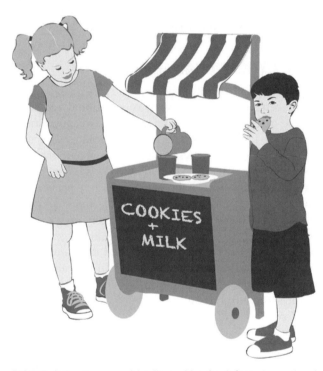

FIGURE 8-4 A young girl sells cookies (an informal vocational activity) to her friend.

3. A method to practice survival skills, and
4. An attitude or mood.[7]

More recent theories assert that play provides the stimulation needed to satisfy a physiologic need for optimal arousal.[23] Theorists describe play in terms of the development of cognitive, emotional, social, language, and motor skills.[25] These theorists propose that play develops as children learn necessary skills. For example, Piaget proposed that children's play developed from sensorimotor (practice) play to symbolic play to games with rules as the child acquires cognitive skills.[24] Table 8-3 describes Piaget's stages of play. McCune-Nicolich proposed that children engage in more make-believe play as their language skills develop.[25] (Table 8-4 provides a description of the progression of symbolic or make-believe play.) Figure 8-5 shows an 18-month-old toddler playing "dress-up" with her mother's shoes. Early theorists such as Erikson and Freud believed that children work out emotional conflicts during play.[25]

Psychoanalysts also theorized that play could be used to evaluate conflicts. Developmental theorists described the changes in play in terms of motor skill progression.[15,24] In doing so, they divided play into the categories of functional (sensorimotor), constructive (manipulative), dramatic ("pretend"), and formal (rule governed).[24] Parham identified the social aspects of play as progressing from solitary to parallel to group

TABLE 8-3

Piaget's Stages of Play

AGE (y)	STAGE
0–2	*Sensorimotor:* Practices games, exploratory behaviors, reflexive behaviors, repetition
2–6	*Symbolic:* Uses imaginary objects, pretend play
6–10	*Games with rules:* Participates in team sports, activities with flexible rules, goals

TABLE 8-4

Symbolic Play

AGE (mo)	PLAY CHARACTERISTICS
12	Play directed toward self Imitation of pat-a-cake and other movements Simple pretend play directed toward self (eating, sleeping) Imitation of familiar actions
18–24	Role-playing with objects (such as feeding a doll) Use of nonrealistic objects in pretend
24–36	Engagement in multistep scenarios (such as giving doll a bath, dressing the doll, and putting the doll to bed)
36–48	Use of language in play Advance plans and development of stories Acting out sequences with miniatures
48	Imaginary play Role-playing entire scenarios Creation of stories with "pretend" characters

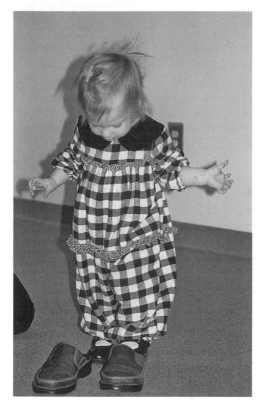

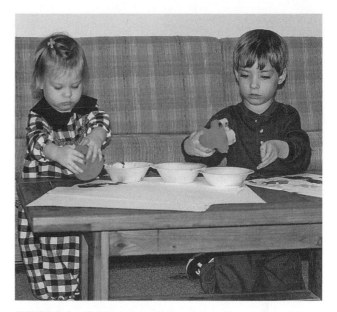

FIGURE 8-6 Children share their paints as they create pictures. They are absorbed in the play process.

FIGURE 8-5 A toddler enjoys playing "dress-up" wearing her mother's shoes, a typical activity for an 18-month-old.

play.[24] Figure 8-6 shows two children engaged in cooperative play. Play encompasses a variety of skills and occupies much of the child's day. Thus OT practitioners must have a firm understanding of its complexities. The Occupational Therapy Practice Framework defines play or leisure activities as "any spontaneous or organized activity that provides enjoyment, entertainment, amusement, or diversion."[2] OT practitioners work with children to facilitate and remediate play skills. The following section discusses OT theorists who made significant contributions to the study of play in OT practice.

Occupational Therapy Theorists and Their Contributions to Play

Reilly

Mary Reilly, a noted occupational therapist and researcher, described play as a progression through three stages: exploratory behaviors, competency, and achievement.[25] Exploratory behaviors are intrinsically motivated and are engaged in for their own sake.[25] Infants engage in exploratory behaviors that focus on sensory experiences.[25] The second stage of development, competency, occurs when children search for challenges, novelty, and experimentation. In this stage, they often want to do everything alone and "their

way."[25] This stage is observed in early and middle childhood. The achievement stage of play emphasizes performance standards (such as winning) and competition. Children at this stage of development take more risks in their play.

Takata

Occupational therapist Nancy Takata developed *play history*, a format that helps OT practitioners obtain information about a child's play.[25] The interview format helps describe a child's play skills. OT practitioners with a solid knowledge of typical play patterns can use this information to design intervention plans.

Knox

The Knox Preschool Play Scale (PPS) was constructed by occupational therapist Susan Knox and is based on Piagetian cognitive stages and Parham's social stages.[24] The revised Knox PPS divides play into four domains: space management, material management, imitation, and participation. The scale provides age equivalents for each domain and an overall play age. This scale is easy to administer and provides information on the motor skill requirements for play.

Bundy

Professor and occupational therapist Anita Bundy designed the Test of Playfulness (ToP) to objectively measure playfulness.[6,7] Bundy found that a child's attitude about and approach to activities (i.e., playfulness) provide valuable information to OT practitioners. Some children who do not possess the skills for play may still be playful. Others have the skills but do not

TABLE 8-5

Toys and Play Activities for Various Ages

AGE (y)	TOYS AND ACTIVITIES
0–1	*Manipulative, sensory:* rattles, musical sounds, bells, swings, soft toys, boxes, pots and pans, wooden spoons, books
1–2	*Movement, manipulative, sensory:* push–pull toys, balls, pop-beads, pop-up toys, toy phones, musical books, noisy toys, ride-on toys, trucks, cause and effect toys
2–4	*Pretend play, movement, manipulative, sensory:* dolls, trucks, action figures, Play-Doh, markers, water play, balls, blocks, Lego, books, dress-up toys, hats, shoes, clothes, tricycles
4–6	*Pretend play, craft activities, movement:* swings, gyms, bicycles, scooters, ball games, beads, painting, Play-Doh, arts and crafts, dolls, cooking, group games (e.g., follow-the-leader, tag, red rover)
6–8	*Pretend play, craft activities, movement:* gymnastic play, jumping rope, coordinated games (e.g., keep-away with ball), arts and crafts, wood kits, model airplanes, painting, drawing, skating, bike riding, swimming
8–10	*Movement, group games, manipulative:* basketball, baseball, soccer, bike riding, skateboarding, tennis, swimming, volleyball, arts and crafts requiring more skill, cooking, collecting
10	*Movement, games that challenge, skilled manipulative resulting in products:* competitive sports, sewing, knitting, woodworking, bowling, walking, going to the beach, flying kites, boating, camping, reading

appear to be having fun. The ToP examines the context in which children perform play activities.[6,7] For example, two 4-year-old boys playing "Godzilla" may engage in rough and tumble "fighting." Because the context of the fighting is play, the children are not being mean spirited or hurtful. They are clearly playing and not fighting.

Play Skill Acquisition

Children acquire play skills as they mature and develop, and play affords opportunities for development. For example, a child needs balance and coordination to ride a bike. At the same time, riding the bike improves the child's balance and coordination. Table 8-5 provides an outline of toys and play activities suitable for different age groups.

Infancy

Infants explore the environment and learn through their senses.[14] They enjoy visual, tactile, auditory, and movement sensations.[6] Toys with bells and noise encourage infants to explore the environment.[15] Play should focus on enhancing their capabilities while furnishing new opportunities for exploration. OT practitioners and caregivers must allow children to repeat activities until they have mastered them.[24] Infant play encourages body awareness. They typically explore their hands and feet spontaneously. Playing games such as pat-a-cake helps them understand that their bodies are fun, as does face-to-face play with an adult.[14] Peek-a-boo is a favorite game at this age. Enjoyable toys encourage mobility, elicit actions, increase motor skills, and facilitate natural creativity.

Parents and caregivers establish bonds with infants by playing comfortably with them. Adults must respond to the infants' cues. Cues that indicate stress include crying, hiccups, gaze aversion, yawning, finger splaying, and tantrums.[5] When infants cry or show signs of stress, they should be comforted and the type of play changed. OT practitioners should remember that play is fun.

Early Childhood

Continued exploration and the development of friendships accentuate childhood play.[6,14] Play provides children with opportunities to learn negotiation, problem-solving, and communication skills. Figure 8-7 shows children challenging their skills in play. Play in early childhood helps children develop and refine motor skills.[6,14] Consequently, adults should be cautious about intervening too quickly during play. Children need opportunities to work out differences among themselves.

Children enjoy manipulative play, imitation, games, and social play with other children of the same sex.[6] They enjoy dramatic and rough and tumble play.[6,25] Role-playing scenarios that facilitate dramatic play stimulates a child's imagination, creativity, and problem-solving abilities.

Middle Childhood

Middle childhood is a time of refinement of skills, such as speed, dexterity, strength, and endurance. Children become more competent in play activities. They enjoy games with rules and competition. Childhood is a time for them to experiment with many play activities. Some of these activities are easy, whereas others are difficult. Children should be encouraged to play, have fun, and realize that everyone has different talents. This is all part of growing up and finding their identities.

Adolescence

Adolescents are in search of independence.[5] Parents need to facilitate socially appropriate play and leisure activities.

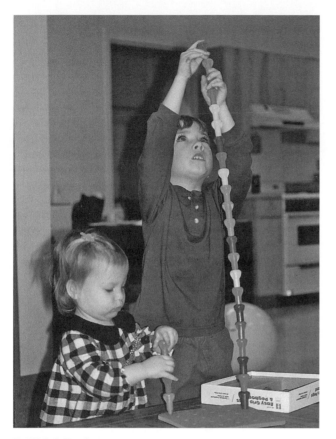

FIGURE 8-7 Children challenge their motor, social, and cognitive skills during play. They must use their fine motor skills to build a tower.

Adolescents enjoy activities in which they can participate with peers.[5,14] They may wish to participate in school or community clubs. OT practitioners and parents need to listen carefully to adolescents to help them discover their goals and talents. At this stage of development, play is beneficial in the establishment of independence.

Developmental Relevance of Play and Leisure

Play is important in each stage of development. It provides children with opportunities to develop motor, social–emotional, cognitive, and language skills. Play also allows children to interact with others, challenge themselves, and identify their own strengths and weaknesses; therefore, play contributes to the quality of life. Play and leisure remain important throughout a person's life. People engage in play and leisure activities because they enjoy them and are intrinsically motivated to participate in them.

SOCIAL PARTICIPATION

Social participation includes organized patterns of behavior expected of a child interacting with others within a given social system, such as the family, peer group, or community.[2] Children with disabilities or special needs are members of a family system. Interventions that have an impact on one member of the family system do so on all members of that system. Therefore it is important for OT practitioners to understand the family system. (Chapter 2 provides a detailed description of the patterns associated with the family system.) Likewise, peers can positively or negatively influence a child's willingness to perform a task.[27] For example, if peers ridicule an adaptive device, it will not be used by the child. Consideration of the child's social routines and cultural and physical contexts is critical in determining the appropriate intervention techniques. Understanding the issues faced by children with disabilities or special needs may help OT practitioners to better address social participation needs. Children may experience limited access to activities because of a disability. Many parents cite lack of adequate supervision or trained staff as factors that prevent them from allowing their children with special needs to participate in afterschool events. As children develop a desire to socialize with peers away from the family, new issues arise. For example, competitive sports and activities become more valued in the middle school and high school years. Children with special needs may, however, be excluded from these activities. OT practitioners who are aware of leisure and social events that include all children are a great resource for children and families. Other issues interfering with social participation of children with disabilities include lack of transportation, excessive costs, and inaccessibility of the event. For example, children who are in wheelchairs require special transportation that may not be readily available in rural communities. When asked about his social life in middle school, one adolescent remarked, "I can go to dances after school; a special bus brings me home. That's cool—I like that." However, he later remarked, "But I can't go to the store with the other kids and my brother on the weekends. My mom won't let me ride my wheelchair on the road. There is no good sidewalk for me, and the cars drive too fast."

SUMMARY

The ADLs of feeding and eating, dressing and undressing, personal hygiene and grooming, and toilet hygiene are the most basic tasks learned by children as they grow and mature. The IADLs of home management, community mobility, and caring for others are critical to the child's development and ability to be active outside the home. The specific age at which young children develop independent ADL and IADL skills varies according to the family's cultural expectations, opportunities for practice, and the child's motivation for independence. OT practitioners are in an excellent position to teach parents and teachers ways to facilitate the development of self-care skills in children.

Education, work, sleep, and rest are considered occupations addressed by OT practitioners. Although all children and adolescents participate in educational tasks, great variability exists in the ways they participate in home management activities, the care of others, and vocational activities. Children must develop readiness skills (both motor and psychosocial) for work. Sleep and rest patterns are essential occupations to maintain performance and health.

Play and leisure activities provide the foundation for problem solving, skill development, social interaction, and negotiating. OT practitioners can play a key role in teaching parents, teachers, and peers ways to play and be playful with children with special needs. OT practitioners assist children who have disabilities in developing play skills so they may reach their potential.

OT practitioners must have firm knowledge of the occupational areas of daily living, education, work, play and leisure, rest and sleep, and social participation to effectively work with children and their families. OT practitioners use their knowledge of the contexts in which activities occur to design appropriate interventions. Finally, the ability to analyze each of the areas of occupation through activity analysis is essential to effectively work with children and adolescents.

References

1. *American Heritage Dictionary* (2011). (5th ed.). Boston: Houghton Mifflin.
2. American Occupational Therapy Association. (2014). Occupational therapy practice framework: domain and process (3rd ed.). *Am J Occup Ther*, 68(Suppl. 1), S1–S48.
3. American Occupational Therapy Association. (2007). Specialized knowledge and skills in feeding, eating, and swallowing for occupational therapy practice. *Am J Occup Ther*, 61.
4. Bazyk, S., & Cahill, S. (2015). School-based occupational therapy. In J. Case-Smith, & J. O'Brien (Eds.), *Occupational therapy for children and adolescents* (7th ed.). (pp. 664–703). St. Louis, MO: Mosby.
5. Berger, K. S. (2011). *The developing person through the lifespan* (9th ed.). New York: Worth Publishers.
6. Bundy, A. C. (1993). Assessment of play and leisure: delineation of the problem. *Am J Occup Ther*, 47, 217.
7. Bundy, A. C. (2010). Play and playfulness: What to look for. In L. D. Parham, & L. S. Fazio (Eds.), *Play in occupational therapy for children* (2nd ed.). St. Louis, MO: Mosby.
8. Case-Smith, J. (2004). Self-care strategies for children with developmental deficits. In C. Christiansen, & K. Matuska (Eds.), *Ways of living: self-care strategies for special needs* (3rd ed.). Bethesda, MD: American Occupational Therapy Association.
9. Clark, G. F. (1993). Oral-motor and feeding issues. In C. B. Royeen (Ed.), *AOTA Self-study series: classroom applications for school-based practice.* Rockville, MD: AOTA.
10. Johnson-Martin, N. M. (2004). In *The Carolina curriculum for infants and toddlers with special needs* (3rd ed.). Baltimore, MD: Paul H. Brookes.
11. Klein, M. D. (1999). *Pre-dressing skills: skill starters for self-help development.* Tucson, AZ: Communication Skill Builders.
12. Klein, M. D., & Delaney, T. A. (2006). *Feeding and nutrition for the child with special needs: handouts for parents.* Tucson, AZ: Therapy Skill Builders.
13. Korth, K., & Rendell, L. (2015). Feeding intervention. In J. Case-Smith, & J. O'Brien (Eds.), *Occupational therapy for children and adolescents* (7th ed.). (pp. 389–460). St. Louis, MO: Mosby.
14. Linder, T. W. (2008). *Transdisciplinary play based assessment* (2nd ed.). Baltimore, MD: Paul H. Brookes.
15. Kids Health. (n.d.). All about sleep. http://kidshealth.org/parent/growth/sleep/sleep.html?tracking=P_RelatedArticle.
16. Reference deleted in proofs.
17. Lorens, L. A. (1976). *Application of a developmental theory for health and rehabilitation.* Rockville, MD: AOTA.
18. Lowman, D. K., & Lane, S. J. (1999). Children with feeding and nutritional problems. In S. Porr, & E. B. Rainville (Eds.), *Pediatric therapy: a systems approach.* Philadelphia: FA Davis.
19. Lowman, D. K., & Murphy, S. M. (1999). *The educator's guide to feeding children with disabilities.* Baltimore, MD: Paul H. Brookes.
20. Morris, S. E., & Klein, M. D. (2000). *Pre-feeding skills: a comprehensive resource for mealtime development* (2nd ed.). Tucson, AZ: Therapy Skill Builders.
21. Murphy, S. M., & Caretto, C. (1999). Anatomy of the oral and respiratory structures made easy. In D. K. Lowman, & S. M. Murphy (Eds.), *The educator's guide to feeding children with disabilities.* Baltimore, MD: Paul H. Brookes.
22. Murphy, S. M., & Caretto, C. (1999). Oral-motor considerations for feeding. In D. K. Lowman, & S. M. Murphy (Eds.), *The educator's guide to feeding children with disabilities.* Baltimore, MD: Paul H. Brookes.
23. Orelove, F. P., Sobsey, D., & Silberman, R. (2004). *Educating children with multiple disabilities: a collaborative approach* (4th ed.). Baltimore, MD: Paul H. Brookes.
24. Parham, L. D., & Primeau, L. (2010). Play and occupational therapy. In L. D. Parham, & L. S. Fazio (Eds.), *Play in occupational therapy for children* (2nd ed.). St. Louis, MO: Mosby.
25. Reilly, M. (1974). *Play as exploratory learning: studies in curiosity behavior.* Beverly Hills, CA: Sage.
26. Rubin, K., & Fein, G. G. (1983). Play. In P. H. Mussen (Ed.), *Handbook of child psychology* (4th ed.). New York: Wiley.
27. Santrack, J. W. (2011). In *Life span human development* (7th ed.). Florence, KY: Cengage Learning.
28. Shepherd, J. (2015). Activities of daily living and sleep and rest. In J. Case-Smith, & J. O'Brien (Eds.), *Occupational therapy for children and adolescents* (7th ed.). (pp. 416–460). St. Louis, MO: Mosby.

REVIEW *Questions*

1. Describe the developmental sequence of oral motor control, feeding, and eating skills.
2. Which foods and utensils are appropriate for children at various ages?
3. List the developmental sequences of dressing and undressing, toilet hygiene, grooming, bathing and showering, and oral hygiene.
4. What are the sleep and rest patterns for infants and children?
5. Provide examples describing the progression of play skills.

6. Which terms describe play?
7. Describe the contributions of Reilly, Takata, Knox, and Bundy to the study of play in occupational therapy.
8. What is the difference between formal and informal work and productive activities? Give an example of each.
9. List the readiness skills expected of a child entering kindergarten. Why are these skills important?

SUGGESTED *Activities*

1. In a small group, list and discuss examples of how different cultural expectations might affect the development of self-care skills.
2. Visit a local child-care center.
   a. Observe preschool children of different ages eating lunch. What similarities and differences do you notice?
   b. Note all the different ways you see children putting on their coats.
   c. Visit a day-care class of 2 year olds. How many children are in diapers? How many are toilet trained?
3. Participate in play with an infant, a child, and an adolescent. Describe the ways their play differed.
4. Watch a child playing for 15 minutes. Describe the way Reilly, Knox, Takata, and Bundy would describe the child's play.

5. Describe your favorite play activities as a child, adolescent, and adult. Record the setting, materials, group members, and feelings. Share your activities with classmates. How are the activities similar? Different?
6. In a small group, discuss your recollections of your formal education. In what ways do your stories differ and at what age?
7. Make a log of home management, care of others, and vocational activities that you remember engaging in as a child and adolescent. Compare logs with classmates.
8. Research different sleep routines and develop a variety of home programs. Describe the aspects of sleep and rest that must be considered when developing a plan.

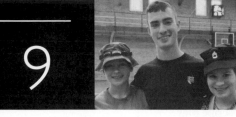

9

KERRYELLEN G. VROMAN

Adolescent Development: Becoming an Adult

CHAPTER *Objectives*

After studying this chapter, the reader will be able to accomplish the following:

- Describe the physical, cognitive, and psychosocial development of adolescents.
- Recognize the interrelationship between health and adolescent development.
- Identify the role and responsibilities of the occupational therapy practitioner in facilitating the adolescent client's healthy transition to young adulthood.
- Apply knowledge of development to the choice of therapeutic activities, interventions, and strategies used with adolescent clients.

CHAPTER *Outline*

Occupational therapy (OT) practitioners working with adolescents in the 21st century find their role both rewarding and frustrating. There are times when one is surprised, saddened, delighted, distressed, but seldom bored. Flexibility, a sense of humor, the capacity to see strengths before weaknesses, and the ability to recognize and validate positive change and acquisition of occupational performance skills, and to constructively and consistently establish boundaries, are desirable attributes when working successfully with adolescents. Equally important is the clinical reasoning required to identify and integrate an adolescent's developmental and health needs into OT evaluation and occupation-based interventions.

Today's American adolescent population is diverse (Box 9-1).[68] This chapter describes adolescent development and the occupations that are vital to an adolescent's transition from childhood to early adulthood. Case studies illustrate the role of cognitive, physical, and psychosocial development in the choice and delivery of OT services. The practitioner integrates all these areas of development to view adolescence as a dynamic interrelated process of growth. The practice guidelines included in this chapter assist the reader in applying the principles of adolescent development. It is essential to consider the unique work setting and to individually apply this information to each adolescent.

ADOLESCENCE

Most definitions of adolescence attempt to capture the distinct physical, emotional, and social changes that characterize this turbulent stage of human development. Writing in her diary, young Anne Frank voiced her experience of adolescent angst.

"They mustn't know my despair, I can't let them see the wounds which they have caused, I couldn't bear their sympathy and their kind-hearted jokes, it would only make me want to scream all the more. If I talk, everyone thinks I'm showing off; when I'm silent they think I'm ridiculous; rude if I answer, sly if I get a good idea, lazy if I'm tired, selfish if I eat a mouthful more than I should, stupid, cowardly, crafty, etc. etc."[22]

Adolescents experience a full spectrum of emotions: elation and joy; overwhelming loneliness; laughter and fun; seemingly unbearable emotional pain, anger, and frustration; and embarrassment. Supreme confidence and a sense of immortality contrast with moments of hopelessness, which they perceive as lasting an eternity. They experience the closeness of friendships and discover the pleasure of intimacy. They have intense passions, often reinforced and heightened by the mass media for music, video games, sports, or other interests, which for a week, a month, or a year are all absorbing.

Adolescents also have remarkable creativity, energy, compassion, and potential. The teenage years are a time of exploration, idealism, and cynicism. They will make some of the most important decisions of their lives. Ideally, they will plan and prepare for their futures, develop positive attitudes and make healthy, safe, behavioral choices.

STAGES OF ADOLESCENT DEVELOPMENT

The term *adolescence* defines the psychosocial development that occurs during puberty. However, there is little agreement about the ages at which adolescence begins

---

BOX 9-1

Quick Facts: U.S. Teenagers

- In the United States (2012 Census), there were 20.6 million teens between the ages of 10 and 14 years and 21.2 million between the ages of 15 and 19 years. One third of the U.S. population (31.2 million) are adolescent-young adults
- The adolescent population is increasingly becoming more diverse racially and ethnically than the profile of the general population. White non-Hispanic adolescents make up 52.2% and this figure is expected to drop below 50% by 2050; 16.5% are Hispanic; 13.6% are black non-Hispanic; 3.9% are Asian; and 0.9% are American Indian/Alaskan Native (www.census.gov/ipc/www/usinterimproj/).
- More than half of all adolescents live in suburban areas of the United States; the highest percentage of adolescents aged 10 to 19 live in the South (35.6%), followed by the Midwest, West, and East at 23.5%, 22.7%, and 18.1%, respectively.
- In 2004, 10.3% of adolescents between the ages of 16 and 24 years were not enrolled in school and did not have a high school credential. More boys (12%) than girls (9%) dropped out of high school (2004).
- One-third of high school students are working.
- Almost 16% of all adolescents aged 10 to 17 years lived in families with incomes below the poverty threshold ($19,971 per year in 2005, for a family of four). An additional 20% of adolescents lived in families near poverty. Black and Hispanic adolescents are more likely to experience poverty.
- In 2005, 25% of white non-Hispanic adolescents, 60% of non-Hispanic black adolescents, and 35% of Hispanic adolescents lived with a single parent (mother or father).

Data from: U.S. Census Bureau, Current Population Survey, Annual Social and Economic Supplement, 2012, Internet release data December 2013. http://www.census.gov/population/age/data/2012comp.html U.S. Census Bureau. (2012, December 12). U.S. Census Bureau projections show a slower growing, older, more diverse nation a half century from now. census.gov/newsroom/releases/archives/population/cb12-243.html. U.S. Department of Health and Human Services, Health Resources and Services Administration, Maternal and Child Health Bureau. (2013). Child Health USA 2012. mchb.hrsa.gov/chusa12/pc/pages/ruc.html.

and ends. This chapter uses the most commonly agreed on period of adolescence, 10 to19 years. By age 19, most young people have completed high school; they are experiencing living outside the family home; and they are pursuing divergent paths (e.g., work, college, parenting, or military service) to adulthood. However, the transition to adulthood often continues through the ages of 20 to 24, and these years of young adult life often are included as part of a continuum of adolescence. Therefore the chapter also includes some data related to this age group.

Physical maturation and psychosocial development shape the adolescent's capacities to think, relate, and act as a future adult. This development affects and is influenced by adolescents' choices of occupations and the quality of their occupational performance. The end of adolescence is marked by the legal status of adulthood with all its rights and responsibilities. OT practitioners understand development as a maturational process, which is observed in the age-related tasks and occupational performance challenges that adolescents undertake. These developmental tasks include seeking independence from parents; learning and adopting the norms and lifestyles of peer groups; accepting the physical and sexual development of one's body; and establishing sexual, personal, moral, and occupational identities. If successfully achieved, these developmental tasks result in a sense of well-being, whereas failure leads to further life difficulties.[37] For example, the adolescent is proud to graduate high school and make plans about the future (Figure 9-1).

However, developmental tasks do not stand alone, and they are best understood when viewed in the context of adolescents' sociocultural and economic environments. Table 9-1 provides an overview of the physical cognitive, and psychosocial development that occurs in adolescence.

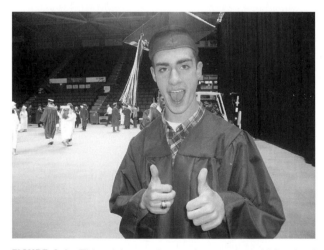

FIGURE 9-1   This adolescent is proud to graduate high school and make decisions about his future.

TABLE 9-1

Summary of Adolescent Development

TYPE OF DEVELOPMENT	DESCRIPTION
Physical	Skeletal growth spurt
	Growth in muscle mass and strength
	Growth and maturation of reproductive organs
	Growth of secondary sex characteristics; pubic and body hair
	Advanced motor and coordination skills
	Boys:
	Significant increased muscle mass
	Onset of sperm production and ejaculation
	Girls:
	Development of female body shape, including breast development
	Menarche
Cognitive	Increased capacity for abstract thinking—logical thinking
	Advanced reasoning— hypothetical deductive reasoning
	Development of impulse control— emotional self-regulation
	Increased ability to assess risks and consequences versus rewards
	Increased problem-solving skills
	Improved use and manipulation of working memory
	Improved language skills, especially in girls
	Future-oriented planning and goal setting
	Increased capacity to cognitively regulate emotional states
	Emergence of moral reasoning—conventional level of morality
	Greater ability to perceive others' perspectives
	Focus on role obligations and how one is perceived by others
	Questioning of values of parents and institutions
Psychosocial	Emotional separation from parents
	Exploration of interests, ideas, and roles
	Experimentation related to interests and preferences
	Formation of personal identity
	Identification with a peer group
	Exploration of romantic relationships
	Development of a sense of one's sexuality
	Developing sexual orientation
	Establishing occupational identity for future worker role

Adapted from Hazen, E., Schlozman, S., & Beresin, E. (2008). Adolescent psychological development: a review. *Pediatr Rev, 29*, 161.

PHYSICAL DEVELOPMENT AND PUBERTY

Physical development is the result of significant biological changes. Adolescents gain approximately 50% of their adult weight and 20% of their adult height during this rapid period of physical growth. This dramatic increase in height and weight and changes in body proportions occur as the result of a complex regulatory process, involving pituitary gland initiation of the release of growth and sex-related hormones from the thyroid, adrenal glands, and ovaries or testes.[14]

Due to individual differences, growth varies in onset and duration. The average growth period lasts about 4 years. It can begin as early as when the child is 9 years old, and in some adolescents, it may continue to around age 17. In the United States the average peak of growth for girls occurs around age 11, and they usually reach their full height 2 years after they begin menstruating. In boys, age 13 is typically the time of peak growth. Skeletal growth and muscle development result in an overall increase in strength and endurance for physical activities. Bones grow; increase in length, width, strength; and change in composition. This skeletal growth is not consistent; head, hands, and feet reach their adult size earliest. Bones calcify, replacing the cartilaginous composition of bones making them denser and stronger.

During this period of bone growth, muscles also increase in size and strength. Strength is greatest around 12 months after an adolescent's height and weight have reached the peak. The related development in coordination and endurance results in an overall improvement in skilled motor performance.[14] These gains in muscle mass and increased capacity in heart and lung functions are greatest in boys, and their performance peaks around 17 to 18 years of age.[12] The difference between the sexes in strength and gross motor performance continues throughout adulthood.

Girls show an increase in motor performance earlier, around the age of 14 years. It also includes enhanced speed, accuracy, and endurance. However, motor performance changes in girls are highly variable. A complex interaction of physical and social factors such as their musculoskeletal development and menses as well as their interest, motivation, participation, and attitude toward physical activities influence their motor performance and response to their physical abilities.[12]

Many adolescents find social confidence in fitting within the "typical" pattern of physical development. They derive comfort in being similar to their peers, but there are also advantages in physical competence in sport activities that build **self-esteem** and enhance social status. Rappelling is a challenging activity that may help adolescents develop self-esteem (Figure 9-2). In particular, early-maturing boys are more likely to be described as being popular, well adjusted, and leaders at school and in social groups. These adolescents often are more concerned about being liked and adhering to rules and routines than later-developing boys. However, there is a downside to early physical development; it brings about the expectations of coaches, parents, and peers to excel in physical activities. This unwelcome pressure can lead to anxiety. In contrast, late-maturing boys are reported to feel self-conscious about their lack of physical development.[56] A comparable pattern of early physical competence and increased social status is not observed in girls.

Puberty

Puberty, the biological process of sexual reproductive maturity that occurs with the rapid physical growth of adolescence, is controlled by a complex interactive feedback loop involving the pituitary gland, hypothalamus, and the gonads (ovaries in girls and testes in boys). Similar to physical growth, the age of puberty varies by as much as 3 years.[51,56]

In puberty, specific changes occur in the sex organs. Menstruation begins in girls; the penis and testicles increase in size in boys. Race, socioeconomic status, heredity, and nutrition influence menarche in girls. Ovulation typically starts 12 to 18 months after menarche and at the peak period of physical growth.[56,58] In boys, in addition to primary sexual growth changes such as increase in the size of the penis, spermarche (first ejaculations) generally occurs between 12 and 13 years of age. At the same time that secondary sex

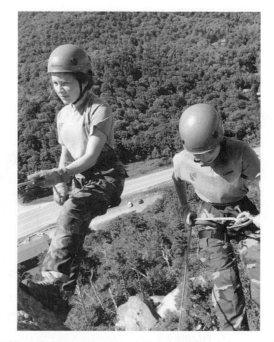

FIGURE 9-2 Rappelling is a challenging activity that may help adolescents develop self-esteem.

characteristics develop, boys experience the development of facial hair and a lower voice, and girls experience the development of breasts and areolar size changes; pubic hair develops over a 3- to 4-year period in both sexes. Many adolescents will also experience acne, but it is more common in boys (70%–90%) due to the effect of testosterone.[25,51]

Only minimal research has been conducted on puberty in adolescents with developmental and physical disabilities. Therefore little specific information exists to assist these adolescents, their caregivers, or their health professionals in understanding how puberty may differ for them.[55] Some research suggests that in girls with moderate to severe cerebral palsy, sexual maturation begins earlier or that it ends much later than in the general population.[71] Another retrospective study involving women with autism spectrum conditions reported that menstruation begins 8 months earlier (i.e., around the age of 13 years) or ends later than is typical.[36]

OT practitioners who work with adolescents, including those with disabilities and chronic conditions, need to be receptive to teen-initiated discussions and be willing to talk to them and their parents on topics ranging from physical development, sexual expression, and contraception. Referral to counselors and health care providers who offer counseling or are specialists in women or men's reproductive health can be beneficial. In addition, OT practitioners need to recognize the signs of sexual abuse (see Box 14-2 in Chapter 14).

Implications of Physical Growth and Sexual Maturation for Adolescents

An adolescent's adjustment to his or her physical and sexual development influences global self-esteem.[5,58] Family, friends, and available information are important factors that contribute to a healthy adjustment. Some adolescents accept their physical development easily, with a degree of pride, considering it a welcomed sign of their transition to adulthood. For others, these changes can be a source of confusion, anxiety, or emotional turmoil.[75]

Psychosocial development accompanies puberty, integrating physical and physiologic changes into a positive **body image.** The perception of one's own image affects a person's emotions, thoughts, and attitudes toward self and others. It influences choice of behaviors and relationships, especially intimate relationships.[10] Helping adolescents learn about their bodies, understand their feelings, express their thoughts about their bodies, and recognize that many of their peers share their experiences can contribute significantly to reducing anxiety (Figure 9-3).

Adolescents compare their bodies and appearances with "ideal masculine and feminine" images (Box 9-2). This social comparison is a significant dimension of body image perception and attitude toward one's body. It is pervasive in the media and manipulated by marketing (e.g., advertisements, teen magazines, TV shows, music videos, and the fashion industry). These images bear little relationship to the ethnic or physical appearance of the diverse population of American teens or their lifestyles. Therefore it is not surprising that many adolescents struggle with their physical images and are critical of their bodies.[9,13]

CLINICAL *Pearl*

Information about sex education as it relates to people with disabilities can be found at sites such as www.sexualhealth.com and the National Information Center for Children and Youth with Disabilities (NICHCY) (http://www.parentcenterhub.org/repository/sex-ed-deaf-blind/ and https://nationaldb.org/library/list/61).

CASE *Study*

Alisha is an attractive 14-year-old girl, 5 ft. 3 in. tall. Her outward appearance to her friends, family, and teachers is that of a successful adolescent. She achieves good grades, plays in the high school band, and is a member of the dance team. However, in the past 6 months she has become increasingly

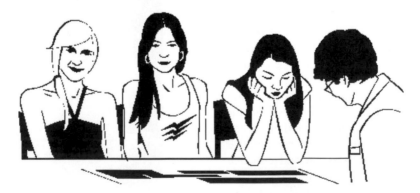

FIGURE 9-3 Adolescent girls take part in a group to develop body awareness, understand feelings, express thoughts and feelings, and recognize that others share their feelings. (From O'Brien, J., Solomon, J. (2012). *Occupational analysis and group process.* St. Louis: Mosby.)

BOX 9-2

Healthy Development of Body Image

The practitioner may observe the following behaviors in the early and middle years of adolescence. These behaviors are typical of an adolescent concerned with developing a positive body image.

EARLY ADOLESCENTS

- Evaluate physical attractiveness and explore self-identity with single mindedness.
- Make comparisons between their bodies/appearances with those of others, especially those portrayed in the media.
- Have interest in and anxiety about their sexual development.

MIDDLE ADOLESCENTS

- Have achieved most of the physical changes associated with puberty and are developing an acceptance of their bodies.
- Are less preoccupied with their physical changes, and their interest now is oriented on developing their appearance, grooming, and "trying to be attractive."
- Eating and other body image—related disorders develop and are established.

Adapted from Radizik, M., Sherer, S., Neinstein, L. (2002). Psychosocial development in the normal adolescent. In L. S. Neinstein (Ed.), *Adolescent health: a practical guide*. Philadelphia: Lippincott Williams & Wilkins.

self-conscious, especially about her developing body and about the fact that she does not have a boyfriend like her friends do. To her delight, Alisha quickly loses weight on a diet program. However, her dramatic weight loss does not change her belief that she is overweight and unattractive. She withdraws from her friends and increases her exercise routine. When Alisha's mother finds her purging after eating, she becomes concerned and takes Alisha to a psychiatrist. The psychiatrist diagnoses Alisha's condition as anorexia nervosa, a disorder characterized by a distorted self-image and a dysfunctional pattern of restricting food intake, purging, or both. (See chapter 14 for further discussion of anorexia nervosa.)

Negative body image, such as Alisha's view of herself, reflects low self-esteem. Both often are associated with mental health problems. Depression, anxiety, and body image disorders (e.g., dysphoria and anorexia nervosa) are common among adolescents. It is estimated that between 40% and 70% of girls, especially in early adolescence, are dissatisfied with two or more aspects of their physical appearance.[26] When listening to conversations among teenage girls, one is likely to hear comments such as "Do you think my backside looks too big in these jeans?" or "I'm too fat, I need to lose weight." Studies of body image report that body dissatisfaction is universal and that most girls, regardless of ethnicity, express a desire to be thin.[42]

Boys also experience dissatisfaction with their bodies. Their internalized perception of how they "should" be in relation to the images of masculinity involves greater muscle definition and muscle mass, typically in the upper body (i.e., shoulders, arms, and chest).[74]

Adjusting to these physical changes and developing a healthy body image contribute to a positive **self-concept.** This is a process of self-evaluation related to other abilities and competencies in physical activities (e.g., competitive sports). It also involves experimenting with changing one's physical appearance to express individuality. This can be simple and temporary, such as dying or cutting one's hair, or a more permanent statement such as body piercing and tattoos.

Adolescents with disabilities do not always have opportunities to make choices about their appearance and to experiment with change as part of their adolescence experience. Exploring self-image and body image is more difficult for them because they may depend on others for their self-care, may not have their own money, and often lack independence in community mobility. Maintaining their childlike status, rather than adjusting to the emotional and psychological changes and demands of adolescence, may be more comfortable for their parents. Within the framework of therapy, OT practitioners can facilitate experimentation and also support parents in their attempts to encourage typical adolescent activities.

Another dimension of physical maturation is sexual identity. Adolescents explore their sexuality and learn to form intimate relationships (Figure 9-4). Similar to physical development in strength and motor performance, early sexual maturity has social consequences. An outward appearance of sexual maturity can make adolescents seem older than their actual age, resulting in demands and expectations from peers and adults that they are not psychologically prepared to handle. As mentioned earlier, physically mature adolescents are more likely to have concerns about being liked than their later-maturing peers. Despite these concerns, they often are popular and are successful in heterosexual relationships, whereas late-maturing boys are more likely to develop inappropriate dependence, feel insecure, exhibit disruptive behaviors, and abuse substances.[25,74] Some late-maturing boys find validation in academic pursuits and nonphysical competitive activities, especially those from middle and upper socioeconomic families that value such achievement.[28] However, studies report that early-maturing girls do not fare as well as their male counterparts. They have lower self-esteem and poorer body image, and are more likely to experience psychological difficulties such as eating disorders and depression than their average maturing peers.[75] Like late-maturing boys, they also are more likely to have lower grades, engage in substance abuse (alcohol, drugs), and exhibit behavioral problems.

With sexual maturation of the body, adolescents also develop further awareness of their gender and sexual

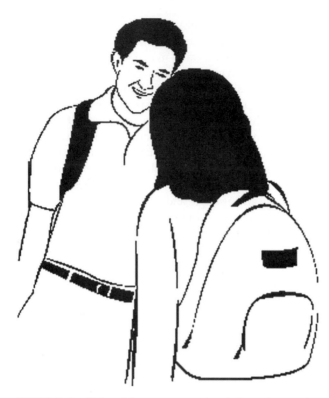

FIGURE 9-4 Older adolescents may explore intimacy in opposite-sex relationships. (From O'Brien, J., Solomon, J. (2012). *Occupational analysis and group process.* St. Louis: Mosby.)

orientation. *Gender identity* refers to a person's perception of and identification with being either masculine or feminine, which is not the same as being biologically female or male. Gender identity is subjective and internal to the individual; it is expressed through personality and how a person presents himself or herself to others.

Sexual orientation refers to a person's preference pattern of physical and emotional arousal, and sexual attraction toward others of either the opposite sex or the same sex/gender.[23] Adolescence is a time of sexual exploration, dating, and romance, and this period heightens awareness of one's sexual orientation.

Most adolescents identify their sexual orientation as heterosexual, whereas about 15% of teens in midadolescence experience an emotional and/or sexual attraction to their same sex. Approximately 5% of teens will identify themselves as gay or lesbian, but they often delay openly identifying their sexual orientation until late adolescence or early adulthood.[57] This postponement of identification as gay or lesbian is attributed to lack of support and acceptance among peers, prejudicial attitudes, and experiences of verbal and physical harassment in high school.[23]

Openness as well as willingness to discuss emerging sexuality and sexual and gender orientation is important to all OT practitioners. This openness includes using gender-neutral language (e.g., *partner* rather than *boyfriend* or *girlfriend; protection* rather than *birth control*),

inquiring if they suspect violence in intimate relations, and providing nonjudgmental support.

COGNITIVE DEVELOPMENT

The quality of thinking evolves in adolescence. Cognitive development is the evolution of mental processes: higher-level thinking, construction, the acquisition and use of knowledge, as well as perception, memory, and the use of symbolism and language.[54] Piaget, the most notable theorist of cognitive development, referred to this phase as *formal operations*, the development of logical thinking.

The development of formal operation varies among adolescents. Their ability to think becomes more creative, complex, and efficient (speed and adeptness). It is more thorough, organized, and systematic than it was in late childhood.[12] Adolescents' ability to problem solve and reason becomes increasingly sophisticated, and they develop the capacity to think abstractly (i.e., they do not require concrete examples). Initially, they are less likely to apply this more sophisticated thinking to new situations.[35,74]

The distinction between preadolescent thinking, which is characterized by consideration of possibilities as generalizations of real events, and logical thinking is the realization that the world is one of possibilities, imagined as well as real.[54] This process of thinking about possibilities without the use of concrete examples is referred to as *hypothetical–deductive reasoning* and is essential for problem solving and arguing. This type of reasoning makes it possible for a person to identify, imagine, and theoretically explore potential outcomes to determine the most likely or best one. With this newly acquired abstract thinking, adolescents develop the ability to make decisions about their behaviors that integrates values and weighs options. For the first time in their lives, adolescents begin to develop a perspective of time that is future oriented. They see the relationship between their present actions and the future consequences of these actions.

Some gender differences are present in cognitive development. On average, girls exceed boys in verbal abilities, possibly because they acquire language skills earlier. In contrast, boys tend to outperform girls in tasks that use visual–spatial skills, especially manipulating images (e.g., mental rotation). In the area of math performance, boys demonstrate skills in geometry and word problems, whereas girls excel in computational tasks.[56]

As advanced cognitive abilities become established, adolescents achieve independence in thought and action.[11] The quality of performance in academic learning activities (i.e., educational achievement) improves, and adolescents begin to consider and develop occupational skills that will translate into career and work. Personal, social, moral, and political values that denote membership in adult society also evolve. Figure 9-5 illustrates two adolescents who enjoy being part of the

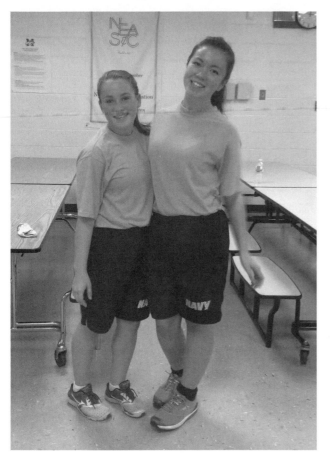

FIGURE 9-5 Organizations can help adolescents learn about political and societal values. These adolescents enjoy taking part in Navy Junior Reserve Officers Training Corps activities.

BOX 9-3

Strategies for Working with Adolescents with Cognitive Impairments

- Identify how each teen learns best. Ask the teen, family, or teachers.
- Identify strengths and build from existing skills.
- Offer specific choices ("Which of these three things would you like to do?") rather than an open-ended choice ("What would you like to do?").
- Select activities that match the teen's abilities, needs, and interests. Offer activities that are age related but are within the teen's performance level (e.g., themes that deal with developmental needs such as relationships, appearance, grooming, and self-identity).
- Break down activities into simple steps that are achievable, but still provide a challenge.
- Keep instructions simple.
- Present only one instruction or step at a time.
- Increase instructions only if the client consistently follows current directions.
- Present directions systematically.
- Use many methods of instruction (e.g., verbal instructions, demonstrations, visual cues such as pictures, step-by-step diagrams, and the hand-over-hand technique).
- Help the client develop and learn a new skill in a familiar setting before using the skill in novel settings (e.g., the community).
- Give specific feedback with concrete examples. Describe the correct or incorrect skill or behavior demonstrated. "Good" is an example of encouragement; it does not give clear feedback on performance.
- Be consistent, and use repetition.
- Do not introduce variety without a reason. Change can mean new cognitive demands for the teen and can increase the stress of learning. Flexibility and behavioral and cognitive adaptations are difficult for adolescents with cognitive impairments.

Navy Junior Reserve Officer Training Corps at school. Kohlberg, an important moral development theorist, described this level of thinking as *postconventional*.[31] It refers to the ability to base one's moral judgment on one's own values and moral standards. Adolescents comprehend the bases of laws, the principles that underpin right and wrong, and the implications of violating these principles. This development of moral and social reasoning enables them to deal with concepts such as integrity, justice, truth, reciprocity, and ambiguity.[31]

Cognition informs occupational performance. One dimension of cognition is **self-regulation**, the ability to control and monitor one's behavior and emotions relative to the situation and social cues.[1] Impulsive, ill-conceived behaviors with little or no consideration of the consequences are more characteristic of junior high school or early high school students.[34] Adolescents with mild to moderate cognitive impairments associated with head injuries, severe mental health disorders, and mild intellectual disabilities also exhibit impulsive and poor behavioral self-monitoring. They sometimes fail to comprehend the consequences of their actions or to recognize the subtle social cues used as feedback to modify responses. Difficulty in processing social cues (nonverbal body language and facial expressions) adversely influences the quality of their social interactions and ability to maintain relationships.[60] Their cognitive impairment also may result in limited problem-solving skills and poor insight as to the implications of behaviors and decisions. Box 9-3 lists some strategies for working with adolescents with cognitive impairments.

PSYCHOSOCIAL DEVELOPMENT

Psychosocial development is the essence of adolescence. There are three characteristic phases of psychosocial development:[2,56]

- Phase 1 is early adolescence during the middle school years between the ages of 10 and 13

TABLE 9-2

Typical Characteristics of Psychosocial Development

PHASE	CHARACTERISTICS
Early adolescence	Being engrossed with self (e.g., interested in personal appearance)
	Emotional separation from parents (e.g., reduced participation in family activities); less overt display of affection toward parents
	Decrease in compliance with parents' rules or limits, as well as challenging of other authority figures (e.g., teachers, coaches)
	Questioning of adults' opinions (e.g., critical of and challenging their parents' opinions, advice, and expectations); seeing parents as having faults
	Changing moods and behavior
	Mostly same-sex friendships, with strong feelings toward these peers
	Demonstration of abstract thinking
	Idealistic fantasizing about careers; thinking about possible future self and role(s)
	Importance of privacy (e.g., having own bedroom with doors closed, writing diaries, having private telephone conversations)
	Interest in experiences related to personal sexual development and exploring sexual feelings (e.g., masturbation)
	Self-consciousness, display of modesty, blushing, awkwardness about self and body
	Ability to self-regulate emotional expression; limited behavior (e.g., not thinking beyond immediate wants or needs, therefore, being susceptible to peer pressure)
	Experimenting with drugs (cigarettes, alcohol, and marijuana)
Middle adolescence	Continuation of movement toward psychological and social independence from parents
	Increased involvement in peer group culture, displayed in adopting peer value system, codes of behavior, style of dress and appearance, demonstrating individualism and separation from family in an overt way
	Involvement in formal and informal peer groups, such as sports teams, clubs, or gangs
	Acceptance of developing body; sexual expression and experimentation (e.g., dating, sexual activity with partner)
	Exploring and reflecting on the expressions of own feelings and those of other people
	Increased realism in career/vocational aspirations
	Increased creative and intellectual ability; growing interest in intellectual activities and capacity to do work (e.g., mentally and emotionally)
	Risk-taking behaviors underscored by feelings of omnipotence (sense of being powerful) and immortality; engaging in risky behaviors, including reckless driving, unprotected sex, high alcohol consumption, and drug use
	Experimenting with drugs (cigarettes, alcohol, marijuana, and other illicit drugs)
Late adolescence	More stable sense of self (e.g., interests and consistency in opinions, values, and beliefs)
	Strengthened relationships with parents (e.g., parental advice and assistance valued)
	Increased independence in decision making and ability to express ideas and opinions
	Increased interest in the future; consideration of the consequences of current actions and decisions on the future; this behavior leads to delayed gratification, setting personal limits, ability to monitor own behavior, and reach compromises
	Resolution of earlier angst at puberty about physical appearance and attractiveness
	Diminished peer influence; increased confidence in personal values and sense of self
	Preference for one-on-one relationships; starting to select an intimate partner
	Becoming realistic in vocational choice or employment, establishing worker role, and working toward financial independence
	Definition of an increasingly stable value system (e.g., regarding morality, belief, religious affiliation, and sexuality)

Data from Radizik M., Sherer S., Neinstein L. (2002). Psychosocial development in the normal adolescent. In L. S. Neinstein (Ed.), *Adolescent health: a practical guide*. Philadelphia: Lippincott Williams & Wilkins.

- Phase 2 is middle adolescence during the high school years between the ages of 14 and 17
- Phase 3 is late adolescence between the ages of 17 and 21 in the first years of work or college

Table 9-2 outlines common characteristics of each of these phases.

The critical task of adolescence is achieving a stable, multidimensional self-identity. It involves reflection to identify and integrate one's values, beliefs, and perceptions into a view of one's self as an autonomous and valued member of society. This egocentric process of self-absorption has cognitive and psychosocial dimensions. A cognitive component is the adolescents' belief that others are just as concerned about and interested in their appearances, behaviors, and activities as they are themselves. It involves thinking one is special and invulnerable. The risks and poor decisions with regard to personal safety taken by adolescents are a reflection of this egocentric thinking.

The middle years comprise the most intense period of psychosocial development during adolescence. Family activities are less interesting to adolescents, whereas peer relationships become all important (Figure 9-6). Peers become increasingly influential in the adolescent's life, which makes acceptance into peer groups highly desirable and conformity to the opinions of friends and peers likely.[56]

Late adolescence is a period of consolidation. In this phase, adolescents ideally become responsible young adults who are able to make viable decisions, have a stable and consistent value system, and can successfully take on adult roles such as worker or even parent. It is the stable, positive sense of self and awareness of one's own abilities that enables late adolescents and young adults to establish healthy relationships. In this transition from emotional and physical dependency on parents, familial relationships are reframed to reflect the adult status.

An increased vulnerability to most mental health disorders is present in adolescence. Difficulty or failure in successfully navigating psychological and social developmental tasks can have far-reaching health and social consequences. The problems an OT practitioner might observe include deterioration in school performance, dropping out of school, suicide attempts, withdrawal from social participation, self-criticizing, and self-harm. Early recognition and effective intervention are crucial.

Theoretical Stages of Identity

The hallmark of psychosocial development is the quest for self-identity. From birth, infants begin this process by establishing themselves as separate entities from their

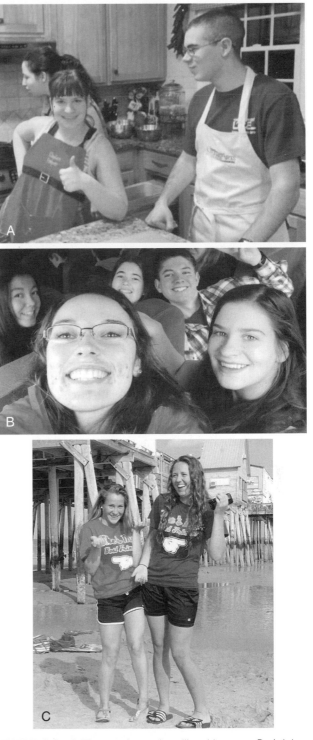

FIGURE 9-6   **A.** Teens enjoy acting silly with peers. **B.** Adolescents enjoy spending time together. **C.** Teens have special friends and enjoy socializing together.

mothers. Throughout childhood and across adult life, a person's sense of self continues to evolve, but the process is most intense in adolescence.[12]

Self-identity has two components: an individual component—"who am I as a person?"—and a contextual component—"where and how do I fit into my world?" The contextual component is one's understanding of one's relationship to others and the world.[38] The individual component is the persona from which a person relates to others and his or her environment.[44] Outwardly, a person's **identity** is visible in his or her values, beliefs, interests, and commitments to work, and the social role he or she assumes, such as daughter or parent.[44] When people believe that others value the qualities and characteristics that define them, they are more likely to experience emotional well-being.

Identity Formation: "Who Am I?"

Erik Erikson was the first developmental theorist to propose that acquiring a sense of identity (identity formation) was the foremost psychosocial task of adolescent development.[44] He theorized that one's self-identity develops through the recognition of one's abilities, interests, strengths, and weaknesses and continues to dictate how identity formation is viewed in research and clinical practice.[44] He described identity formation as crisis resolution and commitment to an identity through a complex process. The outcome, self-identity, is a composite of spiritual and religious beliefs, intellectual, social, and political interests, and a vocational or occupational commitment. It also includes gender orientation, identification with culture and ethnicity, and perceptions of one's personality traits (e.g., introverted, extroverted, open, conscientious).

Adolescents' quest for self-identity is a frequent theme in films and literature and is the angst expressed in the lyrics of popular music. Daydreams and fantasies about real and imagined selves energize and motivate adolescents as they attempt to make sense of their world. To achieve this, they experiment; they try different roles, express a variety of opinions and preferences, and make choices. They try out different activities and lifestyles before eventually settling on a set of values, moral perspectives, and life goals. Adolescents engage in introspection (internalized thinking about the self and making social comparisons between themselves and peers) and self-evaluation. They also evaluate how their family and friends view them. They set goals, take action, and resolve conflicts and problems.[38] All of these behaviors help them identify what makes them individuals.

Promoting psychosocial development is implicit in all adolescent OT services. Meeting an adolescent's psychosocial needs requires recognition of the dimensions of identity and the activities that encourage identity formation. This recognition assists OT practitioners in planning therapy interventions that encourage exploration and resolution of identity-related challenges appropriate to an adolescent's developmental state.

Adolescents' behaviors, thoughts, and emotions may seem contradictory, particularly in those between the ages of 13 and 15. Adolescents may choose healthy behaviors, become vegetarians, or participate in sports, but they may also experiment with alcohol, tobacco, street drugs, or junk food. They may explore different belief systems and argue passionately against their parents' ideological views. They may express disinterest in relationships with the opposite sex and then hang out exclusively with a girlfriend or boyfriend.

CASE *Study*

Sam has body piercings and recently got a tattoo. He frequently breaks his parents' curfew rules and is increasingly argumentative. Lately, he has been skipping classes and is talking about dropping out of his high school basketball team. At the same time, Sam has a job at his uncle's car dealership; he dresses appropriately for work and is reliable. He gets along well with his uncle, takes directions, and shows initiative.

Today's permissive and tolerant society permits adolescents a period of experimentation and exploration. To cite an example, when a teen's parents commented on her recent behavior, she retorted indignantly, "I don't have to be responsible. I am an adolescent." However, adolescents are expected to become young adults whose thinking, emotions, and behaviors are congruent with and reflect the prevailing social norms and values of their communities.

Building on Erickson's theory, developmental theorists describe identity as a series of states. They pose it as an ongoing process of negotiation, adaptation, and decision making. Marcia illustrates this perspective by describing four states of identity—*identity diffusion*, *identity moratorium*, *identity foreclosure*, and *identity achievement*—whose characteristics are different dimensions of exploration of or commitment to stable future goals.[44]

Identity diffusion, common in early adolescence, is the least defined sense of personal identity. In this identity state, an adolescent avoids or ignores the task of exploring his or her identity and has little interest in exploring options. These adolescents have yet to make a commitment to choices, interests, or values. The question "Who am I?" is not a significant issue. They tend to avoid or have difficulties meeting the day-to-day demands of life, such as completing schoolwork or participating in sports or extracurricular activities.[11] In a state of identity diffusion, adolescents seldom anticipate or think about the future. Those who continue to experience identity diffusion well into their middle and late adolescent years may demonstrate impulsivity, disorganized thinking, and immature moral reasoning.[12] Identity diffusion is associated with lower self-esteem; a negative attitude; and dissatisfaction with one's life, parents' lifestyle, and school.[12] Because they have not explored their interests or considered their strengths in relation to work, they sometimes have problems finding employment.

Identity moratorium in early and middle adolescence is emotionally healthy. It can continue into late adolescence, particularly in college students. Adolescents in this state openly explore alternatives, strive for autonomy, try out different interests, and pursue a sense of individuality. Adolescents experiencing a prolonged state of identity moratorium are likely to be undecided about the major course of study and their goals for the future and to still be actively exploring options. When the uncertainty of the moratorium state continues for too long, it is associated with anxiety, self-consciousness, impulsiveness, and depression.[13]

Adolescents who choose to avoid experiencing an identity crisis by prematurely committing to an identity, experience identity foreclosure. These adolescents do not engage in the process of self-exploration and experimentation. Without considering other possibilities, they typically accept their parents' values and beliefs and follow family expectations regarding career choices. Foreclosure is associated with approval-seeking behaviors and a high respect for authority. Compared with their peers, these adolescents are more conforming and less autonomous.[12] They prefer a structured environment, are less self-reflective, have few intimate relationships, and are less open to new experiences.[12] However, foreclosure on an identity makes them less anxious than many of their peers, who struggle with identity issues throughout adolescence.

Identity achievement, following identity moratorium, is an exploration of possibilities and the healthy resolution of the quest. It is reached in the final years of high school, in college, or in the first years of work. It is characterized by a commitment to interests, values, gender and sexual orientation, political views, career or job, and a moral stance. This relatively stable sense of self enhances self-esteem. Adolescents and young adults who attain identity achievement are autonomous, exhibit mature moral reasoning, and are independent. In resolving their identity issues, they are able to change and adapt in response to personal and social demands without undue anxiety because they are less self-absorbed, self-conscious, and less vulnerable to peer pressure. They are open and creative in their thinking.[12] A sense of identity also gives a person greater capacity for intimacy and self-regulation. Identity achievement represents congruency between a person's sense of identity, self-expression, and behavior (Box 9-4).[51]

In late adolescence, the inability to achieve a stable positive identity is associated with lack of confidence and with low self-esteem. As adults, adolescents with this issue

---

BOX 9-4

Behavioral Indicators of Self-Esteem

POSITIVE SELF-ESTEEM
- Expresses opinions
- Mixes with other teens (e.g., interacts with social group of teens)
- Initiates friendly interactions with others
- Makes eye contact easily while speaking
- Faces others when speaking with them
- Maintains comfortable, socially determined space between self and others
- Speaks fluently in first language without pauses or visible discomfort
- Participates in group activities
- Works collaboratively with others
- Gives directions or instructions to others
- Volunteers for tasks and activities

NEGATIVE SELF-ESTEEM
- Avoids eye contact
- Is overly confident; for example, brags about achievements or skills
- Acts as class clown; seldom contributes to class constructively
- Is verbally self-critical; makes fun of self as a form of humor; puts self down
- Speaks loudly or dogmatically to avoid listening to others' responses
- Is submissive and overly agreeable to others' requests or demands
- Is reluctant to give opinions or views, especially if it will draw attention to him or herself
- Monitors behaviors; for example, hypervigilant of surroundings and other people
- Makes excuses for performance; seldom evaluates personal performance as satisfactory
- Engages in putting others down, name calling, gossiping, and, at worst, bullying

---

tend to have difficulties in many areas of their lives, such as work and intimate relationships. They are challenged by the countless responsibilities and stresses of adult life.

Social Roles

A person's roles are closely associated with self-identity. Social roles have characteristics and expectations assigned to them, and are universal to a particular cohort (i.e., a group of people with similar attributes, such as age and cultural affiliations). Therefore the roles of adolescents place demands and constraints on their behaviors and define the occupational performance skills needed to successfully fulfill them. The relative importance of roles varies with age. Some roles provide social status, whereas others need to be assumed in order to transition to early adulthood; therefore, these roles influence social development, self-esteem, and identity. Examples of adolescent-specific roles that are associated with identity are sports related (e.g., jock, hockey player, cheerleader); academic (e.g., geek, nerd); have negative connotations (e.g., dork), or are associated with sexual or racial slurs. All of these roles have inferences to various sets of common behaviors, characteristics, and expectations, and they assign group membership.

Adolescents receiving OT services may have disabilities or disorders that marginalize or stereotype them. To some degree, these disabilities or disorders are roles, implying identities, and become barriers to others in recognizing adolescents' characteristics and qualities. An example is the characteristics that are stereotypical of "being disabled." Therefore a goal associated with occupational therapy is to assist adolescents with disabilities to avoid internalizing these labels as integral to their identities and to help them define themselves by their interests, values, and competencies in social and occupational roles. This is achieved by providing adolescents with choices, building skills through individualized interventions and strategies that support inclusion, and advocating for community support.[47]

Adolescents with physical disabilities deal with the paradox of striving to achieve the typical adolescent independence while remaining physically dependent on their parents or caregivers. However, an identity as a self-determining autonomous person is subjective and does not require an adolescent to be physically independent. An adolescent with a physical disability may attain emotional and psychological independence by employing an attendant caregiver, taking on the responsibility to provide instructions about meeting needs, and determining the organization of his or her own daily routine. It may involve moving out of the family home and driving a modified vehicle.

OCCUPATIONAL PERFORMANCE IN ADOLESCENCE

In this section, we discuss the occupations: work, instrumental activities of daily living (IADLs), leisure, sleep/rest, and social participation.[1] Through their participation in occupations, adolescents explore activities that capture their curiosity and reflect their values, interests, and needs. They will take on the values associated with these activities while learning new skills or improving performance skills.[19] The competence they achieve enhances their peer acceptance, social status, and self-esteem.

Work

Work that includes paid employment and volunteer activities contributes to adolescents' developing interests and values.[37] It is a setting in which adolescents interact with adults on a more equal level, have opportunities to assume responsibilities, learn work behaviors and values, and develop preferences for future areas of work/careers. Work also develops other life and social skills such as managing money, organizing time, developing a routine, working collaboratively with other people, and communicating with social groups outside family and school. The earned disposable income gives some adolescents discretionary spending and a sense of economic independence. Other adolescents assume the responsibility for contributing to family income. In late adolescence, work is a recognized societal indicator of adulthood.

Studies of work patterns report that approximately 70% of adolescents work and attend school.[4] However, regulations state that they cannot work more than 4 hours on a school day and that the evening hours of work are restricted. Although some part-time work is beneficial, excessive hours of work (i.e., more than 20 hours a week) can be detrimental. It takes time away from academics, recreation and social activities, and participation in sports, and it increases the risk for work-related injuries. It is also associated with emotional distress, sexual activity, and substance abuse at an early age.[6,72] Despite the adverse consequences, approximately 18% of high school students work 20 or more hours per week.[49] In addition to their paid employment, 26% of high school students participated in volunteer activities.[66,67] Studies have shown that adolescents who volunteer do better in school, feel more positive about themselves, and avoid risky behaviors such as substance abuse.[29]

OT programs can help adolescents effectively deal with the transition from school to work through prevocational readiness evaluations, establishment and maintenance of routines, work-site coaching, managing community mobility, and building social skills. This takes care of one aspect of the transition. Adolescents also engage in a process of developing an **occupational identity**, which combines their interests, values, and abilities in the pursuit of a realistic choice of a job or a career path. This process optimally results in a work choice that integrates psychosocial identity and matches skills, values, and interests with job requirements.

Occupational identity begins to develop in early adolescence. As abstract thinking and the capacity to think about the future develops adolescents start to fantasize about their future work. Initially, these fantasies are idealistic and combine aspirations and dreams about a possible adult self. By middle adolescence, the aspirations are more realistic, and by late adolescence, their work goals combine their interests and values with a realistic match between their performance abilities and actual job demands. Attending college or university can defer the determination of an occupational identity as it delays the transition to work.

Instrumental Activities of Daily Living

To gain competency in the instrumental activities of daily living (IADLs), adolescents gradually take on more responsibilities. It starts with personal or simple family chores, for example, cleaning one's room or emptying the dishwasher, and develops into tasks that contribute to the management of the household (e.g., mowing the lawn, doing laundry, cleaning the car, and cooking). As adolescents become more independent in these routines, they prepare meals for themselves and learn to drive or use public transport so that they can move about the community independently. Still with some parental oversight, they take on their own health management, such as taking medications, learning about health risks, and making decisions about health behaviors (e.g., smoking, having protected sex, nutrition, and personal hygiene routines).[1] They develop money management skills, beginning with activities such as shopping, and progressing to planning how and when to spend money, paying bills, or managing a credit card.

By middle adolescence, some adolescents will take on responsibilities of caring for children by babysitting and assisting with coaching or lifeguard work. With these tasks, they develop knowledge and awareness of safety and emergency procedures.[1] These roles and associated responsibilities extend their skills repertoire.

Cognitively able adolescents with physical disabilities, who are physically dependent, face unique challenges in the area of IADLs. If they are to live independently, their IADL learning involves decision making and problem solving to enable them to manage their health and finances and to acquire skills to instruct and oversee attendant caregivers who maintain their physical care and their environment. OT practitioners, along with parents, can assist these adolescents to take on these responsibilities.

An increasingly time consuming IADL of adolescents is the use and maintenance of a wide variety of communication technologies. A study of Canadian adolescents recommended that their use of technologies be seen as a continuum of personal communication (telephone and cell phone), social communication (e-mail, instant messaging, chat, and bulletin boards), interactive environments (websites, search engines, and computers), and unidirectional sources (television, radio, and print).[61] Much of adolescents' social and emotional development is associated with Internet and phone. Media literacy and positive social uses of media may enhance knowledge, connectedness, and health.[64] Data suggest many adolescents used the information communication technology applications at school and at home as resources for health care information. Furthermore, many trusted the online information, and it was reported that nearly one-fourth modified their behavior in response to information obtained.[25]

Although television remains the main medium of adolescents, research data shows that using some forms of technology especially social media is a routine occupation for children and adolescents.[65] Adolescents between the ages of 12 and 17 years engage in social networking through a variety of information communication technology platforms such as Facebook, texting, Instagram, Twitter, Snapchat, YouTube, Pandora, iTunes, and Facebook messenger. The Pew Internet project, Teen and Technology 2013, reported the following data:[65]

- 78% of adolescents own a cell phone, and 47% own smartphones
- 23% have a tablet computer, a level comparable to the general adult population
- 93% of adolescents have a computer or have access to one at home.
- 22% of adolescents log on to their favorite social media site more than 10 times a day and 50% log on to at least one social media site per day.[43]

Adolescents have digital contact with adults such as teachers and coaches via e-mail and social network sites. Girls dominate most of the content created online by adolescents; 35% of girls blog, whereas only 20% of boys do; 54% of girls post photos on the Internet compared with 40% of boys; but boys post video content more often than girls do.[41]

Adolescents have access to a vast amount of information and are connected to people beyond their immediate social network and geographic location. The benefits of the enjoyment of social networking and the use of the Internet have to be weighed against the risks involved in these activities. The use of technology integrates cognitive skills, values, and interests. Adolescents make moral decisions about the information they will access or share and the values of other teens and adults they interact with. It is important that they protect their personal identities and maintain privacy. However, they are of an age when risk taking is more likely, anticipation of consequences is underdeveloped, and problem-solving skills are inconsistent. There are negative outcomes associated with information communication technology use. Offline behaviors are also exhibited online, poor judgment and impulsivity (sexting, privacy, posting of inappropriate images and content), cyber bullying, cliques, Internet addiction especially with games, and sleep deprivation arising from excessive use or disrupted sleep.[64]

OT practitioners working with adolescents need to be comfortable with technology and familiar with social media trends. In developing an occupational profile—social media use will be a significant component. Similarly, information communication technology and technology-based activities are an appropriate for vehicle for intervention strategies, building social, cognitive, and motor occupational performance competencies, a means of expression, and social participation.[20]

Leisure and Play

American adolescents spend more than half their waking hours in free time and **leisure** activities, and the choices they make in these situations are important to their development.[39] Adolescents can use leisure activities to explore and try out new behaviors and roles, establish likes and dislikes, socialize, and express themselves within peer groups. Outside the structured school and work settings, adolescents can assess their strengths, values, interests, and positions in the social context differently through leisure activities.[70] Often in these activities, adolescents experience more personal choice, more scope for creativity, and fewer performance expectations from parents. An OT study of teens' views of leisure reported that they engage in leisure for enjoyment and describe it as "freedom of choice" and "time out."[62]

Not all leisure activities are equal. Some provide a constructive use of time and participation in organized leisure activities and promote the development of physical, intellectual, and social skills.[19] Structured leisure activities that are part of extracurricular school programs (e.g., sports teams, school band or orchestra, drama club, and cheerleading) or community-based activities such as scouts and music and dance classes involve goal-directed challenges but are also fun. These programs promote healthy development and teach skills that are associated with higher academic performance and occupational achievement.[19,30] Other outcomes for adolescents involved in extracurricular activities include an increased likelihood of attending college, better interpersonal skills, greater community involvement, and lower alcohol and drug use and antisocial behavior.[19,30] For example, boys from low socioeconomic backgrounds who exhibit low to moderate academic performance but play sports are more likely to finish high school.

Participation in physical leisure activities have long-term health advantages and are predictive of adult physical activity levels.[70] The increase in obesity and chronic health conditions in the U.S. population highlights the importance of adolescent physical activity.[36] Many high school, college, and community programs actively promote participation in physical activity as a public health objective. Despite these initiatives, the number of adolescents who engage in sports and physical activities has declined overall. Although a number of studies have identified the many factors (parents, teachers, peers) that influence an adolescent's physical activity level, friends are one of the most influential.[70] Boys are more likely to participate in and have a positive attitude toward physical activities than are girls because of the relationship between masculine identities, sports, and competition.[70]

Adolescents spend much of their unstructured time watching television and playing computer games, and these passive leisure activities have little benefit. The main

criticism is that they contribute to boredom, which is associated with a greater risk for dropping out of school, drug use, and antisocial or delinquent activities.[70] Another risk factor is the development of a lifelong pattern of sedentary leisure activities, which is associated with obesity and increased incidence of chronic health problems.

Leisure activities are a valuable therapeutic area of OT practice. Enhancing leisure and related skills, especially those related to social behavior, has other beneficial outcomes. For example, an improvement in skills related to a leisure activity may enable an adolescent to join and succeed in extracurricular school activities. Successful participation in these popular age-related groups can transfer beyond the context of therapy by building **self-efficacy** and autonomy. Furthermore, as mentioned

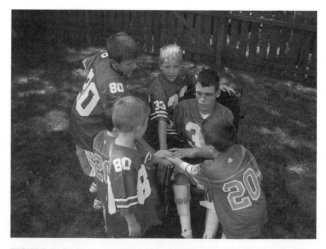

FIGURE 9-7   Adolescents with physical disabilities benefit from participating in sports with same-aged peers. (From Case-Smith, J. & O'Brien, J. (2015). *Occupational therapy for children and adolescents* (7th ed.). St. Louis: Elsevier.)

previously, extracurricular activities are positively associated with healthy life choices.

CLINICAL *Pearl*

Adolescents with disabilities have the challenge of achieving a sense of identity that constructively integrates their differences into a coherent and healthy self-concept. Labeling adolescents by using their disorder to describe them (e.g., "disabled teens") is not acceptable. Client-centered occupational therapy identifies adolescents by their abilities. Like most of their peers, self-conscious and acutely aware of themselves, adolescents with disabilities or chronic health problems want to be "like everyone else," namely, other teenagers in their social groups. The OT practitioner's role is to assist adolescents with disabilities develop personal identities that do not make their disabilities a central or defining characteristic of how they view themselves. For example, labeling Jane "the cerebral palsy student" or Doug "the disruptive student" or "the clumsy student" can encourage adolescents to shape their identities around the labels they hear. As a consequence of this behavior of others, they will set limits on themselves rather than focus on their abilities and characteristics that make them more like other adolescents. Identifying and developing performance skills enhance self-efficacy and self-esteem, which, in turn, promotes a positive sense of self.

Sleep and Rest

In the Occupational Therapy Practice Framework, sleep is identified a distinct area of occupations. Sleep is a vital biological and physiologic process to the health and well-being at all ages.[2] However, despite a need for sleep in adolescence, social, psychological, and biological factors interact resulting in many adolescents experiencing a sleep deficit and some experiencing sleep problems.[45] Lack of sleep has an accumulative effect. Short sleep duration, long sleep-onset latency (difficulty getting to sleep), insomnia, and apnea are problems reported in the adolescent population.[33] Problems with sleep are reflected in reduced occupational performance in daytime functioning, especially executive functioning, mood, and disorganization that affect performance in school activities.[16,29] Other concerns are the link between lack of sleep and car accidents or mental health problems.[29]

CASE *Study*

Luc is a 14-year-old student on the autism spectrum in the second semester of his freshman year of high school. Recently his mother has noticed that he is increasingly irritable and has emotional outbursts. He is having more difficulty organizing himself to get ready for school and his teachers report that he is less focused in the classroom. At his mother's request Luc sees the occupational therapy practitioner who is on his team and contributes to IEP. He assisted Luc and his parents with his school transitions in the past, especially his organization skills and emotional self-regulation. During the initial appointment, the team determines that Luc's sleep patterns have changed. He stays up later, sleeps less during the week, and sleeps in on the weekend, a pattern typical of adolescent boys.[18,34] As the initial step in working on his sleep routines, they decide that Luc will keep log for 1 week of his mood and outbursts and their intensity and a record of his hours of sleep.

Occupational therapy practitioners are unlikely to receive a referral for sleep/rest issues in isolation. But rather, the practitioner working with adolescents who is providing services for primary health conditions such as attention deficit-hyperactivity disorder, depression, eating disorders, autism spectrum disorder, or transition programming, will evaluate and identify sleep routines in their holistic approach. Hours of sleep needed is an individual parameter, but when the OT practitioner becomes aware of changes in behavior and mood paired with dysfunction or unhealthy sleep patterns, the approach is to work with the adolescent to self-identify the problem (e.g., a sleep diary, assistance in establishing a sleep/rest routine, and assistance in their sleep hygiene routine to achieve optimum sleep environment). According to the National Sleep Organization adolescents require 8½ to 9¼ hours of sleep daily to be healthy.[50] Because volition is important in all behavioral change, adolescents will need to be ready to change and identify their sleep habits as unhealthy before they are likely to engage in activities such as meditation, relaxation, changing patterns of information communication technology use, and in-take of stimulates (caffeine-based drinks after 4 PM) before sleep. Turning off the cell phone and other electronic devices and removing TVs from the bedroom are recommended. Similarly, creating a work-study area outside the bedroom is another beneficial strategy.

Social Participation

Social participation, which involves patterns of behavior and activities expected of an individual, is an important area of occupational performance. Social integration, a sense of belonging, acceptance, and friendships, all play a significant role in an adolescent's emotional adjustment.[74] By engaging in a spectrum of social activities, adolescents explore and develop social roles and relationships.[69,70] These roles and relationships provide adolescents with social status and a social identity separate from that which is associated with their roles within their families and expands their sources of emotional and social support to include friends and nonfamily adults.[7,11]

Being part of cliques is one form of social participation (Figure 9-8). Cliques are small, cohesive groups of adolescents and have a somewhat flexible membership. They meet the personal needs of their members, who share a broad range of activities and modes of communication. They provide a normative reference for comparison with peers and significantly influence the development of social attitudes and behaviors.[7] The transition from junior high school to high school is easier with membership in supportive and peer-recognized cliques.

In early and middle adolescence, the membership of cliques initially develops spontaneously around common interests, school activities, and neighborhood affiliations. The cliques in junior high school are usually same-sex groups; in middle to late adolescence, the cliques expand to include the opposite sex. In late adolescence, cliques weaken, and loose associations among couples replace this social structure.[11]

Exclusion from social cliques has a cost. Adolescents experience exclusion as rejection, social isolation, lack of social status, and loss of opportunities to participate in the array of identity-developing activities. An adolescent who does not find his or her niche in a clique or social group is more likely to be depressed, be lonely, and have psychological problems.[11] One explanation for some adolescents joining less-constructive peer groups, such as gangs or groups that engage in illegal or antisocial activities, is their exclusion from desired social cliques or the lack of alternatives for peer-group experiences.

Marginalized adolescents excluded from social groups may experience bullying. Although the occurrence of verbal abuse is consistent across grades, physical bullying peaks in middle school and declines during high school.[32] Newer trends in bullying involve social networking sites like Facebook and other computer-mediated communication modes such as texting and e-mail. Signs than an adolescent is being bullied are loneliness, deterioration in performance (grades), and avoiding school or even dropping out.[15]

In 2000, the U.S. Department of Education issued an official statement regarding disability harassment in school.[32] That same year, the National Center on Secondary Education and Transition provided strategies for school interventions and educational programs to address and deter bullying (http://www.ncset.org). Improving an adolescent's social skills and facilitating participation in social and extracurricular activities can reduce his or her vulnerability to bullying.

Friendships are different from peer groups or clique relationships. Friendships involve openness and honesty and are equally important in an adolescent's development. Adolescents with friends are more emotionally intense and less concerned about social acceptance.[12] Friends share common characteristics: ethnicity, interests, age, sex, and behavioral tendencies. Girls generally have more friends and their friendships are closer; they perceive greater support and intimacy (sharing) than boys.[11] Boys' friendships are congenial relationships established around shared interests such as sports, music, or other common activities.

Adolescent friendships evolve over time and reflect cognitive and psychosocial development.[11] Initially adolescent friendships are between individuals of the same sex and develop around shared activities and possessions and from a closeness of mutual understanding. In middle adolescence, friendships develop around shared loyalty and an exchange of ideas. During these years, emotional intensity and sharing of confidences heighten the vulnerability in peer relationships.[12] By the latter years of adolescence, friendships evolve to incorporate both autonomy and interdependence; dependence on friends diminishes, and sharing of all activities is no longer an essential aspect of the relationship. This is partly because the focus of late adolescents shifts to developing meaningful, intimate relationships (Figure 9-9).

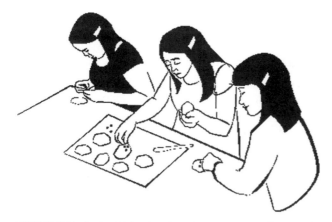

FIGURE 9-8 Junior high school students are more likely to be in same-sex cliques. (From O'Brien, J., Solomon, J. (2012). *Occupational analysis and group process*. St. Louis: Mosby.)

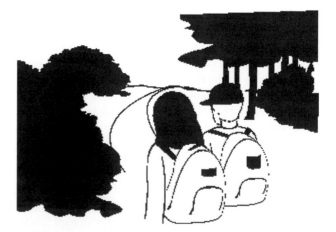

FIGURE 9-9 Intimate relationships involve private conversation. (From O'Brien, J., Solomon, J. (2012). *Occupational analysis and group process*. St. Louis: Mosby.)

Close friendships are important for self-esteem and are associated with less anxiety and depression in adolescence.[12] Social participation and closeness provide intimacy and social and emotional adjustments, which contribute to adult interpersonal skills. Adolescents talk to their friends, share concerns and fears, and learn from each other. This is important because this is a time of emotional separation from parents for most adolescents when they are apt to claim, "My parents don't understand me."

Contrary to popular opinion, major conflicts between parents and adolescents are not a normal part of the adolescent–parent relationship.[40] Stability and security provided by parents or significant adults are critical in adolescence, and for the most part, they continue to maintain a loving and respectful relationship with their parents, provided it existed even before adolescence. The physical and emotional separation from parents and the questioning of parents' values and beliefs are healthy, especially if the family context includes parental positive regard, constructive limit setting, and emotional stability. Although peer influence is mostly around tastes, interests, and lifestyle, parents' influence continues to inform goals, personal values, and morals. When child–parent conflicts exist, they occur mostly in early adolescence and are about autonomy or control. Therefore it is not surprising that adolescents in families with an authoritative parenting style exhibit competitive behaviors.

Quality relationships with adults who are not family members are beneficial to healthy adolescent development. Structured out-of-school activities, such as nonacademic extracurricular and leisure activities, provide the venue for relationships with nonfamilial adults. Adults often reflect on those positive influential experiences with coaches, adult leaders, and teachers who gave them attention during their adolescence. These activities and interactions facilitate problem solving, provide social support outside the family, increase self-esteem, and promote skill acquisition.[17] Research shows that high-risk adolescents benefit from nonfamilial relationships and that they participate less in risky behaviors (e.g., carrying a firearm or using illegal drugs).[9] A number of studies have demonstrated the value of mentoring programs such as Big Brothers and Little Sisters and participation in extracurricular activities.

THE CONTEXT OF ADOLESCENT DEVELOPMENT

This chapter, as does the OT literature, uses the terms *context* and *environment* interchangeably. These terms refer to the settings and the characteristics of the settings in which adolescents live, work, and play. The relationship between an adolescent and his or her context is reciprocal; it has an effect on what is done and how it is done. Salient contexts influence occupational performance by encouraging or supporting development. Others may compromise adolescents' development by being unsafe or by not offering the necessary resources for learning healthy behaviors and acquiring skills.

Social context comprises friends, team members, other students, parents, siblings, extended family, coaches, and teachers, who have expectations, provide support and resources, and are positive or negative role models. Physical context involves the adolescent's school, home, and community, including the socioeconomic factors and the resources that are available. Culture and ethnicity also shape the social and physical contexts.[54] Culture represents the beliefs, perceptions, values, and norms of the group. The dominant culture (mainstream American) can sometimes conflict with family culture, particularly for adolescents who belong to minority groups or immigrant families that have their own cultural, ethnic, or religious beliefs. The values of both the dominant culture and the minority culture have an internalized component related to identity and an externalized component that takes the form of expectations. Adolescents can feel torn between the desire to belong to a peer group within the dominant culture and the desire to identify with and respect the family's culture.[53]

OT practitioners working in diverse settings need to understand the social and cultural norms and expectations of adolescents' ethnic and sociocultural backgrounds. Cultural factors may influence their choices of activities and interests, self-esteem, and the expectations of their families.[53] Cultural perceptions of a disability or a disorder also may influence the family's and adolescent's therapy goals. The expectations of the adolescent's social peer context and family cultural context will together shape his or her "adaptive social and emotional development."[7]

The influence of activities on development varies because contexts may determine the relative importance and value of the activities.[30] For example, in low-income communities, success in high school sports defines a "good student," whereas in higher-income communities that value academic achievement, other types of extracurricular activities will also define a "good student."[30]

Social contexts, for example, a low-income or disorganized family, increase the likelihood of deviant or high-risk behaviors.[46] Similarly, adolescents from disadvantaged or marginalized groups may have limited access to resources and fewer positive and healthy opportunities to develop self-esteem and complex cognitive skills.[5,46] Therefore, school, therapy, and extracurricular activities may play a significant role in meeting their needs and alleviating the harmful effects of their social and home contexts. Client-centered occupational therapy can facilitate development by providing a variety of choices and opportunities for decision making; this will foster a sense of personal control and provide constructive feedback. Likewise, a therapeutic milieu can offer

TABLE 9-3

*Contextual Factors That Contribute to Healthy Adolescent Development**

CONTEXTUAL FACTOR	CHARACTERISTICS
Support	Family support, including positive parent–adolescent communication
	Parental involvement in school activities and schoolwork
	Constructive relationships with other adults
	Caring neighborhood and school environment
Empowerment	Community valuing the youth
	Adolescents given useful and valued roles in the community
	Community involving adolescents in community service activities and valuing their contributions
	Safe home and community environments
Boundaries and expectations of adolescents	Family boundaries that include rules and consequences
	School and neighborhood boundaries that include rules, consequences, and community monitoring of behavior
	Adult role models
	Positive peer influences
	High expectations—family, friends, and school expect adolescent to do well

*For additional information, see http://www.search-institute.org/content/40-developmental-assets-adolescents-ages-12-18.

adolescents opportunities for self-directed exploration in a safe, stable, and supportive environment. Acceptance, positive regard, and opportunities to make mistakes and self-correct without negative consequences (e.g., emotional or physical abuse) are all-important contextual characteristics for healthy development. Table 9-3 lists some of the contextual factors that foster adolescent self-development and skill acquisition.

NAVIGATING ADOLESCENCE WITH A DISABILITY

The estimated 23% to 35% of U.S. adolescents with chronic health conditions or special care needs experience the same development as adolescents without disabilities.[21,52] They will make the same adjustments to physical growth, puberty, psychological independence from parents or caregivers, and social relationships with the same

and opposite sexes and seek to acquire a sense of identity. However, their chronic health conditions, disabilities, and physical dependence on others create additional challenges for these adolescents and their families. Undertaking these developmental tasks such as the prerequisite of choosing a job, being out of school, working and living outside the family home are more complicated.[14,27] Parents also can find the transition challenging. Many have been the primary supports and caregivers for their adolescents and have advocated vigorously for their children's needs. However, the time has come for them to let go of the role that has dominated their lives.

Adolescents with disabilities have fewer opportunities to engage in typical adolescent experiences; to make their own choices; to engage in social relationships; or to explore the world of ideas, values, and cultures different from those of their families.[8,64,73] Yet, they need opportunities to experience and learn from successes and failures they initiate to develop a sense of self-efficacy and determine realistic goals for themselves.[63,73]

Adolescents with disabilities or chronic illnesses (e.g., cancer, diabetes) deal with additional issues: negative self-perceptions, lower expectations, and social isolation. Some confront stigma associated with their disabilities, discrimination, and environmental barriers such as lack of resources, and community accessibility.[17]

Adolescents with physical disabilities report experiencing more loneliness and feeling more isolated than their peers without disabilities. They struggle with social acceptance from peers in and out of the school setting.[18,64] Adolescents without disabilities consider their peers with physical disabilities less socially attractive and report that they are less likely to interact with them socially.[24] Even adolescents with disabilities who have good social relationships in school have less contact with friends outside the school setting than their peers without disabilities.[24]

Although most adolescents strive to be included in peer groups, those with physical disabilities may experience role marginalization. Because they are unable to perform the tasks of many typical age-related roles, they sometimes lack clear roles among their peers.[48] For example, in early and middle adolescence, the basis of social interaction often is physical play and leisure activities, which excludes adolescents with disabilities.[3] However, success in academic activities can promote better social acceptance for adolescents with disabilities.[48] Another factor is how teens with disabilities view themselves. Self-perceptions of social attractiveness and value can be a self-imposed barrier to seeking friendships or group participation. Doubt and McColl shared this account of a student whose positive self-perception promoted his inclusion in a team.[18]

"I approached the [hockey team] about being a statistician because I really wanted to get involved in the team. This is probably the closest without playing ... that I could ... plus I'm doing work for them too, so I am useful and that's a good way to get involved … and it really gives me a chance to be one of the guys finally; a secondary guy, but one of the guys, nonetheless"[18] (p. 149).

Social status among adolescents often is acquired through personal characteristics such as excelling in sports and physical attractiveness. For adolescents with disabilities, the typical access points for social inclusion and status are limited. Additionally, the personal challenge of self-evaluation based on social comparison, which is typical of all adolescents, is also present. For example, body image includes comparison with the "ideal," which is characterized by physical perfection in appearance and athletic performance. This is unrealistic for many adolescents, but especially so for those with obvious physical disabilities or motor disorders. Accepting their bodies is an important step in feeling competent in social and eventually intimate relationships. One strategy to "fit in" employed by adolescents with disabilities is an attempt to mask their disabilities, to make fun of them or themselves, or to self-exclude themselves from social groups. Their underlying motive is to make their peers without disabilities more comfortable with them despite their disabilities.

Adolescents with emotional and behavioral problems or disabilities and those from socially and economically lower backgrounds also can lack supportive environments for healthy development. Violence, poverty, school failure, sexual and emotional abuse, and discrimination negate healthy adolescent development.[73] For example, at-risk teens can have pseudoindependence (i.e., a false sense of independence). Their circumstances lead them to be prematurely independent from the support and nurturing of adults and to be without a safe and stable environment. They assume responsibility for themselves without the skills or the cognitive and psychological maturity to competently meet the demands associated with independence.

OT PRACTITIONER'S ROLE AND RESPONSIBILITIES

All adolescents from the ages of 3 to 21 with special needs are eligible for OT services under the 1975 Public Law 94-142, Education of All Handicapped Children's Act; Part B. Under the 1997 Public Law 105-17, Individuals with Disabilities Education Act (IDEA), every adolescent receiving special education services when he or she reaches age 14 requires an individualized transition plan in his or her IEP; by age 16, it should include a statement of the needed transition services, objectives, and activities. Furthermore, an amendment to the IDEA (PL105-17) expanded the scope of alternative education programs for at-risk students to include all those with disabilities and behavioral issues that need be addressed outside the mainstream educational system. The 2004 Individuals with Disabilities Improvement Education Act sought to ensure that schools and parents have the

resources they need to promote academic achievements and life skills in students with disabilities.

Mainstream as well as alternative school systems have identified the need for OT services for adolescents with cognitive deficits; sensory impairments; and physical, communicative, and behavioral disabilities who attend high schools.[14,64] Specific areas of occupations that have been identified are students' decreased participation in leisure activities and hobbies, poor time management, and poor coping skills such as self-regulation of anger and stress and unhealthy lifestyle behaviors.[14] However, the current role of the OT practitioner in the high school system often is one of consultation or periodic review and monitoring. The transition from high school provides an excellent opportunity to advocate the need for OT reassessment and collaborative interdisciplinary program planning in life and vocational readiness (prevocational) skills. The OT practitioner working in the school system or a in health care setting has an important role in assisting adolescents to participate fully in the social and academic opportunities provided by the school and the community. They work collaboratively with students, their families, and teachers to establish students' strengths and therapy needs in order to assist them to develop the life and coping skills they will need in the future.

CASE *Study*

Tom is a 15-year-old African-American youth with Down syndrome. Psychological test scores place him in the mildly intellectually disabled group under the guidelines of the fifth edition of the *Diagnostic and Statistical Manual (DSM-V)*.[3] Until he started high school, Tom had participated well in mainstream school activities, with some accommodations. However, as the cognitive demands of education increased, he began spending most of his day in a special class setting. The prioritized goals of Tom's recent IEP facilitate his transition from high school to the community and to work.

Tom and adolescents like him who have special needs require assistance to achieve most developmental milestones. OT programs within the comprehensive education plan help these adolescents acquire the performance skills needed to transition from an educational setting to the community and to a work environment. The objective is independence appropriate to their abilities. Programming would involve understanding their physical challenges and adapting their self-care routines appropriately, and training them in the IADLs. Training in social skills is particularly important because these skills are the basis for forming friendships and maintaining appropriate work relationships.[53]

In working with adolescents with cognitive impairments, an OT practitioner needs to identify the cognitive functional level of each adolescent and how this affects his or her ability to perform everyday activities. For example, in the case of Tom, his cognition affects his understanding of basic information and his ability to learn new information, which determines the number and the complexity of instructions he can follow. An adolescent's cognitive ability influences how well he or she is able to recall information, and it will determine the strategies the OT practitioner should use for teaching new skills. The goal of the OT practitioner is to optimize each adolescent's functioning at his or her full capacity. Therefore the skilled OT practitioner develops expectations, goals, and treatments that include just the "right" amount of challenge while still ensuring success. Targeting tasks appropriately to an adolescent's level includes modifying the demands of the environment to help him or her function effectively. Examples of modifications to improve function include a list of the steps to complete an activity or the use of a color-coding system for medication.

SUMMARY

Although growing up and making the transition from childhood to young adulthood is challenging, most U.S. adolescents do become healthy young adults.[59] Fundamental to an adolescent's growth and well-being is the formation of social relationships and the development of a sense of competency through participation in all areas of occupational performance. OT practitioners have the expertise and responsibility to promote the healthy development of the adolescent in the school system as well as in the health care setting. However, it will be only through the active recruitment of OT practitioners who specialize in the high school setting that adequate OT services will be provided to meet the unique needs of adolescents with special needs or disabilities.[47,62]

References

1. *American Child and Adolescent Psychiatry.* (2013). http://www.aacap.org/aacap/Families_and_Youth/Resource_Centers/Resource_Center/Home.aspx.
2. American Occupational Therapy Association. (2014). Occupational therapy practice framework: domain and process (3rd ed.). *Am J Occup Ther, 68*(Suppl. 1), S1–S48.
3. American Psychiatric Association. (2013). *Diagnostic and statistical manual of mental disorders* (5th ed.). Washington, DC: American Psychiatric Association.
4. Arnett, J. J. (2000). Emerging adulthood: a theory of development from the late teens through the twenties. *Am Psychol, 55,* 469.
5. Arnold, P., & Chapman, M. (1992). Self-esteem, aspirations and expectations of adolescents with physical disability. *Dev Med Child Neurol, 34,* 97.
6. Bachman, J. G., & Schulenberg, J. (1993). How part-time work intensity relates to drug use, behavior, time use and satisfaction among school seniors: are these consequences or merely correlates? *Dev Psychol, 29,* 220.
7. Bagwell, C. L., et al. (2000). Peer clique participation and social status in preadolescence. *Merrill-Palmer Quart, 46,* 280.
8. Brollier, C., Shepherd, J., & Markey, K. F. (1994). Transition from school to community living. *Am J Occup Ther, 48,* 346.
9. Cash, T. F., & Smolak, L. (2012). *Body image, A handbook of science, practice, and prevention* (2nd ed.). New York: The Guilford Press.
10. Cech, D. J., & Martin, S. (2002). *Functional movement development across the life span* (2nd ed.). Philadelphia: Saunders.
11. Coleman, J. C., & Hendry, L. (1990). *The nature of adolescence* (2nd ed.). New York: Routledge.
12. Conger, J. J., & Galambos, N. L. (1997). *Adolescence and youth: psychological development in a changing world* (5th ed.). New York: Longman.
13. Croll, J. (2005). Body image and adolescents. In J. Strang, & M. Story, M. (Eds.), *Guidelines for adolescent nutrition services, Center for Leadership, Education, and Training in Maternal and Child Nutrition.* www.epi.umn.edu/let/pubs/adol_book.htm.
14. Davis, S. E. (1985). Developmental tasks and transitions of adolescents with chronic illness and disabilities. *Rehabil Counseling Bull, 29,* 69.
15. Deshler, D., Schumaker, J. B., Bui, Y., & Vernon, S. (2005). *High schools and adolescents with disabilities: challenges at every turn.* http://www.corwinpress.com/upm-data/10858_Chapter_1.pdf.
16. Dewald, J. F., Meijer, A. M., Oort, F. J., Kerkhof, G. A., & Bogels, S. M. (2010). The influence of sleep quality, sleep duration and sleepiness on school performance in children and adolescents: a meta-analytic review. *Sleep Med Rev, 14,* 179–189.
17. Dirette, D., & Kolak, L. (2004). Occupational performance needs of adolescents in alternative education programs. *Am J Occup Ther, 58,* 337.
18. Doubt, L., & McColl, M. A. (2003). A secondary guy: physically disabled teenagers in secondary schools. *Can J Occup Ther, 70,* 139.
19. Eccles, J. S., et al. (2003). Extracurricular activities and adolescent development. *J Soc Issues, 59,* 865.
20. Ettel, G., Nathanson, I., Ettel, D., & Wilson, C. (2012). How do adolescents access health information? And do they ask their physicians? *Perm J, 16,* 35–38.
21. Foundation for Accountability. (2001). *A portrait of adolescents in America 2001: a report from the Robert Wood Johnson Foundation national strategic indicator surveys.* Portland, OR: Foundation for Accountability.
22. Frank, A. (1993). *Anne Frank: the diary of a young girl 1942-1945.* New York: Bateman Books.
23. Frankowski, B. L. (2004). Committee on adolescence: sexual orientation and adolescents. *Pediatrics, 113,* 1827.
24. Frederickson, N., & Turner, J. (2002). Utilizing the classroom peer group to address children's social needs: an evaluation of the circle of friends intervention approach. *J Special Educ, 36,* 234.
25. Ge, X., Conger, R., & Elder, G. (2000). The relation between puberty and psychological distress in adolescent boys. *J Res Adolesc, 11,* 70.
26. Gilligan, C., Lyons, N. P., & Hanmer, T. J. (1990). *Making connections: the relational worlds of adolescent girls at Emma Willard School.* Cambridge, MA: Harvard University Press.

27. Goldberg, R. T. (1981). Towards an understanding of the rehabilitation of the disabled adolescent. *Rehab Lit, 42,* 66.

28. Graber, J. A., Seeley, J. R., Brooks-Gunn, J., & Lewinsohn, P. M. (2004). Is pubertal timing associated with psychopathology in young adulthood? *J Am Acad Child Adolesc Psychiatr, 43,* 718.

29. Gradisar, M., Gardner, G., & Dohnt, H. (2011). Recent worldwide sleep patterns and problems during adolescence: a review and meta-analysis of age, region, and sleep. *Sleep Med, 12,* 110–118.

30. Guest, A., & Schneider, B. (2003). Adolescents' extracurricular participation in context: the mediating effects of schools, communities, and identity. *Sociol Educ, 76,* 89.

31. Hazen, E., Schlozman, S., & Beresin, E. (2008). Adolescent psychological development: a review. *Pediatr Rev, 29,* 161.

32. Hoover, J., & Stenhjem, P. (2003). *Bullying and teasing of youth with disabilities: creating positive school environments for effective inclusion.* http://www.ncset.org/publications/issue/NCSETIssueBrief_2.3.pdf. 15.03.24.

33. Hysing, M., Pallesen, S., Stormark, K., Lundervold, J., & Sivertsen, B. (2013). Sleep patterns and insomnia among adolescents: a population-based study. *J Sleep Res, 22,* 549–556.

34. Keating, D. P. (1991). Cognition, adolescents. In R. M. Lerner, A. C. Petersen, & T. Brooks-Gunn (Eds.). *Encyclopedia of adolescence:* (vol. 1). London: Garland Publishing.

35. Kemper, H. C. G. (2002). The importance of physical activity in childhood and adolescence. In L. Haynan, M. M. M. Mahon, & J. R. Turner (Eds.), *Health behavior in childhood and adolescence.* New York: Springer Publishing.

36. Kirkpatrick, J. M. (2002). Social origins, adolescents' experiences and work value trajectories during the transition to adulthood. *Soc Forces, 80*(4), 1307.

37. Knickmeyer, R. C., Wheelwright, S., Hoekstra, R., & Baron-Cohen, S. (2006). Age of menarche in females with autism spectrum conditions. *Dev Med Child Neurol, 48,* 1007.

38. Kunnen, E. S., Bosma, H. A., & VanGeert, P. L. C. (2001). A dynamic systems approach to identity formation: theoretical background and methodological possibilities. In J. E. Nurmi (Ed.), *Navigating through adolescence: European perspectives.* New York: Routledge Falmer.

39. Larson, R., & Verma, S. (1999). How children and adolescents spend time across the world: work, play and developmental opportunities. *Psychol Bull, 125,* 701.

40. Laursen, B., Coy, K. C., & Collins, W. A. (1998). Reconsidering changes in parent-child conflict across adolescence: a meta-analysis. *Child Dev, 69,* 817.

41. Lenhart, M., et al. (2007). *Teens and social media: the use of social media gains a greater foothold in teen life as they embrace the conversational nature of interactive online media.* http://www.pewinternet.org/PPF/r/230/report_display.asp.

42. Levine, M. P., & Smolak, L. (2002). Body image development in adolescence. In T. F. Cash, & T. Putzinsky (Eds.), *Body image.* New York: Guilford.

43. Madden, M., Lenhart, A., Guggan, M., Cortesi, S., & Gasser, U. (2013). *Teens and technology.* http://www.pewinternet.org/2013/03/13/teens-and-technology-2013/. 15.03.24.

44. Marcia, J. E. (1991). Identity and self-development. In R. M. Lerner, A. C. Petersen, & T. Brooks-Gunn (Eds.). *Encyclopedia of adolescence* (vol. 1). London: Garland Publishing.

45. Matricciani, L., Olds, T., & Petkov, J. (2012). In search of lost sleep: secular trends in the sleep time of school-aged children and adolescents. *Sleep Med Rev, 16,* 203–211.

46. Mechanic, D. (1991). Adolescents at risk: new directions. *J Adolesc Health, 12,* 638.

47. Michaels, C. A., & Orentlicher, M. L. (2004). The role of occupational therapy in providing person-centered transition services: implications for school-based practice. *Occup Ther Int, 11,* 209.

48. Mpofu, E. (2003). Enhancing social acceptance of early adolescents with physical disabilities: effect of role salience, peer interaction, and academic support interventions. *Int J Disabil Dev Educ, 50,* 435.

49. National Adolescent Health Information Center. (2008). *Fact sheet on demographics: adolescents & young adults.* nahic.ucsf.edu//downloads/Demographics08.pdf.

50. National sleep foundation. (nd). Teens and sleep. www.sleepfoundation.org/sleep-topics/teens-and-sleep

51. Neinstein, L. S., & Kaufman, F. R. (2002). Normal physical growth and development. In L. S. Neinstein (Ed.), *Adolescent health care: a practical guide* (4th ed.). Philadelphia: Lippincott Williams & Wilkins.

52. Newacheck, P. W., & Halfon, N. (1998). Prevalence and impact of disabling chronic conditions in childhood. *Am J Public Health, 88,* 610.

53. Oetting, E. R., & Beauvais, F. (1991). Orthogonal cultural identification theory: the cultural identification of minority adolescents. *Subst Use Misuse, 25,* 655.

54. Overton, W. F., & Byrnes, J. P. (1991). Cognitive development. In R. M. Lerner, A. C. Petersen, & T. Brooks-Gunn (Eds.), *Encyclopedia of adolescence.* London: Garland Publishing.

55. Quint, E. (2008). Menstrual issues in adolescents with physical and developmental disabilities. *Ann NY Acad Sci, 1135,* 230.

56. Rathus, S. (2008). *Childhood and adolescence voyages in development* (3rd ed.). Belmont, CA: Thomson Wadsworth.

57. Rotherman-Borus, M. J., & Langabeer, K. A. (2001). Developmental trajectories of gay, lesbian, and bisexual youth. In A. R. D'Augelli, & C. Patterson (Eds.), *Lesbian, gay, and bisexual identities among youth: psychological perspectives.* New York: Oxford University Press.

58. Santrock, J. W. (2003). *Adolescence* (9th ed.). New York: McGraw-Hill Higher Education.

59. Scales, P. C., & Leffert, N. (2004). *Developmental assets: a synthesis of the scientific research on adolescent development* (2nd ed.). Minneapolis: Search Institute.

60. Simmons, C. D., & Griswold, L. (2010). Evaluation of social interaction in a community based program for persons with traumatic brain injury. *Scand J Occup Ther, 17,* 49–56.

61. Skinner, H., Biscope, S., Poland, B., & Goldberg, E. (2003). Adolescents use technology for health information: implications for health professionals from focus group studies. *J Med Internet Res, 5,* e32.

62. Spencer, J. E., Emery, L. J., & Schneck, C. M. (2003). Occupational therapy in transitioning adolescents to postsecondary activities. *Am J Occup Ther, 57,* 435.

63. Steele, C. A., et al. (1996). Lifestyle health behaviours of 11- to 16-year-old youth with physical disabilities. *Health Ed Res Theory Pract, 11*, 173.

64. Stewart, D. A., Law, M. C., Rosenbaum, P., & Willms, D. G. (2001). A qualitative study of the transition to adulthood for youth with physical disabilities. *Phys Occup Ther Pediatr, 21*, 3.

65. Strasburger, V. C., Jordan, A. B., & Donnerstein, E. (2010). Health effects of media on children and adolescents. *Pediatrics, 125*, 756–767.

66. U.S. Bureau of Labor Statistics: Economic news release: volunteering in the United States. bls.gov/news.release/volun.htm.

67. U.S. Census Bureau. (2012, December 12). U.S. Census Bureau projections show a slower growing, older, more diverse nation a half century from now. census.gov/newsroom/releases/archives/population/cb12–243.html.

68. U.S. Department of Health and Human Services, Health Resources and Services Administration, Maternal and Child Health Bureau. (2013). *Child health USA 2012*. mchb.hrsa.gov/chusa12/pc/pages/ruc.html.

69. Vilhjalmsson, R., & Krisjansdottir, G. (2003). Gender difference in physical activity in older children and adolescents: the central role of organized sport. *Soc Sci Med, 56*, 363.

70. Widmer, M. A., Ellis, G. D., & Trunnell, E. R. (1996). Measurement of ethical behavior in leisure among high and low risk adolescents. *Adolescence, 31*, 397.

71. Worley, G., Houlihan, C. M., Herman-Giddens, M. E., O'Donnell, M. E., Conaway, M., Stallings, V. A., et al. (2002). Secondary sexual characteristics in children with cerebral palsy and moderate to severe motor impairment: a cross-sectional survey. *Pediatrics, 110*, 897.

72. Wynn, J. R. (2003). High school after school: creating pathways to the future for adolescents. *New Dir Youth Dev, 97*, 59–74.

73. Zajicek-Faber, M. L. (1998). Promoting good health in adolescents with disabilities. *Health Soc Work, 23*, 203.

74. Zastrow, C. H., & Kirst-Ashman, K. K. (2004). *Understanding human behavior* (6th ed.). Belmont, CA: Brooks/Cole, Thomson Learning.

75. Zehr, J. L., et al. (2006). Early puberty is associated with disordered eating and anxiety in young adults. *Front Neuroendrocrinol, 27*, 139.

REVIEW *Questions*

1. What physical changes occur in adolescence?
2. What cognitive changes occur in adolescents? Give examples of how these developments are seen in an adolescent's occupational performance.
3. With the maturation of the reproductive systems, what changes occur in body image?
4. What are some of the psychosocial issues for each stage: early, middle, and late adolescence?
5. What are some behavioral indicators of positive and negative self-esteem?
6. What are the characteristics of play/leisure and social participation in adolescence?
7. What are some of the issues that children with special needs may face in adolescence?

SUGGESTED *Activities*

1. Interview a teen to learn about interests, hobbies, concerns, and occupations that are important to him or her.
2. Read some teen magazines, and discuss how the themes and images in them might influence an adolescent reader.
3. Make presentations to each other on current teen trends, such as music, dress, styles, and social behaviors. Discuss cultural differences.
4. Develop a list of activities that teens enjoy that might be used in occupational therapy, and identify the relevant developmental learning of task associated with each activity.
5. Spend time alone with a teenager for a few hours, in a group and at home. How does he or she show individuality? How does his or her behavior change with context? How does he or she "fit in" in each setting?
6. View *Breakfast Club* or a similar movie that explores adolescence. Examples of other movies are *16 Candles, Angus, Can't Buy Me Love, Juno, Can't Hardly Wait, Dead Poet's Society, Fast Times at Ridgemont High, Pretty in Pink, Say Anything, St. Elmo's Fire*, and *The Outsiders*. Identify the roles, developmental stages, and tasks identified in the chosen movie. How does this movie exemplify adolescent development?
7. Compare adolescent or teen culture in the United States with that in another part of the world.

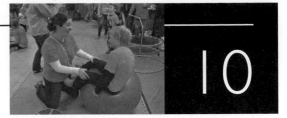

The Occupational Therapy Process

CHAPTER *Objectives*

After studying this chapter, the reader will be able to accomplish the following:

- Describe different pediatric frames of reference and practice models.
- Explain the way in which assessment informs intervention planning.
- Differentiate among long-term goals, short-term objectives, and mini-objectives.
- Apply activity analysis to intervention(s) with children and adolescents.
- Define and describe therapeutic use of self.
- Be aware of the importance of family-centered intervention and cultural diversity.
- Discuss the preparation for and process of discharge planning or discontinuation of occupational therapy services.
- Understand the top-down approach to intervention.
- Describe the tools of practice for working with children and adolescents.

CHAPTER *Outline*

The authors describe the occupational therapy (OT) process by first presenting the role of the OT practitioner and providing an overview of a variety of practice models. The OT process begins with referral, screening, and evaluation and moves from goal setting, intervention planning, and implementation, to reevaluation and discharge planning. A discussion of specific frames of reference used in pediatric practice is illustrated through case examples.

ROLES OF THE OCCUPATIONAL THERAPIST AND THE OCCUPATIONAL THERAPY ASSISTANT IN THE OCCUPATIONAL THERAPY PROCESS

The roles of the occupational therapist and the occupational therapy assistant (OTA) in the OT process differ. The occupational therapist is responsible for the selection of assessments used during evaluation, interpretation of results, and development of the intervention plan. The OTA may gather evaluative data under the supervision of the occupational therapist using an approved structured format but is not responsible for the interpretation of assessment results; he or she may contribute to the process by sharing knowledge of the client gained during the assessment process.

MODELS OF PRACTICE

A model of practice (MOP) helps OT practitioners organize their thinking.[6,10,12,13] For example, practitioners using the Model of Human Occupation (MOHO) know that they will gather information about volition (e.g., the child's or parents' goals and priorities or occupational choices), habituation or routines (e.g., how the child spends the day), performance (e.g., the physical skills and abilities of the child), and environment (e.g., the physical layout of the home). Practitioners using the Person–Environment–Occupational-Performance model will organize their thinking into information about the child (e.g., the child's physical abilities), the environment (e.g., where the child attends school), and occupational performance (e.g., how the child is performing his or her daily occupations). Other commonly used pediatric models of practice include Occupational Adaptation and the Canadian Occupational Performance Model.

MOPs provide practitioners with a framework for thinking about and arranging their materials. They help practitioners focus on factors that influence functioning. MOPs are developed from OT theory and philosophy. As such, they fit with the Occupational Therapy Practice Framework (OTPF) in its emphasis on occupation.[4] (Table 10-1 provides an overview of selected MOPs.)

REFERRAL, SCREENING, AND EVALUATION

The referral, screening, and evaluation aspects of the OT process are concomitantly referred to as the *evaluation period*. During this period, the OT practitioner meets the child, the family, or other referral sources (e.g., teacher, early interventionist) to collect information that will

TABLE 10-1

Models of Practice

MODEL	AUTHOR(S)	COMPONENTS	PREMISES
Model of Human Occupation (MOHO)	Kielhofner	Volition Habituation Performance Environment	The human is an open system. Volition drives the system. The clinician's role is to understand the client in terms of these systems (and subsystems) and intervene to facilitate engagement in occupations.
Canadian Occupational Performance Model	Occupational Therapy Association Townsend et al.	Spirituality Occupation Context (institutional included)	The worth of the individual is central to this model. Spirituality is the core of a person. Thus occupational therapy practitioners must understand the client's spirituality to facilitate engagement in occupations. Performance of occupations takes place within social, physical, and cultural environments.
Person–Environment–Occupational-Performance Model	Law et al.	Person Environment Occupation	Looks at the person in terms of physical, social, and emotional factors. The environment (context) influences the person and occupations. The environment includes culture. Occupations are the everyday things people do.

Data from Kielhofner, G. (2008). *A model of human occupation: Theory and application* (4th ed.). Baltimore, MD: Lippincott, Williams & Wilkins; Law, M., Cooper, B., Stewart, D., et al. (1996). The person-environment-occupation model: a transactive approach to occupational performance. *Can J Occup Ther, 63, 9*; Townsend, E., Brintnell, S., Staisey, N. (1990). Developing guidelines for client-centered occupational therapy practice. *Can J Occup Ther, 57, 69.*

assist in setting goals and developing an activity configuration for the child.

Referral

Children are usually introduced to occupational therapy by means of a **referral**. The reason for a referral depends on the individual state licensure laws or regulations within the area of practice. It is the responsibility of the OT practitioner to know the laws and regulations that govern his or her area of practice setting. A physician or a nurse practitioner generally gives the referral, depending on the state's laws; it is called physician's referral or doctor's orders.

According to the *Standards of Practice for Occupational Therapy* published by the American Occupational Therapy Association (AOTA), only occupational therapists may accept a referral for assessment.[2] Appendix 10-A provides a list of available assessments used with children and youth. The OTA, if given a referral, is responsible for forwarding it to a supervising occupational therapist and educating "current and potential referral sources about the scope of occupational therapy services and the process of initiating occupational therapy referrals."[2] OTAs may acknowledge requests for services from any source.[1,2] However, they do not accept and begin working on cases at their own professional discretion without the supervision and collaboration of the occupational therapist.

Screening

Clients may first be introduced to OT through a **screening**. Screenings provide a general overview of a child's functioning to determine whether further evaluation is needed. Both occupational therapists and OTAs can conduct such screenings. For example, an OTA may be hired to screen children in a well-baby clinic or an incoming kindergarten class to determine the need for additional evaluation before entering school. Once the OTA has identified the need for a more complete evaluation, the occupational therapist determines the specific evaluation or format to be used. The data gathered by the OTA are interpreted by the occupational therapist. An OTA "may contribute to this process under the supervision of a registered occupational therapist."[2]

Evaluation

The **evaluation** is a critical part of the OT process. The occupational therapist is responsible for determining the type and scope of evaluation. An evaluation includes assessments of an individual's areas of performance (e.g., activities of daily living [ADLs], instrumental ADLs [IADLs], work, education, play/leisure, rest and sleep, social participation), client factors (e.g., neuromusculoskeletal, specific and global mental functions, body system), performance skills, performance patterns, contexts, and activity demands.[4] According to AOTA, an entry-level OTA "assists with data collection and evaluation under the supervision of the occupational therapist."[1,2] An intermediate- or advanced-level OTA "administers standardized tests under the supervision of an occupational therapist after service competency has been established."[1] Although the OTA may participate in the evaluation process, the occupational therapist is responsible for interpreting the results and developing the intervention plan.

Levels of Performance

The evaluation provides the OT practitioner with a picture of the child's occupational needs as well as the child's strengths and weaknesses. This occupational profile consists of a description of the level of performance at which the child functions. Box 10-1 provides an overview of the information gained from the profile. A child's level of function may differ in relation to task, pattern, and context. For example, a child may feed himself or herself independently at home after setup but be unable to do so at school in the time provided while sitting at the table because of the loud noises and confusion of the lunchroom.

Functional independence refers to the completion of age-appropriate activities with or without the use of assistive devices and without human assistance (e.g., eating independently with an offset spoon; Figure 10-1, A).

Assisted performance refers to a child's participation in a specific age-appropriate task with some assistance from the caregiver (e.g., washing one's hands; Figure 10-1, B).

BOX 10-1

Components of the Occupational Profile

- Who is the client?
- Why is the client seeking services?
- What is the reason for referral?
- What occupations and activities are successful or are causing difficulties?
- What contexts and environments support or hinder desired outcomes?
- What is the client's occupational history?
- What are the client's priorities and targeted outcomes?

Adapted from American Occupational Therapy Association. (2014). Occupational therapy practice framework: Domain and process (3rd ed.). *Am J Occup Ther, 68*(Suppl 1), S1–S48.

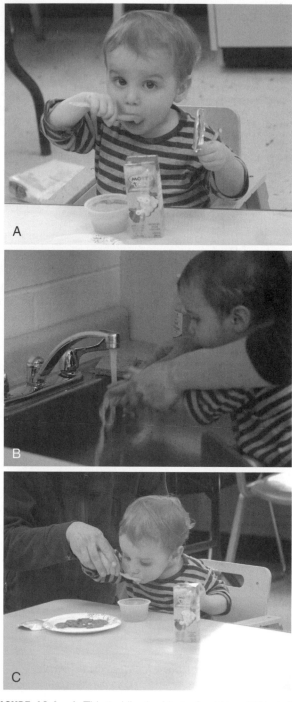

FIGURE 10-1   **A,** This toddler is able to feed himself. He is *independent* after set-up. **B,** The OT practitioner provides *some assistance* to help the child wash his hands. **C,** The OT practitioner provides hand-over-hand assistance so the child can bring the spoon to his mouth. The child is *dependent* on the practitioner to feed himself.

Dependent performance occurs when a child is unable to perform an age-appropriate task. A caregiver is required to perform the task for the child (e.g., holding the spoon for a child; Figure 10-1, *C*).

INTERVENTION PLANNING, GOAL SETTING, AND TREATMENT IMPLEMENTATION

Intervention Planning

The occupational therapist develops an **intervention plan** after the evaluation has been completed. The evaluation includes parental concerns, the client's strengths and weaknesses, a statement of the client's rehabilitation potential, long-term goals, and short-term objectives. The plan describes the type of media (i.e., specific types of materials) and modalities (i.e., intervention tools) that will be used and the frequency and duration of treatment. The plans for reevaluation and discharge as well as the level of personnel providing the intervention are also included.[1,2] (See Chapter 23 for more information on the use of media in practice.)

The intervention plan is based on a selected model of practice or a frame of reference (FOR). The FOR provides guidelines and intervention strategies. The OTA uses knowledge of the selected FORs, activity analysis, and the selection, gradation, and adaptation of activities to carry out the intervention plan.

Frames of Reference

Once practitioners have gained information by using a MOP, they must decide how to intervene. FORs are used to direct occupational therapy intervention. They inform practitioners as to what to do and are based on theory, research, and clinical experience.[6,10] A FOR defines the populations for which they are suitable, describes the continuum of function and dysfunction, provides assessment tools, describes treatment modalities and intervention techniques, defines the role of the practitioner, and suggests outcome measures. A FOR helps the OT practitioner identify problems and develop solutions. Common pediatric FORs in occupational therapy are the MOHO, developmental, sensory integration, biomechanical, sensorimotor, motor control, and rehabilitation.[6,10] (Table 10-2 provides an overview of commonly used pediatric FORs.) MOHO is both a MOP and a FOR because it has numerous assessment tools and intervention strategies. As such, MOHO provides an overall way of thinking and also meets the criteria for an FOR. (See Chapter 26 for a description of MOHO.)

Practitioners may choose to follow a variety of FORs. However, they should be careful to choose an appropriate one and to be clear about the theories and methodologies used with the given FOR. In cases when intervention does not progress as planned, practitioners adhering to one FOR may explore other suggested intervention techniques or change to another FOR. Intervention techniques are based on evidence from research. Given the need for evidence-based intervention, clinicians adhering to a FOR are using techniques investigated and supported through research. Therefore practitioners must

TABLE 10-2

Pediatric Frames of Reference

FRAME OF REFERENCE	REFERENCES	PRINCIPLES	SAMPLE POPULATIONS	TREATMENT MODALITIES
Developmental	Llorens	Development occurs over time and between skills (e.g., gross and fine motor). Some children experience a gap in their development due to physical, emotional, and/or social trauma. The role of occupational therapy is to bridge this gap.	Down syndrome Intellectual disability Failure to thrive Cerebral palsy Pervasive developmental disorder	Identify current level of functioning. Work on the next step to achieve the skill. Intervention includes practice, repetition, education, and modeling of skills.
Biomechanical	Pedretti and Paszuinielli	Improve strength, endurance, and range of motion for occupational performance.	Children with cardiac concerns Brachial plexus Cerebral palsy Juvenile rheumatoid arthritis Down syndrome	*Strength:* Increase weight of toys or repetitive use of objects. *Endurance:* Increase time engaged in occupation. *Range of motion:* Repetitively provide slow, sustained stretch to increase end range.
Sensory integration	Ayres	Children with sensory integration dysfunction have difficulty processing sensory information (vestibular, proprioceptive, tactile). Improvements in sensory processing lead to improved engagement in occupations.	Sensory integrative dysfunction Developmental coordination disorder Sensory modulation disorder Pervasive developmental disorder	Provide controlled sensory input to improve the child's ability to process sensory stimuli. Use suspension equipment and the "just-right challenge." Provide activities that are child directed.
Motor control	Shumway-Cook	Acquisition of motor skills is based on dynamic systems theory. (All systems, including sensory, motor, and cognitive, interact with each other for movement to occur.)	Cerebral palsy Developmental coordination disorder Down syndrome	*Task-oriented approach:* Children learn motor skills best by repeating the occupations in the most natural settings, varying the requirements. They learn from their motor mistakes.
Neuro-developmental	Bobath, Schoen, and Anderson	Children learn motor patterns when they "feel" normal movement patterns.	Cerebral palsy Traumatic brain injury	Clinician uses handling techniques and key points of control to inhibit abnormal muscle tone and facilitate normal movement patterns. Children learn through "feeling" normal patterns and thus should not make motor mistakes.
Model of Human Occupation	Kielhofner	Volition Habituation Performance Environment	All diagnoses	The human is an open system. Volition drives the system. The clinician's role is to understand the client in terms of these systems (and subsystems) and intervene to facilitate engagement in occupations.
Rehabilitation	Early, Pendleton & Schultz-Krohn	Children relearn skills lost; develop compensatory strategies; and develop adaptive techniques.	Acquired brain injury Trauma Stroke	Help children regain function for independence in occupations Help children to practice; improve strength, range of motion, and endurance.

Data from Ayres, A. J. (1979). *Sensory integration for the child* Los Angeles, CA: Western Psychological Services; Bobath, B. (1975). Sensorimotor development. *NDT Newsletter, 7,* 1; Early, M.B. (2006). *Physical dysfunction practice skills for the occupational therapy assistant* (2nd ed.). St. Louis, MO: Mosby; Llorens, L. A. (1976). *Application of a developmental theory for health and rehabilitation* Rockville, MD: American Occupational Therapy Association; Shultz-Krohn, W., & Pendleton, H. (2006). Application of the occupational therapy framework to physical dysfunction. In H. Pendleton & W. Shultz-Krohn, (Eds.), *Pedretti's occupational therapy: practice skills for physical dysfunction* (6th ed.). St Louis, MO: Mosby; Schoen, S., & Anderson, J. (2009). Neurodevelopmental treatment frame of reference. In P. Kramer & J. Hinojosa (Eds.), *Frames of reference for pediatric occupational therapy,* Baltimore, MD: Lippincott, Williams & Wilkins; Shumway-Cook, A., & Woolacott, M. (2002). Motor control: issues and theories. In A. Shumway-Cook & M. Woolacott (Eds.), *Motor control: theory and practical applications* (2nd ed.). Baltimore, MD: Lippincott, Williams & Wilkins.

keep themselves informed by reading and critically analyzing current research literature.

The following sections provide an overview and examples of specific FORs used with children.

Developmental Approach

CASE *Study*

Corey is a 2-year-old boy diagnosed with global developmental delays. Corey attends an early intervention center twice weekly for 2 hours of "group" time and 1 hour weekly for direct OT services. Roanna, the OTA, works with Corey and provides activities that can be continued at home with the family. The OT evaluation, which was based on the Hawaii Early Learning Profile, revealed that Corey functions at a level between 16 and 20 months for most skills, with gross motor skills being his strongest area and fine motor and language skills his weakest. Cognitively, Corey recognizes and points to four animal pictures (16–21 months), identifies himself in a mirror (15–16 months), identifies one body part (15–19 months), and searches for a hidden object (17–18 months). Expressive language skills include saying no meaningfully (13–15 months), naming one or two familiar objects (13–18 months), and using 10 to 15 words spontaneously (15–17 months). Gross motor skills are solid to 20 months: Corey picks up a toy from the floor without falling (19–24 months), runs fairly well (18–24 months), and squats when playing (20–21 months). He does not walk upstairs independently (22–24 months) or jump in place (22–30 months). Fine motor skills are scattered to 18 months. Corey builds a tower with two cubes (12–16 months) and scribbles spontaneously (13–18 months). He uses both hands at midline (16–18 months) but has difficulty pointing with his index finger (12–16 months) and placing one round peg in a pegboard (12–15 months). Socioemotional skills include enjoying rough-and-tumble play (18–24 months), expressing affection (18–24 months), and showing toy preferences (12–18 months). Corey has developed self-help skills to 12 months. He holds a spoon and finger feeds himself (9–12 months), naps once or twice each day (9–12 months), cooperates with dressing (10–12 months), and removes a hat (15–16 months).

The OTA designed an intervention plan based on this developmental picture of Corey and the parents' concern that Corey is not "playing like his 30-month-old cousin." The overall goal of the intervention based on the developmental FOR is to facilitate the child's ability to perform age-appropriate tasks in the areas of self-care, play/leisure, education, and social participation. The developmental FOR targets intervention at the level at which the child is currently functioning and requires that the practitioner provide a slightly advanced challenge. Practitioners using the developmental FOR need a clear understanding of the logical progression of skills. A typical therapy session is illustrated by the following SOAP (subjective, objective, assessment, and plan) note.

S

Corey's mother stated that he draws a line now.

O

During the small-group session with three peers, Corey scribbled spontaneously, holding the crayon in a palmar grasp. He imitated a vertical stroke (18–24 months) consistently and a circular stroke one of five times (20–24 months). Corey built a tower of four cubes (18–22 months). He pointed with his index finger on command (two of five times). Corey had difficulty isolating his index finger for finger games. Corey removed his socks (15–18 months), placed a hat on his head (16–18 months), and held a cup handle (12–15 months). He showed difficulty scooping food with a spoon (15–24 months) and continued to drink from a bottle (18–24 months).

A

Corey exhibits fine motor and self-care skills consistently to 18 months. He shows many emerging self-care skills.

Corey is making progress in achieving age-appropriate skills for play, self-care, and academics.

P

Corey will participate in group sessions designed to facilitate social-emotional and play skills.

Corey will continue to receive weekly individual OT services to improve fine motor and self-care skills for play, self-care, and academics. He will practice skills and work on social-emotional and play skills in groups. His parents have been provided with developmental activities for Corey to engage in at home.

Roanna used the developmental FOR to treat Corey. She focused on fine motor and self-care skills because Corey was participating in group sessions to develop social-emotional and play skills. Roanna designed the intervention to be fun and playful and began at the level at which Corey was functioning. She gradually increased the level of difficulty and provided developmentally appropriate activities for his parents to use at home.

Sensory Integration Approach

CASE *Study*

Jamar is a 13-year-old boy with sensory integration dysfunction. His movements are awkward, and he has poor balance and coordination; associated reactions with effort are noted (such as both hands moving when he writes). Jamar shows poor eye–hand coordination, poor rhythmic skills, and poor body awareness. He also shows signs of poor tactile, vestibular, and proprioceptive processing. The occupational therapist classified Jamar's dysfunction as poor motor planning and body awareness due to inadequate processing of vestibular input (vestibular-based somatodyspraxia; see Chapter 25 for more information on sensory integration).

Jamar is an intelligent child who expressed the desire to "be smoother, learn to dance, and not be the last one in every sport in gym." He also reports handwriting difficulties leading to lower grades in school.

Jamar receives OT services from Jackie, an OTA with 10 years of experience in a community-based sports injury clinic. The following SOAP note describes an intervention session. The goal of Jamar's intervention sessions is to improve body awareness, vestibular processing, and overall quality of movement so that he will be more confident in his body. Sensory integration theory postulates that by improving the ability to process sensory information, the body's ability to plan and execute movements will improve. Ayres emphasized movement-related activities with the use of suspended equipment (to get the intensity needed) and the "just-right challenge." [6,10,12]

S

Jamar states that a dance is taking place at school in 2 weeks.

O

Jamar reluctantly participated in a fast-moving tire-swing activity. He quickly became dizzy with the spinning and enjoyed bouncing into objects. Jamar had difficulty getting on new pieces of equipment. He "talked" his way through a difficult five-step obstacle course. Jamar showed difficulty clapping to the rhythm (five beats before an error) while on the trampoline but was able to clap to the rhythm (20 beats without an error) when sitting on the platform swing. On hearing a noise, he jumped into hoops placed randomly on the floor, showing some difficulty in sequencing and planning. Jamar was able to sequence and plan a difficult three-step obstacle course that involved crawling, swinging, and throwing a ball at a target. He completed 10 minutes of the Mavis typing program with a 70% success rate and was able to imitate simple dance moves (from song 1 of the Twister Moves game). Jamar was not able to successfully complete the dance moves and could not stay with the music after song 1.

A

Jamar exhibits difficulty with motor planning, sequencing, and timing of movements, which interferes with his leisure activities (dancing) and academics (writing).

P

Jamar will continue with sensory integration therapy twice weekly (1-hour sessions) for 3 months to improve his processing of vestibular, proprioceptive, and tactile information for quality of movements and educational and leisure activities. Jamar was provided with a homework assignment to select one song from Twister Moves and complete the dance steps from the game. Jamar will complete a Mavis typing program at the eighth-grade level and use a laptop for writing assignments. He will discuss these activities with his parents and teacher.

Jackie, the OTA, used a sensory integration FOR to improve Jamar's motor planning, sequencing, and timing of movements. Jamar chose the activities, and the session was tailored to address his concern about looking "awkward or weird" (i.e., not dancing to the beat of the music) at the school dance. Using goals that children pick themselves empowers and gratifies them. Furthermore, the child will work very hard to achieve these goals, making the likelihood of success greater. In this example, Jackie used suspended equipment to provide the intensity of input needed for a 13-year-old. She also challenged Jamar to participate in a slightly uncomfortable activity. Children gain confidence when they succeed in activities they deem to be slightly "tougher." In this way Jackie worked on Jamar's self-concept as well. Recommending the use of a laptop is not necessarily a sensory integration technique. However, Jamar is 13 years old and needs to be able to communicate in writing for success in school. Therefore Jackie decided that it was time to move away from teaching writing skills and help Jamar perform his educational occupation.

Biomechanical Approach

CASE *Study*

Abigail is a 14-month-old who suffered a left brachial plexus injury (i.e., damage to the nerves that control arm movement) during birth. An occupational therapist treats her once every 2 weeks. Teresa, an OTA, visits Abigail twice a week to work on the goals that have been established by the occupational therapist in collaboration with the child's family. Abigail's long-term OT goals include

1. Increasing active range of motion (AROM) in her left arm,
2. Increasing the functional strength in her left arm, and
3. Increasing her ability to use her left arm during age-appropriate activities such as playing with a toy and self-feeding.

Abigail's intervention sessions with Teresa last 30 minutes. A typical therapy session is shown in the following daily progress note. The goals of therapy sessions using a biomechanical FOR are to increase strength, endurance, and ROM for successful engagement in chosen occupations (e.g., play and self-care). [6,10]

S

Abigail's mother stated that Abigail enjoys the ROM exercises she performs each day. She especially enjoys singing "Row, row, row your boat" during the stretching exercises.

O

Abigail received a 30-minute therapy session in her home. Her mother and older brother were present for the entire session. Stretching and AROM left-arm exercises were performed. Left-shoulder AROM was 0° to 105° and passive ROM (PROM) 0° to 180°. Activities included weight bearing on her extended (straightened) left arm for 1 minute while reaching for toys with her right arm. Abigail also reached for toys with her left arm while bearing weight on her right arm. Abigail spontaneously used her left arm as an assist while playing with a shape sorter.

A

Abigail actively participates in the activities throughout the session. Her ability to sustain weight on her left arm with minimum physical assistance has improved from 20-second to 1-minute intervals. Left shoulder AROM from 0° to 105° has shown an increase of 10° since last month.

P

Abigail will participate in occupational therapy twice weekly to work on improving left upper extremity functioning for play, self-care, and academic work. Her goals include achieving full AROM for the left upper extremity, strengthening her left arm to lift objects, and spontaneously using the left upper extremity as an assist.

Teresa used the biomechanical FOR to treat Abigail. It is used with children who have orthopedic (i.e., bone, joint, or muscle) problems such as hand injuries or lower motor neuron disorders (affecting the nerve connections outside the central nervous system) such as brachial plexus injuries. (Refer to Chapter 13 to review health conditions.) The goals of the biomechanical approach are to

1. Assess physical limitations on the client's ROM, muscle strength, and endurance;
2. Improve ROM, strength, and endurance; and
3. Prevent or reduce contracture and deformities.[10]

This approach focuses on the physical limitations that interfere with the client's ability to engage in the occupational performance areas of ADLs, IADLs, sleep and rest, play and leisure activities, and work and productive activities. Teresa will work on the overall goal of improving Abigail's ability to use both arms for play, self-care, and academics. (Figure 10-2 presents a play activity that promotes use of both arms.)

Neurodevelopmental Approach

CASE *Study*

Raja is a 4-year-old boy who has been diagnosed with spastic right hemiplegia cerebral palsy. A brain lesion caused abnormal muscle tone on the right side of his

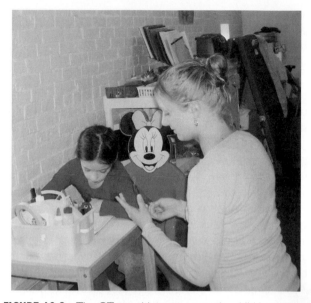

FIGURE 10-2 The OT practitioner engages the child in arts and crafts to promote the use of both hands for play, activities of daily living, instrumental activities of daily living, and education.

body, which prevents him from properly using his right arm and leg. He is receiving outpatient OT services at the local hospital; his mother usually brings him to the clinic. Raja recently had a phenol alcohol nerve block—an injection into the nerves that innervate the arm—to help reduce the increased flexor tone in his right arm. Because of the recent changes in Raja's right arm, Alejandro, the occupational therapist, is currently providing all of the direct OT services. His sessions with Raja typically last 45 minutes. An example of a therapy session is described in the following SOAP note.

The goal of therapy sessions with a neurodevelopmental (NDT) FOR is to normalize muscle tone and to improve movement patterns for occupations (e.g., academics, self-care, and play). (Refer to Chapter 18 regarding NDT treatment techniques.)

S

Raja's mother stated that Raja's right arm is easier to wash and the elbow is straighter since the nerve block.

O

Raja arrived this morning eager to work on the therapy ball. He performed activities on the therapy ball while lying on his stomach and bearing weight on his elbows, followed by bearing weight on his extended arms. Tapping—using fingertips to deliver successive light blows to the muscle belly —over the triceps to facilitate full extension (straightening) of Raja's elbow was performed. (The triceps muscle is primarily responsible for elbow extension.) Raja participated in bilateral hand activities, such as fastening large buttons and creating pictures using finger paint (Figure 10-3). When necessary, the wrist extensor muscles were stroked to encourage

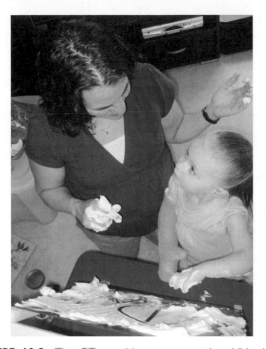

FIGURE 10-3 The OT practitioner engages the child with a hemiplegia in a play with shaving cream to promote use of both hands for activities of daily living and play. This activity promotes movement and range of motion.

maintenance of a functional wrist position (e.g., wrist extension while grasping) during the bilateral tasks. Gentle cueing at the shoulder was used to promote weight shifting on the right. Raja did not spontaneously bear weight on the right during movements. Raja fastened five large buttons in 2 minutes.

A

Raja's ability to use his right arm has improved, as shown by his ability to fasten five large buttons while his wrist is extended.

P

Raja will receive occupational therapy weekly to work on increasing right arm functioning for self-care, academics, and play.

Alejandro is using an NDT FOR to treat Raja. This type of approach involves the use of sensory input to change muscle tone and movement patterns in infants, children, and adolescents who have central nervous system damage.[6,10] Because using an NDT approach requires skill and experience, entry-level occupational therapists and OTAs should be closely supervised while using it.

Motor Control Approach

CASE *Study*

Talasi is a 6-year-old girl who shows a slight intention tremor in her right arm and walks with a wide-based gait. She performs the skills expected of her age, yet the quality of the movement is poor and she falls frequently. She is unable to keep up with her peers on the playground, is slow when getting dressed or undressed, frequently puts her clothes on backward, and spills food and drinks during mealtimes. Her parents are concerned that she is "falling behind" in school because she is forgetful and disorganized. Brian is the OTA responsible for treating Talasi at school. The following SOAP note describes a therapy session with a motor control FOR to improve Talasi's quality of movement for play, academics, and self-care. (See Chapter 24 for more information on motor control/motor learning approach.)

S

Talasi stated that she was having a bad day. She forgot to bring her "show and tell" book from her Grammy.

O

Talasi participated in a game of "dress-up." She put on a sweater and pants, buttoned them, and then removed them. Talasi dressed her doll and played a timed game of dress-up. She played eye–hand games using beanbags, targets, and catching a ball. The placement of the targets, the speed, and her position in relation to the target varied. Talasi balanced herself for 45 seconds on the right foot with eyes open and for 5 seconds with eyes closed. She drank her juice without spilling it but did spill applesauce from a spoon. An intention tremor was noted in her right arm during spoon feeding. Talasi was instructed to hold the spoon closer to the bowl. A weighted spoon eased some of the tremor and resulted in less spilling.

A

Talasi demonstrates poor quality of movement, an intention tremor in her right arm, and slow movements interfering with her functioning in school, at play, and during self-care.

P

Talasi will receive occupational therapy weekly to work on increasing the quality of movement for self-care, academics, and play.

The OTA (Brian) used the motor control FOR to improve Talasi's quality of movement. This FOR follows a task-oriented approach that encourages the repetition of desired movements in a variety of settings and circumstances. For example, Talasi practiced dressing herself with large clothing and dressing a small doll. Both these tasks involve dressing and undressing skills. Motor control theory promotes a practice approach. The clinician provides verbal feedback but allows the child to perform the task and learn from his or her mistakes. For example, Brian allowed Talasi to feed herself, then he instructed her on a different technique, which she practiced. Finally, Brian used a weighted spoon to see if this would decrease the tremor and thus the spilling.

Motor control theories support using activities that motivate the child and have as close a resemblance to the actual task as possible. Imagery and practice are intervention techniques used in the motor control approach.

Rehabilitative Approach

CASE *Study*

Dewayne is a 6-year-old boy whose left arm was amputated below the elbow after a car accident 2 years ago. Dewayne goes to Shriner's Hospital in another town for the fitting of his prosthesis, an artificial limb, and for training in its use. He has outgrown his old prosthesis and is meeting with Missy, an OTA, to work on using and caring for his new artificial arm and to learn activities that will improve his ability to use it functionally. A typical therapy session is shown in the following daily SOAP note.

S

Dewayne said that his new arm felt good.

O

Dewayne was treated in the OT department for prosthetic training and home/family instruction on its care. The department's Prosthetic Checklist was completed during the session. No red areas were noted on the child's arm or hand. Dewayne's father was shown how to don and doff the stump sock and the new artificial arm. Dewayne dressed and undressed himself using the artificial arm. He stabilized a paper with the prosthetic arm and wrote with his right hand.

A

The new artificial arm fits well. Dewayne and his father demonstrated knowledge of proper care, donning and doffing, and using the prosthesis. Dewayne is able to engage in age-appropriate self-care and writing activities while using his prosthesis.

P

Dewayne is discharged from Shriner's Hospital. He will be monitored by an occupational therapist at school.

Missy used the rehabilitative FOR to treat Dewayne. This method is used after an injury or illness to return a person to the highest possible level of functional independence as well as to teach any compensatory methods that may be needed to perform certain activities.[6,10]

Because many children are born with disabilities, OT practitioners are required in some cases to teach new skills (habilitate) instead of teaching previously known skills (rehabilitate). However, for cases in which a child acquires a disability after birth, a rehabilitative approach is appropriate. The methods used during rehabilitation and habilitation include the following:

- Self-care evaluation and training
- Acquisition and training in the use of assistive devices
- Prosthetic use training
- Wheelchair management training
- Architectural and environmental adaptation training
- Acquisition and training in the use of augmentative communication devices and assistive technology
- Play assessment and intervention

An OT practitioner who is using a rehabilitative approach or a habilitative approach focuses on skill acquisition in the occupations of ADLs, IADLs, sleep and rest, play and leisure, education, and work and productive activities.[4]

Model of Human Occupation

CASE *Study*

Peter is an 8-year-old boy with asthma, food allergies, and attention deficit disorder (ADD). Peter has difficulty following rules at school and frequently gets into trouble. He does not do well academically and has few friends. On the playground, Peter tends to play hard and often is "rough" with his friends. His parents are concerned that Peter is not succeeding in school and struggles socially. Peter is on a strict diet and receives medication for his ADD.

S

Peter stated, "I'm fine, I just want to run."

O

Volition: Peter smiled and was easily invested in outdoor active games such as tag, relay races, and swinging. He became agitated while performing reading and writing tasks indoor. However, he enjoyed drawing a picture of outdoor games.

Habits: Peter participated in active games outside at the end of the school day. He followed multistep directions outside and made eye contact with the clinician. Peter was resistant when it was time to come inside. He completed writing tasks reluctantly.

Performance: Peter was able to climb, pump himself on the swing, and played outside for 30 minutes with no evidence of fatigue. Inside, Peter struggled with writing assignments and became frustrated easily. Peter drew a picture of his favorite outdoor play for 10 minutes, using a tripod grasp.

Environment: The playground was equipped with a variety of swings and tires, and many children were playing. The classroom was small, with many children in group sitting arrangement. Peter sat at a table with four other children. At home, Peter has a swing and a trampoline and also plays in the woods. His parents are supportive of his outdoor play.

A

Peter shows strengths in gross motor skills; he has interests in outdoor activities with friends. Peter shows weaknesses in indoor fine motor activities and displays poor attention to details.

P

Peter's enjoyment of gross motor outdoor activity may be used to help him develop academic skills. Consultation with teachers and parents on how to use outdoor activities for schoolwork may prove motivating for Peter and help him succeed in school. Peter will receive occupational therapy for 1 hour weekly during the school year. The OT practitioner used MOHO to guide clinical reasoning. Upon finding out that Peter was volitionally motivated toward active outdoor activities, the clinician planned the intervention around ways to support Peter while working on his poor fine motor skills and his decreased attention to details. Targeting activities that motivate Peter may help him improve his academics. As Peter experiences success in the classroom, his performance capacity may improve. MOHO theory postulates that success leads to the desire to continue to perform and succeed. (See Chapter 26 for more information on MOHO in practice.)

Legitimate Tools

Legitimate tools are the instruments or tools that a profession uses to bring about change.[12] Legitimate tools change over time based on the growing knowledge of the profession, technological advances, and the needs and values of both the profession and society.[12] OT practitioners use occupations, purposeful activities, activity analysis, activity synthesis, and therapeutic use of self as tools to help children in their care.

Occupation

The goal of occupational therapy is to help children participate in their desired occupations. These occupations include social participation, self-care tasks (e.g., feeding, dressing, bathing), educational activities, rest and sleep, IADL, and play. Intervention is designed to help them actively participate to the fullest in these occupations. Therefore OT practitioners analyze occupations to determine why a child is not performing well and use the tools of practice to assist them. Intervention is then designed to remediate the underlying skill deficits that are causing the child's difficulty, to compensate for problem areas, or to adapt the requirements of the skills so that the child may be successful at performing them in a different way.

OT practitioners provide occupation-based interventions. The intervention involves having the child actively participate in the actual occupation with which he or she struggles. For example, an intervention to improve a child's ability to play with others may consist of inviting another child to the therapy session(s) to facilitate playing.

Purposeful Activities

Purposeful activities are defined as goal-directed behaviors or tasks that constitute occupations.[9] An activity is purposeful if the individual is a voluntary, active participant and the activity is directed toward a goal that the individual considers meaningful. OT practitioners use purposeful activities to evaluate, facilitate, restore, or maintain individuals' abilities to function in their daily occupations.

Purposeful activities provide opportunities for individuals to achieve mastery, and successful performance promotes feelings of personal competence. Those involved in purposeful activities focus on the processes required for achievement rather than on the goals. Purposeful activities occur within the contexts of personal, cultural, physical, and other environmental conditions and require a variety of client factors (e.g., neuromusculoskeletal, global, and specific mental functions, and body systems).[4] Purposeful activities are unique to the individual; therefore, the OT practitioner grades or adapts a chosen activity for the individual.[9]

Activity Analysis

Activity analysis is the process of analyzing an activity to determine how and when it should be used with a particular client.[14] It involves the identification of the components or client factors necessary to perform an activity.[1,2] Several methods are used to analyze activities, two of which are discussed in this chapter.

The first method is **task-focused activity analysis**. This method of analyzing activity identifies the physical (sensorimotor), cognitive, and social-emotional (psychological/psychosocial) components involved in a specific task. The OT practitioner uses an activity analysis to describe the materials needed for the activity, the sequential steps of the activity, and safety concerns.[4] Task-focused activity analysis identifies the most and least important performance components needed to complete the activity. The physical, personal, social, and cultural conditions and influences are described.[4] Using this analysis, the OT practitioner identifies how the activity may be graded and adapted for the client. Task-focused activity analysis is used to understand the activity in terms of skills and personal and cultural meanings to help the OT practitioner understand how the activity can be used therapeutically. This type of analysis enables him or her to quickly identify the demand of an activity (Figure 10-4).[5,14]

The second method comprises both **child- and family-focused activity analyses** (Figure 10-5). The OT practitioner analyzes the actual intervention and identifies the child's and family's strengths and weaknesses. The practitioner then identifies the objectives and plans activities that are specifically designed to meet those objectives.[5,14] The practitioner describes the types of materials, supplies, and equipment that will be needed; identifies the position of the child and the OT practitioner during intervention; and documents the expected results or recommendations. Several activities may meet the requirements of the plan.

There is a degree of overlap between the two types of activity analyses. Although each one emphasizes distinct

TASK-FOCUSED ACTIVITY ANALYSIS

CHILD'S NAME: **_Kellie Peralta_**   DATE: **_12/30/16_**

ACTIVITY DESCRIPTION: **_Closing Velcro tabs on shoes_**

SUPPLIES/EQUIPMENT: **_Socks, shoes, chair_**

STEPS OF ACTIVITY:

1) **_Prepare work area with chair, socks and shoes._**

2) **_Position child on small chair or on floor in a quiet area._**

3) **_Demonstrate to child how to put on socks and shoes (allow child to help as much as possible)._**

4) **_Demonstrate how to close tabs._**

5) **_Allow the child to practice closing tabs with hand-over-hand assistance._**

6) **_Allow child to begin practicing closing tabs._**

LIST THE MOST IMPORTANT PERFORMANCE COMPONENTS REQUIRED FOR THIS ACTIVITY:

Sensorimotor	Cognitive	Psychosocial/Psychological
1) Sensory awareness 2) Tactile 3) Proprioception 4) Kinesthesia 5) Fine coordination / dexterity	1) Level of arousal 2) Attention span 3) Sequencing 4) Learning 5) Concept formation	1) Values 2) Interests 3) Role performance 4) Self-expression 5) Coping skills

LIST THE LEAST IMPORTANT PERFORMANCE COMPONENTS REQUIRED FOR THIS ACTIVITY:

Sensorimotor	Cognitive	Psychosocial/Psychological
1) Oral-motor control 2) Reflexes 3) Pain response 4) Olfactory 5) Gustatory	1) Orientation 2) Recognition 3) Categorization 4) Spatial operations 5) Problem-solving skills	1) Self-concept 2) Social conduct 3) Interpersonal skills 4) Time management skills 5) Self-control

ENVIRONMENTAL CONTEXTS:

1. Physical	2. Social	3. Cultural
Activity can be done in the child's room or another room in the home. Area should be well lighted. Child can sit on chair or floor.	Practitioner and child will work together until task is learned. Mother will practice with child.	In own culture, people are expected to wear shoes.

Gradation	Adaptation	Safety Hazards
Method of instruction can vary to accommodate child's learning needs. Task can be taught using hand-over-hand method.	D rings can be placed on tip of tabs to facilitate grasping the tabs.	None

FIGURE 10-4 Task-focused activity analysis form.

CHILD- AND FAMILY-FOCUSED ACTIVITY ANALYSIS

DATE: _12/30/16_

CHILD'S NAME: _Kellie Peralta_   AGE: _2 years, 7 months_

DIAGNOSIS: _Autism-Spectrum Disorder_

SETTING: _Home Based_   FREQUENCY OF OT: _5 times per week_

DURATION: _1 hour per session_

Strengths	Limitations
Strong family support system	*Decreased eye contact*
Enjoys proprioceptive activities	*Delays in fine motor skills*
Enjoys vestibular activities	*Delays in gross motor skills*
	Delay with self-care skills

OBJECTIVE: *Kellie will complete morning self-care task cooperatively (without behavioral outbursts) within 6 months.*

Planned Activities	Materials	Supplies and Equipment
1) Hair brushing *2) Vestibular activities* *3) Dressing activities*		*1) Hair brush* *2) Therapy ball* *3) Clothing, shoes*
Position of Child and Practitioner	**Performance Results**	**Recommendations**
1) Child sits on floor in front of therapist.	*1) Child had difficulty tolerating hairbrushing.* *2) She became agitated after 3 minutes of brushing.*	*1) Continue with deep pressure hairbrushing with corn brush. Allow child to initiate hairbrushing activity.* *2) Limit activity to 3 -5 minutes. Give Kellie a reward after activity (if she does not scream).*
2) Child initially sits on a 9-inch ball. Practitioner is positioned behind child and supports child at hips.	*3) Child was able to remain sitting on ball. She carried out a simple task while sitting on the ball.*	*3) Introduce a 12-inch ball during next session.*
3) Child sits on floor in front of practitioner. Practitioner also sits on floor.	*4) Child was receptive and able to follow directions. Hand-over-hand assistance was required.* *5) Child cooperated for 10 minutes before showing signs of discomfort.*	*4) Mother to practice activity with child everyday. Discrete trial teaching will be used during therapy sessions. Engage child in 5 to 7 minutes of dressing and reward positive behaviors.*

FIGURE 10-5 Child- and family-focused activity analysis form.

aspects of activity, both require that the practitioner understand the needs of the child, a variety of theoretical approaches, and the context of intervention.

Activity Synthesis

Activity synthesis includes adapting, grading, and reconfiguring activities and is considered a legitimate tool used in OT practice.[11]

Adaptation refers to the process of changing steps during an activity so that the client is able to engage in it. An activity is adapted by modifying or changing the sequence of its steps, the way in which the materials are presented, or the way in which the child is positioned, or by presenting the activity in such a way that the child is expected to perform only certain aspects of it. Activities can also be adapted by changing the characteristics of the materials that are used, such as their size, shape, texture, or weight.[11,12] For example, in the case of a child who is fearful of movement and needs to improve or develop righting reactions, the practitioner may have him or her sit on a therapy ball to elicit righting reactions (Figure 10-6). However, because of the child's fear of movement, the practitioner might begin the intervention with a smaller ball that allows the feet to stay on the ground and provides slow, controlled movements. The practitioner can make the activity easier or more difficult to find the right challenge for the child.

Gradation refers to the process of arranging the steps of an activity in a sequential series to change or progress, allowing for gradual improvement by increasing the demand for a higher level of performance as the child's abilities increase.[11,14] For example, the practitioner provides a frame that limits the movement of the ball to help the child feel more comfortable sitting on the ball. Once the child feels comfortable, the practitioner can take away the stabilizing frame. The OT practitioner determines the type and extent of grading based on clinical reasoning.

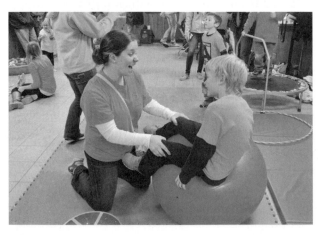

FIGURE 10-6 The practitioner facilitates postural control by playing games on a large ball.

A client's level of performance changes when he or she participates in activities that are graded for his or her needs. Once the practitioner has adapted and graded an activity, it is presented in its "real" form, thus synthesizing the analysis, adaptation, and grading into the activity itself.[11] For example, finger feeding is acceptable while a child is learning self-feeding. The activity is then adapted by the introduction of a utensil. It would be acceptable initially for the child to hold the utensil and attempt to use it to scoop or spear food. The practitioner ultimately expects the child to grasp the utensil, spear the food, and bring it to the mouth, thus synthesizing the activity of self-feeding into the child's repertoire of abilities. The goal of adapting and grading activities is participation in occupations in the given context.[5,12,14]

Activity Configuration

Activity configuration is the process of selecting, on the basis of a child's age, interests, and abilities, specific activities that will be used during the intervention process.[5,12,14] For example, a long-term goal for the child may be the ability to feed himself or herself independently. One short-term objective may be scooping food with a spoon. A session objective may be learning how to control the grasp and release of a spoon. The OT practitioner designs activities specific to the child's intervention goals and based on knowledge of the child's desires. Activities are designed to be flexible, creative, and purposeful to the child. They are age appropriate and challenging, while not being overwhelming.[5,12,14] The OT practitioner considers the methods and media required to allow the child to be successful with each activity.

Therapeutic Use of Self

Therapeutic use of self is the OT practitioner's ability to communicate with the child and the child's family or caregivers while being aware of his or her own personal feelings. OT practitioners use their individual characteristics to relate to families, interact with children, and help them perform occupations. As such, OT practitioners who are aware of their own strengths and weaknesses have insight into how one's use of self can influence intervention, so they may help children and their families more effectively.

Taylor developed the Intentional Relationship Model, which describes six modes of interacting with clients for their benefit.[16] These interpersonal modes include advocating, collaborating, empathizing, encouraging, instructing, and problem solving.[16] OT practitioners may favor one mode over the other, but understanding how to use these modes with different clients can help OT practitioners develop improved therapeutic use of self. Some clients will respond better to certain modes than to others. Becoming mindful of one's use of self in a therapeutic setting benefits clients and strengthens the therapeutic relationship. Taylor provides reflective exercises and examples to help practitioners develop skill and awareness in therapeutic use of self.[16]

In a therapeutic relationship, the OT practitioner helps the child and the family without any expectation of the help being reciprocated.[16] He or she develops and maintains a good relationship with the child and the family.[16] Therefore, OT practitioners must possess a basic knowledge of family dynamics, cultural, and ethnic concepts in the provision of services, and family systems. As Peloquin stated, "concern for the patient as a person remains essential to effective practice."[15]

OT practitioners recognize that a child is treated in the contexts of his or her family, culture, and environment. The OT practitioner's role is to create an atmosphere of freedom and challenge within the structure of the intervention. The intervention should not be so simple that the child becomes bored or so difficult that he or she feels inadequate. The practitioner prepares a setting to meet the child's needs by guiding him or her toward mastery of the skill.[15]

OT practitioners work with the family to guide them as they care for the child. Because families may experience emotional stress associated with the issues of raising a child who has special needs, they may not always be able to participate in the therapeutic process. Clinicians must work with parents where they are and not have unreal expectations or judgments with regard to the parents "getting through" things. (See Chapter 2 on family systems.) Working on goals that are important to a family at a particular time is an effective way to help them. Parents will understand their children's needs better as they work with the OT practitioner to meet the stated goals.

CASE *Study*

Tyrone is an 18-month-old boy with developmental delays; he is unable to walk, speaks very little, and does not manipulate toys. His mother has three other children (ages 9, 7, and 3), lives alone, and receives public assistance. The OT practitioner provides the mother with an extensive home program, which she refuses to carry out. The practitioner documents that the mother is "noncompliant and in denial about her son's diagnosis."

In this scenario, the OT practitioner has failed to examine the context and therefore has too quickly judged Tyrone's mother. The mother may be overwhelmed by this new diagnosis and the demands of caring for four young children by herself on a limited income. She may not be carrying out the home program because she has no time or energy to do it. The OT practitioner has not targeted the goals that support the mother and the family.

Consider the same case with the OT practitioner providing the mother with techniques to include her other children in playing with Tyrone to improve his abilities. This would allow the mother some free time and involve all the children in the activity. The OT practitioner may even provide activities that they could all perform together as "family game time" (e.g., "Simon Says" or finger plays). The OT practitioner may work more closely with the mother in determining how Tyrone's developmental delays impact the family. After identifying that feeding Tyrone is problematic, the OT practitioner may target feeding issues. Targeting the parent's primary issues of concern is the best way to involve them in the intervention process. OT practitioners who target parental concerns seldom find parents who are "in denial" or "noncompliant."

CLINICAL *Pearl*

Examining situations from all angles provides insight that may help OT practitioners working with children.

CLINICAL *Pearl*

The parents may not understand the entirety of the diagnosis, but they generally understand their child. They can learn about their child's strengths and weaknesses during the intervention process. OT practitioners can help parents understand their child better by involving them in goal setting.

CLINICAL *Pearl*

Parents want the best from their children. OT practitioners help them care for their children and play a role in empowering parents.

CLINICAL *Pearl*

Making eye contact, getting to the child's level, and pointing out his or her strengths to the parents help OT practitioners gain trust from the child and from the family. These abilities are considered part of therapeutic use of self.

One way to help parents understand their child better is through modeling behaviors. Parents report that they learn more easily by observing the practitioner work with the child. Being able to observe and ask questions helps them develop skills and routines to care for their child.[6] The OT practitioner models handling techniques, management, and attitudes toward the child. The clinician also models patience, understanding, and acceptance, which, in turn, helps parents show the same. The OT practitioner learns from parents by listening and opening lines of communication; this therapeutic relationship empowers parents. Although the OT practitioner comes into contact with many children with special needs, parents may find this new experience overwhelming. Therefore a clinician who models understanding, caring, and acceptance of the child may teach parents the same, which has an impact on the child and the family in ways that cannot be measured. This is the essence of therapeutic use of self.

Therapeutic use of self requires that OT practitioners be aware of their body language; read parents' verbal and nonverbal cues; and interact in a caring, nonjudgmental manner. Making eye contact, nodding one's head, and using facial expressions to communicate are all aspects of therapeutic use of self that clinicians must understand and use effectively.

Multicultural Implications

CASE *Study*

Maria is a 2-year-old girl diagnosed with spastic quadriplegia. Her parents recently immigrated to the United States from the Dominican Republic. Maria is evaluated at the early intervention center by an occupational therapist, a physical therapist, and a speech therapist. The team decides that Maria needs all the services. The occupational therapist meets with the parents to decide on goals for sessions. The social worker, who speaks Spanish, is present. Using a family-centered approach (mandated by early intervention laws), the OT practitioner asks the parents what their concerns are and what they would like to work on in therapy sessions. The parents are hesitant to respond throughout the meeting. The OT practitioner feels that the parents are not interested in receiving services for their daughter. The OT practitioner and the social worker meet later to discuss the events.

This case study illustrates the need to understand cultural expectations. The OT practitioner does not understand why the parents do not quickly express what they desire for Maria. The practitioner interprets this as lack of caring and interest in the child's progress.

The social worker explains to the OT practitioner that although many American parents feel empowered to discuss their concerns and advocate for their child, parents from the Dominican Republic look to the professional to tell them what to do. Maria's parents have not yet been socialized to the American system. They are not uninterested but, rather, somewhat confused as to why a medical health care professional (e.g., the OT practitioner) would ask them what they wanted. They view health care professionals as the experts and, as such, will follow through with any requirements set forth by the team.

Once the OT practitioner understands this cultural difference, he holds the next meeting in a different way, provides more direction, and gives the parents the

team's recommendations. The team acknowledges that Maria will require OT services when she enters school, and so they will have to help socialize the parents to advocate for their child with professionals. However, the OT practitioner may first have to be more direct than they would need to be with parents already socialized to the American system.

Cultural values have an effect on all areas of family life. OT practitioners need to understand the cultural context of the child in order to meet the child's and the family's needs. Although the OT practitioner may not have direct understanding of each culture, sensitivity and open communication may bridge the gap. Disregard for cultural concerns may interfere with establishing rapport; as a result, the practitioner may find the child or caregiver not investing in the intervention. When this happens, the lack of compliance and satisfaction generally makes the therapy process ineffective.

Goal Setting

The OTA collaborates with the occupational therapist and the family on the development of long-term goals and short-term objectives for any child they are treating.[3,5] Through this collaborative process, the occupational therapist, the OTA, and the family agree on the needs of the child as well as the appropriate priorities for intervention. This makes the intervention process more efficient and effective and leads to a better understanding of the child. Based on the evaluation and discussion of needs, realistic goals for the child can be established.

Long-Term Goals

Long-term goals are statements that describe the occupational goals the client should achieve after intervention. These goals should be measurable, observable, clear, and written in behavioral terms.[3,7,14] Goals need to be very specific and address the problems that have been identified. A practitioner can use the mnemonic device referred to as the **RUMBA criteria** to write up the goal statements (Box 10-2).[7]

Short-Term Goals

Short-term goals are the steps the client needs to achieve so that long-term goals can be met.[3,7,14] They are statements that describe the skills that should be mastered in a relatively short period. For example, consider a client whose long-term goal is independent dressing. The short-term objectives for this client may include developing the pincer grasp for buttoning, learning to button, and developing sequencing skills for dressing.

Treatment Implementation

Treatment implementation (intervention) involves working within the system through which the child is

BOX 10-2

RUMBA Criteria

R (RELEVANT)
A relevant goal reflects the client's current life situation and future possibilities. Everyone involved in the client's care (client, therapist, family, and members of other disciplines) should agree on the goal.

U (UNDERSTANDABLE)
An understandable goal is stated in clear language. Jargon and very specialized or difficult words should be avoided.

M (MEASURABLE)
A measurable goal contains criteria for success.

B (BEHAVIORAL)
A behavioral goal focuses on the behavior or skill that the client must eventually demonstrate.

A (ACHIEVABLE)
An achievable goal describes a behavior or skill that the client should be able to accomplish in a reasonable period.

Adapted from Early, MB (1993). *Mental health concepts and techniques for the occupational therapy assistant* (2nd ed.). New York: Raven Press.

receiving therapy, working with the family, and working directly with the child. Working with the child involves planning each session, developing and analyzing activities, and then grading and adapting those activities as necessary. This process is geared toward reaching the short-term objectives first and then the long-term goals.

Intervention includes the methods used to work toward meeting the goals, the media or activities used during the intervention, and documentation of the child's progress or lack of progress.

Session or Mini-objectives

Session or mini-objectives are the goals the practitioner has set for an intervention session. They are planned before the session in collaboration with the child and parents. Sometimes mini-objectives will remain for several sessions because it may take more than one intervention to meet them. Once the session objectives are identified, the OT practitioner analyzes the activities that will facilitate meeting the objectives.

REEVALUATION AND DISCONTINUATION OF INTERVENTION

Reevaluation

Although the occupational therapist determines whether a reevaluation is indicated, the OTA is responsible for reporting any change in the child's condition to the supervisor.[3] Therefore, if the OTA observes changes, the

changes are brought to the attention of the occupational therapist, and the OTA may suggest a reevaluation. The OTA participates in the reevaluation in collaboration with and under the supervision of the occupational therapist.[3]

Discontinuation of Intervention

In pediatric OT practice, discharge planning or discontinuation of intervention may be mandated by laws that govern the type of system in which the child receives OT services. Regardless of the system, the discontinuation process is the responsibility of the occupational therapist. The OTA collaborates in the discontinuation process under the supervision of the occupational therapist by reporting on the child's progress and making suggestions regarding future needs.

Services are typically discontinued once the child has met the predetermined goals and achieved maximum benefit from occupational therapy or when the parents and the child decide that the child no longer wants to receive occupational therapy. Services may be discontinued when the child moves away or enters another system. The OTA may recommend discontinuation of services to the occupational therapist when any of the conditions mentioned above exist. Discontinuation plans should include a plan for follow-up when indicated. Figure 10-7 provides a summary of the OT process from referral to the follow-up plan.

Although many systems do not allow for children to be discharged and readmitted, this may, in fact, be the best method. For example, a child who is no longer receiving OT services may need occupational therapy periodically in junior high school to help him or her successfully adjust to physical changes or to advanced requirements.

OCCUPATION-CENTERED TOP-DOWN APPROACH

Because OT practitioners are interested in helping children engage in their occupations, evaluation and intervention focusing on occupations are recommended. Fisher proposed a model for OT evaluation and intervention using a client-centered, occupation-based, **top-down approach** called the **Occupational Therapy Intervention Process Model (OTIPM)**.[8]

The following case study illustrates how this translates to practice. The focus of this evaluation and the OTIPM is on the child's occupations.[8] Later in the process, the OT practitioner determines the client factors or components that are interfering with performance. However, goals for intervention can be developed on the basis of overall performance. As highlighted in this case study, OT practitioners are encouraged to address the concerns of parents, caregivers, and teachers when designing an intervention that focuses on occupational performance. OT practitioners are encouraged to read Fisher's work for additional information.[8]

The following case illustrates the top-down approach to OT intervention.

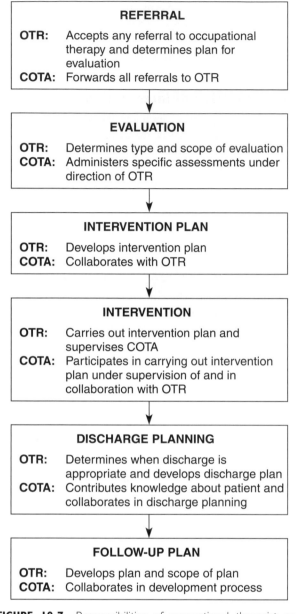

FIGURE 10-7 Responsibilities of occupational therapist and OTA in OT intervention process.

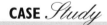

CASE *Study*

Hannah is a 31-month-old girl with a diagnosis of pervasive developmental disorder. She was referred to an early intervention program for evaluation by the pediatrician.

Parental Concerns

Hannah's parents express concern that she does not talk as clearly as her cousin does and never has; becomes agitated very easily and screams, especially during bath time; and does not play with her cousins and sisters. Furthermore, her mother is concerned about the lack of variety in her diet. Hannah's parents are concerned that she is not developing like her sisters (ages 5 and 1), and they are unsure how to manage her behaviors. Her mother is "worried about Hannah's lack of interest in her mother, father, or siblings."

Occupations
Activities of Daily Living

- *Feeding.* Hannah is currently able to drink from a bottle but does not like to drink from a cup. She is very particular about the food she eats and likes only very soft, almost liquid-type foods. Her food preferences currently include Cheerios with milk, pasta, soup, and bland mashed potatoes. Hannah sometimes eats very ripe bananas.
- *Dressing.* Hannah does not yet dress or undress independently. Her mother reports that she likes to wear only long-sleeved shirts and leggings and refuses to walk around barefoot. Hannah is able to remove her socks. She is able to remove mittens, hats, and coats after they are unzipped. She is unable to remove slip-on shoes or unlace or unbuckle other shoes. She is unable to put on or take off pants, skirts, or shirts.
- *Bathing.* Hannah often hides and becomes tearful when her mother announces that it is bath time. She cries, has tantrums, and hits others when placed in the tub. She hates having her face washed; however, her mother reports that sometimes Hannah will rub her face with a washcloth on her own.
- *Toileting.* Hannah wears diapers and does not indicate when she is wet or soiled and shows no signs of discomfort.
- *Sleep.* Hannah sleeps through the night. She goes to bed around 9 PM and wakes up around 7 AM She takes a 2-hour nap during the day.

Play

Hannah does not interact with others when playing; instead she plays alone quietly. She likes balls and stares at them for long periods of time. Hannah sometimes enjoys going to the playground, especially when there are few or no other children around. She goes up and down the slide, sometimes as often as 30 times in an hour. She is terrified of the swing and refuses to go in the sandbox. Hannah enjoys roughhousing with her father.

Social Participation

Hannah's mother reports that Hannah prefers watching children's TV programs and does not play with toys. She does not respond to her name when called despite having had a normal audiologic examination. Hannah's eye contact is limited; she does not look at her mother when asking for things. She does not verbalize her needs but, instead, takes her mother's hand to guide her to whatever she wants. Hannah does not initiate conversation with her sisters or parents.

Habits/Routines

Hannah stays at home with her mother and younger sister; her older sister attends morning kindergarten. Hannah's family lives in a two-story house in the country. Hannah has a swing and sandbox in the yard. She has a variety of toys. Hannah eats breakfast around 8 AM, lunch at noon, and dinner at 6 PM. She takes a 2-hour nap after lunch. Hannah bathes once a week, although her mother would like her to do it more often. The family enjoys taking hikes and spending time together. The children go to gymnastics classes once a week. Hannah frequently does not participate in classes.

The family gets together at the grandmother's house on Sundays for dinner and socializing. Many children are playing there. Hannah finds it difficult to be around them and frequently goes to a quiet room in the house. The family leaves early on many occasions when she has tantrums.

Assessment

Hannah's family established routines in which she is able to participate. She experiences some difficulty at family gatherings but has also demonstrated the ability to adapt (e.g., finding a quiet space). Hannah is able to convey her needs by pulling on her mother's hand, which indicates that she has motivations and desires.

Hannah is demonstrating delays in all areas of self-care, play, and social participation. She shows signs of sensory modulation difficulties that interfere with these occupations.

Plan

Hannah will attend an early intervention program three mornings a week, which will include OT services for improving her ability to play with others, dress and feed herself, and get along with family members.

Abbreviated Intervention Plan

The goals and objectives were designed to meet parental concerns (Box 10-3). The first goal of dressing will help Hannah's parents see that she can participate in daily tasks, and this may empower them to set other goals. Other goals and objectives center around parental concerns that Hannah does not play with other children and shows a lack of interest in her family. Because play is so important in a child's life, the OT practitioner decided to start there. Furthermore, her mother repeatedly expressed concern that Hannah is not interested in the family. Therefore helping the child become part of the family will benefit everyone.

BOX 10-3

Goals and Objectives

1. Hannah will dress herself with verbal prompting within 6 months.
   * Hannah will be able to button a shirt with demonstrative prompts three out of four times.
   * Hannah will unbutton a shirt independently three out of four times.
   * Hannah will show improved bilateral coordination by putting together five pop beads independently four out of six times.
2. Hannah will play with her sisters for 15 minutes, sharing toys at least twice during a 45-minute session.
   * Hannah will engage in parallel play with her sister and cousin (both 5 years old) for 5 minutes without interfering in the play.
   * Hannah will play "pass the ball" with her sister (5 years old) for 5 minutes without becoming upset.
   * Hannah will dance with her sisters for 3 minutes as part of family game night.
3. Hannah will seek her mother's help at least five times a day.
   * Hannah will indicate her desires to her mother by pointing to the objects she wants three out of five times.
   * Hannah will hold her mother's hand to lead her to the objects she wants at least twice during the session.
   * Hannah will make eye contact with her mother twice while playing peek-a-boo.

Because Hannah already gets her mother's attention to show her what she wants, the OT practitioner will build on this skill. This will help the parent and child feel successful early on, build a trusting relationship between parent and child as a way of meeting other goals, and reinforce the connections between Hannah and other family members. Children with a diagnosis of pervasive developmental disorder may not express themselves in the same ways as typically developing children. Therefore grabbing her mother's hand and expressing her desires by means of pointing at pictures near her mother may be Hannah's way of staying close to her. This may cause her mother to feel needed and thus connected to her. Once Hannah is accustomed to pointing to pictures, the OT practitioner may give the pictures to the father, sisters, and teachers.

When the family has seen some progress and Hannah's behaviors are more under control, the OT sessions may focus on the underlying components, such as fine motor skills. For example, once Hannah is able to play with her sisters at home with a large ball, the practitioner may recommend coloring activities or other activities that are more challenging for her. The OT practitioner knows that targeting family issues has the greatest effect on the child's performance. The goal of the sessions is not that Hannah becomes "normal"; instead, the goal is for her to fit in with the family so that other family members can begin to understand her better and make the necessary accommodations.

Frame of Reference

A sensory integration FOR will be used to help Hannah modulate sensory information. The OT practitioner will work with the family to determine Hannah's sensory needs and to provide home strategies for the parents that will help manage Hannah's behaviors more easily.

A developmental FOR will also be used to help Hannah participate in everyday play activities at home. The OT practitioner will provide other family members with simple, easily implemented goals to help them relate to and better understand Hannah. Hannah will learn how to play better through practice and rewards (e.g., sensory or verbal).

Intervention Strategies

Intervention strategies are tailored to meet the needs of the child and the family and thus require creativity, analysis, and reflection on how the activities are meeting the goals. Because children change, intervention strategies must also be fluid.

Hannah's sessions may focus on sensory modulation activities, including brushing programs and tactile exploration (e.g., playing with sand, water, or rice). Many children with pervasive developmental disorder benefit from a sensory integration approach that includes child-directed experiences on suspended equipment, requiring adaptive responses. (See Chapter 25 for more treatment suggestions.)

The OT practitioner carefully adapts and grades activities while reading the child's cues so that the child can succeed. Occasionally including the parents and siblings in the sessions helps model how to promote positive behaviors and provides the parents with strategies to use at home. Because the goal of the sessions is to improve play skills, intervention resembles play and may include small playgroups with other children. The OT practitioner gives the child a reward for positive behaviors (e.g., sharing), which could be a sticker, positive verbal praise, or an extra turn.

To help the child ask for assistance from her mother, the clinician sets up a picture board with the activities of the day and teaches the child how to point to the next activity. Hannah will eventually learn to pick out the activities by pointing. This same strategy can be implemented at home by placing pictures on the refrigerator, from which she may choose. The clinician may decide to give the mother an apron with pictures on it so that Hannah has to go to her to choose a picture. Each intervention session includes a variety of play activities, strategies for parents, and successful performances from Hannah. The OT practitioner pays close attention to Hannah and her family's needs.

SUMMARY

OT services are provided to children from birth to 21 years of age. Before engaging in pediatric practice, the practitioner must be familiar with the profession's tools, the OT intervention process, and federal and state laws to be able to effectively design services. Pediatric OT practitioners work not only with the children but also with the families and caregivers. Specialized training in intervention techniques, family dynamics, and cultural considerations are beneficial. OT practitioners help children participate in everyday occupations. Therefore a top-down approach focusing on occupations as the means and ends and emphasizing client-centered care is recommended.[8]

References

1. American Occupational Therapy Association. (2009). Guidelines for supervision, roles, and responsibilities during the delivery of occupational therapy services. *Am J Occup Ther, 63,* 797–803.
2. American Occupational Therapy Association. (2010). Standards of practice for occupational therapy. *Am J Occup Ther, 64*(Suppl. 1), S106–S111.
3. American Occupational Therapy Association. (2013). Guidelines for documentation of occupational therapy. *Am J Occup Ther, 67*(Suppl), S32–S38.
4. American Occupational Therapy Association. (2014). Occupational therapy practice framework: domain and process (3rd ed.). *Am J Occup Ther, 68*(Suppl. 1), S1–S48.
5. Blesedell-Crepeau, E. (2003). Activity analysis: a way of thinking about occupational performance. In M. E. Neistadt, & E. B. Crepeau (Eds.), *Willard and Spackman's occupational therapy* (10th ed.). Philadelphia: Lippincott.
6. Dunbar, S. (2007). Theory, frame of reference and model: a differentiation for practice considerations. In S. Dunbar (Ed.), *Occupational therapy models for intervention with children and families* (pp. 1–10). Thorofare, NJ: Slack.
7. Early, M. B. (1999). *Mental health concepts and techniques for the occupational therapy assistant* (3rd ed.). Philadelphia: Lippincott Williams & Wilkins.
8. Fisher, A. (2005). *OTIPM: a model for implementing top-down, client-centered, and occupation-based assessment, intervention, and documentation.* Durham, NH: University of New Hampshire.
9. Hinojosa, J., Sabari, J., & Pedretti, L. W. (1993). Purposeful activities. *Am J Occup Ther, 47,* 1081.

10. Kielhofner, G. (2009). *Conceptual foundations of occupational therapy practice* (4th ed.). Philadelphia, PA: F. A. Davis.
11. Kramer, P., & Hinojosa, J. (2014). Activity synthesis. In M. Blount, & J. Hinojosa (Eds.), *The texture of life: purposeful activities*. Bethesda, MD: American Occupational Therapy Association.
12. Luebben, A., Hinojosa, J., & Kramer, P. (2009). Legitimate tools of pediatric occupational therapy. In P. Kramer, & J. Hinojosa (Eds.), *Frames of reference in pediatric occupational therapy* (3rd ed.). Baltimore, MD: Lippincott Williams & Wilkins.
13. MacRae, N. (2001). *Foundations of occupational therapy*. Portland, Maine: Unpublished lecture notes, University of New England.
14. O'Brien, J. (2013). Activity analysis. In J. O'Brien, & J. Solomon (Eds.), *Occupational analysis and group process* (pp. 16–24). St. Louis, MO: Mosby.
15. Peloquin, S. (1990). The patient-therapist relationship in occupational therapy: understanding visions and images. *Am J Occup Ther, 44*, 13.
16. Taylor, R. (2007). *The intentional relationship: use of self and occupational therapy*. Philadelphia, PA: FA Davis.

REVIEW *Questions*

1. In what way does assessment of a child guide the OT practitioner in the processes of intervention planning and implementation?
2. Define and differentiate among long-term goals, short-term objectives, and mini-objectives.
3. What is included in an activity analysis?
4. Describe models of practice and frames of reference used in pediatric practice.
5. Provide examples of the strategies used with specific models of practice and frames of reference.
6. What are the principles for selected models of practice and frames of reference?
7. How does RUMBA inform goal writing?
8. What are some examples of using a top-down approach to OT intervention with children?

SUGGESTED *Activities*

1. Using the task-focused activity analysis form as a guide, analyze the specific daily routines that you personally perform, such as brushing your teeth, getting dressed, and preparing lunch.
2. Visit a day-care center or observe a neighbor's child performing specific tasks. Analyze what you observe using the task-focused activity analysis.
3. Choose an activity in which you typically engage and experiment by changing your position and the materials used for the activity. For example, eat a bowl of ice cream while sitting at the table and then do the same thing on your stomach in front of the television. Try different sizes of bowls and spoons. Write down how the change in position or in the bowl and spoon made a difference in your performance.
4. Identify at least one long-term personal goal. Write short-term objectives about the way you plan on reaching your goal(s). Consider what methods you will use in attaining the objectives and ultimately your goal(s). The goal(s) should be attainable within 12 months. Use the RUMBA criteria when writing up your goal(s).
5. Ask some parents what they would like for their children in the near future. Write these as measurable goals. Describe the trends you observed and what you have learned that may help you in practice.
6. Read a case study and view a video clip provided on the Evolve learning site. Develop goals and intervention strategies specific to the case and based on a selected model of practice or frame of reference.
7. Find a recent research article describing an intervention based on a selected model of practice or frame of reference.

APPENDIX 10-A*

A Sample of Pediatric Assessments

ASSESSMENT	DESCRIPTION
Beery-Buktenica Developmental Test of Visual-Motor Integration, Sixth Edition (Beery VMI; Beery et al., 2004)	The *Beery VMI* assesses the degree to which visual processing skills and finger-hand-wrist movements are well coordinated. The Beery VMI is a developmental sequence of geometric forms to be imitated or copied using paper and pencil. The Beery VMI series also provides supplemental visual perception (motor-free) and motor coordination tests.
Behavior Rating Inventory of Executive Function (BRIEF 2; Gioia et al., 2013)	The *BRIEF* consists of questionnaires for parents and teachers to complete that enables professionals to assess executive function behaviors in children and adolescents ages 5 to18 years. There are two indices: the Behavior Regulation Index (BRI) and the Metacognition Index (MCI). A Global Executive Composite is derived from the BRI and MCI. The subdomains for the BRI are: 1. Inhibit: ability to resist or not act on impulse and ability to stop one's own behavior at the appropriate time 2. Shift: ability to freely move from one situation or activity as circumstances demand, e.g. make transitions, alter attention, change focus from one topic to another 3. Emotional control: self-regulation of behaviors; ability to modulate emotional responses, e.g. self-calming behaviors, ability to respond appropriately to unexpected negatively perceived events The subdomains for the MCI are: 1. Initiate: ability to start tasks; ability to generate ideas or problem-solving strategies 2. Working memory: capacity to hold information in mind to complete tasks 3. Plan and organize: ability to manage current and future-oriented task demands, e.g. imagining, sequencing; ability to organize oral and written expression 4. Organization of materials: orderliness of play, work and storage spaces; manner in which one orders or organizes their world and belongings 5. Monitor: work-checking habits; monitor and evaluate behavior
Bruininks-Oseretsky Test of Motor Proficiency, Second Edition (BOT™-2; Bruininks & Bruininks, 2005)	The *BOT-2* is a reliable tool for assessing both the fine motor and gross motor skills (combined or separately) of children ages 4 to 21. It can be used to measure the motor proficiency of those who are typically developing to those with moderate motor-skill deficits. The tool is comprised of eight tests: fine motor precision, fine motor integration, manual dexterity, bilateral coordination, balance, running speed and agility, upper limb coordination, and strength.
Evaluation Tool of Children's Handwriting (ETCH; Amundson, 1995)	The *ETCH* evaluates the manuscript and cursive handwriting skills of students in grades 1 to 6. It assesses handwriting speed and legibility in writing tasks similar to those required of classroom students. Its focus is to assess a student's legibility and speed of handwriting tasks similar to those required of students in the classroom. ETCH tasks include alphabet and numerical writing, near-point and far-point copying, dictation, and sentence generation. It assesses legibility components, pencil grasp, hand preference, manipulative skills with the writing tool, and classroom observations.
Jordan Left Right Reversal Test 3rd edition (Jordan-3; Jordan, 1991)	The *Jordan-3* is designed to identify children and adolescents who have difficulty recognizing correct orientation of letters and numbers or who may reverse words or other letter sequences.
Motor-Free Visual Perception Test, Third Ed. (MVPT-3; Colarusso & Hammill, 2003)	The *MVPT-3* is designed for ages 4 to 85 years. The MVPT-3 assesses visual perception without copying tasks. Tasks include matching, figure-ground, closure, visual memory, and form discrimination. Stimuli are line drawings. Answers are presented in multiple-choice format. Responses may be given verbally or by pointing. It is particularly useful with those who may have learning, cognitive, motor, or physical disabilities.
Peabody Developmental Motor Scales-2 (PDMS-2; Folio & Fewell, 2000)	The *PDMS-2* is designed to assess the motor skills of children from birth through 5 years of age. It is an early childhood motor development program that provides in-depth assessment of a child's gross and fine motor skills. It is composed of six subtests that measure interrelated motor abilities that develop early in life.

*We acknowledge Mashelle Painter for contributions to this appendix.

ASSESSMENT	DESCRIPTION
Schoodles Pediatric Fine Motor Assessment (PFMA; Frank & Wing, 2011)	The *Schoodles PFMA* is a tool designed to obtain detailed, individualized information/data about fine motor skills required to be successful in school. It is used to evaluate fine motor skills in students aged 3 through 18 years. The assessment is divided into two skills sets: classroom skills and supporting or underlying skills
School Function Assessment (SFA; Coster et al., 1998)	The *SFA* is used to measure a student's performance on functional tasks that support participation in the academic and social aspects of an elementary school program (grades kindergarten to 6). The SFA is comprised of three parts: participation, task supports, and activity performance.
Sensory Processing Measure (SPM; Parham et al., 2007)	The *SPM* is a set of rating forms that enables assessment of social participation, sensory processing abilities or issues, and motor planning skills in children. The school form is completed by a rater who has taught the child on a regular basis for at least 1 month. The purpose of the SPM is to gain insight about how the child responds to input from senses such as touch, movement, sight, and hearing. The items rate how frequently behaviors occur with or without assistance or environmental modifications. The areas rated are: social participation, vision, hearing, touch, taste and smell, body awareness, balance and motion, and planning and ideas.
Sensory Processing Measure-Preschool (SPM-P; Miller Kuhaneck et al., 2010)	The *SPM-P* is a set of rating forms that enables assessment of social participation, sensory processing abilities or issues, and motor planning skills in children of preschool age (2–5 years old). The SPM-P consists of two rating forms, i.e., home and preschool (day-care or other community settings) with interpretation companion forms. The home form is completed by the parent(s) or guardian (s). The school form is completed by a rater who has cared for the child on a regular basis for at least 1 month.
Sensory Profile 2 (Dunn, 1999)	The *Sensory Profile 2* is a group of assessments that help identify a child's sensory processing patterns in the context of home, school, and community-based activities. Questionnaires are used to determine sensory processing patterns by identifying strengths and potential areas of challenge. Questionnaire forms are completed by caregivers and teachers through observation of the child's response to sensory interactions that occur throughout the day.
Test of Visual Perceptual Skills (TVPS-3; Martin, 2006)	The *TVPS-3* can be administered to individuals ages 4 to 18 years. Assesses the ability to mentally manipulate what is seen without requiring a motor response. There are seven subtests: visual discrimination, visual memory, spatial relations, form constancy, sequential memory, visual figure-ground, and visual closure.
The Print Tool (Olsen & Knopton, 2006)	The *Print Tool*, a companion to the Handwriting Without Tears program, is an assessment used to evaluate and remediate capital letters, lowercase letters, and numbers. Students complete writing samples that are then scored. It can be administered to individual students or to entire classes in the fall and spring to compare results over the course of a school year.

MODEL OF HUMAN OCCUPATION ASSESSMENTS (these can be administered by occupational therapy assistants).

Assessment of Communication and Interaction Skills (ACIS); Forsyth, Salamy, Simon & Kielhofner, 1998)	The *ACIS* is an observational assessment that evaluates communication and interaction skills used to accomplish daily occupations. It contains 20 items divided into physicality, information exchange, and relations. Items are rated on a 4-point scale. The occupational therapist observes the child interacting with others for 15 to 45 minutes and completes the scale following guidelines outlined in the manual.
Child Occupational Self Assessment (COSA; Keller, tenVelden, Kafkas, Basu, Federico & Kielhofner, 2005)	A self-report that asks young client's to report their sense of competence when performing and values for everyday activities in their school, home, and community. The COSA takes 15 to 20 minutes to complete; children rate their performance competency and the importance of item. The therapist discusses the results with the child to design intervention based on the child's priorities.
Occupational Therapy Psychosocial Assessment of Learning (OTPAL; Townsend et al., 2001)	This assessment uses observation and interviews to evaluate a student's volition (the ability to make choices), habituation (roles and routines), and environmental fit within the classroom setting. The manual includes reproducible assessment and data summary forms.
Pediatric Volitional Questionnaire (PVQ; Basu, Kafkes, Schatz, Kiraly, & Kielhofner, 2008)	The *PVQ* is an observational assessment designed to evaluate a young child's volition, including motivation, values, and interests, and effect of the environment. The PVQ consists of a 14-item rating scale. The therapist observes the child for 15 to 30 minutes in a variety of contexts and completes the scale. Each item is rated spontaneous, involved, hesitant, or passive, based on the child's performance.

Continued

School Setting Interview (SSI; Hemmingsson, Egilson, Hoffman, & Kielhofner, 2005)	The *SSI* is a semistructured interview that is designed to assess student–environment fit and identify the need for accommodations in the school setting. The SSI consists of 16 items and takes about 40 minutes.
Short Child Occupational Profile (SCOPE; Bowyer, Kramer, Ploszai, Ross, Schwarz, Kielhofner, & Kramer, 2008)	*SCOPE* is a self-report that explores the client's performance, habits, roles, volition, interests. The manual includes reproducible assessment and data summary forms.
Worker Role Interview (WRI; Braveman et al., 2005)	The *WRI* is a semistructured interview used to evaluate injured workers in the areas of personal causation, values, interests, roles, habits and perception of environmental support. The WRI may provide transition assistance for adolescents.
Work Environment Impact Scale (WEIS; Moore-Corner, Kielhofner, & Olson, 1998)	*WEIS* is a semistructured interview that evaluates features in the work environment that support or impede occupational performance, and the effect on a person's performance, satisfaction, and well-being. WEIS may be used with adolescents.

Appendix References

Amundson, S. J. (1995). *Evaluation tool of children's handwriting.* Homer, AK: OT KIDS.

Basu, S., Kafkes, A., Schatz, R., Kiraly, A., & Kielhofner, G. (2008). *The Pediatric Volitional Questionnaire (PVQ), version 2.1.* Chicago: MOHO Clearinghouse, University of Illinois.

Beery, K. E., Buktenica, N. A., & Beery, N. A. (2004). *Developmental test of visual motor integration* (5th ed.). Los Angeles: Western Psychological Services.

Bowyer, P., Kramer, J., Ploszai, A., Ross, M., Schwarz, O., Kielhofner, G., et al. (2008). *The Short Child Occupational Profile (SCOPE). Version 2.2.* Chicago: MOHO Clearinghouse, University of Illinois.

Braveman, B., Robson, M., Velozo, C., Kielhofner, G., Fisher, G., Forsyth, K., et al. (2005). *Worker Role Interview (WRI) (Version 10.0).* Chicago: MOHO Clearinghouse Department of Occupational Therapy, University of Illinois.

Bruininks, R. H., & Bruininks, B. D. (2005). *Bruininks-Oseretsky Test of Motor Proficiency* (2nd ed.). *Manual* Circle Pines, MN: AGS Publishing.

Colarusso, R., & Hammill, D. (2003). *MVPT-3: Motor-Free Visual Perception Test* (3rd ed.). Novato, CA: Academic Therapy Publications.

Coster, W., Deeney, T., Haltiwanger, J., & Haley, S. (1998). *School function assessment.* San Antonio, TX: Psychological Corporation.

Dunn, W. (1999). *Sensory profile user's manual.* San Antonio, TX: Psychological Corporation.

Folio, M. R., & Fewell, R. R. (2000). *Peabody developmental motor scales* (2nd ed.). Austin, TX: Pro-Ed.

Forsyth, K., Salamy, M., Simon, S., & Kielhofner, G. (1998). *The assessment of communication and interaction skills (ACIS). Version 4.* Chicago: MOHO Clearinghouse: University of Illinois.

Frank, M., & Wing, A. (2011). *Schoodles Pediatric Fine Motor Assessment: an OT's guide for assessing children ages 3 and up* (3rd ed.). Marshall, MN: Authors.

Gioia, G. A., Isquith, P. K., Guy, S. C., & Kenworthy, L. (2013). *Behavior rating inventory of executive function professional manual.* Odessa, FL: PAR.

Hemmingsson, H., Egilson, S., Hoffman, O., & Kielhofner, G. (2005). *The school setting interview (SSI) version 3.0.* Chicago: MOHO Clearinghouse: University of Illinois.

Jordan, B. A. (1991). *Jordan left-right reversal test* (3rd ed.). Los Angeles: Western Psychological Services.

Keller, J., tenVelden, M., Kafkes, A., Basu, S., Federico, J., & Kielhofner, G. (2005). *Child occupational self assessment. Version 2.1.* Chicago: MOHO Clearinghouse: Occupational Therapy Department, College of Applied Health Sciences, University of Illinois.

Martin, N. (2006). *TVPS-3: test of visual perceptual skills* (3rd ed.). Novato, CA: Academic Therapy Publications.

Miller Kuhaneck, H., Ecker, C., Parham, L. D., Henry, D. A., & Glennon, T. J. (2010). *Sensory processing measure – preschool (SPM-P): manual.* Los Angeles: Western Psychological Services.

Moore-Corner, R., Kielhofner, G., & Olson, L. (1998). *Work environment impact scale (WEIS) (version 2.0).* Chicago: MOHO Clearinghouse, Department of Occupational Therapy, College of Applied Health Sciences, University of Illinois.

Olsen, J., & Knopton, E. (2006). *The print tool evaluation & remediation package.* Cabin John, MD: Handwriting Without Tears.

Parham, L. D., Ecker, C., Kuhanek, H. M., Henry, D. A., & Glennon, T. J. (2007). *Sensory processing measure manual.* Los Angeles: Western Psychological Services.

Townsend, S. C., Carey, P. D., Hollins, N. L., Helfrich, C., Blondis, M., Hoffman, A., et al. (2001). *The occupational therapy psychosocial assessment of learning (OTPAL), version 2.0.* Chicago: MOHO Clearinghouse, Department of Occupational Therapy, University of Illinois, Chicago.

JEAN WELCH SOLOMON

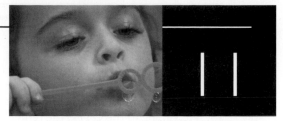

Anatomy and Physiology for the Pediatric Practitioner

11

KEY TERMS

Skeletal system
Muscular system
Integumentary system
Cardiovascular system
Respiratory system
Nervous system
Endocrine system
Digestive system
Urinary system
Lymphatic system
Immune system
Reproductive system

CHAPTER *Objectives*

After studying this chapter, the reader will be able to accomplish the following:

- Distinguish between two branches of biology: anatomy and physiology.
- Understand and describe the hierarchy of organization of the human body.
- Describe the anatomic position.
- Understand and define the descriptive and movement terminology.
- Understand the cardinal planes and axes.
- Describe the structures and functions of the organ systems of the human body.
- Provide examples of pediatric health conditions or disorders of the organ systems of the human body.
- Understand and describe the relationship among body structures, the function of body structures, and one's successful engagement in daily occupations.

CHAPTER *Outline*

Terminology, Planes, and Axes

Skeletal System

Muscular System

Integumentary System

Cardiovascular System

Respiratory System

Nervous System

Endocrine System

Digestive System

Urinary System

Lymphatic System

Immune System

Reproductive System

Relationship Between Body Structures
  and Functions and Occupational
  Performance

Summary

The Occupational Therapy Practice Framework (OTPF) describes the domains and processes inherent to the profession of occupational therapy. According to the OTPF, the term *client factors* refers to those components that influence actions or occupations.[1] For example, a child's neuromuscular status is considered a client factor. Client factors include both body structures and functions (Table 11-1). The term *body structures* refers to the parts that make up the human body.[5] For example, the structure of the hand includes bones, muscles, tendons, nerves, and blood vessels. A child with a missing thumb would have a deficient body structure that may interfere with his occupational performance. The term *body functions* refers to how the body part, organ, or organ system works.[5] In the former example, body function would include the child's hand strength or coordination. Deficits in body functions also may result in poor occupational performance. Because body functions and body structures are essential to understanding occupational performance, this chapter provides an overview of the structures in each body system. The chapter also provides an overview of how body structures and body functions influence occupational performance.

TABLE 11-1

Client Factors

CATEGORY AND DEFINITION	EXAMPLES
VALUES, BELIEFS, AND SPIRITUALITY	
Values: Principles, standards, or qualities considered worthwhile or desirable by the client who holds them	Honesty with self and others
	Personal religious convictions
	Commitment to family.
Beliefs: Cognitive content held as true	He or she is powerless to influence others
	Hard work pays off
Spirituality: Individual search for meaning and purpose, way person experiences connectedness	Daily search for purpose and meaning in one's life
	Guiding actions from sense of value beyond the personal acquisition of wealth or fame
BODY FUNCTIONS	
Mental Functions (Affective, Cognitive, Perceptual)	
Specific Mental Functions	
Higher-level cognitive	Judgment, insight
Attention	Awareness, sustained, selective, attention
Memory	Short-term, long-term, and working memory
Perception	Discrimination, spatial, and temporal relationships
Thought	Recognition, categorization, generalization
Mental functions of sequencing complex movement	Execution of learned movement patterns
Emotion	Coping, adapting
Experience of self and time	Body image, self-concept, self-esteem
Global Mental Functions	
Consciousness	Level of arousal, level of consciousness
Orientation	Orientation to person, place, time, self, and others
Temperament and personality	Emotional stability
Energy and drive	Motivation, impulse control, and appetite
Sleep	
Sensory Functions	
Visual	Detection/registration, modulation, and integration of sensations from the body and environment
Hearing	
Vestibular	Visual awareness
Taste	Sensation of securely moving against gravity
Smell	Association of taste and smell
Proprioceptive	Awareness of body position and space
Touch	Comfort with the feeling of being touched by others
Pain	Localizing pain
Sensitivity to temperature and pressure	Thermal awareness

Continued

TABLE 11-1

Client Factors—cont'd

CATEGORY AND DEFINITION	EXAMPLES
Neuromusculoskeletal and Movement-related Functions	
Functions of joints and bones	Joint range of motion
Joint mobility	Maintenance of structural integrity throughout the body
Joint stability	
Muscle Functions	
Power	Strength
Tone	Degree of muscle tone (e.g., flaccidity, spasticity, fluctuating)
Endurance	Endurance
Movement Functions	
Motor reflexes	Righting and supporting
Involuntary movement reactions	Eye–hand/foot coordination, bilateral integration
Control of voluntary movement	Walking patterns and impairments
Gait patterns	
Cardiovascular, Hematologic, Immunologic, and Respiratory System Functions	
Cardiovascular system function	Blood pressure functions (hypertension, hypotension, postural
Hematologic and immunologic system function	hypotension), and heart rate
Respiratory system function	Rate, rhythm, and depth of respiration
	Physical endurance, aerobic capacity, stamina, and fatigability
Voice and Speech Functions	
	Voice functions
	Fluency and rhythm
	Alternative vocalization functions
Digestive, Metabolic, and Endocrine System Functions	
	Digestive system function
	Metabolic system and endocrine system functions
Genitourinary and Reproductive Functions	
	Urinary functions
	Genital and reproductive functions
Skin and Skin-related Structure Functions	
Skin functions	Protective functions of the skin—presence or absence of
Hair and nail functions	wounds, cuts, or abrasions
	Repair function of the skin—wound healing
BODY STRUCTURES	
Structure of the nervous system	Note: OT practitioners have knowledge of body structures
Eyes, ear, and related structures	and understand how structures influence occupational
Structures involved in voice and speech	performance
Structures of the cardiovascular, immunologic, and respiratory systems	
Structures related to the digestive, metabolic, and endocrine systems	
Structures related to the genitourinary and reproductive systems	
Structures related to movement	
Skin and skin-related structures	

Note. Some data adapted from the ICF (WHO, 2001). World Health Organization. (2001). *International classification of functioning, disability, and health (ICF).* Geneva, Swizerland: WHO.
Adapted from Table 2 (pp. S22–S24) American Occupational Therapy Association. (2014). Occupational therapy practice framework: domain and process (3rd ed.). *Am J Occup Ther, 68*(Suppl. 1), S1–S48; Moyers, P.A., & Dale, L. M. (2007). *The guide to occupational therapy practice* (2nd ed.). Bethesda, MD: AOTA Press.

TABLE 11-2

Major Tissues of the Body

TISSUE TYPE	STRUCTURE	FUNCTION	EXAMPLES IN THE BODY
Epithelial	One or more layers of densely arranged cells with very little extracellular matrix May form either sheets or glands	Covers and protects the body surface Lines body cavities Movement of substances (absorption, secretion, excretion) Glandular activity	Outer layer of skin Lining of the respiratory, digestive, urinary, reproductive tracts Glands of the body
Connective	Sparsely arranged cells surrounded by a large proportion of extracellular matrix often containing structural fibers (and sometimes mineral crystals)	Supports body structures Transports substances throughout the body	Bones Joint cartilage Tendons and ligaments Blood Fat
Muscle	Long fiberlike cells, sometimes branched, capable of pulling loads; extracellular fibers sometimes hold muscle fiber together	Produces body movements Produces movements of organs such as the stomach, heart Produces heat	Heart muscle Muscles of the head/neck, arms, legs, trunk Muscles in the walls of hollow organs such as the stomach, intestines
Nervous	Mixture of many cell types, including several types of neurons (conducting cells) and neuroglia (support cells)	Communication between body parts Integration/regulation of body functions	Tissue of brain and spinal cord Nerves of the body Sensory organs of the body

From Patton, K.T., & Thibodeau G. A. (2016). *Anatomy and physiology* (9th ed.). St. Louis: Mosby.

Successful engagement in daily occupations is dependent on the interactions of many client factors including one's values, beliefs, and spirituality. However, the focus of this chapter is on the client factors related to body structures and functions.

Anatomy is the branch of biology that studies the structures of the human body. Physiology is the branch of biology that studies the functions of the structures of the human body. The human body comprises living matter. A unifying concept in biology is that structure or shape determines function in all living matter. One's successful engagement in chosen daily occupations may be impaired if specific client factors related to body structures and functions are impaired or abnormal.

The organization of the human body is hierarchical. *Atoms* are the smallest unit of matter. By definition, *matter* is anything that takes up space and has mass or weight. Atoms of different elements have unique masses and space requirements. The most abundant elements found in living matter are carbon, hydrogen, oxygen, nitrogen, and phosphorus. Atoms link together (bond) to form *molecules*. For example, two hydrogen atoms bond with one oxygen atom to form one molecule of water (H_2O). Molecules come together to form *cells*. Cells are the smallest units of living matter. Eukaryotic cells are those found in the human body. They have a membrane-bound nucleus that contains a person's genetic information, for example, DNA and genes. Cells come together to form *tissues*. There are four basic types of tissue found in the human body: epithelial, connective, muscle, and nervous (Table 11-2). Tissues come together to form organs. Organs, (e.g., the heart) are made of two or more types of tissues. Organs come together to form organ systems, for example, the cardiovascular system, or the circulatory system, which consists of the heart and associated vessels. Organ systems come together to form organisms. The human body has numerous organ systems that work together to allow one's active participation in chosen daily occupations.

The occupational therapy (OT) practitioner needs to understand the interrelatedness of various organs and organ systems in the human body. Knowledge of the terminology that is used in the study of the human body's structures and functions also is necessary. The anatomic position is used as a reference point when studying the anatomy and physiology of the human body. By definition, the term *anatomic position* refers to a person standing upright with the arms resting at the side of the body, palms forward, and the head and feet pointing forward. The fingers of both hands are adducted (not spread apart; Figure 11-1). The human body has bilateral (two-sided) symmetry, that is, the right side of the body is a mirror image of the left side of the body.[3,4] The human body is divided into front (anterior/ventral) and back (posterior/dorsal) cavities. Organ systems are located in specific regions of the ventral and dorsal cavities. The ventral cavity is subdivided into thoracic, abdominal, and pelvic cavities. The dorsal cavity is subdivided into cranial and spinal cavities (Figure 11-2).

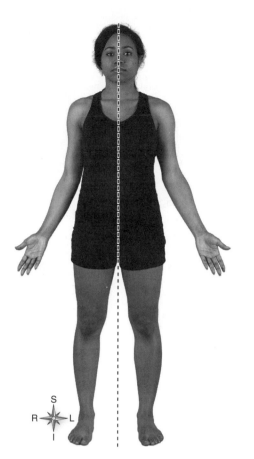

FIGURE 11-1 Anatomic position and bilateral symmetry. (From Thibodeau, G. A., & Patton, K. T. (2016). *Anatomy and physiology* (9th ed.). St. Louis: Mosby.)

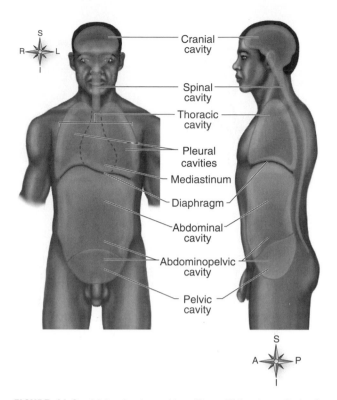

FIGURE 11-2 Major body cavities. (From Thibodeau, G. A., & Patton, K. T. (2016). *Anatomy and physiology* (9th ed.). St. Louis: Mosby.)

TERMINOLOGY, PLANES, AND AXES

In the course of their work, OT practitioners use their knowledge of terminology to examine and understand the structures and functions of the human body. The terms *anterior* or *ventral* refer to the front of the body. The eyes are located in the sockets found on the anterior surface of the head. The terms *posterior* or *dorsal* refer to the back of the body. The spinous processes of the vertebra are found on the posterior surface of the neck and trunk. The terms *superior* or *cephalad* refer to the head, or "above." The nose is superior to the lips. The terms *inferior* or *caudal* refer to the tail/foot, or "below." On the face, the lips are inferior to the nose. *Proximal* means "closer to the body," whereas *distal* means "farther away from the body." The shoulder is proximal to the hand, and the hand is distal to the elbow. *Medial* means "closer to the midline" or to the "midsagittal plane of the body." *Lateral* means "farther away from the midline of the body." With a person standing in the anatomic position, the styloid process of the ulna is medial to the styloid process of the radius.

Knowledge of the three cardinal planes and their axes is important to understand the anatomy and physiology of the human body, especially when analyzing the cross-sections of structures and movements at individual joints. (1) The *sagittal plane* divides the body into left and right sides. If the body is divided into equal left and right parts, then the plane is called the *midsagittal plane*. The axis for the sagittal plane is the *frontal axis*, which is perpendicular to the sagittal plane. (2) The *frontal plane* divides the human body into anterior and posterior parts. The axis for the frontal plane is the *sagittal axis*. (3) The *horizontal* or *transverse plane* divides the body into upper and lower parts. The axis for the horizontal plane is the *vertical axis*. Specific movements occur in each of the three cardinal planes, and the axes are the points about which a body part rotates. For example, bending of the elbow occurs in the sagittal plane. The elbow joint rotates about the frontal axis. Understanding these concepts is crucial to the analysis and measurement of the range of motion (ROM) of joints (Figure 11-3).

Knowledge of terms that are used to describe movements is useful when studying the muscular and skeletal systems to analyze the activity demands and client factors necessary for occupational performance. *Flexion* is the bending at a joint, which decreases the angle of the joint. *Extension* is the straightening of a joint, which increases the angle of the joint. Flexion and extension occur in the sagittal plane, with rotation about the frontal axis. *Abduction* is movement *away* from the midline of the body, whereas *adduction* is movement *toward* the

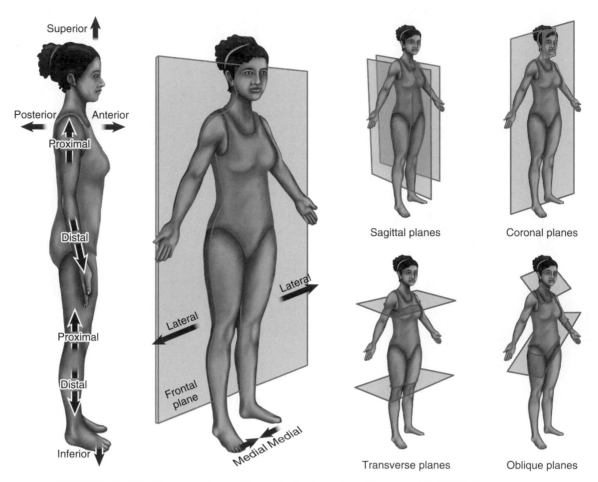

FIGURE 11-3 Directions and planes of the body. (Redrawn from Muscolino, J. E. (2012). *Know the body: muscle, bone, and palpation essentials,* St. Louis: Mosby.)

midline of the body. Abduction and adduction occur in the frontal plane, with rotation about the sagittal axis. Horizontal abduction and adduction, for example, moving the arm across the chest or toward the back of the body, are movements that occur in the horizontal plane. Internal (medial) and external (lateral) rotations, that is, movements of the head of the humerus in and out of the glenoid fossa, occur in the transverse plane. Forearm supination is turning palms up. Forearm pronation is turning palms down so that the palms of the hands face the floor. *Supination* and *pronation* occur in the transverse or horizontal plane, with rotation about the vertical axis. All of these movements are possible only with intact skeletal and muscular organ systems.

CLINICAL *Pearl*

To remember the definition of *supination,* think about how you carry a bowl of soup, palm up; *pronation* is the opposite.

SKELETAL SYSTEM

The **skeletal system** consists of bones, cartilage, ligaments, and joints. The two major subdivisions of the skeletal system are the axial and appendicular systems. The *axial skeletal system* consists of the bones, cartilage, ligaments, and joints of the neck and trunk. The *appendicular skeletal system* consists of the bones, cartilage, ligaments, and joints of the arms and legs (upper and lower extremities; Figure 11-4).

CLINICAL *Pearl*

To remember the number of vertebra in the first three regions of the vertebral column, know that breakfast is at 7 in the morning, lunch is at noon, and dinner is at 5 in the afternoon. This translates into 7 cervical vertebrae, 12 thoracic vertebrae, and 5 lumbar vertebrae. The vertebrae of the sacrum and coccyx are fused, and the number of vertebrae can be variable.

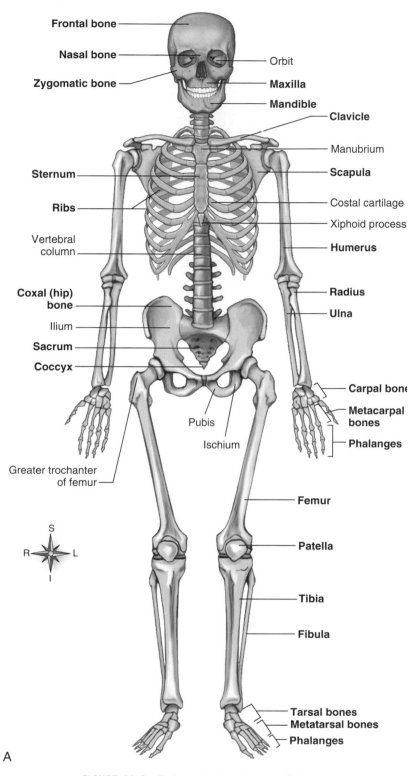

Frontal bone

Nasal bone

Zygomatic bone

Orbit

Maxilla

Mandible

Clavicle

Manubrium

Sternum

Scapula

Ribs

Costal cartilage

Xiphoid process

Vertebral column

Humerus

Coxal (hip) bone

Radius

Ilium

Ulna

Sacrum

Coccyx

Carpal bone

Metacarpal bones

Pubis

Phalanges

Ischium

Greater trochanter of femur

Femur

Patella

Tibia

Fibula

Tarsal bones

Metatarsal bones

Phalanges

A

FIGURE 11-4 Skeleton. **A,** Anterior view. Skeleton.

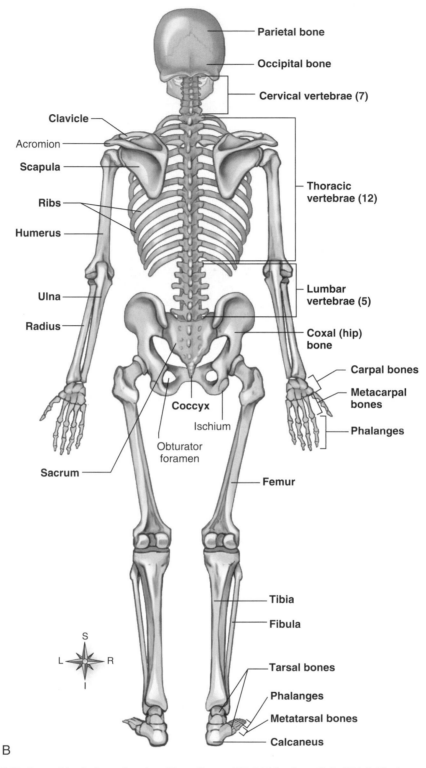

Parietal bone

Occipital bone

Cervical vertebrae (7)

Clavicle

Acromion

Scapula

Ribs

Humerus

Thoracic vertebrae (12)

Ulna

Radius

Lumbar vertebrae (5)

Coxal (hip) bone

Carpal bones

Metacarpal bones

Coccyx

Ischium

Phalanges

Obturator foramen

Sacrum

Femur

S

L R

I

Tibia

Fibula

Tarsal bones

Phalanges

Metatarsal bones

Calcaneus

B

FIGURE 11-4, cont'd   B, Posterior view. (From Patton, K.T., & Thibodeau, G. A. (2014). *The human body in health & disease* (6th ed.). St. Louis: Mosby.)

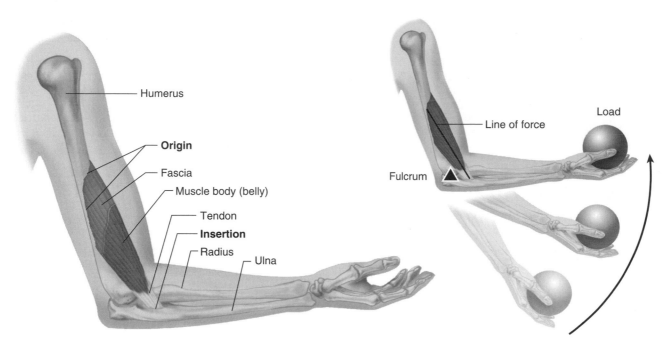

FIGURE 11-5   Attachments of the skeletal muscle. (Adapted from Muscolino, J. E. (2006). *Kinesiology*, St. Louis: Mosby.)

The primary functions of the skeletal system are support of the human body and protection of internal vital organs. In concert with the muscular system, the skeletal system allows movement at joints (articulations between two or more bones) or supports movement-related functions in the human body.[1] Different types of joints are found in the human body. Shoulder and hip joints are called *ball and socket joints*, which are freely movable in all three of the cardinal planes. During typical development, bones fully ossify and provide stability. Examples of disorders of the skeletal system include fractures and congenital amputations. See Chapter 13 for a discussion of disorders and health conditions of the skeletal system.

MUSCULAR SYSTEM

The three types of muscle in the **muscular system** are cardiac, smooth, and skeletal muscles. *Cardiac muscle* is found in the heart; it contracts to maintain blood circulation throughout the body. Cardiac muscle contracts involuntarily and is controlled by its own pacemaker. *Smooth muscle* is found in the internal organs of the body and is not under conscious control. For example, smooth muscle in the organs of the digestive system contracts to move nutrients through the digestive tract. The third type of muscle is *skeletal* or *striated muscle(s)*. The contraction and relaxation of skeletal muscle is under conscious control. Skeletal muscle has at least two attachments to bone—the origin and the insertion, which consist of bands of connective tissue called *tendons*. Between the origin and the insertion is the *muscle bulk* or *muscle belly* (Figure 11-5).

Skeletal muscle contracts to create movement at joints. Skeletal muscles have a role in *thermoregulation* (regulating the temperature of the body) and *osmoregulation* (regulating the amount of water in the human body). Skeletal muscles function as agonists or antagonists when contracting to create movement at a joint. The *agonist* is the prime mover muscle that shortens, producing movement at a joint. The *antagonist* is the muscle that lengthens to allow movement at a joint (Figure 11-6). An example of a minor disorder of the muscular system is a sprain. See Chapter 13 for a discussion of health conditions and disorders associated with the muscular system.

CLINICAL *Pearl*

Skeletal muscles are named in a variety of ways that include the location, the action, and the shape of the muscle. Extensor carpi radialis is located on the radial or thumb side of the forearm (radialis) and extends (extensor) the wrist (carpi). Pronator quadratus is shaped like a rectangle with four sides (quadratus) and pronates (pronator) the forearm.

CLINICAL *Pearl*

Agonists and antagonists simultaneously shorten and lengthen because of reciprocal innervation that results in the coactivation (simultaneous contraction) of both muscle groups.

CLINICAL *Pearl*

Co-contraction is a term used to describe agonistic and antagonistic muscle groups contracting simultaneously at a joint to provide stability proximally or distally to support movement. For example, when you brush your hair, the muscles of the shoulder and wrist contract to stabilize these joints, whereas the elbow straightens and bends moving the brush through your hair.

INTEGUMENTARY SYSTEM

The structures of the **integumentary system** are the skin, hair, nails, and sebaceous glands. The skin is the largest organ in the human body. Skin has two primary layers: the epidermis and the dermis. The *epidermis* is the thin outer layer that is composed of epithelial cells. Epithelial tissue or thin skin also lines the internal organs.

The *dermis* is the deeper, thicker layer of skin that consists of dense connective tissue. The skin functions as the body's first line of defense against potential invading microbes, acting as an external barrier associated with the immune system (immunologic function within the OTPF). It also functions in *homeostasis*, that is, thermoregulation (relatively stable internal body temperature) and osmoregulation (balance among water and electrolytes). The skin also has a role in sensory functions and pain.[1] Acne, typically seen in adolescents and young adults, is a disorder involving the skin and its associated structures. Decubitus ulcers (pressure sores) can be a serious disorder involving the integumentary system. Decubitus ulcers develop from extended pressure on bony prominences that causes skin cells to die. OT practitioners can help prevent decubitus ulcers by recommending a variety of positioning options. Additional information on positioning can be found in subsequent chapters.

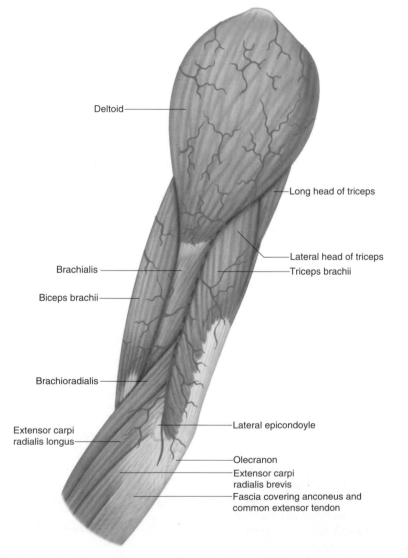

FIGURE 11-6   Muscles of the left upper arm. (From Standring, S. (2004). *Gray's anatomy: the anatomical basis of clinical practice* (39th ed.). Philadelphia: Churchill Livingstone.)

CARDIOVASCULAR SYSTEM

The **cardiovascular system** consists of the heart, blood, blood vessels (arteries, veins, and capillaries), and bone marrow (which is the site of blood cell formation). The cardiovascular system functions in the transport and exchange of oxygen, nutrients, and waste products. It also has hematologic (blood) function. Three circuits of blood flow are found in the cardiovascular system: pulmonary, systemic, and coronary paths. The *pulmonary circuit* allows transport and exchange between the heart and lungs. Oxygen-poor blood is pumped from the right atrium to the right ventricle into the left and right pulmonary arteries going to the capillary beds at the alveoli of the lungs. Carbon dioxide diffuses out of the cardiovascular system and oxygen diffuses in. The pulmonary veins return the oxygen-rich blood to the left atrium of the heart.

In the *systemic circuit,* blood is pumped into the left ventricle and then into the aorta to the entire body. The blood returns to the heart via the superior and inferior vena cavae (Figure 11-7).

The *coronary circuit* transports and exchanges oxygen, nutrients, and waste products between heart cells and the pulmonary system. Table 11-3 lists normal values for vital signs. Common disorders or health conditions associated with the cardiovascular system are presented in subsequent chapters.

RESPIRATORY SYSTEM

The structures of the respiratory (pulmonary) system are the nose, mouth, pharynx, larynx, trachea, diaphragm, and lungs. The nose and mouth are the organs of entrance and exit of materials transported and exchanged with the environment by the **respiratory system**. Breathing,

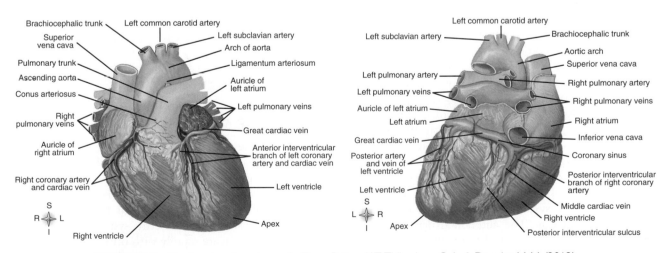

FIGURE 11-7   The heart and great vessels. (From Patton, K.T., Thibodeau, G.A., & Douglas, M.M. (2012). *Essentials of anatomy & physiology.* St. Louis: Mosby.)

TABLE 11-3

Normal Values for Vital Signs in Infants, Children, and Adults

PARAMETER	INFANT	CHILD	ADULT
Heart rate (bpm)	120	70–110	60–80
Blood pressure (mm Hg)	75/50	95/56	120/80
Respiratory rate (breath/min)	20–40	20–30	12–18

the primary function of the respiratory system, involves ventilation and respiration. *Ventilation* is the movement of gases into and out of the lungs. *Respiration* involves an exchange of gases between the alveoli (plural for alveolus) of the lungs and the capillaries of the cardiovascular system. The diaphragm is the major muscle of ventilation. It is a dome-shaped muscle that sits below the lungs separating the thorax from the abdomen of the body. When the diaphragm contracts, the vertical volume increases, thus allowing air to come in (inspiration). When the diaphragm relaxes, the vertical volume decreases, thus forcing air out of the lungs (exhalation). The two major categories of diseases of the respiratory system are obstructive and restrictive diseases. *Obstructive diseases* cause a decrease in airflow. *Restrictive diseases* cause a decrease in the volume or the amount of air that is able to enter the respiratory system. Asthma and cystic fibrosis are examples of obstructive diseases. Kyphoscoliosis is an example of a restrictive respiratory disease.[2] Respiratory distress syndrome is a health condition associated with prematurity. Other pediatric disorders associated with the pulmonary system are presented in subsequent chapters.

NERVOUS SYSTEM

The **nervous system** is further described as one of the two organ systems in the human body that functions in communication and control throughout the body, integrating the functions of all other organ systems. It functions in rapid communication. Refer to Chapter 12 for detailed information on the nervous system. The nervous system has a primary role in mental, sensory, neuromuscular, and movement-related functions.[1] The structures of the nervous system include the brain, spinal cord, cranial nerves, peripheral nerves, and the special sense organs. The two major subdivisions of the nervous system are the central nervous system (CNS) and the peripheral nervous system (PNS). The CNS consists of the brain and the spinal cord. The PNS consists of the network of peripheral nerves, the autonomic nervous system, and the special sense organs such as eyes and ears. The autonomic nervous system consists of the sympathetic (flight or fight) and parasympathetic (rest and digest) nervous systems. The neuron is the basic unit of the nervous system. There are efferent

(motor) and afferent (sensory) neurons. Motor nerves carry electrical messages to effectors such as muscles. Sensory nerves carry sensory information from the periphery to the CNS for processing. Most neurons consist of cell body, dendrite, and axon. The capacity of neurons to communicate rapidly is dependent on the myelin sheath. In certain health conditions, for example, Guillain-Barré syndrome, demyelination occurs and results in temporary paralysis of the muscles innervated by the affected nerves. The disorders associated with the nervous system are presented in subsequent chapters.

CLINICAL *Pearl*

The nervous system stimulates skeletal muscles to contract in order to create movement at the joints. The agonist shortens while the antagonist lengthens because of reciprocal innervation.

CLINICAL *Pearl*

The lower motor neuron (LMN) system includes the cell bodies of the anterior horn of the spinal cord and the spinal and cranial nerves that effect target muscles. The upper motor neuron (UMN) system includes nerve cells in the spinal cord (excluding the cells located in the anterior horn) and all superior structures. Disorders of the LMN system result in flaccidity, decreased or absent deep tendon reflexes, and muscle atrophy. Disorders of the UMN system result in spasticity, exaggerated deep tendon reflexes, and the emergence of primitive reflexes.

ENDOCRINE SYSTEM

The **endocrine system** is the second organ system that functions in communication and control and integrates the functions of other organ systems throughout the human body. The endocrine system is responsible for digestive, metabolic, and hormonal function. Unlike the nervous system, the endocrine system does not necessarily communicate rapidly with other organ systems. The endocrine system contains glands that secrete hormones, which travel to target cells. The circulatory

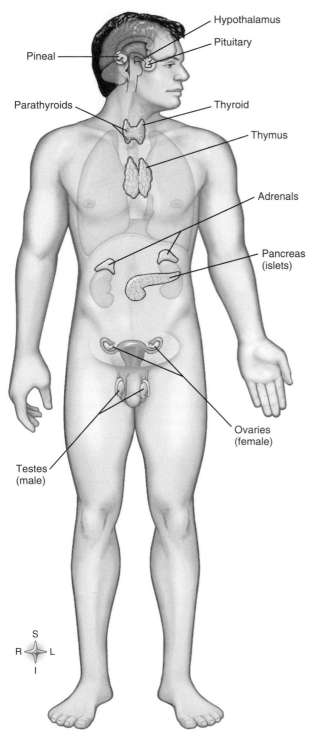

FIGURE 11-8 Locations of some major endocrine glands. (From Patton, K.T., Thibodeau, G. A., & Douglas, M. M. (2012). *Essentials of anatomy and physiology.* St. Louis: Mosby.)

system is the primary means of transport of hormones throughout the body. The endocrine system has hormones that act as agonists and antagonists. Most agonistic and antagonistic hormones function via negative feedback mechanisms. Negative feedback involves the presence of one synergistic hormone signaling another

not to be released. The glands of the endocrine system are widespread throughout the body (Figure 11-8). The nervous and endocrine systems often work in concert with one another. A comparison of the two systems is depicted in Table 11-4. Cushing's syndrome, in which there is redistribution of body fat resulting in a moon face and reddening of the skin, is an example of a disorder of the endocrine system.

DIGESTIVE SYSTEM

The structures of the **digestive system** are the mouth, pharynx, esophagus, stomach, small intestine, large intestine, and accessory organs. The *mouth*, or *oral cavity*, is composed of the teeth, mandible, maxilla, hard and soft palates, and the muscles of the tongue. Certain muscles of facial expression create movement of the lips and the temporomandibular joint (jaw, or the articulation between the maxilla and mandible). Solid, semisolid, or liquid food enters the digestive system through the mouth. Solids are chewed and mixed with saliva to form a bolus in preparation for the food to be digested throughout the digestive system (oral preparation phase of swallow). There are three phases of swallow: oral preparation, oral transit, and pharyngeal phases. The oral transit phase of swallow involves the bolus being actively moved from the front of the mouth to the back. Both the oral preparation and oral transit phases of swallow are voluntary. After the bolus passes into the pharynx, the movement of the bolus is involuntarily controlled by smooth muscles. The movement of food through the digestive system is caused by the involuntary contraction and relaxation of smooth muscle. This movement is known as *peristalsis*. The bolus goes from the pharynx into the esophagus, into the stomach, into the small intestine, and then into the large intestine. The food continues to be chemically digested by these organs. Most of the nutrient resorption occurs in the small intestine, whereas most of the water resorption occurs in the large intestine. Waste products are eliminated though the anus by defecation. Examples of disorders of the digestive system are dysphagia and gastroesophageal reflux disease. *Dysphagia* means difficulty swallowing. Some children and adolescents who have special needs have sensory impairment in the structures of the digestive system. Subsequent chapters further explain how the digestive system is associated with secondary impairments in children and adolescents with special needs.

CLINICAL *Pearl*

Children with low muscle tone often are hyposensitive to tactile and other sensory input. Children with high muscle tone tend to be hypersensitive to input. Hyposensitive children may be unaware of bumps and bruises. Hypersensitive children typically overrespond to input.

TABLE 11-4

Comparison of the Endocrine System and Nervous System

FEATURE	ENDOCRINE SYSTEM	NERVOUS SYSTEM
Overall function	Regulation of effectors to maintain homeostasis	Regulation of effectors to maintain homeostasis
Control by regulatory feedback loops	Yes (endocrine reflexes)	Yes (nervous reflexes)
Effector tissues	Endocrine effectors: virtually all tissues	Nervous effectors: muscle and glandular tissues only
Effector cells	Target cells (throughout the body)	Postsynaptic cells (in muscle and glandular tissue only)
Chemical messenger	Hormone	Neurotransmitter
Cells that secrete the chemical messenger	Glandular epithelial cells or neurosecretory cells (modified neurons)	Neurons
Distance traveled (and method of travel) by chemical messenger	Long (by way of circulating blood)	Short (across a microscopic synapse)
Location of receptor in effector cell	On the plasma membrane or within the cell	On the plasma membrane
Characteristics of regulatory effects	Slow to appear, long lasting	Appear rapidly, short lived

URINARY SYSTEM

The **urinary system** is also known as the *genitourinary system*. The structures of the urinary system are the kidneys, ureters, urinary bladder, and urethra. The functional unit of the kidney is the nephron. The ureters connect the kidneys with the urinary bladder. The urinary bladder is the storage organ for urine. Urine is excreted from the body through the urethra. The primary functions of the urinary system are filtering blood plasma and excreting urine. A developmental hallmark is a toddler's gaining control of the urinary bladder. The sphincter muscle that prevents urine from flowing from the urinary bladder into the urethra must be intact for a child to be able to become toilet trained. An example of health conditions involving the urinary system is incontinence. Disorders of this system can have a significant effect on occupational performance and self-esteem. Toilet hygiene is covered in detail in the chapter on activities of daily living (ADL).

LYMPHATIC SYSTEM

The **lymphatic system** is closely associated with the cardiovascular, or circulatory, system. The primary structures of the lymphatic system are the tonsils, spleen, thymus, lymph, lymphatic vessels, and lymph nodes. The lymph, or lymphatic fluid, is a watery substance that is similar to the fluid found in the spaces between cells throughout the human body. The lymph circulates freely through the lymphatic vessels. The lymphatic system is critical in maintaining homeostasis, or the relatively stable internal environment, within the human body. The second primary function of the lymphatic system is fighting microbes disease-causing organisms in concert with the immune system (immunologic function). An example of a disorder of the lymphatic system is tonsillitis.

CLINICAL *Pearl*

If a word ends in "-itis," it means that inflammation is present in the organ whose name mostly forms the word root. For example, *tonsillitis* means inflammation of the tonsils; *pericarditis* means inflammation of the pericardium of the heart.

IMMUNE SYSTEM

The **immune system** does not have a distinct structure. Blood cells, skin cells, brain cells, and many other cells support the function of the immune system. The primary function of the immune system is to maintain homeostasis of the body and to fight diseases and disorders. Immunity is either nonspecific or specific. *Nonspecific immunity* mechanisms provide a more general defense. The skin is the body's first line of defense against potentially harmful microbes. *Specific immunity* involves different types of mechanisms that target only certain foreign agents called *antigens*. Examples of specific immunity cells are phagocytes and natural killer cells. An inflammatory response occurs when there is injury. The cardinal signs of an inflammatory response are swelling, redness, pain, decreased movement, and warmth to touch (heat). An allergy is a hypersensitivity to a particular substance that is relatively harmless.

Allergens are antigens that cause an allergic response. Juvenile rheumatoid arthritis is an example of a disease of the immune system.

REPRODUCTIVE SYSTEM

The **reproductive system** is necessary for sexual reproduction, but not for other forms of reproduction, for example, mitosis (cell division) or budding (reproduce a new organism from a single parent from a bud). The structures of the human male and female reproductive systems are different. However, both men and women have essential organs known as *gonads*, which produce *gametes* (sex cells that are haploid, i.e., have half the amount of genetic information of the parent cell).

The structures of the male reproductive system include the testes (male gonads), accessory reproductive glands, and supporting organs such as the scrotum and the penis. The function of the male reproductive system is to produce and store gametes. During sexual intercourse, ejaculation of sperm occurs, and subsequently fertilization of the ovum (egg) can occur in the female.

The structures of the female reproductive system include the ovaries, fallopian tubes, uterus, vagina, and accessory reproductive glands. The ovaries are the organs that produce the female gametes, or eggs. The female reproductive system has a cycle between the years of onset of menstruation (menarche) and cessation of menstruation (menopause). The typical menstrual cycle is 28 days, with menstruation lasting approximately 5 days. During menstruation, the outer layer of the uterine wall is shed in preparation for the implanting of a fertilized egg, should it occur.

In the event that a sperm fertilizes an egg, the resulting embryo will implant itself into the endometrium of the uterine wall within several days after fertilization. The fertilized egg is called a *zygote* (diploid cell), which has the same amount of genetic information as each parent. The embryo goes through cell division, or *mitosis*, for approximately 9 months, during which cells, tissues, and organs grow and specialize. The sequence of fetal development is predictable and well documented. During the first trimester, the tactile (touch) system responds to stimuli, the vestibular system begins to develop, and the fetus begins to move inside the womb. During the second trimester, the tactile receptors begin to differentiate and specialize. The fetus begins to process visual and auditory stimuli. The fetus has a wake–sleep cycle. The movement patterns of the fetus are reciprocal and symmetric. During the third trimester, the muscles of the fetus mature. The fetus has tactile, olfactory, and gustatory discrimination. The fetus exhibits primitive reflexes such as rooting and palmar grasp reflexes. Following 36 to 42 weeks of gestation (the average being 40 weeks), a neonate is born. The development from birth through adolescence

was discussed in previous chapters, and genetic disorders are discussed in subsequent chapters.

CLINICAL *Pearl*

Identical twins have identical genetic information but different finger- and footprints. Finger- and footprints develop as a result of the tactile experiences of the fetus in the womb.

RELATIONSHIP BETWEEN BODY STRUCTURES AND FUNCTIONS AND OCCUPATIONAL PERFORMANCE

This chapter provides a discussion of the structures and functions of organ systems from the perspective of a biologist. OT practitioners use this knowledge to better understand how body structures and body functions influence occupational performance and to provide interventions to address areas of deficit. For example, the OT practitioner examines a child's hands to determine whether the structure of the hand (e.g., congenital deformity, edema, or structural anomaly) interferes with the child's performance. The intervention may focus on improving the structure, if possible (e.g., splinting to increase range of motion), or on compensating for the deficit, as might be the case for a child with a congenital anomaly of missing digits.

The OTPF defines body functions according to World Health Organization and includes the following categories:

- Mental functions;
- Specific mental functions;
- Global mental functions;
- Sensory functions;
- Neuromuscular and movement-related functions;
- Muscle functions;
- Movement functions;
- Cardiovascular, hematologic, immunologic, and respiratory system functions;
- Voice and speech functions;
- Digestive, metabolic, and endocrine system functions;
- Genitourinary and reproductive functions; and
- Skin and related structures functions.[1]

The OT practitioner also determines how specific body functions are influencing a child's occupational performance. For example, the OT practitioner examines neuromuscular and movement-related functions such as joint mobility ROM, muscle power (strength), and control of voluntary movements (eye–hand coordination and oculomotor control). If the child's structures are intact, their functions may be influencing the ability of the child to engage in his or her occupations. For example, a child with hypertonicity may have adequate body structures in that the muscles, bones, and joints are within normal limits, but the child may be experiencing difficulty with body functions, including ROM, muscle tone, and control of voluntary movements.

Functions of the cardiovascular and respiratory systems include aerobic capacity and endurance. Again, the OT practitioner uses his or her knowledge of the involved structures to determine the best way to intervene. For example, a child may show decreased endurance secondary to prolonged inactivity, not due to structural dysfunction of the cardiac or respiratory system, such as might be observed when a child has a cardiac abnormality. Thus the OT practitioner acknowledges that the child is showing difficulty in terms body function of the cardiovascular system and that it is interfering with the child's ability to play with peers on the playground, complete ADLs, and perform other occupations.

An immunologic response may be inflammation. Children who have juvenile rheumatoid arthritis may have inflammation in the joints of the wrists and hands that interferes with their occupational performance. OT practitioners observe responses to activities and may provide these children with techniques to lessen the workload, thus reducing inflammation. Subsequent chapters discuss specific joint protection and energy-conservation techniques.

Functions of the digestive, endocrine, genitourinary, reproductive, and integumentary systems have been discussed above. *Metabolism* is the term that sums up all chemical reactions that occur in the human body. Metabolism is important to the maintenance of homeostasis.

OT practitioners examine children's performances in the following occupations: ADLs, instrumental ADLs, rest and sleep, education, work, play, leisure, and social participation. ADLs may also be referred to as *basic ADLs*, or *personal ADLs*. Practitioners analyze children's ability to perform occupations taking into consideration the structures and functions of the associated body systems. For example, eating is an ADL that involves the digestive system and the neuromuscular movement-related system. The OT practitioner considers the body structures by evaluating the child's oral motor structures (e.g., palate, tongue) and consulting with the child's physician to rule out an abnormality in the digestive system function or structure. The OT practitioner analyzes the movement-related functions of the child's oral motor structures and their ability to prepare food to be digested through the digestive tract.

OT practitioners analyze children's ability to perform occupations in light of their body structures and body functions. OT practitioners understand that these occupations occur in a variety of environments (e.g., home, school, community) and contexts (e.g., culture, periods, lifespan) and that many factors influence the child's performance.

SUMMARY

This chapter presented an overview of human anatomy and physiology to help OT practitioners understand how body structures and body functions influence occupational performance. The chapter reviewed basic terminology and planes and their associated axes. Following general information about the organs and organ systems of the human body, body functions from an OT perspective was presented. The chapter concluded by describing the relationship between body structures and functions to occupational performance.

References

1. American Occupational Therapy Association. (2014). Occupational therapy practice framework: domain and process (3rd ed.). *Am J Occup Ther*, 68(Suppl. 1), S1–S48.
2. Moore, A. (2009). *Respiratory lecture*. Charleston, SC: Trident Technical College, OTA Program.
3. Patton, K. T., & Thibodeau, G. A. (2013). *Anatomy and physiology* (8th ed). St. Louis, MO: Mosby.
4. Patton, K. T., & Thibodeau, G. A. (2013). *Mosby's handbook of anatomy and physiology* (2nd ed). St. Louis, MO: Mosby.
5. World Health Organization. (2001). *International classification of functioning, disability, and health*. Geneva, Switzerland: Author.

Recommended Reading

Daniels, P., et al. (2007). *Body: the complete human*. Washington, DC: National Geographic Society.
Chamley, C. A., et al. (2005). *Developmental anatomy and physiology of children: A practical approach*. St. Louis, MO: Mosby.

REVIEW *Questions*

1. What is the difference between anatomy and physiology?
2. Describe the hierarchy of organization of the human body.
3. What *is anatomic position*?
4. What are the structures and functions of the organ systems of the human body?
5. How do body structures and functions impact a child's or adolescent's occupational performance?

SUGGESTED *Activities*

1. Make a table of the organ systems of the human body with three columns for each system: structure, function, and potential effect on occupational performance.
2. Design a three-dimensional model representing planes and axes.
3. Demonstrate the movements of the upper extremity (arm).
4. Conduct an activity analysis carefully describing movement for a given activity.
5. Choose one system and describe how it develops over time. Present this to classmates through a creative project.

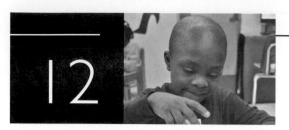

KAREN S. HOWELL

Neuroscience for the Pediatric Practitioner

CHAPTER *Objectives*

After studying this chapter, the reader will be able to accomplish the following:

- Distinguish between the three divisions of the nervous system: central, peripheral, and autonomic.
- Understand the development of the human nervous system and describe common pathologies that occur in neuroembryology.
- Describe the functional areas of the cerebral cortex and anatomic differences in the right and left hemispheres.
- Understand input to the brain and how sensation and perception are integrated.
- Understand output from the brain and the basics of motor control: ascending and descending pathways, cerebellum and basal ganglia.
- Describe the structures and functions of the nervous system that are involved in successful engagement in occupations.
- Provide examples of pediatric conditions that relate to areas of central and peripheral nervous system pathology.
- Understand the structure and function of neurons and the concept of neuroplasticity.

CHAPTER *Outline*

It is simply amazing how a brain, a 3-pound organ that comprises only 2% of our body weight, works to provide the most vital role over our ability to function while also uniquely defining who we are. This chapter will help practitioners gain insight into the fascinating and complex human nervous system. It is big picture information that will hopefully increase your understanding of the nervous system and your ability to help apply that knowledge to treat children who have neurologic conditions that adversely affect occupational performance. Although engagement in occupation is affected by many different client factors, the emphasis in this chapter is to describe the client factors related to the body structures and functions of the nervous system.

THREE DIVISIONS OF THE NERVOUS SYSTEM

The human nervous system can be divided into three parts: the **central nervous system** (CNS), the **peripheral nervous system** (PNS), and the **autonomic nervous system** (ANS) (Figure 12-1). The CNS is comprised of the brain and the spinal cord. The PNS includes the lower **motor neuron**s (LMNs) that leave the ventral horn of the spinal cord and the cranial nerves. These two systems are anatomically distinct from each other. However, the ANS exists both centrally and peripherally with structures such as the hypothalamus and sympathetic and parasympathetic neurons. The ANS is primarily involved in maintaining homeostasis by innervating targeted organs throughout the body.[2,3,4]

When working with a child with a neurologic condition the first task in clinical reasoning for an occupational therapy (OT) practitioner is to determine whether the pathology is a CNS, PNS, or ANS condition. The signs and symptoms the child will display are very different depending on the system involved. See Table 12-1 for signs and symptoms.

CNS damage results in upper motor neuron (UMN) pathology, which is characterized by hyperactive deep tendon reflexes, and spastic paralysis or weakness. Pediatric examples include cerebral palsy (CP), developmental dyspraxia, hydrocephalus, shaken baby syndrome or other reasons for traumatic brain injuries, and spina bifida. Spina bifida is an exception to the rule in

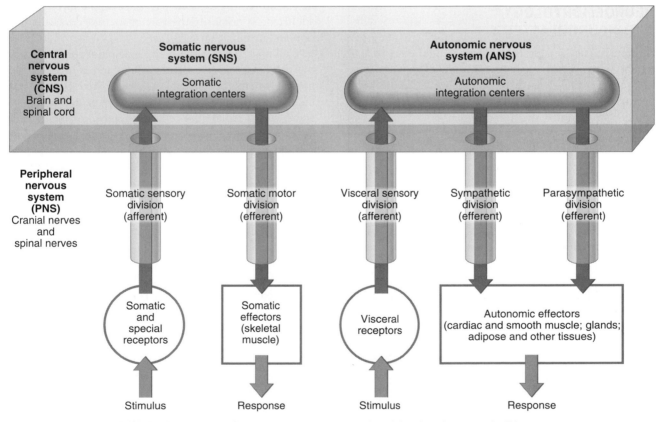

FIGURE 12-1 Three parts of the nervous system: central, peripheral and autonomic. Diagram summarizes the scheme used by most neurobiologists in studying the nervous system. Both the somatic nervous system (SNS) and the autonomic nervous system (ANS) include components in the central nervous system (CNS) and peripheral nervous system (PNS). (From Patton, K. T., Thibodeau, G. A., & Douglas, M. M. (2012). *Essentials of anatomy & physiology.* St. Louis: Mosby.)

regard to UMN pathology because the deficit can result in flaccid or spastic musculature. In contrast PNS damage results in LMN pathology, which is characterized by hypoactive deep tendon reflexes and flaccid weakness or paralysis.[3] Pediatric examples include obstetric brachial plexus injuries such as Erb's palsy and Klumpke's palsy. (See Chapter 13 for a discussion on pediatric health conditions.)

CLINICAL *Pearl*

CP most often occurs with UMN damage to the neurons of the pyramidal tract that transmit the message for voluntary movement or the basal ganglia, which involuntarily help in the execution of complex movements. The child with CP therefore has the clinical manifestations of UMN damage characterized by spasticity and hyperactive deep tendon reflexes. Far less often CP results from damage to the cerebellum. In this situation the motor deficit is manifested as ataxia or postural instability with jerky, uncoordinated movements.[3] (See Chapter 17 for more on CP.)

NEUROEMBRYOLOGY AND NEUROPLASTCITY

The nervous system starts to develop at the end of the second week of embryonic life. This development occurs in five stages: development of the neural tube, proliferation of neurons, migration of neurons, addition of axons and dendrites, and formation of synapses.[4]

The very first event in stage 1, the development of the neural tube, is a thickening in the ectodermal layer of embryonic cells that becomes neuroectoderm. This thickened area begins to form a tube that eventually develops into all of the components of the CNS. A group of cells at the edge of the tube, the neural crest cells, will develop into the entire PNS. The ends of the tube stay open for a week and are referred to as the anterior and posterior neuropore.[4]

TABLE 12-1

Upper and Lower Motor Neuron Signs and Symptoms

UPPER MOTOR NEURON	LOWER MOTOR NEURON
Hyperactive reflexes	Hypoactive reflexes
Increased muscle tone	Decreased muscle tone
Weakness	Weakness
No muscle fasciculations	Muscle fasciculations present
No atrophy	Atrophy

If these openings do not fully close, neurologic problems will occur. Most commonly the problem is the failure of the posterior neuropore to close off completely, resulting in varying degrees of spinal dysraphism: spina bifida occulta, meningocele, and meningomyelocele. (Figure 12-2 illustrates the conditions; see Chapter 13 for more information.) If the anterior neuropore does not close, the brain will not fully develop. This condition is known as anencephaly.[2] In another week the tube differentiates into sections that will eventually contain all of the derivatives of the brain, brainstem, and spinal cord. It also develops flexures that give the brain the perpendicular arrangement of the brain to the spinal cord.

Stage 2, cell proliferation, occurs after closure of the neural tube. These cells, called neuroblasts, once formed pushed externally within the tube to form three zones: ependymal, intermediate (mantle), and later the marginal zone. The ependymal layer borders the spaces of the brain and spinal cord, the ventricles, and central canal. The intermediate layer becomes gray matter or nuclei within the nervous system and the marginal zone; the white matter primarily **ascending and descending pathways**. In this stage close to 85 billion neurons are produced and for the most part, this period ends when the new neurons are produced. The growth in brain size until adulthood is primarily the role of increased vascularization and myelination.[4]

Cell migration for the brain and spinal cord occurs as the third stage in **neuroembryology** and it involves the process where the neuroblasts reach their correct and final location. To correctly migrate, the neuroblast cooperates with a radial glial cell, a transient supporting cell, by allowing the neuroblast to use the radial glial cell as a template to migrate around it to reach its destination. Similar types of migration processes occur in the brainstem and the PNS. Defective migration patterns can lead to several types of congenital deficits such as developmental dyslexia. In addition, microencephaly, a small brain, or lissencephaly, a smooth brain can occur when there are complications with cell migration. These conditions often result in serious motor and cognitive delays or slowing.

Stage 4 is cell differentiation, which is when the neuron develops its axon and then the dendrites. In many regions once a neuron reaches its final destination, the trailing process of the migrating neuron becomes the axon. The final stage is the development of synapses or synaptogenesis, the circuitry for neurons to communicate. The presynaptic axon terminal develops the ability to release neurotransmitters into the synaptic cleft and the postsynaptic cell must develop the ability to receive the neurotransmitters. These connections can be neuron to neuron or neuron to muscle fiber or target organ.[4]

Neuroplasticity, is a term used to describe the dynamic and ever-changing nature of the brain. The brain is use-dependent, meaning that the way an individual uses it is

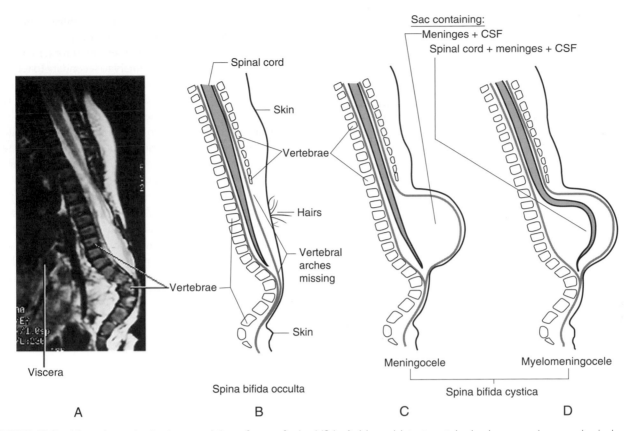

Sac containing:
Meninges + CSF
Spinal cord + meninges + CSF

Spinal cord

Skin

Vertebrae

Hairs

Vertebral arches missing

Skin

Vertebrae

Viscera

Meningocele

Myelomeningocele

Spina bifida occulta

Spina bifida cystica

A   B   C   D

FIGURE 12-2   Normal vertebral column and three forms of spina bifida. **A,** Normal: intact vertebral column, meninges, and spinal cord. **B,** Spina bifida occulta: bony defect in vertebral column. **C,** Meningocele: bony defect in which meninges fill with spinal fluid and protrude through an opening in the vertebral column. **D,** Myelomeningocele: bony defect in which meninges fill with spinal fluid, and a portion of the spinal cord with its nerves protrude through an opening in the vertebral column. (From Haines, D. E. (2013). *Fundamental neuroscience for basic and clinical applications* (4th ed.). St. Louis: Elsevier.)

reflected in its structural and functional architecture. The brain of a pianist will have far more cortical representation for the fingers than that of a prima ballerina. Changes take place throughout a person's lifetime in neurons, vasculature, glia, and other supportive neural structures. However, this plasticity is age-dependent. Take, for example, the acquisition of language. The brain is far more supportive or plastic for the development of language in a young child than in the older adult. It is because of neuroplasticity that there is hope for improvement after there has been CNS damage.[3] Although the neurons that have been destroyed cannot be replaced with new ones, the functions that the damaged neurons had can be relearned through the development of new synapses. Synaptogenesis, the ability to gain new synapses, is a function that stays with us throughout our lives.

CLINICAL *Pearl*

When the brain of a child is damaged, such as from CP, surrounding healthy neurons can take on the functions of the damaged neurons. One factor that will enhance this plasticity is repetition of the task that is being learned.[3]

CEREBRUM: HEMISPHERES, LOBES, AND VASCULATURE

The **cerebrum** is comprised of right and left cerebral hemispheres. One of the first features to note about the cerebrum is that it is not smooth, but is convoluted with the hills called gyri and the grooves called sulci. Most of the surface area of the cerebrum is within the sulci.

In the vast majority of humans the left hemisphere is the dominant hemisphere providing motor control for the right side of the body and specializing in functions such as receiving and expressing speech. In half of the individuals who are left-handed the dominant hemisphere is still the left hemisphere. The right hemisphere specializes in perception and creativity (Table 12-2 describes these functional asymmetries of the left and right cerebral hemispheres).[3,4]

The **cerebral cortex** is the layer of gray matter that surrounds each **hemisphere**. Each hemisphere is divided into five **lobes**: the frontal, parietal, occipital, and temporal on the lateral side and the limbic lobe on the medial side (Figure 12-3). The frontal lobes house personality, judgment, insight, and motor control.

TABLE 12-2

Functional Asymmetries of the Cerebral Hemispheres

LEFT HEMISPHERE DOMINANCE	RIGHT HEMISPHERE DOMINANCE
Language and verbal skills	Singing
Hearing and comprehension	Perceptual abilities
Academics	Spatial relationships, visualizing a way through a maze
Analytical, sequential, logical thinking	Intuitive, creative thinking
The details	The gestalt
Control of the right hand/handwriting	Processing of emotions

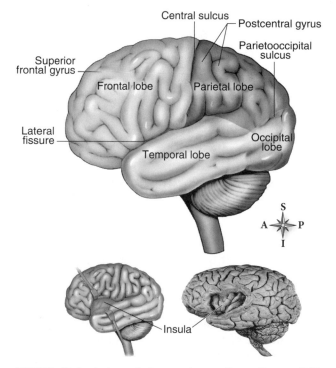

FIGURE 12-3 Lobes of the cerebrum. (From Patton, K. T., Thibodeau, G. A., & Douglas, M. M. (2012). *Essentials of anatomy & physiology.* St. Louis: Mosby.)

The primary function of the parietal lobes is to make sense out of the sensations coming from the body that relate to touch, pressure, tactile discrimination, and conscious proprioception. The occipital lobe receives and makes sense from what one is seeing and the temporal lobe from what one is hearing. The limbic lobe processes memories and is responsible for emotions.

Areas of the cortex have been given names, numbers, and functional designations (Figure 12-4).

The brain processes incoming sensory information in a hierarchical manner using a primary to secondary to tertiary sequence.[2,3,4] Sensory information such as touch, vision, or hearing comes to the primary area in that lobe to start the process of making sense of the sensation. It then goes to the secondary association area to add more detail to the information received from the primary area and finally to a tertiary association area to complete the process. For example, a practitioner places a quarter in a child's hand and asks the child if he or she can tell what it is by touch alone. The first cortical information the child uses to determine the answer is from the primary cortical area that begins to give details of the object such as cold, metal, or round. Next the secondary area puts the information together to let the child identify the item as a quarter and finally the tertiary area ties the quarter to past experiences and gives the quarter meaning in regard to exactly what it is and what it is worth.[2,3,4]

CLINICAL *Pearl*

The exception to the usual pattern for processing of data by the cortex is in the frontal lobe where information about motor planning flows from tertiary areas, formulating a plan to move, to secondary, putting together the details of the movement to primary, executing the plan for the individual contraction of muscles to result in that movement.

When pathology occurs it can damage the cerebrum in any lobe or structures within the lobes throughout the brain. The child with CP, a traumatic brain injury, or a brain tumor will have the signs and symptoms related specifically to where the condition has affected the brain. Injuries to the frontal lobe interfere with the child's ability to initiate movement in the arm, leg, or face opposite to the side of the pathology. Cognitive, psychological, and behavioral problems can occur with damage in the frontal lobe such as poor attention span, errors in judgment, or impulsiveness. Parietal lobe pathology can result in sensory deficits like astereognosis, a person's inability to tell what an object is in his or her hand without seeing it. Perceptual problems also occur with parietal lobe pathology such as deficits with spatial relations, figure-ground discrimination, or body image problems. Occipital lobe pathology can range from cortical blindness if the primary area is damaged to visual agnosia, the inability to recognize what an object is by sight alone, when secondary and tertiary visual association areas are damaged. Pathology in the primary area of the temporal lobe could result in cortical deafness. In secondary areas the child would have difficulty understanding language, receptive aphasia. Memory and emotional disturbances occur with damage to the limbic lobe.

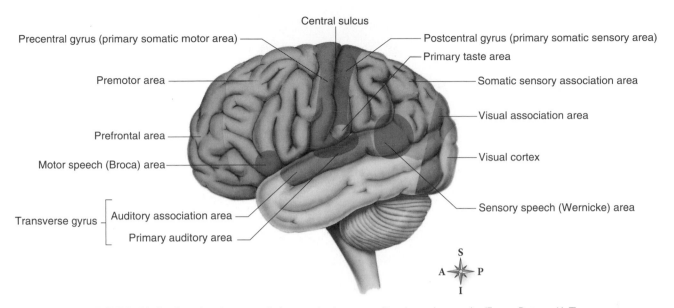

Central sulcus

Precentral gyrus (primary somatic motor area)

Postcentral gyrus (primary somatic sensory area)

Primary taste area

Premotor area

Somatic sensory association area

Visual association area

Prefrontal area

Visual cortex

Motor speech (Broca) area

Transverse gyrus — Auditory association area

Sensory speech (Wernicke) area

Primary auditory area

S
A —★— P
I

FIGURE 12-4 Functional areas of the cerebral cortex (Brodmann's areas). (From Patton, K. T., Thibodeau, G. A., & Douglas, M. M. (2012). *Essentials of anatomy & physiology.* St. Louis: Mosby.)

Uninterrupted flow of oxygen and glucose to the lobes of the cerebral hemispheres is essential because the brain has limited ability to store these life-sustaining resources. The **vasculature** of the brain is designed to meet these high-energy oxygen demands. Two primary systems supply the brain with blood. The anterior system is supplied by the internal carotid arteries and the posterior system is supplied by the vertebrobasilar arteries. The final branches from these two systems are the anterior and middle cerebral arteries from the internal carotids and the posterior cerebral arteries from the vertebrobasilar arteries. The Circle of Willis involves communicating arteries that allow the anterior and posterior blood supply to connect to each other. Figure 12-5 shows the pattern of distribution for these three blood vessels. Cerebrovascular accidents from occlusions or hemorrhages of these vessels will result in predictable deficits. For example, the primary motor and sensory gyri are organized by body parts. This organization is called the motor and sensory homunculus (Figure 12-6). Therefore a child with occlusions in the middle cerebral artery has more involvement in the arm and the child with anterior cerebral artery occlusions has more involvement in the leg.

BRAINSTEM AND CRANIAL NERVES

The brainstem connects the spinal cord to the brain and is the conduit for the **cerebellum** to participate in motor functions. There are three sections of the brainstem from superior to inferior they are called the midbrain, pons, and the medulla (Figure 12-7). Each section contains structures such as **cranial nerve** nuclei; cardiovascular, respiratory, and consciousness nuclei; and ascending and descending pathways. If an individual decides to move his or her foot, the message leaves the primary motor cortex in the frontal lobe and the majority of those neurons carrying that message travel through the brainstem into the spinal cord to then be transmitted to the muscles that can accomplish that motion.[3,4] The movement in the ankle sends sensory messages from joint receptors up to the spinal cord and through the brainstem to the primary sensory cortex in the parietal lobe.

Because the brainstem is roughly the size of one's thenar (thumb) eminence and it contains many basic survival structures, damage to the brainstem results in much worse pathology than the cerebrum.[2] Interruption of the motor pathways can cause paralysis. It is in the medulla that the fibers for motor control cross to the opposite side. This area is known as the pyramidal decussation, and only after the medulla would the paralysis be ipsilateral to (on the same side as) the damage. Above the medulla the paralysis would be contralateral or on the opposite side from the damage. Damage to the pathways carrying sensory information would result in a child's inability to feel sensations such as touch or movement. Damage to the nuclei in the brainstem for consciousness could result in a coma or death. Similarly, damage to the

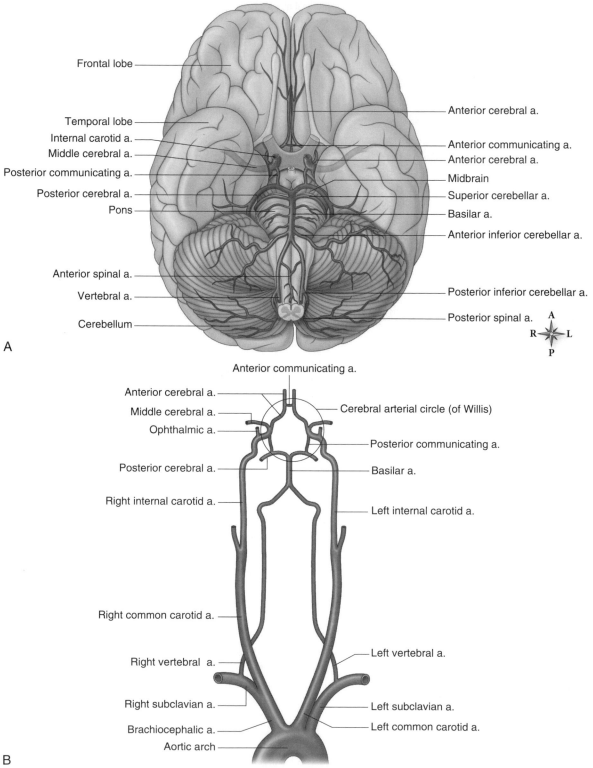

Frontal lobe

Temporal lobe
Internal carotid a.
Middle cerebral a.
Posterior communicating a.
Posterior cerebral a.
Pons

Anterior spinal a.
Vertebral a.
Cerebellum

Anterior cerebral a.

Anterior communicating a.
Anterior cerebral a.
Midbrain
Superior cerebellar a.
Basilar a.
Anterior inferior cerebellar a.

Posterior inferior cerebellar a.

Posterior spinal a.

A

Anterior communicating a.

Anterior cerebral a.
Middle cerebral a.
Ophthalmic a.

Cerebral arterial circle (of Willis)

Posterior communicating a.

Posterior cerebral a.

Basilar a.

Right internal carotid a.

Left internal carotid a.

Right common carotid a.

Right vertebral a.

Left vertebral a.

Right subclavian a.
Brachiocephalic a.
Aortic arch

Left subclavian a.
Left common carotid a.

B

FIGURE 12-5 Arterial distribution. **A,** Diagram shows the cerebral arterial circle (of Willis) and related structures at the base of the brain. (Note the arterial anastomoses). **B,** Origins of blood vessels that form the cerebral arterial circle. (From Patton, K., & Thibodeau, G. (2016). *Anatomy and physiology* (9th ed.). St. Louis: Mosby.)

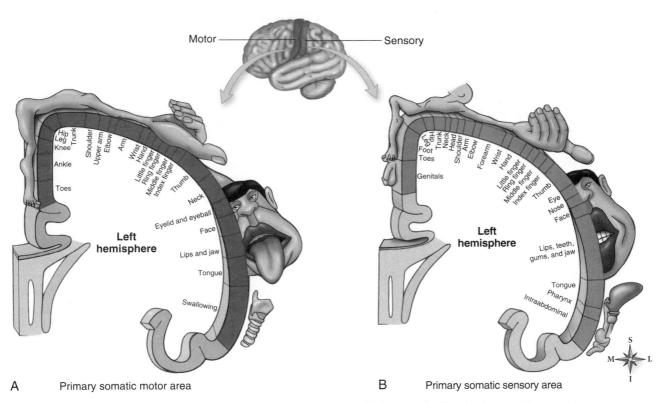

Motor — Sensory

Left hemisphere

Left hemisphere

A   Primary somatic motor area

B   Primary somatic sensory area

FIGURE 12-6   Primary somatic motor (**A**) and sensory (**B**) homunculus. The body parts illustrated here show which parts of the body are "mapped" to specific areas of each cortical area. The exaggerated face indicates that more cortical area is devoted to processing information to and from the many receptors and motor units of the face than of the leg or arm, for example. (From Patton, K. T., Thibodeau, G. A., & Douglas, M. M. (2012). *Essentials of anatomy & physiology*. St. Louis: Mosby.)

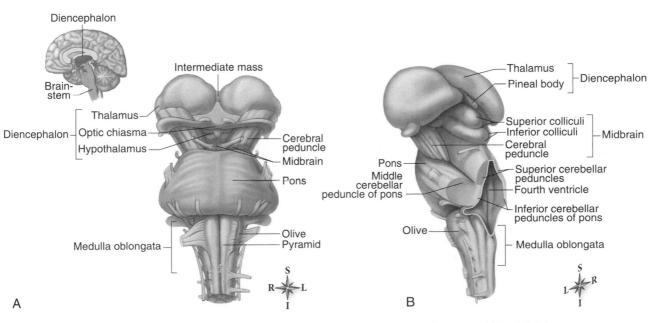

A

B

FIGURE 12-7   Brainstem and diencephalon. **A**, Anterior aspect. **B**, Posterior aspect (shifted slightly to lateral) (From Patton, K. T., Thibodeau, G. A., & Douglas, M. M. (2012). *Essentials of anatomy & physiology*. St. Louis: Mosby.)

nuclei for respiration or cardiovascular control could result in death.

There are 12 pairs of cranial nerves with two primary functions. One is to bring sensory information from the special senses (eyes, ears, smell, taste, movement from the vestibular system) and somatic senses (touch and pain) from the face and head into the brain. The other is to send messages to the muscles of the head and neck and to the viscera. Children with head injuries can have pathology within any of the cranial nerves and OT practitioners evaluate their function and treat when there is dysfunction. The pathology that is particularly emphasized in regard to cranial nerve function with children treated by OT practitioners includes vestibular pathology, oculomotor difficulties, and dysphagia.

The vestibular system is designed to subconsciously maintain equilibrium and visual fixation. It is located within the inner ear and has receptors for linear movement, the otoliths (utricle and saccule) and for rotary movements (the three semicircular canals). Children can have hypoactive or hyperactive vestibular systems. The child with the hypoactive vestibular system may crave movement, be hyperactive and unable to sit still. The child with a hyperactive vestibular system may avoid movement, have poor balance and show excessive nystagmus (back and forth movement of the eyes) when they rotate their heads.

Oculomotor difficulties can result from damage to cranial nerve III, IV or VI, the oculomotor, trochlear and abducens respectively.[4] These cranial nerves control eye movements and reactions of the pupils in response to light. A major input into these cranial nerves comes from the vestibular system. This input allows the eyes to stay fixed on an object when the head is moving in rotation. The eyes will turn opposite to the direction of the rotary movement of the head. OT practitioners can use this relationship to evaluate the intactness of the vestibular system by spinning a child and looking for the oculomotor reaction. Nystagmus, that involuntary back and forth, rhythmic movement of the eyes, is a normal reaction to rotation. Children who show little or no nystagmus may have a hypoactive vestibular system and children who show excessive movement may have a hyperactive vestibular system.

Eating is an essential basic activity of daily living and swallowing is a critical component of this everyday survival task. Occupational therapists evaluate and design intervention for dysphagia, which is difficulty with swallowing. A normal swallow involves many structures including the cerebrum, brainstem, cervical nerve segments, muscles, and six cranial nerves.[2,3] The cranial nerves include the trigeminal (V), facial (VII), glossopharyngeal (IX), vagus (X), accessory (XI), and hypoglossal (XII). A swallowing assessment will include an evaluation of the muscles in the face used to chew, to control the lips and tongue, and to stabilize the neck for swallowing.

CLINICAL *Pearl*

Equilibrium is a three-part process with reliable input needed from proprioceptors in the body, the visual system, and the vestibular system. When testing equilibrium by asking a child to close his or her eyes, the child with pernicious anemia will not be able to maintain equilibrium because the condition damages proprioceptive ability.

SPINAL CORD

The spinal cord is the extension of the brainstem to the body. The tube is not much bigger in circumference than one's index finger, yet it contains all of the pathways that allow the body to send afferent messages to the brain and to receive efferent messages from the brain.[4] There are 31 pairs of spinal segments, 8 cervical, 12 thoracic, 5 lumbar, 5 sacral and 1 coccygeal (Figure 12-8). These segments are named when afferent neurons come into the cord on the dorsal surface and efferent neurons that leave the cord from the ventral surface come together outside of the cord to form a spinal nerve (Figure 12-9). The body is divided into dermatomes, the area of the skin supplied by the **sensory neuron** in a single spinal nerve (Figure 12-10). The efferent component of the spinal nerve is distributed to the muscles that it innervates and this segmental innervation of muscles is the myotome pattern.

There are two areas that are larger in circumference than the rest of the spinal cord. They are the cervical and lumbar enlargements and they house the many efferent LMNs that supply the muscles of the upper extremity and lower extremity respectively. The spinal cord tapers to an end, which is called the conus medullaris. The end of the cord is found around the L2 vertebral body and the LMNs after L2 have to travel a distance to exit beneath their corresponding vertebra. This mass of LMNs looks like a horse's tail and is called the cauda equine (see Figure 12-8).

Internally, the cord has a gray matter "H or butterfly shape" center, which is composed of nuclei, command centers, surrounded by the ascending and descending white matter pathways or tracts (see Figure 12-9).[4] The gray matter is divided into horns and the white matter into columns. The dorsal horn and column functions are primarily sensory and the ventral horn and column functions primarily motor. The lateral horn is related to ANS functions and the lateral column a mix of sensory and motor pathways.

The spinal cord may be damaged by trauma or by disease. Examples of trauma can be from the shearing force of a motor vehicle accident, diving into a shallow

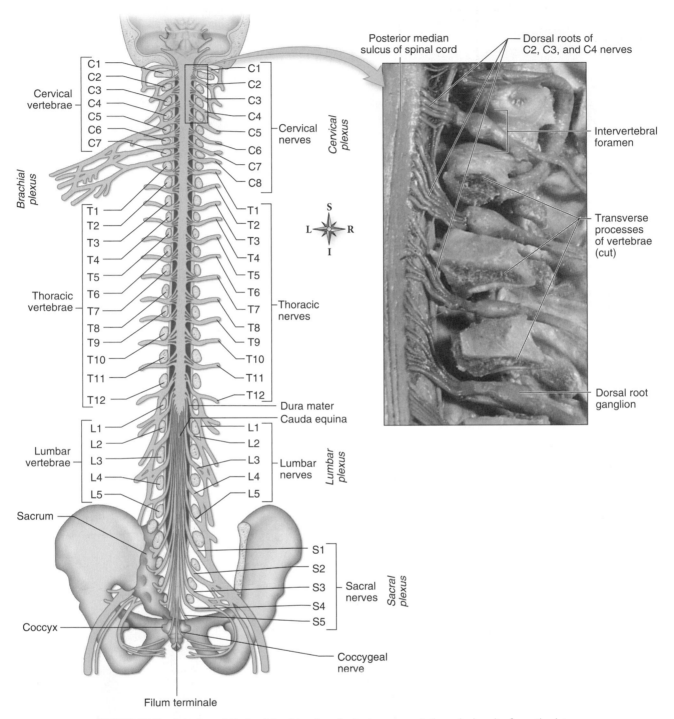

FIGURE 12-8 Spinal cord. Each of the 31 pairs of spinal nerves exit the spinal cavity from the intervertebral foramina. The names of the corresponding spinal nerves are on the right. The inset shows a dissection of the cervical region, showing a posterior view of cervical spinal nerves exiting intervertebral foramina on the right side. (From Thibodeau, G. A., & Patton, K.T. (2012). *Structure & function of the body* (14th ed.). St. Louis: Mosby.)

pool, or a penetrating injury such as from gunshot or a knife wound. A resulting injury can be classified as complete with loss of all sensation and motor function below the injury or incomplete, which would involve partial loss and sparing of some motor and sensory function below the level of the lesion. When both the upper and lower extremities are involved, the injury is described as tetraplegia and is usually in the cervical segments.[2,3] It is paraplegia if the injury is in the thoracic and lumbar areas of the spinal cord. Examples of

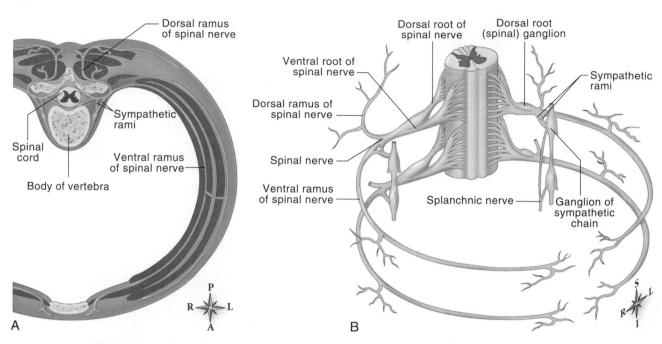

FIGURE 12-9 Cross-section of the spinal cord with spinal nerve. (From Patton, K., & Thibodeau, G. (2016). *Anatomy and physiology* (9th ed.). St. Louis: Mosby.)

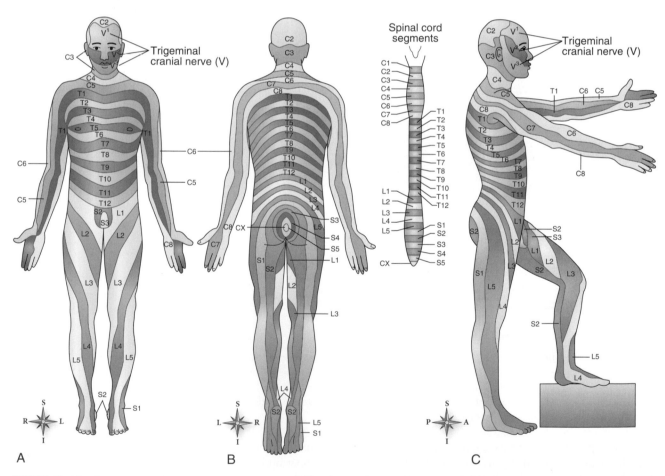

FIGURE 12-10 Dermatome distribution of spinal nerves. **A,** The front of the body's surface. **B,** The back of the body's surface. **C,** The side of the body surface. The inset shows the segments of the spinal cord connected with each of the spinal nerves associated with the sensory dermatomes shown. *T,* Thoracic segments and spinal nerves; *L,* lumbar segments and spinal nerves; *S,* sacral segments and spinal nerves. (From Patton, K., & Thibodeau, G. (2016). *Anatomy and physiology* (9th ed.). St. Louis: Mosby.)

diseases that impact the spinal cord include multiple sclerosis, amyotrophic lateral sclerosis, poliomyelitis, and Guillain-Barré syndrome. (See Chapter 13 on pediatric health conditions.)

CLINICAL *Pearl*

A lumbar puncture procedure is done to remove cerebrospinal fluid for testing or to introduce an analgesic agent. Because the spinal cord tapers to an end roughly equivalent to the L2 vertebra in an adult the procedure should be done around the L4 interspace to avoid possible damage to the spinal cord.

ASCENDING AND DESCENDING PATHWAYS

The ascending pathways send various sensations coming from the body to the brain and the cerebellum. One of the primary ascending pathways is the dorsal column medial lemniscus.[4] This pathway carries touch, vibration, tactile discrimination, and stereognosis, which is the ability to identify objects placed in the hand using only tactile clues. Without this pathway being intact, a client may have poorer motor control because the sensory information is inadequate. Think of trying to pick up small pegs while wearing a pair of gloves. A second important sensory pathway is the lateral spinothalamic tract. This pathway carries information about pain and temperature. The pain function serves to protect an individual by alerting him or her if there has been tissue damage and that the individual needs to take action to avoid more damage. It is a vital pathway for survival signaling that something is wrong.[3]

For these two pathways there are three neurons (first, second, and third order) that carry information from the sensory receptor in the periphery to the brain. The first-order neuron carries the sensory experience into the spinal cord and for these ascending pathways the second-order neuron crosses to the opposite side. Sensation, therefore, on the right side is received and interpreted by the left cerebral hemisphere. The third-order neuron runs from the **thalamus** to the portion of the brain that will begin the integration of the sensation, which results in the person making sense out of the sensation.

There are also pathways that carry movement sensation to the cerebellum. They are called the dorsal and ventral spinocerebellar pathways. They keep the cerebellum constantly apprised of the position of joints and their movements. Without these pathways being intact the resulting motor deficit is ataxia, which is the inability to coordinate movement resulting in jerkiness and ineffective motor control.[3]

The descending pathways can be divided into two categories: one that initiates voluntary movement and those that support the success of these movements but do not cause conscious movements to occur. The lateral corticospinal pathway initiates voluntary movement. It starts in the frontal lobe in the precentral gyrus where the motor homunculus exists. The pathway then flows down through the brainstem and into the medulla in an area called the pyramids. It is in the pyramids that the majority of the fibers cross to the opposite side. This crossing, called the pyramidal decussation, is why the right side of the brain controls the left side of the body and vice versa. Descending pathways that lie outside the pyramids are referred to as extrapyramidal.[4] They alter muscle tone and support the success of the voluntary movement initiated by the lateral corticospinal pathway. These pathways include the rubrospinal, tectospinal, reticulospinal, and vestibulospinal. The rubrospinal comes into play when the movement involves dexterity and it helps to support fine motor control. The tectospinal comes into play if there is a visual or auditory stimulus by beginning the process of reflexively turning your head to orient to the stimuli. The reticulospinal is for altering muscle tone in relationship to one's state of consciousness. The more alert a person is, the more extensor tone and the more asleep a person is, the more flexor tone is facilitated.[2,3] The vestibulospinal responds to gravity and movement by increasing the extensor tone in your body. Think of being on a roller coaster and the body needing to increase your ability to be upright against gravity as a result of this movement.

CLINICAL *Pearl*

When an object like a quarter is placed in a child's hand and the child is asked to tell what it is by using tactile sensation only, the child's stereognosis is being tested. Astereognosis or the inability to determine what an object is through tactile input can occur when there is pathology in any area of the parietal lobe or in the dorsal column medial lemniscus pathway.

CEREBELLUM AND BASAL GANGLIA

The complexity of voluntary motor control cannot be considered complete without description of how the cerebellum and **basal ganglia** contribute to the process. The cerebellum is involved in the success of motor control in many important ways. Chapter 24 provides information on motor control and motor learning. When the motor cortex initiates a movement say to pick up a pencil and write one's name in a small box on a form, the cerebellum plays a critical role in the successful execution of this task. It helps some motor units to relax while others contract making the movement smooth. The cerebellum helps control the speed of the movement and makes adjustments so one can write in the correct space with the correct size print for the space. It monitors the position of the body and therefore plays a huge role in keeping one balanced in the position or postures needed for walking, running, sitting, and so on. It also has an important role in motor learning the complex sequences necessary for a successful motor task and it is especially critical when the motor task requires speed and dexterity.

The cerebellum can be organized into three functional subdivisions: vestibulocerebellum, spinocerebellum, and cerebrocerebellum (Figure 12-11).[4] The most medial section is the vestibulocerebellum, which functionally provides one with balance and equilibrium reactions. In addition it is intricately involved in coordinating head and eye movements. The most lateral section is the cerebrocerebellum, which is important in initiating movement and in motor planning. Pathology in this section can result in apraxia, which is the inability to motor plan.[2,3] The intermediate section is the spinocerebellum , which functionally coordinates the timing and success of rapid movements and corrects for deviations in unintended movements. Pathology can result in ataxia or jerky movements; dysmetria, or difficulty correctly judging the distance for a movement; or dysarthria, which involves motor speech problems.[2,3]

The basal ganglia are a group of gray matter nuclei located deep in the cerebral hemispheres, diencephalon, and midbrain of the **brainstem**. These nuclei are interconnected with many different types of neurotransmitters involved in numerous circuits through the various structures of the basal ganglia. Destruction of any of the

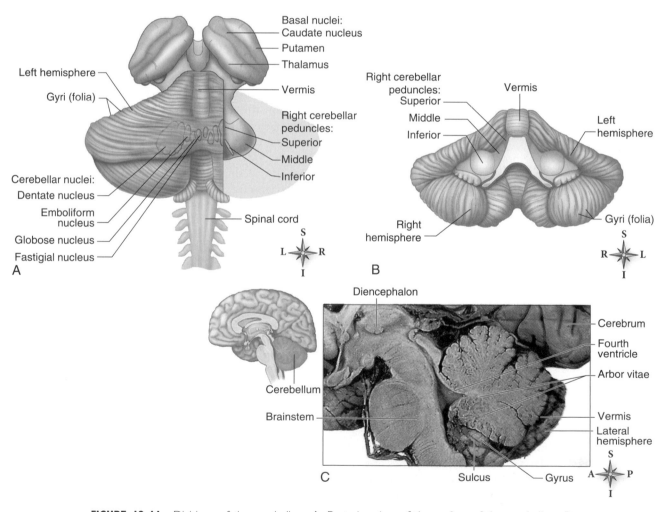

FIGURE 12-11 Divisions of the cerebellum. **A,** Posterior view of the surface of the cerebellum. **B,** Anterior view of the cerebellum (with brainstem removed). **C,** Photograph of midsagittal brain section shows internal features of the cerebellum and surrounding structures of the brain. (From Patton, K., & Thibodeau, G. (2016). *Anatomy and physiology* (9th ed.). St. Louis: Mosby.)

basal ganglia will result in motor dysfunctions, which can be categorized as resulting in too little movement (e.g., bradykinesia and rigidity) or too much movement (e.g., dyskinesia and tics). Although the most common pathology involving the basal ganglia is Parkinson's disease, there are conditions that affect children. Examples of these disorders include spasmodic torticollis, a type of dystonia with rotation and lateral flexion of the neck; athetosis where the excess involuntary movements are slow and writhing; and tics, a random repeated contract and relax spasm.

There are four circuits involving the various basal ganglia. The first two include a motor circuit that helps assure the success of complex movements; an oculomotor circuit helps with saccadic or rapid eye movement. The last two circuits are the association and limbic. The association circuitry helps to establish motor memories and the limbic circuitry, which is involved in limbic regulation of emotions and motivation.

CLINICAL *Pearl*

Because successful speech involves intricate patterns of coordinating muscle contractions with the appropriate sequence and speed, children with cerebellar damage will often have speech problems such as dysarthria or slurred speech.

PERIPHERAL NERVOUS SYSTEM

The PNS consists of the 12 pairs of cranial nerves, 31 pairs of spinal nerves, and associated structures such as sensory receptors, ganglia and supporting cells. The peripheral or sensory receptors are categorized as those that respond to various touch sensations, pain, temperature, movement, light energy, and changes internally (e.g., glucose levels). The tactile receptors, also called mechanoreceptors, lie within the dermis and transmit an impulse when physical contact with the skin alters the receptor. The altered receptor sends a generator potential, which may not be significant enough to jump the first node of Ranvier on the sensory neuron. If it does jump the node of Ranvier it becomes an action potential, which will be transmitted to the brain as it follows the all-or-none phenomena.[4]

Pain receptors are also called free nerve endings or nociceptors. They are widespread and respond when there has been tissue damage that releases bradykinin, histamine, or other substances that stimulate the pain receptor. The fiber that carries this impulse can be either an Aδ–size fiber or a C fiber. The A fiber has more myelin than the C fiber and therefore transmits a message quicker than the C fiber. The A fiber, therefore, carries acute, sharp, and well-localized pain, whereas the C fiber carries chronic, dull, and more generalized pain information.[4]

Accurate interpretation of movement starts with receptors such as the muscle spindles, Golgi tendon organs, and several of the tactile mechanoreceptors. By far, the most used receptor for position sense especially in midranges of the joint is the muscle spindle. As a muscle contracts, a person needs continuous information on the length, tension, and speed of the contraction. Every striated muscle contain numerous of these spindle-shaped receptors that lie parallel with the main contractile element of a muscle, the extrafusal muscle fibers. Muscle spindles have tendons that merge with the tendons or fascia of the muscle that surround the spindles. The sensory part of the spindle is sensitive to tension, which can be applied by the lengthening of the extrafusal muscle fibers or by the contractile portion that lies within the spindle itself. It is, however, not the role of the spindle to cause a muscle to contract. Contraction occurs only when extrafusal muscle fibers shorten.[4]

Ganglia are collections of cell bodies that lie within the PNS. One example is the dorsal root ganglia, which are the cell bodies for the sensory neurons. They divide this neuron into a peripheral branch from the receptor to the dorsal root ganglia and a central branch, which enters the **spinal cord**. Supporting cells for the peripheral nervous system include Schwann cells, which surround peripheral nerve fibers and contain the myelin that speeds conduction of an impulse along axons that are myelinated.

THE NEURON

Neurons, like any cell, have a nucleus and cytoplasm, which includes the typical complement of intracellular organelles necessary for the metabolic functions of the cell (Figure 12-12). The three regions of the neuron include the cell body (soma), dendrites, and an axon.[4] The soma contains the nucleus and the organelles and has large attachments that branch repeatedly from it known as the dendrites. The principle function of the dendrites is to increase the surface area for the neuron to receive most of its synaptic connections. Neurons have one specialized axon. Axons are thinner but longer than dendrites. Axons have three regions: the initial segment, the axon proper, and the terminal bouton.[4] The initial segment is a transition area from the soma to the axon proper. In most neurons the terminal bouton has secretory vesicles that contain neurotransmitters that can be released into the synaptic cleft. This segment is the presynaptic component, which is specialized to release neurotransmitters into the synaptic cleft, which are then received by the postsynaptic component of a neighboring neuron.[4]

Most of these synapses occur between axons and dendrites (axodendritic) although synapses can occur elsewhere, for example, between axons and other axons

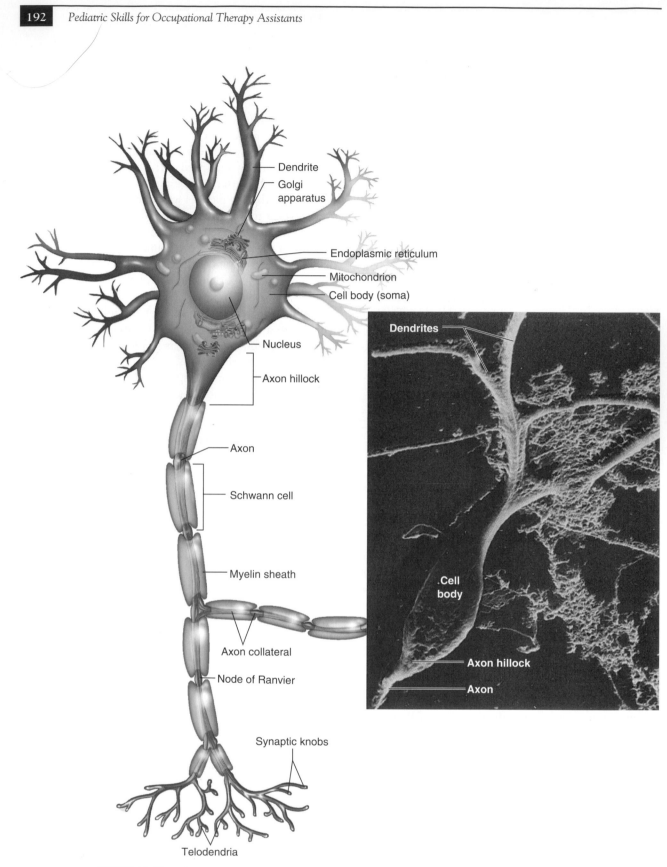

FIGURE 12-12 Neuron. (From Patton, K., & Thibodeau, G. (2016). *Anatomy and physiology* (9th ed.). St. Louis: Mosby.)

TABLE 12-3

Important Neurotransmitters

ACETYLCHOLINE	DOPAMINE	GABA	GLUTAMATE	NOREPINEPHRINE	SEROTONIN
Most common neurotransmitter. Facilitates muscle contractions and modulates synaptic plasticity. Also used in ANS	Primarily inhibitory and a neuromodulator through basal ganglia and limbic functions	Inhibitory neurotransmitter through entire CNS	Facilitates neurotransmission and modulates synaptic plasticity	Neuromodulator; used by ANS in response to stress	A neuromodulator for mood and sleep functions

ANS, Autonomic nervous system; *CNS*, central nervous system

(axoaxonic) or between axons and cell bodies (axosomatic). The neurotransmitters (Table 12-3) that are used to send messages across the synapses can be classified into two types. One group communicates quickly between neurons either resulting in facilitation or inhibition. The other group is involved in neuromodulation, which communicate slower and involve regulating neuronal growth or synaptic transmission. Think of neurotransmitters as the language of the nervous system.

Supporting cells also exist in the CNS and PNS. The supporting cells of the CNS are known as glial cells.[4] The most numerous of these cells are the astrocytes, star-shaped neuroglial cells that encase blood the surfaces of the brain and its blood vessels and the oligodendrocytes, myelin forming neuroglial cells. The supporting cells of the PNS are the Schwann cells, which were discussed earlier.

CLINICAL *Pearl*

Acetylcholine is considered the major neurotransmitter for the PNS and plays an important role in the CNS being known as the primary transmitter for the neuromodulation involved in memory.

OCCUPATIONAL PERFORMANCE RELATIONSHIP

This chapter provided a discussion of the structures and functions of the human nervous systems. Understanding how the central and peripheral components of the nervous system influence occupational performance allows the OT practitioner to select the appropriate evaluation and treatment interventions for his or her client with a neurologic deficit.

The Occupational Therapy Practice Framework describes the core, foundational concepts that guide the practice of occupational therapy.[1] In every aspect of the domain the human nervous system plays a vital role in the assessment and consideration of intervention strategies that promote participation in client-centered occupations.

Our domain is occupation, such as the child's engagement in activities of daily living or rest and sleep, which is heavily influenced by function and dysfunction within the nervous system. For example, sleep is regulated by reticular nuclei within the brainstem. The effectiveness of the neurotransmitters that facilitate or inhibit these nuclei can promote normal or abnormal sleep patterns. These same nuclei also allow an individual to attend and focus on a task or be easily distracted by competing sensory stimuli.

Client factors include body and sensory functions, and structures that relate to the nervous system. For example, the OT practitioner examines a child's neuromuscular function when evaluating a child's muscle tone to determine whether there is too little tone, hypotonicity or too much tone, hypertonicity. The intervention may focus on improving the child's muscle tone perhaps through handling techniques or weight bearing or by compensating for the deficit with positioning equipment. Reflexes, posture, balance reactions, and eye and hand coordination are all components of a neuromuscular evaluation. Cranial nerves are assessed when looking at the child's vision, hearing, vestibular, and taste or smell functions. Ascending pathways are examined when assessing a child's proprioceptive, touch, and pain functions.

Body functions develop into performance skills when neurologic development is normal. However, when neurologic dysfunction prevents normal development, motor and process skills are delayed, which in turn affects social interaction skills. Neurologic systems for motor control such as the cerebellum and basal ganglia impact performance skills such as reaching with precision and a smooth and fluid arm movement or being able to successfully stabilize and coordinate movements. Process skills such as attending to the task, sequencing, or problem solving involve many areas of the CNS including all lobes of the brain but especially the frontal lobe.

Social interaction skills rely heavily on the limbic system. Appropriate social initiation, gestures, or touching are adversely affected by functional or structural damage to the limbic system.

To complete occupations successfully the child needs to engage in performance patterns. Habits, routines, rituals, and roles all need to be developed and examined if a child is not effectively engaging in occupations. Finally, occupations happen within a context and environment unique to the individual, and these factors (such as culture) and where the child is temporally need to be considered in order to complete a holistic evaluation of functional or dysfunctional engagement in occupation.

SUMMARY

This chapter presented an overview of neuroscience to assist OT practitioners in understanding how the CNS and PNS influence occupational performance. The chapter reviewed the organization and function of the CNS from cerebrum and brainstem to the spinal cord. The fundamentals of the PNS and the mechanism for sensation to be sent to the brain and motor control

to descend from the brain were described. The chapter concluded by describing the relationship between neurologic structures and functions to occupational performance.

References

1. American Occupational Therapy Association. (2014). Occupational therapy practice framework: domain and process (3rd ed.). *Am J Occup Ther*, 68(Suppl. 1), S1–S48.
2. Blumenfeld, H. (2010). *Neuroanatomy through clinical cases* (2nd ed.). Sunderland, MA: Sinauer Associates, Inc.
3. Cohen, H. (1999). *Neuroscience for rehabilitation* (2nd ed.). Philadelphia: Lippincott.
4. Young, P. A., Young, P. H., & Tobert, D. L. (2008). *Basic clinical neuroscience* (2nd ed.). Philadelphia: Lippincott.

Recommended Reading

Arnadottir, G. (1990). *The brain and behavior: assessing cortical dysfunction through activities of daily living.* St Louis: Mosby.

REVIEW *Questions*

1. What is the difference between the central, peripheral, and autonomic nervous systems?
2. What are the stages of neuroembryology?
3. What are the functions associated with the five lobes of the brain?
4. How is the right hemisphere of the brain different from the left?
5. How does the brain integrate sensation?
6. How do the brain, cerebellum, and basal ganglia influence motor control?
7. Why is neuroplasticity critically important to occupational therapy practitioners and the clients whom they treat?

SUGGESTED *Activities*

1. Make a conscious effort to observe people whom you see with neurologic deficits in everyday places and determine whether their condition would be classified as upper or lower motor neuron pathology from watching them move.
2. Test light touch by swiping a cotton ball along your partner's arms or legs and asking them to indicate when and where they were touched by tactile sensation only. Check your dermatome chart to match the areas you tested to the correct dermatome.
3. Evaluate the integrity of the vestibular system by having your partner sit in a chair that will rotate. With his or her head slightly flexed and eyes open, spin them completely around 10 times in 20 seconds. When you stop his or her rotary movement have them look forward and count the amount of beats of nystagmus and how long it takes before the back and forth movement of the eyes stops.

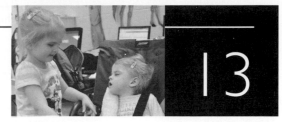

Pediatric Health Conditions

KEY TERMS

Contusion

Crush wound or injury

Dislocation

Sprain

Fractures

Closed fracture

Open fracture

Joint protection
techniques

Energy conservation
techniques

Central nervous system

Peripheral nervous
system

Cortical blindness

Visual perception

American Sign Language

Total body surface area
(TBSA)

Partial-thickness burns

Acute medical
management

Rehabilitation

Universal precautions

CHAPTER *Objectives*

After studying this chapter, the reader will be able to accomplish the following:

- Describe the characteristics of a variety of pediatric conditions.
- Describe the signs and symptoms of pediatric orthopedic, genetic, neurologic, developmental, cardiopulmonary, neoplastic, sensory, and environmentally induced conditions.
- Describe the types and classification of burns.
- Describe treatment precautions associated with specific pediatric conditions.
- Summarize the ways in which different conditions affect children's and adolescent's occupational performance.
- Describe general intervention principles and strategies associated with pediatric health conditions or diagnoses.

CHAPTER *Outline*

Orthopedic Conditions
ACQUIRED MUSCULOSKELETAL DISORDERS
AMPUTATION
ARTHROGRYPOSIS
CONGENITAL HIP DYSPLASIA
JUVENILE RHEUMATOID ARTHRITIS
OSTEOGENESIS IMPERFECTA
GENERAL INTERVENTIONS

Genetic Conditions
ACHONDROPLASIA
DUCHENNE MUSCULAR DYSTROPHY
FRAGILE X SYNDROME
PRADER-WILLI SYNDROME
TRISOMY 21 (DOWN SYNDROME)
GENERAL INTERVENTIONS

Neurologic Conditions
ERB'S PALSY (BRACHIAL PLEXUS INJURY)
SEIZURES
SPINA BIFIDA
SHAKEN BABY SYNDROME
TRAUMATIC BRAIN INJURY
GENERAL INTERVENTIONS

Developmental Conditions
ATTENTION DEFICIT HYPERACTIVITY DISORDER
AUTISM SPECTRUM DISORDERS
DEVELOPMENTAL COORDINATION DISORDER
RETT SYNDROME
GENERAL INTERVENTIONS

Cardiopulmonary System
CARDIAC DISORDERS
PULMONARY DISORDERS/CHRONIC RESPIRATORY
 DISORDERS
HEMATOLOGIC CONDITIONS

Sensory System Conditions
VISION IMPAIRMENTS
HEARING IMPAIRMENTS
GENERAL SENSORY DISORGANIZATION
LANGUAGE DELAY AND LANGUAGE IMPAIRMENTS
GENERAL INTERVENTIONS

Other Pediatric Health Conditions
BURNS

Neoplastic Disorders
LEUKEMIA

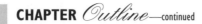

CHAPTER *Outline*—continued

This chapter describes the major characteristics, signs and symptoms, and intervention strategies of a variety of pediatric conditions encountered by occupational therapy (OT) practitioners. Knowing the course and characteristics of each of these conditions serves as a framework for assessment, evaluation, and intervention planning. Additionally, precautions specific to health conditions are also reviewed to ensure safety as OT practitioners provide intervention. Knowledge of the disease process and prognosis enables the OT practitioner to be a valuable member of the intervention team. Box 13-1 lists some potential members of the pediatric team.

A brief description of the major characteristics of each condition is presented and is followed by intervention principles that are useful in OT practice. Case examples are provided to describe OT interventions. This chapter presents an overview of conditions in orthopedics, genetics, neurologic, developmental, cardiopulmonary, neoplastic, sensory system integrity, and environmentally induced conditions.

Across all diagnostic categories, the OT goals of intervention for infants and youth are to optimize occupational performance, facilitate ongoing developmental progress, help the infant and child be able to interact in their environment, and provide parent education and support. All areas of occupational performance may be addressed with children and adolescents with components of work performance being applicable with adolescents. For children with degenerative diseases such as Duchenne muscular dystrophy or Friedrich ataxia, the goal is to optimize occupational performance, provide adaptations and compensatory strategies as needed, and avoid activities that could worsen the disease process.

As a child grows and matures, the focus of therapy shifts. When working with infants, toddlers, and preschoolers, OT practitioners may emphasize developmental processes and facilitate development. As a child moves into school age and adolescence, the practitioner emphasizes enabling the child to be functional in school settings and with activities of daily living, instrumental activities of daily living, play, and social participation. The OT practitioner may also address the following:

- Behavioral modification techniques to develop socially appropriate behaviors
- Task-specific activities to teach child-specific skills for daily living
- Adaptations or compensation for deficits in motor, cognition, emotional, or social functioning
- Sensory processing strategies to enhance self-regulation and learning.

BOX 13-1

Potential Team Members

- Behavior specialist
- Cardiologist
- Cardiac surgeon
- Child life specialist
- Dietitian
- Emergency medical technician
- Geneticist
- Neonatologist
- Neurologist
- Neuropsychologist
- Neurosurgeon
- Nurse
- Occupational therapist
- Occupational therapy assistant
- Orthopedist
- Orthopedic surgeon
- Orthotist
- Physical therapist
- Physical therapy assistant
- Physician
- Physiatrist
- Prosthetist
- Psychologist
- Pulmonologist
- Respiratory therapist
- Speech language pathologist

- Volition and feelings of self-efficacy to increase participation in occupations
- Success in educational and leisure activities despite missing opportunities due to illness
- Successful achievement to develop self-concept and positive self-esteem

Parent/caregiver education and support is important at each stage. Parents act as advocates for their children and OT practitioners can facilitate this with their knowledge of systems, development, and the individual child. Case-Smith[13] researched parent perspectives in dealing with children with chronic health needs. Parents described stressors specific to the care of the child with chronic health needs, the risk for isolation, dependence on health care workers for social connections, and also the joy of being advocates for and seeing changes in their children. OT practitioners remain sensitive to parents' perspective.[13]

In this chapter, common pediatric conditions are reviewed. The author describes specific precautions and intervention guidelines specific to health conditions. The author presents common diagnoses encountered in the pediatric population and provides strategies to address related issues.

ORTHOPEDIC CONDITIONS

Orthopedic or musculoskeletal conditions involve bones, joints, and muscles. The musculoskeletal system consists of the skeletal and muscular systems. The skeletal system consists of bones, joints, cartilage, and ligaments. The muscular system consists of muscles, tendons, and the fascia covering them. Tendons, which are bands of tough, inelastic fibrous tissue, connect muscles to bones. Muscles are activated by the nervous system and move bone(s) to create movement at a joint. Ligaments are bands of inelastic fibrous tissue that provide stability to joints. Fascia is connective tissue surrounding muscles and organs, providing support and also allowing movement.

Congenital disorders of the musculoskeletal system include arthrogryposis, congenital hip dysplasia, juvenile rheumatoid arthritis, and osteogenesis imperfecta (brittle bones). Box 13-2 lists signs and symptoms of orthopedic conditions. Children may be born with missing digits or limbs (amputations). Acquired orthopedic disorders include fractures and sprains. Chapter 28 discusses interventions for orthopedic conditions.

CLINICAL *Pearl*

Therapy for an older child who has lost a limb as a result of trauma or surgery is different than therapy for a child with a congenital amputation. A child who loses a limb later in childhood benefits from having a prosthesis fitted as soon as possible for psychological and rehabilitation reasons.

BOX 13-2

Musculoskeletal Disorders: Signs and Symptoms

- Misalignment of joints
- Swelling
- Pain
- Warmth to touch
- Immobility
- Discoloration (redness, blueness, whiteness)

Children with congenital upper extremity amputations may adapt to limb abnormalities more easily and use prostheses less than children with acquired amputations. Daily prostheses usage time and the child's experiences with the prostheses may determine function. Children with orthopedic conditions may experience difficulties in the performance of daily occupations such as activities of daily living (ADLs), instrumental ADLs (IADLs), play and leisure, and work and productive skills.

Acquired Musculoskeletal Disorders

Acquired musculoskeletal disorders are conditions that are not present at birth and involve injury or trauma to the skeletal and/or muscular systems. Soft tissue injuries and fractures require the attention of an orthopedist, a medical doctor who specializes in diseases of the musculoskeletal system.

CLINICAL *Pearl*

To avoid causing fractures, use care when handling and doing range of motion (ROM) exercises with severely affected, inactive children. Maintaining good joint mobility with daily careful passive stretching and proper positioning initiated during infancy helps maintain optimal joint alignment and provides comfort.

Soft Tissue Injuries

Soft tissue injuries involve damage to muscles, nerves, skin, and/or connective tissue and include contusions, crush injuries, dislocations, and sprains. A **contusion** is an injury that does not disrupt the integrity of the skin and is characterized by swelling, discoloration, and pain. In the absence of any complicating health conditions, contusions heal with time and do not require medical or therapeutic intervention.

A **crush wound or injury** is a break in the external surface of the bone caused by severe force applied against tissues (e.g., a finger caught in a door). This type of injury may require medical or occupational therapy (OT) intervention if alignment and immobility are necessary for the injury to heal. Untreated crush injuries may result in permanent deformity and pain of the joint(s) involved. The permanent misalignment of a body structure may have functional implications.

A **dislocation** is the displacement of a bone from its normal articulation at a joint. Dislocations of the shoulder and hip joints are frequently seen in infants and young children, as these joints are freely movable. The shallowness of the shoulder joint increases the likelihood of dislocation occurring at this structure.

A **sprain** is a traumatic injury to the tendons, muscles, or ligaments around a joint and is characterized by pain, swelling, and discoloration. Sprains can occur when children or adolescents lose their balance and consequently use a protective response that makes the wrist and ankle the most vulnerable joints for injury. Sprains are most frequently seen in the ankles and wrists. Most do not require emergency medical attention or OT intervention.

CLINICAL *Pearl*

Immediately apply ice to a soft tissue injury for a minimum of 20 minutes or until the area becomes pain free. The application of ice will reduce swelling at the involved site and relieve pain.

Fractures

Fractures are breaks, ruptures, or cracks in bone or cartilage. They may be defined as closed or open. A **closed fracture** has no open wounds from the broken bone penetrating the skin, whereas an **open fracture** involves an open wound, where complications are more common. Fractures require immediate realignment followed by immobilization to allow the bone(s) to heal. Immobilization requires casts, orthoses, pins, or other external fixations. Children often require occupational and physical therapy during the acute stage of injury following the fracture with focus on mobility, independence with ADLs such as dressing, toileting, and bathing, and provision of adaptive equipment such as a bath bench. For example, families may use a plastic outdoor chair as a shower seat since adaptive equipment is needed only for a short time.

Amputation

An infant born missing all or part of a limb has a congenital amputation. A traumatic amputation is the result of an accident, infection, or cancer. Each year, approximately 26 of 10,000 children in the United States are born missing all or part of a limb. The types of amputations vary greatly (Table 13-1). Thumb and below-elbow amputations are the most common types of upper extremity congenital amputations.[9] Children who have traumatic amputations need to heal the area involved

TABLE 13-1

Types of Congenital Upper Extremity Amputations

TYPE OF DEFICIENCY	MISSING SKELETAL PARTS
TRANSVERSE AMELIA	
Forequarter amputation	All or most of the arm is missing from the shoulder and below
TRANSVERSE HEMIMELIA	
Below-elbow amputation	All of the arm is missing from the elbow and below
LONGITUDINAL HEMIMELIA	
Partial amputation	One of the long bones of the forearm is missing
	Fingers or thumb may or may not be missing
PHOCOMELIA	
	Bones of the upper or lower arm are missing
	All or part of the hand remains

Data adapted from Rothstein, J. M., Roy, H. R., & Wolf, S. L. (1998). *The rehabilitation specialist's handbook* (2nd ed.). Philadelphia, PA: FA Davis.

in the trauma and then begin the rehabilitation process. Fingers and thumbs are the most common amputations and accidents with lawn mowers.[17]

Children with congenital amputations are often fitted with a passive prosthesis by 6 months of age to encourage use of the prosthesis during movement, to build foundational skills for bilateral upper extremity use, and to ease the transition for more sophisticated devices such as myoelectric prostheses.[27] Additionally, early use of prostheses decreases the risk for cumulative trauma syndromes.[37] OT practitioners analyze the activities that the child with an amputation will engage in and determine how to compensate for or adapt the task so that the child can be successful. In some cases, use of technology or prosthesis may be prescribed to help the child engage in daily activities.[27] The OT practitioner considers the child's age and the type of amputation and works with a team of professionals to determine the course of treatment.[17]

CASE *Study*

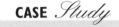

Beth was born with an above the elbow amputation. The occupational therapist completed a developmental evaluation at 3 months and determined that Beth was achieving all her developmental milestones. The attending physician, occupational therapist, physical therapist, and social worker discussed the pros and cons of prosthesis with Beth's parents. The team explained that most children with congenital upper extremity amputations choose to use a prosthesis as a tool some of the time, but they learn adaptive techniques for performing many activities without it. Very young children often use the sensations in their residual limb to learn about their environments. The OT practitioner provided the parents with some informational books as well as the phone numbers of other parents who had children with congenital upper extremity amputations; the OT practitioner suggested that Beth's parents spend some time talking to other parents with experience raising a child with an upper extremity amputation.

Beth's parents decided to wait to have her fitted with a prosthesis until she was 2 years old because she could then begin to understand its use as a tool. They also thought that at 2 years her language skills would make it easier for her to learn to use the prosthesis. They felt that Beth would gradually learn when to do things with or without the prosthesis.

Beth's first prosthesis had a rubber mitt and a friction elbow that did not lock. Later, an adept hand, which was made of plastic and had one C-shaped "finger" with an indentation in which the end for the opposing "thumb" could be fit, was added. The adept hand would remain open until Beth chose to close it by pulling on a cable attached to a shoulder harness.

Beth is now 7 years old. She has had two surgeries to the end of the bone in her stump. Every year she has a prosthesis revision, and small details are added or changed. Now that she is older, Beth's parents include her in the decisions for changes. The family learned that Beth usually knows what works for her better than anyone on her treatment team. Whenever a change is made, the occupational therapy assistant (OTA) spends a few OT sessions with Beth exploring the new uses and operation of the updated prosthesis. During these sessions, the occupational therapist and the OTA work closely together; Beth's training requires specific understanding of the ways in which the components of the prosthesis work and function.

Fitting a prosthesis on a child with a congenital amputation at a very young age allows the child to reach developmental milestones in a timely manner and for the prosthesis to become a part of the child's body image. A prosthesis is more likely to be rejected when the child is older. In the case of a less severe congenital amputation, a child often does well without a prosthesis. The use of a prosthesis depends on the severity of the amputation and whether one or both arms are involved. See Box 13-3 for stump and prosthesis care.

Arthrogryposis

Arthrogryposis is sometimes genetic but is also attributed to reduced amniotic fluid during gestation or central

---

BOX 13-3

Care of the Residual Limb and Prosthesis

- Decreased skin surface may result in overheating.
- Bandages must be dry and monitored.
- Examine the stump site for excessive redness, irritation, or swelling when the prosthesis is removed each night.
- Report any discomfort, redness, or pressure areas to the occupational therapist immediately.
- Wash the residual limb daily with soap and water, rinse, and dry carefully. Do not soak it.
- Cleanse the residual limb at night, ensuring enough time for it to dry thoroughly.
- Do not shave or apply lotions or moisturizers to the residual limb.
- Check the correct fitting of the prosthesis, and make sure there are no pressure areas.
- Change the stump socks daily, and wash them by hand using mild soap and water.
- Keep the leather parts, liners, and webbing of the prosthesis clean and dry. Inspect for wear.
- Check the mechanical parts or components frequently.

Adapted from NSW Artificial Limb Service: Care of the residual limb and prosthesis. http://www.monash.edu.au/rehabtech/pub/reports/CAREOFPR.PDF.

---

nervous system (CNS) malformations.[10,45a] Arthrogryposis can range from mild to severe, depending on the number of joints involved and the amount of muscle tissue missing. In the classic form of arthrogryposis, all the joints of the extremities are stiff, but the spine is not affected. In addition to contractures, muscles are often thin, weak, or missing. Arm posture with children with arthrogryposis often includes internal rotation, elbow extension with limited flexion, and flexed wrists with ulnar deviation. Contractures in the lower extremities are noted with typical posture including hip abduction and external rotation, knee extension or knee flexion contractures, and foot deformities. Arm and leg muscles are small, with webbed skin covering some or all of the joints. Infants are born with significant contractures that improve with aggressive ROM exercises during infancy.[8] In typical cases, all the joints of the arms and legs are fixed in one position, partly due to muscle imbalance or lack of muscle development during gestation (Figure 13-1).

Ongoing occupational and physical therapies help children with arthrogryposis meet educational, self-care, and play needs. Children with arthrogryposis can have many physical limitations that interfere with all areas of occupational performance. OT practitioners may enable children with arthrogryposis to participate in occupations by maintaining or increasing ROM necessary for activities. They also promote children's independence

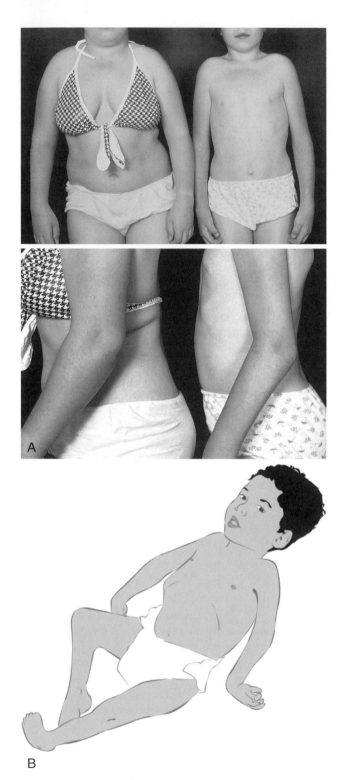

FIGURE 13-1   Child with arthrogryposis. **A,** Note the assymetrical posture, flexed elbows, and curvature of spine. **B,** Note wrist and ankle postures. (**A** from Zitelli, B. J., & Davis, H.W. (2012). *Atlas of pediatric physical diagnosis* (6th ed.). St. Louis: Mosby.)

in occupations by adapting activities. OT practitioners may elect to use technology to help children with arthrogyporosis engage in ADLs, IADLs, play, education, and social participation (See Chapter 27 for information on assistive technology.) Due to the multiple issues associated with arthrogryposis, OT practitioners consult with family members and school personnel to provide the best intervention. The following case example illustrates some intervention principles.

CASE *Study*

Courtney is a 4-year-old girl, who has a large vocabulary. Her arms and legs have a tubular shape; the skin between her fingers and in the folds of her knees and elbows is webbed. During the first 2 years of life, Courtney could not sit on the floor to play because she could not bend her hips and knees, and her feet turned in so much that the soles faced each other (i.e., she had clubbed feet). To get from place to place, she rolled along the floor using the normal movement of her trunk. Her arms are internally rotated with back of hands touching her trunk and wrists flexed. She has very limited elbow flexion. She currently cannot bend her elbows, and her wrists are permanently flexed. She has limited and weak finger movement. The palms of her hands are narrow and almost fold together.

Courtney had surgery at the age of 2 to repair clubbed feet to enable her to place the soles of her feet on the floor. Before surgery, she stood, taking weight on lateral side of feet; after surgery, she can now stand with dorsum of foot in contact with floor surface. Although she can stand with support of braces on knees and ankles, she cannot transition into standing position. To keep her legs stable while standing, she wears braces on her knees and ankles. Seated at a table of the right height, Courtney can move toys that are moderately sized and not too heavy. She grasps small things by pressing them between the backs of her wrists.

Courtney has received occupational and physical therapies since birth. OT intervention consists of performing ROM, stretching, and play activities to maintain and improve Courtney's movement for all activities and providing supportive positioning to promote arm use so she can participate in a daily activities, education, play, and social participation. The OT practitioner provided Courtney's parents with home programs of fun activities to promote social interaction and play; integrated stretching activities into the morning dressing routine so as to not overwhelm the parents; and fabricated wrist extension orthoses to encourage functional wrist and hand positioning. The OT practitioner provided soft fabric bands to help Courtney keep her elbows flexed (and not outstretched) for 10 to 15 minutes at a time.

CLINICAL *Pearl*

Parents of a newborn with arthrogryposis have much to learn in a short period. Functional gains are made in the early months of the infant's life. To maintain the gains in joint movement made during therapy, a clearly written home program should be created so that the parents can have easy-to-follow guidelines. The program includes specific exercises, precautions, and a clearly written orthotic-wearing schedule.

CLINICAL *Pearl*

A dynamic elbow flexion orthosis for an infant with arthrogryposis can be made with elastic and orthoplast. The elbow straightens against the pull of the elastic; the elastic then pulls the elbow into flexion, allowing hand-to-mouth movement. The dynamic elbow flexion orthosis allows infants to do activities such as eating finger food or blowing bubbles.

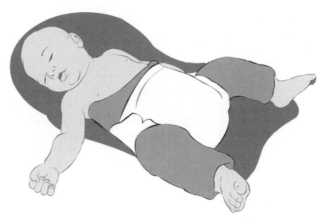

FIGURE 13-2 Infant positioned in a spica cast.

Congenital Hip Dysplasia

Congenital hip dysplasia (or dislocation of the hip) may be caused by genetic or environmental factors. An infant may be genetically prone to instability of one or both of the hip joints, and stretching of an unstable hip or prolonged time in a position that makes the hip vulnerable may cause a dislocation.[14,44] In addition, infants who are tightly swaddled with legs extended and adducted are at increased risk for hip dislocation.[16] Medical intervention at an early age is critical to preventing permanent physical or body structure damage. Surgery may be necessary. Less invasive procedures, such as bracing and casting, may promote proper hip alignment and stability (Figure 13-2).

OT practitioners may work with infants and children who have casts to support hip alignment. Helping parents and children with ADLs during this period involves simplifying activities and providing adaptive equipment to ensure successful engagement in activities. For example, it may be necessary to provide a bath seat in which a child can be positioned for a sponge bath. These children may need seating that is adapted to accommodate the cast. Those children who are in a full-body brace will not be able to explore their environments, so the OT practitioner may adapt developmentally appropriate activities to help these children to explore.

Juvenile Rheumatoid Arthritis

There are three types of juvenile rheumatoid arthritis (JRA): Still's disease (20% of cases), pauciarticular arthritis (40% of cases), and polyarticular arthritis (40% of cases; Table 13-2).[5] Children with JRA experience exacerbations and remissions of symptoms. During exacerbations, or flare-ups, symptoms worsen, and the joints become hot and painful; joint damage can occur. During remissions, or pain-free periods, children with JRA may resume typical activities. Joint protection techniques and energy conservation techniques are encouraged at all times so that these strategies become a habit (Box 13-4).

By the time they are adults, 75% of individuals with JRA have permanent remission.[9] However, these children may have functional limitations due to contractures and deformities. The OT practitioner helps educate children with JRA on how to protect their joints, compensate for decreased ROM during exacerbations, and complete activities with less stress on the joints (**joint protection or energy conservation techniques**). Furthermore, the OT practitioner provides children with stretching and movement activities to maintain the functioning of the joints and prevent contractures (Box 13-5). The OT practitioner may prescribe adaptive equipment or technology to help children engage in everyday activities.

CASE *Study*

Five-year-old Amber, a cheerful kindergartener, loves riding her bike. Amber has pauciarticular arthritis and as a result her joints periodically become painful, hot, and swollen. The OT practitioner provides Amber with a home program of passive and active stretching and strengthening activities and suggests that Amber do these activities right before playing outside or riding her bike. The OT practitioner stresses that stretching will help Amber ride more easily without getting injured. The OT practitioner measured all of Amber's joints with a goniometer to ensure that Amber's ROM is not deteriorating and adapted her bicycle to include built-up handle bars, making it easier for Amber to grasp them without causing damage to her wrist and finger joints.

TABLE 13-2

Three Types of Juvenile Rheumatoid Arthritis

TYPE	LIMB INVOLVEMENT	FUNCTIONAL IMPLICATIONS
PAUCIARTICULAR (FEW JOINTS)		
Affects ≤4 joints Comprises approximately 40% of JRA cases	Only a few unmatched joints are affected. Leg joints are usually affected, but elbows can also be affected. Children often recover in 1-2 y. Children can develop an eye inflammation called iritis, which can lead to blindness unless treated early.	Pain and joint stiffness may limit activities. Contractures can develop. Orthoses may be needed. Work simplification may be necessary. Adaptive equipment may be needed. Climbing stairs may be difficult.
POLYARTICULAR (MANY JOINTS)		
Comprises approximately 30% of JRA cases Five or more joints affected Girls more commonly affected than boys	Symmetric joints of legs, wrists, hands, and sometimes the neck are affected.	Fast onset. Functional implications are the same as those for pauciarticular arthritis but also include the following: Activities can be limited by fatigue. There is difficulty with fine motor activities.
STILL'S DISEASE		
Affects joints as well as internal organs Comprises approximately 20% of JRA cases	Speed of onset and affected limbs are the same as those for polyarticular arthritis. Other organs, for example, the spleen and lymph system, may also be affected. Bone damage may affect growth.	Functional implications are the same as those for polyarticular arthritis but also include the following: Rash and fever may develop, last for weeks, and require bed confinement.

Data from Rogers, S. (2010). Common conditions that influence children's participation. In J. Case-Smith, & J. O'Brien (Eds.), *Occupational therapy for children* (6th ed., pp. 153–154). St. Louis: Mosby; Arthritis Foundation. http://www.arthritis.org/disease-center.php?disease_id=38&df=effects. *JRA*, Juvenile rheumatoid arthritis.

BOX 13-4

Rules of Joint Protection for Children with Juvenile Rheumatoid Arthritis

- If the joints are warm and swollen, encourage the child to use them carefully during all activities and to continue to do range-of-motion exercises as much as possible.
- Because tired muscles cannot protect the joints, teach the child that he or she should not remain in the same position, such as holding a pencil to write, for long periods without stretching or taking a break.
- Larger muscles are found around the big joints, thus teach the child the correct way to use the big joints for heavy work; for example, balancing a lunch tray on the forearms, wearing a backpack on both shoulders, or carrying a purse over the shoulder rather than in the hand.
- If the child becomes tired or is in pain, stop the activity.
- Proper positioning prevents contractures and deformities. Teach the child that he or she should always use good posture.

BOX 13-5

Intervention for Juvenile Rheumatoid Arthritis

- Orthoses to prevent development of contractures and support optimal joint alignment
- AROM and PROM exercises to maintain ROM
- Carefully monitor each joint to maintain functional level and to prevent deformity
- Provide exercises to maintain or increase strength
- Teach the importance of joint protection during all activities to prevent deformities or contractures

AROM, Active range of motion; *PROM*, passive range of motion; *ROM*, range of motion

OT practitioners working with children with JRA frequently provide adaptations to activities to help their clients perform activities. This may include providing built-up handles on items such as spoons or hair brushes (adaptive equipment), showing children how to perform activities more easily (e.g., energy conservation), or instructing them in an alternative method to perform an activity (e.g., using a computer instead of writing as a means of written expression).

Osteogenesis Imperfecta

Osteogenesis imperfecta (OI) is a genetic condition in which collagen fails to form and blocks the scaffolding of bone mineral on the collagen base.[25] Healthy growing children lay down 7% more bone than they resorb, whereas children with OI form only 3% more bone than they resorb. Consequently, children are prone to fractures with typical handling and movement. They are at high risk for developing scoliosis during childhood. Children with OI also have secondary osteoporosis.

Osteoporosis may also co-occur with other developmental conditions such as cerebral palsy as the child has a lack of weight-bearing activities such as crawling and standing. The bones are weakened as a result of mineral loss; weight-bearing activities and muscles pulling on bones during movement make bones stronger. Children with OI are usually very inactive and unable to stand; their bones can become so brittle that even simple activities such as dressing may cause a fracture.

OT practitioners who work with children with OI and osteoporosis must be gentle when helping them experience play, ADLs, IADLs, education, and social participation. The OT practitioner educates family, teachers, and others on how to handle the child and also educates the child on how best to move through any given space and pay attention to body positions. Weight-bearing activities help develop bone growth and should therefore be encouraged. Children with OI may require orthoses to protect bones and prevent contractures.

CLINICAL *Pearl*

With proper joint management, children can be placed in prone or supine standers for weight-bearing activities. Standing is good not only for bone growth and strengthening but also for body functions such as circulation and digestion.

General Interventions

Children with orthopedic conditions may exhibit difficulty in performing ADLs, IADLs, education, or play because of improper joint alignment. They may even have disruptions in sleep and rest caused by pain or difficulty assuming a comfortable position. For example, children with juvenile rheumatoid arthritis may have difficulty grasping and manipulating objects because of hand pain, edema, deformity, or contractures. They benefit from practice, modification, and adaptation (Table 13-3). They may need work-space modifications (e.g., adapted chairs). Furthermore, their physical stature may interfere with play. Children with JRA may develop contractures that limit their active ROM and interfere with their ability to perform play, leisure, and academic activities

TABLE 13-3

Orthopedic Conditions: General Intervention Considerations

CONSIDERATION	DEFINITION AND EXAMPLE(S)
Promotion of proper joint alignment	Through static (nonmovement) and dynamic (movement) orthotic devices, facilitating the typical alignment of muscles and joints. (Note: In the absence of soft tissue contracture and/or bony deformities)
Application modalities such as ice or moist heat	Placing a moist heat pack or ice pack on the inflamed area
Immobilization with a cast or orthosis	Keeping the involved area in proper alignment
Instruction in proper positioning to reduce edema or swelling	Elevating the involved/inflamed area to increase flow of body fluids back to the trunk
Compensation	Helping the child engage in occupations through changing the ways or techniques used to participate
Modification /adaptation	Helping the child participate in occupations by changing how the activities are performed
Emotional /psychosocial consideration	Addressing emotional/psychosocial issues associated with disorders. Children may need to work on developing a positive self-concept, body awareness, and sense of control
Social participation	Promoting social participation in children

and ADLs. They benefit from stretching exercises and work-simplification techniques. Children with OI may need activity modification to decrease risk for fractures.

OT practitioners help children with orthopedic conditions engage in play, leisure, and educational activities, ADLs, IADLs, and sleep and rest.

OT interventions for orthopedic conditions frequently involve the following:

- Helping children engage in occupation (e.g., play, ADLs, IADLs, education, sleep and rest)
- Developing home programs to facilitate engagement in occupations that easily can be integrated into the child's and family's daily activities

- Providing passive or active stretching exercises to improve ROM for occupations. This may be accomplished through activities, orthoses, or casting. OT practitioners may design orthoses to help with the alignment of joints. Clinicians frequently consult with orthopedists to explore the functional outcome of the orthotic, or procedure
- Providing joint protection/energy conservation techniques to rest inflamed joints and to protect joints
- Adapting equipment to compensate for limited ROM or congenital anomalies
- Providing compensatory techniques to allow children to succeed by performing their occupations differently than peers
- Remediation to strengthen muscles and stability around the joints

GENETIC CONDITIONS

Inherited pediatric health conditions occur in response to changes in the genetic makeup of the fetus. Humans have 23 pairs of chromosomes, which are tiny thread-shaped structures found in each cell of the body. Each chromosome is made up of tiny sections called genes. Half of the genetic information (genome) comes from the mother through her egg, and the other half of the genome comes from the father through the sperm. The offspring's genome is unique to the individual and determines every aspect of a person's characteristics (phenotype or the physical expression of the genotype). Because so many genes (23 pairs of chromosomes per cell multiplied by 250 to 2000 genes per chromosome) and mutations are possible, genetic disorders occur. Sometimes a gene carrying a specific problem can be passed from one or both parents to the child. Problems develop when genes mutate (i.e., a gene that has been damaged or is abnormal in some way) or a genetic problem is passed from parent to child. Genetic conditions cause some disease processes and also characteristic physical features involving body structures and patterns of involvement in body functions that have an effect on one's successful performance in occupations. An understanding of certain genetic conditions helps OT practitioners to design and implement interventions.

Approximately 30% of developmental disabilities are related to genetic conditions; 50% of major hearing and vision problems are caused by genetic syndromes.[9] The descriptions that follow highlight genetic conditions commonly encountered in OT practice. Table 13-4 and Box 13-6 provide an overview of other selected genetic disorders and the signs and symptoms or genetic disorders.

Achondroplasia

Achondroplasia, or dwarfism, is a genetic condition in which cartilage does not ossify into bones, especially long bones of arms and legs. Typical physical features include a large protruding forehead and short, thick arms and legs on a relatively normal trunk. Children with achondroplasia often have elbow flexion contractures and short fingers affecting fine motor development and hand use.

Due to their physical stature and features, children with achondroplasia may require adaptive technology or equipment to perform daily occupations. OT practitioners may provide compensatory strategies to help these children achieve independence despite their small stature and short, yet large, hands. Frequently children with achondroplasia exhibit poor hand coordination and require OT intervention to develop hand skills for occupations. Occasionally, medical intervention might include orthopedic surgery, and the OT practitioner would address ROM and relearning of movements postsurgically.

Duchenne Muscular Dystrophy

One of the more common types of muscular dystrophy (MD) is Duchenne muscular dystrophy (DMD), or pseudohypertrophic (which means "false overgrowth") MD. In children with DMD, muscle lacks a protein called dystrophin and is replaced by fat and scar tissue. The buildup of fat and scar tissue can make the muscles especially those of the calves look unusually large. DMD is seen only in boys because it is an X-linked genetic disorder and boys have only one X chromosome. About 1 in 3300 boys develops the condition.[8] Most children with DMD survive until their 20s, and a few live into their 30s. The cause of death is usually cardiopulmonary system (heart and lung) complications that lead to pneumonia.

Sometimes parents suspect that something is wrong when their infant begins to walk on his toes around 1 year of age (Box 13-7). The diagnosis is usually made by the age of 4 years after a muscle biopsy is performed. By then, the child's calves look large and progressive weakness has begun, especially in the joints closest to the body. Scoliosis (Figure 13-3) can develop because of muscle weakness, especially during growth spurts. Proper wheelchair positioning and support are important to prevent scoliosis. Older children with DMD may have to use a ventilator, thus good body alignment is important for maintaining chest capacity that is vital for breathing. High-resistance exercises and activities should be avoided as they can accelerate muscle cell damage; however, nonresistive exercises such as swimming or walking are encouraged to maintain strength.[25]

CASE *Study*

Kevin has DMD. He is in second grade in a general education classroom. When seated at his desk, he looks like the rest of the students in the class although his arms and legs look "chubby." He is bright, but he has trouble keeping up with

TABLE 13-4

Selected Genetic Conditions

CONDITION AND GENETIC CAUSE	INCIDENCE	COMMON SYMPTOMS AND SIGNS	FUNCTIONAL IMPLICATIONS
TUBEROUS SCLEROSIS			
Autosomal dominant gene or mutation	1 in 20,000 births[16]	Very mild to severe symptoms Tumors in brain; can cause seizures, intellectual disability, delayed language skills, and motor problems, which is rare Tumors in heart, kidneys, eyes, or other organs; can (but may not) cause problems	Possible learning disabilities Possible aggressive or hyperactive behavior Possible inability to speak and need for alternative communication Possible severe delays in gross and fine motor skills Mild to severe delays in self-help skills
ANGELMAN SYNDROME			
Deletion of chromosome 15 from mother[10]	1 in 25,000[13]	Tremors and jerky gait Developmental delays Severe language impairment; nonverbal or severe speech delay Very happy mood (happy puppet syndrome) Possible seizure disorder	Microencephaly Gross and fine motor delays, delayed walking skills Severely delayed self-care skills Inability to speak but possible use of alternative communication Sleep disorders (can be very disruptive to family life) Severe sensory processing problems Behavior problems such as biting, hair pulling, stubbornness, and screaming
PRADER-WILLI SYNDROME			
Deletion of chromosome 15 from father[19]	1 in 15,000[19]	Growth failure related to poor suck–swallow reflex in infancy Obsessed with food, possibly causing obesity (parents must lock all kitchen cabinets as a precaution; the child may eat anything) Developmental delays, low intelligence Hypotonia and poor reflexes Speech problems related to hypotonia Laid-back attitude but possible stubbornness and violent tantrums Severe stress on families resulting from behavior problems	Obsession with eating (can be dangerous during treatment) Gross and fine motor delays Delayed development of self-help skills Difficulty walking resulting from obesity or low muscle tone May need alternative communication Possible benefits from prevocational and vocational training
RETT SYNDROME			
Genetic but undetermined[14]	Seen only in girls	Normal or nearly normal development during first 6–18 mo of life Loss of skills and functional use of hands beginning at approximately 18 mo Loss or severely impaired ability to speak Development of repetitive, almost constant hand movements such as hand washing and wringing, clapping, and mouthing Shakiness in trunk and limbs Unsteady, wide-based, stiff-legged walking	Gross and fine motor problems Delayed or lack of self-help skills Difficulty walking or inability to walk Delayed response to requests, possibly taking up to 2 min to respond Possible need for alternative communication

Continued

TABLE 13-4

Selected Genetic Conditions—cont'd

CONDITION AND GENETIC CAUSE	INCIDENCE	COMMON SYMPTOMS AND SIGNS	FUNCTIONAL IMPLICATIONS
FRAGILE X SYNDROME			
Mutation on X chromosome (most common genetic disease in humans)[11]	1 in 2000 boys and 1 in 4000 girls[1]	Boys more severely affected than girls Possible hyperactivity Low muscle tone Sensory processing problems involving touch and sound Possible autistic behavior Language delays (more common in boys); possible dysfunctional speech Intelligence problems ranging from learning disabilities to severe intellectual disability	Mobility problems; delayed walking skills Gross and fine motor delays Delayed development of self-help skills Possible learning problems ranging from learning disabilities and ADD to intellectual disability Possible need for alternative communication in boys (unusual for girls) Possible benefits from prevocational and vocational training

ADD, Attention deficit disorder.

BOX 13-6

Genetic and Chromosomal Disorders: Signs and Symptoms

- Developmental delays
- Microcephaly
- Impaired cognitive development
- Unusual or excessive eating habits or patterns
- Small body structure
- Congenital anomalies
- Facial features characteristic of syndrome
- Simian crease in hands (characteristic of Trisomy 21 syndrome)
- Failure to thrive

BOX 13-7

Progression of Functional Losses in Children with Duchenne Muscular Dystrophy

LEVEL 1
Initially independent but has progressive functional losses over a period of several years; for example, walks independently but then loses stair-climbing ability and needs leg braces to walk and assistance to get up from a chair

LEVEL 2
In wheelchair: sits erect and is able to roll chair and perform ADLs such as upper extremity dressing, eating, and brushing the teeth in bed or chair

LEVEL 3
In wheelchair: sits erect but is unable to perform ADLs in bed or chair, such as placing equipment conveniently or rolling over without assistance

LEVEL 4
In wheelchair: sits erect with support and can do minimum ADLs such as brushing teeth or eating with adapted equipment

LEVEL 5
In bed: can do no ADLs without assistance

Adapted from Rothstein, J. M., Roy, H. R., & Wolf, S. L. (1998), *The rehabilitation specialist's handbook* (2nd ed.). Philadelphia, PA: FA Davis. *ADLs,* Activities of daily living.

---

his classmates. He struggles to write, and his handwriting is difficult to read. Of late, when he needs to get his pencil, he walks his fingers across the desk. It is hard for him to raise his hand to get the teacher's attention or to get his books out of his desk. When the class goes to other parts of the school for gym or music, Kevin can easily be spotted by his waddling gait. He has lordosis (see Figure 13-3); to keep from falling forward, he carries his shoulders and head back. His gait looks like a slow march because he has to pick his feet up high so that his toes do not drag. He falls often. To rise from the sitting position, he "walks" his hands up his legs (Gower's sign).

The OT practitioner works with Kevin at school on a weekly basis and provides his teacher with suggestions to help meet Kevin's classroom needs. For example, the OT practitioner suggested that Kevin start using a computer for his written work, sit at a larger table, and have all his books within easy reach. The OT practitioner monitors

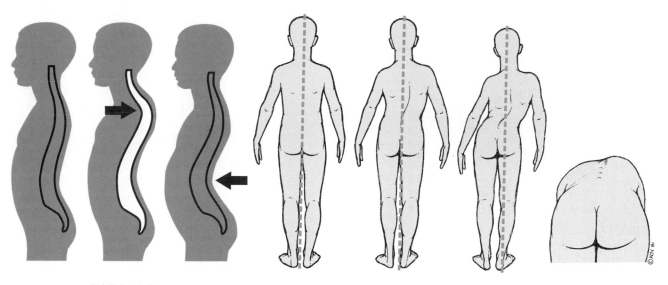

FIGURE 13-3   Scoliosis: curvature of the vertebral column sideways. In severe cases, the ribs are rotated, compressing the lungs and reducing their function; and lordosis—an increased forward curve of the lower back—occurs. The abdomen falls forward and the knees lock backward. The posture shifts weight forward; to balance weight, the child tends to carry his or her head and shoulders back farther than normal. This posture is common in children with hypotonia. (Redrawn from Hilt, N. E., & Schmitt, E. W. (1975). *Pediatric orthopedic nursing.* St. Louis: Mosby for Wilson, D. (2007). *Wong's clinical manual of pediatric nursing* (7th ed.). St. Louis: Mosby.)

Kevin's needs for adaptive equipment. Because Kevin's ability to move has decreased, the practitioner provided Kevin's family with some ROM exercises that will help him keep his joints mobile, which, in turn, will make it easier for the caregiver to dress and bathe him. The OT practitioner taught Kevin's family members about proper body positioning to prevent contractures or scoliosis. Finally, the OT practitioner gave Kevin a list of strengthening exercises that will help him function independently for as long as possible. (By the age of 9 years, most children with DMD require a wheelchair at least part of the time).

Fragile X Syndrome

Fragile X syndrome affects boys more often than girls because it is an X-linked genetic disorder. Children present with limited cognitive development, abnormal skull, joints, and feet structures.[20] They exhibit typical structural features, including elongated faces, prominent jaws and foreheads, hypermobile or lax joints, and flat feet. Children with fragile X syndrome may be intellectually delayed and often present with autistic-like behaviors. OT practitioners often work with children with Fragile X on sensory processing difficulties, social participation, ADLs, and IADLs.

Prader-Willi Syndrome

Prader-Willi syndrome (PWS) involves chromosome 15. Infants often present with significant hypotonia and feeding and swallowing difficulties.[40] As they get older, they have an insatiable appetite and high risk for obesity. Children and adolescents who have PWS exhibit varying degrees of intellectual deficits, overeating habits, and self-mutilating behaviors such as picking sores until they bleed or biting their fists until large calluses develop.[8]

> **CLINICAL** *Pearl*
>
> To avoid excessive weight gain and obesity in children and adolescents who have PWS, a strict diet and eating schedule must be established and maintained.

Trisomy 21 (Down Syndrome)

Children with trisomy 21 have an extra chromosome on the 21st chromosome. Maternal age is a factor. One of every 2000 infants born to women who are younger than 40 years of age and 1 of every 40 infants born to women who are older than 40 years have trisomy 21. About 95% of individuals with Down syndrome have an extra 21st chromosome, 4% have translocation of the extra chromosome and 1% has mosiac form in which some but not all of the cells have the extra chromosome.[42] The extra chromosome comes from the father 25% to 30% of the time.[42]

Children with trisomy 21 have characteristic facial features (slanted eyes, skinfold over nasal corners of eyes, flat nasal bridge, small mouth, protruding tongue),

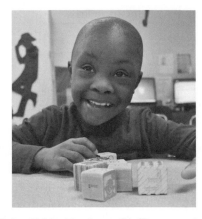

FIGURE 13-4 Child with trisomy 21 (Down syndrome). Note the facial features: slanted eyes, skinfold over nasal corners of eyes (epicanthal fold), flat nasal bridge, and small mouth with tongue (somewhat protruding).

low muscle tone throughout, intellectual disabilities, and simian creases in hands. (See Figure 13-4 and Box 13-8.) Children with trisomy 21 are at risk for medical problems including congenital heart defects, duodenal atresia (incomplete section of the small intestine), hypothyroidism, hearing and vision difficulties, and increased risk for developing leukemia. Additionally, up to 15% of children with trisomy 21 may have C1-C2 instability so the OT practitioner must be cautious with activities such as somersaults.

Early intervention, including occupational, speech, physical, and developmental therapies and special education are an important part of helping children with trisomy 21 reach their full potential. Recent research indicates that early intervention, including teaching families ways to enrich their children's environment, helps reduce developmental delays.[42] As children with trisomy 21 age, the focus of therapy shifts to promoting function in the school setting and later transition to vocational interests.

CLINICAL *Pearl*

Children with trisomy 21 often tongue thrust (i.e., force tongue forward) when eating. Placing food to the sides of the mouth helps them control this forward movement. Caregivers should be encouraged to place small spoonfuls of food to the side of the mouth or two-thirds of the way into the mouth (on the tongue) with slight pressure to encourage lip closure.

CASE *Study*

Dennis, 15 years old, has trisomy 21. When he was 12 years old, the OTA gave him a prevocational assessment at the occupational therapist's request. The occupational

---

BOX 13-8

Physical Characteristics of Trisomy 21

- Shortened limbs and fingers
- Slanted eyes
- Skinfold over nasal corners of eyes (epicanthal fold)
- Small mouth; protruding tongue
- Flat nasal bridge
- Straight line across palm of hand (simian line)
- Heart defects (congenital, high incidence)
- Intellectual disability (usually mild or moderate)
- Atloaxoid instability (important factor for children who engage in sports); can cause quadriplegia after minor neck injuries
- Hypotonia
- Hyperextensibility of joints: lumbar hyperextension, hips, knees, elbows, and fingers
- Sensory processing problems
  - Diffuse tactile discrimination difficulties
  - Tactile sensitivity
  - Gravitational insecurity
  - Hyperactive postrotary nystagmus
  - Poor bilateral motor coordination
- Changes in developmental reflexes in infants (caused by altered sensory processing)
  - Reduced suck reflex
  - Increased gag reflex (eventually resulting in food selectivity or intolerance and chewing problems)
  - Diminished palmar grasp reflex
  - Prolonged and exaggerated startle reflex
  - Prolonged flexor withdrawal and avoidance reactions in hands and feet
  - Delayed placing response in hands and feet
  - Lack of primary standing or air response*
  - Poor optical righting
  - Poor body-on-body righting delayed equilibrium responses, particularly in quadruped and standing positions

*Normally, when infants' feet touch a supporting surface, they support their body weight against the surface with their feet. Infants with Trisomy 21 pull their feet away from the supporting surface.
Data from Crepeau, E. B., & Neistadt, M. E. (Eds.). (1998). *Willard and Spackman's occupational therapy* (6th ed.). Philadelphia, PA: JB Lippincott-Raven.

therapist and the OTA developed a plan of care to improve Dennis's prevocational skills through vocational readiness classes at school. Dennis now works at a local grocery store two half-days a week as part of the vocational training program. His short fingers and hands move slowly when he carefully sorts and places items in grocery sacks. His tongue sometimes protrudes, and it seems large for his mouth. His face is full and round. Behind his glasses is a fold of skin on either side of his nose. Dennis is about 5 feet 6 inches tall. His chest is round. When he pushes grocery carts to customers' cars, he walks with a wide base

TABLE 13-5

Genetic and Chromosomal Disorders: General Intervention Considerations

CONSIDERATION	INTERVENTION EXAMPLE(S)
Failure to thrive	Many genetic disorders have associated feeding difficulties. These may be due to motor, cognitive, or structural functions. The OT practitioner should evaluate and treat them through training, compensation, adaptive technology, or remediation.
Developmental delays	Many genetic disorders have associated delays in motor, social, language, and self-care skills. OT practitioners can help children learn the skills needed for their occupations through intervention.
Cognitive delays	Lower cognitive abilities are frequently a part of genetic disorders. Children may learn skills at a slower rate and may show difficulty in problem solving and with abstract thought and reasoning. Practicing occupations in a variety of contexts helps children generalize skills.
Congenital anomalies	Children with genetic disorders may exhibit certain physical features (short stature, flat hand arches) that interfere with motor skills. OT practitioners can help them compensate or adapt to perform occupations.
Psychosocial/emotional issues	Children with genetic disorders also experience a range of emotional and psychological issues. OT practitioners can help them cope with everyday situations, deal with periods of stress, adapt to life changes, and work with their strengths.
Social participation/behaviors	OT practitioners work with children, families, and communities to help the children engage in occupations. Children with all levels of ability benefit from social participation. OT practitioners can assist them in fitting into groups by helping them develop socially appropriate behaviors.

of support and his feet roll in. He politely chats with the customers he helps. Dennis is a confident young man and enjoys his work.

OT intervention for children with trisomy 21 focuses on helping children engage in ADLs, IADLs, play, education, and social participation. Early intervention services are aimed at enhancing the child's developmental abilities, including improving muscle tone for movement and feeding ability (decreasing tongue thrusting and promoting lip closure). Children with trisomy 21 may require adaptations to participate in regular classrooms. As children with trisomy 21 age, OT practitioners focus on helping them develop healthy lifestyle routines (such as work, sleep and rest, leisure, community mobility).

General Interventions

Often the diagnosis of a genetic disorder is made in infancy and many (but not all) genetic disorders include developmental delays and cognitive problems (Table 13-5). Infants may be referred for early intervention with the focus on parent education and support and facilitating developmental progress. As the child moves to school age, the focus of therapy intervention often shifts to promoting the child's function and participation in the school setting. This may include working on school skills such as handwriting and social participation skills in promoting more socially acceptable behaviors. Often the child with a genetic disorder needs additional assistance and support of OT practitioners to be independent with ADLs such as dressing, grooming and hygiene, self-feeding, toileting and IADLs including assisting in home routines. Adolescents and adults may continue to require support to thrive in the community. They may need assistance with daily living tasks, work or vocational requirements, or socialization. Adolescents may need assistance with making transitions, finding resources, and accessing services.

NEUROLOGIC CONDITIONS

The neuromuscular system includes the nervous system and the muscles of the human body. Chapter 12 provides a more detailed description of the nervous system. The nervous system can be subdivided into the **central nervous system** (CNS), **peripheral nervous system** (PNS), **and autonomic nervous system** (ANS). The CNS includes the brain and spinal cord. The PNS consists of the nerves that originate from the spinal cord and innervate the muscles of the neck, trunk, arms, and legs. The ANS is primarily involved in maintaining homeostasis by innervating targeted organs throughout the body (see Chapter 12). Children born with problems in the brain or spine (CNS) have congenital neurologic conditions.

These conditions also may be acquired from trauma or infection at the time of birth or in the early months of life. Children also can have congenital difficulties with the PNS, such as a brachial plexus injury at birth. The more common neurologic conditions seen by the OT practitioner are discussed in the following sections. Table 13-6 describes other CNS conditions.

Erb's Palsy (Brachial Plexus Injury)

During birth, stretching or tearing of the peripheral nerves in the brachial plexus that supply the arm and shoulder can cause Erb's palsy, injury to the upper fibers of the brachial plexus. Erb's palsy occurs in about 2% of births.[41] Infants who are born feet first or who are too large for the birth canal are at risk for this type of injury. Erb's palsy can generally be diagnosed in the first 24 hours after birth. Infants with Erb's palsy tend to keep shoulder adducted and internally rotated, elbow extended and wrist flexed. The paralysis may resolve, even if untreated, in a few days or weeks (40% of infants); the symptoms get worse in 35% of children. Some children with Erb's palsy have long-term residual problems with innervation and function of the arm. Toddlers with brachial plexus injuries experience delays in the development of gross and fine motor skills.[41]

Early intervention includes joint protection to avoid overstretch of joints, gentle passive ROM and sensory input, and adapted holding and dressing techniques of the infant to ensure the arm with limited innervation is supported. Sometimes infants need a wrist splint to support the wrist in neutral alignment, as it tends to flex because of limited innervation. OT practitioners working with infants who have Erb's palsy begin by examining the infant's movement of the extremity and teaching parents how to support the extremity. This involves holding the arm close to the infant's body and encouraging the infant to touch the extremity and bring his or her hand to the mouth. As the infant develops motor skills, the OT practitioner promotes weight-bearing activities and exercises for ROM and strengthening of the extremity. As movement improves, the OT practitioner facilitates bilateral hand activities. Fabricating an orthosis may help the child support the extremity and regain function. Slings may be helpful as a way to protect the infant's arm (Figure 13-5).

Seizures

Seizures are defined as transient disturbances of brain function resulting from abnormal excitation of cortical neurons. The diagnosis of epilepsy is made if a child has at least two unprovoked seizures at least 24 hours apart. The prevalence of epilepsy is 4 to 10 per 1000 children. It is variable in severity.[8] Epilepsy occurs more often in children than in adults, and many children outgrow these seizures.[4] Seizures are classified as one of three types:

TABLE 13-6

Other Common Central Nervous System Conditions

CONDITION	SYMPTOMS OR SIGNS
AGENESIS OF THE CORPUS CALLOSUM	
Absence or poor development of the central part of the brain that connects the two hemispheres	Deficits ranging from mild learning problems to severe physical and mental problems
	Possible vision or hearing problems
	Possible sensory processing problems
	Possible eye–hand coordination problems
	Intellectual disability and epilepsy (common)
MICROENCEPHALY	
Literally, "small head"	Head that appears small for body
	Moderate to severe intellectual disability
	Moderate to severe motor problems
	Possible seizure disorder

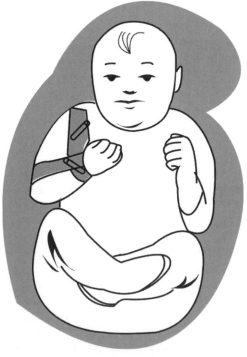

FIGURE 13-5 Sling for infant with Erb's palsy. The sling is made of a cotton stockinette. It is wrapped around the infant's shoulder in a position that keeps the affected hand near the infant's face.

generalized (including grand mal, petit mal, myoclonic, tonic-clonic), partial (focal), and epilepsy syndromes. Most people who have seizures have only one type, which is usually grand mal (Table 13-7). About one-third experience both grand mal and petit mal types.[4,8] Children with developmental disabilities are at greater risk for seizures and it is five times more common in children with cerebral palsy as compared with typically developing children.

OT practitioners should be made aware of their pediatric clients with seizures for several reasons. First, the practitioner needs to know how the seizures present to monitor for any unusual behaviors. If a child has a seizure, the OT practitioner may need to ensure that the child is in a comfortable setting with no dangerous

objects nearby. The child can be placed on his or her side on the floor. The OT practitioner should never place an object in the child's mouth during a seizure. The child may be "postictal" after a seizure and less alert and interactive for a time. Additionally, the OT practitioner may ask parents about side effects of some of the child's medicines. For example, Dilantin can affect the health of the child's gums and influence oral care such as brushing his or her teeth.

Seizures may be provoked by fast spinning movements, flashing lights, and spinning visual stimuli. The OT practitioner who observes a child having a seizure should document the child's behavior before, during, and after the seizure as well as the duration of the seizure. The OT practitioner should contact the parents and the child's physician and provide a description of the event. Some children have frequent unprovoked seizures, which should always be documented. As children get older, they may need more psychosocial support. Seizures can be a source of embarrassment and anxiety and can affect self-esteem. Although children with seizures can participate in most sports and recreational activities, they may need to avoid activities imposing danger such as rock climbing.[8]

TABLE 13-7

Seizures

TYPE OF SEIZURE	CHARACTERISTICS
Grand mal seizures	Possible crying out or mood change before the seizure Loss of consciousness for 2–5 min Falling; shaking of arms, legs, and body Possible loss of control of bowels and bladder Afterward, possible deep sleep, headache, or muscle soreness
Absence (petit mal) seizures	Mostly in children Most likely to occur many times a day Brief loss of consciousness (10–30 sec) Possible eye or muscle fluttering No loss of muscle tone Sudden cessation of activity; restarts a few seconds later
Febrile seizures	Mostly in children 3 mo to 5 y Most common in children with existing neurologic problems In individuals with fever but no brain infection Varying duration; brief or up to 15 min
Infantile spasms ("salaam" seizures)	Seen in children younger than 3 y with obvious brain damage A few seconds in duration but occur several times each day Sudden flexion of arms, extension of legs, and forward flexion of the trunk
Akinetic or drop seizures	Brief and sudden Complete loss of consciousness and muscle tone Danger of head injury because the child will suddenly fall to the ground

Data from Berkow, R. (Ed.). (1999). *The Merck manual* (17th ed.). Rahway, NJ: Merck.

CASE *Study*

Ryan is a 6-year-old diagnosed with right hemiplegic cerebral palsy and a seizure disorder. During a busy day in the clinic, Ryan and Jill (the occupational therapy assistant [OTA]) were working on putting a shirt on Ryan. Ryan was having difficulty putting on his shirt; then he gave a high-pitched cry, his head went back, and he fell off the stool. Jill knew Ryan had a history of uncontrolled seizures and knew right away what happened (Box 13-9). She immediately removed the stool from the area so that his flailing arms and legs would not hit it. She turned his head to the side and tucked a cushion under it. She carefully

BOX 13-9

Caring for a Child Who Is Having a Seizure

- If the child is flailing, make sure nothing is close by that could cause an injury if hit with his or her body.
- Place something soft under the head.
- Do not place anything in the mouth; it may damage the teeth.
- Do not put a finger in the mouth. It will be bitten—hard.
- Roll the child on the side to avoid inhalation of vomitus.
- Call for emergency medical help if the child's skin begins to turn blue.

watched his breathing and skin color, timed the seizure, and waited for it to subside. In a few minutes, Ryan began to regain consciousness but was groggy. Jill knew that the OT session for that day was over and that Ryan needed a nap. She documented the entire seizure episode and informed the parents and physician.

Spina Bifida

Spina bifida, a condition in which one or more of the vertebrae are not formed properly in part because of malformed spinal canal, is the most common type of congenital spinal abnormality.[8] Spina bifida is a neural tube defect that occurs very early in pregnancy when the CNS starts to form. Spina bifida is classified into three types: occulta, meningocele, and myelomeningocele (Figure 13-6). The meninges (the covering of the spinal cord) or both the meninges and the spinal cord push out through an abnormal opening in the vertebra in the meningocele and myelomeningocele types of spina bifida, respectively. With infants who have myelomeningocele, both the meninges and the spinal cord protrude through the opening in the spine. The amount of resulting disability can range from minimal, as in individuals with spina bifida occulta, to severe, as in individuals who have a myelomeningocele. The OT practitioner typically sees children with the myelomeningocele type because their limitations and disabilities are the most severe of the three.

Spina bifida occurs in about 1 of every 1000 births. Its cause may be genetic, or it may result from high maternal body temperatures or insufficient folic acid in the mother's diet. The amount of resulting physical disability is related to the size and location of the defect. The higher the level of the spinal opening, the greater the disability. Eighty percent of children born with spina bifida have

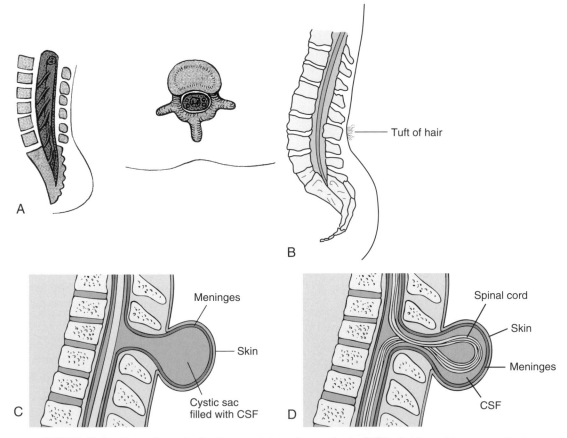

FIGURE 13-6 Normal vertebral column and three forms of spina bifida. **A,** Normal: intact vertebral column, meninges, and spinal cord. **B,** Spina bifida occulta: bony defect in vertebral column. This type of spina bifida can be diagnosed only by x-ray and often goes undetected. **C,** Meningocele: bony defect in which meninges fill with spinal fluid and protrude through an opening in the vertebral column. **D,** Myelomeningocele: bony defect in which meninges fill with spinal fluid and a portion of the spinal cord with its nerves protrude through an opening in the vertebral column. (**A** from Wong, D. L. (1999). *Whaley and Wong's nursing care of infants and children* (6th ed.). St. Louis: Mosby; **B** from Sorrentino, S. A. (2012). *Mosby's textbook for nursing assistants* (8th ed.). St. Louis: Mosby; **C** and **D** from Huether, S. E., McCance, K. L. (2008). *Understanding pathophysiology* (4th ed.). St. Louis: Mosby.)

hydrocephalus caused by blockage of flow of the cerebrospinal fluid into the spinal column. A ventriculoperitoneal (VP) shunt placed in the ventricles of the brain runs down the neck to the abdomen, where the extra fluid drains. Depending on the level of the lesion, infants and children have varying innervation to the lower extremities and may be born with equinovarus (club feet). Scoliosis or kyphosis may be present at birth or may develop later (see Figures 13-3 and 13-7). In the early months of life, proper positioning of the paralyzed legs is important to prevent the development of contractures. Because of their immobility, these children are unable to engage in the normal sensorimotor experiences that influence development. Infants with myelomeningocele are typically referred for early intervention to promote developmental progression. In addition, due to the interruption in innervation to organs, children with myelomeningocele may have difficulty with bowel and bladder control.

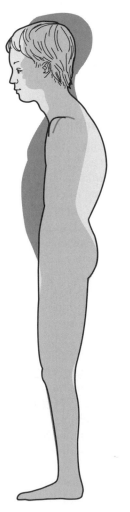

FIGURE 13-7   Congenital kyphosis: a backward rounding of the spine in the chest area that can be caused by malformed vertebrae. Changes in the spine cause the head and shoulders to be carried forward. The front of the body bends forward, compressing the internal organs.

OT practitioners may work with school-age children to become independent with inserting a catheter into the bladder to remove urine.

CASE *Study*

Ten-year-old Niki was on the school playground playing catch when she began to feel ill. When she got off the bus with a fever and headache her father rushed her to the emergency room (Box 13-10). Today, she is in the hospital recovering from surgery to repair a shunt that had been previously placed to control her hydrocephalus. Niki was born with spina bifida and had many surgeries including repair of her spine and opening her back and then several surgeries related to shunt placement and function. She also had surgery to repair her feet alignment (equinovarus). Her legs are paralyzed, and she has no bowel or bladder control. She has learned to use a catheter to empty her bladder and uses a special bowel program to eliminate. When she was younger, Niki walked with crutches and braces but was always frightened of being on her feet. As she got older, she gained weight, which made it difficult for her to walk. Now Niki uses a manual wheelchair to move around.

OT practitioners address the multiple issues affecting the ability of a child with spina bifida to perform daily occupations. Physical issues such as lack of movement, lack of sensation, and positioning, as well as visual perception skills and fine motor skills, are addressed. As these children get older, they are responsible for self-catheterization that requires adequate fine motor skills. OT practitioners address mobility issues in the school and community and also help these children to develop body image and self-concept. OT practitioners help children with spina bifida to meet their requirements at school, play, home, and in the community. Interventions include positioning equipment, adapted technology, compensatory techniques, and developmental strategies. OT practitioners must be aware of the signs of shunt malformations and educate children, family members, and caregivers on signs and symptoms.

BOX 13-10

Signs of a Blocked Shunt

- Headache
- Nausea or vomiting
- Irritability
- Changes in alertness
- Changes in behavior or school performance
- Temperature elevation
- Pallor
- Visual perception difficulties

CLINICAL *Pearl*

Some shunts have magnetically programmable shunt valves. Children with shunts need to be careful regarding iPads, which have embedded magnets. Although the child with a shunt can use an iPad, the device should be kept several inches away from the child's head.

Shaken Baby Syndrome

Infants who are violently shaken by adults sustain serious brain damage, which is referred to as shaken baby syndrome, also known as abusive head trauma (AHT). When an infant is shaken, it causes the brain to hit the inside of the skull so hard that it bruises the brain or causes bleeding and thus can be considered a traumatic brain injury.[1] Box 13-11 lists some of the possible injuries. Retinal hemorrhages may occur and brain damage may be more "diffuse" because of limited myelination. A study analyzing abusive head trauma reported that the incidence is 32 per 100,000 infants, with the peak in hospitalizations occurring between 2 and 4 months.[36] Some instances may be subtle and may go undetected. Many cases of abusive head trauma show that the children have suffered previous abuse. Members of lower socioeconomic groups and younger adults are more likely to shake infants too hard, and the person shaking the infant may have a history of being abused. Only a small percentage of infants who survive a severe shaking regain normalcy after the abuse.[1] Children with disabilities are at greater risk for being abused and neglected; they are at least twice as likely to be mistreated as children without disabilities.[23]

Children with shaken baby syndrome experience neurologic damage that results in developmental delays, visual impairments, mild learning problems, or profound mental impairments. The head trauma may result in loss of muscle control or cerebral palsy (see Chapter 17). Vision problems can stem from injury to the retina, injury deeper in the brain affecting the optic nerve, and also injury to the occipital lobe, which processes visual input. The injury to the eyes may heal within weeks; however, if the visual area of the brain is damaged, children may demonstrate permanent cortical visual impairments or **cortical blindness**. The child with cortical visual impairment functionally does not attend to visual stimuli even if retina and optic nerve are intact.

Infants with abusive head trauma are referred for early intervention services after discharge from the hospital. OT practitioners working with children with shaken baby syndrome evaluate and facilitate the child's development in all areas of occupational performance. OT practitioners examine oculomotor and visual perceptual skills to determine whether the deficits may be

BOX 13-11

Possible Injuries from Shaken Baby Syndrome

- Injuries inside the brain
- Brain swelling
- Diffuse nerve cell damage
- Shear injury
- Bleeding
- Injuries outside the brain
- Retinal bleeding (75–90%)
- Rib fractures
- Bruises
- Abdominal injuries

Adapted from Alexander R. C., & Smith, W. L. (1998). Shaken baby syndrome. *Infants Young Child, 10*(3), 1–9.

interfering with the child's ability to perform daily occupations. The OT practitioner examines the child's motor abilities. The children may have cerebral palsy caused by the brain damage sustained while shaken. A child may exhibit intellectual deficits caused by the brain damage. Children with head trauma often need long-term intervention as they move from early intervention through preschool and school-age programs.

Traumatic Brain Injury

A traumatic brain injury (TBI) is a serious injury to the brain, also known as a closed head injury (CHI) or head injury (HI). TBI results from damage to the CNS as a result of forces coming in contact with the skull. Damage to the nerve tissue occurs both during and after the immediate trauma.[14,47] Recovery can take an extended time. Often children receive therapy services in the acute hospital setting; they may transfer to inpatient and/or outpatient rehabilitation and continue to need support with transition back to the school setting.

Children and adolescents with TBIs are referred for occupational therapy because of their inability to function in the areas of occupation (ADLs, IADLs, education, work, play, and social participation; see Box 13-12). The trauma to the brain typically results in motor, cognitive, and emotional changes. Motor deficits may include abnormal muscle tone (changes in the resting state of a muscle typically resulting in increased muscle tone), hemiplegia (involvement of the arm and leg on one side of the body), and quadriplegia (involvement of both arms and legs). As the swelling of the brain begins to heal, some of the deficits may improve. Children and adolescents with TBI may need to relearn motor patterns. They may have musculoskeletal concerns secondary to muscle tone problems and may require orthoses of the extremities to maintain and improve the ROM. OT practitioners work with children and adolescents who have sustained TBIs to help them relearn movements.

BOX 13-12

Neurologic Disorders: Signs and Symptoms of Traumatic Brain Injury

- Loss of consciousness
- Lethargy
- Vomiting
- Irritability
- Motor: loss of balance, abnormal muscle tone, weakness
- Processing, memory loss
- Communication/interaction impairments: slurred and/or slowed speech, word-finding problems
- Severe headache
- Confusion
- Personality changes
- Flat affect

Data from Rogers, S. (2010). Common conditions that influence children's participation. In J. Case-Smith, & J. O'Brien (Eds.), *Occupational therapy for children* (6th ed.). St Louis: Mosby.

OT practitioners address cognitive changes such as difficulty with attention and concentration, loss of memory, word-finding problems, and poor abstract thinking and reasoning. These children and adolescents may experience perceptual deficits that include lack of awareness of their surroundings and poor sequencing and timing skills. They may experience emotional changes such as lability (moods ranging from happy to tearful or angry), inappropriateness (e.g., cursing, touching, disrobing), and personality changes. Children and adolescents with TBI may demonstrate a "flat" affect, showing little or no emotion. Often, aggressiveness, impulsivity, and irritability occur during recovery.[47]

OT practitioners working with children and adolescents with TBI work closely with their parents and a team of professionals, including speech and language pathologist, physical therapist, rehabilitation specialist, physiatrist, nurse, psychologist, and teacher (Table 13-8). The OT practitioner is a key player on this team and has the responsibility of addressing the child's ability to function in everyday occupations.

CLINICAL *Pearl*

Muscle tone in a child or adolescent who has sustained a TBI is different from that in a child who has cerebral palsy. The abnormally high muscle tone is more resistant to handling and inhibitory techniques. OT practitioners should determine appropriate treatment techniques to address postural control and tone management. Positioning becomes a key therapeutic focus when children have significant tone alterations.

TABLE 13-8

Neurologic Disorders: General Intervention Considerations (Traumatic Brain Injury)

CONSIDERATION	DEFINITION AND EXAMPLE(S)
Preparatory activities	Prepare the child for activities by making him or her more ready to interact with the environment. "Normalize" sensory awareness/response and muscle tone. The child participates in sensory games, rubbing objects with different textures, and awareness activities.
Enabling activities	Build up skills needed for engagement in occupations (e.g., arm strength, visual attention, memory). Examples include weight-bearing and weight-shifting activities and development of arm strength through repetitive activities (e.g., weight training, lifting plates, picking up laundry).
Purposeful activities and occupations	Facilitate performing the actual occupation or activity in an environment closest to the natural one. Examples include unbuttoning the shirt in preparation for evening shower and preparing lunch at the clinic.

General Interventions

OT interventions for neurologic conditions frequently involve the following:

- Motor learning and relearning, including facilitation of more normal tone and postural responses, facilitation of more normal movement patterns, and support of wearing orthoses and ROM to promote engagement in occupations
- Improving hand functioning for occupational performance
- Providing compensation or adaptations to allow children to participate in occupations
- Promoting cognitive functions, including executive functioning, attention, and problem solving for daily living
- Providing resources and support systems to allow the child or youth to engage in occupations at school, home and in the community

DEVELOPMENTAL CONDITIONS

A developmental disorder is a mental and/or physical disability that arises before adulthood and lasts throughout a person's life. Autism spectrum disorders (ASDs) affect a variety of body functions and structures with a wide range of severity. Other examples include Rett syndrome, attention-deficit/hyperactivity disorder (ADHD), and developmental coordination disorder (DCD; Box 13-13).

Attention Deficit Hyperactivity Disorder

ADHD is a prevalent neurobehavioral disorder characterized by developmentally inappropriate levels of inattention and distractibility and/or hyperactivity that impairs adaptive function at home, at school, and in social settings.[8] It occurs in boys three times more often than in girls. Children with ADHD have issues such as difficulty with attention, hyperactivity, distractibility, and impulsivity (Box 13-14). Others include sleep disorders, emotional lability, poor self-esteem, and poor frustration tolerance.[4,8] The prevalence of ADHD is estimated between 7% and 10% in the United States.[4] It is often diagnosed in grade school but symptoms persist through adolescence and adulthood.

Children with ADHD benefit from organization, structure, and being given clear expectations. OT practitioners and psychologists can provide parents with strategies and/or techniques to help their children with behavior problems. Treatment approaches may include cognitive-behavioral therapy, family therapy, coaching, and skill building for interpersonal skills.[8] OT practitioners can provide sensory strategies that help children with ADHD remain calm, focus, and improve concentration. Physical activity may help them modulate their behaviors and pay attention more effectively in class. OT practitioners may consult with the teacher on sensory-based classroom strategies along with providing suggestions regarding classroom environment. In fact, some schools have walking programs for all children before the start of classes.

Autism Spectrum Disorders

The most recent *Diagnostic and Statistical Manual (DSM-V)*[3] defines *autism* by the presence of four diagnostic criteria as follows:

1. Persistent deficits in social communication and social interaction across multiple domains
2. Restricted, repetitive patterns of behavior, interests, or activities. This may include stereotyped motor activities, insistence on sameness, fixed routines and ritualized patterns, highly restricted, fixated interests, and/or altered sensitivity and reactivity to sensory input
3. Symptoms presenting early in life (apparent by 12–24 months but manifest earlier)
4. Symptoms causing significant impairment in social and/or occupational functioning.[3]

The Centers for Disease Control and Prevention (CDC) estimates that four times as many boys than girls are

---

BOX 13-13

Developmental Disorders: Signs and Symptoms

- Delays in motor, processing, and communication/interaction skills
- Impaired body functions
- Limited repertoire of behavior
- Stereotypical behaviors
- Decreased attention to purposeful activities and occupations
- Milestones not met
- Infants show decreased exploration and interest in environment

---

BOX 13-14

Characteristics of Children with Attention-Deficit Disorder or Attention-Deficit/Hyperactivity Disorder

- Active or fidgety; talks nonstop
- Impulsive; acts without thinking about consequences
- Makes careless mistakes
- Lacks focus; daydream
- Difficulty following directions
- Difficulty completing tasks
- Racing thoughts
- May interrupt frequently
- Inattentive during activities they consider boring or unexciting (which often include schoolwork)
- Slow to wake up in the morning; disorganized or grumpy unless anticipating an exciting activity
- Slow to fall asleep
- Spatially dyslexic (write mirror-image reversals of letters; have difficulty with left–right discrimination; have difficulty properly sequencing letters, words, or numbers)
- Episodic temper tantrums that include hitting, biting, and kicking
- Wets the bed
- Inexplicably emotionally negative

Adapted from National Institute of Mental Health. ADHD. http://www.nimh.nih.gov/health/publications/attention-deficit-hyperactivity-disorder/complete-index.shtml#pub2.

diagnosed with autism.[15] The incidence of autism is on the rise with significant changes in prevalence in the past 10 years. Children with autism come from all racial, ethnic, intellectual, and socioeconomic backgrounds.[3,4] Autism affects the child's ability to participate in occupations in varied contexts and settings including home, education, and recreational, and in the community.

Children with autism present with a variety of signs and symptoms that range in severity. The *DSM-V* ranks severity on three levels: level 1 requires support, level 2 requires substantial support, and level 3 requires very substantial support.[3]Although therapy for each child needs to be individualized, certain considerations may be beneficial (Box 13-15). Children with autism require a structured environment and clear expectations.

OT practitioners working with children with autism must be able to read verbal and nonverbal cues

---

BOX 13-15

Signs of Autism

INFANT

- Stiffens when picked up or does not physically conform to the adult's body when held
- Does not calm when held; may prefer to lie in the crib
- Startles easily when touched or when the bed is bumped
- Hates baths, dressing, or diaper changing
- Has poor sucking ability or is hard to feed
- Has poor muscle tone; body feels floppy
- Does not have age-appropriate head control or age-appropriate ability to sit, crawl, or walk

CHILDREN

- Seems unaware of surroundings
- Does not make eye contact
- Has general learning problems
- Does not relate to others
- Only eats certain food textures
- Refuses to touch certain textures (e.g., mud and sand)
- Has sleep problems such as difficulty getting to sleep or staying asleep
- Hyperactivity
- Withdrawn, miserable, anxious, or afraid
- Displays repetitive behavior or speech patterns
- Fixates on one object or body part
- Compulsively touches smooth objects
- Shows fascination with lights
- Flaps arms when excited
- Frequently jumps, rocks, or spins self or objects
- Walks on tiptoes
- Giggles or screams for no apparent reason
- Eats strange substances (e.g., soil, paper, toothpaste, soap, rubber)

---

quickly. Because these children have difficulty expressing themselves verbally, they may experience frustration when OT clinicians do not "listen" to them. This may cause escalation of poor or acting-out behavior. Children with autism experience difficulty processing sensory information; they may benefit from a sensory integration approach (see Chapter 25). The OT practitioner should carefully monitor the child's reaction to activities; it may be difficult for the child to select from several activities. Therefore, asking a child with autism to choose between only two activities facilitates decision making.

Communication with children who have autism may include the use of simple signs, verbal expressions, demonstrations, pictures, and communication systems. OT practitioners will need to consult with speech/language therapists, teachers, parents, and other professionals to determine the most effective way(s) to communicate. OT practitioners work with children with autism to improve their ability to participate in ADLs, IADLs, education, work, play, and social participation (Box 13-16). Because these children typically experience deficits in all of these areas, OT practitioners must prioritize and identify meaningful goals. These goals are most effectively developed by collaborating with parents and/or teachers. For example, holding a spoon during mealtime is easily understood as addressing feeding goals. It would be harder for parents and/or teachers to understand how grasping a cube will help with feeding.

Developmental Coordination Disorder

DCD encompasses a wide range of characteristics, but an essential feature is that the child's motor coordination is markedly below his or her chronologic age and intellectual ability and significantly interferes with activities of daily living.[3] The diagnosis of DCD cannot be the result of physical, sensory, or neurologic impairments.[3] In addition, children are diagnosed with DCD only if the criteria for autism spectrum disorder are not met.[3] If intellectual disability is present, the motor difficulties must be in excess of those usually associated with the level of severity of intellectual disability.

Children with DCD have difficulty forming letters quickly and precisely; this is often manifested in an inability to keep up with classmates and complete assignments efficiently.[29,32] For example, a child with DCD may be able to complete only one simple sentence in the time allotted, whereas other children are able to complete full paragraphs. The extra energy and time that children with DCD spend on the mechanics of writing often interfere with their ability to manage other classroom tasks. They take longer and are less efficient in carrying out everyday self-care tasks, which include such

BOX 13-16

General Intervention Techniques for Children with Autism

- Provide structure and consistency.
- Keep the same routine.
- Read the child's nonverbal as well as verbal cues.
- Communicate through signs, pictures, communication boards, and/or singing.
- Work with the child at his or her level.
- Follow the child's cues.
- Redirect when the child begins self-stimulation.
- Listen to the parent(s) to learn about the child's preferences.
- Provide a quiet setting.
- Allow the child to play with other children.
- Use positive behavioral reinforcers.
- Use sensory integration techniques:
  - Tactile
  - Vestibular
  - Proprioceptive
  - Olfactory
  - Gustatory (children with autism may enjoy very spicy or sour tastes instead of bland tastes)
- Provide the child with choices (may have to start with only two).
- Allow the child time to respond.
- Keep your talking to a minimum; use simple directions.
- Use behavioral management techniques.
- Realize that children have "off days" (you may have to change the plan).
- Realize that practitioners have "off days"; spend some time thinking about what you could have done differently.
- Listen to the parents!
- Work on occupation-centered goals so that therapy is meaningful to the child and to the family.

things as brushing teeth and getting dressed. Tasks that other children accomplish easily (e.g., fastening clothing, tying shoes, or organizing homework) may be problematic for a child who has DCD.[26] These children also often exhibit low self-esteem, show frustration, and begin to expect failure.[19,45] Feelings of low self-esteem develop as early as 6 years of age,[26,45] a time when children with DCD experience difficulty keeping up with their peers and struggle with sports and play activities. The feelings associated with perception of low physical competence and inadequacy in performing tasks that other children take for granted can, and often do, result in emotional problems.[26,32,45]

Many professionals suggest that these children will outgrow their coordination deficits, but evidence indicates that children who have DCD continue to have difficulty in adolescence and adulthood.[29] Losse et al

monitored a group of children for 10 years and reported significant differences in verbal IQ, performance IQ, and academic performance between children with DCD and their peers.[29] Those with DCD experienced more behavioral problems; had more difficulty with handwriting, art design, and technology; demonstrated trouble with home economics; and exhibited lower performance in practical science lessons.

The motor deficits exhibited by children with DCD are many and varied. Among other things, they exhibit poor balance, postural control, and coordination and are more variable in their motor responses.[49] Timing and sequencing deficits and slower movement times have also been reported for children who have DCD.[49] These children tend to rely more on visual than proprioceptive information, fail to anticipate or use perceptual information, and do not use appropriate rehearsal strategies.[49] This, in turn, impairs quality of movement, especially in situations in which the child has to react to a changing environment. According to sensory integration theory, the primary basis for the poor motor performance of children with DCD lies in the central processing of information related to the planning, selecting, and timing of movement. These children have been shown to have difficulty processing tactile, vestibular, and proprioceptive information.[6,12] The treatment of children with DCD may follow a motor control (see Chapter 24) or sensory integration (see Chapter 25) approach.

CLINICAL *Pearl*

Children with sensory processing deficits may experience the signs and symptoms of ADHD. OT practitioners can provide sensory strategies and intervention that may help children modulate their attention and function within the home and the classroom. Diet may also cause ADHD behaviors (this has not been proved, but many parents support this). Overstimulating or anxious environments may cause children to exhibit behaviors of ADHD. Those experiencing emotional trauma may exhibit the signs of ADHD.

CLINICAL *Pearl*

Developmental dyspraxia is a disorder characterized by impairment in the ability to plan and carry out sensory and motor tasks. Children with this problem may have trouble starting or stopping a movement. They may be able to do routine activities but have trouble with new ones. Sometimes the force of their movement is too strong or too weak to be effective, or they may have trouble with balance, vision, or short-term memory.

Rett Syndrome

Rett syndrome is a progressive neurologic disorder that occurs only in girls. It is a genetic disorder with mutation of the X chromosome.[8] The infant or toddler seems to be developing normally until 6 to 18 months of age, at which time regression in all skills is observed. Microencephaly, seizures, abnormal muscle tone, intellectual disability, loss of purposeful hand use, and stereotypical patterns of behavior (especially hand wringing) emerge. Adolescents with Rett syndrome are generally nonambulatory and do not have functional hand use.

General Interventions

OT interventions for developmental disorders (Table 13-9) frequently involve the following:

- Analysis of occupational performance, including the child's strengths and weaknesses and how they influence the child's performance
- Developmental interventions to facilitate achievement of milestones and to promote occupational performance
- Motor development and refinement of abilities
- Cognitive-behavioral techniques to facilitate goal setting and occupational performance
- Interventions to increase coordination and motor planning abilities for occupations
- Sensory diet to help regulate the child's emotional and attentional states
- Successful achievement to develop self-concept and positive self-esteem
- Organizational strategies
- Behavioral modification techniques to develop socially appropriate behaviors
- Task-specific activities to teach child-specific skills for daily living
- Adaptations or compensation for limited problem solving, memory, or generalization

CARDIOPULMONARY SYSTEM

The cardiopulmonary system consists of the cardiac (heart and vessels) and respiratory (trachea, lungs, and diaphragm) systems, which are located in the thoracic area of the human body. The health conditions discussed in this section affect the cardiac and respiratory body structures and consequently one's ability to participate fully in life's roles and occupations (Box 13-17).

CASE *Study*

The OT clinic receives a referral from a physician to evaluate and treat the feeding ability of a 7-month-old child on the

TABLE 13-9

Developmental Disorders: General Intervention Considerations

CONSIDERATION	DEFINITION AND EXAMPLE(S)
Behavior management programs	Provide programs to promote appropriate daily actions by identifying target behaviors, establishing positive reinforcers, and implementing a behavioral plan and follow-up with data collection.
Structured environment	Set up clear routines with consistency to allow the child to understand and practice daily occupations.
Total communication approach	Use a variety of systems to relate to the child, such as a communication board, sign language, verbal language, pointing/gesturing, and facilitative communication.
SI intervention	Use suspended equipment to provide a controlled sensory input so that the child can make an adaptive response. SI theory postulates that this will help with CNS development.
Practice occupations	Repeat skills and occupations such as using backward or forward chaining. Children learn through repetition.
Teach and repeat	Simplify occupations to allow the child to participate and increase ability to reach milestones.
Education	Teach the child how to perform occupations. Educate parents, teachers, and others about the child's condition and techniques to support child's occupations.
Promote interests	Provide novelty to promote interests and exploration.
Emotional/psychosocial issues	Address the child's self-concept, self-awareness, and body awareness by providing opportunities for exploration and success.

CNS, Central nervous system; *SI,* sensory integration.

BOX 13-17

Cardiopulmonary Disorders: General Signs and Symptoms

- Decreased tolerance for exercise
- Increased occurrence of respiratory infections
- Shortness of breath
- Decreased endurance
- Small physical size for age
- Cyanosis (bluish discoloration of skin and mucous membranes)
- Poor distal circulation
- Failure to thrive
- Persistent cough or wheezing
- Pain or discomfort in joints and muscles

---

pediatric cardiac unit. The child has undergone surgery for the repair of a heart defect. The occupational therapist and the OTA, who will be working together, study cardiac disorders so that they can be informed before evaluating the child.

Cardiac Disorders

Cardiac disorders are conditions that involve the heart and/or vessels (Figure 13-8). Congenital heart defects are somewhat common with an incidence in 1 in 85 births. Congenital heart diseases and dysrhythmias are examples of pediatric cardiac health conditions. Congenital heart defects are classified by several factors including the type of defect, presenting symptoms (cyanotic or acyanotic), and the type of repair needed. Additionally, infants can simultaneously have multiple heart defects, making the diagnosis and treatment more complex. The American Heart Association (2007) described 18 common types of congenital heart defects.[39] Infants with acyanotic defects may present with healthy pink coloring yet have significant heart defects. Common acyanotic defects include ventricular septal defects, atrial septal defects (ASDs), patent ductus arteriosus, and coarctation (or aortic narrowing) of the aorta. In contrast, cyanosis presents with a bluish discoloration of the skin due to low oxygen saturation. Some common cyanotic heart defects include transposition of the great vessels and tetrology of Fallot. Infants with cyanotic congenital heart defects often experience low energy, poor endurance, and increased stress because the mixture of oxygenated and deoxygenated blood results in chronic hypoxia. Infants born with narrowing of the aorta or with transposition of the great vessels require surgery immediately after birth but typically recover and have no additional problems. Infants and children with complex heart defects such as tetrology of Fallot or hypoplastic left heart may need multiple surgeries throughout childhood (Figure 13-9).

Children with congenital heart defects allocate more energy for basic physiologic function leaving less energy available for developmental tasks. A referral of children with cardiac disorders to the pediatric OT practitioner is typically based on secondary deficits associated with the child's primary diagnosis. Oral–motor and feeding issues or sensory processing problems may necessitate a referral to a pediatric occupational therapist.[48]

CLINICAL *Pearl*

Older children who know that they have a congenital heart disorder are likely to avoid exercise and activity because of fear and decreased endurance. The OT practitioner can explore volitional activities that help motivate the child to be active, such as yoga or martial arts, which do not stress the cardiopulmonary system.

Dysrhythmias

A normal heart has recurrent expansion and compression of the chest that maintains proper circulation of the blood and respiration, which collectively are known as cardiac rhythm. Dysrhythmias are irregular cardiac rhythms. Examples of dysrhythmias include bradycardia (an abnormally slow heartbeat) and tachycardia (an abnormally fast heartbeat).

Children with cardiac disorders may experience difficulty with activities involving strength (due to weakness), endurance (due to limited endurance—in part from impaired cardiac function), and/or pain or discomfort in the joints and muscles (due to the lack of use or decreased oxygen). These difficulties may result in impaired functioning in the areas of occupation, including education, social participation, play, and self-care (Table 13-10).

CLINICAL *Pearl*

Infants with heart defects may not be able to hold a regular-sized rattle due to poor cardiac endurance. They can successfully hold small, lightweight rattles. OT practitioners may start with these rattles until the child builds up strength and endurance. Additionally, although tummy time is important in typical development, this activity may need to be modified for infants who have cardiac issues.

CLINICAL *Pearl*

Infants and children with congenital heart defects are at risk for slower growth because more resources are required for basic physiologic function. They may benefit from higher-calorie foods and drinks. Consultation with a dietitian is helpful in determining the appropriate food for infants and children. Infants with heart defects may benefit from adapted feeding ideas including supportive positioning, prolonged rests, and supplemental feedings (tube feedings) as they fatigue quickly.

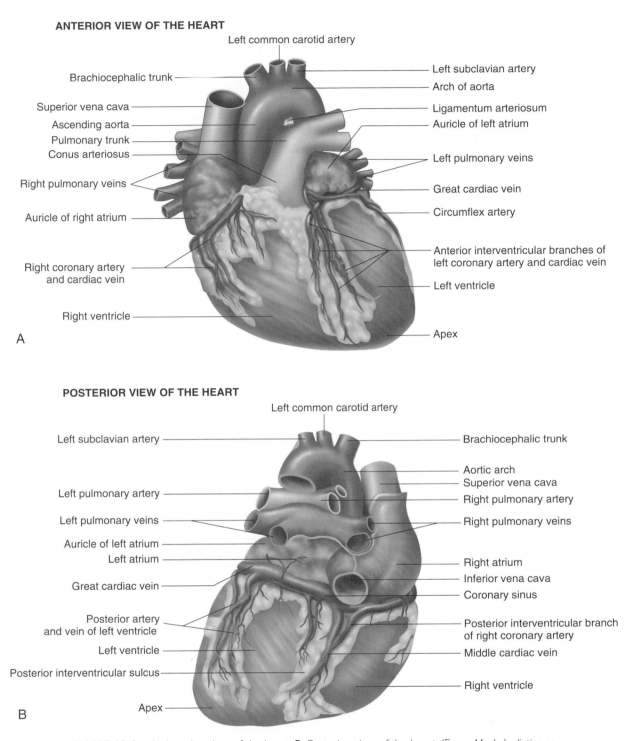

ANTERIOR VIEW OF THE HEART

Left common carotid artery

Brachiocephalic trunk

Superior vena cava

Ascending aorta

Pulmonary trunk

Conus arteriosus

Right pulmonary veins

Auricle of right atrium

Right coronary artery and cardiac vein

Right ventricle

Left subclavian artery

Arch of aorta

Ligamentum arteriosum

Auricle of left atrium

Left pulmonary veins

Great cardiac vein

Circumflex artery

Anterior interventricular branches of left coronary artery and cardiac vein

Left ventricle

Apex

A

POSTERIOR VIEW OF THE HEART

Left common carotid artery

Left subclavian artery

Left pulmonary artery

Left pulmonary veins

Auricle of left atrium

Left atrium

Great cardiac vein

Posterior artery and vein of left ventricle

Left ventricle

Posterior interventricular sulcus

Apex

Brachiocephalic trunk

Aortic arch

Superior vena cava

Right pulmonary artery

Right pulmonary veins

Right atrium

Inferior vena cava

Coronary sinus

Posterior interventricular branch of right coronary artery

Middle cardiac vein

Right ventricle

B

FIGURE 13-8   **A,** Anterior view of the heart. **B,** Posterior view of the heart. (From *Mosby's dictionary of medicine, nursing & health professions* (9th ed.). (2013). St. Louis: Mosby).

Pulmonary Disorders/Chronic Respiratory Disorders

Pulmonary disorders are conditions that involve the lungs and one's ability to breathe. The most common pulmonary diseases affecting children are asthma and cystic fibrosis. Children with pulmonary diagnoses are referred for occupational therapy when they experience problems that interfere with ADLs, IADLs, sleep and rest, education, play, and social participation.

Asthma

Asthma is a chronic respiratory disease that is characterized by bronchial smooth muscle hyperactivity, sudden, recurring attacks of labored breathing, chest constriction,

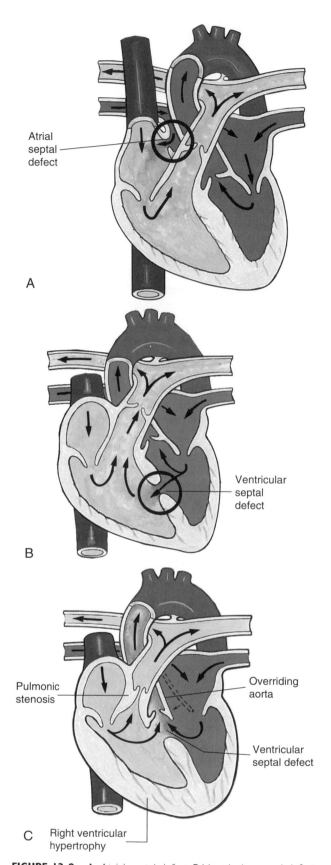

Atrial septal defect

A

Ventricular septal defect

B

Pulmonic stenosis

Overriding aorta

Ventricular septal defect

C Right ventricular hypertrophy

FIGURE 13-9 **A,** Atrial septal defect. **B,** Ventricular septal defect. **C,** Abnormally large right ventricle. (From Hockenberry, M. J. (2013). *Wong's essentials of pediatric nursing* (9th ed.). St. Louis: Mosby.)

TABLE 13-10

Cardiopulmonary Disorders: General Intervention Considerations

CONSIDERATION	DEFINITION AND EXAMPLE(S)
Breathing exercises	Exercises that promote optimal respiration rate by exerting the muscles involved in breathing, including the diaphragm and the oblique muscles.
Relaxation techniques	Techniques such as controlled breathing to promote decreased heart rate, lower metabolism, and decreased respiration rate. Additional relaxation methods include visualization of pleasant experiences, yoga, exercises, and biofeedback.
Energy conservation techniques	Principles and methods that promote using the least amount of energy and movement to perform activities. Sitting rather than standing while making a sandwich is one example of an energy conservation technique.
Balance/pacing of activities	Principles and methods that promote equal consideration between work and rest.
Balanced diet	Eating and drinking food with nutritional value to promote physical health and well-being.
Avoidance of internal and environmental "triggers"	Attempting to lower exposure to internal (e.g., stress, lack of rest) and external (e.g., pollen, smoke, dust) stimuli that initiate a negative cardiopulmonary response.
Strength and endurance activities	Techniques to increase participation time in activities through increased repetition and decreased breaks.
Emotional/ psychosocial issues	Address the child's self-concept, perception of their abilities, interests, and so on. Help children gain an appreciation of their strengths.

and coughing. It is a reactive disease of the small airway structures in the lungs. Risk factors include presence of allergies, family history, frequent respiratory infections, low birth weight, second-hand smoke exposure, and low-income environment.[2] Environmental and internal stimuli can trigger an attack in a child or adolescent with asthma. Examples of environmental triggers include changes in atmospheric pressure, cold air, and cigarette smoke. Examples of internal triggers are exercise and stress. During an asthma attack, the muscular walls of the airway structures undergo spasm, and excessive mucus is secreted. These occurrences result in laborious breathing. Children with asthma have described feeling as if they were drowning in their own saliva and being unable to catch their breath. Most children and adolescents anticipate oncoming attacks and are able to prevent a trip to the emergency room or doctor by following previously prescribed intervention procedures. Medical intervention often involves inhalant and/or drug therapy.[7] Children with asthma may have less energy for play and require more frequent rest periods. School-age children and adolescents may benefit from some more conscious relaxation techniques if they have anxiety regarding breathing. OT practitioners may need to monitor a child's activity level and impose rest as needed. Children may be fearful of overexertion and physical activity that could precipitate an asthma attack.

Cystic Fibrosis

Cystic fibrosis (CF) occurs primarily in whites and is diagnosed during infancy or early childhood. CF is an inherited (genetic) disease that affects the exocrine (externally excreting) glands. The pancreas, respiratory system, and sweat glands are the most affected. The secretions from these glands are abnormally clammy or sticky. Symptoms of CF include frequent greasy stools, failure to thrive (problems in feeding and weight gain), frequent colds, and pneumonia with chronic coughing or wheezing. Chronic obstructive pulmonary disease (COPD) is the most serious complication of CF. Symptoms of COPD include wheezing, infections, and recurrent pneumothorax (partial collapse of a lobe of the lung).

Medical intervention for this pediatric health condition includes antibiotics for infections, inhalant therapy, and supplemental oxygen. Physical therapy may be required to assist with postural drainage, which, in turn, decreases the excessive buildup of sticky mucus in the lungs.

Children with chronic respiratory disease can experience disruption of sleep, difficulty with ADLs and IADLs, and difficulty with gross motor activities requiring endurance.[28] Additionally, children with chronic illnesses need to manage for health care needs including medical visits and hospitalizations and limit time available for play and leisure. Children with chronic respiratory disease also are at higher risk for depression, anxiety, and suicide.[28]

CLINICAL *Pearl*

Children who have cystic fibrosis may benefit from swimming. Care should be taken to provide relaxing swim sessions while still challenging the child. Consultation with the physician and physical therapist is beneficial.

CLINICAL *Pearl*

As part of health management and maintenance, clinicians may help children and adolescents who have cystic fibrosis establish a routine for ensuring that an inhaler is available whenever needed.

Hematologic Conditions

Hematologic disorders are conditions of the blood. Human blood is a fluid that consists of plasma, blood cells, and platelets. The purpose of blood is to carry nutrients and oxygen to the tissues of the body and to carry waste materials away from the tissues. Anemia, a pathologic deficiency in the oxygen-carrying component of the blood, deprives body tissues of necessary nutrients and oxygen. Anemia also leads to a buildup of waste products in human tissue.

Sickle cell anemia is one type of hematologic disorder that occurs in the black people of Africa or those of African descent. The red blood cells of an affected person are crescent shaped. It is characterized by exacerbation (flare-ups) and remission (lack of symptoms). During exacerbation, the person who has sickle cell anemia may experience pain in the joints, fever, leg ulcers, and jaundice (Figure 13-10). Depending on the severity of the disease, secondary complications might arise, including a hemorrhage or cerebrovascular accident (CVA).[21] Children with sickle cell anemia may need to avoid strenuous activity. Discussions of CVA and other potential secondary complications of sickle cell anemia are beyond the scope of this text.

CLINICAL *Pearl*

OT practitioners working in school systems may recruit adolescents with chronic health conditions (such as sickle cell anemia) to lead support groups for the younger children. This helps the adolescent "give back" in a volunteer role that benefits all participants in the group.

SENSORY SYSTEM CONDITIONS

Sensory system conditions include those involving vision impairments (seeing impairments) and auditory system impairments (hearing impairments). Children also may have processing problems or deficits in other sensory systems, including the tactile (touch) system, the vestibular (balance and movement) system, and the proprioceptive (position sense) system (see Chapter 25).

Vision Impairments

About 1 in 4000 children is legally blind. One in 20 has significant but less severe vision problems. One-half to two-thirds of children with developmental disorders

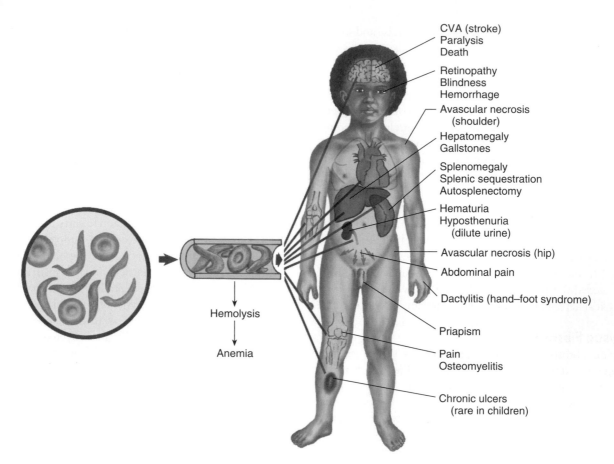

CVA (stroke)
Paralysis
Death

Retinopathy
Blindness
Hemorrhage

Avascular necrosis
(shoulder)

Hepatomegaly
Gallstones

Splenomegaly
Splenic sequestration
Autosplenectomy

Hematuria
Hyposthenuria
(dilute urine)

Avascular necrosis (hip)

Abdominal pain

Dactylitis (hand–foot syndrome)

Priapism

Pain
Osteomyelitis

Chronic ulcers
(rare in children)

Hemolysis

Anemia

FIGURE 13-10 Sickle cell anemia. (From Hockenberry, M. J. (2013). *Wong's essentials of pediatric nursing* (9th ed.). St. Louis: Mosby.)

have a significant ocular disorder.[8] Because a large proportion of children with disability also have vision problems, the vision of all children with special needs should be monitored closely (Box 13-18).

The vision system is complex and visual problems can stem from a number of problems. These may include:

- Abnormal ocular (eyeball) development with difficulties such as glaucoma and cataracts;
- Ocular motility disorders—eye muscle imbalance such as strabismus or amblyopia affecting visual tracking and binocular vision (ability of both eyes to work together—important for depth perception);
- Nerve conduction problems such as optic nerve hypoplasia;
- Retinopathy of prematurity—a disorder specific to infants born prematurely; and
- Damage within the CNS with resultant cortical visual impairment and field cuts.

Discovering vision problems early can alert OT practitioners and family members to the need for appropriate intervention. Additionally, vision develops very quickly

in the first year of life and affects all areas of development so early screening and detection of difficulties can prevent or mitigate later developmental problems. Glasses may ease developmental and motor delays if the problem is detected early. Children who are identified early as having vision problems may be referred to special organizations for help.

Children who are legally blind may be able to see objects if they are close enough. People who are totally blind have no perception of light. Children with cortical blindness have physically functional eyes, but the visual processing part of their brain has been damaged in some way. Less severe vision problems must also be considered during therapy. **Visual perception** is the understanding of what is being seen and is important for eye–hand coordination. Crossed eyes cause double vision because the image seen by each eye does not fuse into one image. A lazy eye (amblyopia) can affect depth perception because only one eye is working at a time. Many of the more minor problems can be improved by performing eye exercises prescribed by a developmental optometrist. Minor problems in vision are identified in 80% of children with reading problems.[35]

The intervention plan for children who have vision impairments depends on the severity of the impairment (Table 13-11). Legally blind children may be able to see quite well with corrective lenses. Legally blind children may have problems with sensory integration, particularly with tactile defensiveness (being extremely sensitive to certain textures) and vestibular processing demonstrating delays in antigravity movement and postural control and often display fear of movement—gravitational insecurity.

The OT practitioner may work with a child to improve postural control, antigravity insecurity, and be more tolerant of movement. To help children who are blind tolerate movement, the practitioner starts with gross motor activities that involve little movement and increase the amount of movement slowly. Many playground toys can be adapted for this purpose by the OT practitioner. Infants and younger children who are blind do not know to reach out for objects in the environment. By tying toys to strollers, chairs, or cribs and guiding infants to feel for objects with their hands, children can be taught to "look" for objects around them. Teaching the children to look for objects in increasingly larger areas enhances this skill (Figure 13-11).

Vision is a learned skill and a child with visual impairment will use any residual vision. The more the child uses the visual pathways, the better the vision becomes. Treating the child in a darkened room with a spotlight on the activity helps him or her see better by reducing other visual distractions.

Children with total blindness often fill the void left by lack of visual stimulation with other forms of sensory self-stimulation called *blindisms*. Blindisms are consistent, repetitive movements that are proportional to the degree of blindness. Blindisms can take the form of body rocking or head shaking, which stimulates the vestibular system, or eye poking, which stimulates the optic nerve. These activities can become socially unacceptable, so more accepted forms of stimulation should be taught to these children.

TABLE 13-11

Suggestions for Working with Children with Vision Impairments

METHOD TO USE	PURPOSE OF THE APPROACH
Use the children's names.	Helps reduce the feeling of isolation; alerts children that they are included in what is going on around them
Explain what is going to occur.	Helps create a relationship as well as helps children understand what is going on
Describe the room.	Helps children associate sounds, smells, and shapes
Walk the children to locations when possible.	Helps children develop space perception
Reduce extra noise.	Helps children identify sound clues
Use touch to introduce new things; brush objects on the back of the hand first.	Helps identify location and function of objects; helps children develop independence; and teaches children that their actions have a cause and effect
Explain new activities and surroundings.	Helps calm children who do not understand a new activity; helps them understand what is going to happen
Talk to the children, not about them.	Prevents underestimating the children's ability to understand what is said to them
Never assume that children with vision impairments see something.	Prevents assuming that children can see you and understand you

Data from Harrell, L. (1984). Touch the baby. Blind and visually impaired children as patients: Helping them respond to care. New York, NY: American Foundation for the Blind.

CLINICAL *Pearl*

It is not unusual for children with cortical blindness to need corrective lenses or glasses because they are nearsighted or farsighted. A developmental optometrist can determine whether glasses would be beneficial.

CLINICAL *Pearl*

All children should have their eyes examined by age 3. A visual-evoked response test that detects brain activity during visual stimulation can be administered to infants who are suspected of having vision problems.

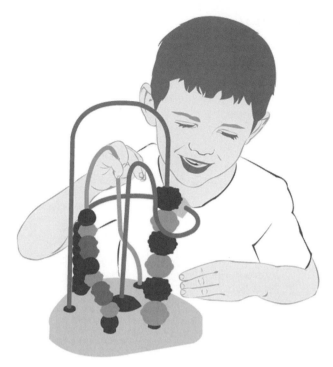

FIGURE 13-11   Child with visual impairment exploring a toy.

Hearing Impairments

The sense of hearing is integral for communication, human interaction, and learning. Hearing difficulties can affect speech and language, literacy, social emotional problems, and learning.[8] About 28 million Americans have hearing loss, and about 2 million are profoundly deaf.[46] Hearing loss can be categorized as conductive (dysfunction in the external or middle ear) or sensorineural (dysfunction in inner ear—cochlea).

Few OT practitioners work with people who are deaf unless those individuals have other disabling conditions. However, individuals with hearing problems also can have vestibular problems in part because of the close linkage of these two systems with the vestibulocochlear nerve. Hearing loss accompanies many developmental problems and can be caused by maternal infection during pregnancy or by medical and environmental effects right after birth. Infections such as cytomegalovirus or meningitis, medications that damage the cochlea, trauma, and excess noise exposure contribute to risk for hearing loss prenatally or in the perinatal period.[8] An undetected hearing loss causes developmental delays. Because a critical period exists for the acquisition of language skills, early detection of a hearing loss is very important.

OT services for individuals with hearing impairments address the related developmental delays. The first 4 years of life are the most important for language development. Impaired language skills affect all other areas of development, including social and environmental interactions and identification of objects. Early detection and treatment of hearing loss are essential for normal development in these areas. Universal hearing screening of all newborns has helped with early identification. A vigilant therapist is aware of and able to identify the signs of hearing loss in children (Box 13-19).[46] Parents often begin to suspect that their infant has a hearing loss when he or she is not awakened by loud noises or does not turn toward a noisy toy. Older infants who do not hear well will not pay attention to simple commands or give feedback to questions. Any infant or child who is suspected of having hearing loss should be referred for hearing testing. This usually includes brainstem auditory-evoked responses, which is a record of brain waves that occur in response to test sounds. Early detection of hearing loss allows for interventions, which may range from early use of hearing aids, to sign language, to cochlear implants. Several methods can be used to communicate with those with hearing impairment. Total communication includes lip reading, use of oral speech, signing, and gestures (Box 13-20).

If the family chooses to use sign language, the OT practitioner can aid this process by using the signs taught in the home and introducing new signs for identifying new objects or activities during therapy. The signs chosen should relate to items or ideas the child understands, such as objects the child can see or touch or actions such as eating and dressing. Constant communication

BOX 13-19

Possible Indications of Hearing Loss in Infants and Children

- Newborn has no startle reflex when hearing a loud noise.
- Three-month-old does not turn his or her head toward toys that make noise.
- Infant stops babbling around 6 months of age.
- Infants between 8 and 12 months do not turn toward sounds coming from behind.
- Two-year-old does not use words.
- Two-year-old does not respond to requests such as "show me the ball."
- Three-year-old's speech is mostly unintelligible.
- Three-year-old skips beginning consonants of words.
- Three-year-old does not use two- or three-word sentences.
- Three-year-old uses mostly vowels.
- Child of any age speaks too loudly or too softly; voice has poor quality.
- Child always sounds like someone with a cold.

Adapted from Russel, E., & Nagiashi, P. (2010). Services for children with visual or hearing impairments. In J. Case-Smith, & J. O'Brien (Eds.), *Occupational therapy for children* (6th ed., pp. 772–774). St. Louis, MO: Mosby.

BOX 13-20

Suggestions for Total Communication

- Face the child at eye level.
- Be directly in front of the child so that your face and hands can be easily seen.
- Get the child's attention.
- Use good overhead lighting.
- Speak in a normal tone of voice.
- Say a word and sign it at the same time.
- Use appropriate pauses.
- Sit close to the child.
- Keep instructions simple.
- Be consistent.
- Talk to the child. Hearing impaired children need to "hear" the same amount of language as an average child.

Adapted from Russel, E., & Nagiashi, P. (2010). Services for children with visual or hearing impairments. In J. Case-Smith, & J. O'Brien (Eds.), *Occupational therapy for children* (6th ed., pp. 772–774). St. Louis: Mosby.

between the OT practitioner and the parents is vital to prevent confusion and to foster language growth in the child and everyone who is working with the child.[46]

Helping a child to accept using a new hearing aid or cochlear implant may be difficult because of tactile defensiveness (a physical and tactile overreaction to objects). The head is often the most sensitive part of a child's body. The younger an infant is when fitted with hearing aids,

the easier the acceptance. The aids must be thought of as clothing—necessary items that are put on each morning. An older child may need to start using new hearing aids during quiet times in speech-related activities. Hearing aids have recently undergone significant changes. Audiologists can now make more precise fittings to accommodate certain types of hearing loss. OT practitioners can screen children for balance and vestibular function.[46] Additionally, sensory processing difficulties should be screened and intervention needs identified.

General Sensory Disorganization

In some conditions, all of the child's sensory systems transmit information poorly, causing the perception of the world to be frightening. Changes in any one of the sensory systems affect development, making it difficult for these children to make sense of gross or fine motor activities or even their surroundings.[6,12] For example, one way that the infant learns about the mother is through the sense of touch; if the perception of touch is not normal, the infant may perceive touch as painful or frightening. If the vestibular system (which detects movement) is not responsive, the infant may be happy only when he or she is moving or when held by someone who is walking. If several sensory systems are not functioning properly, behavior and development can be adversely affected as well as the relationship between infants and their parents or caregivers.[6,12]

Language Delay and Language Impairments

Children develop language problems for many reasons. Children with language difficulties typically understand more (receptive language) than they can talk about (expressive language). Speech is the ultimate of fine motor skills and children may have difficulty with intelligibility. Some children eventually learn to talk, others may learn only a few sentences, and still others may never learn any words at all. Children often are nonverbal because of other developmental problems caused by genetic disorders or because of neurologic conditions such as cerebral palsy. Major language delays seem to occur more often in boys, who often have several areas of sensory processing problems. Children with language delays can develop learning problems later.

OT practitioners model patience with children who do not talk or have trouble understanding speech. Most children use "prelanguage" before they start using speech as a form of communication; they point to an object to indicate that they want it or pull the parent or caregiver, for example, to the cookie jar to indicate they want a cookie. Children who are physically unable to move their limbs may indicate their needs with a smile or a gaze. Language comprehension develops before the child's ability to express himself or herself in words.

Other forms of communication can be used to reduce frustration while verbal skills are developing. Those children with fair or good hand control can learn words in **American Sign Language** to aid in communication. Use of sign language may reduce frustration with children who have limited ways to let their needs be known. Using signs during therapy sessions and at home may be the most convenient way for the child to communicate. The OT practitioner should use signs that have meaning to the child's everyday life. Another alternative for communication is a simple poster board to which are affixed pictures of people and objects commonly encountered in a particular child's everyday life. In the case of young children, green- and red-colored shapes could be substituted for the words "yes" and "no," which are important for indicating choices. A more portable communication system can be created by using a small photo album with a single picture on each page.

CLINICAL *Pearl*

OT practitioners who treat children with language delays often consult with a speech language pathologist regarding use of language during OT intervention. The speech language pathologist may provide ideas such as using gestures, sign language, visual language systems, or simplifying verbal cues to facilitate child understanding of OT treatment ideas. This interprofessional focus helps the child communicate, learn, and achieve developmental goals.

General Interventions

OT interventions for sensory disorders frequently involve the following:

- Analysis of the child's sensory needs and how to regulate his or her behaviors
- Educating family members and caregivers on the child's sensory needs
- Central nervous system strategies to change the child's sensory processing (e.g., calming techniques)

OTHER PEDIATRIC HEALTH CONDITIONS
Burns

Burns are a major cause of a large number of children and adolescents having to undergo prolonged, painful hospitalization. Burns result from accidents involving thermal, electrical, chemical, and radioactive agents.

A thermal burn is caused by hot objects or flames, such as heat from an open fire, an iron, a stove, or the tip of a cigarette. An electrical burn results from skin or other body tissue coming into contact with electricity, such as from lightning or a direct electrical current coming from an outlet or plug. A chemical burn is caused by a chemical substance such as acid or some other poison (i.e., something or some substance that is destructive or

fatal). A radioactive burn is caused by rays or waves of radiation that come into contact with body tissue.

Thermal burns are the most common of the four types.[14] Specific criteria determine the severity and extent of a burn and the prognosis for recovery. The percentage of body area burned is assessed according to the **total body surface area** (TBSA) by the rule of nines in children older than age 10. According to the rule of nines, 9% is assigned to the head and both arms, 18% to each leg, 18% to both the anterior (front) and posterior (back) of the trunk, and 1% to the perineum. The formula is modified for infants and young children because of their proportionately larger head size. (Figure 13-12 presents the percentage of distribution per area of the body.)

The American Burn Association also classifies burns as minor, moderate, and severe.[24] In minor burns, less than 10% of the TBSA is covered with a partial-thickness burn; these burns are adequately treated on an outpatient basis. A moderate burn is considered 10% to 20% of the TBSA covered with a partial-thickness burn; it requires hospitalization. Any full-thickness burn or more than 20% of the TBSA covered with a partial-thickness burn is considered a major burn.[24]

The depth of a burn is assessed according to the number of layers of tissue involved in the injury (Figure 13-13). Superficial or first-degree burns damage tissue minimally and heal without scarring. Second-degree burns are **partial-thickness burns** and involve the epidermis and portions of the dermis. Although second-degree burns will heal, the process can be painful and scarring may be a result. Deep-thickness burns can be third- or fourth-degree (involving muscle) burns and require emergency and ongoing medical intervention. During the **acute medical management** of a child or adolescent who has been seriously burned, the prevention of secondary infections, wound debridement (cleaning), and wound closure are critical along with supporting joint integrity. During the **rehabilitation** phase of intervention, team members work closely to accomplish the outcomes of healing of the body structures involved, correction of cosmetic damage, reduction and management of scar tissue, restoration of function, and reintegration into the child's or adolescent's natural environment (Table 13-12).

OT practitioners working with pediatric and adolescent burn patients begin by providing orthoses to keep the limb immobile, thus optimizing muscle and joint alignment, aiding healing, and later facilitating function. They work closely with physical therapists on debridement and pain management techniques and can help with ways to compensate for physical limitations or regain physical skills. Facilitating play/leisure activities helps children and adolescents with burns recover emotionally and physically and return to their occupations. OT practitioners may address psychological concerns through play, self-concept

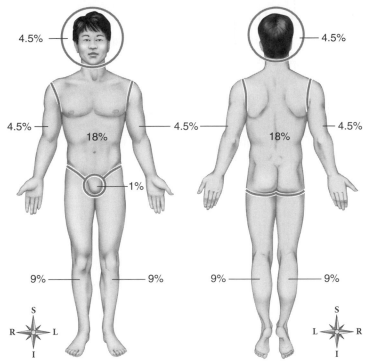

FIGURE 13-12 Estimating body surface area. "Rule of nines." The "rule of nines" is one method used to estimate amount of skin surface burned in an adult. (From Patton, K. T., & Thibodeau, G. A. (2014). *The human body in health & disease* (6th ed.). St. Louis: Mosby.)

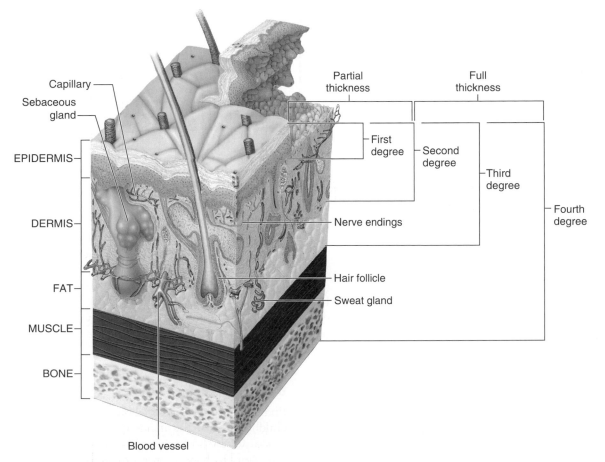

FIGURE 13-13 Classification of burns. Partial-thickness burns include first- and second-degree burns. Full-thickness burns include third-degree burns. Fourth-degree burns involve tissues under the skin, such as muscle or bone. (From Patton, K. T., & Thibodeau, G. A. (2014). *The human body in health & disease* (6th ed.). St. Louis: Mosby.)

TABLE 13-12

Burns: General Intervention Considerations

CONSIDERATION	DEFINITION AND EXAMPLE(S)
Positioning and orthotics	Orthoses in functional position to initially aid in healing and later orthoses to increase function.
ROM	Use passive and active ROM techniques to promote full AROM and PROM.
Engagement in occupations	Provide remediation, adaptation, and modification so that the child may participate in occupations.
Social participation	Help the child return to social situations.
Scar tissue management	Use orthoses, desensitization techniques, and pressure garments to decrease scarring.
Edema management	Use retrograde massage, gentle ranging, and elevation to manage edema.
Self-concept	Help the child participate in occupations to develop positive self-concept.
Psychological/emotional issues	Provide a range of activities to help the child work through emotional difficulties associated with burns. Children with burns may have issues with body image.

AROM, Active range of motion; *PROM,* passive range of motion; *ROM,* range of motion.

activities, and discussion and help children and adolescents with burns learn, through participating in everyday occupations, how they may function in the aftermath of the burns.

NEOPLASTIC DISORDERS

A neoplasm is an abnormal new growth of tissue (a tumor). It may be localized (in one place) or invasive (in multiple tissues and organs). It may be benign (not immediately life threatening) or malignant (possibly cause death). Tumors are named for location, type of cellular makeup, or the person who first identified it.[4]

Leukemia

Leukemia comprises a group of pediatric health conditions involving various acute and chronic tumor disorders of the bone marrow. A child or adolescent with

BOX 13-21

Neoplastic Disorders: General Signs and Symptoms

- Weight loss
- Night sweats
- Chronic fatigue
- Recurrent headaches
- Vomiting
- Behavior changes
- Pain
- Lumps
- Misalignment of bones or joints
- Evident growths on bone

leukemia may experience an abnormal increase in white blood cells; enlargement of the lymph nodes, liver, and spleen; and impaired blood clotting. These body function deficits can cause pain, fatigue, weight loss, recurrent infections, excessive bruising, and/or hemorrhaging (Box 13-21). Medical interventions may include treatment with antibiotics, chemotherapy, and blood transfusion. Referral to an occupational therapist is made because of secondary disorders and/or complications. Focus of treatment includes strength and endurance activities as the child may be debilitated by the disease process, hospitalization, and effects of some of the medications.

Tumors of the Central Nervous System

Tumors of the CNS (i.e., those located in the brain and/or spinal cord) are the most common solid tissue tumors in children and adolescents.[9] The causes of central nervous system tumors are unknown. Medical interventions vary with differential diagnoses. Depending on the location of the tumor in the brain, the child may have difficulty with motor control, sensory responses, and overall function because of impingement of the tumor on vital brain centers. Additionally, the tumor may be surgically removed and OT practitioners can assist in the acute and ongoing rehabilitation following brain surgery. As with any injury to the brain, the OT practitioner should intervene if the child presents with tone concerns, postural control, motor relearning, sensory processing, and cognitive functioning.

Bone Cancer and Tumors

Primary (first to develop) bone tumors are rare during childhood, with the incidence peaking during adolescence. Often bone cancer results from metastasis, or spreading, to bone from a primary tumor(s) located in a different body structure. Medical interventions may

TABLE 13-13

Neoplastic Conditions: General Intervention Considerations

CONSIDERATION	DEFINITION AND EXAMPLE(S)
Energy conservation	Children with neoplastic conditions may benefit from learning ways to perform occupations with less physical stress. For example, sitting down while getting ready for school conserves energy.
Compensation techniques	Children may experience physical symptoms and require strategies to perform everyday tasks (e.g., using the left hand instead of the right for eating).
Psychosocial/emotional issues	Children may miss school and feel "left out." They may experience the full range of emotions and stress of a life-threatening illness. Families may be in turmoil over the illness. These children may feel alone and require intervention to help them deal with the illness so that they may engage in their occupations.
Adaptive equipment	Adaptive equipment may be recommended to assist these children in their occupations. For example, positioning young children on a bath seat may make bath time easier for the caregiver.
Engagement in occupations	Children may feel "left out" of regular activities and require participation in occupations to regain a sense of being. OT practitioners can help the children return to school, home, and play activities through education, assistive technology, and compensation techniques.

include surgery, radiation therapy, or chemotherapy. Children with neoplastic disorders may require OT interventions to help the child catch up with schoolwork after missing a number of days due to surgery or other medical interventions (Table 13-13). Children with bone tumors may experience physical symptoms including weakness, difficulty with alignment, and pain from the tumor. OT interventions focus on rehabilitation, strengthening, and compensatory strategies, particularly if the child undergoes a surgical amputation. OT practitioners may address the emotional needs of the children and their families by acknowledging stressors, incorporating play activities, and helping the child gain a sense of control in the medical setting.

IMMUNOLOGIC CONDITIONS

The immune system depends on the interaction of many organ systems in response to inflammations or infection. Immunologic conditions affect the immune system and interfere with the ability of the body to fight viruses.

Human Immunodeficiency Virus

Human immunodeficiency virus (HIV) causes the immune system to shut down, which results in many different problems as early as the first 1 or 2 years of life. Early symptoms may be failure to thrive (FTT), fever, and diarrhea. Half of all HIV-infected infants develop full-blown AIDS by the age of 3.[34] A woman infected with HIV can pass the virus on to her infant during pregnancy, delivery, or while breast-feeding. Infants born to women who are infected before or during pregnancy and who receive no medical treatment have about a 25% chance of being born with the HIV infection. Medical treatment with zidovudine (AZT) during pregnancy and

BOX 13-22

Precautions for Working with Children

- Wear gloves when coming into contact with blood or secretions.
- Mix 1 oz of bleach with 10 oz of water, and use this solution to disinfect surfaces.
- Dress all cuts and sores.
- Wash your hands and/or body parts immediately after contact with blood.
- Use sharp instruments only when necessary.

Adapted from the Centers for Disease Control. http://www.cdc.gov/mmwr/preview/mmwrhtml/rr5811a1.htm..

labor may reduce the risk for infant infection to about 1 in 12. Mothers with HIV infection may pass the virus through breast-feeding. Treating infants with AZT for the first several weeks of life can reduce but not prevent the risk for infection.[34]

Children with AIDS may have delayed motor or cognitive development. They may not meet developmental milestones or attain certain intellectual skills and may develop microencephaly.[34] The loss of social skills and language occurs in about 20% of children with AIDS. Paralysis, tremors, spasticity, and balance problems can also develop, and major organ systems are damaged. Half of the infants born with AIDS develop pneumonia by 15 months, a common cause of death.[4] Children with AIDS-related complex have HIV infection and some symptoms but no serious infections.[4] In the United States, 2% of all individuals with AIDS are children or adolescents. In 90% of pediatric AIDS cases, children have been infected at birth by receiving the virus from their mothers (Boxes 13-22 and 13-23).[9]

BOX 13-23

Transmission of HIV

HIV does not survive well in the environment. Simply drying a surface contaminated with HIV kills 90% to 99% of the virus. HIV exists in different concentrations in the blood, semen, vaginal fluid, breast milk, saliva, and tears. Infection occurs when blood or body secretions that could contain visible blood, such as urine, vomit, or feces, come into contact with an open wound or mucous membranes, which are found inside the mouth, nose, eyes, vagina, and rectum. The concentration of the virus in saliva, sweat, and tears is low, and no case of HIV infection through these fluids has been documented.

Adapted from the Centers for Disease Control. http://www.cdc.gov/mmwr/preview/mmwrhtml/rr5811a1.htm.

CLINICAL *Pearl*

Monitoring for developmental delays is one of the main goals of occupational therapy for children with AIDS. Because their mothers may be ill as well, the OT practitioner coordinates care for the mothers and their children.

ENVIRONMENTALLY INDUCED AND ACQUIRED CONDITIONS

Environmentally induced and acquired conditions can develop before or after birth and are directly related to factors found in the environment. Contributing factors include drugs, toxic chemicals, allergens, and viruses.

Latex Allergy

Between 18% and 40% of children with spina bifida or frequent surgeries and those who use catheters for congenital urinary tract problems are likely to develop sensitivity to latex.[43] However, anyone who has frequent exposure to latex through work or surgery can develop an allergy. A reaction can occur after breathing latex dust from an open package or contact between latex and skin, mucous membranes, open lesions, or blood. Coming into contact with a person or object that has just been in contact with latex can cause a reaction. Symptoms include watery eyes, wheezing, hives, rash, and swelling. Severe reactions can result in anaphylaxis, a system-wide body reaction that affects heart rate and the ability to breathe, which can be fatal.[43]

More children are developing allergies to latex since the institution of **universal precautions**, which require the use of latex gloves to prevent the spread of infection; latex is also used in many health care products, such

BOX 13-24

Most Common Foods Associated with Allergies

- Wheat
- Soy
- Corn
- Eggs
- Peanuts
- Milk
- Citrus items
- Tree nuts
- Shellfish

Adapted from University of Maryland Medicine. http://www.umm.edu/pediatric-info/food.htm.

as tapes, bottle nipples, and catheters. Exposure to latex increases the chance for an allergy.

OT practitioners can avoid using latex in the clinic by substituting Mylar balloons for latex balloons and by wearing vinyl gloves instead of latex gloves. OT practitioners and parents should check the labels of tapes or any other substances that may contain rubber products. The OT practitioner should caution parents and caregivers about possible allergies and educate parents on the symptoms of allergies.

CLINICAL *Pearl*

Children who are allergic to latex also may be allergic to bananas, avocados, and kiwi fruit because they are all from the same plant family. Being around latex and consuming any of these fruits may heighten the reaction.

Allergies to Foods and Chemicals

The use of art supplies, construction materials, and various foods during pediatric occupational therapy should be carefully assessed so that children's developing bodies are not unnecessarily exposed to toxic chemicals, toxic materials, and allergy-producing foods. OT practitioners should always check with parents or guardians about their children's food allergies before any food item is used for an art project or feeding therapy (Box 13-24). Many children have gluten intolerance and peanut allergies so OT practitioners need to adhere to careful practice with food preparation.

Toxic chemical fumes or materials may cause asthma, skin irritation, anaphylaxis, or other unseen damage that can accumulate over time.[2,7] OT practitioners should always ensure that the materials used in therapy are nontoxic. They should avoid using latex products when a substitute is available.

BOX 13-25

Signs of Failure to Grow

- Weight persistently <3% on growth charts
- Weight <80% of ideal for height and age
- Progressive loss of weight to below third percentile
- Decrease in expected growth rate compared with previous pattern
- Decreased speed of growth
- Crossing three channels on the growth chart.

Data from Berkow, R. (Ed.). (1999). *The Merck manual* (17th ed.). Rahway, NJ: Merck.

Failure to Grow

CASE *Study*

Josie is a 15-month-old toddler diagnosed with feeding and growth concerns and referred to an interdisciplinary feeding team. In reviewing her history, Josie was born slightly prematurely at 36 weeks and had slow growth in utero. Her birth weight was 4 pounds 6 ounces. Her mother struggled with breast-feeding and eventually transitioned to bottle-feeding when Josie was 2 months old. Josie had difficulty tolerating formula and frequently vomited after feeding. She had difficulty transitioning to spoon foods. During the evaluation, Josie's mother described stressors around feeding. Doctors emphasized the importance of weight gain and talked about a gastrostomy. Josie refuses spoon foods and gags easily. She uses primarily sucking motions with food in her mouth and does not chew food. Family members are pressuring Josie's mother to wean her from the bottle.

Failure to grow (also referred to as failure to thrive [FTT]) can be a symptom of another acute or chronic condition or can be a condition in itself. Children who have difficulty getting adequate nutrition typically falter in weight gain initially, then slowed linear growth (length), and finally head circumference with prolonged poor nutrition. Weight gain is the most accurate indicator of an infant's nutritional status (Box 13-25).[11]

Infants can have growth problems for a variety of reasons, both medical and psychosocial.[11] Medical and physical problems care categorized as organic FTT and psychosocial causes of growth problems are referred to as nonorganic FTT. An infant may have medical issues such as gastrointestinal problems including reflux (gastroesophageal reflux disease), pyloric stenosis, short gut, respiratory problems such as cystic fibrosis, neurologic difficulties affecting oral motor efficiency, or congenital heart defects. Psychosocial causes may include limited financial resources, neglect, parental stressors or medical problems such as maternal depression, difficulty with reading infant cues of hunger, or excessively passive babies who do not cue parents to feed them.

Children with failure to grow present with feeding issues such as poor suck–swallow–breathe synchrony, tactile sensitivity, delayed oral–motor skills, and decreased variety of foods and textures in their diets. OT practitioners provide evaluation and interventions in these areas. An important aspect of the treatment of failure to grow includes parental or caregiver training on feeding issues. Children who need to gain weight may require frequent high-calorie snacks throughout the day. Therefore, consultation with a dietitian is warranted. Children with failure to grow may require interventions aimed at improving sensory processing with feeding with careful review of food textures, efficiency of feeding, and positive mealtime experiences. Occupational therapists work closely with families and caregivers to help children with failure to grow, providing support in a sensitive parenting area.

CASE *Study (continued)*

Although Josie has sensory and behavioral concerns with feeding with restricted food intake, the first focus of therapy is on encouraging optimal food intake. Liquids and soft spoon foods have more calories. The OT practitioner can focus on positive mealtime experiences and encourage increased food intake. The OT practitioner can encourage skill development of chewing during one snack a day until Josie has better nutritional status. Dietitians and OT practitioners can work closely with children with feeding and growth concerns and their parents to ensure optimal growth and positive feeding experiences.

Fetal Alcohol Syndrome Disorders

The use of alcohol during pregnancy is the most common cause of birth defects. Fetal alcohol syndrome (FAS) occurs in 2 to 6 births out of 1000.[8,9] Children may not have all the markers of FAS yet still have milder sequelae. This group is said to have alcohol-related neurodevelopmental disorder.[8] The infants of chronic drinkers are the most severely affected. Alcohol consumption during pregnancy causes intellectual disability, microencephaly, small facial features, low body weight, poor development of the corpus callosum, and heart defects. Characteristic facial features include a turned-up nose and small jaws, thin upper lip and absent philtrum, and close set, smaller eyes. Infants with FAS may also experience failure to thrive and be fussy (Figure 13-14). Children with FAS are frequently hypotonic, have poor coordination, and may have sensory processing difficulties.[9] Infants or children with alcohol-related neurodevelopmental

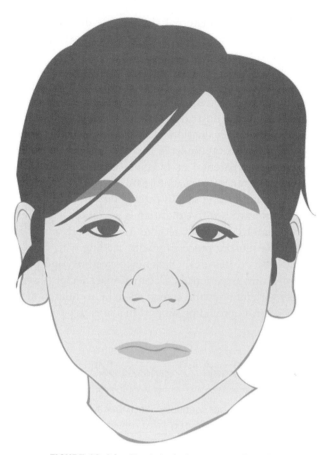

FIGURE 13-14   Fetal alcohol spectrum disorder.

disorder may be referred for OT treatment for hyperactivity caused by a sensory processing disorder. As they age, the children may develop learning problems. Children with FAS or alcohol-related neurodevelopmental disorder usually have difficulty with executive function and this becomes more problematic once in school and in adolescence when greater cognitive function is expected. They present with poor memory, reasoning, and judgment skills. Children with FAS have difficulty sequencing tasks such as bathing and dressing, often have difficulty with attention and distractibility, and require supervision with IADLs.

Prenatal Drug Exposure

Infants with prenatal drug exposure have risks for development problems. Knowledge of how the drug affects the infant's brain during the fetal period is essential in understanding how the drug can affect development. Family support, maternal sensitivity, and home environment have a big effect on a baby's development and can mitigate risk factors. Long-term studies are difficult to perform with these populations. Often mothers take more than one drug during pregnancy, may not report drugs taken, and can have multiple social and psychological risk factors.

Environmental factors associated with substance abuse may supersede the biological effects of the substance.[33]

Infants are exposed to narcotics in utero when mothers take anything from prescription pain medications to methadone to morphine to heroin. Infants with narcotic exposure undergo the difficult process of withdrawal in the newborn period. They are at a slight increased risk for sudden infant death syndrome. Longer-term studies indicate that development can be within normal ranges when the child is in a nurturing environment.

Cocaine acts as a stimulant and causes vasoconstriction of the blood vessels. As a result, infants exposed to cocaine in utero are at risk for growth restriction with limited oxygen and nutrients, smaller brain volume, and strokes. Long-term studies show conflicting results. Some studies indicate that prenatal cocaine exposure is correlated with developmental delays, adverse social-emotional interactions, and difficulty with school performance. Other studies show the child can develop more typically depending on family and social factors.

Children exposed to marijuana in utero are at risk for cognitive and social concerns including hyperactivity, impulsivity, inattention symptoms, and externalization. One study indicated marijuana exposure in utero is correlated with memory deficits.

Methamphetamine works similarly to cocaine and infants are at risk for growth problems. It also affects neurotransmitters and dopamine receptors. Researchers have also identified changes in brain structures deep in the brain (hippocampus, putamen, globus pallidus; see Chapters 11 and 12). Methamphetamine exposure in utero has been correlated with regulatory and sensory concerns in infants, lower IQ in preschool children, and difficulty with peer interactions in grade school-aged children. A recent study showed that children with methamphetamine exposure have difficulty with school performance and cognition during school years but did not display problems with ADHD as reported by previous studies.[18]

Maternal tobacco use has been correlated with smaller infant size and some irritability associated with nicotine withdrawal in the newborn period. Children with prenatal tobacco exposure are at more risk for respiratory infections and asthma.

Lead Poisoning

It is estimated that about 4 million children in the United States have high enough lead levels that their development will be slowed.[22] Although many environmental toxins exist, lead is the one that most commonly affects children. Children living in older homes have a greater risk for exposure to lead in peeling paint (which children sometimes eat) and to lead used in plumbing. Lead is no longer used in these materials; however, children can eat or breathe lead from contaminated air, food, water, and soil as well. Some industries, such as battery manufacturing, produce higher air and dust levels of lead than do others. Parents working in these industries can carry lead home on their clothing. Mothers with high lead levels can pass it to their infants during gestation. Mild lead toxicity produces muscle aches and fatigue, and moderate levels cause fatigue, headaches, cramping, vomiting, and weight loss. High toxicity levels in infants causes intellectual disability, behavior problems, seizures, and sometimes death. Even low toxicity levels can affect intelligence and behavior.[3,8,9]

SUMMARY

This chapter presented an introduction to various pediatric health conditions. The author provided descriptions of the general signs and symptoms and general intervention considerations for a variety of conditions. Working with children can be a rewarding experience for OT practitioners. OT practitioners must not only meet the needs of their clients, but they must also educate their clients' families and caregivers and work as part of an interprofessional team. Knowing the common characteristics of children's health conditions allows OT practitioners to complete a thorough initial assessment and intervention plan. Although conditions have some common characteristics, the needs of each child and his or her family are unique.

References

1. Alexander, R. C., & Smith, W. L. (1998). Shaken baby syndrome. *Infants Young Child, 10,* 1–9.
2. American Lung Association. (2014). *Asthma and children fact sheet.* http://www.lung.org/lung-disease/asthma/resources/facts-and-figures/asthma-children-fact-sheet.html.
3. American Psychiatric Association. (2013). *Diagnostic and statistical manual of mental disorders* (5th ed.). Washington DC: American Psychiatric Publishing.
4. Anderson, D. M. (2002). *Mosby's medical, nursing, and allied health dictionary* (6th ed.). St. Louis, MO: Mosby.
5. Arthritis Foundation. *Juvenile arthritis.* http://www.kidsgetarthritistoo.org/about-ja/the-basics/.
6. Ayres, A. J. (1972). *Sensory integration and learning disorders.* Los Angeles: Western Psychological Services.
7. Barnhart, S. L., & Czervinche, M. P. (1995). *Perinatal and pediatric respiratory care.* Philadelphia: Saunders.
8. Batshaw, M., Roizen, N. J., & Lotrecchiano, G. R. (Eds.). (2013). *Children with disabilities* (7th ed.). Baltimore: Brookes.
9. Blackman, J., MacQueen, J. C., & Biehl, R. I. (Eds.). (1997). *Mosby's resource guide to children with disabilities and chronic illness.* St Louis, MO: Mosby.
10. Boyd, S. A. (2014). *Arthrogryposis multiplex congenita.* http://www.merckmanuals.com/professional/pediatrics/congenital_craniofacial_and_musculoskeletal_abnormalities/arthrogryposis_multiplex_congenita.html.
11. Bruns, D., & Thompson, S. D. (2013). *Feeding challenges in young children.* Baltimore: Brookes Publishing.
12. Bundy, A., Lane, S., & Murray, E. (2008). *Sensory integration: theory and practice* (3rd ed.). Philadelphia: FA Davis.
13. Case-Smith, J. (2004). Parenting a child with a chronic medical condition. *Am J Occup Ther, 58,* 551–560.
14. Case-Smith, J., & O'Brien, J. (2015). *Occupational therapy for children and adolescents* (7th ed.). St Louis, MO: Mosby.
15. Centers for Disease Control and Prevention. (2014). *About autism spectrum disorder.* http://www.cdc.gov/ncbddd/autism/facts.html.
16. Clarke, N. M. P. (2014). Swaddling and hip dysplasia: an orthopaedic perspective. *Arch Dis Child, 99,* 5–6.
17. Conner, K. A., McKenzie, L. B., Xiang, H., & Smith, G. A. (2010). Pediatric traumatic amputations and hospital resource utilization in the United States. *J Trauma, 68,* 131–137.
18. Diaz, S. D., Smith, L. M., LaGasse, L. L., Derauf, C., Newman, E., Shah, R., et al. (2014). Effects of prenatal methamphetamine exposure on behavioral and cognitive findings at 7.5 years of age. *J Pediatr, 164,* 1333–1338.
19. Fox, A. M., & Lent, B. (1996). Clumsy children: primer on developmental coordination disorder. *Can Fam Physician, 42,* 1965–1971.
20. Fragile-X National Foundation. (nd). Fragile X. http://www.fragilex.org/.
21. Gould, B. E. (2006). *Pathophysiology for health professions* (3rd ed.). Philadelphia: Saunders Elsevier.
22. Haan, M. N., Gerson, M., & Zishka, B. A. (1996). Identification of children at risk for lead poisoning: an evaluation of routine pediatric blood lead screening in an HMO-insured population. *Am Acad Pediatr, 97,* 84.
23. Hibbard, R., Desch, L. W., and the Committee on Child Abuse & Neglect and Council on Children with Disabilities. (2007). Maltreatment of children with disabilities. *Pediatr, 119,* 1018.
24. Kagan, R. J., Pack, M. D., Ahrenholz, D. H., Hickerson, W. L., Holmes, J., 4th, Korentager, R., et al. (2013). Surgical management of burn wound and use of skin substitutes: an expert panel white paper. *J Burn Care Res, 34,* e60–e79.
25. Kang, P. B. (2013). Muscles, bones and nerves. In M. L. Batshaw, N. J. Roizen, & G. R. Lotrecchiano (Eds.), *Children with disabilities* (7th ed.). Baltimore: Brookes.
26. Klein, S., & Magill-Evans, J. (1998). Perceptions of competence and peer acceptance in young children with motor and learning difficulties. *Phys Occup Ther Pediatr, 18,* 39–52.
27. Korkmaz, M., Erbahçeci, F., Ulger, O., & Topuz, S. (2012). Evaluation of functionality in acquired and congenital upper extremity child amputees. *Acta Orthop Traumatol Turc, 46*(4), 262–268.
28. Lorenzo, R. F., & Metz, A. E. (2013). Occupational therapy practitioners' knowledge and perceptions of childhood asthma and cystic fibrosis. *Occupational Therapy in Health Care, 27*(3), 256–270.
29. Losse, A., et al. (1991). Clumsiness in children—do they grow out of it? A 10-year follow-up study. *Dev Med Child Neurol, 33,* 55.
30. Reference deleted in proofs.
31. Reference deleted in proofs.

32. Missiuna, C., & Polatjko, H. J. (1995). Developmental dyspraxia by any other name. *Am J Occup Ther*, *49*, 619.

33. National Abandoned Infants Assistance Resource Center. (April, 2008). *Fact Sheet: Prenatal Substance Exposure*. UC Berkeley. Retrieved from http://aia.berkeley.edu/media/pdf/2008_perinatal_se.pdf.

34. National Institute of Allergy and Infectious Diseases. (2000). *Backgrounder: HIV infection in infants and children*. Retrieved June 16, 2015 from http://aidsinfo.nih.gov/news/507/backgrounder—hiv-infection-in-infants-and-children.

35. Optometrists Network: What is vision therapy? Retrieved June 16, 2015 from: http://www.children-special-needs.org/vision_therapy/what_is_vision_therapy.html.

36. Parks, S., Sugerman, D., Xu, L., & Coronado, V. (2012). Characteristics of non-fatal abusive head trauma among children in the USA, 2003–2008: application of the CDC operational case definition to national hospital inpatient data. *Inj Prev*, *18*(6), 392–398.

37. Peterson, J. (2012). The prosthetic habilitation of a congenital, transradial limb deficient child: a Case Study analyzing the functional effectiveness and the benefits of early prosthetic fitting, appropriate prosthetic equipment, and consistent caregiver follow up. *ACPOC News*, *18*(2), 17–24.

38. Reference deleted in proofs.

39. Pierpont, M., Basson, C. T., Benson, D. W., Jr., Gelb, B. D., Giglia, T. M., Goldmuntz, E., et al. (2007). Genetic basis for congenital heart defects: current knowledge: a scientific statement from the American Heart Association Congenital Cardiac Defects Committee, Council on Cardiovascular Disease in the Young; endorsed by the American Academy of Pediatrics. *Circulation*, *115*(23), 3015–3038.

40. Prader-Willi Syndrome Association. What is Prader-Willi syndrome? www.pwsausa.org.

41. Pronsati, M. P. (1991). Erb's palsy. *Adv Occup Ther*, *7*, 19.

42. Roizen, N. (2013). Down syndrome (Trisomy 21). In M. L. Batshaw, N. J. Roizen, & G. R. Lotrecchiano (Eds.), *Children with disabilities* (7th ed.). Baltimore: Brookes.

43. Romanczuk, A. (1993). Latex use with infants and children: it can cause problems. *Matern Child Nurs*, *18*, 208.

44. Salter, R. B., & Dudos, J. P. (1974). The first fifteen years' experience with innominate osteotomy in the treatment of developmental hip dysplasia and subluxation of the hip. *Clin Orthop*, *98*, 72.

45. Schoemaker, M. M., & Kalverboer, A. F. (1994). Social and affective problems of children who are clumsy: how early do they begin? *Adapt Phys Activ Q*, *11*, 130.

45a. Shriners Hospitals for Children: Arthrogryposis. Available at: http://www.shrinershq.org/sitecore/content/Hospitals/LosAngeles/Services/Arthrogryposis.aspx?sc_database?master.

46. Stancliff, B. (1998). Silent services: treating deaf clients. *OT Practice*, *3*, 27.

47. Trovato, M. K., & Schultz, S. C. (2013). Traumatic brain injury. In M. L. Batshaw, N. J. Roizen, & G. R. Lotrecchiano (Eds.), *Children with disabilities* (7th ed.). Baltimore: Brookes.

48. Wiener, A. S., Long, T., DeGangi, G., & Battaile, B. (1996). Sensory processing of infants born prematurely or with regulatory disorders. *Phys Occup Ther Pediatr*, *16*(4), 1–17.

49. Williams, H. G., Woolacott, M. H., & Ivry, R. (1992). Timing and motor control in clumsy children. *J Mot Behav*, *24*, 165.

REVIEW *Questions*

1. Provide an overview of the signs and symptoms of a variety of pediatric health conditions. What are some general intervention strategies associated with specific conditions?

2. What are the three types of juvenile rheumatoid arthritis? Describe them. What functional limitations does each type cause?

3. Name the four spinal conditions discussed in this chapter. How does each affect the functional performance of the child?

4. Describe the reason an OTA must have a good understanding of the symptoms and signs of a child's condition before performing the initial assessment. How does this aid in treatment?

5. Describe two genetic syndromes. Explain the ways they affect a child's ADL skills.

6. Using information you have learned about sensory systems, explain why it is important to treat sensory system problems early.

7. What are the differences between legal, total, and cortical blindness? How are they the same? How can you make learning easier for a child with vision impairments?

8. How does an undetected hearing loss affect a child's early development?

9. Name three avoidable environmental factors that affect infants either before or after birth. How do these factors cause developmental delays?

10. Describe arthrogryposis. How can it affect a child's daily functioning?

11. What are the four types of burns? Define each, and identify the most common.

12. Describe intervention strategies used for children with various pediatric conditions.

SUGGESTED *Activities*

1. Visit a class of children with special needs and observe them at work. During your visit observe and keep a list of how each child's condition affects his or her ability to do schoolwork. Later, make a list of suggestions you think might improve each child's ability to do schoolwork.

2. Spend some time at an outpatient clinic observing children who are receiving OT services. Make a list of characteristics observed in individual children. Later, try to identify each child's possible condition or which of the systems is/are involved.

3. Spend some time observing a child with a disability at play. Write down ways that the child's condition affects his or her ability to play.

4. Talk with family members of a child with a disability. Before the interview, use the knowledge you have gained from this chapter to make a list of how you would expect the child's disability to affect the family. During the interview, make notes about the family's comments. Later, compare your initial list with the family's comments. How accurate were your expectations?

5. Interview a firefighter to consider the different types of fires, burns, and client factors in the persons he or she has rescued.

6. Interview a family member of a child with a diagnosis presented in this chapter. Develop a handout on the particular diagnosis for the child's siblings.

7. Using the tables as your guide, develop activities related to each type of pediatric condition described in this chapter.

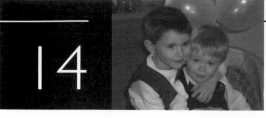

KERRYELLEN G. VROMAN
JANE CLIFFORD O'BRIEN
JEAN WELCH SOLOMON

Childhood and Adolescent Psychosocial and Mental Health Disorders

CHAPTER *Objectives*

After studying this chapter, the reader will be able to accomplish the following:

- Define psychosocial occupational therapy practice for children and adolescents.
- Recognize the signs and symptoms of behavioral and mental health disorders seen in children and adolescents.
- Have knowledge as to how the occupational therapy assistant assists the occupational therapist in the evaluation process.
- Recognize assessments used by the occupational therapy practitioner to develop intervention.
- Use evaluation results to guide psychosocial and mental health practice.
- Be familiar with the frames of reference that direct intervention in psychosocial and mental health practice.
- Select activities that support evidence-based practice.
- Be familiar with the types of occupational therapy group interventions used with children and adolescents who have psychosocial and mental health disorders.

CHAPTER *Outline*

Occupational therapy (OT) practitioners employed in pediatric settings (e.g., early intervention programs, rehabilitation programs, and school systems) provide **psychosocial occupational therapy** to address children's mental health as physical and emotional well-being support occupational participation. Performance problems associated with psychosocial and mental health disorders include regulating and controlling behaviors, interacting and collaborating with other children, forming and maintaining friendships, relating to and taking directions from adults, and attending to tasks.[9] Children diagnosed with mental health disorders may also have difficulties regulating their emotions, organizing their thoughts, and demonstrating appropriate behaviors.

This chapter provides a description of psychosocial and mental health disorders with associated behavioral problems that present in childhood and adolescence consistent with the diagnostic criteria of the Diagnostic and Statistical Manual of Mental Disorders (DSM-V).[3] Understanding the physical, mental, and behavioral signs and symptoms associated with each disorder may help OT practitioners design effective interventions. We outline frames of references that guide individual and group OT interventions. Case examples and intervention strategies are provided throughout. In addition, topics such as bullying and suicide risk are discussed.

UNDERSTANDING PSYCHOSOCIAL AND MENTAL HEALTH DISORDERS

One of every five children has a mental health problem or disorder that is likely to disrupt his or her ability to perform age-related activities (Box 14-1). These disorders include major depression, bipolar disorder, anxiety disorders, disruptive behavioral disorders, and schizophrenia spectrum. In adolescence, the risk for mental health disorders increases significantly; eating disorders, aggressive and antisocial behaviors, and substance abuse are more prevalent than they are in younger children.[26] Effective treatment for mental health problems in childhood and adolescence is crucial because these disorders as well as behavioral problems disrupt learning and social development, which, in turn, can have an effect on adult functioning.[4,14,16,20] For example, disorders that develop in adolescence are associated with poorer occupational performance and adaptation in adulthood.

Multidisciplinary pediatric services for children and adolescents with mental health and psychoemotional and behavioral problems are provided in a variety of settings, including psychiatric units in acute care hospitals, independent psychiatric hospitals, day treatment centers, and community mental health centers. Public schools provide psychiatric and mental health services as well. Furthermore, some community activities benefit children with mental health needs (i.e., teen support groups). Many adolescents with mental health problems are also under the care of services such as the social welfare department or juvenile justice system and may live in a residential facility, group home, or foster care home.

In children and adolescents, mental health disorders often present as behavioral problems and/or as difficulty performing everyday activities. They are the result of the interaction of biological, sociocultural,

BOX 14-1

Quick Facts About Child and Adolescent Mental Health

- In the United States, one in five children has a diagnosable mental, emotional, or behavioral disorder (SAMHSA, 2009). However, 70% of children do not receive mental health services.
- Children and teens with a chronic illness, endure abuse or neglect, or experience other trauma have an increased risk for depression (NIMH, 2000).
- ADHD is one of the most common mental disorders in children. About 2 million children in the United States have been diagnosed with this disorder (NIMH, 2009).
- Autism and related disorders develop in childhood and affect an estimated 3.4 per 1000 children in the United States (NIMH, 2001). It is four times more common in boys (NIMH, 2008). Girls tend to present with more severe symptoms and have greater cognitive impairments (NIMH, 2008).
- It is estimated that 1 in every 33 children and 1 in 8 adolescents may have depression (Center for Mental Health Services, 1998). This is between 10% and 15% of all children and teenagers in the United States (SAMHSA, 2009).
- Depression is more common in teenage girls than boys (NIMH, 2001). Children with a parent who has depression are at an increased risk (SAMHSA, 2009).

- Approximately 750,000 children in the United States have bipolar disorder. If not treated, bipolar disorder puts children at an increased risk for drug abuse, school failure, and suicide (SAMHSA, 2010).
- Anxiety disorders are the most common mental, behavioral, and emotional conditions to affect children and adolescents. Approximately 13 of every 100 children aged 9 to 17 years in the United States have some form of anxiety disorder (SAMHSA, 2010).
- About 50% of children and teens with an anxiety disorder have a comorbid second anxiety or a mental or behavioral disorder, often depression (SAMHSA, 2010).
- Throughout the average life span, about 0.5% to 3.7% of females in the United States will develop anorexia and around 1.1% to 4.2% bulimia. Females are more at risk for developing an eating disorder than are males, but binge-eating disorders are more common in males (NIMH, 2010).
- Suicide is the third leading cause of death for 15- to 24-year-olds and the sixth leading cause of death for 10- to 14-year-olds in the United States.[1]
- Approximately 20% of the youths in juvenile justice facilities in the United States have a serious emotional disturbance, and most have a diagnosable mental disorder. An additional 30% of the youths in these facilities have substance abuse disorders or concurrent substance abuse disorders (OJJDP, 2000).

Data from the National Mental Health Association 2009-2010: www.nmha.org/infoctr/factsheets; National Institute for Mental Health: www.nimh.nih.gov/publicat/numvbers.cfm, or http://www.nimh.nih.gov/health/publications/the-numbers-count-mental-disorders-in-america/; United States Department of Health and Human Services: Substance Abuse and Mental Health Services Administration 2007-2009: http://mentalhealth.samhsa.gov/, Surgeon General's Report on Mental Health, 1999, Office of Juvenile Justice and Delinquency Prevention, [OJJDP] 2000.

psychological, and social factors (Figure 14-1). Family history of mental illness, or sexual, physical, or emotional abuse or stresses associated with lower socioeconomic circumstances such as poverty or parental unemployment increase the risk for mental illness. Box 14-2 provides warning signs that suggest possible sexual abuse. OT practitioners pay attention to these signs and report any observations. A biological predisposition or genetic component may make a child vulnerable to a mental health disorder, but the child will only develop a disorder when other factors are also present. Therefore an integrative model that considers biological, behavioral, psychological, and sociocultural dimensions is typically used to understand each child's mental health disorder.[30]

The biological dimension includes genetics, and the structures and functions of the brain such as the role of neurotransmitters, sensory processing, and the endocrine system (refer to Chapters 12 and 13). Some disorders have explicit genetic causes that are present at birth. These conditions often are those with multiple

symptoms, including intellectual disabilities. Other disorders have genetic or biological origins that are less clearly identified (e.g., depression, anxiety disorders, and autism spectrum disorders). The psychological dimensions encompass cognitive, emotional, and personality factors, namely, characteristics of personality, learning abilities, emotional arousal, coping abilities, self-concept, and self-esteem. The social dimension includes relationships of family, friends, and other significant adults (such as teachers and extended family), whereas the sociocultural dimension encompasses such factors as gender orientation (see Chapter 5), ethnicity, culture, religion, and socioeconomic status.

NEURODEVELOPMENTAL DISORDERS

Neurodevelopmental disorders are characterized by developmental deficits that interfere with successful engagement in personal, social, academic, or occupational functioning. The onset of these disorders is during the developmental period. This category includes

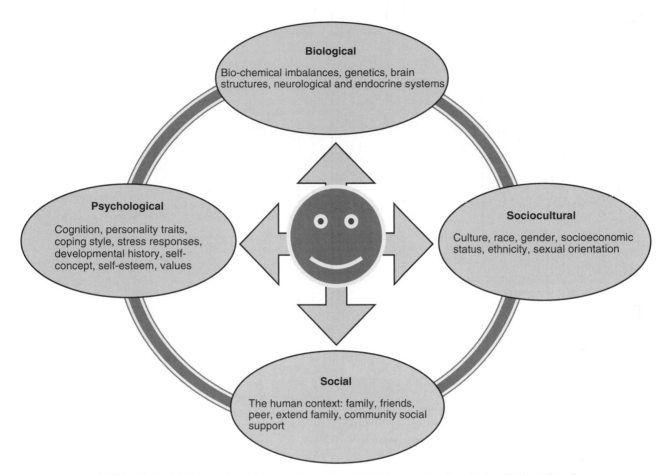

FIGURE 14-1   Multidimensional factors of mental health. (Adapted from Sue. D., Sue D. W., & Sue, S. (2010). *Understanding abnormal behavior* (9th ed.). Boston: Wadsworth Cengage Learning.)

attention-deficit/hyperactivity disorders, motor disorders, and specific learning disorders.

Attention-Deficit/Hyperactivity Disorder

Attention-deficit/hyperactivity disorder (ADHD) is the most common developmental behavioral and cognitive disorder diagnosed in childhood in the United States.[6] There are two presentations: inattentive and hyperactivity-impulsivity. A diagnosis of ADHD relies on an experienced multidisciplinary health care team that determines that the symptoms interfere with the child's ability to perform activities of daily living (ADLs), sleep/rest, and instrumental ADLs (IADLs; see Chapters 19 and 20) and that these symptoms are not the result of another medical, psychiatric, or social condition.[3] It is necessary to rule out other reasons why children may have difficulty paying attention in class (such as anxiety, sensory processing difficulties, feeling overwhelmed, fatigue, and boredom). Diet, routines at home, and exercise can also influence a child's ability to pay attention in class. The symptoms must be evident before age 7, last for at least 6 months, and not be associated with an anxiety disorder.[3]

ADHD, Inattention Presentation

CASE *Study*

Seven-year-old Thomas is in a regular grade 2 classroom and is having trouble in school. The teacher describes him as a disorganized child who has "difficulty sustaining attention to assignments and direct instruction, loses things, seems not to listen, has poor time management, and avoids tasks that require sustained mental attention." These symptoms are interfering with his learning. Thomas frequently stares off into space and has difficulty following multistep verbal directions (Figure 14-2). He is shy and quiet. At home, his parents report that he needs frequent reminders to follow through with tasks. Thomas is easily frustrated and becomes bored with tasks quickly. For example, he does not brush his teeth adequately or get himself dressed in the morning. Instead, he gets distracted. His parents describe their frustrations with Thomas, his ability to lose things, forget assignments, and his untidiness.

After a comprehensive evaluation by a team of professionals (an occupational therapist, a physical therapist,

BOX 14-2

Warning Signs of Sexual Abuse

These signs do not mean conclusively that an adolescent or child is being sexually abused. They can also be symptoms of other problems or mental health disorders. However, if these symptoms are present, sexual abuse should be considered a possibility and an appropriate health professional should be consulted to discuss the reasons for these changes in a child or adolescent. All children are at risk for sexual abuse; for example, children with disability have a high risk for sexual abuse.

Warning signs of sexual abuse in children and adults are recent changes, including the following:
- Sleep problems without an explanation (e.g., nightmares)
- Being distracted or distant
- A change in eating habits: refusing to eat, loss of or drastically increased appetite, or trouble swallowing
- A sudden change in mood or fluctuating moods: rage, fear, insecurity, or becoming withdrawn
- A new interest in discussing sexual issues or making sexual comments or exhibiting adult-like sexual behaviors, language, or knowledge
- Disturbing sexual and nonsexual content in stories, art work, or dreams
- Developing new or unusual or excessive fears of people or places
- Becoming secretive or having secrets and refusing to discuss them with an adult or older child

- Having a new friend who is older or having unexplained money or other gifts
- A change in attitude to body: self as bad or body as dirty, or similar
- Complaining of pain while urinating or defecating
- Symptoms of genital infections or discomfort

Signs common in adolescents involve the development of these behaviors or symptoms:
- Self-injury (cutting, burning)
- Decline in personal appearance and hygiene
- Using drugs and alcohol to excess
- Being sexually promiscuous
- Running away from home or withdrawing from activities
- Signs of anxiety or depression, including suicide attempts
- Fear of intimacy or closeness
- Eating disorders: binge eating, anorexia, or bulimia

These symptoms should never be ignored. It may be uncomfortable to initiate a conversation about them, but the best approach is always a calm, matter-of-fact one. An abuser threatens the child or adolescent; therefore, the child needs to feel safe to disclose the secret. He or she needs to know that you will cope with what they say without judgment and that you will listen. Because the abuser is often someone known to the family, the child may feel safe talking to the OT practitioner, who is a person outside the family.

This material was compiled from suggestions listed on the following sites: http://www.stopitnow.com/warning_signs_child_behavior; http://www.protect kids.com/abuse/abusesigns.htm

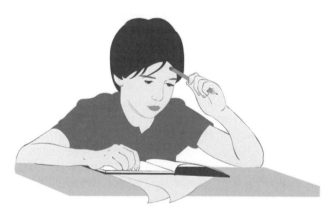

FIGURE 14-2 Children with ADHD may present as quiet, shy, and not paying attention.

a social worker, a psychologist, and a developmental pediatrician) and consultation with the teacher, the parents, and the child, Thomas is diagnosed with ADHD, inattentive presentation. The evaluation includes a classroom visit because one criterion for this diagnosis is difficulty in more than one situation (e.g., home and school).

Interventions for ADHD may include medication (stimulants), behavioral modification techniques, sensory modulation, and learning strategies to help children focus on a task. Positive behavioral support interventions can benefit children with ADHD. Classroom modifications such as low-stimulus sensory areas or assigned individual workspaces may help children focus on their work (Table 14-1).

Hyperactivity/Impulsive Presentation

CASE *Study*

Five-year-old Eugene is always in motion. During calendar circle time, he is not able to sit quietly on his carpet square as do his classmates. He frequently goes from one center to another without permission. Upon arriving at a "new" center, he disrupts the activities of the other children. During direct instruction in mathematics, he blurts out the correct answer before his teacher has the opportunity to call on a student. At recess he breaks in line to climb the ladder up the slide. Eugene enjoys climbing so much that

TABLE 14-1

Classroom Modifications to Improve Attention

SPECIFIC AREA	MODIFICATIONS
General strategies	• Use the child's strengths. • Provide structure and clear expectations. • Use short sentences and simple vocabulary. • Provide supportive opportunities for success to help build self-esteem. • Be flexible in classroom procedures (e.g., allowing the use of recording device for taking notes and tests when students have trouble with written language). • Make use of self-correcting materials that provide immediate feedback without embarrassment. • Use computers for written work. • Reinforce social skills in school and at home. • Provide short breaks by allowing children to move, to stretch, or to verbalize in the classroom. • Mix up the responses required of students (e.g., ask them to clap to the right response, sing the answer, or raise both arms). • Use positive behavior support techniques to reinforce learning.
Helping with schoolwork	• Show an interest in the child's homework. • Ask about homework; ask questions that require answers longer than one or two words. • Help the child organize homework materials. • Establish a regular time with the child to do homework; develop a schedule. • Find a specific place that has plenty of light and space and is quiet where the child can do homework. • Encourage the child to ask questions and look for answers. • Make sure the child justifies answers with facts and evidence. • Practice the skills taught in school and at home. • Relate homework to the child's everyday life (e.g., teach fractions and measurements as you do other therapy activities, such as cooking). • Be a role model: read a book or newspaper, write a letter with the child, or talk about your experiences of these activities. • Praise the child for both the small steps and big leaps in the right direction.
Language	• Have the child sit where he or she can hear you and not be distracted. • Repeat directions; remember to use gentle cuing and helpful reminders. • Provide visual cues for where to begin tasks and assignments. • NEVER embarrass students. • Phrase questions so that the student may answer "yes" or "no." • Assign shorter written language assignments. • Provide written and verbal directions for homework (so that the child does not miss assignments).
Memory	• Use mnemonic strategies: use rhyming games; allow children to mouth or whisper reading assignments in class. • Allow the child to underline in book or circle key words. • Use a recording device for taking notes. • Older children may enjoy using their iPod to keep track of their schedule and assignments. • Have the child practice memorization before bedtime. • Elaborate on information, and relate it to prior knowledge. • Allow the child extra time on tests and assignments. • Use visual or verbal learning. • Use active learning such as role-playing and hands-on experiences. • Divide information into categories for the child.
Sensory integration: coordination	• Allow the child to move around the classroom. • Ensure that the child goes to recess. • Provide the child with movement experiences. • Provide the child with quiet space when he or she is overly aroused. • Have the child sit in the back of the room, with few distractions. • Allow for breaks. • Provide noncompetitive games to help make all the children successful. • Work on the proximal control needed for handwriting skills. • Provide strengthening and endurance games. • Work on perceptual skills through gross motor activities (e.g., obstacle course).

Continued

TABLE 14-1

Classroom Modifications to Improve Attention—cont'd

SPECIFIC AREA	MODIFICATIONS
Sequential processing	• Repeat instructions slowly and provide word or picture lists of steps. • Allow them to talk through or whisper the order of the steps during a task. • Anticipate difficulties. • Use a whole-word approach to reading.
Visual processing	• Provide graph paper or grid, which may help the child focus on the page. • Use tactile cues such as raised lines to help the child.
Organizational skills	• Establish routines. • Provide written as well as verbal instructions for assignments (e.g., a study guide for reading or task completion). • Outline the steps with the child so that he or she can learn the skill. • Develop strategies for taking notes (e.g., highlight key words or tasks). • Make lists, and check off the items (e.g., give the child a day planner; electronic day planners can be cool!). • Break long-term projects into small chunks.

the tops of the bookshelves have become his preferred seat. However, Eugene rarely sits on top of the bookshelf for more than a minute. Eugene was recently diagnosed with ADHD, hyperactivity/impulsivity presentation.

Children who have excessive energy and motor activity are diagnosed with ADHD, hyperactivity/impulsiveness presentation. This disorder is more common in boys than girls (2:1 ratio).[3] Signs of ADHD, hyperactivity/impulsivity include fidgeting, squirming, talking excessively, and impulsive behavior (e.g., difficulty waiting one's turn, and interrupting others who are talking). Other features associated with ADHD include sleep disorders, mood fluctuation, emotional hypersensitivity (i.e., emotional lability), poor self-esteem, and low frustration tolerance. It is common for children with ADHD to experience difficulties relating to other children.

As in the case example of Eugene, a child with ADHD, hyperactivity/impulsivity presentation receives a comprehensive evaluation before being diagnosed. The team of health care and educational personnel determines whether there are any other causes for the impulsive/hyperactive behaviors. An OT practitioner observes and evaluates the child in the classroom, at home, and in the community to provide information on how his or her behaviors affect daily functioning, especially during play and learning tasks. The OT practitioner provides strategies and modifications to help the child regulate his or her emotional arousal and manage sensory distractions. Interventions include sensory integration therapy, accommodations and modifications in the classroom and home environment, self-regulation strategies, positive behavioral support, cognitive-behavioral therapy (CBT), and monitoring the behavioral outcomes of medication. OT practitioners work with teachers to develop therapy goals

for an individualized education program (IEP). Their work with family involves developing parenting strategies to create an environment that supports the child's ability to modify and regulate his or her behavior. The work with families and teachers is likely to involve positive behavior support strategies based on an applied functional behavioral analysis frame of reference (Table 14-2).[15]

CLINICAL *Pearl*

A variety of assessments based on the Model of Human Occupation (MOHO)[20] theory may provide structure to learn about the child and help design effective intervention. For example, the Pediatric Volitional Questionnaire can be used by OT practitioners to better understand a child's volition (e.g., motivation, desires, and belief in efficacy).[7] The Short Child Occupational Performance Evaluation (SCOPE) can provide data on volition, habituation (habits and roles), performance capacity, and environment.[12] The information gained from these occupation-based assessments can inform intervention and provide the OT practitioner with useful tools to better understand children.

CLINICAL *Pearl*

Applied behavioral analysis examines three components of behavior to develop the intervention plan. These components are: antecedent (what happens before observed behavior); observed nonpreferred behavior; and consequences of the behavior (adult response to the nonpreferred behavior). Intervention is aimed at changing antecedents or consequences to promote desired behaviors.

TABLE 14-2

Psychosocial Frames of Reference

PSYCHOSOCIAL FRAMES OF REFERENCE	PRINCIPLES	STRATEGIES
COGNITIVE-BEHAVIORAL THERAPY		
This frame of reference assumes that maladaptive or faulty thinking patterns adversely influence emotions and contribute to dysfunctional behavior. Examples of this faulty thinking include overgeneralizing (i.e., if it is true in one situation, it is always true) or catastrophizing (i.e., always thinking the worst possible outcome). The greatest improvement occurs when a child or adolescent decreases his or her negative and faulty thinking. This is not achieved by changing negative thoughts to positive ones.	How one thinks and what one believes influence behavior and emotions (e.g., a child's positive or negative view of him or herself and his or her view of the world as threatening or safe, caring, and supportive). A change in thinking can lead to improvement in function and can reduce emotional distress. The basic core and conditional beliefs are learned and become the personal rules that guide life (e.g., "if I do this [rule] the consequences are..."). It is a way of making sense of cause-and-effect relations. Focus on the present problems. Time-limited individual or group therapy focuses on a specific difficulty, condition, or skill acquisition.	Interventions include teaching a person about the relationships among their thinking, behavior, and emotions. Interventions: With the use of media and activities, the following techniques and skills are developed: • Identifying patterns of thinking and core beliefs and being aware of how thinking affects feelings and behavior (e.g., "I always fail") and leads to anxiety in new situations and not trying new activities because of the fear of failure. • Cognitive restructuring, also called reframing thinking. This involves changing beliefs and thinking patterns. • Self-monitoring and self-talk • Learning skills to reduce stress, such as relaxation • Developing problem-solving skills to address client-identified problems • Homework assignments to consolidate learning and transfer it beyond the therapy setting
SKILL ACQUISITION		
This frame of reference emphasizes that learning, practicing, and acquiring skills help children and adolescents function in social, academic, work, and family occupations.	Children develop self-efficacy, a sense of success, and skills through practice. Acquiring foundational skills can help children perform in home, school, and community settings. Skill acquisition is based on teaching-learning principles. Learning can be achieved through a therapist's instruction or in an experiential group setting through peer modeling and observation. Skill refinement occurs through specific behavioral feedback. Skills are acquired sequentially (i.e., simple to complex).	Interventions are designed to develop, modify, and refine specific skills for functional occupational performance through instructional methods such as role-playing, experiential skill-based groups, practice and generalization of skill performance, modeling, and feedback on skill performance.
BEHAVIOR MODIFICATION		
This frame of reference changes or develops behaviors required for occupational performance. The OT practitioner identifies target behaviors and shapes these behaviors using reinforcement schedules. Applied behavioral analysis is a widely used frame of reference in health and education.	Children and adolescents exhibit behaviors that can be identified and reinforced. Changing or developing behaviors will improve occupational performance. Behavior can be modified by external forces (e.g., reward or punishment schedules).	Interventions are designed to develop, modify, and refine specific behaviors. Interventions follow strict protocols that are targeted to a specific behavior to be increased or decreased (e.g., increase eye contact from a child with autism or decrease head banging in such a child). Identify behaviors to be shaped, changed, or developed. Teach, demonstrate, and practice behavioral strategies. Increase desired behaviors with rewards (e.g., praise, tokens such as stars that can later be redeemed for a toy or an activity of one's choice). Intermittent reinforcement strengthens a behavior.

Continued

TABLE 14-2

Psychosocial Frames of Reference—cont'd

PSYCHOSOCIAL FRAMES OF REFERENCE	PRINCIPLES	STRATEGIES
PSYCHOEDUCATIONAL GROUP THERAPY		
The purpose of the psycho-educational group is to share information along a common focus and learn from the experiences and knowledge of group members. This process facilitates change and/or the development of skills. This approach is often used in school-based programs to develop or improve social, communication, or coping skills.	Through knowledge comes change. To develop knowledge and skills for coping with crisis events, developmental transitions, mental health disorders, or current situational challenges (e.g., parental divorce, adolescent difficulties, depression, or bullying) Draws from cognitive-behavioral principles Education is a significant component. Focuses on the here and now. Intentional use of group experience for mutual and vicarious (by the examples of others and observation) learning as well as support.	Time-limited and theme-focused groups of children and adolescents with similar needs or difficulties. A well-developed curriculum with sequential instructional sessions in which a variety of teaching methods are used, such as videos, handouts, PowerPoint presentations, and blackboards. Interactive and experiential learning strategies are important components. The techniques consist of brief lectures or presentations, small-group discussions, written exercises, role-playing and behavior rehearsal, peer-group modeling and learning from others, and homework tasks to reinforce learning and transfer it to everyday settings.
APPLIED BEHAVIORAL ANALYSIS		
Positive support behavior: This approach consists of systemic and individualized strategies for achieving social and learning outcomes. The goal is preventing problem behavior.[15]	All behavior has a purpose for a child, and behavior is related to context. Challenging behaviors are symptoms. Interventions respect the child's preferences, dignity, and goals. Relationships are the building blocks of prosocial behaviors Learning new skills takes time.	Teach skills directly. Ask why a child is acting the way he or she is acting, because there is always a reason. Identify patterns of behavior; if problems are predicted, they can be prevented. A-B-C model: Identify the **A**ntecedent behavior or event that precedes the child's behavior. Identify the **B**ehavior that is to be acquired or decreased, and establish **C**onsequences and teach skills.
COACHING MODEL		
The premise is that children will be more successful at reaching the goals that they develop themselves. Children will learn lifelong strategies through setting goals and take progressive steps toward meeting goals successfully. This child-directed model requires that the OT practitioner provide direction, support, advice, and strategies. This takes the form of coaching and mentoring.	Children and adolescents will be more successful meeting goals that they develop. Children will develop lifelong strategies as they learn to analyze the steps toward goals. Providing children with support and encouraging them will facilitate progress toward goals. Children may need "coach" support or mentorship to develop abilities to meet goals. Teach children to self-evaluate and problem-solve.	Children develop goals with support from OT practitioners. Analyze the steps to meet goals. Children set realistic tasks to meet goals. Support children in addressing steps and learning skills to meet goals. Get children to practice skills. Use cueing and reminders. Act as the children's "coach" or "mentor" with weekly or daily "check-ins."

TABLE 14-2

Psychosocial Frames of Reference—cont'd

PSYCHOSOCIAL FRAMES OF REFERENCE	PRINCIPLES	STRATEGIES
MODEL OF HUMAN OCCUPATION[20]		
The premise of MOHO is that children will engage in those activities that they find meaning. This process is dynamic and involves an interaction between personal factors (volition, habituation, performance capacity) and the environment. Understanding the child and family allows OT practitioners to intervene in meaningful ways.	Occupational actions, thoughts, and emotions always arise out of the dynamic interaction of volition, habituation, performance capacity, and environmental context. Change in any aspect of volition, habituation, performance capacity, and/or environment can result in a change in the thoughts, feelings, and doing that make up one's occupation. Volition, habituation, and performance capacity are maintained and changed through what one does and what one thinks and feels about doing. Children will maintain a particular pattern of volition, habituation, and performance capacity as long as the underlying thoughts, feelings, and actions are repeated in a supportive environment.[20]	• Validating • Identifying • Giving feedback • Advising • Negotiating • Structuring • Coaching • Encouraging • Providing physical support

CBT, Cognitive behavioral therapy; *OT,* occupational therapy.
Data compiled from Furr, S. R. (2000). Structuring the group experience: a format for designing psycho-educational groups. *J Specialists Group Work,* 25, 29; Jones, K. D., & Robinson, E. H. (2000). A model for choosing topics and experiences appropriate to group stage. *J Specialists Group Work,* 25, 356; Kramer, P., & Hinojosa, J. (1999). *Frames of reference for pediatric occupational therapy* (2nd ed.). Baltimore, MD: Lippincott, Williams & Wilkins; Sommers-Flanagan, R., Barrett-Hakanson, T., Clake, C., et al. (2000). A psycho-educational school-based coping and social skills group for depressed students. *J Specialists Group Work,* 55,170; Stein, F., & Culter, S. K. (2002). *Psychosocial occupational therapy: A holistic approach* (2nd ed.). New York, NY: Delmar; Crone, D., & Horner, R. (2003). Building positive behavior support systems in schools. New York, NY: The Guildford Press; Kielhofner, G. (2008). *A model of human occupation: theory and application* (4th ed.). Philadelphia: Lippincott, Williams, & Wilkins.

The behaviors associated with ADHD, hyperactivity/impulsivity presentation can frustrate parents, teachers, and other children in the family or classroom. Because these behavioral difficulties often are the presenting problem that precedes referral to the health care team, children with ADHD sometimes are regarded as "difficult," "problematic," or "stupid." These negative labels can make children feel inferior and create low self-esteem. They experience difficulties succeeding in school tasks and making friends, which also affects self-esteem. As time goes on and even when others may have ceased to identify these children as problems, they may still identify themselves with the negative labels, which influences their behaviors and motivation for learning. They avoid trying because they have experienced failure.

The OT practitioner can help by explaining to parents and teachers how to work with the child to address his or her comprehensive needs in ways that will build confidence and self-esteem. Activities are graded (i.e., changed in some manner) so the level of difficulty is gradually increased to encourage success. Parents and children alike can benefit from support groups. Children can gain skills and confidence from participation in summer camps or community activities that are able to accommodate or adjust expectations for children with special needs.

CLINICAL *Pearl*

Teachers frequently mention to parents that their child has problems paying attention in class. This alone does not necessarily mean that the child has ADHD. The child may demonstrate attention problems for a variety of reasons. OT practitioners assist team members in determining whether the attention problems are secondary to environmental, social, or sensory conditions. OT practitioners working in school systems play a role in educating teachers concerning the strategies and modifications that help children succeed.

Motor Disorders

Motor disorders are characterized by deficits in the acquisition and execution of coordinated movements.[3] As a result of these deficits the child is clumsy and slow to perform daily occupations. Movements may be stereotypic and purposeless interfering with social, academic, and adaptive functioning.

Tic disorders are neurologic and characterized by stereotypical, repetitive, involuntary, recurrent movements or vocalizations. They are classified as motor, phonic, vocal, or complex tics, which may involve talking to oneself, facial grimacing, or using obscene words (coprolalia). Common motor tics are eye blinking, neck jerking, coughing, shoulder shrugging, facial grimacing, foot stomping, touching objects, and excessive grooming. Common vocal tics are throat clearing, grunting, sniffing, snorting, barking, hiccupping, yelling, and the repetition of others' words (echolalia). Tics often increase in stressful situations and due to fatigue or anxiety, and they can decrease during sleep or absorbing activities such as computer games.[3] Tourette's syndrome is the most common tic disorder for which occupational therapy services are sought.[3,8]

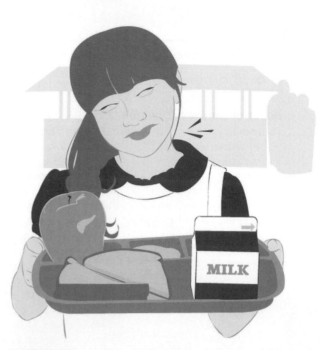

FIGURE 14-3 A child with Tourette's syndrome exhibits involuntary movements and noises that may distract others.

Tourette's Syndrome

CASE *Study*

Kyle is a 7-year-old third grader. Recently he has started to jerk his neck to the side and make strange faces and grunting noises (Figure 14-3). These behaviors occur intermittently throughout the day. Kyle is embarrassed that he is unable to control these movements and noises. His parents and teacher are concerned by these behaviors. Kyle's classmates are annoyed when he cannot stop and have started to avoid and tease him. His school performance is suffering because the jerks and noises distract him.

Kyle's symptoms are consistent with Tourette's syndrome. The typical onset of Tourette's syndrome is between 6 and 7 years of age and is more prevalent in boys. Tourette's syndrome is viewed as a genetic disorder involving repetitive involuntary motor and vocal tics. The tics may occur many times a day and must occur consistently for 1 year or more before the age of 18 for a diagnosis of the syndrome. Related comorbidity occurs with ADHD, behavioral problems, specific learning disabilities, or obsessive-compulsive disorder (OCD).[3] Although it is typically a chronic disorder, some children experience improvement during adolescence and early adulthood.

Tics may disrupt a child's schoolwork and participation in social activities, ADLs, sleep/rest, IADLs, and play/leisure activities. Many children are not significantly affected by their tics and do not require treatment. Others may require medication (antipsychotic medications,

selective serotonin reuptake inhibitors [SSRIs], and benzodiazepine), but the response to medications varies. Behavioral, anxiety, and anger management benefit some children, especially when the disorder occurs with other disorders such as OCD.

Other associated challenges are social. Kyle's experience, especially his vocal tics, is an example of how this disorder can isolate a child. The strange and obvious nature of verbal and motor tics makes children vulnerable to discrimination, and they often experience bullying or teasing.[11] It is important that the OT practitioner is aware of the bullying and includes goals for social participation in the IEP of children with this problem. (See Box 14-3 for strategies to prevent bullying.)

Specific Learning Disorders

CASE *Study*

Greg is a cooperative 8-year-old in grade 3. He is reluctant to ask questions in class and avoids activities that require reading in front of other students. Although the school psychologist reports Greg's IQ is 110, well within the normal range, his performance on writing and reading tasks falls well below his grade-level expectations. During a classroom exercise, the occupational therapy assistant (OTA) observed Greg struggling to write one sentence during "free writing," whereas his classmates were able to complete paragraphs. The teacher, using positive

BOX 14-3

Strategies for Responding to Bullying

Children with mental health disorders and disabilities, especially those that affect their social skills, are vulnerable to bullying and teasing. Bullying is often underreported, minimized, or unacknowledged in schools. In 2000 the U.S. Department of Education issued an official statement regarding harassment of those with disabilities in school. That same year, the National Center on Secondary Education and Transition provided advice and strategies on school interventions and educational programs to address and deter bullying. It specifically targeted the prevention of disability harassment (http://www.ncset.org).

OT practitioners working in the schools system can:

- Contribute to a school environment that is aware of and sensitive to disability concerns and harassment
- Report any identified bullying to the appropriate school services
- Be open to discussing bullying during therapy
- Have a zero-tolerance policy toward teasing and bullying in the OT department
- Teach children and adolescents constructive strategies to stop any bullying they experience
- Encourage parents, students, employees, and community members to discuss harassment of those with disabilities and to report it when they become aware that it is happening
- Recommend that victims and perpetrators of harassment seek counseling
- Participate in the school team that assesses and modifies existing harassment policies and procedures to ensure effectiveness

From Hoover, J., & Stenhjem, P. (2003). Bullying and teasing of youth with disabilities: Creating positive school environments for effective inclusion. *National Center on Secondary Education and Transition Issue Brief*, 2(3), 1-5. http://www.ncset.org/publications/viewdesc.asp?id=1332.

behavioral support, commented to Greg, "I can see you are working hard."

Greg has a specific learning disability in the areas of reading and written expression. The school team met to develop an IEP to provide special education and related services with accommodations that would facilitate Greg's success at school. These accommodations included preferential seating in close proximity to the teacher, additional time for writing assignments, access to a keyboard to type his assignments, and small-group oral administration of all state-required standardized tests in the area of written expression. In his general and special education classrooms, teacher expectations and student responsibilities are clearly posted and reviewed daily.

Of school-aged children, 5% to 15% experience a specific learning disorder in the academic domains of reading, mathematics, and written expression.[3,8] These children often are aware of their differences and difficulties, although when they are young, they may not understand or be able to describe it. A **specific learning disorder** is present if the child experiences difficulty with learning key academic skills during the developmental period; performance is well below the average compared with same aged peers; learning difficulties are apparent in early school years and the difficulties are not due to intellectual disabilities or global developmental delay or general external factors (e.g., economic disadvantage, excessive absenteeism, neurologic condition).[3] A child may have a specific learning disorder in one or more of the academic areas of reading, mathematics, and written expression. The levels of severity of learning disorders[3] can be described as follows:

- **Mild:** The child experiences some difficulties learning skills in one or two academic areas, but is able to compensate and function well with accommodations, special education services, resource support, and/or related services.
- **Moderate:** The child demonstrates marked difficulty learning skills in one or more of the core academic areas such that he or she is not likely to succeed without intensive support through special education and related services outside of the general education classroom and with small-group specialized direct instruction.
- **Severe:** The child shows severe difficulty learning skills in several academic areas requiring ongoing and intensive individualized and specialized instruction in a special education self-contained classroom setting with related services specific to his or her specific needs.[3]

Children with specific learning disorders often are referred to occupational therapy for difficulties with sensory processing, motor planning, organization, or handwriting. They may experience behavioral issues related to poor performance and, therefore, can benefit from modifications to allow them to be successful and develop positive self-esteem. OT practitioners evaluate to determine the child's current skills and abilities as well as assess for the possible underlying causes specific to the child's difficulties. Assessment tools are used to identify present levels of performance, learning styles, and strengths and weaknesses. The occupational therapist determines which assessments are appropriate to use and may assign the administration and scoring of such to the OTA (see Appendix 10-A for a summary of assessments used in practice). OT practitioners use select frames of references and strategies such as sensory integration, coaching techniques, cognitive-behavioral therapy, or a compensatory approach to enable children with specific learning disorders to succeed in class (see Table 14-2).

DISRUPTIVE, IMPULSE-CONTROL, AND CONDUCT DISORDERS

Disruptive, impulse-control, and conduct disorders are conditions characterized by socially disruptive behaviors. The child or adolescent cannot self-control his or her emotions or behaviors. These disorders are manifested by behaviors that violate the rights of others through aggression or property destruction that bring the individual into significant conflict with societal norms and/or authority figures (Figure 14-4).[3] The underlying causes of these disorders can vary greatly. These disorders are dependent on problems in two types of self-control: emotions (e.g., anger and

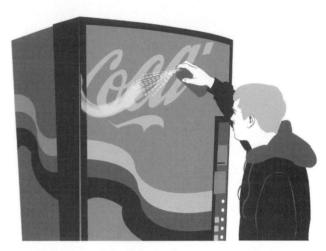

FIGURE 14-4 A child with disruptive impulse control and conduct disorder may violate the rights of others and vandalize property without feeling bad.

irritation) and behaviors (e.g., aggression, argumentativeness, defiance). These disorders tend to be more common in boys than girls and have first onset during childhood or adolescence. Many of the symptoms that define these disorders can occur to a lesser degree in typically developing children and adolescents. The frequency, persistence, and pervasiveness across environments of these behaviors as well as the associated impairments in daily occupational performance is critical to accurately diagnosis an individual as having a disruptive, impulse-control, or conduct disorder.[3] Conduct disorder, oppositional defiant disorder (ODD), and intermittent explosive personality disorder are examples of conditions in this category that are frequently seen in children and adolescents.

Conduct Disorder: Childhood Onset

CASE *Study*

Rodney is a 10-year-old who has difficulty getting along with other children. His parents describe him as an irritable baby, a difficult toddler who had tantrums, and a young child who was disruptive in the family and did not adjust easily to preschool. Now, he is inclined to bully other children, and neighbors complain about his behavior (e.g., throwing rocks at windows, fighting with other children, and stealing). Particularly distressing is his cruelty to animals and, more recently, his fascination with fire. His parents feel powerless because he does not respond to their attempts to discipline him; of late, he has started hurting his younger sister. At school, he is doing poorly in grade 3; he was suspended recently for stealing money from his teacher's desk. The school called a parent conference to discuss his aggressive behavior and poor school performance.

Rodney's behaviors are characteristic of a conduct disorder, characterized by long-standing behaviors that violate the rights of others and the rules of society. The following behaviors characterize conduct disorder in children and adolescents[3,11]:

- Physical aggression toward other people or animals
- Participation in mugging, purse snatching, shoplifting, or burglary
- Destruction of other people's property (e.g., setting fires)
- Breaking rules (e.g., running away from home or skipping school)
- Impaired school performance, especially verbal and reading skills
- Suspensions from school for behavioral problems

Boys with conduct disorder are likely to be involved in behaviors such as vandalism, stealing, and fighting, whereas girls with the disorder tend to be sexually permissive (e.g., prostitution), and engage in manipulative behaviors such as lying or running away. Other problems associated with conduct disorder are abuse of addictive substances, reckless behavior, and temper outbursts. Children diagnosed with conduct disorders exhibit a lack concern for others, and they show no feelings of guilt or remorse. However, despite this image of toughness, they often have poor self-esteem and experience anxiety, depression, and suicidal thoughts.

Children with conduct disorder are at high risk for poor outcomes, including dropping out of school, unemployment, and engaging in criminal behaviors and substance abuse. If left untreated, many will develop antisocial personality disorder as adults (i.e., in approximately 40% of cases, childhood-onset conduct disorder develops into antisocial personality disorder).[29] Antisocial personality disorders are associated with serious crimes, including rape, physical assault, and homicide.[3]

CLINICAL *Pearl*

It is important to praise or recognize a child when he or she is working on or exhibiting desired behaviors. This recognition should be clear, and should label the behavior of the child, for example, "Well done, you are working quietly on the task." This is better than saying, "Nice work!" This strategy helps the child feel validated and shapes his or her behavior.

Oppositional Defiant Disorder

CASE *Study*

Dwayne is a 9-year-old grade 3 student. His mother says that he has always been a somewhat "difficult, angry" child,

but his behavior has worsened over the past 19 months. He argues constantly with his parents and older sisters, loses his temper over seemingly trivial issues, and has uncontrollable rage. He blames others, refuses to obey his parents' rules, and deliberately annoys other people. He says that he hates school and his sisters and that his classmates "suck." His parents find it very difficult to set limits for him.

The primary symptoms of ODD are negative, hostile, and defiant behaviors that are uncharacteristic of typical children.[1,3] Children and early adolescents with ODD display outbursts of temper, argue, defy adults, and are especially hostile to authority figures.[1] These children seem to be angry all the time and resent rules; they become easily annoyed and readily blame others for their mistakes. Behaviors that might be observed are frequent temper tantrums; mean, hateful talking; revenge-seeking behaviors; and deliberately annoying others. These behaviors differ in duration and intensity from the occasional "difficult" periods some children and adolescents may experience.[1,3] Ongoing oppositional behavior and stormy relationships with teachers and other children result in poor academic performance in school and few friendships.[8] Children with ODD may eventually grow out of it, especially if the onset occurs in preschool years. Adolescents diagnosed with ODD are more likely (75%) to have symptoms that persist into adulthood.[2]

ODD may also be an indication of underlying childhood depression or an inability to cope effectively with anger and other uncomfortable feelings. ODD differs from conduct disorder in that these children do not seriously violate the rights of others or ignore their feelings.[1] Furthermore, they rarely engage in activities that cause physical harm to others, and as a rule, they do not engage in criminal activity.

Intermittent Explosive Personality Disorder

CASE *Study*

Jaylen is a second-grade student who receives special education services in a self-contained classroom. For the past 4 months, Jaylen has had aggressive, behavioral outbursts at least twice a week at school. During his behavioral outbursts, Jaylen throws chairs and other furniture at his classmates, making it dangerous for them to remain in the room. The teacher's assistant quickly takes all of his classmates to the media center when he has an outburst. His teacher documented that these outbursts are preceded by minor issues (e.g., someone sitting in his preferred space or being unable to find his pencil). Jaylen's outbursts typically last for 20 to 30 minutes, after which it is safe for his classmates to return to class.

Jaylen has intermittent explosive personality disorder. The primary symptoms of an intermittent explosive personality disorder are:

1. Recurrent aggressive behavioral outbursts;
2. Magnitude of outburst significantly out of proportion to the provocation;
3. Not premeditated; and
4. Impulsive and/or anger-based outbursts.[3]

Intermittent explosive disorder is more common among younger individuals. Its onset is typically in late childhood (6 years or older) and adolescence. Because of the impulsive and aggressive outbursts, the individual with this disorder has social, academic, and adaptive functioning deficits. If the aggressive behavior is against person or property, the outburst may result in criminal charges.

ANXIETY DISORDERS

About 13 of every 100 children and adolescents have an **anxiety disorder**. Anxiety disorder is more common among girls than boys (2:1 ratio).[3] It is important to recognize that anxiety is a normal adaptive response to stress, involving feelings of apprehension and arousal of the autonomic nervous system (e.g., palpitations, perspiration, chest pain, stomach discomfort, restlessness, and/or headache).[21] It energizes and prepares an individual to handle a situation, especially a new one.

However, anxiety is not adaptive when anxious feelings become distressing and interfere with everyday functioning. A nonadaptive stress response involves physiologic arousal (high cortisol levels, raised blood pressure, and increased heart rate), physical sensations and symptoms (e.g., vomiting), and negative thoughts. An anxious child or adolescent may experience cognitive symptoms such as shame, or a distorted or inaccurate view of the threat of a situation.[3] Children will describe having symptoms such as headaches, a sick feeling, sweating hands, butterflies in their stomach, nervousness, or fear.[13] They may experience difficulty making decisions, learning, concentrating, and accurately perceiving situations (e.g., seeing safe situations as threatening). Children with anxiety disorders exhibit poor school attendance, low self-esteem, and adjustment difficulties. Their social interactions are affected by poor social skills, and as they become adolescents, they are more likely to use alcohol and other drugs. Anxiety disorders are distinguished from one another by the types of objects or situations that induce fear, anxiety, avoidance behaviors, and the associated cognitive ideation.[3]

Generalized Anxiety Disorder

Generalized anxiety disorder (GAD) is diagnosed in 0.9% of the adolescent population in the United States and is more prevalent in girls than boys.[3] Symptoms include excessive anxiety and worrying (e.g., about future events, school performance, family health, and world events) on most days without a specific trigger event or social situation.[26,27] Children with GAD cannot control their fear of situations and activities, and these fears manifest as irritability, tiredness, inability to relax (i.e., feeling on edge), restlessness, apprehension, negative self-image, difficulty concentrating, and disrupted sleep.[21] The physical symptoms described previously can also occur with other anxiety or mood disorders (e.g., panic attacks, phobias, or dysthymia).[21] Not surprisingly, these children will have difficulty in school, social situations, and all areas of occupational performance.

Separation Anxiety Disorder

CASE *Study*

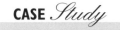

Caitlin is a tentative, shy 5-year-old. She prefers to be at home, and she follows her mother around the house. She will not fall asleep at night unless her mother lies with her on the bed. She awakens during the night with "bad dreams," which have a common theme of finding herself left behind in the supermarket. Caitlin does not want to go to preschool. She cries hysterically and becomes so distressed that she vomits. At preschool, she stays close to one teacher and does not play with the other children.

Although separation anxiety is normal in infants and very young children, it is not appropriate for children of Caitlin's age. Caitlin has separation anxiety disorder, which is characterized by extreme anxiety when anticipating separation or separating from home or her mother (Figure 14-5). It is a disorder experienced by about 4% of children.[26] Children or adolescents with this disorder may experience extreme distress traveling away from home or may refuse to go to school or visit or sleep over at a friend's home. In severe cases, children may refuse to attend school or participate in social and recreational activities.[3] The diagnostic criteria includes repeated nightmares involving the theme of separation, reluctance or refusal to sleep without a significant person nearby, and persistent worrying about separation or harm to major attachment figures (e.g., mother or father).[3] Separation or the anticipation of separation may trigger physical (somatic) symptoms that include headaches, dizziness, palpitation, stomachache, nausea, and vomiting.[21,27] Typically there are exacerbations and remissions with this disorder.[3] Children with separation anxiety disorder exhibit delayed social development, refusal to attend school, and anxiety while at school, all of which result in poor academic performance.[11] Separation anxiety disorder will usually

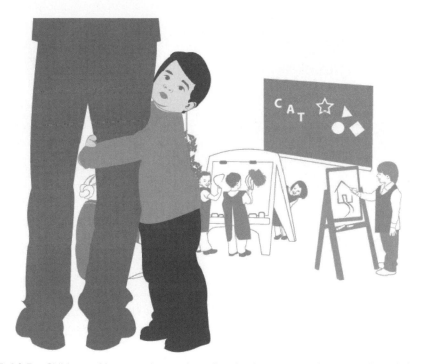

FIGURE 14-5 Children with separation anxiety disorder become overly upset when their parent leaves them (even for a short time).

resolve or decrease in severity with time, but it may also be a precursor to other conditions such as panic disorder.

Social Anxiety (Social Phobia) Disorder

Phobias refer to intense irrational fears of things or situations, (e.g., dogs, injections, blood, storms, or heights). Young children become very distressed, have tantrums, cry, or cling to parents when near an object or in the situation that causes the fear. The response to the object or situation is one of panic. Adolescents and adults may experience anxiety resulting in panic attacks associated with phobias.

Social anxiety (social phobia) disorder refers to symptoms of specific, persistent, and recurring fears when in social situations. Older children and adolescents with social phobia are extremely self-conscious, easily embarrassed, afraid of being humiliated, and overly concerned about whether they are presenting themselves appropriately in social or public situations. Consequently, they withdraw from or avoid social contact, which further limits social development and relationships with peers. Social anxiety disorder symptoms do not occur in situations with family members or familiar people with whom they have good relationships. Depending on the number and intensity of the phobia, this disorder disrupts routines and restricts children's experiences.

With all phobias, the avoidance of the object or the situation is the behavior that becomes disabling. The longer the child or adolescent avoids social situations the more intense the phobia becomes. Treatment involves medication (e.g., SSRIs or benzodiazepines) combined with cognitive-behavioral therapy and relaxation strategies. OT practitioners enable children to address their fears and learn how to manage anxiety by engaging children in structured play and creative activities at the right level. CBT can be integrated easily into the OT session so that the child chooses goals, develops positive evaluations of his or her performance, and makes desired changes. The OT practitioner may grade the social aspects of intervention by beginning with activities that the child completes with the practitioner and building to a new group activity. To help manage the anxiety the practitioner may engage the child in role-playing and practice the group task so the child is successful. The OT practitioner may also grade the social components of the activity by starting out with a 3-minute activity with a peer and building up to 30 minutes.

OBSESSIVE-COMPULSIVE AND RELATED DISORDERS

Obsessive-Compulsive Disorder

Obsessive-compulsive disorder (OCD) is characterized by recurring, disruptive, intrusive thoughts that cause anxiety and compulsive, ritualistic, repetitive patterns of behavior that reduce the anxiety.[27] These behaviors become essential to the child, and if he or she tries to resist them, the anxiety increases. The anxiety is a product of persistent obsessive thoughts, which often are irrational concerns or fears, for example, disgust with dirt, germs, or bodily waste; or thoughts about terrible things happening to self or parents, friends, and siblings. There can be a preoccupation with orderliness,

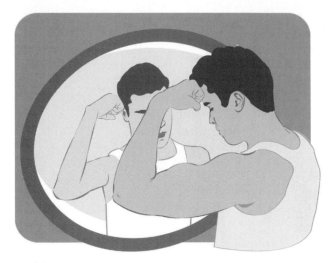

FIGURE 14-6 Young men with body dysmorphic disorder see themselves differently than they actually present.

excessive praying, magical thinking (e.g., lucky and unlucky numbers), and forbidden yet intrusive (sexual) thoughts or images.[21] The compulsive behaviors of children and adolescents include ordering and rearranging, excessive or ritualistic hand washing or bathing routines, and checking locks or switches that may be performed with the intention to prevent harm coming to family members or self. In severe cases, this disruptive and time-consuming disorder interferes with routine daily activities. Because of the preoccupation with obsessive, intrusive thoughts, concentration and task completion are also impaired.

Body Dysmorphic Disorder

Body dysmorphic disorder is characterized by one being preoccupied with perceived physical flaws or defects that drive the person to perform excessive, repetitive acts such as looking in the mirror or touching/feeling a specific body part. The preoccupation causes impairment in social, occupational, academic, and daily living performance. Muscle dysmorphic disorder occurs in males only. Males with this disorder have normal-looking or very muscular looking bodies, but perceive that their bodies are too small or insufficient (Figure 14-6). The onset of this disorder is during adolescence with the most common age of onset at 12 to 13 years of age.

Hoarding Disorder

CASE *Study*

Sarah is a sixth grader who receives special education instruction in a resource classroom for written expression and math. Recently her resource teacher contacted the

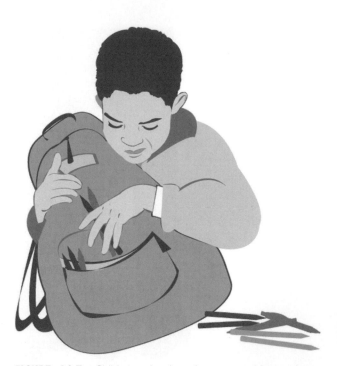

FIGURE 14-7 Children who hoard are not able to throw objects away, despite their actual value.

school-based OT practitioner because of his concerns that Sarah could not find anything in her book bag because of all of the pencils piled into it. Sarah told the OT practitioner she collected pencils because she hated to write. Her thoughts were if she collected the pencils, then she would not have to do written work (Figure 14-7).

A child or adolescent with a hoarding disorder has a long-standing difficulty throwing away, selling, giving away, or recycling specific possession(s) regardless of the actual value of the items.[3] The saved items clutter the person's living space and/or book bag/backpack. The objects are typically piled together in disorganization. Associated features include indecisiveness, avoidance, procrastination, and distractibility. The prevalence of hoarding disorders is 2% to 6% affecting both males and females. Symptoms typically emerge between 11 and 15 years. The behaviors start to significantly interfere with daily functioning by the mid-20s.[3]

Trichotillomania (Hair-Pulling) Disorder

CASE *Study*

Mikaila is a 6-year-old girl who was recently adopted and moved from Bulgaria to North Carolina. The first 4 years of her life were spent primarily in a crib in an orphanage. She recently started school and is in a self-contained classroom for students with moderate to severe intellectual disabilities. Recently Mikaila began pulling her hair out of the back of her head. She created a large bald spot on the back of her head and now is pulling her hair out on the sides. The OT practitioner suggested that a large, stretch head band be used to discourage Mikaila from pulling hair out from the sides of her head.

Trichotillomania (hair-pulling) disorder is recurrent pulling out of one's hair resulting in significant hair loss. The hair may be pulled from any region of the body in which hair grows (e.g., eyebrows, scalp, axillary) and has negative effects on the individual.[3] Females are more affected by this disorder than males with a ratio of 10:1.[3]

CLINICAL *Pearl*

Having the child who suffers from trichotillomania wear a scarf or hat may decrease the pulling out of the head hair.

Excoriation (Skin-Picking) Disorder

CASE *Study*

For the past several months, the OT practitioner noticed four to five lesions on both of Marlene's forearms. Upon questioning, Marlene explained that her arms itched so she scratched them. Frequently, during his weekly intervention, the OT practitioner observed Marlene picking at her sores seemingly unaware of her behavior. The practitioner asked Marlene to stop picking at the sores and to clean her hands with disinfectant. Marlene complied and continued to work on her project. Marlene has an excoriation disorder.

Excoriation (skin-picking) disorder is recurrent picking at one's skin resulting in skin lesions. This disorder occurs much more frequently in females than males with the typical onset coinciding with the onset of puberty.[3]

TRAUMA- AND STRESSOR-RELATED DISORDERS

Trauma- and stressor-related disorders are characterized by traumatic or stressful events that result in anxiety-based and/or fear-based behaviors that interfere with an individual's active and successful engagement in daily occupations.

Reactive Attachment Disorder

Reactive attachment disorder of infancy and childhood is characterized by a pattern of markedly delayed attachment behaviors in which the child minimally turns to primary caregiver for comfort, support, protection or nurturance. It is a rare clinical diagnosis primarily seen in toddlers and children who have been exposed to severe neglect.[3]

Disinhibited Social Engagement Disorder

Disinhibited social engagement disorder of childhood is characterized by a pattern of behavior in which the child is overly familiar with relative strangers. A diagnosis of this disorder cannot be made before the developmental age of 9 months, at which time selective attachments can be formed.[3]

Posttraumatic Stress Disorder

CASE *Study*

Chantrelle, her sister, and her parents moved to the United States from Haiti 1 month after an earthquake destroyed their home and took the lives of her grandparents and brother. Chantrelle, who is 6 years old, has been attending a local school. Her parents hoped that the routine of school and living away from the chaos created by the earthquake would help her recover from the experience. However, Chantrelle is no longer the outgoing girl she was before the earthquake. She has not made friends, often reports feeling sick, and has little interest in food. Most nights she wakes up crying because of "bad" dreams. Chantrelle was diagnosed with posttraumatic stress disorder (PTSD) and referred to a child psychologist who specializes in trauma disorders in children.

Acute stress disorder (ASD) and PTSD are both anxiety disorders that develop in response to a traumatic event such as natural disasters (e.g., hurricane or earthquake). Other events associated with stress disorders are serious accidents, acts of terrorism, war, and physical and sexual abuse. Children separated from parents during traumatic event(s) are most vulnerable to PTSD. ASD is an immediate stress response to exposure to trauma that lasts approximately 1 month. If the symptoms continue for longer than a month, the diagnosis is PTSD.

Unlike adults, symptoms of ASD and PTSD persist longer and become more intense with time for children.[17] Children experience recurring nightmares, repeated memories of the event, difficulty sleeping, changes in eating habits, and physical symptoms (e.g., sick feeling, headaches). They are likely to have problems focusing on activities and schoolwork. Some children may become stoic about the event, withdraw from society, isolate from other children, or engage in more risk-taking behaviors. The most common comorbid disorders are panic attacks and substance abuse.

DEPRESSIVE DISORDERS

Depressive disorders are a common feature of feeling sadness, emptiness, or an irritable mood.[3]

Disruptive Mood Dysregulation Disorder

A child or adolescent between 7 and 18 years of age who has a disruptive mood dysregulation disorder is angry and irritable all of the time. The child or adolescent experiences verbal or behavioral outbursts across environments at least three times a week. Typically, the behavioral outbursts involve aggressive, destructive acts against property, self, or others. The child or adolescent has chronic, persistent irritability or an angry mood between the outbursts throughout the day nearly every day.[3]

Major Depressive Disorder

CASE *Study*

Wendy is a 12-year-old seventh grader. She lives with her mother and her 14-year-old brother. Typically she is a pleasant, cooperative child, but she has been irritable and withdrawn lately. Her teacher describes her as a good student but somewhat anxious. Over the past several weeks, Wendy's schoolwork deteriorated, and she stopped spending time with her friends at school. Instead of playing with friends, she comes home after school, watches TV, and goes to sleep early. Her mother noticed that she is not interested in food and that she stopped participating in activities she previously enjoyed (e.g., playing computer games and having friends over to play). She complains of headaches, stomachaches, and being tired. Her 18-year-old cousin recently was admitted to the hospital following a suicide attempt.

The most common of the mood disorders are major depression, minor depression, and brief recurrent depression. At any particular time, it is estimated that 15% of children and adolescents have some depressive symptoms, and between 3% and 5% meet the criteria for major depression.[10] In young children, depression reportedly is more common in boys. This changes in adolescence, and by the age of 14 years, twice as many girls as boys will have depressive disorders. Wendy's presentation is consistent with major depression, with the common symptoms of irritability and physical (somatic) complaints such as headaches and stomachaches. Other symptoms are anxiety and social withdrawal. In adolescents, the symptoms of depression are more consistent with those reported by adults. Adolescents will experience thoughts of suicide (suicidal ideation), guilt, feelings of worthlessness and shame, and changes in sleep patterns and appetite.

CLINICAL *Pearl*

Never be reluctant to ask the child or adolescent in a straightforward manner, "Are you thinking about hurting yourself?". If the answer is affirmative, ask whether he or she has a plan and, if so, the details of the plan. It is important that you ask these questions even at the risk for upsetting the child. If asked directly, a child will be more likely to respond honestly, and you can take the necessary steps to make him or her safe.

Wendy's depressive symptoms are typical. She is experiencing an overall state of unhappiness, she is dissatisfied with her life, feels pessimistic, and has lost interest and pleasure in almost all her activities.[28] The objective signs of depression are changes in weight (either gain or loss); inability to sleep or excessive sleeping; feeling tired; slowed motor activity; and agitation. Low self-esteem, poor body image, and feelings of lack of personal control, as well as phobias, substance abuse, sexual promiscuity, and absences from school, are also associated with depression.

CLINICAL *Pearl*

Depression can lead to aggressive feelings toward others, including homicidal thoughts. Talking about suicide with adolescents needs to include questions about whether the teen has a desire to hurt other people, such as parents or peers at school. Depression is often an underlying problem in many children who commit violent crimes against family members, teachers, or peers.

The multidimensional model in Figure 14-1 is useful to understand depression. No single known cause for depression exists. However, biological, sociocultural, social, and psychological factors increase the likelihood of depression. Biological factors include chronic childhood illnesses (e.g., diabetes) and a family history of depression, especially in the mother. Psychosocial and cultural factors that increase the risk for depression are physical, emotional, and sexual abuse; neglect; lack of affection and support; and stress caused by factors such as poverty.[32] The presence of other mental health disorders (e.g., ADHD, learning disabilities, or eating disorders) also increases the risk for depression. Other negative events such as parents' divorce, bullying, or the death of a family member can also increase the risk.

OT practitioners need to be aware of functional difficulties associated with depression, including poor concentration, not completing tasks, learning difficulties, and aggressiveness toward others. Because children and adolescents experience apathy and fatigue, they may neglect basic ADLs such as personal hygiene and grooming. When the child or adolescent loses interest and stops participating in previously enjoyed group activities, the ensuing social isolation impairs social development and development of a positive sense of identity.[3,11]

> ## CLINICAL *Pearl*
>
> Depression and depressive symptoms are common and cause occupational performance deficits. Even children and adolescents with subclinical symptoms of depression (i.e., insufficient to meet the criteria for diagnosis) have significant difficulties.

OT practitioners need to be able to assess suicide risk because it is the third leading cause of death among 15 to 19 year olds and the fourth leading cause of death among the 10- to 14-year-old age group.[1] A child or adolescent expressing suicidal thoughts or exhibiting a preoccupation with death should receive professional psychiatric help immediately and be monitored closely. Figure 14-8 provides a checklist of suicidal risk signals. The OT practitioner should immediately report signs of self-mutilating behavior or suicidal ideation to the parents and/or to a supervisor or other appropriate team member (e.g., nurse, psychologist, or mental health counselor) and document this on the child's chart. Supervision and a safe environment (e.g., no access to medications and supervision of use of tools) is the best protocol when working with children who are depressed.

A child or adolescent who has recently started therapy with antidepressants can have an increased risk for suicide. The therapeutic response to a widely used antidepressant medication (e.g., an SSRI such as Prozac or Zoloft) usually takes 2 to 3 weeks before a marked improvement in mood occurs. However, ironically, the gradual improvement in energy and mood due to the medication may actually push the child or adolescent who is still depressed to act on his or her suicide thoughts. Therefore the OT practitioner should be suspicious of sudden elation or energy in a child or adolescent diagnosed with depression. This sudden unexplained improvement is known as a "flight into health" and can signify that the decision to end one's life has been made. Other warning signs of impending suicide include getting organized, subtle good-bye gestures, and giving away personal items.

Bipolar Disorder

Bipolar disorder in children and adolescents has received more attention in the past decade and presents with symptoms similar to ADHD, anxiety disorders, childhood psychosis, and delinquency. Although its prevalence in adolescents is about 1% to 1.5% of the population in the United States, its incidence in younger children is unknown. The characteristics of this disorder are the two extremes of mood: depression and mania. A child or adolescent with **bipolar disorder** will experience symptoms of major depression alternating with episodes of mania or hypomania (milder form of mania) characterized by excessive elation and energy, aggressive and disruptive behaviors, low frustration tolerance, and impulsive behavior. In both states, children may experience delusions, which are irrational beliefs.

Although a strong genetic predisposition and usually a family history are present, the onset of bipolar disorder is multidimensional and thus requires a comprehensive treatment approach. This disorder interferes significantly with development, and although it can be managed with mood stabilizing medication, it remains a lifetime condition. The OT practitioner works with the health care team to minimize the effects of the disorder on functional abilities in occupation. The OT practitioner can also assist with diagnosis by paying attention to children who are "out of control," irritable, excitable, or have mood swings (e.g., exhibiting extreme energy and elation at one time and at other times being irritable, short tempered, sad or confused, or unable to concentrate). During manic episodes, adolescents with bipolar disorder might describe themselves being frightened because they feel "out of control," or they might not understand that a problem exists because they are feeling "high on life." They may be impulsive, take excessive risks, or have an increased interest in sex. Younger children do not always have the language to describe their emotions and instead will say that they are bored, angry, or restless; hate school; or do not like the friends they previously did. The children may be defiant, show poor judgment, or talk excessively. Parents may report that their children experience sleeplessness and that they see changes in weight, appetite, and social activities. The cyclic pattern, even when the positive and negative mood swings are not extreme, is an important indicator of bipolar disorder. The associated functional problems include poor school performance, few social relationships, disorganization, difficulty regulating behavior, and poorer long-term outcome. Early recognition and intervention are essential.

SCHIZOPHRENIA SPECTRUM AND OTHER PSYCHOTIC DISORDERS

Schizophrenia and other psychotic disorders are characterized by abnormalities in one or more domains: delusions, hallucinations, disorganized thinking (speech),

Suicidal Risk Signals

If you can answer "Yes" to any of the following questions about a young person, they may be thinking about suicide. Questions highlighted in bold are particularly concerning and require follow-up from a mental health professional. Be sure to document your concerns and the professionals you notified (e.g., parents, school nurse, or counselor, or teacher). Be sure that the child or adolescent is in a safe supervised situation.

Yes **No**

☐ ☐ **Depression:**
— — Does this child/adolescent appear sad, irritable, or worthless?
— — Is this child/adolescent exhibiting symptoms of depression?
(Symptoms of depression include insomnia, anorexia, withdrawn from others, decreased ability to concentrate, and fatigue.)
— — Is the child/adolescent acting out or abusing alcohol or drugs?
(Depression can be masked by substance abuse, aggressive or risk-taking behavior.)

☐ ☐ **Preoccupation with death and dying:**
— — Has this child/adolescent been drawing pictures or writing poems or stories about death and suicide?

☐ ☐ **Talking about suicide:**
— — Has this child/adolescent been expressing a desire to die?
— — Has this child/adolescent been making suicidal threats?
— — Has this child/adolescent been listening to music with negative themes?
— — Has this child/adolescent been joking about suicide?
— — Does this child/adolescent have a plan of how he or she would carry out suicide?

☐ ☐ **Hopelessness about the future:**
— — Can this child/adolescent tell you about plans for the next week or next month?
— — Has this child/adolescent been "putting affairs in order?"
— — Has this child/adolescent given away special possessions or written a will?

☐ ☐ **Changes in life situation:**
— — Have there been any major recent changes such as death of a parent, separation or divorce of parents, school problems, or boyfriend or girlfriend problems?

☐ ☐ **Previous suicide attempts:**
— — Has this child/adolescent previously attempted to commit suicide?
— — Is there evidence of self-injurious behavior (e.g., scratches, cutting)

☐ ☐ **Lack of support from family and friends:**
— — Has this child/adolescent expressed feeling unloved or unwanted?

☐ ☐ **Excessive use of drugs or alcohol:**
— — Has this child/adolescent begun or increased use of substances?

☐ ☐ **Risk-taking behavior:**
— — Does this person engage in dangerous behavior, such as driving too fast or walking in the middle of the road rather than on the sidewalk?

FIGURE 14-8 Suicide risk signals. (From Hafen, B. Q., & Frandsen, K. J. (1984). *Youth suicide: depression and loneliness.* Evergreen, CO: Cordillera; Hermes, P. (1987). *A time to listen: preventing youth suicide.* San Diego: Harcourt Brace Jovanovich.)

grossly disorganized motor behavior, and/or negative symptoms such as decreased emotional expression.[3] Symptoms include the following:

- Delusions: fixed beliefs that do not change irrespective of conflicting evidence. Delusions may be persecutory, referential, grandiose, erotomanic, nihilistic or somatic.[3]

- Hallucinations: vivid and clear perceptions of experiences without an external stimulus.[3]
- Disorganized speech: speech that involves switching topics or answering unrelated questions.[3]
- Disorganized motor behavior: behavior manifests itself in a variety of ways from unpredictable agitation to silliness.[3]

Brief psychotic disorder is a sudden onset (within 2 weeks) of positive psychotic symptoms.[3] Schizophrenia with a childhood or adolescent onset typically involves avolition or reduced drive to actively engage in daily occupations.[3] **Schizophrenia spectrum** is a serious chronic condition that is difficult to diagnose and has a significant genetic predisposition. Poor school performance and developmental delays in speech and motor skills associated with schizophrenia are not due to intellectual disability.[21] It can present with symptoms of severely disturbed behavior similar to autism. It is more common in boys and can develop as early as 5 or 6 years of age.[3,27] Schizophrenia of the disorganized type is seen most commonly in males in their late adolescence or early adulthood.

Early recognition of severe mental illness and intervention are critical for long-term outcome. Before the first acute psychotic episode, an early stage of schizophrenia when the symptoms begin to develop occurs. In this prodromal stage, children and adolescents may begin to withdraw from activities and social contacts because of difficulty functioning in groups such as the classroom or group social settings. They may self-medicate with alcohol or illegal drugs, which can trigger the onset of their schizophrenia.

An acute psychotic state at the onset of schizophrenia is characterized by positive symptoms; extremely disorganized thinking, behaviors, and speech (e.g., rapid or incomprehensible speech); perceptual disturbances (e.g., hallucinations); and thought disturbances (e.g., delusions). Hallucinations involve the senses, and in children they are usually simple; nevertheless, they can be frightening. For example, auditory hallucinations involve hearing voices, which are often critical or instruct the adolescent to harm self or others, whereas visual hallucinations involve seeing changes in faces, seeing distortions of light, or seeing people who are not there. A sign of hallucinations can be the expression of emotions that do not match the situation, such as giggling without being able to explain the reason. Delusions in children can present as "magical thinking."

With the onset of schizophrenia, there is a marked deterioration in function (i.e., occupational performance). The psychotic episode and the positive symptoms typically resolve with medication, but the child or adolescent is likely to continue to have negative symptoms of schizophrenia, which are debilitating, as they affect the ability to communicate and to interact socially and interfere with motivation to engage in everyday activities. The negative symptoms of schizophrenia include lethargy, blunted affect (i.e., the lack of visible emotional expression in relation to a situation), poor skills in understanding social cues and body language, disorganized thinking, poor concentration, and apathy.

Negative symptoms are highly correlated with poor functioning and outcome in adulthood because they affect learning and interfere with normal development necessary to transition from adolescence to adulthood.[3,27] Therefore the focus of occupational therapy is age-related skill development, especially social and life skills. This is provided within a multidisciplinary team, using groups and individual therapy based on one of the following frames of reference: psychiatric rehabilitation, MOHO, cognitive disability, psychoeducation, or illness recovery and management (see Table 14-2).

FEEDING AND EATING DISORDERS

Feeding and eating disorders occur primarily in later childhood, adolescence, and early adulthood. If untreated, dysfunctional eating behaviors result in serious physical health problems and even death.[3] For example, approximately 10% of adolescents with anorexia nervosa will die of starvation or electrolyte imbalance.[3]

The most common eating disorders are anorexia nervosa (AN) and bulimia nervosa (BN); other eating disorders are binge eating, and body dysmorphic disorder. Although they present more in girls, the clinical presentation for girls and boys is similar across all eating disorders. Occupational performance is generally unaffected in children and adolescents with eating disorders. They perform well in school and work settings, and ADLs are primarily intact, except for eating, food-related behaviors, and exercise routines. Social participation becomes impaired with the duration of the disorder as a preoccupation with weight and fear of rejection interferes with social relationships and participation in age-related activities. Fearing others will identify their eating disorder or finding eating with others stressful, children and adolescents may spend their leisure time on weight-reducing activities and may avoid leisure situations that involve food.[11,24]

Adolescents with eating disorders have low self-esteem; their sense of worth has an externalized component based on their concerns of how other people judge them and their appearance and their overall self-evaluation is influenced by how they perceive their bodies and body shapes.

Anorexia Nervosa

CASE *Study*

Jen is a 13-year-old high school junior. She has very good grades, is popular, and participates in extracurricular activities such as gymnastics and cheerleading. Despite her outward appearance, she exhibits poor self-esteem and is somewhat anxious. During the past 6 months, her parents have become worried about her health. They notice that Jen skips meals and is very particular about what she eats. She has lost weight and looks thin. She wears baggy clothes and loose tops with sleeves.

Despite her weight loss, Jen thinks she looks fat when she looks at herself in the mirror. She has always been critical of her body, but she started dieting 6 months ago to make the varsity gymnastics squad. In addition to her cheerleading and gymnastics practices, she does aerobic exercises at least 3 hours a day. Jen has not menstruated in more than 4 months and takes laxatives every day.

The two types of AN are restrictive and binge eating with purging. Jen has the characteristics of the restrictive type of AN. She limits her food intake, uses activity and exercise to control her weight, and shows a distorted perception of her body.

AN typically develops in early adolescence (around 13 years of age).[22] However, it can present in younger children or older adolescents and adults. AN is characterized by an intense fear of being overweight, although most often weight for age and height is well below the average. The condition is characterized by active pursuit of thinness, inability to realistically perceive the risks of weight, and self-denial of weight loss.[3,22] When confronted by parents or concerned friends, adolescents with AN deny or minimize the severity of the problem and resist treatment efforts. They have a distorted body image and see themselves as overweight in all or some body parts regardless of how thin or emaciated they are. Jen is critical of her body and genuinely sees herself as fat when looking in a mirror. The patterns of behavior associated with AN include binging on food, vigorous exercising, use of laxatives and diuretics, and purging (self-induced vomiting). The later defines AN of the binge eating purging type. Adolescents with AN are preoccupied with food, and they can enjoy preparing meals for others, although they eat little of the food themselves.[3] See Figure 14-9.

Daily food consumption may consist of fat-free yogurt and several diet drinks, and as a result AN can lead to serious medical problems associated with malnutrition. These include cessation of menstruation (amenorrhea), hypothermia (decreased body temperature), and cardiovascular impairments (e.g., bradycardia, hypotension, and arrhythmia). Decreased renal function can be impaired, leading to electrolyte imbalance. Vomiting of stomach acid can cause dental erosion, and osteoporosis may result from the insufficient intake of calcium and estrogen-containing foods.

Therapeutic interventions for eating disorders include medication, individual counseling, family therapy, and group programs, some of which are based on cognitive-behavioral or cognitive models. Intervention aims to address both dysfunctional eating behaviors and their

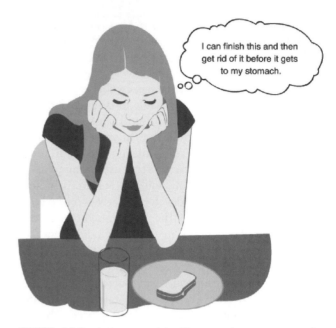

I can finish this and then get rid of it before it gets to my stomach.

FIGURE 14-9 A teenage girl with anorexia nervosa worries constantly about food and her weight.

associated psychological problems.[22] Hospitalization may be necessary to stabilize the medical condition when weight loss is severe. Short-term success of therapy is reported to be as high as 76%; however, long-term recovery rates are much lower.[22]

CLINICAL *Pearl*

In cooking and eating activities with clients who have eating disorders, the OT practitioner needs to be aware of problems with food that these children or adolescents may have. They may choose to hide food or purge after eating. Be aware of a teen who uses the restroom during or shortly after eating. Individuals with AN may enjoy cooking. It may be a way to feel in control of situations involving food; they do not perceive any pressure to eat, as it may not be a requirement for being involved in a cooking group.

Bulimia Nervosa

CASE *Study*

Kim, a high school sophomore, is slightly overweight. She seldom says anything positive about herself and lacks confidence when interacting in social groups. Her friends are concerned about her. They noticed that she vomits in the school bathroom immediately after lunch. Kim buys cookies and other junk food and hides them. Sometimes she fasts, but when she is alone, she eats a lot of food rapidly, cramming it into her mouth in big chunks. Immediately after she has eaten excessively, she is overwhelmed with guilt and feels disgusted with herself. In an attempt to feel better, she makes herself vomit. Recently the dental hygienist noted enamel erosion on her teeth and told her that frequent vomiting will cause this to happen.

Kim has the primary characteristics of BN. Adolescents with BN tend to have normal to above-average weight for their height and are aware that their eating patterns are abnormal.[22] For example, Kim has episodes of binge eating (e.g., eating larger than normal amounts of food, usually very rapidly) and feels she is unable to control how much she eats during these binges. Later, she becomes anxious about gaining weight and feels disgusted with herself for binging. Therefore her binge eating is combined with drastic steps to lose weight by using laxatives, fasting, excessive exercise, and self-induced vomiting.[22] Unlike adolescents with AN, those with BN do not purge on a regular basis.

Bulimia nervosa (BN) shares many of the psychosocial symptoms characteristic of AN; feelings of inadequacy, low self-worth, poor body image, and depression. The adolescent's sense of emptiness and loneliness or the overwhelming anxiety prompts eating excessive amounts of food, usually alone. This leads to feelings of anxiety, shame, guilt, and fear. Purging temporarily eases these feelings and has a calming effect. As a result, the pattern of eating and purging becomes a way to regulate mood and cope with emotions. Adolescents with BN usually want to stop the pattern of binging and weight loss behaviors but feel unable to change it.

Pica Disorder

Pica is characterized by the eating nonfood and non-nutritive substances for more than 1 month. A child diagnosed as having a pica disorder is older than 2 years of age to rule out developmentally appropriate mouthing of objects (Figure 14-10). A child who is developmentally delayed, lacks supervision, or is neglected is more likely to develop a pica disorder. Pica disorders are more prevalent and severe in children with intellectual disabilities.

CASE *Study*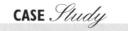

Lamika has a moderate intellectual disability. While working with the OT practitioner, she eats play dough and theraputty during weekly OT interventions. Because of the practitioner's concerns about this pica behavior she decides to make homemade edible play dough to decrease the risk for gastrointestinal problems.

Rumination Disorder

A child with a rumination disorder regurgitates food repetitively. Once the food is regurgitated, it may be re-chewed, swallowed, or spit out. These behaviors occur typically daily and may result in significant weight loss

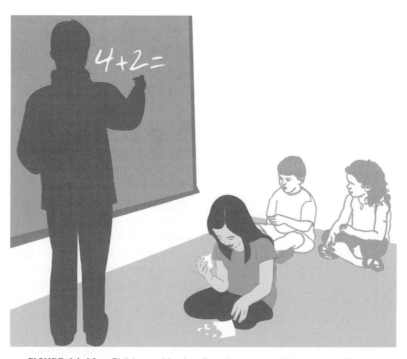

FIGURE 14-10 Children with pica disorder may eat little scraps of paper.

and/or malnutrition. The onset of a rumination disorder is from infancy throughout adulthood.

ELIMINATION DISORDERS

Elimination disorders are conditions that involve the voluntary or involuntary repeated voiding of urine or feces into inappropriate places. The diagnosis of an elimination disorder is based on chronologic as well as developmental age. The minimum chronologic and equivalent developmental age is 4 (encopresis) to 5 (enuresis) years.

Enuresis

CASE *Study*

Jacob

Jacob is a 6-year-old first-grade boy. He was recently invited to an overnight birthday camp-out party. On the Friday morning of the sleep over, Jacob fakes a stomachache so that he will not have to go to school. His mother calls the friend's mother to let her know that Jacob is sick and will not be spending the night for her son's party. Later during the day, his mother takes Jacob for a follow-up appointment with his clinical psychologist to discuss his bed-wetting behaviors while he sleeps. Jacob has recently been diagnosed as having enuresis.

Aisha

Aisha recently was removed from her mother and placed in emergency foster care. She was enrolled in the school of residency near the group home in which she was placed. In her first-grade classroom when she became frustrated she would urinate through her clothes onto the floor. After 4 weeks in the group home she was moved to a foster home that had a different school of residency. Aisha began urinating not only in her home classroom but also during OT sessions. The attending OT practitioner (both schools) discussed the increased inappropriate behaviors with the team leader, who scheduled a special review meeting. During the special review team meeting, it was decided that the following interventions would be implemented:
- Social stories at home and during OT and speech therapy sessions (at least three times per week)
- Preferred activity reward throughout her school day as a part of a positive behavior intervention plan
- Increased opportunities to go to the restroom throughout the school day
- Moving the entire class to a classroom with a restroom.

Enuresis is characterized by repeated elimination of urine involuntarily or intentionally in inappropriate places. To diagnose a child with enuresis, there must be at least

two occurrences per week for at least 3 months and they must result in distress with impairment in active engagement in daily occupations. For Jacob, the enuresis is involuntary and is interfering with his attending school and participating with his preferred peers. For Aisha, the enuresis is intentional and a means of releasing anxiety.

Encopresis

CASE *Study*

Erick is a 5-year-old kindergartener who is having difficulty at school. For the past 4 months Erick has bowel movements in his pants during recess. Each time this happened Erick's mother went to his school with a change of clothes and helped her son clean himself and change his clothes. Because of the effect on both Erick and his mother, the school nurse recommended that he be seen by his pediatrician. During the most recent doctor's visit, Erick was referred to a clinical psychologist for evaluation of the possibility that Erick has encopresis.

Encopresis is characterized by repeated elimination of feces in inappropriate places. To diagnose a child with encopresis, there must be at least one occurrence each month for least 3 months. The behavior cannot be a result of a physiologic response to a substance such as a laxative. Most often the behavior is involuntary; however, when it is intentional, it is typically associated with a psychological reason (such as anxiety or opposition).

> **CLINICAL** *Pearl*
>
> If possible, the best time to give a child a laxative is on a Saturday morning so that the result of the substance does not interfere with participation in school.

SLEEP–WAKE DISORDERS

See Chapter 19 for additional information relative to OT interventions for sleep/rest issues. OT practitioners examine the roles and routines of infants, children, and adolescents. Sleep and rest is considered an occupation.[2] Infants engage in sleep and wake routines that may be established by caregivers. Determining the infant's routines and cycles allows the OT practitioner to provide consultation regarding techniques to establish healthy routines that fit within the family system.[20] Toddlers engage in more of the routine and may benefit from structured nap and bedtime routines. Identifying factors that may influence sleep and wake routines allows the OT practitioner to provide effective intervention. Collaborating with families is necessary when addressing sleep and wake routines.

The *DSM-V* defines **sleep-wake disorders** as conditions in which an individual has poor quality, timing, and amount of sleep.[3] Sleep–wake disorders result in poor performance of daily occupations resulting in daytime distress. Depression, anxiety, and cognitive changes are often associated with sleep–wake disorders.

Insomnia

CASE *Study*

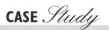

Jeannie has been waking up between 3:30 and 4 a.m. for the past 8 months. Although she does not go to the bus stop until 7:45 a.m. she cannot seem to go back to sleep until her alarm rings at 5:50 a.m. Jeannie is experiencing late insomnia.

Insomnia is characterized by difficulty going to sleep or staying asleep. Because of the lack of quantity and quality of sleep, the individual experiences distress that affects the ability to successfully engage in social, occupational, and educational activities. The disruption of sleep typically causes behavioral manifestations such as inattentiveness or negative disposition. Insomnia can occur at different times of the sleep cycle (i.e., initial, middle, late). Initial insomnia involves difficulty falling/going to sleep. With middle insomnia, the individual wakes up frequently for prolonged awakenings throughout the night. In late insomnia, the individual has an early awakening and cannot go back to sleep.

Breathing-Related Sleep Disorders

Breathing-related sleep disorders frequently diagnosed in children and adolescents are obstructive sleep apnea-hypopnea syndrome (OSAHS) and sleep-related hypoventilation. Children who experience these disorders may be tired during the day. They may require medical interventions to assist them in sleeping through the night.

Obstructive Sleep Apnea-Hypopnea Syndrome

OSAHS is characterized by repeated episodes of obstruction of the pharyngeal airway.[3] It is the most common breathing-related sleep disorder. The child may experience apnea (absence of airflow) or hypopnea (two missed breaths in children). Obstructive sleep hypopnea occurs in 1% to 2% of children.

CASE *Study*

Velocity is a 3-year-old preschooler who has a medical diagnosis of Down syndrome. She was recently hospitalized to have a sleep study. Upon the analysis of her sleep study the medical team determined that Velocity required a series of surgical procedures to improve her sleep–wake disorder. During the next 12 months Velocity will have her adenoids surgically removed and portions of her middle tongue excised. Before and after each surgical procedure, Velocity will be seen in the hospital's pediatric outpatient clinic weekly. Kayla who is a certified occupational therapist will be a part of the medical team (see Chapter 3 on the medical system) who will provide services to Velocity and her family. Velocity has an obstructive sleep apnea hypopnea syndrome.

Sleep-Related Hypoventilation

Sleep-related hypoventilation in children typically exists comorbidly as a result of another medical condition such as muscular dystrophy, obesity, and cervical spinal cord injuries.[3]

CASE *Study*

Alex is an extremely obese 7-year-old. His parents have begun to notice that he has episodes of shallow breathing throughout the night. He complained to his parents that he wakes up often throughout the night. In the mornings he has a headache before going to school. During the past month, his teacher commented that he shows signs of excessive sleepiness throughout the school day. Alex had a sleep study (polysomnography), which revealed that Alex has sleep-related hypoventilation. Alex and his family have decided that reducing his weight will reduce this and other potential health conditions associated with obesity (see Chapter 15). His elementary school has an after-school program that focuses on proper diet and exercise. The program was designed and implemented by OTA students who attend a local community college. The OTA faculty supervises the students. In addition to planned activities for 2 hours three times a week. There are parent educational and support meetings each month in the evenings. The second-year nursing students come to the program monthly to monitor and record height, weight, blood pressure, pulse, breaths per minute resting and then after an aerobic activity led by the OTA students. This data, in addition to the OTA students' data, are used to monitor individual progress. Within 6 weeks Alex lost 4 pounds and was able to actively engage in an aerobic activity from 4 to 7 consecutive minutes.

Parasomnias

Parasomnias are characterized by abnormal behavioral, experiential or physiologic events that occur while sleeping. Examples of the types of behaviors that can occur when an individual has a parasomnia disorder include sleepwalking, sleep terrors, nightmares, and restless legs. Sleepwalking is rising from bed and walking about being nonresponsive. A sleep terror involves an abrupt awakening with signs of autonomic arousal.

SUBSTANCE-RELATED AND ADDICTIVE DISORDERS

The *DSM-V* defines **substance-related and addictive disorders** as the misuse of drugs, toxins, and medications.[3] The terms *substance abuse* and *substance dependence* describe the severity of substance use. Substance abuse classifies a pattern of use that results in adverse consequences, such as drinking alcohol and driving, or absence from school due to use of drugs or alcohol, or relationship difficulties related to drug use. *Addiction* is a term associated with substance-related disorders and refers to the intense physiologic and psychological craving for the substance being abused.[23] The terms dependence and addiction are essentially synonymous. Substance dependence classifies substance use that involves physical dependency on a substance (e.g., alcohol, cocaine, and other street drugs or prescription medications). In substance dependence, there is a pattern of continued use despite serious cognitive, behavioral, and physiologic symptoms and that has seven characteristics/symptoms.[3] At least three of the seven symptoms of the following must be present for a diagnosis of substance dependence:[3]

1. The development of tolerance (the need to use larger amounts of the substance to obtain the desired effect)
2. Unpleasant withdrawal symptoms when use is decreased or stopped
3. Use of the substance in increasing amounts or for increasingly longer periods of time
4. A desire to stop as well as failed attempts to stop using the substance
5. Excessive time spent in acquiring, using, and recovering from the substance
6. Neglect and a decline in occupational performance (e.g., work, leisure, ADLs)
7. Continued use despite the presence of problems caused by the substance

Children and adolescents may abuse substances such as alcohol, amphetamines (uppers), cannabis (marijuana), hallucinogens (e.g., ecstasy and other club drugs, such as GHB and LSD), opioids (e.g., heroin, cocaine), phencyclidines (e.g., PCP, angel dust), sedatives, hypnotics, anxiolytics (e.g., Valium, Librium), steroids, and inhalants (e.g., nitrous oxide, acetone). Young people with substance dependence and abuse disorders can spend much of their time acquiring, using, and recovering from the substance.[23] As their dependence on and need for a

drug grow, adolescents may become involved in illegal activities that often place them at further risk for harm (e.g., prostitution or selling drugs). Using and acquiring drugs has significant health risks, and children and adolescents entering treatment programs for substance dependence or abuse often have poor physical health and sometimes contract life-threatening conditions such as HIV or hepatitis from sharing needles. A strong association exists between alcohol use and suicide.

The extensive resources that are available identify specialized interventions for young people with substance abuse and dependence problems. There are residential programs that combine intensive therapy with the development of life skills and vocational skills and promote engaging in healthy activities. This chapter highlights one form of substance abuse: the use of inhalants, which is more common in children and adolescents than in adults, as these substances are easily accessible at relatively low costs.

Inhalant-Related Disorder

CASE *Study*

Michael, a 15-year-old high school student, was found semiconscious in a local park and was hospitalized. In the preceding 6 months, Michael's parents noticed changes in his behavior. He appeared "spaced out and distracted and became disinterested in his personal hygiene." They suspected that he and his friends were drinking and smoking. More recently, his mother noticed a rash around his nose and mouth; he became less outgoing and avoided family activities. Furthermore, Michael failed two subjects last semester. He no longer played basketball with neighborhood boys after school and on the weekends; instead, he now spent his time "just hanging." Although he received a generous allowance, he no longer seemed to have money. Michael's admission to the hospital was the result of respiratory complications from inhalant use. His level of use may have already caused permanent brain damage.

The highest rates of inhalant use are among adolescents and children who live at or below the poverty level, and the majority of emergency consultations for inhalant-related problems are males.[3] Users refer to inhaling toxic substances as "huffing" or "sniffing." Substances commonly inhaled include gasoline, nail polish remover, solvent-based glue, paint thinner, spray paint, dry erasers and permanent markers, correction fluids, and aerosol propellants. Inhalant abuse leaves a common telltale rash around the nose and mouth and sometimes a runny nose, as noticed by Michael's mother. A cloth soaked in fluid inhalants (e.g., gasoline and paint thinner) is held over the mouth and nose and inhaled. This leaves a smell of paint or solvent on the teen's clothes, whereas aerosol substances are sprayed into a paper or plastic bag and inhaled with the bag over the mouth and nose.

The inhalant is rapidly absorbed into the bloodstream to create an almost immediate, intense "high." Psychotic experiences including auditory, visual, and tactile hallucinations (sensory perceptions incompatible with reality, such as the feeling of insects crawling beneath the skin) and delusions (beliefs incompatible with reality, such as believing parents are poisoning them) are common. Vomiting, dizziness, generalized weakness, and abdominal pains and/or nausea are other symptoms of inhalant abuse.[3] The chronic use of inhalants can cause anxiety, depression, and permanent and occasionally lethal respiratory, cardiac, kidney, and liver problems.[3] Whatever the inhalant, its frequent use leads to significant impairment in all areas of occupational performance. Adolescent inhalant users neglect self-care, and decreased attendance and performance in school or work can occur. Changes in leisure interests such as dropping out of school activities and spending more time partying or participating in aimless activities, as with Michael's habit of "just hanging," is typical. Socially, the adolescent may stop spending time with friends who do not use substances and will develop relationships with those peers who do. In severe cases, irreversible brain damage with cognitive deficits may occur, causing long-term disability.

IMPLICATIONS FOR OCCUPATIONAL PERFORMANCE

Children and adolescents with psychosocial or behavioral disorders experience deficits in occupations (ADLs, sleep/rest, IADLs, work, education, social participation, and play/leisure).[2] OT practitioners examine performance patterns (i.e., habits, routines, and roles) associated with the occupational performance.[2,20] For example, does the child or teen engage in self-care, attend school regularly, and participate in extracurricular activities with peers? The examination of performance patterns is combined with analysis of performance skills (i.e., motor, processing, and social interaction). For example, basic sharing, following rules, and peer communication skills are considered. Table 14-3 describes the effect of specific disorders on occupational performance, which is dependent on intact client factors, which are divided into mental (global and specific), neuromusculoskeletal, sensory, and systemic (i.e., cardiovascular, hematologic, immunologic, and respiratory) functions.[2]

The OT practitioner also considers the influence of context on performance. For example, with whom does the child or adolescent play? Do they feel safe at home and school or in other environments? Are the parents supportive physically as well as emotionally? In addition to considering the physical and social contexts, it is vital to bear in mind the child and family's cultural background. For example, there are differences in individual level of comfort with therapy and school. Differences in culture and experience may mean practitioners having to spend extra time explaining and connecting with parents so that they feel more comfortable participating with their children in the therapy settings and following recommendations. For example, parents who themselves did not have positive school experiences or did not attend school in the United States may be tentative in expressing their needs or knowing what is expected of them and their child. By demonstrating a willingness to listen and taking time for explanations, OT practitioners can help bridge cultural differences and reduce the anxiety of families. Furthermore, by creating an open and trusting relationship, practitioners may advocate for the children and their families in accessing needed resources and services. The goal is that with experience and increased knowledge, parents will become their child's advocate.

Although OT practitioners examine all the client factors required to perform occupations, those working with children and teens experiencing psychosocial or mental health disorders pay close attention to global and specific mental functions. Global mental functions refer to consciousness, orientation, sleep, temperament and personality, and energy and drive.[2] Specific mental functions refer to attention, memory, perception, thought, higher-level cognition, the mental functions of language, calculation, mental functions of sequencing complex movements, psychomotor ability, emotion, and experiences of self and time.[2]

Children with global mental function impairments may present with low self-esteem because of frequent failure or frustration. They may have difficulty expressing themselves through language and may show lability of emotions (frequent fluctuations in mood), which typically affects their social participation. Specific mental functions may be manifested as difficulties with memory needed for academic and ADL tasks. Similarly, specific mental functions are required for organization (e.g., dressing and other ADLs). Children with these impairments may also show poor attention to detail, resulting in errors in academic work.

The OT practitioner should analyze the child's ability to perform the occupation, paying careful attention to the global and specific mental functions that may be interfering with the child's ability to be successful. On the basis of a frame of reference, the OT practitioner should design remedial, developmental, and compensatory interventions for occupational performance problems.

TABLE 14-3

Impact of Selected Mental Disorders on Occupational Performance

PSYCHOSOCIAL DISORDER	FUNCTIONING IN ACTIVITIES OF DAILY LIVING/INSTRUMENTAL ACTIVITIES OF DAILY LIVING	SCHOOL AND WORK FUNCTIONING	PLAY AND LEISURE FUNCTIONING	SOCIAL FUNCTIONING
DISRUPTIVE BEHAVIOR DISORDERS				
Attention deficit disorder	Inattention to detail	Tardiness, absence, and neglect of school or work assignments and homework	Poor concentration, inattention, and disorganization	Inability to read social cues
ADHD	Refuses to comply with rules	Poor concentration, inattention, and disorganization	Difficulty with activity completion	Aggressive behavior toward others
Conduct disorder	Difficulty following directions	Restless and off-task behaviors	Lack of personal responsibility	Destruction of others' property, deceitfulness, and lack of remorse and guilt
ODD	Disorganization and forgetfulness	Education potentially disrupted when suspension results from defiant behavior at school or work (e.g., stealing, bullying)	Engaging in reckless activities (e.g., joining gangs) Lack of constructive leisure activities Physically aggressive or bullying Tendency to defy rules of games or sports Solitary leisure activities may not be affected	Annoys others by being argumentative, losing temper, and blaming others for own mistakes
Learning disorders	Seldom has problems with ADL skills, IADL skills may be disrupted by poor academic skills, disorganization, and lack of ability to maintain routines	Specific disorder deficits (e.g., reading, writing, math) interfere with school or work performance Low frustration tolerance Poor self-efficacy in performance Additional time required for academic and work activities	Associated poor self-esteem Avoidance of sophisticated games dependent on scholastic abilities due to poor self-efficacy	Associated poor self-esteem Additional time required for academic work may interfere with social activities Feelings of low self-efficacy may result in avoidance of new social situations
TIC DISORDERS				
Tourette's syndrome	Motor tics: may interfere with movement during ADL/IADL Vocal tics: may avoid public places due to social stigma Vocal and motor tics: may interfere with safety because of distraction and unexpected movement	Motor and vocal tics interfere with concentration, visual scanning, writing, and communication Motor and vocal tics interfere with participation in group learning activities Difficulty finding an accepting employment/school setting	Avoidance by others Motor tics interfering with physical abilities Vocal and motor tics may interfere with safety because of distraction and expected movement Leisure activities that are engrossing and performed alone often unimpaired; in fact, the tics may decrease or disappear	Avoidance by adults and children Socially disruptive nature Embarrassment (self-imposed social withdrawal)

ANXIETY DISORDERS

Separation anxiety disorder	Anxiety inhibiting beginning ADLs and IADLs	Anxiety inhibiting beginning tasks	Separation anxiety in attending group activities, after school activities, or play groups	Limiting relationships to significant and familiar persons
Generalized anxiety disorder	Fear of failure	Separation anxiety in attending school or work	Reluctance to take risks	Poor social self-efficacy
Phobic and social anxiety disorder	Perfectionism	Fear of failure	Anxiety inhibiting the startup of tasks	Fear of embarrassment
Obsessive-compulsive disorder	Phobias Ritualistic behaviors Inability to attain transition Intrusive thoughts	Poor self-efficacy in scholastic activities Perfectionism Phobias Ritualistic behaviors Intrusive thoughts Inability to transition Reluctance to take risks	Fear of failure Poor self-efficacy in new activities Perfectionism Phobias Ritualistic behaviors Intrusive thoughts Inability to transition or join in new groups	Reluctance to take risks Anxiety initiating social interaction Hypervigilance to social cues or oversensitivity and misinterpretation of cues Poor self-esteem Phobias Ritualistic behaviors Intrusive thoughts Lack of spontaneity

MOOD DISORDERS

Major depressive disorder	Decreased energy and apathy Sleep and appetite disturbances Difficulty initiating and completing activities Lethargy (psychomotor retardation) Disinterest in appearance Poor self-esteem and self-loathing Somatic (physical) illness	Decreased energy and apathy Sleep and appetite disturbances Difficulty initiating and completing activities Lethargy (psychomotor retardation) Decreased concentration Difficulty with memory and following directions Difficulty with problem solving Somatic (physical) illness	Decreased energy and apathy Sleep and appetite disturbances Difficulty initiating and completing activities Lethargy (psychomotor retardation) Decreased concentration Inability to derive pleasure Lack of spontaneity Lack of adaptive, imaginative, playfulness	Decreased energy and apathy Difficulty initiating social contact Self-imposed isolation Lethargy (psychomotor retardation) Decreased concentration Inability to derive pleasure Lack of spontaneity Poor self-esteem Slowed cognitive processing Preoccupation with ruminating thoughts

Continued

TABLE 14-3

Impact of Selected Mental Disorders on Occupational Performance—cont'd

PSYCHOSOCIAL DISORDER	FUNCTIONING IN ACTIVITIES OF DAILY LIVING/INSTRUMENTAL ACTIVITIES OF DAILY LIVING	SCHOOL AND WORK FUNCTIONING	PLAY AND LEISURE FUNCTIONING	SOCIAL FUNCTIONING
Schizophrenia	Poor concentration and inattention Disorganized thoughts Preoccupation with internal stimuli (e.g., hallucinations) Lack of awareness of reality Distractibility interferes with completing ADL/IADLs Overall lack of awareness of personal needs	Poor concentration and inattention Disorganized thoughts Preoccupation with internal stimuli (e.g., hallucinations) Lack of awareness of reality Distractibility interferes with school and work activities Tardiness, absence, and neglect of school or work assignments and homework Physical restlessness and agitation Off-task behaviors Gaps in learning Frequent hospitalization interfere with school and work performance	Poor concentration and inattention Disorganized thoughts Preoccupation with internal stimuli (e.g., hallucinations) Lack of awareness of reality Distractibility interferes with play and leisure performance	Poor concentration and inattention Disorganized thoughts making conversations difficult Preoccupation with internal stimuli (e.g., hallucinations) Lack of awareness of reality Tangential thinking Distractibility interferes with developing social relationships Sometimes inappropriate behavior Inattentive to external cues in social situations
EATING DISORDERS				
Anorexia nervosa	ADL and IADL performance generally not affected with the exception of eating	Performance generally not affected unless physical health is compromised	Anorexia nervosa causing a focus on weight-controlling behaviors such as exercise	Avoids social contact for fear of having the disorder discovered
Bulimia nervosa	Inappropriate food consumption	Hospitalization leading to work and school absence	Poor body image	Poor self-esteem
Obesity	Time spent on health-related behaviors (e.g., dieting, laxative use, exercising)	Fatigue Poor concentration	Overweight teens may restrict sport and leisure activities Lack of cardiovascular fitness	Poor self-concept Avoids social events involving food (e.g., going to a restaurant with friends)
SUBSTANCE-RELATED DISORDERS				
Substance-related disorders	Risky behaviors (e.g., use of illegal substances and promiscuity)	Cognitive impairment	Replacing activities with individuals who do not use substances with those associated with substance use	Limits social network to substance-using peers
Inhalant abuse	Apathy about hygiene and appearance Neglect of proper nutrition Time and money spent on substance	Tardiness, absence, and neglect of school or work assignments and homework Poor concentration Substance-induced state Consequence of poor physical health (e.g., fatigue, nausea, drug dependency symptoms) Education potentially disrupted when suspension results from criminal activity and use of illegal substances Unreliable in work setting or stealing from employer to support substance use	Dropping out of extracurricular activities to spend time "hanging out" or partying Money spent on substance Substance use dominates activities	Self-imposed social withdrawal from family

ADL, Activities of daily living; *IADL,* instrumental activities of daily living; *ODD,* Oppositional defiant disorder.

DATA GATHERING AND EVALUATION

The OT practitioner has the ultimate responsibility of interpreting evaluation information. He or she determines the specific areas of evaluation and specific assessment methods and tools. Once an OTA achieves service competency, specific aspects of the information-gathering process may be given to him or her, including review of records, interviews, observations, and structured assessments. Many methods may be used to gather information about the child or adolescent's current level of functioning. OT practitioners may be assigned the task of reviewing the client's records. Inpatient and outpatient settings typically maintain medical records that provide information about the client's age, sex, academic level, family situation, cultural background, diagnosis, medical history, psychiatric history, medications, and current symptoms. In the school setting, educational records are reviewed.

CLINICAL *Pearl*

Observation skills are developed by practice. Take every opportunity to observe typical children in their areas of occupation. This provides a comparison for observing children with special needs.

Interviews with the child or adolescent and family members provide information about the individual's home environment, performance of self-care tasks, relationships with family members, and participation in leisure activities. Other members of the treatment team may provide valuable insight (verbally and as documented in the client's records) into the child's or adolescent's occupational performance. For example, in an inpatient setting, nursing staff can identify the client's specific problems with ADLs. In the school setting, teachers may be able to identify specific problems that interfere with learning and academic performance.

Observation is one of the most important evaluation tools of the OT practitioner. Much can be learned about specific client factor deficits by observing the individual's performance in ADLs, IADLs, work, education, leisure/play, and social participation. For example, by observing the child or adolescent during a classroom activity, the OT practitioner can identify specific problems in concentration, attention span, work skills (e.g., neatness and rate of completion), and behavioral deficits that interfere with learning. Observation of the child or adolescent during recess provides information about social skills, including the amount and appropriateness of interaction with peers and participation in available leisure activities. Observation is also the ongoing data-gathering process for monitoring improvement. The OTA can play a significant role in the evaluation process because he or she is the practitioner who has regular contact with the child or adolescent.

Structured evaluation tools may be used to assess the occupational performance of children and adolescents.[5,27] For example, the Piers-Harris Scale is used to determine a level of self-concept among children.[24] Many of the assessments based on the MOHO[20] provide a structured means of learning about children's and adolescents' psychosocial challenges. The Child Occupational Self-Assessment[19] explores an adolescent's values and how he or she perceives performance and competencies. The Pediatric Volitional Questionnaire[7] provides practitioners with information about what the child finds motivating and the Assessment of Communication and Interaction Skills[18] provides information on the child's interactions and communication with others. The SCOPE[12] provides an overview of the child's volition, habituation, performance capacity, and environment that informs practice and helps the practitioner establish a therapeutic relationship. These assessments may be administered by OTAs and interpreted by the occupational therapist. Many OT departments have developed facility-specific assessments by modifying and combining available tools to meet the needs of a specific setting and client population.

INTERVENTION

Planning

Occupational therapy is guided by frames of reference and the best practice guidelines for the child or adolescent presenting with occupational performance difficulties (see Table 14-2). Intervention planning involves collaborating with the child or adolescent, family, and other individuals, such as the members of a health care team or an educational team. Planning considers the strengths and weaknesses of the individual to develop long- and short-term goals and determine interventions (e.g., purposeful activities and strategies or techniques for implementation) as well as the frequency and duration of intervention activities. The OT practitioner capitalizes on a child's psychological, social, and behavioral strengths to determine intervention activities that will meet therapeutic goals. The goals and activities are based on the client's needs, interests, culture, and environment. The OTA should contribute to this intervention planning and implementation.

Long-term psychosocial goals identify the desired treatment outcome, and short-term goals identify the steps necessary to achieve the long-term goals. For example, increased social participation is a common desired outcome of therapy. Such an outcome improves the child or adolescent's ability to develop competence in age-appropriate occupational roles. Tyrone's story provides an example of one long-term and three short-term goals.

CASE *Study*

Nine-year-old Tyrone has been living in a foster care home with his two younger brothers since the death of their mother from a drug overdose. Tyrone has become extremely withdrawn and fearful over the past 6 months. In school, he is aggressive and socially isolated. His academic performance has dropped significantly. Tyrone was diagnosed with depression and prescribed medication. He attends a before- and after-school program for children at risk. The OT practitioner working at the school and the team developed the following goals:

Long-term goal: At discharge, Tyrone will demonstrate positive social behaviors during peer group activity.

Short-term goal 1: By the end of week 1, Tyrone will verbally interact one on one with a peer at least twice during a 30-minute group play activity.

Short-term goal 2: By the end of week 2, Tyrone will initiate conversation with peers a minimum of two times during a 30-minute group activity.

Short-term goal 3: By the end of week 1, Tyrone will demonstrate collaborative behaviors, as demonstrated by sharing materials with peers and taking turns at least three times in a 30-minute play activity.

Implementation

An effective intervention follows a set of principles and uses techniques and strategies that are based on a selected frame of reference. The purpose of following a frame of reference is to ensure that the outcomes are related directly to the method of treatment used. For example, medication combined with CBT may be the most effective intervention for the treatment of depression.[4,28] This combination of interventions relieves symptoms and prevents relapse. Table 14-2 shows some of the frames of reference that direct psychosocial OT interventions.

Most OT interventions with children and adolescents occur in groups and provide opportunities to learn and practice skills.[4] Well-designed OT groups create an optimal environment for achieving the child's or adolescent's goals, facilitating interpersonal interactions, and developing competence in a broad range of skills. Regardless of whether interventions occur individually or in groups, they typically include structure, consistency, and positive experiences. Intervention activities promote the acquisition of appropriate behavioral skills and address specific areas of occupational performance in which children perform poorly. These activities for children emphasize play and may include toys, games, and crafts that are developmentally appropriate, interesting, fun, and challenging. For adolescents, the activities have a peer-group focus and may involve a variety of creative arts and role-playing.[16] The emphasis often is IADLs, self-care, and social activities that facilitate transition to adulthood.

Group interventions generally address specific problem areas tailored to a particular age group. For example, in a school setting, the OT practitioner may design a task group for children in grades 1 to 3 who have difficulty attending to a task or demonstrate poor work skills. Children can develop or improve the skills needed to complete tasks effectively by working on individual craft projects in a structured small-group setting away from the distractions of the busy classroom. During group sessions, the OT practitioner can adapt the planned activities to ensure success and to extend the skill level of the children. Additional therapeutic benefits also intentionally addressed are age-appropriate social skills (e.g., sharing equipment and materials, keeping the workspace tidy, and asking for assistance) and coping skills (e.g., dealing with frustration). Table 14-4 provides examples of psychosocial OT groups.

For many group interventions, a number of well-developed protocols and programs are available.[4,14,16] Education, social work, occupational therapy, outdoor education, and psychology all have developed structured programs that have been shown to achieve the identified goals. This is particularly true for social skills, coping skills, assertiveness training, childhood fitness, and self-esteem and self-awareness programs. The OT practitioner should identify and use these resources when planning group interventions.

THERAPEUTIC USE OF SELF

The benefits of an empathic (i.e., conveying to another individual that you have an appreciative sense of that individual's experience), positive relationship between a child or adolescent and adult are well recognized and are the basis of many health and educational mentoring programs (e.g., Big Brothers and Big Sisters). In the relationship between the OT practitioner and the child or adolescent, the interaction and rapport developed is dependent on the OT practitioner's capacity to facilitate effectively a positive validating relationship and use communication and interpersonal skills in a therapeutic manner.

In a relationship with a child, the challenges include being empathetic and consistent and setting boundaries to create a safe and supportive environment while remaining flexible. Implicit in this relationship is respect for the child or adolescent. It is essential to give feedback that makes it clear that it is the behavior that is unacceptable or disliked not the child.

Awareness and mindfulness of how OT practitioners relate to clients is important in the OT process, and being conscious and intentional in all interactions is a necessary dimension of the therapeutic relationship. Taylor's Intentional Relationship Model describes six modes used in therapeutic relationships: advocating, collaborating, empathizing, encouraging, instructing, and problem solving.[31] OT practitioners have their own favorite

TABLE 14-4

Sample Occupational Therapy Groups for Children or Adolescents with Psychosocial Dysfunction

GROUP	PURPOSE	METHODS	OUTCOMES
IMAGINATIVE PLAY GROUP Population/group membership: Children and adolescents with difficulty enjoying or participating in play, interacting with others, problem solving, or feeling good about themselves. Imaginative games may help children/adolescents decrease stress and connect with others. Play groups can be used to work on many psychosocial issues. They help children and adolescents learn flexibility and problem solving and may teach clients how to adapt and cope with different situations.	Provide social opportunities to improve the following: • Social participation • Playfulness • Adaptability and flexibility • Problem solving • Imagination • Taking turns • Sharing	Develop a "play" in small groups that is later presented. Members discuss the play. Depending on the age of the children, pretend clothing may be used, different scenarios or role-playing. Children may be asked to act out a story or work as a team. Group storytelling Puppetry Props Music	Increased self-expression Increased playfulness (one's approach to activities) Opportunities to role-play may help with reading cues, understanding oneself and others, and dealing with issues. Improved social participation Improved stress reduction
TASK SKILLS GROUP Population/group membership: Children and adolescents experiencing difficulty performing occupations (e.g., ADLs, IADLs, school, work, leisure, social participation). Task skills group helps clients learn, practice, and refine the skills needed to accomplish occupations. Members receive support from the group while developing and refining the skills needed for living.	Provide opportunities to improve the following task skills: Task organization, planning, and implementation such as preparation of materials and cleanup of work area. Ability to follow directions On-task behaviors Task completion Recognition of errors and problem-solving skills Ability to work with others Ability to identify steps of projects	Develop a plan as a group and carry out selected tasks. Work together toward completion of the tasks. Engage in group and individual tasks required for ADLs, IADLs, work, education, and leisure/play. Types of groups include meal planning, events (e.g., dance, field trip), crafts, and planning a party.	Improve social participation, sense of belonging, efficacy, and self-confidence through completion of selected tasks as part of a team. Improve the organizational, planning, and problem-solving skills needed to complete selected tasks. Develop skills for ADLs, IADLs, education, work, leisure, and social participation.

Continued

TABLE 14-4

Sample Occupational Therapy Groups for Children or Adolescents with Psychosocial Dysfunction—cont'd

GROUP	PURPOSE	METHODS	OUTCOMES
LIFE SKILLS			
Population/group membership: Typical children and adolescents with significant physical or intellectual disabilities living in a residential setting such as a group home. Groups focusing on IADL skills are provided to older adolescents with psychiatric, intellectual, or cognitive disabilities. These adolescents may or may not be in a residential setting. Many may be undergoing transition from the home to a community residential setting such as a group home.	Teach and promote independence in basic life and self-care skills in the following areas: • Personal care of hygiene, grooming, etc. • Dressing • Money management • Functional mobility • Community mobility • Health maintenance • Medication routines • Functional communication • Emergency response • Sexual expression Teach and promote independence in IADLs. These skills overlap with basic life skills but also include the ability to care for oneself and one's environment. These skills include meal preparation, home management, caregiving, care of clothes, more complex money management beyond immediate personal use, and safety procedures.	Methods include task analysis, role-playing, and behavior rehearsal. Educational model advocates teaching, demonstrating, guiding, and practicing with supervision, followed by independent practice. Experiential learning that involves gradual skill development is a key component in these groups. The setting can be the group home, school, or clinic.	Develop life skills Gain age-appropriate independence
SOCIAL SKILLS			
Population/group membership: All children and adolescents Groups work the most effectively if children or adolescents have similar developmental and cognitive/intellectual levels as well as common problem areas. These groups are often divided into skill areas to include specific groups in communication, relationships and supporting others, problem solving in relationships, and self-monitoring in social situations.	Develop the skills required for interacting and "getting along" with others. Develop the skills required for effective verbal and nonverbal communication. Learn and practice socially appropriate behaviors (e.g., manners, sharing). Learn and practice cooperation and teamwork. Develop positive attitudes toward others (e.g., peers, family, teachers, and authority figures such as the police). Groups can focus on coping with specific problems such as shyness or loneliness.	Concrete activities demonstrate and practice social skills and are often based on a psychoeducational, educational, or sociocognitive model. These structured groups use a variety of learning techniques that combine knowledge and practice of the social skills learned. Methods include pen and paper, role-playing, practical skill demonstration sessions, films, behavior rehearsal, guided practice, homework tasks, experiential learning, and imitation.	Improvement in personal and social relationships Increased verbal participation in classroom setting Positive participation in group activities Increased social interaction with peers Increased inclusion in peer activities Reduction in inappropriate social behavior

COPING SKILLS

Population/group membership: Children and adolescents with no significant intellectual disabilities. Groups work the most effectively if the children or adolescents have similar developmental and cognitive/intellectual levels as well as common problem areas.	Provide opportunities to improve or learn coping skills including self-regulation in the following problem areas: • Poor impulse control • Excessive motor activity • Distractibility • Low frustration tolerance • Difficulty in delaying gratification • Depression, anxiety, or hostility The groups can focus on coping with specific problems such as grief and stress. Reflection on the techniques and/or alternatives used to perform occupations helps children and adolescents learn coping skills. Strategies for working on specific areas may benefit children and adolescents, such as stress management, homework strategies, massage, and writing assignments. The methods include pen and paper, role-playing, practical skill demonstration sessions, films, behavior rehearsal, guided practice, homework tasks, experiential learning, and imitation.	Increased self-esteem and positive self-image Increased self-efficacy in one's ability to manage emotions in a variety of situations Improvement in one's ability to interact in social settings Improvement in one's ability to share space and materials in a group setting and one on one Decrease in self-destructive behaviors and aggressive or acting-out behaviors

SELF-AWARENESS

Population/group membership: Adolescents with no intellectual disabilities. Adolescents are able to function in group settings and cope emotionally and cognitively with personal exploration.	Provide activities that increase insight and self-awareness. Facilitate self-reflection and self-evaluation in a supportive and safe context. Facilitate the resolution of inner conflicts. Develop a constructive self-concept and build self-esteem. Methods used in self-awareness groups usually involve an activity after which the product or experience is used in a process of self-reflection. Thoughts and feelings are explored and discussed in the group setting to help the adolescents confront and gain insight into their inner feelings and conflicts. Process of self-discovery leads individuals to make connections between past experiences and current feelings, difficulties, and behaviors. Activities can be group collaborative or competitive exercises and projects as well as individual activities including art, ceramics, sculpture, dance, movement "ropes" courses and/or exercises, games, massage, writing, poetry, and drama. Discussions that are facilitated by the activity can address themes such as who am I, caring about myself and others, understanding and confronting my problems, taking responsibility for myself, understanding the consequences of my actions, and making connections between past events and current feelings.	Reduction in symptoms (e.g., depression) Behavioral change: Reduction in self-destructive, aggressive, or antiauthority behavior Reduction in suicidal thoughts Improvement in self-worth and ongoing development of positive self-concept Improvement in academic performance Improvement in the quality of interpersonal relationships

Data compiled from Cara, E., & MacRae, A. (2005). *Psychosocial occupational therapy: a clinical practice*. Albany, NY: Delmar; Stein, F., & Cutler, S. K. (2002). *Psychosocial occupational therapy: a holistic approach* (2nd ed.). Albany, NY: Delmar.

ADL, Activities of daily living; IADL, instrumental activities of daily living.

modes, but it is possible to use multiple modes.[31] Certain modes will be more effective for some clients than for others. Overuse of a particular mode may work against the therapeutic relationship. For example, a practitioner who solely uses the instructing mode may find that the teen stops listening. Because teens frequently rebel against authority figures, the instructing mode may make them feel like they are being "lectured at." OT practitioners working with teens may have more success using the collaborating or advocating modes.

OT practitioners must realize that all behavior has meaning, including that of their own behavior as the health care professional. Children and adolescents will ascribe meaning to the OT practitioner's actions. Individuals with poor self-esteem and low self-worth easily misinterpret interpersonal cues. For example, if the OT practitioner is consistently late for appointments, the child may feel that he or she is not important even though thoughts and feelings are not necessarily obvious or expressed verbally. Instead, OT practitioners may observe them in the child's behaviors, affect (mood), or responses.

The therapeutic use of self requires that an OT practitioner be self-reflective, open to feedback, and aware of the influence of personal disposition, values, and culture. Although working with children and families is rewarding, it is also emotionally demanding and at times stressful. Therefore, supervision and peer support are beneficial. Having a supportive working environment, participating in continuing education, and taking care of one's own well-being will ensure the OT practitioner's capacity to have therapeutic relationships with children or adolescents with whom they work.

SUMMARY

Children and adolescents can have psychosocial and mental disorders that affect areas of occupational performance impeding their development. Knowledge of the signs and symptoms of these disorders helps the OT practitioner design effective interventions. The goal of intervention is to provide the child or adolescent with the appropriate tools to engage effectively in occupations, be able to feel successful, and develop independence. This chapter presented the OT practitioner with practical clinical information for treating children and adolescents with psychosocial and mental health disorders.

References

1. American Academy of Child and Adolescent Psychiatry. (2013). *Oppositional defiant disorder.* http://www.aacap.org/aacap/Families_and_Youth/Resource_Centers/Oppositional_Defiant_Disorder_Resource_Center/Home.aspx.

2. American Occupational Therapy Association. (2014). Occupational therapy practice framework: domain and process (3rd ed.). *Am J Occup Ther,* 68(Suppl. 1), S1–S48.

3. American Psychiatric Association. (2013). *Diagnostic and statistical manual of mental disorders* (5th ed.). Washington, DC: American Psychiatric Association.

4. Arbesman, M., Bazyk, S., & Nochajski, S. M. (2013). Systematic review of occupational therapy and mental health promotion, prevention, and intervention for children and youth. *Am J Occup Ther,* 67, e120–e130.

5. Asher, I. E. (2007). *Occupational therapy assessment tools: an annotated index* (3rd ed.). Bethesda, MD: AOTA Press.

6. Banerjee, T. D., Middleton, F., & Faraone, S. V. (2007). Environmental risk factors for attention-deficit hyperactivity disorder. *Acta Paediatrica,* 96, 1269.

7. Basu, S., Kafkes, A., Schatz, R., Kiraly, A., & Kielhofner, G. (2008). *The Pediatric Volitional Questionnaire (PVQ), Version 2.1.* Chicago, IL: MOHO Clearinghouse, University of Illinois.

8. Batshaw, M. L. (2012). *Children with disabilities* (7th ed.). Baltimore: Brooks Publishing.

9. Bazyk, S. et al. Occupational therapy and school mental health: American Occupational Therapy Association facts sheet. http://www.towson.edu/etu/insider/110409/images/OT_sheet.pdf.

10. Bhatia, S. K., & Bhatia, S. C. (2007). Childhood and adolescent depression. *Am Fam Physician,* 75, 73–79.

11. Bonder, B. R. (2014). *Psychopathology and function* (5th ed.). Thorofare, NJ: Slack.

12. Bowyer, P., Kramer, J., Ploszai, A., Ross, M., Schwarz, O., Kielhofner, G., et al. (2008). *The Short Child Occupational Profile (SCOPE). Version 2.2.* Chicago, IL: MOHO Clearinghouse, University of Illinois.

13. Brain Behavior Research Foundation. (2013). Bipolar disorder. https://bbrfoundation.org/frequently-asked-questions-about-bipolar-disorder.

14. Conduct Problems Prevention Research Group. (2007). Fast track randomized controlled trial to prevent externalizing psychiatric disorders: findings from grades 3 to 9. *J Am Acad Child Adoles Psychiatry,* 46, 1250–1262.

15. Crone, D., & Horner, R. (2003). *Building positive behavior support systems in schools.* New York: The Guildford Press.

16. Daykin, N., Orme, J., Evans, D., McEachran, M., & Brain, S. (2008). The impact of participation in performing arts on adolescent health and behavior: a systematic review of the literature. *J Health Psychology,* 13, 251–264.

17. Silove, D., & Bryant, R. (2006). Rapid assessments of mental health needs after disasters. *JAMA,* 296, 576.

18. Forsyth, K., Salamy, M., Simon, S., & Kielhofner, G. (1998). *The Assessment of Communication and Interaction Skills (ACIS). Version 4.* Chicago, IL: MOHO Clearinghouse, University of Illinois.

19. Keller, J., tenVelden, M., Kafkes, A., Basu, S., Federico, J., & Kielhofner, G. (2005). *Child Occupational Self Assessment. Version 2.1.* Chicago, IL: MOHO Clearinghouse, Occupational Therapy Department, College of Applied Health Sciences, University of Illinois.

20. Kielhofner, G. (2008). *A model of human occupation: theory and application* (4th ed.). Philadelphia: Lippincott, Williams, & Wilkins.

21. Masi, G., et al. (2004). Generalized anxiety disorder in referred children and adolescents. *J Am Acad Child Adolesc Psychiatr, 43,* 752.

22. Neistein, L. S., & Mackenzie, R. G. (2002). Anorexia nervosa and bulimia nervosa. In L. S. Neistein (Ed.), *Adolescent health care: a practical guide* (4th ed.). Philadelphia: Lippincott Williams & Wilkins.

23. Patton, G. C., et al. (2004). Puberty and the onset of substance use and abuse. *Pediatrics, 114,* e300.

24. Piers, E. V. (1984). *Piers-Harris children's self-concept scale (rev ed.).* Los Angeles: Western Psychological Service.

25. Polatajko, H. J., & Mandich, A. D. (2004). *Enabling occupation in children: the cognitive orientation to daily occupational performance (CO-OP) approach.* Ottawa: Canada: CAOT Publications ACE.

26. Robins, L. N., & Regier, D. A. (Eds.). (1991). *Psychiatric disorders in America: the epidemiologic catchments area study.* New York, NY: The Free Press.

27. Sadock, B. J., Sadock, V. A., & Ruiz, P. (2014). *Kaplan and Sadock's synopsis of psychiatry: behavioral sciences/clinical psychology* (11th ed.). Baltimore, MD: Lippincott, Williams & Wilkins.

28. Sarles, R. M., & Neistein, L. S. (2002). Adolescent depression. In L. S. Neistein (Ed.), *Adolescent health care: a practical guide* (4th ed.). Philadelphia: Lippincott Williams & Wilkins.

29. Searight, H. R., Rottnek, F., & Abby, S. L. (2001). Conduct disorder: diagnosis and treatment in primary care. *Am Fam Physician, 63,* 1579.

30. Sue, D., Sue, D. W., & Sue, S. (2010). *Understanding abnormal behavior* (9th ed.). Boston, MA: Wadsworth Cengage Learning.

31. Taylor, R. (2007). *The intentional relationship: use of self and occupational therapy.* Philadelphia: FA Davis.

32. Warner, V., et al. (1999). Grandparents, parents, and grandchildren at high risk of depression: a three generational study. *J Am Acad Child Adolesc Psychiatr, 38,* 289.

Recommended Reading

Early, M. B. (2009). *Mental health concepts and techniques for the occupational therapy assistant* (4th ed.). Philadelphia: Lippincott Williams & Wilkins.

Early, P. (2006). *A father's search through America's mental health system: Crazy.* New York, NY: The Berkley Publishing Group.

Taylor, R. (2007). *The intentional relationship: use of self and occupational therapy.* Philadelphia: FA Davis.

REVIEW *Questions*

1. What is a mental health disorder?
2. What is the *DSM-V,* and how does the OT practitioner use it?
3. Briefly describe three symptoms of each of the following disorders: conduct disorder, oppositional defiant disorder, separation anxiety disorder, Tourette's syndrome, anorexia nervosa, bulimia nervosa, and major depressive disorder.
4. Describe symptoms that indicate depression in adolescents and how these symptoms would present in therapy.
5. What are five strategies you would teach to a child to help him or her cope with anxiety?
6. Describe how the symptoms of each of the disorders in question 3 affect school performance.
7. What are the principles of psychoeducational groups, and when would you use them?
8. Describe important considerations when designing OT intervention for children with ADHD.

SUGGESTED *Activities*

1. Visit a day-care center and observe children engaged in educational and play activities. Respond to the following questions:
   a. Who is playing alone? What activities are the children engaged in (e.g., is the play imaginative, repetitive, creative, or educational?)?
   b. How do children transition between tasks and follow the teacher's instructions?
   c. What social interactions are happening between children as they play and work?
   d. Record age-appropriate psychosocial behaviors. Do not draw conclusions about children; just observe behaviors that are functional or less functional (e.g., collaborative, aggressive, and inability to attend to play activities).

2. Visit a place where adolescents gather, such as a mall. Observe the social interaction among the adolescents, and consider their dress and choice of activities in relationship to their age.

3. Many videos that depict mental disorders in children and adolescents are available through the university or college library or health services. Watch videos on the disorders discussed in this chapter, and imagine the way you would feel if the child or adolescent were a member of your family. List the questions and concerns that come to mind. Movies and documentaries that you might watch include *Precious* (2009), based on the book Push; Thin, an HBO documentary (2006) about eating disorders; or Phoebe in Wonderland, a movie about a young girl with Tourette's syndrome.

4. Contact the National Alliance for the Mentally Ill (1-800-950-6264) for information on family support.

5. Look at self-help sites for parents and teens. What are the concerns and questions that parents and teens express? Answer these questions using the chapter and other sources of information.

6. Visit the website of at least three mental health organizations (e.g., those of childhood depression, ADHD, schizophrenia). Discuss your findings in a small group.

KERRYELLEN G. VROMAN

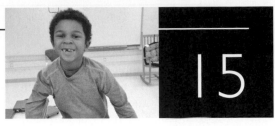

Childhood and Adolescent Obesity

CHAPTER *Objectives*

After studying this chapter, the reader will be able to accomplish the following:

- Describe the factors that contribute to obesity in children and adolescents.
- Recognize the behavioral and psychosocial factors that may be associated with childhood and adolescent obesity.
- Identify individual and group interventions for preventing obesity at individual, family, school, and community levels
- Plan and implement intervention with occupational therapy team members and other health and educational professionals that address and prevent childhood and adolescent obesity such as a comprehensive school program that promotes physical activity, healthy lifestyle patterns, and self-efficacy for healthy behaviors.
- Plan and implement intervention with occupational therapy team members and other health and educational professionals that is specifically targeted to address and prevent childhood and adolescent obesity among children and adolescents with disabilities and other conditions that increase the risk for weight gain.

CHAPTER *Outline*

"*O*verweight and *obese*—those words don't tell the full story because this isn't about inches and pounds, and it's not about how our kids look ... it's about how our kids feel, and it's about how they feel about themselves. It's about the impact that this issue [obesity] is having on every aspect of their life."[49]

Obesity interferes with occupational performance in everyday activities, play, and social participation. Children and adolescents who are obese enjoy and participate in fewer physical activities (sport) than their peers who are not overweight. They report joint discomfort and problems with breathing, and they particularly dislike intense physical activity such as running.[20] Many social activities are not enjoyable for children who are obese, such as shopping for clothes, eating out with friends, or dancing.[72] Furthermore, they often find themselves marginalized and excluded from social activities and consequently denied the developmental growth in psychosocial skills associated with peer relationships.

Childhood obesity is a national public health issue with short- and long-term health consequences. First lady Michelle Obama first raised national awareness of the significance of childhood obesity and its negative social, emotional, and health consequences with her Let's Move Campaign initiative in 2010.[47] Since then there have been meaningful changes designed to improve and promote the health of U.S. children. Child-focused corporations, such as Disney, have changed their policy about marketing of foods and beverages high in fats and sugars; there are initiatives at the national and community levels to involve more children and adolescents in physical activities; school meals programs have been required to include healthier food choices (e.g., Health Hunger-free Kids Act 2010), communities are working on environmental changes that will better support safe physical and play activities, and large-scale grocery chains have made a commitment to open stores in communities that have limited access to healthy foods. Despite these initiatives, childhood and adolescent obesity continues to increase.[50]

The growing national awareness of the need to proactively address and prevent childhood obesity has been mirrored in the occupational therapy (OT) profession. OT researchers, practitioners, and the American Occupational Therapy Association have increased attention to childhood and adolescent obesity. We are challenged by both the short- and long-term medical and psychosocial consequences and recognize the dynamic interaction of excessive weight, occupational performance, and capacity for successful participation in age-related occupations. The response has been initiatives within the profession to develop effective prevention and health promotion strategies and services to address the sequelae of obesity for children with and without disabilities.[3]

This chapter addresses issues of obesity and OT services for both typical children and adolescents and those with disabilities and conditions. The author provides an overview of the biopsychosocial factors that contribute to obesity and identifies conditions associated with weight gain and obesity. The implications of prejudicial **anti-fat** and **stereotypical attitudes** in OT practice are discussed. These earlier topics provide foundational information for planning and implementing programs, strategies, and resources that an OT practitioner can use within occupational therapy to manage and prevent weight gain.

CHILDHOOD AND ADOLESCENT OBESITY: CONTRIBUTING FACTORS

Obese describes the weight status of 18% of children in the United States and more than 33% meet the criteria for being classified as overweight or obese.[50] *Overweight* and *obesity* are the terms used to describe weight that is well above normal for height and build. The National Institutes of Health uses **body mass index** (BMI) to determine body-to-fat ratio. Although BMI correlates with the amount of body fat, it is not a direct measure of body fat. A BMI of 30 kg/m^2 or greater is the criteria for a diagnosis of obesity (Box 15-1). However, in determining the weight status of children and adolescents, differences in body fat between boys and girls and age-related difference are taken into account.[55] A child or adolescent is generally considered overweight if he or she is more than 20% over the ideal weight.

Additional methods used to estimate body fat and body fat distribution include measurements of skinfold

---

BOX 15-1

Obesity and BMI

Body mass index (BMI; [weight in pounds/height in inches] × 703]) is a reliable method used to measure body fat. It correlates highly with direct measures of body weight (e.g., underwater weighing displacement).

After a child's BMI is calculated, the score is plotted on the BMI for age growth chart for sex to obtain the child's percentile ranking. This ranking rates the child relative to children of the same age and sex. Some practitioners prefer to use degrees of overweight because the term *obesity* is regarded as a stigmatizing term. Others use ranges of obesity from mild to severe because this method is more informative. If the BMI index is used, the following classification is used to classify children's weight:

Underweight—<5th percentile
Healthy weight—5th to <85th percentile
Overweight—85th to <95th percentile
Obese—≥95th percentile

thickness and waist circumference, calculation of waist-to-hip circumference ratios, and procedures such as ultrasonography and computed tomography.[55]

Weight gain is a result of a physiologic process that results from an energy imbalance, namely, energy intake (i.e., food) is greater than energy expenditure (physical activity).[74] Figure 15-1 shows children engaging in healthy activity to promote wellness. However, this simplistic equation does not capture the complexity of the causal and/or contribute mechanisms that underpin obesity. Obesity is an outcome of the interactions among biological, genetic, sociocultural, economic, and environmental factors (Box 15-2).[34] For example, genetic predisposition, diet, eating behaviors, low physical activity patterns, and a sedentary lifestyle may explain the positive correlation between the weights of parents and their children. Excessive weight gain is further complicated by medical and congenital disorders such as diabetes, thyroid imbalance, Down syndrome, or Prader-Willi syndrome.

Biological and Genetic Factors

In their guidelines for the management of overweight and obese adults, the American College of Cardiology, American Heart Association, and the Obesity Society recommended the classification of obesity as a disease.[30] It is from this biomedical paradigm that children who are overweight or obese are identified. Early identification means children can receive personalized interventions (pharmacologic, lifestyle, and diet measures) or preventive health care that will potentially decrease their vulnerability to chronic health disorders (e.g., diabetes, orthopedic abnormalities, and cardiovascular disease).[66]

Research studies, especially those based on genomes, have identified that there is family susceptibility to obesity.[37] Children and adolescents who are genetically predisposed to obesity will gain weight when exposed to a suboptimal diet-and-exercise pattern (e.g., poor diet and lack of exercise). The studies identifying chromosomes related to being overweight are ongoing, the findings are best viewed as preliminary work.[37] Further evidence of heritable factors and the scope of knowledge of biological factors related to excessive weight gain will become more comprehensive with time.

Early-onset obesity is a symptom that occurs in some chromosomal syndromes, including the Mendelian syndrome, Prader-Willi syndrome, Albright hereditary osteodystrophy, and Bardet-Biedel syndrome.[38] Associated characteristics with weight gain in these syndromes are small stature, low activity levels, low muscle tone (hypotonia), and intellectual disability. In other chromosomal disorders, weight gain is a secondary problem. For example, children with Down syndrome often are overweight or obese due to low intensity of activity and other physical factors such as low muscle tone, heart defects (restricting participation in and endurance for physical activity), and hypothyroidism.[73]

Because hormonal, metabolic, and neuronal factors regulate weight, the body seeks to maintain a baseline weight, and the desire for food is adjusted accordingly through a feedback system involving the interaction of peripheral hormones, gastrointestinal peptides, and neuropeptides.[38] OT practitioners need to be aware of the biological and genetic factors that may be contributing to a child's weight. For example, hypothyroidism slows metabolic rate, and children with this disorder will need to perform high-intensity activities.

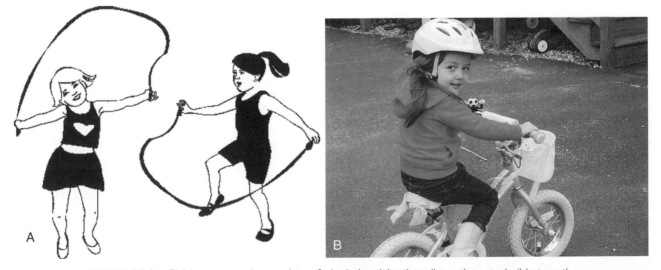

FIGURE 15-1 Children engage in a variety of physical activity that allows them to build strength, endurance and physical abilities. **A,** Children enjoy jump roping. **B,** Riding a bicycle develops strength and coordination, and allows children to be active. (**A** from O' Brien, J., & Solomon, J. (2013). *Occupational analysis and group process.* St. Louis: Mosby.

BOX 15-2

Factors Associated with Childhood and Adolescent Obesity

Obesity is the outcome of multiple factors interacting. These include:

- Biological/physiologic factors
  - Genetic disorders, medical conditions
  - Hormonal or endocrine disorders (e.g., hypothyroidism, diabetes)
- Diet
- Limited physical activity and sedentary lifestyle
- Personal contexts: family, friends, and peer networks
- Family stressors
- Parent education, ethnicity, and socioeconomic status
- Parents' limit setting concerning food choices
- Family physical activity patterns, interests and leisure activities
- Family preference for sedentary activity patterns
- Factors associated with health (e.g., medications, chronic health conditions, such as asthma, that restrict participation in physical activity)
- Environment: unsafe urban settings (e.g., playgrounds with poorly maintained equipment, or used as meeting places by adults engaging in criminal activities), underresourced schools, high-density communities with limited access to fresh produce and healthy food choices, limited community resources for participating in physical activities
- Access to affordable health care services across the life span (e.g., prenatal and postnatal care, early childhood screening)

From Minihan, P. M., Fitch, A. N., & Must, A. (2007). What does the epidemic of childhood obesity mean for children with special health needs? *J Law Med Ethics, 35,* 61.

Behavioral Factors: Activity and Diet

Genetic, demographic, family, sociocultural, and physical factors collectively influence activity pattern and diet. Patterns around food type and intake and exercise are first learned within the family (Box 15-3). However, diet, sedentary behaviors, and lack of physical activity are modifiable causal factors of childhood and adolescent obesity. For example, insufficient physical activity is a recognized risk factor for obesity and related chronic conditions, whereas engaging in physical activity from an early age (toddlers) protects children from excessive weight gain.[29,66] These physical activity patterns established in childhood positively influence later activity patterns. Unfortunately, for many, especially girls, participation in physical activity declines across childhood and into adolescence.[61] The Centers for Disease Control and Prevention Youth Media Campaign Longitudinal Study found that 61.5% of children between the ages of 9 and 13 years did not participate

BOX 15-3

Diet and Physical Exercise Factors Associated with Obesity in Children

- Foods used as a reward or to soothe a child
- Inexpensive foods are cheaper, often easy to prepare, but high in calories
- Lack of healthy role modeling (eating and physical activity, and nutrition)
- Lower socioeconomic status
- Family's ethnicity, dietary choices less nutritional
- Inconsistent meals or access to healthy foods
- Limited education related to healthy nutrition and physical activity
- OT reimbursement does not include interventions for obesity: IEP goals are based on function or motor planning, and developing gross motor skills for academics
- Absence of a comprehensive approach to obesity that addresses the problems on an individual, family, school, and the community level
- Lack of effective interventions and policies

in any organized physical activity in nonschool hours, and 22.3% did not participate in any free-time activity.[15]

Low physical activity and sedentary behaviors are interrelated. However, healthy children and adolescents have a balance of low and high physical activities and derive benefits developmentally from both. For example, a child may be an avid reader, play sports, go hiking with his or her family, and watch TV and maintain a healthy weight. The growth in technology-based leisure pursuits such as watching TV, playing video games, and engaging in multiple forms of computer-mediated communication have contributed to sedentary behaviors and the resultant rise in obesity.[4] The problem is not that **sedentary activities** require a low expenditure of energy. Rather, sedentary activities may displace high physical energy activities, and children who engage in sedentary activities end up with a lower metabolic rate than their physically active peers.

CLINICAL *Pearl*

Experts recommend that children watch no more than 2 hours of TV per day. This recommendation can also be applied to other information communication technology-based passive activities (e.g., iPad and computer Internet games and social media use). Children and adolescents with TVs in their bedrooms watch TV more than those who do not have TVs in their rooms. Watching less TV can lead to a reduction in a child's weight, but it is most effective when replaced by physically active leisure.[1]

Numerous client factors as well as environmental contexts interact to result in a child and family leading predominantly sedentary, less than healthy, lifestyles. Poverty also contributes to higher levels of sedentary activities and poor diet. This should not necessarily be viewed as a matter of choice. Lower socioeconomic communities often lack resources such as grocery stores or markets with fresh produce, safe play and walking areas, and affordable sports and leisure activities.[41] Similarly there is a relationship between sedentary activity pattern and higher food intake and/or unhealthy eating patterns. Children and adolescents who are physically active are more likely to have a healthy diet.[62] Conversely, TV viewing means advertisements promoting fast foods, snacks, and drinks. This targeted advertising is designed to encourage snacking on prepared foods that are often high in sugar and fats. Eating while watching TV is unfocused eating resulting in higher consumption, whereas sitting down at the table for a family meal models healthy eating patterns and helps children monitor food intake and portion size. Furthermore, family meals are associated with a higher intake of vegetables and a lower intake of items such as sodas and fried foods.[24]

Dysfunctional **habits** and **routines** contribute to low activity and poor diet patterns among children, adolescents, and their families. Eating patterns, in relation to diet and food preferences, in households where a parent is obese differ from households in which neither parent is obese.[5,61] Therefore family-centered interventions are the basis of many programs to address childhood obesity. Effective behavioral dietary and physical activity interventions have been shown to address weight issues and the psychosocial problems associated with obesity.[66] Families that provide healthy snack choices (Figure 15-2) help children gain lifestyle skills. Interventions for children who have parents with their own challenges around diet and weight are less successful; therefore interventions particularly need to address the habits, routines, and patterns of the entire family. [62]

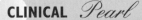

CLINICAL *Pearl*

Introducing family meal times without television can be an attainable goal that will benefit all family members. It can be an initial tangible strategy for changing a family's routines associated with food. Change comes gradually and family meal times do not need to be immediately associated with dietary changes. Changes can be made gradually and families can aim for success rather than create additional demands that may lead to further stress. Advantages of the family eating together include the need to prepare only one meal (instead of several for different family members at different times) and an increase in family interaction.

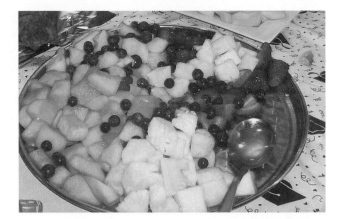

FIGURE 15-2 Having fruit readily available allows children to make healthy choices.

Environment: Economic, Cultural, Physical, and Social Contexts

Family and peer relationships, attitudes, **education**, ethnicity, behaviors, school/community environments, and societal attitudes are the socioeconomic, cultural, and physical factors that influence activity patterns, eating behaviors, and attitudes toward food, physical activity, leisure choices, and personal weight (e.g., body image).[51,70] Therefore, these factors can contribute positively or negatively to a child's or adolescent's weight.[62] For example, environmental factors may support and encourage a healthy active lifestyle, whereas others can be barriers to positive behavioral change. Figure 15-3 illustrates children engaging in physical activity in a supportive environment. A 2-year study of households that restricted certain foods, especially when it involved a mother's dietary restriction, found that an increase in the weights of the children.[19] An explanation for this finding may be that when these children managed to get access to the restricted foods, they ate more of them. In contrast, the availability of healthy foods (e.g., fruits and vegetables) in the home and the healthy eating patterns modeled by parents (and grandparents) positively influence food preferences and eating behaviors that will persist when children begin to make their own choices about the foods they will eat.[21] See Figure 15-4 for examples of interventions to increase healthy diets in families. See Box 15-4 for an example of a fun healthy recipe that can help families change eating habits.

Because family context significantly affects eating and exercise patterns, it is important to establish healthy eating and exercise habits early, before parental control over diet diminishes during adolescence.[22] Adolescents are more likely to purchase foods outside the home that are often foods of convenience, high in sugars and fats, and of questionable nutritional value. If paired with an increase in sedentary activity level (e.g., homework, fewer physical extracurricular activities),

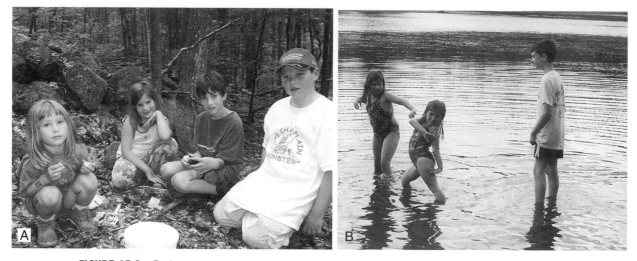

FIGURE 15-3 Environments can support physical activity. **A,** Hiking or playing in the woods provides children with a healthy environment to explore. **B,** Children exert much energy playing in the water. (**A** from O' Brien, J., & Solomon, J. (2013). *Occupational analysis and group process.* St. Louis: Mosby.)

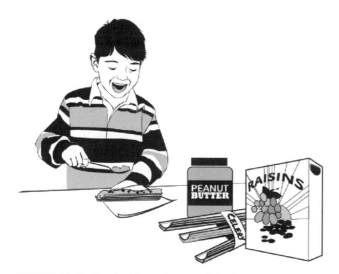

FIGURE 15-4 Fun healthy recipes can help families change eating habits. Making "ants on a log" is a fun and easy way to enjoy healthy snacks.

BOX 15-4

Banana Sushi

Wheat bread
Banana
Peanut butter, soy butter, apple butter or Nutella

1. Roll out wheat bread into thin slice with a rolling pin.
2. Spread with peanut butter, soy butter, Nutella, and/or apple butter.
3. Place banana on edge and roll bread around it.
4. Press tightly so bread stays around banana.
5. Cut into small "sushi"-sized bites

From O' Brien, J., & Solomon, J. (2013). *Occupational analysis and group process.* St. Louis: Mosby.

---

the change in diet can lead to weight gain in adolescents. Adolescence brings challenges associated with weight, diet, and exercise. It is the peak time for dysfunctional eating patterns and psychopathology. At the same time, peer and the media are influential forces in relation to behaviors and attitudes concerning weight, body image, and choices about exercise and use of discretionary time.

Physical and economic contexts influence activity levels and choice of activities. Children in low-income communities in metropolitan areas have an increased risk for obesity. Regardless of community, parents report being concerned about their children's safety, especially in urban settings. The outcome of parental concerns are that children are less likely to walk or cycle to school,

and spend less free play time in outdoor settings such as parks leading to less creative and less vigorous physical play.[10] Parents prefer to supervise their children in public spaces or have them involved in extracurricular activities. At the same time, intense marketing of sedentary computer-mediated games and a decline in the availability of community and school sports and physical education for a range of abilities continue to occur.

Fewer students at the elementary and high school levels are participating in any form of organized physical activity.[64] Sports activities progressively recruit and retain the athletically able children with an expectation of increased skills with age. Additionally, early in childhood, sport activities potentially exclude economically disadvantaged children because of the cost of equipment, transportation costs, the lack of resources in their communities, and the need for parents to work in positions with little to no flexibility, which makes it difficult for them to take their children to sports and other extracurricular physical activities (e.g., dance classes, judo, or karate) difficult. The national "Let's Move" initiative and many state initiatives seek to reverse this trend by increasing child and family activity levels (Figure 15-5), providing education to improve children's nutrition, and improving the content of school meals.

PSYCHOSOCIAL CONSEQUENCES OF GROWING UP OBESE

A significant relationship exists between obesity and psychological difficulties.[55] Failure to recognize and intervene in a child's weight issues not only increases the risk for adult obesity and its associated morbidity and mortality,[2,63] it heightens the risk for depression, low self-esteem, eating disorders, poor academic achievement, and difficulties with social relationships.[72] Inclusion of intervention for psychosocial problems should be an integral component of OT intervention for children who are obese. It is a secondary concern to weight reduction and engagement in physical activities. If psychosocial problems are not explored and addressed, they will undermine behavior-change initiatives. Healthy behaviors, body image, self-esteem and positive self-concept are constructs applicable to all children regardless of size.[60]

It is wrong to assume all children or adolescents who are overweight or obese will have psychological problems.[8] Lower self-esteem is particularly prevalent among children and adolescents who believe that they are themselves responsible for their overweight, and those who think that being overweight interferes with their social relationships.[52] Dissatisfaction with physical appearance is significantly associated with obesity, namely, poor **body image**, as well as psychosocial problems.[28] Poor body image in girls has been shown to predict poor psychological function, depression, and binge eating.[15,45] Furthermore, a lower level of participation in physical activities is associated with poor psychological functioning. It is an iterative challenge; children who are obese report less enjoyment in sports, especially high-energy activities such as running. Inactivity increases the likelihood of weight gain, body dissatisfaction, lower self-esteem and **self-efficacy** in physical occupations. Given these factors it is difficult for children and adolescents to expect success in activities that would promote greater health and reduction in weight.

Although social context has a contributory role in childhood obesity, it also is a significant factor in the psychosocial well-being of children and adolescents who are obese. Peer victimization is an experience of children who are obese. Body size is the most stigmatizing physical

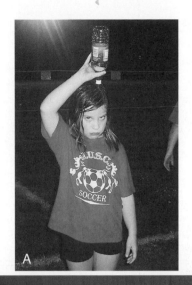

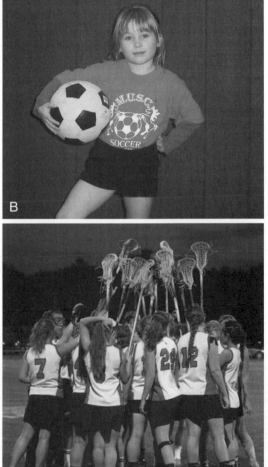

FIGURE 15-5 Children enjoy playing on sports teams, but the opportunity to do so may not be available to all children. Some teams become more exclusive as children age and some children may not be able to participate due to transportation or economic issues. **A,** Alison is tired after a nighttime soccer game. **B,** Molly is proud of her accomplishments. **C,** High school lacrosse players celebrate a lacrosse victory!

BOX 15-5

Weight-Based Bullying

The one out of three Americans between the ages of 2 and 19 years old who are overweight or obese are vulnerable to weight-based bullying. They are subject to teasing, discrimination, and social exclusion.[56,57,70] For example, in one study, 45% of children with weight issues reported being teased, compared with 15% of children with normal weights.[26] Weight-related teasing and poor body image are significant issues among elementary school children who are obese.[27] In addition to the painful experiences of being teased or bullied, these children also experience psychological, attitudinal, and behavioral negative outcomes. Children who experience weight-related criticism are likely to express negative attitudes toward sports and to engage less in physical activities. Similarly, adolescents who reported weight-related teasing are more likely to have dysfunctional patterns of weight control, such as smoking, purging, using laxatives and diuretics, and fasting, than do their peers without weight-related problems. Because of the high incidence of weight-related teasing and anti-fat prejudicial attitudes, practitioners should assume that children who are overweight might be experiencing victimization (e.g., bullied). At all times, the practitioner needs to be sensitive to any comments about weight. Weight reduction is not an OT outcome and neither can it be written as an occupation-based goal. Prioritizing weight reduction reinforces negative weight stereotypes and negative body image.[70]

Health and education professionals including OT practitioners need to understand that the consequences of weight-based peer stigmatization is complex and must be addressed on multiple levels. They should take the following steps (no order is implied by the numbering) to reduce weight-based victimization:

1. Honestly examine one's own biases and stereotypes related to weight. We must examine our attitudes and stereotypical beliefs concerning obesity and how these attitudes and beliefs influence our approaches to interventions for children and adolescents who are obese. OT practitioners are not excepted to have stereotypical attitudes regarding obesity.[70] The attitudes of many health care professionals are consistent with the stereotypical anti-fat attitudes prevalent in society.[23,70] One study showed that OT students were more likely to negatively evaluate and show discriminatory attitudes toward clients who were obese than toward those who were not. The OT students reported they were less likely to choose to work with clients who are obese, to view these clients as deserving of sympathy and understanding. They did not believe it would be easy to be empathetic toward these clients.[70] Similarly, OT students ranked obesity as one of the hardest disabilities to live with.[11] Despite the ethical guidelines of the OT profession, which unequivocally states that all people are entitled to equal and compassionate care, anti-fat attitudes will negatively influence OT practitioners' relationships with children and adolescents who are overweight. Therapists must provide a nonjudgmental therapeutic climate.

2. Recognize that changing attitudes of peers will not resolve the social isolation of children who are obese. Before children who are obese can successfully participate in peer social and physical activities, the negative consequences of past exclusion needs to be addressed. Building social and physical occupation performance competencies and self-esteem will facilitate their successful social participation.

3. Work with educational and health professionals to change educational/school climate, beginning with play groups and preschools. Attitudes are formed early. School bullying program curriculum needs to include content that deals with weight-based stereotypes and the role of physical appearance in discriminatory attitudes. Weight and gender generate the most bullying in schools.

characteristic after race. These children are marginalized by their peers, bullied, and teased (Box 15-5).[56,57] Comparison with the Western ideal of physical attractiveness, which idealizes thinness for women and muscular physiques for men, individuals who are obese are considered unattractive.[13,42] Stereotypical characteristics such as laziness, self-indulgence, unreliability, untrustworthiness, and lack of self-discipline are attributed to individuals who are obese.[12,60,69] Children as young as 3 years old have been found to describe children who are obese as "ugly," "stupid," and "dirty."[26] These negative attitudes are not limited to children; 20% of high school teachers and health care workers stated that they thought obese individuals were more emotional, less tidy, less likely to succeed at work, and had personalities different from those of nonobese individuals.[26]

CLINICAL *Pearl*

Make positive behavioral comments, including appearance. All children need positive feedback and praise. More often than not, children who are overweight or obese hear mostly negative comments, or positive comments are omitted. Listen to the comments made to the children who are not overweight and ask yourself whether you provide similar comments or encouragement to children in the group who are overweight.

OCCUPATIONAL THERAPY: PREVENTION, INTERVENTION APPROACHES, AND STRATEGIES

The need for health care practitioners and families to be mindful of children's weights and levels of physical activity is not a new concern, and the primary strategies to address obesity have not changed significantly. Dr. R. S. Solomon, a family doctor in rural South Carolina, wrote the following in his 1960s newspaper column:[65]

> "One fact is established, and that is that the time to treat it [obesity] is during childhood and adolescence. The prescription is relatively simple—more exercise, the right diet, and watchful parental–doctor [health care professional] supervision. ... The human machine, like any other, functions on intake and output but must have an emotional stability in self and parent."

Similar words could easily have been written in 2016. The following sections of this chapter explore individual and group programs and strategies occupational therapy practitioners can use to promote health for children and interventions that holistically address obesity.

No longer is obesity an emerging practice domain. Today, many OT practitioners who work with children and adolescents acknowledge that evaluation and interventions associated with obesity are incorporated into their everyday practice. The evidence of this shift to pediatric OT services for obesity being more mainstream practice is reflected in the increase in OT articles related to childhood obesity being published in the past 5 years, national conference presentations, and American Occupational Association sponsored activities (e.g., the AOTA Tip Sheet: Addressing Childhood Obesity and Childhood Obesity resources materials in the School Mental Health Kit).[3]

OT interventions for children and adolescents who are obese or at risk for becoming obese can be divided into two broad categories:

1. Health promotion with children at risk for obesity who are overweight and/or obese and typical children. Dwyer and colleagues (2009) advocated that OT practitioners and physical therapy practitioners "embrace a broad perspective of physical activity and extend children's therapeutic and health promotion programs to include assessment of habitual level of physical activity and sedentary behaviors and promotion of recommended levels of physical activity" (p. 28).[16]
2. The evaluation and interventions to promote occupational performance and participation. This category of therapy includes children whose performance is compromised by weight and children already receiving OT services for other disorders such as developmental, motor coordination, and sensory processing disorders; genetic or metabolic disorders; congenital disabilities; or learning and functional problems. Children with diabetes and cardiac issues are also among those receiving occupational therapy for weight-related problems. In this population being overweight or obese is often secondary to the primary disorders, making a focus on health promotion integral to all pediatric services. For example, children with spina bifida or muscular dystrophy may be overweight because they are only minimally physically active due to limited mobility.

Obesity is more prevalent among children and adolescents with physical and cognitive disabilities than among those without disabilities.[29] In the case of children with special needs, excess weight further exacerbates their occupational performance difficulties (e.g., mobility).[39] The chronic and secondary problems associated with obesity in adolescents who are disabled can compromise their independence and limit their opportunities to participate in a variety of occupations.[58] Similarly, it is now recognized that fine as well as gross motor skills are affected in children for whom obesity is a primary disorder.[40,25]

Obesity in Youth with Existing Disorders

OT practitioners who work with children who have disabilities need to understand the mechanisms and consequences of obesity in children with disabilities and existing childhood and adolescent disorders. Effective programs and individual interventions begin with an awareness of the behavioral and environmental factors that are precursors and contributory factors to weight gain.[43] The outcome is comprehensive family-centered OT intervention plan and implementation.

Obesity in Youth with Intellectual or Developmental Disorders

CASE *Study*

Sean, a 5-year-old boy, is short in stature, overweight, clumsy, and has mild intellectual impairment. Sean has Prader-Willi (PWS) syndrome. He receives OT services and his therapist and parents share a concern about his weight gain. The basis of his weight gain is physiologic and behavioral. Typical of children with PWS, Sean is preoccupied with food. His overeating started as a toddler (around 2 years old) and as he has grown older his behavior has escalated to stealing and hoarding food. The family has placed locks on the refrigerator and kitchen cupboards to reduce Sean's access to food. However, his preschool is struggling with Sean's food-seeking behaviors (e.g., taking food from other children and eating Play-Doh and crayons).

PWS is a genetic disorder and the most common syndrome form of obesity[11] (see Chapter 13). Children with PWS have low muscle tone and low levels of sex hormones. They constantly feel hungry because the area of the brain that controls feelings of fullness or hunger does not work properly. There is no effective medication for this eating-appetite disorder. As these children develop, their stature, poor motor skills associated with low muscle tone, and patterns of overeating lead to obesity. Other problems associated with PWS are sleep disorders, mild intellectual disability, and behavior problems. Challenging behaviors include temper tantrums, obsessive-compulsive symptoms, and trouble regulating their emotions.

Sean's therapy needs are similar to many children and adolescents with genetic syndromes and chromosomal abnormalities that include low muscle tone as an infant, poor and delayed motor development, and behavioral problems. Obesity in the pediatric population is typically due to factors such as dysfunctional food or eating behaviors, sedentary or low activity levels, and metabolic disorders associated with their primary disorders. For example, nearly half of children with Down syndrome are obese or overweight because of low activity levels and poor motor skills.

The approach for Sean is child- and family-centered therapy that includes his health and educational service providers. As mentioned, it requires a comprehensive approach to address this complex disorder. A behavioral frame of reference is the most effective approach in designing and implementing individual interventions to address Sean's behavioral problems (poor emotional regulation, temper tantrums, and food seeking) to promote inclusive participation in a group setting. The most common model used is applied behavioral functional analysis or positive behavioral support (see Chapter 14). A skill acquisition and/or developmental frame of reference is also required to promote his overall development in occupation (e.g., activities of daily living [ADLs], play). Because specific impairments such as low muscle tone and motor coordination affect his motor skills, the OT practitioner examines these areas to promote Sean's competence and participation in physical activities to achieve a healthy ratio of food intake and physical activity.

For Sean and children like him, effective communication between school and home is paramount. A certified occupational therapy assistant (COTA) who works with the parents and in the school setting may be central to ensuring the consistency of these children's behavioral programs across settings. A health care or educational practitioner who specializes in applied behavioral analysis can develop a behavioral program, but the implementation will become the task of everyone who has contact with the child. It should be written into a child's individualized education plan (IEP) and reflected in the OT goals. OT services for these children include occupation-based interventions to improve and promote age-appropriate performance. Although therapy sessions and goals are performance focused, due to underlying motor impairments and overall fitness, the OT practitioner should also include activities that improve physical strength, agility, coordination and endurance that follow the principles of a biomechanical frame of reference (e.g., resistance, repetition, and frequency). The development of lean muscle mass and increased physical activity will maintain and potentially reduce weight. Prevention of obesity is an overall health and wellness goal, as it will further limit occupational performance and developmental gains.

Obesity in Youth with Limited Functional Mobility

CASE *Study*

Twelve-year-old Gary has spina bifida. His lesion is in the lower lumbar area. Since starting middle school, he has used a wheelchair for functional mobility. He found transitioning between classes was too slow when he walked with his crutches. Coinciding with his wheelchair use and the new school environment, Gray gained weight and is at the 92nd percentile on the BMI scale for his age. His increased weight and growth have not only reduced his ambulation, they are also making transfers difficult. His increased dependence on assistance is reducing his opportunities to participate in out-of-school activities with peers.

Spina bifida is a neuroskeletal structural abnormality of the spine (see Chapter 13). Like children with physical and neurologic disorders, such as cerebral palsy, muscular dystrophy, and spina bifida, weight gain with age can become a problem. Weight gain can be due to a number of reasons. As children age, the demands of age-related activities increase, so they use more efficient, less physically demanding means of functional mobility (e.g., a power chair replaces a manual chair or crutches). The physical demands of walking or the manual operation of the chair make the activity a high-intensity one that expends more energy, providing a caloric exercise balance. However, strength and motor skills of children with disabilities become more problematic as their bodies mature and moving a larger skeletal frame often paired with weight gain is more challenging. For others, adolescence is associated with deterioration of their condition (e.g., Duchenne muscular dystrophy). The physical growth, maturation, and changes in condition often coincide with a decline in therapy exercises, physical play, and participation in organized activities (such as sports). Inclusion in school physical education decreases with age. As a result sedentary academic activities and the reduced physical activity lead to weight gain.

Obesity in Youth as a Primary Problem

Increasingly, school and community settings are seeking obesity prevention and health promotion programs and individual interventions from OT practitioners. Children and adolescents may be referred to OT services because occupational performance and social participation is compromised by their weight. Obesity, in this population needs to be approached as a complex physical, social and psychological disorder.[14] Psychosocial problems and/or mental illness may be a precursor (anxiety, depression, eating disorders) or consequence of the child's or adolescent's obesity (e.g., bullying/victimization, low self-esteem, depression). Furthermore, children who are obese have been identified as having poorer gross and fine motor skills, motor planning, coordination, and executive functioning performance than their peers.[7,25] Another high incidence of weight problems is in students with specific learning disabilities. Bandini and colleagues found that girls with learning disabilities were twice as likely to be overweight as their peers without these disabilities.[5] In the adolescent population referred to occupational therapy with weight problems, a notable subgroup experiences mental health problem especially eating disorders (e.g., binge eating or bulimia nervosa).

CASE *Study*

Gina is 16 years old. She has always been on some kind of diet because her weight is slightly above average for her height, but lately she has gained weight. In the past 8 months, she developed a pattern of compulsive overeating when she is stressed or unhappy about her parents' separation and pending divorce, her schoolwork, or not getting along well with her friends. She secretly and rapidly eats large amounts of food several times a week and then feels disgusted with herself. She feels she has no control over this behavior. Unlike individuals with bulimia nervosa, she does not purge; as a result, she is rapidly becoming obese.

Gina's, obesity is due to binge eating. Binge eating accounts for 2% to 25% of individuals who are obese. The American Psychiatric Association classifies binge eating as a distinctive disorder characterized by recurring episodes of consuming a large amount of food in a short time. Their excessive eating and inability to control the binging causes distress. Similar to other eating disorders, secrecy, shame, and guilt are among

the symptoms experienced.[4] Gina's obesity is related to her psycho-emotional difficulties; therefore a psychosocial frame of reference such as **cognitive-behavioral therapy**, illness management and recovery and/or participation in psychoeducational group would become the primary approach for occupational therapy intervention. The OTA works with the team to implement individual and group interventions/activities that support Gina's function-based occupational performance goals.

OT practitioners working with children and adolescents seeking intervention for weight issues will be members of an interprofessional team that may include a physician, nutritionist, social worker, exercise specialist, teacher, and psychologist. OT programs for children for whom weight is compromising occupational performance, are comprehensive and occupation-based and emphasize occupational performance skills in age-related activities. The OT goals for this population are to improve functioning, manage weight, and develop a healthy lifestyle through behavioral change and adaptation. Based on a functional and cognitive evaluation, individualized OT interventions are based on frames of reference that effectively promote the following:

- Development of age-appropriate performance skills that support optimal functioning in all domains of occupations (e.g., ADLs, instrumental ADLs, education, social participation)
- Behavioral change to establish a healthy lifestyle through educational cognitive-behavioral and/or experiential learning strategies that include participation in peer and family group programs or individual interventions
- Participation in activities that support and reinforce weight loss
- Strategies to promote occupational activities that will enhance and improve motor skills, motor planning, coordination, and executive functioning
- Expand repertoire of play and leisure activities and build competencies
- Development of skills that include emotional self-regulation, stress management skills, social skills, and communication skills to achieve self-efficacy in social participation. Through a multifaceted approach, self-esteem can be increased, and body image and a positive sense of self can be established. Psychosocial frames of reference will guide assessment and intervention and play an important role in maintaining healthier eating patterns, physical activity level, routines, and habits

In extreme cases when children or adolescents are morbidly obese, compensatory approaches such as assistive devices may be provided (e.g., ADLs). Obesity limits children's motor skills and motor planning; therefore, opportunities to engage in age-appropriate occupations with peers and to function at their optimal performance level is always the overarching goal and desired outcome, regardless of weight.

THERAPEUTIC APPROACHES

The approaches and models that guide therapy interventions are frames of reference. These are templates for therapy and following an evidence-based frame of reference ensure effective interventions. An eclectic approach seldom results in effective replicable interventions. One or more of the following frames of references (approaches) can be used to plan and implement programs and individual interventions for obesity:

- Health education
  - Acquisitional–habilitation–developmental models
- Behavioral change theory (e.g., transtheoretical theory of behavioral change also commonly known as stage change theory)
- Behavioral approaches (e.g., positive behavioral support)
- Cognitive-behavioral therapy
- Social learning theory, or social cognition theory (a model of group therapy commonly used with adolescents)
  - Psychoeducational model (effective as a family and/or individual intervention)
  - Model of Human Occupation to promote intervention aimed at volition, habituation, performance capacity, and environment. [33]

As a team, the occupational therapist and the COTA identify the approach that is effective with their population and will achieve the desired outcomes. The OT process begins with thorough evaluation and assessment of the client to identify the problem and individualize goals, interventions, and therapy priorities.

INDIVIDUAL INTERVENTION STRATEGIES
Prevention: Individual Strategies for Infants with Special Needs

Often an OT practitioner's first contact with children with specials needs is as infants as the practitioner works on feeding. This early phase is a crucial stage for establishing healthy eating patterns and routines as well as food preferences. The first decision is whether to promote breast milk or formula. Children with feeding difficulties may be bottle- rather than breast-fed. When possible, breast milk is preferable even with bottle- or tube-fed infants because breast milk and breastfeeding appear to have some protective effects against obesity. When introducing solids in a feeding program, the OT

practitioner should provide education about healthy choices as part of the program. There is a tendency to give children who are difficult to feed or fussy eaters their preferred foods, which are often sweet.

CLINICAL *Pearl*

Some children with special needs will not be at risk for obesity. Children with cerebral palsy characterized by high or fluctuating muscle tone need a high caloric intake because of the energy expenditure due to their muscle tone or constant movement patterns. However, preference for healthy foods remains a priority.

In early childhood, eating routines in structured settings will begin to establish patterns and attitudes concerning food.[24] The OT practitioner works with families on setting eating patterns and how food will be viewed. For example, never using food as a reward avoids the later necessity for children having to unlearn this behavior when they become overweight. It is better that they develop healthy snack choices that accommodate their food challenges or special needs. Meals at structured times in a high chair will also develop a habit of eating being associated with sitting at the table. Eating randomly while playing is the beginning of unhealthy snacking habits.

CLINICAL *Pearl*

Encourage parents to offer their young children foods that vary in taste and texture, especially fruits and vegetables, to limit prepared snacks (e.g., sweet cereals, chips) and to avoid using foods as incentives or rewards or to comfort. Children develop likes and dislikes of foods and eating patterns (when and how much) in the first 5 years of life.[6]

Managing and Preventing Obesity

Helping children or adolescents and their families address issues of obesity requires an examination of the children's habits and routines (Box 15-6). OT practitioners gather information on children or adolescents' developmental, physical, psychosocial, and cognitive performance and seek to understand cultural, familial, and physical contexts. This information is used to set child- and family-centered achievable goals. When setting goals, weight reduction may be a desired benefit but is not the focus or goal. OT practitioners develop comprehensive intervention plans to target the psychosocial consequences (e.g., poor self-esteem) and **behavioral change** to develop healthy activity patterns, dietary habits and routines, and improvement of occupational performance through remedial strategies, which may or may not include weight management. Short-term, achievable goals motivate children and families.

Managing and Preventing Obesity

- Set goals that are obtainable, simple, and easy to measure.
- Set one short achievable goal at a time.
- Make goals very concrete so the child sees progress. For example, provide the child with a pedometer to measure distance walked. Have simple short-term goals, such as walk to best friend's house or walk to the nearest store.
- Develop goals with the child or adolescent. Have the child set his or her own reward system.
- Keep goals positive; for example, have the child walk to the end of the street every other day rather than every day; have the child pick a day of the week to not watch TV.
- Involve friends and family in goals.
- Minimize the number of breads, sweets, soda available to the child and replace them with healthy choices such as fruit, vegetables, and water at home.
- Do not completely deny the child occasional sweets or soda. Otherwise, the child may crave them and eat more when they are available.
- Address issues of health rather than weight.
- Focus on the child's volition (interests, motivation and desires) to engage in a variety of activities.
- Build on existing physical and healthy routines and habits.
- Consistently repeat new behaviors until they become part of the child's everyday behaviors.
- Encourage the child to get regular sleeping hours.
- Involve the child in chores that require physical effort (e.g., sweeping, taking out garbage, raking, running errands).

Sample goals:
- Mark will eat a vegetable at each meal.
- Diane will play outside with her family or friends for 1 hour each day.
- Jose and his family will drink water instead of soda on the weekend.
- Rochelle will try Frisbee and tee ball (two new activities) at least three times.
- Sajay will help his parent prepare a low-fat, low-carbohydrate meal (once a week).

After identifying factors that interfere with occupational performance, OT practitioners develop strategies to improve or enhance performance. Goals are developed with children, adolescents, and families. The OT practitioner works closely with them to develop family-based initiatives focusing on sustainable healthy behaviors and routines while diminishing unhealthy eating and activity habits. The individualized attention received in working with a therapist has been found to support positive outcomes. In using online technology behavioral weight management programs, researchers reported that

individuals who received organized and structured interventions with weekly meetings and individual critiques lost more weight than those who solely used the links provided online.[68] A monitoring–mentoring role is one ideally suited to the OTA.

The interventions may follow the principles of behavioral approaches by using age-appropriate **incentives** to shape and reinforce positive behaviors (see Chapter 14). Allowing the children or adolescents to participate in choosing the incentives reinforces motivation and enables them to feel a sense of control. Sense of personal control and autonomy may become an important component of therapy when the child or adolescent feels unable to control his or her weight, eating, or emotions. A cognitive-behavioral approach helps children identify the dysfunctional thinking and behaviors that may be interfering with making healthy lifestyle choices or exercising and the relationship between thoughts, feelings, and events and excessive eating (see Chapter 14). It is necessary that children's cognitive abilities are adequate for insight that will enable them to comprehend the relationships among their thoughts, feelings, and behaviors.

Social cognitive theory may serve as the model for group interventions on an individual level and proposes that gaining personal motivation and self-efficacy about the ability to perform skills increases the ability to plan and carry out behavioral change.[9] Understanding a child's motivation is fundamental in designing and grading group and individual interventions. For example, individually developing motor skills, which can be applied in age-related sports, will give a child confidence to participate in extracurricular physical activities. A sense of competency promotes engagement, which in turn can be reinforcing and may further strengthen and expand related occupational performance skills. Additional benefits (social and academic) are associated with participation in extracurricular activities.[17]

As OT practitioners individually focus on bringing about behavioral changes that shift children toward healthy physical activity and nutrition, an educational approach involving teachers, parents, children, and adolescents is an effective parallel approach. All approaches require that activities and programs be graded so that they are not burdensome to the family, child, or adolescent. Self-identified doable expectations and gradual changes are more likely to be sustainable. For example, although a goal may be to provide intervention to promote high-intensity physical activity, it may start with a short walking program, such as walking home from school, and once established increase the distance, frequency, or intensity. Change is a gradual iterative process—OT practitioners should be sure that children and adolescents have realistic expectations of themselves and that lapses are part of the change process. Another example would be making one or two changes to a family's dietary patterns, such as

BOX 15-7

Recommendations for Physical Activity for All Children at Their Ability Levels

- Perform daily vigorous physical activity for at least 1 hour.
- Engage in play and activities that involve physical activity in a variety of settings: home, school, and community.
- Participate in physical activity with parents; parents can set an example and encourage physical activity as part of everyday life.
- Explore a variety of activities and choose an activity of interest.
- Participate in enjoyable, fun, and motivational activities that promote long-term activity.
- Participate in activities with peers and siblings; peers and siblings can act as role models for physical activity and make it fun.
- Try new activities.

introducing one vegetable at a time to weekend dinners or replacing one high-caloric meal per week or ending post-evening meal snacks.

Home follow-up programs and social support systems (i.e., family, friends, and peers) are significant to the success of individual interventions and should be components of any program (Box 15-7). Programs such as the buddy system are effective in increasing and maintaining physical activity and can increase the children's participation in afterschool free play and involvement in physical activities such as baseball and soccer.

Cultural, social, and community factors exert strong influences on a child and must be integrated into OT interventions.[71] As mentioned previously, obesity rates are higher in inner cities where fresh produce or green space (to play) may be minimal.[18,43,54,67] Practitioners need to be knowledgeable about community resources so that they can make appropriate and feasible recommendations (e.g., recreational departments, local YMCA, afterschool programs, facilitate a school garden program).

Increasing Physical Activity

Children and adolescents should be encouraged to participate in 1 hour of vigorous physical activity every day (www.letsgo.org). Children or adolescents with disabilities are naturally likely to engage in sedentary activities.[58] Similarly, children or adolescents who are obese may have preexisting or acquired motor difficulties that discourage them from engaging in physical activities. When physical activity is difficult, lacking in enjoyment and competence, it is natural that children are drawn to sedentary activities (e.g., watching TV, playing computer

games) where they experience enjoyment and/or success.[58] Increasing physical activity levels includes examining and modifying time use and rewards derived from sedentary activities.

CLINICAL *Pearl*

If a child has a disability, should he or she be physically active? Physical activity is important for all children. There are appropriate types and amount of physical activities for children with disabilities. A physical activity routine should be a component of a child's IEP. Group physical activities in a school setting can offer important social inclusion for a child with a disability.

By understanding client factors associated with obesity, the OT practitioner can target intervention to facilitate movement and engagement in physical activity within the children's ability levels with the "just right" challenge to promote skill development and enjoyment. By analyzing the steps to activities and making the necessary modifications, children and adolescents may experience success in physical activities and gain confidence. Success and enjoyment in physical activities motivates engagement in more activities. Practitioners may design simple steps to increase a child's or adolescent's physical activity level at home by developing programs that involve walking or helping with daily household tasks and that encourage movement (such as dance or retaining some ambulation skills at home or in the classroom and using wheelchairs for outdoor functional mobility). When physical activity can be built into an everyday routine it is more likely to be integrated in the child's and family's routine activity patterns.

Planning use of time and providing incentives is beneficial to maintaining behavioral changes. Sedentary behaviors patterns are addressed in conjunction with increasing physical activity.

CLINICAL *Pearl*

Take an active role in identifying opportunities for physical activity within supportive environments (e.g., teams and physical fitness programs that accommodate children with all levels of ability). Children and adolescents also experience a variety of physical activities and gain physical skills in other settings such as summer camps and community group activities (e.g., scouts). These programs have additional social and emotional benefits.

Children and adolescents are more likely to change exercise patterns if the family is proactive and involved in the process. Encouraging families to make changes, such as turning off the television and having a family evening

BOX 15-8

Recommendations for Promoting Healthy Food Choices for Families

- Make a weekly menu.
- Use a grocery list when shopping.
- Involve children in grocery shopping and meal preparations.
- Eat meals together when possible.
- Limit the amount of soda and candy in the house.
- Establish a nutritional and/or physical goal as a family.
- Make slow transitions when changing food habits so that the changes are achievable.
- Plan and prepare meals in advance to avoid getting take-out foods when pushed for time.
- Limit availability of unhealthy choices in the home, and increase the variety of healthy snacks.
- Avoid associating unhealthy foods with fun and celebrations.
- Do not restrict sodas and candy entirely so that they become "special" foods.

doing alternative activities, reducing computer time, and participating in physical activity together, may all help improve the child's as well as family members' health. Family members can support each other and encourage success. OT practitioners working to make changes in the family system begin by suggesting simple, concrete steps toward goals that the family values. Asking children, adolescents, and families to complete just one of the steps of the program at a time will seem less overwhelming and help them experience success. For example, adolescents who drink large amounts of soda may be able to swap one soda a day for a glass of water. This goal is more achievable than not drinking any soda at all. Family members who support the adolescent by trying to increase their own water intake (over soda) can help him or her develop healthy nutritional patterns in a more effective way. See Box 15-8 for ideas to promote healthy family nutrition.

GROUP AND COMMUNITY INTERVENTIONS

Increasingly, descriptions of programs that target childhood obesity, health, nutrition, and physical activities are appearing in the occupational and educational literature. See Table 15-1 for a description of sample programs addressing obesity for children. The philosophies and emphasis of the programs vary, but the core principles consistently address the following:

- Moderate to high-intensity physical activity
- Social participation
- Nutritional activities and education

- Health education
- Behavioral change and volition
- Self-directedness in spontaneous play and physical activities
- Occupational performance skills

To promote follow-through, many programs involve team models and the education of teachers and parents. Other programmatic goals include promoting sports and extracurricular activities, encouraging hobbies, and involving families and friends in a more active lifestyle.[46] Importantly, programs emphasize setting realistic goals as key to successful outcomes. The outcomes are not measured solely by the amount of weight loss, but generally include child, adolescent, family, or school satisfaction; increased knowledge of nutrition and exercise; improvement in healthy eating habits; increased levels of physical activity; and increased participation in social activities. Figure 15-6 provides examples of low-cost, noncompetitive activities that children and their families may enjoy as part of an intervention plan.

There are a number of OT programs that have a health promotion–obesity prevention agenda or that take a health and fitness approach including weight reduction. There are many ways to design programs. Some programs use environmental design to meet the needs of all children. The playfulness of children has been applied innovatively to provide occupational therapy to children who are obese by introducing novel physical activity toys to Australian playgrounds.[10] The premise of the approach applied by Bundy and colleagues is that play has become too "safe." The hypervigilance and protectiveness of adults is limiting children's creativity and the intensity of their activities, except in organized contexts such as a sports team, which becomes more limited as children age and sports become increasingly competitive. In a randomized control study, novelty play items (e.g., tires, hay) were introduced to selected schools. Although adults provided supervision, they were trained to support children's play without interruption unless their safety was at risk.[10] The children who received this intervention in these schools (when novelty materials were on the playground) were more physically active and playful and were described as "social," "creative," and "resilient," compared with those in the control schools where no changes were introduced to the school playground.[10] This program models an inexpensive preventive approach to changing the play environment to increase children's physical activity levels, with the additional benefits of playfulness and creativity. Another similar OT model of creative outdoor adventure play that is gaining international recognition is the Timbernook program started by occupational therapist Angela Hanscom (http://www.timbernook.com/our-philosophy).

TABLE 15-1

Sample Programs for Children

NAME	DESCRIPTION OF PROGRAM	KEY FEATURES OF PROGRAM
HeartPower! http://www.americanheart.org American Heart Association	The Heart Power! program is a preventive health education project geared to children ages 4–7. It teaches children about heart disease risk factors, which may help reverse current adult trends.	HeartPower! Online is the American Heart Association's collection of free educational materials for preschool, elementary, and middle school students. Printable lesson plans, activity sheets, and teaching ideas can be used for grades K–2, 3–5, and 6–8. These science-based online resources can introduce students to healthy habits and encourage them to live long, healthy lives by making smart choices.
Let's Go! http://www.letsgo.org/ Maine-based program	Let's Go! is a community-based initiative to promote healthy lifestyle choices among children, youth, and families in 12 greater Portland communities. The goal is to increase physical activity and healthy eating in children and youth—from birth to 18 years.	*5, 2, 1, 0 slogan:* 5 fruits and vegetables 2 hours of screen time 1 hour of physical activity 0 sugar Materials and handouts are available.
Be Active Kids North Carolina http://beactivekids.org/bak/Front/Default.aspx	Be Active Kids is an innovative, interactive physical activity, nutrition, and food safety curriculum for North Carolina preschoolers ages 4 and 5 years.	The program uses colorful characters, interactive hands-on lessons, and bright visuals to teach children that physical activity, healthy eating, and food safety can be fun!
Let's Move http://www.letsmove.gov/	Let's Move! has an ambitious but important goal: to solve the epidemic of childhood obesity within a generation.	The program will give parents the support they need, provide healthier foods in schools, help children to be more physically active, and make healthy, affordable food available in every part of the country.
ReCharge! Energizing After School http://www.actionforhealthykids.org/recharge/about/ Action for Healthy Kids and the National Football League	ReCharge! Energizing After-School is an afterschool program designed to help students in grades 2–6 learn about and practice good nutrition and physical activity habits through fun, team-based strategies. It focuses on 4 core concepts: 1. "Energy In" (nutrition) 2. "Energy Out" (physical activity) 3. Teamwork 4. Goal setting	The program addresses national education standards. It is designed to be practical, feasible, and adaptable to a variety of settings and programs.

There are programs that are based on change through education. Munguba et al applied an OT nutrition education program in a municipal school setting.[44] The authors developed both a video game and a board game based on nutritional education and compared the effectiveness of these strategies for learning nutritional information. Two hundred children played the video game and the board game; 27% preferred the video game, and 6% preferred the board game. The children learned facts about nutrition from both games, which suggests that play-based activities are potentially an effective tool in nutritional education. As OT practitioners are skilled at examining and addressing play in children and adolescents, they are encouraged to use games and pretend play to educate children and adolescents on healthy lifestyles.

There are a number of school- and community-based programs.[31,32,53] Increasingly, practitioners who work with children and adolescents who are obese or at risk for obesity are developing school and community-based programs, especially those that focus on nutrition and physical activity choices and promoting health lifestyles.

1. Suarez-Balcazar and colleagues introduced system changes in Chicago schools as a way to help children

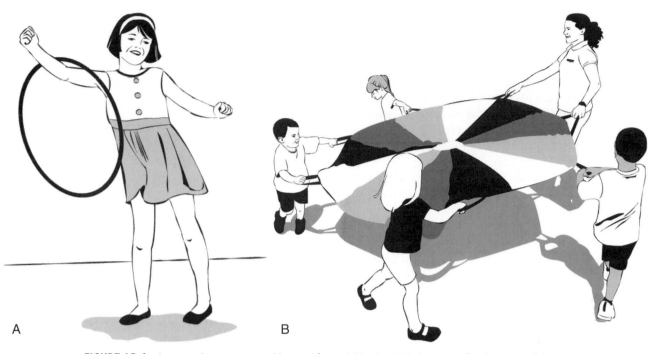

A

B

FIGURE 15-6   Inexpensive, noncompetitive, and fun activities in which the whole family can participate. **A,** Hula-hooping is a great exercise. **B,** Parachute games are fun for all, introduce novelty, and keep children physically active. These activities can easily be graded to accommodate a variety of skill levels.

and adolescents lead healthier lifestyles.[44,67] The authors described many factors involved in the school system (including students, teachers, food vendors, as well as the institution, community, and social and policy structures). They examined the barriers to system changes and implemented strategies to facilitate change. In an effort to make system changes, the authors developed new school initiatives to offer healthier choices in the vending machines and introduced the Cool Food initiative (salad bar wagons). The systems changes were paired with nutrition education sessions for students.

2. Kuo and colleagues used a service-learning model with graduate OT students to offer an interprofessional culturally sensitive weight prevention and intervention weight management program to 8- to 15-year-olds in Indiana.[35] The S.T.O.P. (Stop Taking On Pounds) 12-week program focused on fitness, nutrition, and behavioral management. The main goals were to teach families how to eat nutritious foods in the right amount, to teach them fun ways to be physically active together, and to change behaviors that may lead to weight gain.[35] The program offered hands-on educational sessions that included participating in physical activities and working on weekly nutrition and fitness goals with positive social support and weekly incentive prizes. A bilingual (Spanish and English) version of the program was offered after 1 year. A template of this successful intervention program is provided by Kuo et al.[35]

3. Lau and colleagues developed several programs.[36] The most recent, Healthy Choices for Me, was a 12-week urban elementary school program for children from two lower socioeconomic schools. It was designed to provide children experiences with physical activity and healthy foods to promote self-efficacy in healthy lifestyle behaviors.[36] Children in the afterschool program, which was implemented by OT students, demonstrated positive changes in food behavior, food self-efficacy, and vegetable consumption.

4. Children with developmental coordination disorder (DCD) are a high-risk group for excessive weight gain. These children's poor motor skills are associated with low levels of fitness and being overweight.[59] Missiuna and colleagues offer a tiered model of intervention, which is based on a partnership between OT practitioners, teachers, and parents.[40] The focus is capacity building; this is not a fitness-health style prevention promotion program. An example is included here to demonstrate that participation and gains in motor-based occupational performance that builds self-efficacy is an alternative approach to address health-related concerns that are associated with an existing disorder or disability. The design is a collaborative and coaching model that employs strategies to enhance the child with DCD school experience. Principles of universal learning design and awareness of facilitating motor skills in classroom activities changes the classroom environment (physical and social) to promote

occupational performance. Children with specific occupational performance–related needs receive specific instructional assistance, strategies that facilitate their learning and accommodations as required. Effective interventions promote inclusion for children with DCD and prevent likelihood of problems with physical health (unhealthy increases in weight and lack of fitness), social and mental health problems, and deterioration in academic performance.

These examples provide OT practitioners with strategies at the individual, group, and system levels that help children and adolescents lead healthier lives. The short-term consequences of childhood obesity are significant (e.g., type 2 diabetes, cardiac disease, asthma, apnea, and limited mobility); therefore OT practitioners must join efforts by health and educational colleagues to reduce the incidence of obesity. The studies mentioned here offer models of effective programs and intervention strategies such as games based on nutrition, introducing novel toys to the playground, and increasing healthy nutritional choices at school that have made a difference in the health of children and adolescents with weight issues. The case study presented here offers an in-depth look at one of the programs.

CASE *Study*

The "FUN" Maine Program

OT practitioners consider the complex nature of obesity when designing a program to improve engagement in healthy occupations and routines as a way to prevent obesity and promote health. Typically, programs emphasize helping children develop attitudes for overall wellness, that is, thoughts, feeling, and beliefs toward health.[25] Without attitude and behavioral change the newly acquired knowledge and activity patterns will not be generalized and sustained as the child develops.

The Maine FUN Program used the Model of Human Occupation (MOHO) as a frame of reference for designing an effective program.[33] The explicit use of an OT frame of reference was a distinct feature of this health and fitness afterschool rural program. Kielhofner suggested that engaging children in volitionally oriented activities helps them sustain activity over time, which makes a difference in their overall health.[33] This model is applicable and addresses the multiple factors associated with childhood obesity and, thus, informs a practitioner in designing and implementing multisystem interventions.

O'Brien and colleagues designed and conducted a community afterschool intervention (Fitness, yoU, and Nutrition [FUN] program) to target children's volition, habits, and performance (Figure 15-7).[48,49] See Box 15-9 for an overview of the program. The aim of the FUN program was to develop healthy habits and encourage children to journal their eating patterns, engage in a variety of play activities, and exercise weekly. The children in the FUN program received incentives (such as hula-hoops) to continue to play actively.

The program measured outcomes in terms of interest in activity (volition), habits (habituation), and performance (physical fitness, BMI). Children received workbooks with weekly goals to enhance the program, which expanded

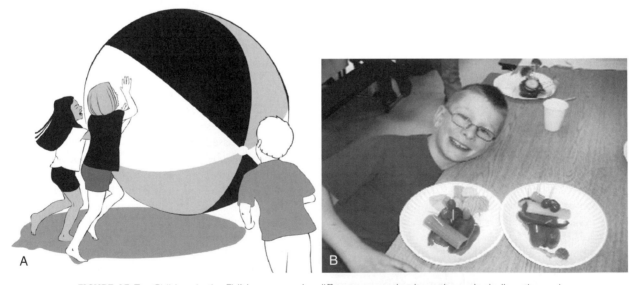

FIGURE 15-7 Children in the FUN program play different games that keep them physically active and having fun. These games are motivating and interesting to children. **A,** Space day includes games with a giant ball (the moon)! **B,** Zander is proud of his "alien" vegetables. Children in the FUN program try nutritious foods while making interesting recipes. Making nutritional education fun and playful helps children learn.

to include more parental input and family follow-through. Children enjoyed engaging in fun activities after school with friends. Parents reported that children ate more varieties of food, paid attention to the food they were eating, drank more water, and played outside using incentives (e.g., hula hoops, jump ropes).

BOX 15-9

Fitness, yoU, and Nutrition (FUN)[48,49]

Focusing on fun afterschool activities, the authors of the program encouraged children in grades 3 and 4 to participate in physical activities and take steps toward healthy nutrition. OT students designed and implemented creative weekly sessions based on selected themes and emphasizing healthy nutrition and physical activity. Participants learned about healthy nutritional choices (e.g., the five food groups, variety in diet, importance of water, protein, grains, vegetables, and fruits). Children received incentives, such as hula-hoops, jump ropes, and Frisbees. One hundred children from the Waterboro Elementary School in Waterboro, Maine, participated in the 2-year program.

The overall objectives of the FUN program include:

- *Volition:* Increase child's motivation and interest in physical activity and healthy nutrition.
- *Habituation:* Develop healthy nutritional and physical activity habits and routines.
  - Children will engage in physical activity for 1 hour daily.
  - Children will show improved nutritional habits, such as drinking water instead of soda, and eating more vegetables.
- *Performance:* Achieve healthy BMI; succeed in the Presidential Physical Fitness Test.
- *Environment:* Parents will be engaged in effort to improve nutritional and physical activity habits and routines.

The FUN program will provide a free afterschool program in the child's community.

SAMPLE FUN WEEKLY SESSION

Theme: Beach Day
Goal: Drink water instead of soda. Play outside with friends!
Physical Activity: Children enjoyed playing beach-type games, such as directing a "fish" into the water. This game involved holding newspapers and using arm movements to move construction-paper fish into the hula-hoops (water). Other games included hula-hoop contest to beach music and playing with the 8-foot beach ball.
Snacks and Drinks: Fruit kabobs (introduce children to something they might not have tried).
Incentive: Children took home with them bottled water, fresh fruit, and hula-hoops.

SUMMARY

A child's capacity to participate in meaningful occupations is affected by obesity.[3] OT practitioners are in a unique position to address the multitude of factors contributing to this serious issue. Along with physical limitations such as limited movement, decreased endurance, lack of strength, and poor mobility, obesity may harm a child's or adolescent's psychosocial well-being; children and adolescents who are obese often suffer from bullying, teasing, and low self-esteem. Environmental influences may present barriers to the ability of the child, adolescent, and family to engage in occupations. OT practitioners can help remove these barriers by introducing programs that address healthy physical and nutritional habits and routines for all children. Social afterschool programs help children achieve lifestyle changes within their own communities and serve as educational and behavioral models for change. A review of the biological, physical, and psychosocial issues present in this population includes the development of self-efficacy, self-esteem, and body awareness for children and adolescents who are overweight or obese. The contributing factors to obesity, strategies for intervention planning, and sample programs to promote healthy routines and habits in children and adolescents were presented. Case examples illustrated key concepts.

References

1. American Academy of Pediatrics. (2001). Children, adolescents, and television. *Pediatrics, 107,* 423.
2. American Academy of Pediatrics. (2003). Prevention of pediatric overweight and obesity. *Pediatrics, 112,* 424.
3. American Occupational Therapy Association (AOTA). (2011). *Occupational therapy's role in mental health promotion, prevention, and intervention with children & youth: childhood obesity.* Bethesda, MD: Author.
4. Anderson, P. M., & Butcher, K. E. (2006). Childhood obesity: trends and potential causes. *Future Child, 16,* 19.
5. Bandini, L. G., et al. (2005). Prevalence of overweight in children with developmental disorders in the continuous National Health and Nutrition Examination Survey (NHANES) 1999-2002. *J Pediatr, 146,* 738–743.
6. Birch, L. L., & Davidson, K. K. (2001). Family environmental factors influencing the developing controls of food intake and childhood overweight. *Pediatr Clin North Am, 48,* 893.
7. Boeka, A. G., & Lokken, K. L. (2008). Neuropsychological performance of a clinical sample of extremely obese individuals. *Arch Clin Neuropsychol, 23,* 467–474.
8. Britz, B., et al. (2000). Rates of psychiatric disorders in a clinical study group of adolescents with extreme obesity and in obese adolescents ascertained via a population based study. *Int J Obes Relat Metab Disord, 24,* 1707–1714.
9. Budd, G. M., & Volpe, S. L. (2006). School-based obesity prevention: research, challenges, and recommendations. *J School Health, 76,* 485.

10. Bundy, A. C., et al. (2008). Playful interaction: occupational therapy for all children on the school playground. *Am J Occup Ther, 62*, 522.

11. Butler, M. G., Hanchett, J. M., & Thompson, T. (2006). Clinical findings and natural history of Prader-Willi syndrome. In M. G. Butler, P. D. K. Lee, & B. Y. Whitman (Eds.), *Management of Prader-Willi syndrome*. New York: Springer.

12. Carr, D., & Friedman, M. (2005). Is obesity stigmatizing? Body weight, perceived discrimination, and psychological well-being in the United States. *J Health Soc Behav, 46*, 244.

13. Davidson, M., & Knafl, K. A. (2006). Dimensional analysis of the concept of obesity. *J Adv Nurs, 54*, 342.

14. Delin, C. (1995). Perceptions of disability by students, the formerly obese and general community. *Psychol Rep, 76*, 1219.

15. Duke, J., Huhman, M., & Heitzler, C. (2002). Physical activity levels among children aged 9-13 years—United States. *MMWR Morb Mortal Wkly Rep, 52*, 785.

16. Dwyer, G., et al. (2009). Promoting children's health and well-being: broadening the therapy perspective. *Phys Occup Ther Pediatr, 29*, 27.

17. Eccles, J. S., et al. (2003). Extracurricular activities and adolescent development. *J Soc Issues, 59*, 865.

18. Evans, G. (2004). The psychological environment of childhood poverty. *Am Psychol, 59*, 78.

19. Faith, M. S., et al. (2004). Parental feeding attitudes and styles, and child body mass index: prospective analysis of a gene-environment interaction. *Pediatrics, 114*, 429.

20. Faith, M. S., et al. (2002). Weight criticism during physical activity, coping skills, and reported physical activity in children. *Pediatrics, 110*, 23.

21. Field, A. S., & Kitos, N. R. (2009). Social and interpersonal influences on obesity in youth: family, peers and society. In L. J. Heinberg, & J. K. Thompson (Eds.), *Obesity in youth: causes, consequences, and cures*. Washington, DC: American Psychological Association.

22. Fisher, J. O., Sinton, M. M., & Birch, L. L. (2009). Early parental influences and risk for the emergence of disordered eating. In L. Smolak, & J. K. Thompson (Eds.), *Body image, eating disorders, and obesity in youth: assessment, prevention and treatment*. Washington, DC: American Psychological Association.

23. Foti, D. (2005). Caring for the person of size. *OT Practice, 10*, 9.

24. Gillman, M. W., et al. (2000). Family dinner and diet quality among older children and adolescents. *Arch Fam Med, 9*, 235–240.

25. Gill, S. V., & Hung, Y.-C. (2014). Effect of overweight and obese body mass on motor planning and motor skills during obstacle crossing in children. *Res Dev Disabil, 35*, 46–53.

26. Haines, J., & Neumark-Sztainer, D. (2009). Psychosocial consequences of obesity and weight bias: implications for interventions. In L. J. Heinberg, & J. K. Thompson (Eds.), *Obesity in youth: causes, consequences, and cures*. Washington, DC: American Psychological Association.

27. Haines, J., Neumark-Sztainer, D., & Thiel, L. (2007). Address weight-related issues in an elementary: what do students, parents, and school staff recommend? *Eat Disord, 15*, 5.

28. Herbozo, S., & Thompson, J. K. (2009). Body image in pediatric obesity. In L. J. Heinberg, & J. K. Thompson (Eds.), *Obesity in youth: causes, consequences, and cures*. Washington, DC: American Psychological Association.

29. Hill, J. O., et al. (2003). Obesity and the environment: where do we go from here? *Science, 299*, 853.

30. Jensen, M.D., et al. (2013). AHA/ACC/TOS guideline for the management of overweight and obesity in adults. Available at: http://circ.ahajournals.org.

31. Johnston, C. A., Moreno, J. P., El-Mubasher, A., Gallagher, M., Tyler, C., & Woehler, D. (2013). Impact of a school based pediatric obesity prevention program facilitated by health professionals. *J School Health, 83*, 171–182.

32. Khambalia, A. Z., Dickinson, S., Hardy, L. L., Gill, T., & Baur, L. A. (2011). Obesity Prevention: A synthesis of existing systematic reviews and meta-analyses of school-based behavioural interventions for controlling and preventing obesity. *Obes Rev, 13*, 214–233.

33. Kielhofner, G. (2008). In *Models of human occupation: theory and application* (4th ed). Baltimore, MD: Lippincott Williams & Wilkins.

34. Koplan, J. P., Liverman, C., & Kraak, V. I. (Eds.). (2005). *Preventing childhood obesity*. Washington, DC: National Academies Press.

35. Kuo, F., Goebel, N. A., Satkamp, N., Beauchamp, R., Kurrasch, J. M., Smith, A. R., et al. (2013). Service learning in a pediatric weight management program to address childhood obesity. *Occupational Therapy In Health Care, 27*, 142–162.

36. Lau, C., Stevens, D., & Jia, J. (2013). Effects of an Occupation-Based Obesity Prevention Program for Children at Risk. *Occup Ther Health Care, 27*, 166–175.

37. Lyon, H. N., & Hirschhorn, J. N. (2005). Genetics of common forms of obesity: a brief overview. *Am J Clin Nutr, 82*(suppl), 215S–217S.

38. Markward, N. J., Markward, M. J., & Peterson, C. A. (2009). Biological and genetic influences. In L. J. Heinberg, & J. K. Thompson (Eds.), *Obesity in youth: causes, consequences, and cures*. Washington, DC: American Psychological Association.

39. Minihan, P. M., Fitch, A. N., & Must, A. (2007). What does the epidemic of childhood obesity mean for children with special health needs? *J Law Med Ethics, 35*, 61.

40. Missiuna, C. A., Pollock, N. A., Levac, D. E., Campbell, W. N., Whalen, S. D., Bennett, S. M., et al. (2012). Partnering for change: an innovative school-based occupational therapy service delivery model for children with developmental coordination disorder. *Can J Occup Ther, 79*, 41–50.

41. Morland, K., Wing, S., Roux, A. D., & Poole, C. (2002). Neighborhood characteristics associated with the location of food stores and food service places. *Am J Prev Med, 22*, 23–29.

42. Morrison, T. G., & O'Connor, W. E. (1999). Psychometric properties of a scale measuring negative attitudes towards overweight individuals. *J Soc Psychol, 139*, 436.

43. Morland, K., et al. (2002). Neighborhood characteristics associated with the location of food stores and food service places. *Am J Prev Med, 22*, 23.

44. Munguba, M. C., Valdes, M. T., & da Silva, C. A. (2008). CAD: the application of an occupational therapy nutrition education programme for children who are obese. *Occup Ther Int, 15*, 56.

45. Neumark-Sztainer, D., Levin, M. P., & Paxton, S. (2006). Prevention of body dissatisfaction and disordered eating: what next? *Eat Disord, 14*, 265.

46. Nowicki, P. (2007). Physical activity—key issues in treatment of childhood obesity. *Acta Paediatr, 96*, 39.

47. Obama, M. (2010). Remarks of First Lady Michelle Obama. Available at: http://www.whitehouse.gov/the-press-office/remarks-first-lady-michelle-obama.

48. O'Brien, J., et al. (2010). *FUN program (Phase II): parent involvement and behavioral changes to improve wellness in elementary school children.* Portland, ME: University of New England.

49. O'Brien, J., et al. (2010). *FUN program (Phase I): development of the Fitness, yoU, and Nutrition (FUN) after school program to improve wellness in elementary school children.* Portland, ME: University of New England.

50. Ogden, C. L., Carroll, M. D., Kit, B. K., & Flegal, K. M. (2014). Prevalence of childhood and adult obesity in the United States, 2011-2012. *JAMA, 311*, 806–814.

51. Pieper, J. R., & Whaley, S. E. (2011). Healthy eating behaviors and the cognitive environment are positively associated in low-income households with young children. *Appetite, 57*, 59–64.

52. Pierce, J. W., & Wardle, A. (1997). Cause and effect beliefs and self-esteem of overweight children. *J Child Psychol Psychiatr, 38*, 645–650.

53. Pizzi, M., Vroman, K., Lau, C., Gill, S., Bazyk, S., Suarez-Balcazar, Y., et al. (2014). Occupational therapy and the childhood obesity epidemic: research, theory and practice. *J Occup Ther Sch Early Interv, 12*, 87–105.

54. Powell, L., Slater, S. A., & Chaloupka, F. (2004). The relationship between physical activity settings and race, ethnicity, and socioeconomic status. *Evid-Based Prev Med, 1*, 135–155.

55. Centers for Disease Control and Prevention. (2009). *Overweight and obese.* Available at: http://www.cdc.gov/obesity/defining.html.

56. Puhl, R. M., Peterson, J. L., & Luedicke, J. (2013). Strategies to address weight-based victimization: youths' preferred support interventions from classmates, teachers, and parents. *J Youth Adolesc, 42*(3), 315–327.

57. Puhl, R. M., Luedicke, J., & Heuer, C. (2011). Weight-based victimization toward overweight adolescents: observations and reactions of peers. *J School Health, 81*, 696–703.

58. Rimmer, J. H., Rowland, J. L., & Yamaki, K. (2007). Obesity and secondary conditions in adolescents with disabilities: addressing the need of an underserved population. *J Adolesc Health, 41*, 224.

59. Rivilis, I., Hay, J., Cairney, J., Klentrou, P., Liu, J., & Faught, B. E. (2011). Physical activity and fitness in children with developmental coordination disorder: a systematic review. *Res Dev Disabil, 32*, 894–910.

60. Russell-Mayhew, S., McVey, G., Bardick, A., & Ireland, A. (2012). Mental health, wellness, and childhood overweight/obesity. *J Obes.* http://dx.doi.org/10.1155/2012/281801.

61. Sallis, J. F., Prochaska, J. J., & Taylor, W. C. (2000). A review of correlates of physical activity in children and adolescents. *Med Sci Sports Exerc, 32*, 963.

62. Sallis, J. F., Rosenberg, D., & Kerr, J. (2009). Early physical activity, sedentary behavior, and dietary patterns. In L. J. Heinberg, & J. K. Thompson (Eds.), *Obesity in youth: causes, consequences, and cures.* Washington, DC: American Psychological Association.

63. Serdula, M. K., et al. (1993). Do obese children become obese adults? A review of the literature. *Prev Med, 22*, 167 1993.

64. Shanklin, S., et al. (2008). CDC: Youth Risk Behavior Surveillance—selected steps communities, United States, 2007. *MMWR, 5–7*(SS-12), 1–27.

65. Solomon, J. W. (1960). *Childhood obesity.* Post and Courier: Charleston, SC.

66. Sorof, J., & Daniels, S. (2000). Obesity, hypertension in children: a problem of epidemic proportions. *Hypertension, 40*, 441.

67. Suarez-Balcazar, Y., et al. (2007). Introducing systems change in the schools: the case of school luncheons and vending machines. *Am J Community Psychol, 39*, 335.

68. Tate, D. F., Wing, R. R., & Winett, R. A. (2001). Using Internet technology to deliver a behavioral weight loss program. *JAMA, 285*, 1172–1177.

69. Teachman, B. A., & Brownell, K. D. (2001). Implicit anti-fat bias among health professionals: is anyone immune? *Int J Obes, 25*, 1525.

70. Vroman, K., & Cote, S. (2011). Prejudicial attitudes toward clients who are obese: measuring implicit anti-fat attitudes of occupational therapy students. *Occup Ther Health Care, 25*(1), 77–90.

71. Warren, J. M., et al. (2003). Evaluation of a pilot school programme aimed at the prevention of obesity in children. *Health Promotion Int, 18*, 287.

72. Warschburger, P. (2005). The unhappy obese child. *Int J Obes, 29*, S127.

73. Whitt-Gover, M. C., O'Neill, K. L., & Stettler, N. (2006). Physical activity patterns in children with and without Down syndrome. *Pediatr Rehabil, 9*, 158.

74. Woods, S. C., & Seeley, R. J. (2005). Regulation of appetite, satiety, and energy metabolism. In J. Antel, et al. (Ed.), *Obesity and metabolic disorders.* Amsterdam: IOS Press.

Recommended Reading

Heinberg, L. J., & Thompson, J. K. (Eds.). (2009). *Obesity in youth: causes consequences and cures.* Washington, DC: American Psychological Association.

Smolak, L., & Thompson, J. K. (Eds.). (2009). *Body image, eating disorders, and obesity in youth: assessment, prevention and treatment.* Washington, DC: American Psychological Association.

Resources

www.aota.org/-/media/Corporate/Files/AboutOT/consumers/
Youth/obesity.pdf
American Occupational Association Tip Sheet *Addressing Childhood Obesity*
www.aota.org/Practice/Children-Youth/Mental%20Health/
School-Mental-Health.aspx
Strongly recommends these informative resources materials for occupational therapists.

- Occupational Therapy's Role in Mental Health Promotion, Prevention, & Intervention with Children & Youth: Childhood Obesity.
- Occupational Therapy's Role in Mental Health Promotion, Prevention, & Intervention with Children & Youth: Bullying Prevention and Friendship Promotion
- Occupational Therapy's Role in Mental Health Promotion, Prevention, & Intervention with Children & Youth: Recess Promotion

- Occupational Therapy's Role in Mental Health Promotion, Prevention, & Intervention with Children & Youth - The Cafeteria: Creating a Positive Mealtime Experience

www.timbernook.com/our-philosophy
An innovative nature-based developmental program, established by a pediatric occupational therapist, designed to foster creativity, imagination, and independent play in the great outdoors. It offers camps that give children the right combination of space and resources to build, create, and explore nature to promote a child's healthy development.
www.whitehouse.gov/blog/2010/02/09/making-moves-a-healthier-generation.
This web site is the Let's Move campaign site with updates of programs and activities to decrease obesity and promote health in America's children.
www.mypyramid.com.
This web site describes healthy food and activity habits and routines for children. Printable and lessons for nutrition and activity for children are provided on this site.

REVIEW *Questions*

1. Explain to another colleague/student the factors that contribute to obesity in children and adolescents and how these factors interact?
2. What are the principles of interventions for preventing obesity?
3. What are the client factors that may be influenced by obesity in children who have special needs?
4. Describe anti-fat attitudes and stereotypes and how they might influence the OT practitioner–client relationship and treatment effectiveness.
5. How might obesity interfere with the occupational performance of children and adolescents?
6. How do interventions for preventing obesity differ in the following settings: family, school, and community?
7. What is the COTA's role in promoting physical activity, healthy lifestyle patterns, and self-efficacy for healthy behaviors?

SUGGESTED *Activities*

1. Go to www.implicit.harvard.edu/implicit/demo, the web site for the Implicit Attitude Test (IAT), which measures one's attitudes toward those who are obese. Take the test to find out what your attitudes are toward people who are obese. Reflect on the findings, and discuss how you will use this information in practice.
2. Develop a physical activity and nutritional lesson plan for children or adolescents. Include handouts.
3. Keep a food and exercise diary for a week, including the weekend. What did you learn about your eating and exercise patterns? Did you meet the criteria for a healthy diet? In the following week, eat one more fruit or vegetable each day, and at the end of the week, review your success with this behavioral change. What were the barriers, and what supported you to make this dietary change?
4. Measure the height and weight of 10 children. Determine each child's age. Calculate each child's BMI and percentile and categorize the findings. Describe your findings, and report what percentage of the children would meet the criteria for being obese or overweight.
5. Explore resources in your area for physical activities for children. Compile a list of resources, and share it with your classmates. Are any of these resources also available to children or adolescents who have disabilities?

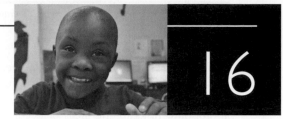

16

JEAN WELCH SOLOMON

Intellectual Disabilities

CHAPTER *Objectives*

After studying this chapter, the reader will be able to accomplish the following:
- Identify possible causes of intellectual disabilities.
- Differentiate the classifications of intellectual disabilities.
- Identify adaptive functioning for each level of intellectual disabilities.
- Identify the amount of support needed for each level of intellectual disabilities.
- Explain the roles of the occupational therapist and the occupational therapy assistant in assessments of and interventions with children who have intellectual disabilities.

CHAPTER *Outline*

A child diagnosed with **intellectual disability** (ID) has impaired cognitive functioning that interferes with his or her ability to perform age-appropriate tasks in the areas of occupation, including social participation, education, activities of daily living (ADLs), instrumental ADLs (IADLs), and play/leisure. A child diagnosed with ID may or may not have an associated secondary disability, such as cerebral palsy or a speech and language impairment, that interferes with the acquisition of performance skills. Infants, toddlers, school-age children, and adolescents with ID benefit from occupational therapy (OT) interventions to promote performance in occupations. Adults with ID also benefit from OT interventions to successfully participate in occupations over the life span.

DEFINITION

The former term *mental retardation* has been replaced by the current term *intellectual disability* to describe the condition in which a child has cognitive impairments that interfere with adaptive skills. The term *intellectual disability* will be primarily used in this chapter; the term *mental retardation* will be referred to when describing the classification of children with the type of disability or when referring to past sources that use this term.

ID is a neurodevelopmental disorder that occurs before the age of 18 years and is characterized by significantly below-average intellectual functioning as well as deficits in two or more adaptive skill areas (e.g., ADLs, communication, social participation, education, play/leisure, homemaking skills, and skills required to attain and maintain independence).[1] See Table 16-1 for summative descriptions of conceptual, social, and practical adaptive behaviors for specific levels of severity of the ID.[1]

Children with IDs may look different. Some children have secondary conditions or syndromes (e.g., trisomy 21) and present with certain physical features. Other children may exhibit no atypical physical characteristics. In general, parents and professionals suspect ID when a child fails to meet developmental milestones. Some children with mild disability may not be identified until they begin school. Unlike a learning disability, which affects one area of learning (e.g., math or reading), ID affects learning in all areas of one's occupation.

The diagnosis of ID involves consideration of the child's cultural, linguistic, behavioral, sensory, motor, and communication abilities and, in particular, how those abilities may influence intelligence testing. Professionals consider the child's age, strengths, and weaknesses, along with the limitations in intelligence when examining how these factors influence adaptive functioning.[2] Health care professionals not only provide the diagnosis, they are also interested in providing information to develop an individualized plan of needed supports that will improve the child's ability to participate in occupations.[8]

TABLE 16-1

Severity Levels for Intellectual Disability (Intellectual Developmental Disorder)

SEVERITY LEVEL	CONCEPTUAL DOMAIN	SOCIAL DOMAIN	PRACTICAL DOMAIN
Mild	For preschool children, there may be no obvious conceptual differences. For school-age children and adults, there are difficulties in learning academic skills involving reading, writing, arithmetic, time, or money, with support needed in one or more areas to meet age-related expectations. In adults, abstract thinking, executive function (i.e., planning, strategizing, priority setting, and cognitive flexibility), and short-term memory, as well as functional use of academic skills (e.g., reading, money management), are impaired. There is a somewhat concrete approach to problems and solutions compared with agemates.	Compared with typically developing agemates, the individual is immature in social interactions. For example, there may be difficulty in accurately perceiving peers' social cues. Communication, conversation, and language are more concrete or immature than expected for age. There may be difficulties regulating emotion and behavior in age-appropriate fashion; peers notice these difficulties in social situations. There is limited understanding of risk in social situations; social judgment is immature for age, and the person is at risk for being manipulated by others (gullibility).	The individual may function age appropriately in personal care. Individuals need some support with complex daily living tasks in comparison with peers. In adulthood, supports typically involve grocery shopping, transportation, home and child-care organizing, nutritious food preparation, and banking and money management. Recreational skills resemble those of agemates, although judgment related to well-being and organization around recreation requires support. In adulthood, competitive employment is often seen in jobs that do not emphasize conceptual skills. Individuals generally need support to make health care decisions and legal decision, and to learn to perform a skilled vocation competently. Support is typically needed to raise a family.

Continued

TABLE 16-1

Severity Levels for Intellectual Disability (Intellectual Developmental Disorder)—cont'd

SEVERITY LEVEL	CONCEPTUAL DOMAIN	SOCIAL DOMAIN	PRACTICAL DOMAIN
Moderate	All through development, the individual's conceptual skills lag markedly behind those of peers. For preschoolers, language and preacademic skills develop slowly. For school-age children, progress in reading, writing, mathematics, and understanding of time and money occurs slowly across the school years and is markedly limited compared with that of peers. For adults, academic skill development is typically at an elementary level, and support is required for all use of academic skills in work and personal life. Ongoing assistance on a daily basis is needed to complete conceptual tasks of day-to-day life, and others may take over these responsibilities fully for the individual.	The individual shows marked differences from peers in social and communicative behavior across development. Spoken language is typically a primary tool for social communication but is much less complex than that of peers. Capacity for relationships is evident in ties to family and friends, and the individual may have successful friendships across life and sometimes romantic relations in adulthood. However, individuals may not perceive or interpret social cues accurately. Social judgment and decision-making abilities are limited, and caretakers must assist the person with life decisions. Friendships with typically developing peers are often affected by communication or social limitations. Significant social and communicative support is needed in work settings for success.	The individual can care for personal needs involving eating, dressing, eliminations, and hygiene as an adult, although an extended period of teaching and time is needed for the individual to become independent in these areas, and reminders may be needed. Similarly, participation in all household tasks can be achieved by adulthood, although an extended period of teaching is needed, and ongoing supports will typically occur for adult-level performance. Independent employment in jobs that require limited conceptual and communication skills can be achieved, but considerable support from co-workers, supervisors, and others is needed to manage social expectations, job complexities, and ancillary responsibilities such as scheduling, transportation, health benefits, and money management. A variety of recreational skills can be developed. These typically require additional supports and learning opportunities over an extended period of time. Maladaptive behavior is present in a significant minority and causes social problems.
Severe	Attainment of conceptual skills is limited. The individual generally has little understanding of written language or of concepts involving numbers, quantity, time, and money. Caretakers provide extensive supports for problem solving throughout life.	Spoken language is quite limited in terms of vocabulary and grammar. Speech may be single words or phrases and may be supplemented through augmentative means. Speech and communication are focused on the here and now within everyday events. Language is used for social communication more than for explication. Individuals understand simple speech and gestural communication. Relationships with family members and familiar others are a source of pleasure and help.	The individual requires support for all activities of daily living, including meals, dressing, bathing, and elimination. The individual requires supervision at all times. The individual cannot make responsible decisions regarding well-being of self or others. In adulthood, participation in tasks at home, recreation, and work requires ongoing support and assistance. Skill acquisition in all domains involves long-term teaching and ongoing support. Maladaptive behavior, including self-injury, is present in a significant minority.

MEASUREMENT AND CLASSIFICATION

Formal testing procedures are used to diagnose children with ID. The diagnosis is made using information from interviews with parents, observations of the child, and completion of norm-referenced tests. The following criteria suggest the diagnosis of ID:

1. Deficits in intellectual function (e.g., abstract thinking, problem solving, academic learning) as confirmed by clinical assessment and individualized, standardized testing.

2. Deficits in adaptive behavior that require ongoing support to be successful in daily life across multiple environments as confirmed by clinical assessment. Because adaptive functioning determines the level of support an individual needs, the level of severity of ID is defined by adaptive functioning that is a more reliable indicator of intensity of

TABLE 16-2

Categories of Intellectual Disability Based on IQ Scores

RANGE OF IQ SCORES	INTELLECTUAL DISABILITY CATEGORY
55–69	Mild
40–54	Moderate
25–39	Severe
<25	Profound

IQ = intelligence quotient

support compared with intellectual quotient (IQ) measures.[1]

3. "Onset of intellectual and adaptive deficits during the developmental period."[1, p. 33]

Intelligence Testing

An **intelligence quotient** (IQ) is a score derived from one of several different standardized tests designed to assess intelligence. Scores from tests of intelligence are primary tools for identifying children with IDs. Intelligence tests are scored on a scale of 0 to 145, with the average score of 100 and a standard deviation of 15 points. Table 16-2 describes the categories of intellectual disability according to IQ scores.[5]

Scores between 85 and 115 are considered within normal limits (average IQ). Children who score between 70 and 84 fall within the borderline ID range; a score between 55 and 69 represents mild ID; a score between 25 and 39 is considered severe ID; and children with scores lower than 25 are classified as having profound ID.[5]

IQ tests such as the revised Wechsler Intelligence Scale (WISC-R),[16] Stanford-Binet Intelligence Scale,[13] McCarthy Scales of Children's Ability,[10] and Bayley Scales of Infant Development[4] are administered by a qualified psychologist. These tests include sections on motor and verbal abilities. Administering IQ tests to children with severe disabilities can be challenging; any changes in how the test is administered tend to interfere with standardization and the results. Therefore, OT clinicians must view the results of IQ tests cautiously. Because infant and child IQ tests require motor responses, those who are physically unable to perform certain motor tasks may receive lower scores.

Along with intelligence testing, children must exhibit a deficit in two or more areas of adaptive functioning to be diagnosed with ID. Understanding the areas in which a child is able to function provides OT practitioners with information for planning interventions and providing support services.

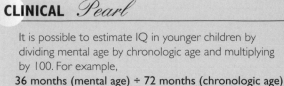

CLINICAL *Pearl*

It is possible to estimate IQ in younger children by dividing mental age by chronologic age and multiplying by 100. For example,
36 months (mental age) ÷ 72 months (chronologic age) × 100 = 50.
The child in this example has an IQ of 50. (Note: This is considered an estimate.)

Adaptive Functioning

Adaptive functioning refers to the conceptual, social, and practical abilities that children rely on to adapt to changing environments and to function in their everyday lives. Conceptual skills include receptive and expressive language, reading and writing, money concepts, and self-direction. Social skills refer to self-esteem, social problem solving, and the ability to follow rules, obey laws, and avoid being victimized. Practical skills include ADLs, occupational skills, health care, travel/transportation, schedules/routines, safety, use of money, and use of the telephone.[3] Limitations in these areas significantly interfere with a child's ability to navigate through everyday situations.[1,2]

To measure adaptive behavior, OT practitioners look at what a child can do in comparison with other children of the same age. Adaptive skills are evaluated in many different settings, with input from the caregiver or teacher as well. A variety of scales are available to measure adaptive functioning:

- The Vineland Adaptive Behavior Scale uses parental input to evaluate adaptive behavior in terms of communication, daily living, socialization, and motor skills.[12]
- The School Functional Assessment uses input from the teacher to assess the child's ability to perform the occupational tasks necessary in the school setting.[7]
- The Support Intensity Scale (SIS) measures the pattern and level of support required for an adult with ID to lead a normal, independent life.[14] Subscales of the SIS are home living activities, community and neighborhood activities, school participation, school learning, health and safety, social, and advocacy. The SIS measures the support required in the medical, behavioral, and life activity areas and also addresses the frequency, time of day, and type of support required. This is beneficial when developing support plans and can assist with resource allocation and financial planning.[11]

Mental Age

Mental age refers to the age level at which the child is functioning, whereas chronologic age refers to the child's actual age. For example, a 5-year-old child who is only able to perform tasks that a typical 3-year-old performs would be considered to have a mental age of 3. Mental age is based on and determined by performance on standardized tests. These tests allow the child's performance to be equitably compared with the chronologic age standard.

ETIOLOGY AND PREVALENCE

The prevalence of ID in the general population is approximately 1%.[1] Causes include genetic factors, problems during pregnancy, difficult births, and health problems. In many cases, the cause remains unknown. Children with ID can also have physical and psychological disabilities. These deficits can include visual impairments, hearing loss, muscle tone problems, seizures, and sensory disorders. Physicians often categorize the causes of ID on the basis of when they occur. Prenatal causes occur before birth, perinatal causes occur at birth, and postnatal causes occur from birth to 3 years of age.

Prenatal Causes

Prenatal (before birth) causes of ID include genetics, disturbances in embryonic development, and acquired causes (e.g., maternal toxins).

Genetic Causes

ID may be caused by errors occurring when genes combine, by genes changing during the process (i.e., mutations), or by inheriting impaired genes from parents. Each human cell contains 23 pairs of chromosomes. Genes on these chromosomes contain DNA, the material that contains the unique physical and genetic plans for each individual. The store of DNA information on each of the genes is called the genetic code. The first 22 pairs are called autosomes and the 23rd pair the sex chromosomes. During reproduction, 23 chromosomes come from the mother and 23 from the father, resulting in a cell with 46 chromosomes. When too many or too few chromosomes are present (e.g., 47 instead of 46) or an abnormal gene exists, the developing fetus is negatively affected. Genetic disorders may be inherited or caused by errors in cell division. Two common examples of genetic conditions associated with ID are trisomy 21 and fragile X syndrome. Trisomy 21 (also known as Down syndrome) is a condition in which individuals have three copies of chromosome 21 instead of a pair. Individuals with fragile X syndrome have an abnormal, or "fragile," X chromosome that contains a weak area. See Chapter 13 for more on these health conditions.

Acquired Causes

A teratogen is any physical or chemical substance that may cause physical or developmental complications in the fetus.[6] Teratogens can include prescription medications, lead, alcohol, or illegal drugs consumed by the mother; maternal infections; and other toxins. The effects of teratogens on the fetus range from congenital anomalies (defects) to ID. The type of agent, the amount of exposure, and the point at which exposure occurs during embryonic and fetal development play important roles in the outcome. Exposure to teratogens during the first 12 weeks of pregnancy can have the most dangerous consequences because it is during this time that the fetal brain, spinal cord, most internal organs, and limbs develop.

Perinatal Causes

ID may occur during birth (perinatal) as a result of lack of oxygen (anoxia) to the neonate or due to brain trauma (e.g., bleeding) caused by undue stress on the neonate during the birthing process. Infants born prematurely or at low birth weights may experience complications that result in intellectual deficits.

Prematurity

Infants born before completion of week 37 of gestation are considered premature.[15] Numerous factors may cause prematurity, such as poor nutrition, lack of prenatal care, toxemia, multiple fetuses, a weak cervix, numerous previous births, and adolescent mothers.[9] Although prematurity does not necessarily mean that a disability will develop, some complications caused by prematurity may result in intellectual disability. For example, prematurity can cause respiratory distress syndrome, a condition in which the premature infant's lungs are not yet producing surfactant, a chemical on the surface of the lungs that helps keep the lungs from collapsing. Another complication of prematurity is apnea, a condition in which the infant stops breathing; apnea can last from seconds to minutes. Anoxia refers to a total lack of oxygen, while hypoxia refers to a decreased amount of oxygen.[15] ID can result when either condition affects the brain. The severity of brain dysfunction depends on (a) the location and size of the area deprived of oxygen; (b) the amount of time the area is without oxygen; and (c) the metabolic changes that take place in the body as a result of cell death in that area of the brain. Anoxia or hypoxia can occur during labor because of a small birth canal, which can result in bleeding around the baby's brain, compression of the umbilical cord, tearing of the placenta (placenta previa), or breech birth (i.e., the child is born with the buttocks presenting first instead of the head as in normal births).

Prematurity can also cause hydrocephalus, a condition in which the cerebrospinal fluid accumulates in the brain and can cause the head to grow disproportionately large (Figure 16-1). The extent of the infant's prematurity and associated complications affects the severity of the impairment (if any develops). Premature brain development puts infants at risk for brain hemorrhages (bleeding).

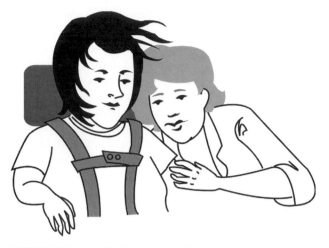

FIGURE 16-1   Adult with disproportionately sized head caused by hydrocephalus that was not shunted.

Postnatal Causes

Postnatal causes of ID include infection, trauma, tetragons, and neglect that occur after birth.

Infections

Infections can cause brain damage and resulting ID in infants and children. Viral meningitis is a condition in which a virus attacks the protective covering around the brain and spinal cord, known as the meninges.[7] Several different viruses cause meningitis, including chickenpox virus. In small children and infants, meningitis may cause permanent brain damage that results in intellectual disability, the severity of which depends on the extent of brain damage. Inflammation of the brain, known as encephalitis, may be caused by complications from the mother contracting chickenpox, rabies, measles, influenza, and other diseases.[15] The severity of any resulting ID varies depending on the area and amount of the brain damaged.

Trauma

Any traumatic injury to the brain, including those sustained from an automobile accident, falls, bicycle accidents, near-drowning, and physical abuse can cause brain injuries and thus intellectual impairments in the child. Physical abuse to a pregnant mother can also cause harm to the growing fetus.

Teratogens

Toxins are poisonous substances that cause particular problems when ingested.[15] Because infants and small children often place objects and substances in their mouths, certain common household substances can pose serious and life-threatening problems. For example, older homes often have lead-based paint on the walls. Inhaling, licking, or eating peeling paint can cause lead poisoning, resulting in developmental problems. Once diagnosed, lead poisoning can be treated, but residual permanent damage may exist. Other common household toxins include mercury in thermometers and cleaning agents.

Neglect

Poor nutrition and environmental deprivation (e.g., lack of physical, emotional, and cognitive support required for growth, development, and social adaptation) during infancy and early childhood may cause ID. Lack of stimulation, starvation, or poor nutrition may interfere with early brain development in children and result in intellectual deficits.

PERFORMANCE IN AREAS OF OCCUPATION

The capacity of a child with ID to perform in areas of occupation varies depending on the severity of ID and the presence of additional deficits. Regardless of ID, "all people need to be able or enabled to engage in the occupations of their need and choice, to grow through what they do, and experience independence or interdependence, equality, participation, security, health and well-being."[11]

CLINICAL *Pearl*

Do not judge a book by its cover! A child with even the most profound ID may be more capable than you think (Figure 16-2). Randy is severely physically handicapped, requiring full support for his body; however, he showed great success in using an augmented communication system.

Children with ID experience significant delays in meeting age-appropriate motor and cognitive milestones. Although learning speed may be slower for these children than it is for those who are developing typically, all children are capable of learning. OT practitioners are interested in determining how the child's limitations interfere with functional skills in occupations.[3] Performance ability is related to the severity of the intellectual delay. The following case examples provide readers with a general description of expected capabilities based on the level of ID.

CLINICAL *Pearl*

The parents or primary caregivers of children who are intellectually disabled have valuable information concerning the children's abilities and the activities that they enjoy. This information will assist OT practitioners in developing interventions for the child and the family.

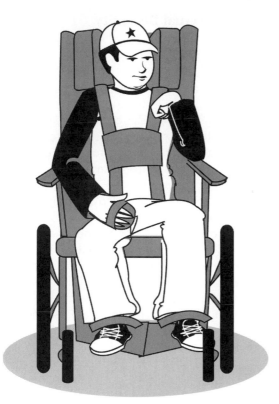

FIGURE 16-2   Adolescent with multiple disabilities and intellectual disability.

Mild Intellectual Disability

CASE *Study*

Sarah is 9 years old and is in second grade. When she was born, her parents found that she was "floppy" (an indicator of low muscle tone) and "weak." She had difficulty breastfeeding. Since she could not sustain a sucking pattern, a gastrostomy tube (g-tube) was placed in her stomach at 1 month. The tube was removed when Sarah was 2 years old, and she currently eats a regular diet with Ensure supplements. Sarah received early intervention services, including occupational therapy, physical therapy, and speech/language therapy until she was 3 years old. Currently, Sarah receives 2 hours of resource help daily for reading and math. Sarah has made a close friend and is able to follow daily classroom routines. Sarah reads sight words and books at a first grade level. Handwriting is a challenge for Sarah because she is unable to remember how to form letters, but she is able to copy print from a model. Each day Sarah's teacher has her write her name, address, and phone number three times in a designated area to promote increased speed and fluency. Sarah's individualized educational program includes adaptations of preferential seating, a modified workload, oral testing, the use of a word processor, and extra time for completion of

work as needed. For writing assignments, she uses the computer/word processor with Co: Writer and Write: OutLoud programs, which audibly read the words on the screen and provide a list of words from which she can select. Sarah is independent in school- and home-related self-care tasks but requires extra time to complete them. At home, Sarah's mother encourages her to bathe on her own and select her clothing the night before. In the future, Sarah would like to be a teacher's aide and help take care of children.

Sarah has mild intellectual disability.

Individuals with **mild intellectual disability** have IQ scores of 55 to 69 and may be further classified as "educable." Children in this category may not seem significantly different from others until they attempt to attain higher levels of cognitive skills and perform tasks that require significant abstract thinking. These children can develop social and communication skills and usually master academic skills from grades 3 to 7; however, it takes them longer than average to attain them.

They are able to achieve the following academic skills:

- Reading at the grade 6 to 7 level
- Writing simple letters or lists, such as a grocery list
- Performing simple mathematical functions such as multiplication and division
- Using the computer and the Internet to perform simple research or to communicate with others

As adults, their social, vocational, and self-help skills are usually sufficient to allow them to partially or completely support themselves financially through employment. Therefore they can live independently or in a minimally supervised setting in the community.

Moderate Intellectual Disability

CASE *Study*

Daniel is 7 years old and is enrolled in a self-contained classroom for children with moderate intellectual disability. He is mainstreamed with typically developing peers during lunch, recess, and special areas. He is nonverbal but indicates his needs by gesturing and pointing to pictures on a simple communication board. Daniel uses a visual schedule to follow daily classroom routines. He is sensitive to certain clothing and food textures. Daniel requires minimum to moderate assistance to put on clothing, especially to get them correctly oriented. He requires moderate assistance to button and zip clothing because of inattention and the inability to follow multistep processes. He feeds himself with a fork but is a very picky eater. He is able to print his first name and sort items by size, shape, and color. An occupational therapist recommended that Daniel participate in a classroom and home sensory program to decrease his hypersensitivity. Following a consultation between the occupational therapist and the occupational therapy assistant (OTA) with regard to the intervention plan, the OTA provides direct therapy and periodically consults with the school staff and the family to promote sensory modulation and oral desensitization. After 3 months, the staff and family have a better understanding of what upsets Daniel. He has begun eating a variety of foods at school and at home.

Daniel has moderate ID.

Individuals with **moderate intellectual disability** have IQ scores of 40 to 54; they may also be considered "trainable." These children need support regularly and are likely to have deficits in academic, communicative, and social skills. With special education, individuals with moderate ID are usually able to attain the skills of a first- or second-grade student, including the following:

- Writing name
- Reading simple texts and emergency words
- Remembering home phone number
- Understanding written numbers and quantities (e.g., being able to select three apples from a pile of apples as directed)
- Understanding basic concepts of money

Children and adolescents with moderate ID require supervision but are able to follow a series of simple verbal directions. They may learn recurring actions, such as making a sandwich for lunch. They may be able to participate in simple leisure activities. Children and adolescents with moderate ID can communicate their desires and preferences and thus should be provided with opportunities to make choices. Adolescents and adults with moderate ID may require supervision to complete ADLs and IADLs. These individuals can do some meaningful work in sheltered workshops or community-supported employment settings. Numerous adults with moderate ID live successfully in supervised living arrangements. OT practitioners can provide support and strategies to caregivers to facilitate physical routines and adapt IADLs and work activities.

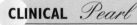

CLINICAL *Pearl*

Family, caregivers, and teachers are instrumental in helping children with ID succeed. Encourage them to share their expertise with you.

Severe Intellectual Disability

CASE *Study*

Thomas is a 9-year-old boy who attends a self-contained class at his local elementary school. He is short, has low muscle tone, and appears to be unsteady when he moves about the classroom. He is able to walk, loves to eat, and has mastered feeding himself independently with a fork but is unable to open ketchup packets or milk containers. Thomas is on a toileting schedule at home and at school. He counts to 2, recognizes colors, and responds to his name. In class, he scribbles on paper but tends to color the table or another student's paper if an adult is not supervising him. He is a dependent worker and requires verbal cues with supervision to stay on task. He has learned to sort silverware with a model but will stop working if not directed to continue by an adult. His favorite things to do are banging objects on the table, rocking back and forth, and taking off his shirt when he has nothing to do. His language is very limited, but he is able to point to the items he wants and use some picture symbols to indicate basic needs (e.g., food, bathroom, favorite toy, and computer). He requires constant adult supervision when on the playground or walking to the lunchroom or he will roam away from the class.

Thomas has severe intellectual disability.

Individuals with **severe intellectual disability** have an IQ score between 25 and 39 and therefore require support in all areas of occupational performance on a regular basis. Functional independence depends greatly on their associated physical limitations. Habitual basic self-care skills such as feeding and hygiene tasks may be learned because of the recurring nature of these activities. Children with severe ID have difficulty generalizing skills and perform best with routine and consistency. For example, the child might be able to unzip his or her school bag but not an unfamiliar jacket.

Desires and needs can be communicated verbally or nonverbally by using communication boards or other methods. As adolescents and adults, those with severe ID may be successful in supervised prevocational training activities. They require extensive supervision and support in order to live independently. It is unlikely that these individuals will achieve any particular academic grade level in school because tasks such as reading and writing are extremely difficult for them.

With special education, the child with severe ID can do the following:

- Recognize his or her photograph
- Perform self-care skills that are routinely done (e.g., feed oneself with a spoon, pull pants up/down)

- Learn how to follow simple classroom rules that are done consistently (hang up backpack when entering classroom)

Children and adolescents with severe ID frequently also have physical disabilities, including cerebral palsy, seizure disorder, visual impairment, hearing loss, and communication disorder. OT practitioners must evaluate and address the physical demands of activities along with the global and specific mental function demands. Family members who are caring for the child may require education on handling techniques and behavior management. OT practitioners work with other family members to help them understand so that they may interact and socialize and enjoy each other.

CLINICAL *Pearl*

Nonverbal children with severe ID can point to pictures mounted on a place mat to indicate their wants and needs during mealtime. For example, they can point to a picture of a cup to let caregivers know that they want more milk.

Profound Intellectual Disability

CASE *Study*

Jamie is a 5-year-old girl who is very frail. She is unable to sit or stand because she has poor head, neck, and trunk control. She depends on others for all her care needs, including eating, toileting, and dressing. She eats pureed food and sips from a straw. Jamie drools because of her poor oral motor control. She smiles when she hears a familiar voice or music. Her eye fixation is inconsistent, and she is unable to move her body on command or respond to simple yes or no questions.

Jamie has profound intellectual disability.

An IQ score below 25 classifies individuals as having **profound intellectual disability**. Because of the numerous physical disabilities that may accompany profound ID, these individuals often have difficulty progressing developmentally and require constant support occupations. Depending on the extent of their physical limitations, individuals with profound ID may learn to communicate and perform basic or routine self-care activities, such as hygiene and grooming tasks. Extensive assistance is required for all other ADL skills, and continuous support is needed in living arrangements. Maintenance of the physical skills required for everyday occupations assists in preserving the overall health of the child. OT practitioners working with children with profound ID concentrate on basic skills required for occupations.

For example, the goals of therapy may include such tasks as the following:

- Smile on approach
- Indicate food preference
- Feed oneself with a spoon
- Make visual contact
- Allow caregiver to bathe them
- Allow caregiver to touch them
- Cooperate with dressing or self-care

CLINICAL *Pearl*

Children with profound ID have preferences for certain people, toys, and food and typically have a sense of humor. The OT practitioner must respect their preferences and try to discover what motivates them.

CLIENT FACTORS: FUNCTIONAL IMPLICATIONS AND OT INTERVENTIONS

Client factors refer to the specific abilities, characteristics, or beliefs that may affect performance in occupations and include values, beliefs and spirituality, body functions, and body structures.[3] The following provides examples of how client factors may be manifested in children and adolescents with ID and provides suggestions for intervention.

Mental Function

Global mental functions are frequently delayed or absent in children and adolescents with intellectual deficits. Deficits in cognitive function and learning styles characteristic of children with ID include poor memory, slower learning rates, attention problems, difficulty generalizing what they learn, and lack of motivation. Furthermore, these children may lack orientation to person, place, time, self, and others. Children with ID may not make eye contact or attend to activities (consciousness level). Temperaments and personalities of these clients vary, and they may experience emotional instability (e.g., quickly change from one emotion to another). OT practitioners may find that clients have difficulty choosing activities (energy and drive), have few preferences (interests), or have difficulty with impulse control.

Intervention

Intervention is not aimed at improving intelligence (it is not possible to reverse the condition); instead, it is aimed at helping the child or adolescent develop performance patterns, including habits, roles, and rituals used in the process of engaging in meaningful activities. Each client should be assessed in terms of his or her strengths and

BOX 16-1

Sample Goals Showing a Variety of Functional Levels

- Using a built-up handled spoon, Greg will feed himself independently at dinner within 2 weeks.
- Sandy will initiate a simple conversation with another adolescent during the school picnic.
- After demonstration and with minimal assistance, Ira will sort white and dark clothes into two separate containers within 1 month.
- In 1 month, given minimal verbal cues, Amy will cooperate with dressing and undressing by extending her arms.
- Given two choices, Faye will turn her head right or left to identify her food preferences for each meal, within 2 months.
- Jerry will follow a 4-step handwashing routine, with the use of a visual schedule, by 1 month.

weaknesses. OT practitioners focus on the occupations that the child or adolescent hopes to perform as goals. (Box 16-1 presents sample goals.)

CASE *Study*

A typical second grade health objective requires that students be able to identify the five food groups. Once students are able to identify the five food groups, teachers hope that they will make healthy food choices. Eight-year-old Reinhardt has moderate ID. The school staff would like him to eat a more balanced diet because he only eats sweets and foods with a crunchy texture. Therefore the OT practitioner rewrote Reinhardt's health goal to read: "The student will eat at least one bite of two food groups." In this case, rewriting the goal to include the exact occupational behavior needed is more functional and meaningful to the child and to the school staff. The intervention session would emphasize the importance of consuming at least a small portion of fruits or vegetables, bread, dairy products, or meat. The OT practitioner may decide to use a positive reinforcer (in this student's case, dessert) after she accomplishes this. (It is not wise to use food as a reinforcer in all cases. However, during mealtime, it is easy to allow dessert after the meal as a reinforcer.)

Specific mental functions that children with ID may demonstrate include the following:

- Shorter attention span
- Difficulty storing and retrieving information (memory)
- Difficulty recognizing direction and relation of objects to one another (perception)

- Slower learning ability (thought)
- Inability to recognize objects or people (thought)
- Difficulty making sense of stimuli (perception)
- Difficulty with problem solving and critical thinking (higher-level cognition)
- Difficulty generalizing information and mastering abstract thinking (thought)
- Slow, delayed, or absent language skills
- Difficulty with adding and subtracting (calculations)
- Poor motor planning (sequencing complex movements)
- Inappropriate range and regulation of emotions; self-control (emotional)
- Difficulty with body image, self-concept, and self-esteem (self and time)

Language Functions

As with physical milestones, it can take longer for children with ID to reach speech and language milestones. These children are slower to use words, put words together, and speak in complete sentences. Their social development is sometimes slow because of cognitive impairment and language deficiencies. For example, shorter memory and attention span could make recalling and retrieving words difficult, whereas difficulties with abstract thinking may make it challenging to mentally grasp certain concepts. The language and speech of children with ID may be related to associated physical problems such as inadequate oral–motor muscle tone, which results in unclear articulation, difficulty taking deep breaths, and difficulty moderating one's speech (i.e., speaking too softly or loudly). Speech therapists specifically address language function during regularly scheduled intervention sessions. The OT practitioner collaborates with the speech therapist to incorporate alternative means of communication into individual and/or group OT intervention sessions.

Behavioral/Emotional Functions

Children with ID are likely to exhibit behavior that may be related to specific situations that compound an impaired ability to communicate. Children with intellectual deficits may have difficulty accepting criticism, managing self-control, and displaying appropriate behaviors. They may show aggression toward others or engage in self-injurious or self-stimulating behaviors, such as hand flapping, biting, and hitting, that make them stand out in typical settings. They may suck on clothing, make repetitive noises, or hop on their toes.

Children with ID may exhibit hyperactivity (impulsiveness and excessive activity that result in difficulty functioning in social situations), excessive shyness (withdrawing during familiar group activities), and distractibility (difficulty paying attention to one task). These behaviors interfere with their functioning and ability to participate in social or academic occupations. These children attain their social skills later than other children and thus may often misbehave or act in a manner much younger than what is appropriate for their chronologic age.

During adolescence, children with ID may behave inappropriately socially or sexually. Some of these children may develop psychosocial disorders such as depression, obsessive–compulsive disorder, or attention-deficit disorder.

Intervention

OT practitioners use a behavioral approach (the ABC approach) to facilitate positive behaviors in children with ID. Box 16-2 provides the techniques used in this approach. The occupational therapist and the OTA can be instrumental members in designing a behavioral modification plan. First, data are collected to identify the behavior(s) that need to be changed. Then practitioners collect data on the antecedent behavior(s), referred to as "A," that represent the events and behaviors that occur before target behavior. They identify the target behaviors, referred to as "B" (i.e., the behavior to be modified or changed). Practitioners establish consequence(s), "C," of the target behavior (e.g., the child receives desired adult attention, the child does not to complete undesired task). OT practitioners use their expertise to describe these behaviors and analyze them to determine why they are occurring using an ABC approach. The occupational therapist determines the child's strengths and weaknesses so that the team may establish an appropriate award system. The OTA reinforces the system and checks with the school staff daily to see if there are any new concerns. OT intervention is aimed at reinforcing positive behaviors as well as working on other established goals.

CLINICAL *Pearl*

Children with ID establish friendships and other relationships. They may experience the full range of emotions, although they may not be able to express these feelings. OT practitioners can help children and adolescents with ID deal with feelings of grief, sadness (when losing someone), intimacy, and love.

CLINICAL *Pearl*

Children with ID may enjoy participating in athletic events such as the Special Olympics. These events allow children to develop feelings of success by working toward an athletic goal. Children experience teamwork, achievement, and the benefits of physical activity. Events such as these promote a positive self-concept and self-esteem.

BOX 16-2

Developing a Behavioral Modification Plan

1. Identify behaviors that interfere with learning, socialization, or engagement in occupations.
2. Collect data on each behavior. Consider the following when analyzing the behavior: When does the unacceptable behavior occur? How often does it occur? Under which circumstances does it occur? In what setting (quiet, noisy, dark, etc.) does the behavior occur?
3. Prioritize the behaviors that should be addressed first. Behaviors that involve safety issues are priorities.
4. With the team (e.g., parent, caregiver, teacher, staff), create a plan to reduce the behavior. The OT practitioner provides a task analysis of the behavior and identifies reinforcers or provides insight into why the behaviors occur. The plan must be simple enough to work for a variety of people with limited training. Behavioral objectives must be stated very specifically and in observable and measurable terms. Plans should be simple so that the student can incorporate them into his or her daily schedule.
5. Implement the plan. OT practitioners may be responsible for training the staff on the implementation of the plan. OT practitioners may adapt or suggest changes to the plan after a careful task analysis. Writing effective behavioral objectives requires practice. Be prepared to reflect on your objectives and learn from them. You will soon find out what works and what does not work.
6. Collect data on the behavior. Evaluate the outcome, and discuss it with the team. All team members are responsible for documenting the outcome of the plan.
7. Make modifications to the behavior plan as needed to impact positive outcomes.

CASE *Study*

A referral was made by the school to determine why a student was throwing his tray on the floor at lunchtime. The occupational therapist met with the staff, reviewed the charts, and observed the child during lunch. The OTA then observed the child at breakfast. The OTA and the occupational therapist met and compiled their observations, discussed possibilities, and brainstormed solutions. During mealtimes, the student sat at a table with three other students with severe ID, who required one-on-one assistance to eat. The OT team used the ABC method to analyze the behaviors.

A: This student was able to feed himself with the proper setup. He was positioned in his wheelchair at the table. He ate slowly, with a tremor. The staff was busy with other clients and did not speak to this student during the meal. The student was nonverbal but was able to point or gesture to communicate.

B: On completion of his meal, the student threw his entire tray on the floor.

C: The staff rushed to his side, picked up the tray, cleaned up the student, and took him back to the classroom.

The staff was frustrated with this student's lunchroom behavior but met his needs quickly when he threw his tray down. Getting quick attention thus reinforced this behavior. Both the occupational therapist and the OTA noticed that the student looked around right before he threw his tray down. They decided that the cause of the behavior was that the student was trying to communicate his need for some help and attention. Consequently, the staff changed their behavior by periodically checking to see if the student was done eating, taking the tray from him when he was ready, and bringing him back to his classroom where he enjoyed a few minutes of downtime with a few friends. The student was now getting his needs met, and the staff was reinforcing meal completion and appropriate behaviors.

Other suggestions to make mealtime more enjoyable for this student included the following:

- Limiting the number of students (with aides) at the table
- Limiting talking among aides and encouraging interaction among students
- Assigning a peer (from the regular education class) to join the student at lunch

The OTA consulted with the staff weekly. Caregivers were willing to try new strategies because the OT practitioners listened to them, addressed their concerns, and actually made their jobs easier.

Sensory Functions and Pain

Children with ID may experience and process sound, taste, touch, and auditory information differently. Screenings and evaluations by health care professionals help rule out any medical problems. These children may experience adverse reactions to sensory experiences and consequently respond in an unexpected manner in certain situations. OT practitioners may be asked to evaluate children's reactions to taste, smell, touch, movement, and body position to determine sensory preferences. OT practitioners assess sensory needs and make recommendations to help the children adapt to their environments. For example, a child may not want to eat food of a certain texture. The staff may assume that the child is not hungry when, in fact, the child does not like the texture of the food. Children with tactile sensitivity (or defensiveness) usually dislike being touched softly on areas of their bodies and/or may avoid contact with certain textures. Some children have difficulty with the modulation or self-regulation of sensory input that they receive during the day. A sensation that calms one child may excite

or disturb another. Frequently, when the children cannot handle all of the sensations bombarding them during the day, they might act out, become hyperactive or aggressive, or even withdraw from the situation.

Intervention

OT practitioners frequently provide teams with information concerning the sensory processing abilities of children who have intellectual disability. A thorough analysis of these children's responses to a variety of sensory experiences provides insight into behaviors interfering with occupations. For example, some children with tactile defensiveness may overreact to bathing. They may dislike the feeling of water on the skin, but the staff or caregivers may interpret this reaction as uncooperative or aggressive behavior. The OT practitioner may be able to prepare the client for the bathing experience by means of a sensory program. This may be as simple as changing the time of the bath, regulating the temperature of the water, changing the soap, or establishing a brushing protocol before the bath. Other sensory modulation issues may be addressed by providing the caregiver and the child more time to accomplish the occupations; both the clients and the caregivers feel frustrated when they are rushed.

CASE *Study*

A staff member at a residential setting was responsible for waking, toileting, dressing, and feeding three adolescents with severe ID before they were transported to school. The staff member stated that giving them breakfast was an impossible task; the adolescents would not cooperate with her and frequently spat out their food. On observation, the OTA realized that the staff member was hurried, the adolescents were stressed, and they were unable to express their food preferences. One adolescent was spitting out food because of a motor deficit (tongue thrusting); the others were being served foods that they did not like. Intervention consisted of the OTA assisting the staff member in the morning until a routine was established. The OTA modeled the correct feeding techniques to help decrease tongue thrusting in the one adolescent and helped the staff identify the food preferences of the other two. The three adolescents were instructed on how to indicate their preferences instead of spitting out the food. A system change was implemented in that two staff members became responsible for the morning routines of the three individuals. This was accomplished by having one staff member come in early, which worked for her in light of her own personal/family responsibilities.

The importance of examining sensory processing can be observed as the children with ID respond to loud noises with exaggerated reactions (startle). A startle reaction may cause some children to fall or have a seizure, which is not common in typically developing children. Children with ID may have sensory problems related to body movement and muscle coordination (vestibular and proprioceptive), which lead to further motor deficits. They may not express pain proportionate to the stimuli; therefore, OT practitioners must be sensitive and perceptive to what may be perceived as pain by the child or adolescent. Children with intellectual deficits may not understand procedures and may be fearful of new people, making their feelings of pain more intense. Familiar people providing medical preparation and comfort during procedures may help.

CLINICAL *Pearl*

Create opportunities for success and independence. Remember that pullover shirts, pants with elastic waistbands, and shoes with Velcro make dressing easier.

CLINICAL *Pearl*

When teaching a new task to a child with ID, divide the task into small steps. Demonstrate the steps. Have the child practice the steps, one at a time. Provide assistance when necessary and immediate feedback. Practice the task in its natural context for the best carry over.

Movement-Related Functions

Children with ID often reach major physical milestones (e.g., roll, sit, stand, walk) later than usual. In fact, many infants are referred for OT because of motor delays before being diagnosed with ID. These infants and children typically exhibit low muscle tone and can exhibit a range of motor problems related to brain damage and difficulty learning complex motor tasks.

Intervention

Intervention is aimed at developing motor function and helping children with ID adapt to or compensate for their movement problems. OT practitioners working on movement-related problems must remember that clients with intellectual deficits have difficulty finding ways to adapt to physical challenges. Because they are not able to problem solve or use cognition as readily as their peers without disability can, they will show slower progression in movement. They require extended practice, repetition, simple directions, and modification and/or adaptation of the requirements to succeed (see Chapter 24). Specific motor intervention is designed to address the physical problems associated with secondary diagnoses.

System Functions

OT practitioners working with children with ID must have knowledge of how body systems affect functional ability. Children may be susceptible to cardiac, pulmonary, blood, digestive, metabolic, urinary, reproductive, and skin disorders. For example, children with trisomy 21 experience ID and may be at risk for cardiac disorders. Food allergies and the adverse effects of medicines may affect these children. OT practitioners must be keen observers of behavior and knowledgeable about their clients' medical histories.

CLINICAL *Pearl*

Order simple and uncomplicated adaptive/positioning equipment for children and adolescents who have intellectual deficits so children, family and/or staff understand how to use or adjust it. The staff and family members may misplace items and become frustrated with complicated equipment demands.

ROLES OF THE OCCUPATIONAL THERAPIST AND THE OCCUPATIONAL THERAPY ASSISTANT

OT practitioners provide individualized services and supports to help children with ID develop independence by performing meaningful activities. The process includes a comprehensive evaluation that focuses on developing an occupational profile and analysis of the occupational performance (e.g., the ability to carry out ADLs, IADLs, work, play/leisure, sleep and rest, education, and social participation).[3,7] The American Association on Intellectual Disabilities recommends that an individual's needs be assessed in nine key areas:

1. Human development,
2. Teaching and education,
3. Home living,
4. Community living,
5. Employment,
6. Health and safety,
7. Recreation,
8. Living environments, and
9. ADLs.[2]

These key areas all fall within the scope of OT practice. The occupational therapist interviews the child's parents, primary caregivers, and teacher to gain information on the child's strengths and weaknesses and the contexts in which the occupations occur (e.g., physical, social, personal, cultural, temporal, spiritual, and virtual environments). The OTA may administer standardized tests after the establishment of service competency and at the discretion of the supervising occupational therapist. The OTA and the occupational therapist work together constantly to reevaluate and monitor the child's needs as he or she grows and learns. Infants, children, and adolescents with ID are treated in the home and at day-care centers, outpatient clinics, schools, and residential settings. Knowledge of the contexts, including community resources and environmental supports, is essential to the intervention process.

CLINICAL *Pearl*

Children with ID learn through repetition. For example, learning how to dress, bathe, or brush teeth may best be accomplished by performing the task when it naturally falls within the context of the day.

SUMMARY

Children with ID exhibit deficits in a range of cognitive skills that interfere with their ability to engage in occupations. OT practitioners evaluate the child's ability to perform occupations by analyzing the specific demands and client factors associated with the occupations in which the child engages. The intervention plan is designed to maximize the child's strengths and work on his or her weaknesses. Children with ID will learn, but at a much slower rate, and exhibit lifelong deficits in occupational performance. The developmental and behavioral frames of references are effective in helping children develop abilities within their potential. The goal of OT intervention is to help children or adolescents participate in occupations such as ADLs, IADLs, play/leisure, work, education, and social participation. OT practitioners work with team members and families and consider the overall goal of increasing the children's ability to participate in occupations. Toward this end, activities must frequently be adapted and modified to help children succeed. OT practitioners working with children with ID need to be aware of community agencies for respite, social opportunities, housing, and assistance. Furthermore, children with ID may experience physical limitations that interfere with their occupations. OT practitioners educate and empower caregivers to care for their children and facilitate independence. The role of the OT practitioner in working with children and adolescents with ID is complex. They must use creativity, OT knowledge, and life skills to assist the children, adolescents, and their families in reaching the desired goals.

References

1. American Psychiatric Association. (2013). *Diagnostic and statistical manual of mental disorders* (5th ed.). Washington, DC: Author.
2. American Association on Intellectual Disabilities. (2010). *Intellectual disabilities: definition, classification, and system of supports* (10th ed.). Washington, DC: Author.
3. American Occupational Therapy Association. (2014). Occupational therapy practice framework: domain and process (3rd ed.). *Am J Occup Ther*, 68(Suppl. 1), S1–S48.
4. Bayley, N. (1993). *Manual for Bayley scales of infant development* (2nd ed.). San Antonio TX: The Psychological Corporation.
5. Case-Smith, J. (1998). *Pediatric occupational therapy and early intervention* (2nd ed.). Stoneham, MA: Butterworth-Heinemann.
6. Case-Smith, J., & O'Brien, J. (2015). *Occupational therapy for children and adolescents* (7th ed.). St. Louis: Mosby.
7. Coster, W. J., Deeney, T., Haltiwanger, J., et al. (1998). *School function assessment*. San Antonio, TX: PsychCorp.
8. Schell, B. B., Gillen, G., & Scaffa, M. (2013). *Willard and Spackman's occupational therapy* (12th ed.). Philadelphia: Lippincott Williams & Wilkins.
9. Mader, S. (2004). *Understanding human anatomy and physiology* (5th ed.). Dubuque, IA: William C. Brown.
10. McCarthy, D. (1972). *Manual for the McCarthy scales for children's abilities*. San Antonio, TX: The Psychological Corporation.
11. Smith, R. (1993). *Children with mental retardation: a parent's guide*. Bethesda, MD: Woodbine House.
12. Sparrow, S. S., Cicchetti, D. V., & Balla, D. A. (2005). *Vineland Adaptive Behavior Scales* (2nd ed., Vineland-II). Circle Pines, MN: American Guidance Service.
13. Roid, G. H. (2003). *Stanford-Binet Intelligence Scales* (5th ed.). *Technical manual*. Itasca, IL: Riverside Publishing.
14. Thompson, J. R., et al. (2003). *Supports intensity scale*. Washington, DC: American Association on Mental Retardation. Available at www.aaidd.org.
15. Venes, D. (Ed.). (2009). *Taber's cyclopedic medical dictionary* (21st ed.). Philadelphia: FA Davis.
16. Wechsler, D. (1991). *Wechsler Intelligence Scale for Children*—Third Edition. San Antonio, TX: The Psychological Corporation.

Recommended Reading

Beirne-Smith, M., Patton, J., & Kim, S. (2006). *Mental retardation: an introduction to intellectual disability* (7th ed.). Upper Saddle River, NJ: Prentice Hall.

Bernstein, J. (2007). *Rachel in the world: a memoir*. Champagne, IL: University of Illinois Press.

Drew, C., & Hardman, M. L. (2006). *Intellectual disabilities across the lifespan* (9th ed.). Upper Saddle River, NJ: Prentice Hall.

Osbune, A. G., & Russo, C. J. (2006). *Special education and the law: a guide for practitioners* (2nd ed.). Thousand Oaks, CA: Corwin Press.

REVIEW *Questions*

1. How is ID diagnosed and categorized?
2. What are some causes of ID?
3. What is the role of the registered occupational therapist and the certified occupational therapy assistant in the intervention for children with ID?
4. What are some behavioral strategies for working with children who have intellectual deficits?

5. What are the functional implications of being classified as having mild, moderate, severe, or profound ID?
6. What frames of reference work well with this population, and why?
7. How do behaviors interfere with learning in children with ID?

SUGGESTED *Activities*

1. Volunteer at a facility that specializes in working with children with ID.
2. Attend a Down syndrome support group to learn about the challenges faced by the families and caregivers of individuals with this syndrome.
3. Volunteer your time in a school system or early intervention program. Ask to see a sample of the individual family service plan or individualized educational program.
4. Volunteer to babysit or provide respite care for a child who has ID.

5. Volunteer in a special education classroom that has children with a variety of disabilities. How do the children interact? What types of structure is provided? How do the professionals (e.g., teacher, aide) adjust activities to accommodate to each child?
6. Volunteer in a day-care center and screen the children's developmental skills. Observe the different behaviors.
7. Analyze the cognitive and motor tasks of a daily activity to determine the steps. How would you make the activity easier or more challenging?

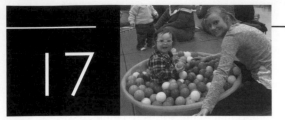

PATTY COKER-BOLT
TERESSA GARCIA REIDY
ERIN NABER

Cerebral Palsy

KEY TERMS

Cerebral palsy
Postural mechanism
Primitive reflex patterns
Righting reactions
Equilibrium reactions
Protective extension
    reactions
Muscle tone
Hemiplegia
Diplegia
Quadriplegia
Spasticity (hypertonicity)
Dyskinesias
Athetosis
Ataxia
Hypotonicity

CHAPTER *Objectives*

After studying this chapter, the reader will be able to accomplish the following:

- Describe the frequency, pattern, types, and classification of cerebral palsy.
- Identify the impaired progression of movement associated with cerebral palsy.
- Describe the components of normal postural control and movement in children who have cerebral palsy.
- Recognize the differences among motor development, motor learning, and motor control.
- Explain ways in which normal muscle tone and impaired muscle tone influence movement.
- Identify the role of the certified occupational therapy assistant in the assessment and intervention of movement disorders in children who have cerebral palsy.
- Describe the range of interventions used with children who have cerebral palsy, including medical, constraint-induced movement, complementary and alternative medicine, and splinting and casting.

CHAPTER *Outline*

*Progression of Atypical Movement
    Patterns*

Primary and Secondary Impairments

Frequency and Causes

*Posture, Postural Control, and
    Movement*

*Righting, Equilibrium, and Protective
    Reactions*
    MUSCLE TONE
    PRIMITIVE REFLEXES

*Postural Development and Motor
    Control*
    REFLEX-HIERARCHICAL MODELS
    DYNAMIC SYSTEM MODELS

Classification and Distribution

*Functional Implications and
    Associated Problems*
    MUSCLE AND BONE
    COGNITION, HEARING, AND LANGUAGE
    SENSORY PROBLEMS
    HAND SKILLS AND UPPER EXTREMITY FUNCTION
    VISION
    PHYSICAL AND BEHAVIORAL MANIFESTATIONS

*Roles of the Occupational Therapist
    and the Occupational Therapy
    Assistant*
    ASSESSMENT
    INTERVENTIONS

Summary

Cerebral palsy (CP) is a term used to describe a range of developmental motor disorders arising from a nonprogressive lesion or disorder of the brain (Box 17-1).[3] Associated brain damage is characterized by paralysis, spasticity, or abnormal control of movement or posture. Although the injury to the brain is considered static, the pattern of motor impairment may change over time, affecting development in all daily occupations of childhood. The motor disorders associated with CP are often accompanied by disturbances of sensation, cognition, communication, perception, and/or a seizure disorder.[4] The lesion or damage in the brain may cause impairment in muscle activity in all or part of the body. CP typically affects the development of sensory, perceptual, and motor areas of the central nervous system (CNS). This can cause the child to have difficulty integrating all of the information that the brain needs to correctly plan and direct the skilled, efficient movements in the trunk and extremities that are used in everyday interactions with the environment. The muscles shorten and lengthen in uncoordinated, inefficient ways and are unable to work together to create smooth, effective motion.

PROGRESSION OF ATYPICAL MOVEMENT PATTERNS

Children with CP have difficulty achieving and maintaining normal posture when lying down, sitting, and standing because of impaired patterns of muscle activation.[3,17] These abnormal patterns result from the decreased ability of the CNS to control coactivation and reciprocal innervation of select muscle groups. Coactivation of muscle is the result of a co-contraction of agonist and antagonist muscle groups around a joint. Simultaneous contraction of agonist and antagonist muscle groups provide stability around a joint and also affect overall body posture. Reciprocal innervations in muscle groups occur when excitatory input directs the agonist muscle to contract while inhibitory input directs the antagonist muscle to remain inactive.[17,32] These reciprocal innervations allow for movement to occur around a joint and in the body. Children with CP may develop abnormal movement compensations and body postures as they try to overcome these motor deficits to function within their environments. Over time, movement compensations and atypical motor patterns create barriers to ongoing motor skill development. Instead of freely moving and exploring the world, as children with a normally developing sensorimotor system do, children with CP may rely on early automatic reflex movement patterns as their primary means of mobility. These early automatic reflexive movements occur without conscious control of the child and are typically elicited by a specific sensory motor action.

PRIMARY AND SECONDARY IMPAIRMENTS

Children with CP manifest primary impairments that are the direct result of the lesion in CNS. Primary

BOX 17-1

Definition of Cerebral Palsy

Cerebral palsy is a movement disorder affecting smooth and coordinated movements of the body needed for participation in everyday activities such as play and self-care. Disordered movement patterns are seen in the head/neck, arms, legs, and trunk. Impairments can be seen in one or more areas of development, including fine motor, gross motor, language/communication, and overall adaptive functions.

impairments are an immediate and direct result of the cortical lesion in the brain. The nervous system damage that causes CP can occur before or during birth or before a child's second year, the time when myelination of the child's sensory and motor tracts and CNS structures rapidly occurs. CP is described as nonprogressive, nonhereditary, and noncontagious.[17] As a nonprogressive condition, the original defect or lesion occurring in the CNS typically does not worsen or change over time. However, because the lesion occurs in immature brain structures, the progression of the child's motor development may appear to change. Normal nervous system maturation shifts control of voluntary movement to increasingly higher and more complex areas of the brain. The child with CP exhibits some changes in movement ability that results from the expected progression of motor development skills, but these changes tend to be delayed relative to age and often show much less variety than those seen on the normally developing child.

Children with CP develop secondary impairments in systems or organs over time due to the effects of one or more of the primary impairments.[3,33] These secondary impairments may become just as debilitating as the primary impairments. For example, a child with CP may have a primary impairment such as hypertonia and a muscle imbalance across a joint. This abnormal muscle tone may cause poor alignment across a joint, further muscle weakness, and eventually a contracture in the joint. The resulting muscle contractures, poor body alignment, and poor ability to initiate movement would be considered secondary impairments. It is important to understand this because a diagnosis of CP means that a child has a static nonprogressive lesion in the brain. Although the initial brain injury remains unchanged, the results or the secondary impairments are not static and change over time with body growth and attempts to move against gravity. Children with CP may continue to rely on automatic movement patterns because they are unable to direct their muscles to move successfully in more typical motor patterns (Figure 17-1). The atypical patterns used to play or complete functional activities may become repetitive and fixed. The repetition of

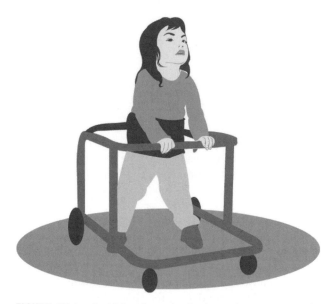

FIGURE 17-1 A child with cerebral palsy and upper extremity spasticity and tightness in her shoulders and arms as well poor proximal stability in her trunk.

the atypical movement patterns prevents children with CP from gaining independent voluntary control of their own movements and can lead to diminished strength and musculoskeletal problems. The combination of impaired muscle coactivation and the use of reflexively controlled postures may lead to future contractures in muscles, tendons, and ligamentous tissues, causing the tissues to become permanently shortened. Bone deformities and alterations of typical posture or spinal and joint alignment may also occur.

FREQUENCY AND CAUSES

The prevalence of CP has remained stable since the 1950s, although prenatal and perinatal care have improved dramatically over the past 4 decades.[17,33,35] A diagnosis of CP is approximately 1.5 times more common in boys and is higher among non-Hispanic African American children, and children from low- to middle-income families.[17] According to the United Cerebral Palsy (UCP) Foundation, approximately 800,000 children and adults in the United States live with one or more symptoms of CP.[35] The origin of brain injury may occur during the prenatal, perinatal, or postnatal period, but evidence suggests that 70% to 80% is prenatal in origin.[33]

It is increasingly apparent that CP results from the interaction of multiple factors and, in many cases, a single cause cannot be identified.[17,33] Prenatal maternal infection, premature birth, low birth weight, and multiple pregnancies have been associated with CP.[35] Prenatal factors may include genetic abnormalities or maternal health factors such as stress, malnutrition,

exposure to damaging drugs, and pregnancy-induced hypertension. Some gestational conditions of the mother, such as diabetes, may cause perinatal risks to the developing infant and prematurity and low birth weight significantly increase an infant's chance of acquiring a CP diagnosis.[17] Medical problems associated with premature birth may directly or indirectly damage the developing sensorimotor areas of the CNS. In particular, respiratory disorders can cause the premature newborn to experience hypoxemia, which deprives brain cells of the oxygen needed to function and survive. Typical postnatal causes of cerebral palsy include conditions that result in significant damage to the developing CNS such as hypoxic ischemia encephalopathy resulting from lack of oxygen to the brain. Postnatal causes include infections or exposure to environmental toxins. Box 17-2 provides an overview of some of the postnatal causes of CP.

POSTURE, POSTURAL CONTROL, AND MOVEMENT

To understand the functional movement problems that develop in children with CP, the occupational therapy (OT) practitioner must be familiar with the ways that people normally control their bodies and execute skilled movements. The term *posture* describes the alignment of the body's parts in relation to each other and the environment. The ability to develop a large repertoire of postures and change them easily during an activity depends on the integration of several automatic, involuntary movement actions referred to as the **postural mechanism**, which includes several key components:

- Normal muscle tone
- Normal postural tone
- Developmental integration of early, **primitive reflex patterns**
- Emergence of righting reactions, equilibrium reactions, and protective extension reactions
- Intentional, voluntary movements against the forces of gravity
- The ability to combine movement patterns in the performance of functional activities

Disruption in the postural mechanism and the movement problems seen in children with CP are considered secondary impairments, which may be significantly reduced by OT interventions.

RIGHTING, EQUILIBRIUM, AND PROTECTIVE REACTIONS

The functions that aid individuals in maintaining or regaining posture are **righting reactions** and **equilibrium reactions**, often referred to concomitantly as balance reactions. These functions can be thought of as static or dynamic. When people are sitting and not engaged in any activity, they are using static balance. When they bend to pick up an object from the floor, for example, they use dynamic balance to right themselves. Righting reactions are the foundation for all balance responses and help maintain upright postures against gravity during times when the center of gravity is moving off the body's base of support. Righting reactions help sense that the head is out of alignment with the body and produce a motor response to realign the head with the body. This requires the ability to bring the head and trunk back into "normal" skeletal alignment by using only the necessary muscle groups. When righting and equilibrium reactions are not sufficient to regain an upright posture quickly and safely, individuals use another reflexive reaction called the **protective extension reaction**. When people fall, they frequently use this reaction, automatically reaching outward from their bodies to catch themselves or break the fall. A protective response requires the motor ability to quickly bring an extremity (i.e., arm or leg) out from the body to prevent a fall and also the strength to support the body's weight momentarily while bracing.

When movement abilities develop normally, children experience and practice many different movements and positions as they work toward mastering the upright, two-legged stance. Postural stability and the ability to demonstrate righting, equilibrium, and protective responses evolve developmentally through experimentation and play in a variety of developmental positions (e.g., prone, supine, sitting, kneeling, standing).

As children refine their control of specific postures through developmental progression, they develop the stable righting, equilibrium, and protective responses needed for a variety of skills and functional tasks. The majority of functional activities involve combinations of movement patterns of the head and neck, trunk, upper extremities, and lower extremities while moving the center of gravity off the body's base of support. Rarely do activities require isolated movements in one extremity or in a single plane of motion. Through a careful clinical analysis, the possible combinations enabling a functional activity can be described and used as a basis for making intervention decisions. For example, when a person reaches across the dinner table to pass a serving dish, he or she must remain stable in the chair while going through several hand and arm motions to lift the dish, move it across the table, and then carefully release it to the person receiving the dish. Such a task requires the use of the muscles of the trunk and pelvic girdle areas as stabilizers; that is, these muscles provide postural stability as the upper extremity and shoulder girdle muscles perform the skilled movement task. In addition to the different types of muscle activity used for this task, the person must also rely on intact righting and equilibrium reactions to help keep the body upright against gravity and maintain a sitting posture in the chair while the body's weight is being shifted during the reaching task. The person passing the dish will probably lean to the left, right, or forward. In this instance just as in every executed movement, the leaning or moving from the center of gravity requires shifting of the body's weight. Each time a person shifts weight, righting and equilibrium reactions are used to counterbalance the weight shifts during the movements and help regain an upright posture with body parts correctly realigned. Vision, hearing, and other sensory inputs also provide perceptual information about whether the person is moving just the right distance when reaching and whether that person is upright in the context of the immediate surroundings.

Muscle Tone

Muscle tone is the force with which a muscle resists being lengthened and can also be defined as the muscle's resting stiffness. The OT practitioner tests muscle tone by passively stretching the client's muscle from the shortened state to the lengthened state and feeling the resistance offered by the muscle to the stretch. A child's

BOX 17-3

*Common Problems of Motor Development
in Children with Cerebral Palsy*

- Abnormal muscle tone
  - Hypertonicity: increase in resting state of muscle
  - Hypotonicity: decrease in resting state of muscle
  - Fluctuating: muscle tone changes between hypertonic and hypotonic
- Persistence of primitive reflexes
- Atypical righting, equilibrium, and protective responses
- Poor sensory processing
  - Decreased processing of vestibular, visual, and proprioceptive information
  - Distorted body awareness and body scheme
- Joint hypermobility
  - Reduced limb stability and poor co-contraction across joints
- Muscle weakness and poor muscle coactivation
- Delays in typical progressing of motor skills and adaptive function
- Decreased exploration of the environment

ability to perform sequential movements is supported by the ability of muscles to maintain the correct amount of tension (stiffness) and elasticity during the movements. Muscle tone is highly influenced by gravity. Muscles must have enough tone to move against gravity in a smooth, coordinated motion. Emotions and mental states, including levels of alertness, fatigue, and excitement, can also influence muscle tone. Normal muscle tone develops along a continuum, with some variability among members of the typical population.

The qualities of contractility and elasticity are necessary for the muscle's accurate response to changes in stimuli experienced during movement, an event referred to as coactivation. Muscle tone allows muscles to adapt readily to changing sensory stimuli during functional activities. Children with CP resulting from a lesion in the CNS experience disruption in postural control, righting, equilibrium, protective reactions, and atypical muscle tone. Decreased muscle tone, which is defined as hypotonia, can make a child appear relaxed and even floppy. Increased muscle tone, which is defined as hypertonia, can make a child appear stiff or rigid. In some cases, a child may initially appear hypotonic, but the muscle tone may change to hypertonia after several months of life and the influence of movement against gravity. An occupational therapy assistant (OTA) must possess an understanding of the ways in which postural control and muscle tone can affect normal movement patterns and everyday occupations when planning therapeutic interventions for children with cerebral palsy (Box 17-3). This knowledge is imperative for planning functional therapeutic activities that are appropriate for the child's age and physical abilities.

Primitive Reflexes

Much of the early movement patterns seen in newborns appears to be reflexive in nature and can be elicited by specific sensory motor stimulation. These early reflexes may disappear as the CNS matures and are replaced by more purposeful, voluntary, and skilled movements. The presence or absence of early reflexes is used to evaluate the health of infants. For example, when you provide gentle tactile stimulation to the cheek of a newborn, the infant will turn his or her head toward the cheek that is touched. This early reflex, referred to as the rooting reflex, helps newborns find the source of nutrition (i.e., breast or bottle).

POSTURAL DEVELOPMENT AND MOTOR CONTROL

As newborns grow, they are continually developing and refining postural control. As with motor skills, the characteristics of posture vary with age. In the past 20 years, much research has been devoted to understanding motor control so that OT practitioners may provide effective neurologic rehabilitation to persons who have CP and other neurologic disorders. Motor control theory is complex (refer to Chapter 24 for additional material). However, the OT practitioner should be aware of the two main schools of thought on motor control. This knowledge can guide the OT practitioner in seeking information that can contribute to implementing effective therapeutic approaches. The theories can be grouped into two models of motor control: the traditional reflex–hierarchical models, and the more recent systems models.

Reflex-Hierarchical Models

Reflex-hierarchical models propose that purposeful movement is initiated only when the individual experiences a need to move.[32] In reflex-hierarchical models, motor development is based on CNS maturation. Motor development is "wired" in the brain and an infant's first movements reflect lower-level brain centers (i.e., the brainstem) before cortical brain functions mature allowing more controlled movement. These movement patterns are "hardwired" into the human nervous system and do not depend on the application of learned patterns for performing tasks. According to this model, children with CP lack the ability to independently learn to control movement from higher-level brain centers. Their abnormal postural mechanisms and disordered muscle tone cause them to repeatedly use and store in memory those movement patterns that are governed predominantly by the early tonic reflex patterns; these patterns inhibit the functional use of agonist and antagonist muscles during daily tasks (reciprocal innervations and coactivation).

Current research evidence does not support reflex-hierarchical models of intervention.[26] Recently, this theory has been applied to the Masgutova Neurosensorimotor Reflex Integration (RNRI) method, which states that the therapist assumes that motor reflex patterns play a subordinate role in the maturation of more complex motor reflex schemes (i.e., rolling over, sitting up, crawling, etc.). Masgutova's RNRI method is based on the previous principles that integrating reflexes will improve functional movement. However, current research suggests that engaging children in whole meaningful activities will improve functional movement and, consequently, reflexes and tone may improve as a result. The newest research suggests that focusing on the end product or activity is better than the component (e.g., reflex). There are limited published studies on the efficacy of the RNRI method and a recent systematic review on therapies for children with CP did not support the use of RNRI.[26] More rigorous study of the RNRI approach is needed in order to support use in current practice.

> **CLINICAL** *Pearl*
>
> The movement patterns of children with CP may be influenced by primitive reflex activity, including the asymmetric tonic neck reflex, symmetric tonic neck reflex, and the tonic labyrinthine reflex affecting the acquisition of normal developmental milestones such as the ability to roll, sit unsupported, stand, and walk (Figure 17-2).

Dynamic System Models

The dynamic systems approach to understanding motor behavior proposes that postural control is greatly influenced by an individual's many volitional and functional daily tasks and activities.[19] Systems theorists recognize that it is impossible to understand motor control issues without understanding the external and internal forces that affect movement against the forces of gravity. Systems models purport that posture and movement must be flexible and adaptable so that a person can perform a wide range of daily activities, whereas reflex-hierarchical models state that the control of posture and movement is the outcome or product of a process. Dynamic systems models postulate that posture is anticipatory to the initiation of movement. Postural adjustments actually precede movements; they prepare the body to counterbalance the weight shifts that are caused by the movement activity. In this way, less balance disturbance occurs. Dynamic systems theorists also suggest that control of movement occurs due to the interactions of many body systems working cooperatively to achieve a desired movement goal. This concept is called the distributed model of

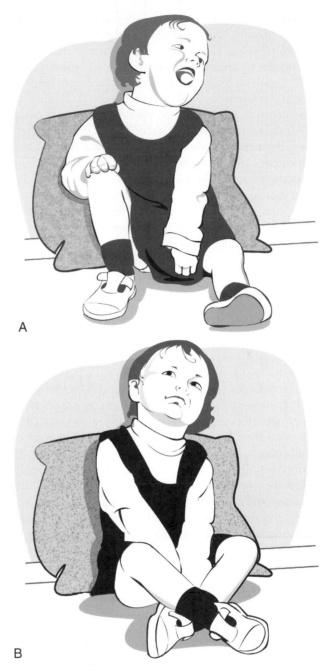

FIGURE 17-2 **A**, Child's head is turned to side stimulating the asymmetrical tonic neck reflex (ATNR) response (flexion on skull side and extension on the other side). **B**, Child is repositioned to help bring hands to midline and decrease the effects of the ATNR.

motor control. Consider this example of a child trying to catch two balls, one of which is a small tennis ball and the other a large, heavy medicine ball. Before catching the balls, the child has used his or her vision to inspect them, used visual perception to make decisions about their sizes and weights, assumed an appropriate postural stance, and positioned the arms forward away from the body to be ready to catch. This anticipatory process is called feed forward.

According to the systems approach, feed-forward actions require that posture be highly variable and subject to being affected by all the factors motivating the person to choose to catch the balls. No one right way to execute movement exists; rather, movement is strongly influenced by many variables. According to this approach, in contrast to reflex–hierarchical models, motor development follows a steplike progression, starting with primitive reflexes and progressing to voluntary movement control through the higher brain centers. The research of systems theorists has shown that motor activity is most often initiated by the interaction of sensory, perceptual, environmental, and other factors leading to task-focused, goal-directed movement.

One other concept from systems model research has important therapeutic implications for the treatment of children with cerebral palsy or other neurologic disorders. Postural control and movement are at their greatest levels of efficiency, flexibility, and adaptability after randomized practice and repetition. Infants attempt to roll, crawl, stand, and walk over several hundred attempts with varied success and failure. Each attempt provides necessary feedback that will feed forward to more skilled motor responses and the eventual mastery of the motor skill. For example, children in elementary school have many opportunities to practice learning to print their names so that the letters are neatly aligned and are of small, equal sizes. Although children practice printing during class, they are also practicing any time they spontaneously write their names during typical childhood activities and games. Over time, this repeated motor pattern develops into a skill; children can adapt the postures and movements used in the activity to fit several different tasks. They can write their names at the top of school papers while seated at their desks or at the bottom of pictures they are drawing while stretched out on the floor. By repeating this task in many different contexts, children gain the skill of motor problem solving. Systems models suggest that children with cerebral palsy need to be challenged with meaningful activities that encourage repetition of motor actions that will develop motor strategies in a variety of play environments.

CLASSIFICATION AND DISTRIBUTION

CP can be defined by the location of the lesion in the CNS and by distribution of abnormal muscle tone in the trunk and extremities. Involvement of one extremity is commonly referred to as monoplegia, upper and lower extremities on one side of the body as **hemiplegia**, both lower extremities as **diplegia** or paraplegia, all limbs as **quadriplegia**, and all limbs and head/neck as tetraplegia. CP is also classified according to four main types of movement disorders: spastic, dyskinetic, ataxic, and mixed (Table 17-1).

TABLE 17-1

Classification of Cerebral Palsy

MOVEMENT DISORDER	AREA OF BODY INVOLVED	PREVALENCE, %
Spastic	Diplegic: legs > arms	32
	Quadriplegic: all 4 extremities	24
	Hemiplegic: one-sided involvement, arm > leg	29
	Double hemiplegic: both sides; one greater than other, arms > legs	24
Dyskinetic	Choreoathetoid	14
	Dystonic Athetoid	
Ataxic		<1
Mixed		Percentages included above

Children with spastic CP demonstrate hypertonia and muscle spasticity. **Spasticity** is defined as a velocity-dependent resistance to stretch.[19] Resistance to range of motion (ROM) will either increase with speed of force or will increase with quick movement. The effects of spasticity are often associated with clonus, an extensor plantar response, and persistent primitive reflexes. As a child with spastic CP attempts to move, excessive muscle tone builds up and is then rapidly released, triggering a hyperactive stretch reflex in the muscle. It may show up at the beginning, middle, or end of a movement range, but the result is poor control of voluntary movement and little ability to regulate the force of movement. Distribution of spasticity in spastic CP can be monoplegia, diplegia, hemiplegia, quadriplegia, or tetraplegia.

The second main type of CP is the dyskinetic type. Dyskinesias include athetoid, choreoathetoid, and dystonic CP. Distribution of muscle tone is typically quadriplegia for all three types. **Dyskinesias** are abnormal movements—most obvious when a child initiates a movement in one extremity—that lead to atypical and unintentional movement of other muscle groups of the body. The child exhibits slow, writhing, involuntary motor movements in combination with abrupt, irregular, and jerky movements. Children with pure **athetosis** demonstrate a fluctuation of muscle tone from low to normal with little or no spasticity and poor coactivation of muscle flexors and extensors. Children with choreoathetosis have constant fluctuations from low to high, with jerky involuntary movement that may be seen more distally than proximally. Dystonic movements are sustained twisted postures that are absent at rest and triggered by movement (action). The movements follow a similar pattern, and these repetitive postures support the diagnosis of dystonia (unlike choreoathetosis, in which movement fluctuations are random).

The third type of CP, **ataxia**, has less effect on muscle tone, but greatly affects balance and coordination. Children with ataxia may show shifts in muscle tone, but to a lesser degree than those with dyskinesias. Distribution of related muscle control issues is typically quadriplegic. Children with ataxic CP are more successful in directing voluntary movements but appear clumsy and may have tremors involuntarily and at rest. They have considerable difficulty with balance, coordination, and maintenance of stable alignment of the head, trunk, shoulders, and pelvis. These children may have poorly developed equilibrium responses and lack proximal stability in the trunk to assist with the control of hand and leg movements.

Children with CP who often show combinations of high and low muscle tone problems are considered to have the mixed type. Those who have spastic CP move their extremities with abrupt hypertonic motions but may also exhibit marked **hypotonicity** in their trunk muscles. The distribution for mixed-type CP is typically quadriplegic.

Knowledge of the degree of muscle tone abnormality and the child's cognitive, sensory, and perceptual status can help the OT practitioner establish realistic and practical therapeutic goals and interventions. The child with mild motor involvement and normal cognition has greater potential to succeed at gaining new motor skills, whereas the child with severe motor involvement and normal cognition may benefit more from assistive technologies that compensate for the absence of motor skills.

CLINICAL *Pearl*

Children with spastic CP may have contractures in one or more joints requiring use of orthoses to help elongate tight muscles and to correct misalignments in thumb web space, wrist, and fingers.

CLINICAL *Pearl*

Children with dyskinetic CP often have average to above-average intelligence. Often when these children attempt to use their arms and legs for play, self-care, or school tasks, the movements are very uncoordinated, which leads to frustration from repeated failed attempts at tasks. Occupational therapy may be successful if it focuses on a specific task (e.g., drinking from a cup) and the movements needed to complete those tasks are properly analyzed. Children should practice all the motor patterns of a task in simulated, fun activities during therapy while also practicing the actual functional activity.

CLINICAL *Pearl*

Children with ataxic CP demonstrate fixing of joints while attempting to reach or move due to poor balance responses. These children may also show some apprehension when trying dynamic activities in which their balance is challenged, such as reaching toward their feet to put on socks and shoes while sitting unsupported on a bench on in a low-back chair.

FUNCTIONAL IMPLICATIONS AND ASSOCIATED PROBLEMS

CASE *Study*

Seventeen-year-old Tammy has been diagnosed with spastic quadriplegic CP. She was recently admitted to a rehabilitation hospital to receive intensive OT and physical therapy (PT) services. She has a history of multiple orthopedic surgeries, including spinal fusion for scoliosis and bilateral tendon lengthening for wrist flexion contractures. She has a percutaneous endoscopic gastrostomy (PEG) tube in place for ingesting liquids, as otherwise she tends to aspirate thin liquids; Tammy also has significant dysarthria. She primarily uses a power wheelchair for mobility in the community. As she has gotten older, her muscle tone has affected the position of her joints and the length of her muscles. Contractures in her hips make it hard for her to stand when completing stand-pivot transfers to and from her wheelchair. Tammy also reports having trouble managing the pain in her hips. Her balance has decreased so much that she is afraid of falling and hurting herself or her grandmother, who is her primary caregiver. Her grandmother reports having trouble bathing Tammy because of her muscle tightness and size. Tammy's muscle tone and contractures have also caused more difficulties with toileting. Due to her hip tightness, it is hard for her to wipe herself and to pull up her pants while standing holding on to the toilet rail; she had been able to do this with just supervision when she was younger. Tammy will be working with the case manager and with the OTA to find resources in the community, such as independent living centers and home health aides, to help Tammy's grandmother with her care.

Muscle and Bone

CP can cause a host of associated changes in body structures and functions, which influence each person's functional potential. Although CP is a nonprogressive condition in terms of changes in the CNS lesion, the resulting motor disorder may cause secondary impairments in the musculoskeletal system over time.

Weakness and abnormal muscle tone and movement patterns can contribute to the development of muscle tissue contractures, bone deformities, and joint dislocations or misalignment. Some joint dislocations or misalignment may require surgical intervention to reposition the joint to a more functional position. As the child grows older, the potential for arthritis in misaligned joints increases, and this pain can additionally impact the person's ability to function. All of these changes further limit functional movement and can decrease the person's ability to complete activities of daily living (ADLs).

Other impairments associated with decreased functional mobility include risk for skin breakdown and decreased bone density. Individuals who are unable to assume more than a few positions or independently shift body weight risk skin breakdown. This is because body weight in these individuals is often concentrated over a few points for prolonged periods. Similarly, decreased time spent standing or ambulating can affect the strength of the individual's bones. Children diagnosed with CP are noted to have decreased bone mineral density and are vulnerable to pathologic fractures.[17,22]

> ### CLINICAL *Pearl*
>
> Positioning and orthotic programs aim to minimize the effect of muscle tone on joint position.

> ### CLINICAL *Pearl*
>
> The child who often keeps his or her hand in a tight fist may have hygiene issues associated with ROM limitations.

Cognition, Hearing, and Language

Due to abnormal muscle tone and musculoskeletal changes associated with CP, children diagnosed with CP may have various problems with speech and language. These potential problems include decreased speech production, poor articulation, and decreased speech intelligibility. *Dysarthria* is the term used to describe a disorder of speech production that is secondary to decreased muscle coordination, paralysis, or weakness.[3] In addition to speech production disorders, children with CP may have changes in the quality of their voice due to decreased strength or control of respiratory and postural muscles. Because CP has the potential to affect areas of the brain outside of the motor system, it can cause decreased expressive and receptive language skills.[28] This means that children with CP have difficulty

processing language-based information or producing responses. Hearing loss, which can also occur in this population, is another factor that inhibits normal speech.[28]

All of these potential impairments can have a significant effect on participation in age-appropriate activities. The child's cognitive and linguistic skill level can play a significant role in his or her ability to benefit from therapeutic and educational interventions, and it can have a great effect on the types of interventions or adaptive equipment an OT practitioner chooses for the child.

Sensory Problems

As many as 50% of children with CP experience sensory problems, including visual impairments such as blindness, uncoordinated eye movements, and eye muscle weakness and 25% have auditory reception and processing deficits.[17] Conductive hearing loss and sensorineural hearing impairments may occur if the child has been affected by a congenital CNS infection. Both vision and hearing should be tested regularly in children with CP.

Additional sensory problems include deficits in the processing of tactile and proprioceptive information. Some children have difficulty with tactile discrimination as well as fingertip force regulation during object manipulation. Children with CP may also demonstrate tactile hypersensitivities (i.e., overreacting to touch, textures, and changes in head position), causing some to become visibly upset when handled or moved by others. Children with multiple sensory processing problems have more difficulty understanding their environments. Some tactile sensation problems are also linked to abnormal oral movement patterns. The disorganized muscular movements that children with CP experience in their arms, legs, and trunk, may also be seen in oral–facial musculature affecting feeding experiences. Many of these children dislike certain food textures and may have problems coordinating their chewing, sucking, and swallowing movements. Those with severe problems in this area may be surgically fitted with a PEG tube for feeding. OT practitioners must consider the child's sensory limitations and strengths while setting intervention goals and determine individually which sensory experiences are likely to improve occupational performance abilities.

Hand Skills and Upper Extremity Function

Children with CP demonstrate problems with upper limb function due to abnormal muscle tone and decreased ability to maintain a stable posture when attempting functional tasks (Figure 17-3).[17] Efficient use of arms and hands depends on the proximal control and dynamic stability of the trunk and shoulder girdle. Children with CP demonstrate weakness in the

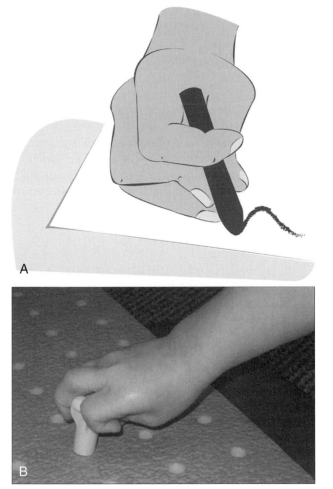

A

B

FIGURE 17-3 Due to thumb tightness and decreased thumb abduction and closed web space, the child is using an atypical grasp between his thumb and middle finger with wrist ulnar deviation as shown in **A** and **B**.

shoulder girdle; may have contractures in their elbow, forearm, wrist, fingers, and thumb due to hypertonicity; or may move the arm and hand in synergistic patterns, as they lack the ability to isolate single joint movements. Postural instability can affect upper extremity movement also, as these children may need to use their upper extremities to support upright postures against gravity. When the upper extremities are fixed and used to help stabilize and compensate for trunk weakness, the arms and hands cannot be used for functional tasks (e.g., playing with toys at the midline of the body while challenged to sit unsupported).

Vision

A wide spectrum of visual issues affects children with CP. Children with more severe cerebral palsy typically have greater visual impairment.[16] Regardless of the child's functional level, issues related to vision should always be taken into consideration during performance

of fine motor tasks, play, and ADLs. Vision plays an important role in the timing of grasp and release, manipulating objects, orienting materials, making eye contact, and finding needed items. Children with visual impairments may use postural adaptations, such as a head tilt or changes to the angle of gaze to compensate for visual deficits. These deficits may be oculomotor in nature, that is, the muscles of the eye do not move smoothly and synchronously or may move involuntarily. The term *strabismus* describes the misalignment of eyes due to muscle imbalance. Functionally, strabismus may cause difficulty attending to visual tasks. The child may have decreased convergence or divergence, decreased depth perception, or double vision. Other terms describing misalignment of the eyes include *exotropia* (one eye drifts temporally), *esotropia* (one eye drifts nasally), *hypertropia* (one eye drifts upward), and *hypotropia* (one eye drifts downward). The term *nystagmus* describes the constant movement of eyes in a repetitive and uncontrolled way. Functional issues associated with nystagmus include reduced acuity, difficulty fixing on a target to maintain balance, reduced target accuracy when reaching or grasping, compensatory head movements, or posturing to compensate for visual deficit. In addition to oculomotor impairments, the child may have deficits in the way the brain processes visual information. Without proper processing, the child may not understand the spatial relationships between objects, may miss part of the visual field, or not identify a partially hidden item, for example, his or her coat inside a closet.

CLINICAL *Pearl*

Children with CP may compensate for their vision problems in a variety of ways. Turning the head to the side to use peripheral vision or fixing the body posture in a way that seems awkward to observers are examples of the adaptations used by these children to utilize the visual fields and abilities they have.

CLINICAL *Pearl*

Placement of materials in the area of the child's strongest visual field can help minimize the postural compensations that children with CP use to visually interact with their environments.

Physical and Behavioral Manifestations

Children with CP may experience problems such as seizures and other medical conditions not directly related to the movement disorder. Abnormal posture and weak muscle activity may compromise cardiac and respiratory functions and prevent these systems from working efficiently. The resulting low endurance and fatigue can influence the child's capacity for activity. The OT practitioner monitors each child's physical endurance and plans therapeutic goals to increase strength and endurance.

Behavioral problems and social delays are not unusual in children with CP. They may become accustomed to receiving assistance from others, and problems such as "learned helplessness" may prevent them from attempting the developmental challenges needed for continued growth and mastery of skills. The inability to manage social and peer interactions can lead to social isolation and immaturity and a repertoire of undesirable social behaviors. The OT practitioner can often assist families and work collaboratively with the child's educational team, which may include teachers, consultants, and administrators, to suggest strategies to enhance the child's social development.

CASE *Study*

Antoine is an 8-year-old boy with a history of a seizure disorder and athetoid CP. He uses a power wheelchair for mobility and an augmentative communication device. He attends elementary school, where he is placed in an age-appropriate classroom with accommodations and related services, including PT, occupational therapy, speech therapy, and assistive technology. Antoine's continuous body movements make it difficult for him to complete fine motor tasks, including accessing his communication device to complete class work. He tends to get frustrated when he knows the answer to a question but is not able to communicate it to his teacher and classmates. His therapy team discovers that a head stick helps Antoine improve his access to his communication device. The OTA has also worked with his art teacher to fasten a holder for tools, such as a paintbrush, to his head stick. Now Antoine is able to creatively express himself through a variety of mediums, including paint and pastels, which do not require a lot of pressure when drawing. Antoine also seems to have improved success in using the device when he can hold on to the armrest of his wheelchair, so his OTA experiments with a bar mounted on Antoine's tray so that he can push against it to improve his trunk stability.

ROLES OF THE OCCUPATIONAL THERAPIST AND THE OCCUPATIONAL THERAPY ASSISTANT

The occupational therapist and the OTA collaborate to provide services to children with CP. The individual needs of the child and the family and the child's chronologic age determine each step in the assessment and intervention processes. During the child's infancy and early childhood, OT practitioners focus on family care and management issues such as feeding and bathing, mobility around the home, sleep and rest, and family participation. During the child's early school years, the occupational therapist and the OTA assist the child with classroom participation, self-care skills, peer socialization, leisure and vocational readiness, and educational and community mobility. In the case of the adolescent with CP, OT services may focus on helping with engagement in work or other productive activities, development of independent living skills, sexual identification and sexual expression, and mobility in the community at large.

Assessment

The occupational therapist and the OTA collaboratively assess each individual child's needs. Together they evaluate areas of performance, client factors, activity demands, and contexts. The occupational therapist may use one or several standardized tests requiring specialized administration and interpretation skills and can provide the team with specific information about reflex development, sensorimotor functioning, motor skills, and developmental skill levels. The experienced, trained OTA may assist in the administration of some tests. Observation is a crucial part of the assessment process because many children with CP cannot easily follow the directions of standardized tests because of their impaired motor skills. Both the occupational therapist and the OTA can observe the child's functional abilities at home, in school, and during leisure activities. Observation of the child's occupational performance provides the OT practitioner with data on factors influencing the child's muscle tone, reflex activity, gross and fine motor skills, sensory systems, cognition, perception, and psychosocial development. The OTA may provide information to plan the most effective OT intervention. Early identification of atypical postures can minimize the use of compensatory and dysfunctional movements that could lead to serious deformities and undesirable behaviors. To help the child make progress in meeting typical developmental milestones, more mature and typical movement patterns can be facilitated by both the OTA and the occupational therapist.

Assessment data create a "picture" of the child's functioning and indicate his or her strengths and weaknesses. The OT practitioner uses this information (along with parental input) to formulate goals to match the child's needs and developmental abilities or potential. Examples include increasing the child's ability to participate in a classroom writing activity and teaching family members ways to reduce the hypertonicity in the child so that they can bathe and feed him or her. Goals for the adolescent might address accessing public transportation or learning ways to perform homemaking skills. Thorough OT assessment data are essential when working as part of a service delivery team. Classroom teachers may rely on the OT practitioner's expertise for help with the establishment and implementation of educational goals. Vocational skills trainers need to know the student's physical performance abilities and attitudes toward new tasks. Families may use OT input to select recreational activities for their children.

The Model of Human Occupation Clearinghouse provides a variety of assessments that examine the child's occupational performance. Interviews such as the Pediatric Volitional Questionnaire[2] provide information on the child's motivation. The Child Occupational Self-Assessment[20] and the Short Child Occupational Profile Evaluation[4] provide an overview of the child's volition, roles, habits, and performance within various contexts. The School Setting Interview[18] and the School Function Assessment[11] provide information on how the child is functioning at school. These assessments and others explore how the child performs his or her occupations. Motor-based assessments include the Alberta Infant Motor Scale and the Gross Motor Function Classification Scale[31] (Table 17-2). See Appendix A in Chapter 10 for an overview of the variety of assessments available. The Alberta Infant Motor Scale is an observational assessment scale that measures the motor skills of infants from birth through the time when they start walking. Weight bearing, posture, and antigravity movements are evaluated. This assessment tool is often used in early intervention settings.[27]

TABLE 17-2

Gross Motor Function Classification System[31]

LEVEL	DESCRIPTION OF FUNCTIONAL ABILITIES
I	Walks without limitations. Performs gross motor skills such as running and jumping, but speed, balance, and coordination may be impaired.
II	Walks with limitations. Includes walking on uneven surfaces, inclines, and stairs, for long distances, or in crowds or confined spaces.
III	Walks using a hand-held mobility device. Walks on even surfaces, indoors, and outdoors with an assistive device; may use manual wheelchair for long distances.
IV	Self-mobility with limitations. May use powered mobility or require assistance from a caregiver; may walk short distances with a mobility device but relies primarily on wheeled mobility.
V	Transported in a manual wheelchair. Has no means of independent mobility and relies on caregiver for all transportation needs.

Interventions

Individuals with CP who receive OT services can experience a sense of empowerment and control when they successfully perform meaningful occupations, within the self-care, instrumental ADLs, sleep and rest, work, education, and leisure domains. OT practitioners develop and implement interventions to promote functional performance within each individual's capacity. Through training and consultation, they also assist caregivers and educators in the provision of interventions that facilitate and support the child's occupational performance. Intervention strategies include positioning and handling. (Chapter 18 provides more information on positioning and handling techniques.) The OT practitioner determines the variety of postures the child can assume, maintain, and achieve independently or with physical assistance. Optimal positions are determined for ADLs. Upright sitting positions are needed for most classroom activities, whereas a relaxed, partially reclined position may be optimal for assisted bathing. Practitioners can also select and recommend specific types of positioning equipment, such as chairs, supine or prone standers, and sidelyers, which support the child during functional activities with the best possible postural alignment, control, and stability. Handling techniques such as slow rocking, slow stroking, imposed rotational movement patterns, and bouncing are used to enhance the child's muscle tone, activity level, and ability for independent movement (see Chapter 18). Techniques such as weight bearing and weight shifting can promote postural alignment and independent movement. A stiff, hypertonic child fixed in a strong extensor posture can be easily positioned in a wheelchair after the OT practitioner has slowly and alternately rotated the shoulders in a forward and backward motion. Handling relaxes the child's muscle tone throughout the body and is used within a neurodevelopmental treatment approach. Each joint can move more easily, and the child can then be placed in the wheelchair with good postural alignment and comfort. Positioning and handling methods are especially important for the child with CP who is unable to move independently. These methods also help the child work toward the achievement of performance-area goals such as increased independence in dressing, feeding, playing, and doing schoolwork. The OT practitioner can learn these treatments in special training programs or under the direction of a skilled occupational therapist. The OTA can implement positioning recommendations, teach them to caregivers, and use handling methods to improve the child's functional performance by following the instructions of the occupational therapist.

Individuals with CP can achieve greater independence in ADLs with the help of assistive and adaptive devices. The OT practitioner may recommend adapted utensils for the child with limited grasp abilities; suggest a large, weighted pen to aid a student who has tremors; or attach a large zipper pull on a coat for a self-dressing activity. The OTA consults with the occupational therapist to determine the safest and most appropriate devices to match each child's abilities. The task is particularly important in the selection of feeding equipment that can ensure safe swallowing. The OTA should become familiar with a number of assistive device vendors so that equipment recommendations can be offered for all appropriate occupational performance areas and budget considerations. With a little creative thinking, an OTA can often fabricate assistive devices from inexpensive materials. PVC plumbing pipe from a hardware store can be assembled to make an inverted U-shaped frame with suspended toys that can be placed in front of the child. This could be one way to help children with limited reaching and grasping abilities engage in a meaningful play activity.

The OTA assists clients with CP in a variety of settings. Intervention programs can occur in the family home, a school setting, or a hospital. In each setting, the OTA is part of an interdisciplinary treatment team whose goal is to maximize the child's health, functional capacities, and quality of life. As an OT specialist, the OTA combines knowledge and skill to help each child accomplish purposeful and meaningful daily living tasks within the home, school, and community settings.

Medical Interventions

A number of medical interventions exist to treat the effects of CP and are often used in conjunction with rehabilitation therapies. Common pharmacologic treatments for spasticity include oral baclofen and injectable botulinum neurotoxin (Botox).[19] Baclofen is an antispasticity medication that may be administered orally or injected into a pump that delivers the medication directly into the cerebrospinal fluid. It is a systemic medication and can reduce muscle tone throughout the person's body. Botox is a more specific approach, with injections delivered directly to a spastic muscle or muscles with the goal of reducing muscle tone. The effects of Botox are short lived, lasting around 3 to 6 months. An injection is often paired with aggressive therapy to increase ROM and splinting to maintain gains in mobility and function. One surgical approach to spasticity management is selective dorsal rhizotomy, which involves cutting the selective sensory nerves that come from the lower limbs to the spinal cord.

Types of orthopedic surgery to address contractures and muscle imbalances include tendon transfer, muscle release, and osteotomy.[23] Tendon transfers move the insertions of muscles to change the action that the muscle produces. For example, the child with weak or paralyzed hand musculature may have a wrist muscle moved to the hand to assist with grasp. Other types of soft tissue surgery include muscle release or lengthening. These procedures lengthen or release tight muscle tissue to allow increased movement of a joint. Often done in conjunction with soft tissue surgery, osteotomies are procedures in which the bone is cut to lengthen it, shorten it, or improve its alignment. All of these surgeries involve a period of immobilization initially, but early movement and physical therapy are important in maximizing functional gains from these interventions.

CLINICAL *Pearl*

To maximize the effect of medications for muscle tone management, a regime of stretching, splinting, and functional strengthening exercises may be recommended by the physiatrist.

CLINICAL *Pearl*

A recent comprehensive review of interventions used with children with CP[26] found the following interventions to be some of the most supported by evidence: functional and goal-directed training, constraint-induced and bimanual training, fitness training, home exercise programs, occupational therapy after botulinum toxin injections, and interventions targeting reduction of pressure ulcers.

Complementary and Alternative Medicine

The term *complementary and alternative medicine* (CAM) refers to those interventions that are not presently considered to be part of conventional medicine (Table 17-3).[25] CAM use in the population overall has grown in recent years, and it is becoming more common for parents of children with CP to seek out alternative therapies. According to the 2007 National Health Interview Survey, which gathered information on CAM use among more than 9000 children aged 17 and under, nearly 12% had used some form of CAM during the past 12 months. Children with multiple health disorders, including CP, were found to be some of the most frequent users of CAM interventions.[8] Majnemer and colleagues reported that 25% of the 166 adolescents with CP in their study used some form of CAM over the course of their lifetime.[22] The most popular of these was massage. Some OT practitioners with training in these methods or advance certifications may use CAM. Ultimately occupational therapists are responsible for the safety of their patients and should use their clinical judgment and the best available evidence to determine use of these intervention techniques to complement their service delivery.[1]

TABLE 17-3

Complementary and Alternative Medicine Programs

CAM PRACTICE	INTERVENTION DESCRIPTION
Hippotherapy	Uses the help of a horse, for example, to help a child develop postural stability
Acupuncture/ acupressure	Stimulation of specific points on the body with pressure or needles
Massage therapy	Soft tissue mobilization
Craniosacral therapy	Mobilization of cranium/sacral bone
Myofascial release	Mobilization of interconnected fascial system
Tai chi	Slow, graceful movement with emphasis on mind–body connection
Yoga	Body positioning, breathing, and meditation
Pilates	Breathing; core control; organization of the head, neck, and shoulders; spine articulation; alignment and posture; and movement integration
Biofeedback	Electronically using information from the body to teach an individual to recognize what is going on inside his or her own body
Dietary supplements	Substances taken by mouth to supplement the diet, including vitamins, minerals, herbs or other botanicals, amino acids, and certain other substances

Commonly used CAM reported by occupational therapists include guided imagery, myofacial release, yoga and meditation.[19]

Constraint-Induced Movement Therapy

Constraint-induced movement therapy (CIMT) is an evidenced-based intervention approach to address functional implications and learned nonuse or developmental disregard of the impaired upper extremity in children with hemiplegia. *Learned nonuse* and *developmental disregard* are terms used to describe how children with hemiplegic CP do not use their affected limbs because of negatively reinforced experiences despite the function that may be available.[8,25] CIMT developed out of basic experimental psychology research by Edward Taub and his colleagues, on sensory contributions to motor learning in nonhuman primates.[6,29,34] CIMT was then used in the rehabilitation of adult patients who had experienced a stroke and later was tested with children.[7,16,29]

CIMT can be defined as either a signature CIMT or modified CIMT (m-CIMT). A signature CIMT approach has five essential components, including the following[29]:

1. Constraint of the unaffected upper limb
2. A high dosage of repetitive task practice (3 to 6 hours of therapy per day over several consecutive days)
3. The use of shaping techniques
4. Therapy provided in a natural setting
5. A transition or post-CIMT program to maintain gains acquired during CIMT program

A typical signature approach provides massed practice and shaping of more mature motor movement for at least two consecutive weeks (14–21 days, dosage 42–128 hours) by a professional with an understanding of rehabilitation techniques to improve motor function.[29,30]

m-CIMT is defined as constraint of the stronger or less affected upper limb combined with less than 3 hours per day of therapy. Most of the five essential elements of the signature approach are provided, but with modifications including variation in where the therapy is provided (e.g., clinic or camp vs individual treatment at home) or a variation in the dosage of therapy (e.g., less concentrated, may be more distributed over several days or weeks).[29] Massed practice may be provided by a professional with training in CIMT, but not necessarily an occupational or physical therapist (e.g., parent, day-care worker, camp counselor). Unlike therapists in adult settings, pediatric therapists using a CIMT embed repetitive task practice in daily functional and play activities. A variety of restraining devices such as mitts, casts, splints, and slings are used in research and clinical protocols.[7,9,10,12,13,29] Current literature describes home-, clinic-, and camp-based models of implementation.[7,9,10,12,13,29] Unlike occupational therapists in adult settings, pediatric occupational therapists using this approach embed repetitive task practice in play activities. Future studies on the outcomes of pediatric CIMT will continue to define optimal parameters of the protocol, including age, level of function, and spillover effects on gait, language, and cognition.[29]

CASE *Study*

Four-year-old Brandon has hemiplegic CP. He has been receiving outpatient OT services weekly. Brandon is working on his upper extremity strength by pulling up his pants with both hands, performing weight-bearing activities, and maintaining grasp with his affected right hand. Brandon is participating in a CIMT program at an outpatient clinic. Brandon attends the program 3 hours a day and wears a cast on his unaffected, stronger arm. Activities that are motivating, such as carrying a bucket loaded with toy cars and picking up the toy cars and putting them on a race track,

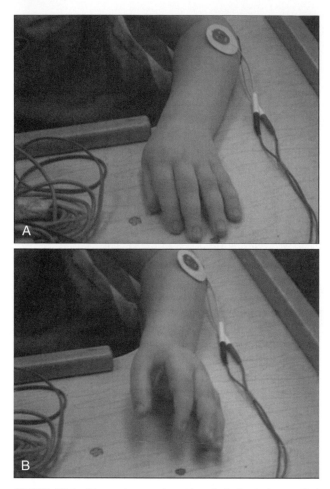

FIGURE 17-4 These pictures show electrical stimulation applied to the supinators of a child's affected upper extremity. **A,** The child's position at rest. **B,** The child's hand supinates in reaction to the electrical stimulation.

are done at a high level of repetition. Imaginary play activities, such as pushing his affected arm through dress-up clothes, help generalize these new skills to play and ADL tasks.

Modalities

Various modalities can be used within OT sessions to improve muscle length and strength and reduce spasticity in children with cerebral palsy. These treatment modalities include hot/cold therapy and electrical stimulation. Heat maybe used in conjunction with ROM programs to improve muscle length and reduce pain, whereas cryotherapy (ice, cold packs) may be used in cases of inflammation associated with arthritis to improve patient comfort. Another modality commonly used with children with motor impairments is electrical stimulation (Figure 17-4). It may be used for a variety of reasons, including strengthening antagonist muscles, muscle reeducation, pain reduction, improving coordination, increasing ROM, and reduction of spasticity.[5,24,37] Electrical stimulation is most effective when paired with

a functional activity, such as grasping finger foods and bringing them to the mouth when stimulating the biceps or releasing toys into a container while stimulating wrist extensors.[20,37]

Robotics

The area of robotics in occupational therapy takes advantage of new technology to enhance motor and cognitive performance in children with CP. Robotic therapy provides a means for repetitive practice of target movements, such as reaching in space.[14,15] These devices typically employ robotic arms, joysticks, or other controllers to measure the patient's performance of the targeted movement. Early studies demonstrate that patients using robotic devices in therapy sessions are motivated and make positive gains.[14,15,19,29]

Robotic devices come in all shapes and sizes. They range from large stationary devices with both gross and fine motor components to glove-based systems with small sensors. See Figure 17-5 for examples of different devices. Most robotic devices are connected to a computer so patients can receive feedback from the game graphics on a screen or monitor.

The literature reports a few large studies and many case reports of using this intervention clinically. Few studies exist with children.

Kinesio Tape

Kinesio taping (also described in Chapter 28) was developed by a Japanese chiropractor Dr. Kenzo Kase in 1973. Kinesio taping gained wide exposure when used by Japanese athletes at the 1988 Seoul Olympics. Originally used by athletes, it is now widely used in hospitals and clinics to treat adults and children with neuromuscular conditions. The kinesio tape is applied directly to the skin and works by increasing stimulation to cutaneous mechanoreceptors that facilitate muscle contraction or inhibition. This occurs due to the stretch properties of the kinesio tape; this is why the amount of stretch can be important for specific muscle tapings. The degree of stimulation is determined by the degree of stretch and inward pressure. When using kinesio taping on children with CP, it is best to select a specific muscle group for rehabilitation and then apply the tape repeatedly to the same muscle group. For example, in the case of a child with CP who demonstrates tightness in wrist flexors and weakness in wrist extensors, the kinesio tape can be applied to facilitate a stronger contraction of the wrist extensors as well as to inhibit the contraction of the overactive wrist flexors. The elastic properties of the tape also can be used to reposition joints to a more appropriate alignment. Due to potential skin sensitivities in these children, it is always important to apply a small "test" strip to the child's skin to see if there is any negative reaction to the properties of the tape before fully taping an extremity.

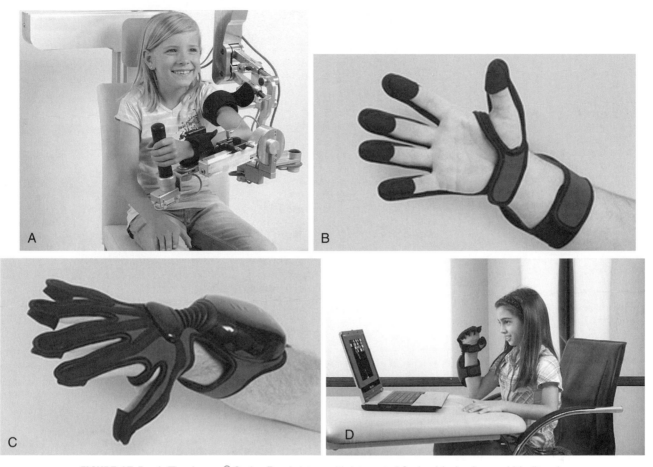

FIGURE 17-5   **A,** The Armeo© Spring Exoskeleton with Integrated Spring Mechanism and Meditouch Hand Tutor, which helps children use their hands and practice. **B, C,** and **D,** Robotics that help children with a variety of activities. (**A** courtesy Hocoma, Switzerland; **B, C, D** courtesy of Meditouch.)

Orthotics and Casting

Static orthoses and casts are used to help children with CP maintain a joint in one position for a variety of different goals (see Chapter 28; Figures 17-7 and 17-8). The overall objective of orthoses or casting is to improve hand function, prevent further joint contracture, improve hygiene, address pain in a specific joint, or to restrict arm and hand movement if the child is using the hands for unsafe behaviors. Serial static orthoses and casts are designed to lengthen tissues and correct deformities through application of gentle forces sustained for extended periods with the goal of reducing tightness

or spasticity in a selected muscle group (e.g., elbow flexors).[30,35,36] A reduction of tightness in the muscles around a joint will allow for greater independent use of the extremity, reduce pain from contracted muscles, and improve ease of bathing and hygiene tasks provided by the caregiver. Casting and orthoses are most effective in applying low-load prolonged stretch to contracted muscle tissues. Orthoses are remolded and casts replaced at intervals, which allows the muscle tissue to respond to the lengthened position. The biomechanical effects of orthoses and casting relate to changes in the length of muscles and connective tissues, and this can reverse the effects that occur when a muscle is maintained in a shortened position. Research has shown that applying orthoses to lengthen tight contracted muscles in children with CP is most effective when applied continuously for periods greater than 6 hours.[36] Casting has additional biomechanical and neurophysiologic effects, although the exact neurophysiologic effects of casting on spasticity are not well defined at this time. It is theorized that inhibition of muscle contractions allowing lengthening of muscle tissues results from decreased cutaneous

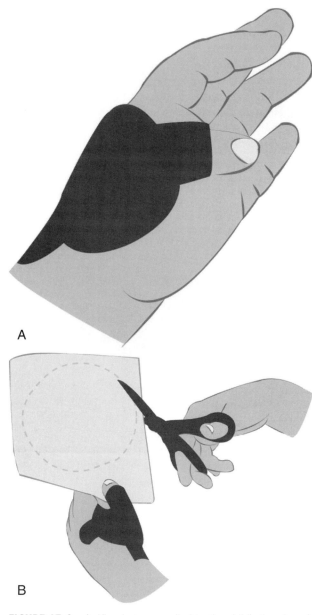

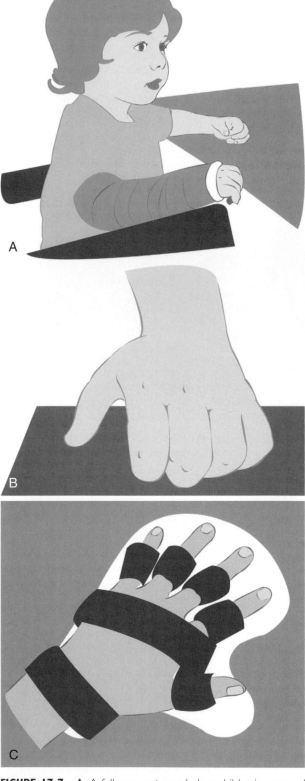

FIGURE 17-6   **A,** Kinesio tape applied to the child's thumb web space opens up the hand so the child can use the hand for activities. **B,** The child can now successfully hold a piece of paper while using scissors in the opposing hand.

sensory input from muscle receptors during the period of immobilization. The effects of neutral warmth and circumferential contact also are believed to contribute to modification of spasticity. A systematic review of splint use in children with CP reported that splint use must be combined with an active therapy program.[26]

Children with CP often wear orthoses to improve overall function. Orthoses are designed to meet specific objectives identified by the child or the parents (Box 17-4). In many instances, orthoses can compensate for functional deficits in hand grasping toys or pointing to get toys, holding eating utensils, holding writing

FIGURE 17-7   **A,** A full-arm cast may help a child gain range of motion. **B,** A child's hand without an orthosis may not allow the child to weight bear completely. **C,** An orthosis can be applied to help the child keep the hand stable and open for activities. The orthosis stabilizes the child's joints so the child can engage in a variety of activities.

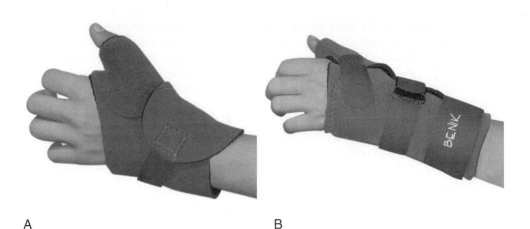

A   B

FIGURE 17-8   BENIK produces prefabricated neoprene orthoses and orthoses that are produced after proper sizing and measurement by an occupational therapist. These orthoses provide stability at the thumb (**A**) and at the wrist (**B**).

Potential Goals and Benefits of Orthoses

- Improve overall function in play, self-care, mobility, and school-related tasks
- Improve position of a joint
  - Decrease joint stiffness and muscle contractures
  - Improve active and passive range of motion in a joint
- Increase access to skin and allow for cleaning and hygiene
- To protect or to help modify behavior
  - For example, use of an elbow orthosis to keep the hands away from the face if the child is biting hands or attempting to pull on tracheostomy or feeding tubes

implements, or accessing computing devices. Examples of this type of orthotic include using a splint to isolate a finger to point and touch a keyboard or augmentative communication device or fabrication of a joystick "goal post" on the toggle switch of a power chair to improve grasp and hand control. Finally, orthoses are also fabricated by OT practitioners to prevent movement from the hand to the mouth in cases where the children may be engaging in self-injurious behaviors or attempting to pull out feeding tubes, intravenous lines, or tracheostomy tubing.

CASE *Study*

Six-year-old Missy had a prolonged period of anoxia during her birth, which resulted in spastic diplegia. Missy has moderate hypertonia throughout her lower extremities and mild muscle tone problems in her upper extremities. These problems cause difficulties with fine motor and in-hand manipulation tasks such as drawing, writing, and brushing teeth. Missy demonstrates good balance reactions from her middle trunk area upward but easily loses her balance when seated on a chair without armrests. She frequently topples over when she tries to bend to retrieve something dropped to the floor. Missy is a bright, happy child with normal intelligence and good vision and hearing abilities. From ages 3 to 6 she attended a special preschool and kindergarten program, where she received OT and PT services. PT practitioners worked with Missy to develop functional mobility skills. She now ambulates independently with a wheeled walker, can lower and raise herself to and from the floor level using an environmental support, and can transfer on and off a preschool-size toilet. OT practitioners helped Missy increase her independence in dressing with the use of Velcro closures and zipper pulls, and they used therapeutic handling and strengthening techniques to improve her manipulation skills with drawing materials and pencils. Because Missy has been so successful in learning self-management skills, her parents and the special education team believe that she is ready to enroll in the regular first-grade class at her local elementary school.

OT consultation services are recommended to assist in Missy's successful school transition. Before she starts school, the OTA and the occupational therapist participate in a team meeting. Missy's parents, her new first-grade teacher, the school's physical education teacher, and the school principal also attend the meeting. The team members decide that the OT team will consult with the classroom teacher to address Missy's seating needs and make sure that she can participate in typical first-grade activities. The school district's occupational therapist reviews the OT documentation from Missy's previous OT practitioners and then schedules a classroom visit for herself and the OTA during the first week of school. During their visit, they note that the classroom desks are too high for Missy. She is not able to maintain a stable, upright posture on a desk chair and loses her balance whenever she leans sideways. Missy also has difficulty keeping her papers firmly on the desk surface when writing and drawing. The occupational therapist and the OTA note two other problems: First, because of her lack of developed balance reactions in the lower body, Missy is unable to remove or put on her coat in the coatroom when she is with the other children of her class. Second, at snack time, Missy has difficulty opening her cardboard juice cartons. The teacher also tells the OTA that each student is expected to perform a daily job, and she would like to get some assistance in selecting one for Missy.

The occupational therapist and the OTA review Missy's functional motor skills and muscle tone problems. They note that she sits in a regular chair with her hips rolled back, her knees and toes pointing inward, and her upper body bent forward because of the lack of postural control and stability in the pelvic area and lower extremities. The occupational therapist instructs the OTA to find a smaller chair with armrests for Missy and discusses ways to determine a good functional seating position.

The following week, the OTA and Missy's teacher locate a chair with armrests that provides Missy with good stability. Now her feet are flat on the floor, and her hips fit on the seat with a 90-degree bend. The OTA places a piece of Dycem, a nonskid rubbery material, on the seat to provide Missy with additional stability so that she can shift her weight and lean somewhat without significant loss of balance. A desk of a suitable height is found, and nonslip grips are placed under the feet of the desk so that Missy can reach a standing position easily by bracing against the desk. The OTA recommends using removable sticky putty to help Missy keep her papers in place and finds a small bench that can be positioned against the wall in the coatroom. Missy can easily manage her coat by sitting on the bench and leaning against the wall. The teacher has learned that Missy enjoys exploring the building but has fewer opportunities to do so than her classmates because she needs additional time to move around with her walker. The teacher believes that Missy would like the job of taking the daily attendance report to the school office but is not certain how she can accomplish it. The OTA suggests attaching an attractive bicycle basket of Missy's choice to her walker. The basket can also be handy for transporting other classroom materials. To solve Missy's snack-time drink problem, the OTA chooses a small piece of brightly colored splinting material and fashions a ring with an inch-long pencil-like protrusion for Missy's middle finger. She can slide on the ring with the protrusion pointing down from her palm and then use the force of her open hand to punch a hole in the juice carton. The basket and ring enable Missy to be as independent as the other children at snack time.

The OTA remembers that the repeated practice of skills in a variety of situations and environments can increase a person's independent motor skills. He contacts Missy's mother, who agrees that Missy can use her ring to manage her drinks at home. After speaking with the OTA, the physical education teacher places a bench against a wall in the area where the children change into their gym shoes. Missy can now independently don and doff her gym shoes that have Velcro closures.

The OTA follows up with Missy's parents and teachers to ensure that she is meeting all the challenges. Later, he administers the Pediatric Volitional Questionnaire to ensure that the team has considered all of Missy's needs.

SUMMARY

The term *cerebral palsy* encompasses a number of postural control and movement disorders resulting from damage to the areas of the CNS that control movement and balance. Common problems associated with CP include limitations in movement options, delays in occupational skill development, muscle tone abnormalities that cause secondary problems such as contractures, and bone or joint deformities. CP can involve total or partial areas of the body, and many individuals with CP are also affected by a number of associated disorders, such as impaired vision, hearing, and communication; below-normal cognition; and seizures.

OTAs can play a vital role in helping children with CP increase their abilities to function independently and expand their repertoire of occupational performance roles. With an understanding of movement control and skill development, OTAs can apply their knowledge of positioning and handling methods to improve an individual's ability to interact with the environment. OTAs can recommend and instruct in the use of assistive devices and specialized equipment to enable children with CP to engage in purposeful activities that match their occupational roles and interests. With guidance from the occupational therapist, OTAs can help the children by using techniques to develop postural control, righting and equilibrium reactions, and controlled movement against gravity. Individual therapy plans incorporate interventions that correspond to each child's unique developmental skills and occupational needs. OTAs offer service in many environmental contexts and find creative ways for each child to engage in meaningful activities at home, in the school, and in the community.

References

1. AOTA. (2005). *Complementary and Alternative Medicine (CAM) Position Paper*. American Occupational Therapy Association. November/December, 59(6).
2. Basu, S., Kafkes, A., Schatz, R., Kiraly, A., & Kielhofner, G. (2008). *The Pediatric Volitional Questionnaire (PVQ), Version 2.1*. Chicago, IL: MOHO Clearinghouse, University of Illinois.

3. Batshaw, M. L. (2013). *Children with disabilities* (6th ed.). Baltimore: Paul H. Brookes Publishing.

4. Bowyer, P., Kramer, J., Ploszai, A., Ross, M., Schwarz, O., Kielhofner, G., & Kramer, K. (2008). *The Short Child Occupational Profile (SCOPE). Version 2.2*. Chicago, IL: MOHO Clearinghouse, University of Illinois.

5. Bracciano, A. G. (2000). *Physical agent modalities: theory and application for the occupational therapist* (2nd ed.). Thorofare, NJ: Slack Incorporated.

6. Brady, K., & Garcia, T. (2009). Constraint induced movement therapy: pediatric applications. *Develop Disabil Res Rev, 15*, 102–111.

7. Case-Smith, J., DeLuca, S. C., Stevenson, R., & Ramey, S. L. (2012). Multicenter randomized controlled trial of pediatric constraint-induced movement therapy: 6-month follow-up. *Am J Occup Ther, 66*(1), 15–23.

8. Centers for Disease Control and Prevention. (2007). *2007 National Health Interview Survey. United States Government.* Available at http://www.cdc.gov/nchs/nhis/nhis_2007_data_release.htm.

9. Charles, J., & Gordon, A. M. (2005). A critical review of constraint-induced movement therapy and forced use in children with hemiplegia. *Neural Plast, 12*, 245–261.

10. Cope, S. M., et al. (2008). Modified constraint-induced movement therapy for a 12-month-old child with hemiplegia: a case report. *Am J Occup Ther, 62*, 430–437.

11. Coster, W. J., Deeney, T., Haltiwanger, J., et al. (1998). *School function assessment.* San Antonio, TX: PsychCorp.

12. Deluca, S. C., et al. (2006). Intensive pediatric constraint-induced therapy for children with cerebral palsy: randomized, controlled, crossover trial. *J Child Neurol, 21*, 931–938.

13. Eliasson, A. C., Bonnier, B., & Krumlinde-Sundholm, L. (2003). Clinical experience of constraint induced movement therapy in adolescents with hemiplegic cerebral palsy—a day camp model. *Dev Med Child Neurol, 45*, 357–360.

14. Fasoli, S. E., et al. (2008). Upper limb robotic therapy for children with hemiplegia. *Am J Phys Med Rehabil, 87*, 929–936.

15. Frascarelli, F., et al. (2009). The impact of robotoic rehabilitation in children with acquired or congenital movement disorders. *Eur J Phys Rehabil Med, 45*, 135–141.

16. Ghasia, F., et al. (2008). Frequency and severity of visual sensory and motor deficits in children with cerebral palsy: Gross Motor Function Classification Scale. *Investigat Ophthamol Visual Sci, 49*, 572–580.

17. Green, L., & Hurvitz, E. (2007). Cerebral palsy. *Phys Med Rehabil Clin North Am, 18*, 859–882.

18. Hemmingsson, H., Egilson, S., Hoffman, O., & Kielhofner, G. (2005). *The School Setting Interview (SSI) Version 3.0.* Chicago, IL: MOHO Clearinghouse, University of Illinois.

19. Henderson, A., & Pehoski, C. (2006). *Hand function in the child* (2nd ed.). St. Louis: Mosby.

20. Keller, J., tenVelden, M., Kafkes, A., Basu, S., Federico, J., & Kielhofner, G. (2005). *Child Occupational Self Assessment. Version 2.1.* Chicago, IL: MOHO Clearinghouse, University of Illinois.

21. Leet, A. I., et al. (2006). Fractures in children with cerebral palsy. *J Pediatr Orthop, 26*, 624–627.

22. Majnemer, A., Shikako-Thomas, K., Shevell, M., Poulin, C., Lach, L., Schmitz, N., et al. QUALA Group. (2013). Pursuit of complementary and alternative medicine treatments in adolescents with cerebral palsy. *J Child Neurol, 28*(11), 1443–1447.

23. McLellan, A., Cipparone, C., Giancola, D., Armstrong, D., & Bartlett, D. (2012). Medical and surgical procedures experienced by young children with cerebral palsy. *Pediatr Phys Ther, 24*, 268–277.

24. Merrill, D. R. (2009). Review of electrical stimulation in cerebral palsy and recommendations for future directions. *Develop Med Child Neurol, 51*(Suppl 4), 153–164.

25. National Institutes of Health National Center for Complementary and Alternative Medicine. *Backgrounder: CAM use and children.* Available at: http://nccam.nih.gov/health/children/#patterns.

26. Novak, I., McIntyre, S., Morgan, C., Campbell, L., Dark, L., Morton, N., et al. (2013). A systematic review of interventions for children with cerebral palsy: state of evidence. *Dev Med Child Neurol, 55*(10), 885–910.

27. Piper, M. C., & Darrah, J. (1994). *Alberta Infant Motor Scale.* Philadelphia: Saunders.

28. Pirila, S., et al. (2007). Language and motor speech skills in children with cerebral palsy. *J Commun Disord, 40*, 116–128, 207.

29. Ramey, S., Coker-Bolt, P., & DeLuca, S. (2013). *A handbook of pediatric constraint-induced movement therapy: a guide for occupational therapy and health care clinicians, researchers, and educators.* Bethesda, MD: American Occupational Therapy Association Press.

30. Reidy, T. G., Naber, E., Viguers, E., et al. (2012). Outcomes of a clinic-based pediatric constraint-induced movement therapy program. *Phys Occup Ther Pediatr, 32*(4), 355–367.

31. Russell, D., Rosenbaum, P., Gowland, C., Hardy, S., Lane, M., Plews, N., et al. (1993). *Gross motor function measure manual* (2nd ed.). Hamilton, Ontario, Canada: McMaster University.

32. Shumway-Cook, A., & Woollacott, M. (2001). *Motor control theory and practical applications* (2nd ed.). Baltimore, MD: Lippincott Williams & Wilkins.

33. Strauss, D., et al. (2007). Survival in cerebral palsy in the last 20 years: signs of improvement? *Develop Med Child Neurol, 49*, 86–92.

34. Taub, T., et al. (2012). Pediatric CI therapy for stroke-induced hemiparesis in young children. *Dev Neurorehabil, 10*, 3–18.

35. United Cerebral Palsy. Cerebral palsy prevalence. Available at: http://www.ucp.org/.

36. Wilton, J. (2003). Casting, splinting, and physical and occupational therapy of hand deformity and dysfunction in cerebral palsy. *Hand Clin, 19*, 573–584.

37. Wright, P., Durham, S., Ewins, D., & Swain, I. (2012). Neuromuscular electrical stimulation for children with cerebral palsy: a review. *Arch Dis Child, 97*, 364–371.

REVIEW *Questions*

1. List and describe the possible causes of cerebral palsy.
2. List and describe the types of CP based on the distribution of abnormal muscle tone.
3. List and describe the types of CP based on the affected body structures.
4. What is muscle tone? How is tone different than muscle strength?

5. How does abnormal muscle tone affect a child's participation in daily occupations?
6. List and describe the types of abnormal muscle tone found in CP.
7. List three types of traditional and nontraditional approaches to intervention when working with a child with CP.

SUGGESTED *Activities*

1. Visit a classroom in which children with CP are enrolled. Interact with the children and request permission to palpate specific muscles to feel the muscle tone and tension in the muscle.
2. Visit a summer camp for children with special needs. Plan a simple craft activity and provide hand-over-hand assistance to children who require help. Palpate the wrist and hand muscles while providing hand-over-hand assistance, noticing the stiffness.

3. Volunteer to assist in a camp that uses CIMT.
4. Palpate your biceps and triceps muscles at rest. Palpate your classmate's biceps and triceps at rest and while bending and straightening the elbow. Note the tension at rest and at work.

PATTY COKER-BOLT

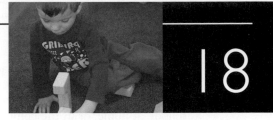

18

Positioning and Handling: A Neurodevelopmental Approach

CHAPTER *Objectives*

After studying this chapter, the reader will be able to accomplish the following:

- Understand the importance of proper positioning to enhance a child's ability to participate in daily activities.
- Describe the variety of positions and transitional movements children use in typical development over the first year of life.
- Describe the characteristics of developmental positions prone, supine, side-lying, sitting, quadruped, and standing.
- Identify positioning and handling techniques occupational therapy practitioners use during treatment of children and adolescents with developmental delays.
- Explain the key concepts and principles of neurodevelopmental treatment.
- Understand the application of therapeutic positioning and handling principles and techniques exemplified through case examples.

CHAPTER *Outline*

Occupational therapy (OT) practitioners consider how proper positioning contributes to a child's ability to successfully engage in activities at school, at home, or in the community. Positioning refers to children's ability to maintain postural control while participating in daily activities. For example, a therapist may help a child sit in an adapted chair that provides additional support at the trunk so that he or she can write more efficiently and effectively in school. Therapeutic handling refers to dynamic techniques used to guide the movements of children or adolescents. Handling techniques may be used to influence the state of muscle tone, promote **postural stability**, or trigger new automatic movement responses for function. The OT practitioner uses therapeutic handling to feel the child's response to changes in **posture** and movement and facilitate postural control and movement in the context of functional tasks. For example, the OT practitioner may gently support a child's shoulder so that the child is able to reach for toys in front of him or her. This chapter begins by providing readers with a description of the variety of positions seen during typical motor development in the first year of life. These positions include the characteristics of positions and examples of equipment that help children engage in their daily occupations in specific positions. An overview of neurodevelopmental treatment (NDT) theory and case study examples illustrate the principles and application of therapeutic **positioning** and **handling** techniques.

TYPICAL MOTOR DEVELOPMENT

CASE *Study*

Two-year-old John loves to play with trucks in his grandmother's hallway. He lies on the floor on his belly, rolls the cars down the hall, jumps up to catch them, and runs down the hallway. Once on the other side, John kneels on one knee (half-kneels) and collects all his trucks. He then sits down, places them all in a line again, and moves on his belly, gently pushing the trucks forward one at a time.

This play scenario illustrates the many different positions that typically developing children assume during play. In this short play activity, John assumed the prone, sitting, half-kneeling, and standing positions. He also ran down the hall. A hallmark of typical development is that children move in and out of a variety of positions with ease. Movements in and out of different positions are called **transitional movements**. For example, John transitioned from the supine position to a standing position to run down the hallway. He then moved from standing to sitting on the floor to prone on his stomach. Typically

developing children assume a variety of positions as they engage in activities of daily living (ADLs), such as feeding, hygiene, bathing, and dressing; instrumental ADLs (IADLs), education, rest and sleep, and play and leisure.

Neonates are born with **physiologic flexion** because of their position in utero. Physiologic flexion passively stretches the extensor muscles of the trunk particularly during the last trimester of pregnancy. Elongation of the neck and trunk extensors prepares the infants for active movement against gravity shortly following birth. The first voluntary movement observed in typically developing infants is neck extension while the infant is in the prone position. As the infant lifts or extends his or her head in the prone position the cervical flexors are then stretched or elongated, which prepares these muscle to become active. Head control is achieved as the infant gains strength and coactivation of the cervical flexors and extensors allowing him or her to support the head at midline.

The infant first accidentally rolls from the prone position to the supine position when the cervical-thoracic extension causes the infant's weight to be shifted too far to the left or right. When this occurs, the infant's whole body will accidentally roll like a log (no segmentation) from the prone position to the supine position. As the infant gains proximal stability in the arms, he or she can assume the prone-on-elbows position. As the infant places and shifts weight onto the shoulders in the prone-on-elbows position, the upper thoracic flexors are elongated. The infant gains proximal shoulder stability and upper body trunk control as the upper thoracic flexors and extensors coactivate and co-contract. This strengthening of neck, shoulder, trunk, pelvis, and leg flexors and extensors will continue as the infant continues to move and play in the environment allowing for more mature postures such as upright sitting, standing, and walking.

In the case of typically developing children, assuming and maintaining a variety of positions leads to the development of more mature movement and overall motor control. Children naturally gain improved motor planning and coordination as they develop postural control in each new developmental position. Practicing new movements in new positions strengthens the large and small muscles and allows for the processing of new sensory input, which drives refinement of new motor actions. Children with special needs, such as those with cerebral palsy (CP), often require interventions to help them develop the postural and muscle control required for skilled functional movements. Positioning and handling techniques are frequently used in OT interventions to help children with abnormal muscle tone receive appropriate sensory input and develop typical movement patterns needed to function in everyday activities.

GENERAL CONSIDERATIONS

The progression of motor development and development of more controlled movement is necessary for engagement in daily activities. The following section describes aspects of motor control and development that OT practitioners consider when using positioning and handling techniques to help children engage in occupations.

Skeletal Alignment

One of the first principles of positioning is to assure that children have the capacity to align head, trunk, and pelvis with extremities approaching midline. The ability to maintain proper body alignment is important for developing postural stability and allows children to participate in daily occupations.[11] When the skeletal system is aligned and children are positioned symmetrically, each side of the body develops adequate muscle strength needed for postural stability. Symmetric alignment helps children maintain the full range of motion (ROM) for movement. Symmetric positioning, with head, neck, trunk, and pelvis aligned, allows children to move their arms and legs efficiently, bring the hands to midline to play with objects, couple the visual system with hand use, and engage the upper and lower body together.[11] Positioning children in symmetric postures with proper alignment of the head, trunk, pelvis and extremities provides physical comfort, reduces fatigue, and promotes postural stability to increase engagement in daily occupations such as feeding, dressing, playing and education. Thus OT practitioners may use positioning devices to support children in good alignment with symmetric positions. Often, providing external support helps children maintain a position to perform daily occupations (Figure 18-1).

Typical Development

A useful guide to help OT practitioners working with children with movement disorders is consideration of the normal progression of typical posture and movement and how it allows children to interact with their environment. OT practitioners provide a variety of therapeutic positions that allow children to experience a full range of life experiences. For example, infants between 7 and 10 months begin to explore their surroundings by creeping and crawling. Therefore a practitioner working with an infant who has difficulty moving, may provide positioning and movement opportunities which promote the prone-on-extended-arms position and support the infant's efforts to crawl. Similarly, infants between 7 and 10 months enjoy sitting and playing with toys, coupling hands and arms together. The OT practitioner may consider special equipment to provide external trunk support to allow the infant to maintain the upright position to use hands to successfully engage in ADLs, IADLs, education, and play activities.

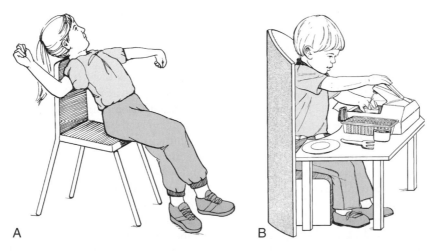

A   B

FIGURE 18-1   **A,** A child in asymmetric position and showing abnormal posture has difficulty reaching for toys. **B,** Using external supports from a chair allows a child to sit in a symmetric position to reach for toys. (From Case-Smith, J., & O'Brien, J. (Eds.). (2009). *Occupational therapy for children.* (6th ed.). St. Louis: Mosby.)

Perception and Body Awareness

Not only does assuming and maintaining various positions promote motor development, the engagement in motor activities also stimulates perceptual development and **body awareness**. For example, moving from the sitting to the standing position provides children with a different viewpoint, engages the vestibular system, and enhances their perception of the surroundings. Each new position provides different opportunities and experiences that help children understand how to move their bodies and to fully engage in their environment. Children develop perception and body awareness as they move into and out of different developmental positions, allowing a new view of their surroundings and environment from different angles.[11] For example, infants' early feeding experiences occur while they are in the reclining position held by parent, whereas toddlers feed in the upright sitting position in a high chair or at a table.

Changing positions and moving into and out of positions stimulates different sensory experiences. For example, weight bearing on hands provides infants with tactile sensations and experiences that are important for later hand development. Children develop body awareness as they experience proprioceptive feedback from their muscles and joints allowing them to learn to understand where their bodies are in space. As children develop the ability to sit upright, they see things at different angles; they feel different sensations; and they develop a sense of balance, which helps promote postural stability for mobility and functional activity (Figure 18-2).

Postural Control for Balance and Functional Activity

Maintaining positions requires postural control, which refers to the ability to sustain the necessary trunk control to use the arms, hands, and legs and efficiently carry out skilled tasks, such as playing, coloring, or feeding. See Box 18-1 for a description of the relationship between stability and mobility. Along with adequate muscle tone and skeletal alignment, children need a sense of balance, or equilibrium, to maintain postural control.[11] The center of gravity is the point where the total body weight is most evenly distributed over the base of support. The center of gravity is also referred to as the center of mass when it relates to the child's center of distribution. Children must first sense changes in the center of mass before they are able to respond to these changes. Children respond to changes in balance through righting and **equilibrium reactions**. **Righting reactions** support midline postures and are those reactions that bring the head back in alignment with the body. For example, righting reactions are present as an infant moves his or her head upright and vertical when tilted to the side (righting the head on the neck). Another example of righting reactions is

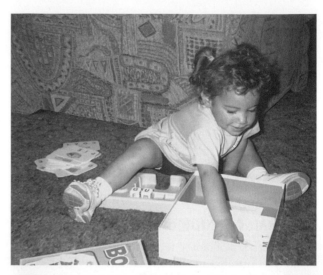

FIGURE 18-2 Child sits upright and plays. She is able to move to reach for objects. (From Parham, L. D. (2007). *Play in occupational therapy for children* (2nd ed.). St. Louis: Mosby.)

BOX 18-1

Stability and Mobility

The ability to control movements occurs within the framework of stability and mobility. Stability is defined as the ability to maintain or stabilize a posture. Mobility is defined as the ability to move into or assume a posture. Infants are born with the ability to move, and mobility will be present before stability. Infants must gain strength and co-contraction between opposing muscle groups (e.g., trunk flexors and trunk extensors) in order to stabilize postures. Once a stable posture is established, an infant can learn to control movements within that position or posture.

---

when the head, trunk, and pelvis rotate on an axis, as seen in rolling to maintain alignment of the body segments (head, trunk, pelvis). This is observed as infants turn their bodies in alignment to roll toward a toy. The infant develops head righting reactions in the first few months of life in response to visual and vestibular sensory input. Equilibrium reactions help one maintain body alignment and balance when the body's center of mass is shifted too far over the base of support. Equilibrium reactions may require the use of the head, trunk, arms, and legs to flex or abduct in order to adjust the body's center of mass over the base of support to prevent a fall. The maturation of equilibrium reactions occurs in an orderly sequence—prone, supine, sitting, quadruped, and standing—as the infant gains antigravity muscle strength and postural control (Figure 18-3). Equilibrium reactions may also involve subtle changes in muscle tone to maintain position. For example, equilibrium reactions can be

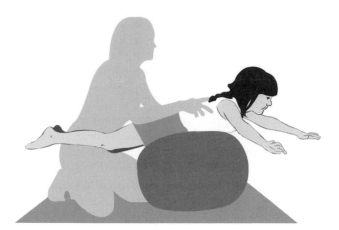

FIGURE 18-3   Playing on an exercise ball can help elicit equilibrium reactions in children.

TABLE 18-1

Postural Reactions

BALANCE REACTIONS	AGE (mo)
RIGHTING REACTIONS	
Neck on body	
Immature	Birth
Mature	4–5
Body on body	
Immature	Birth
Mature	4–5
Body on head	
Prone (partial)	1–2
Mature	4–5
Supine	5–6
Landau	
Immature	3
Mature	6–10
Flexion	
Partial (head in line)	3–4
Mature (head forward)	6–7
Vertical	
Partial (head in line)	2
Mature (head to vertical)	6
PROTECTIVE REACTIONS	
Forward	6–7
Lateral	6–11
Backward	9–12
EQUILIBRIUM REACTIONS	
Prone	5–6
Supine	7–8
Sitting	7–10
Quadruped	9–12
Standing	12–21

Case-Smith, J., & O'Brien, J. (Eds.). (2009). *Occupational therapy for children.* (6th ed.). St. Louis, MO: Mosby.

observed as a child maintains balance when standing on one foot. This involves subtle adjustments in muscle tone to maintain the upright position. **Protective extension** reactions occur when the body's center of mass is shifted too far off the base of support and righting and equilibrium reactions cannot bring the body back to midline. A protective response involves extending an arm or a leg forward to protect oneself when the change in balance is so extreme that a child is unable to correct his or her position to avoid falling. Protective extension can be observed as a child quickly places a hand on the floor to catch him or herself when a change of balance occurs suddenly. (Table 18-1 describes the development of postural reactions.)

All movement requires an initial **weight shift**. The term *weight shift* refers to a change in the center of mass that allows one to move a body part. During a lateral weight shift in the sitting or standing position, the side that accepts the weight will respond with trunk elongation, and the side that is unweighted will respond with trunk shortening. This allows the person to maintain an upright position with the head remaining in proper alignment with the body and avoid falling into gravity during shifts of the body's center of mass. Children may also initiate cephalo-caudal (head to tail) or caudal-cephalo (tail to head) weight shifts. For example, a cephalo-caudal weight shift is required when initiating movement from the supine position to the prone position. Anterior–posterior weight shifts may involve tilting the pelvis forward or backward.

POSITIONING AS A THERAPUETIC TOOL

OT practitioners consider how to position children so that they can actively engage in daily occupations, such as feeding, dressing, bathing, or play. Positioning children in the upright sitting position may promote socialization, independence in feeding, and successful engagement in academics and play. Some children may require external postural support to assume and maintain upright positions. OT practitioners use the principles of positioning to evaluate postures and offer solutions to help children engage in age-appropriate occupations.

The principles of positioning children include the following:

• Provide the child with a variety of positioning options throughout the day.
• Consider positions that enhance function in specific activities.

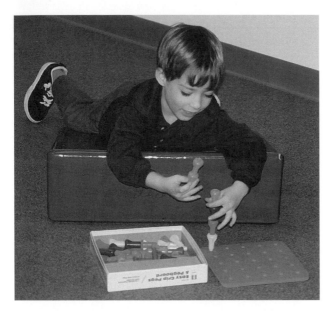

FIGURE 18-4 Child in prone position over a wedge. Note the axillary position, wedge height, and amount of neck extension.

- Avoid positions that restrict the child's ability to move purposefully.
- Provide positions that are comfortable for the child.
- Consider safety when determining optimal positions (e.g., do not leave a child unattended in a positioning device).
- Ensure proper skeletal alignment and body **symmetry** during positioning of the child.
- Recommend positioning equipment that provides external trunk stability to facilitate movement.

As previously stated, generally, children develop movement against gravity in the following sequence of positions: prone, supine, prone-on-elbows, prone-on-extended-elbows/arms, side-lying, sitting, quadruped, half kneel, kneel, standing.[2,7] The following sections describe the development of positions and provide examples of equipment that may be used to help children assume and maintain these positions.

Prone Position

The prone position, in which a child is positioned on his or her tummy, facilitates neck and trunk extension and thus helps the child build muscle strength and stability in the neck, upper back, shoulders, arms, and hands. Once a child develops strength, he or she is able to better stabilize and control upper arm muscle control. Prone position leads to higher-level motor skills such as prone-on-elbows, prone-on-extended-elbows, and quadruped positions.

Placing a firm foam wedge under an infant's upper body, with the edge of the wedge just below the axillary area, encourages the prone-on-elbows or prone-on-extended-elbows position, depending on the height of the wedge. A practitioner can determine the correct degree of incline according to the infant's ability to independently hold his or her head up during the selected activity. Neck extension below a 45-degree angle is recommended, as this prevents the head movement from triggering hyperextension throughout the body. A pillow or towel can be placed between the knees to separate them if necessary (Figure 18-4). A practitioner can use his or her own arms or legs to promote prone positions while working with infants and toddlers. Therapeutic play over a bolster or while on a Swiss (exercise) ball can be used to promote weight bearing and weight shifting in the prone position.

CLINICAL *Pearl*

The prone position is good for elongating and stretching the hip flexors. Place the small child or infant prone across your lap or prone on a play mat and encourage gradual head lifting, hip extension, and lowering of the pelvis to the mat. Make sure that the wedges and rolls are not so high that they cause excessive extensor tone or so low that those with very low muscle tone or strength cannot lift their heads.

Supine Position

Infants develop physiologic flexion in utero and have slightly increased flexor muscle tone when born. Within the first months of life, as cervical and back extension is strengthened during positioning in prone, a reduction of physiologic flexion will be noted. The cervical flexors become elongated during infant play in prone, gaining strength to move against gravity. Once the cervical extensors and flexors have equal strength and are balanced, an infant will demonstrate head control and the ability to keep head in alignment at midline. The supine position, in which an infant is positioned on the back, helps the infant further develop neck and abdominal muscle control. The increased neck strength and subsequent head control allows for an infant to bring the head, hands, and feet to midline. In the supine position, the infant engages in play that encourages downward visual gaze and active head turning. During play activities to maintain head at midline, the infant uses balanced neck flexor and extensor control to couple head and hand movements during play (Figure 18-5). This co-contraction of neck flexors and extensors will provide the stability needed to maintain the head at midline in the supine, prone, sitting, and standing positions.

Infants are frequently held in the supine position when swaddled in a blanket or positioned in a car seat

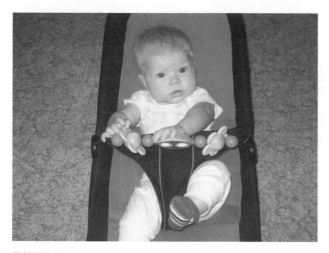

FIGURE 18-5   The supine position requires some neck and leg flexion and helps children develop the abdominal muscles.

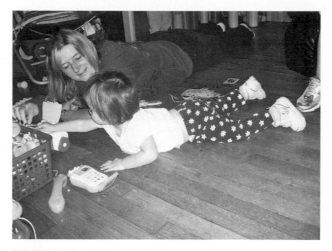

FIGURE 18-6   Children begin to bear weight on elbows before moving to the prone-to-extended-arms position. This position encourages exploration and hand development.

or infant seat. Some seats cradle the infant in the supine position (e.g., in a car seat), whereas other seats (e.g., strollers) require maintaining the supine position. The infant may be positioned on a flat or inclined surface using wedges, pillows, rolls/bolsters, or towels to provide support. OT practitioners promote positioning infants in the supine position with the head at midline and flexed slightly forward for optimal visual exploration of the environment. Rolled towels under the infant's knees encourage hip flexion and are therefore recommended for premature infants (who may have less or diminished physiologic flexion).

CLINICAL *Pearl*

When working with an infant or child who is in the supine position, support the child's head in midline with chin slightly tucked and flexed-forward. An OT practitioner can flex a child's knees and hips to maximize midline and flexed postures and minimize the effects of abnormal extensor tone.

Prone-on-Elbows and Prone-on-Extended-Arms Position

In a prone-on-elbows and prone-on-extended arms position, the infant begins to stretch out the tightness in the hip flexors and develop head control in the prone position. In these positions, the infant begins to shift the center of gravity posteriorly to the pelvis, which allows for greater ranges of head lifting of the head and weight bearing on elbows. As the infant develops improved head and trunk control while maintaining the prone-on-elbows position, he or she is able to complete a greater

posterior weigh shift toward the pelvis and assume the prone-on-extended-arms position. Once in the prone-on-extended-arms position, the infant receives proprioceptive and tactile input to the palms of the hands, important for future development of the arches of the hands. Playing in these positions further encourages weight shifting to right and left to allow the infant to reach with one hand toward objects (Figure 18-6). As with the basic prone position, wedges, rolls, and towels propped under the children's trunk support the prone-on-elbows and prone-on-extended-arms positions and encourage active head lifting and upper extremity weight bearing.

Side-Lying Position

The side-lying position is a natural and comfortable position for children, especially during sleep or playing on a mat. Children who have motor and sensory control issues may require external support to maintain alignment in the side-lying position. A balanced coactivation of the head and trunk flexors and extensors is necessary to maintain this position. The side-lying position encourages children to maintain their head at midline; this promotes hands being placed in the line of vision and toward the midline of the body, which is important for gaining an understanding of the overall body scheme and the relationship of body parts to their functions. Body scheme awareness promotes successful engagement in functional activities, such as bringing the hands to the mouth or manipulating a toy bilaterally (Figure 18-7). Commercially made side lyers (e.g., Tumble forms) are available. Bolsters, wedges, pillows, rolled towels, and benches help children assume the side-lying position.

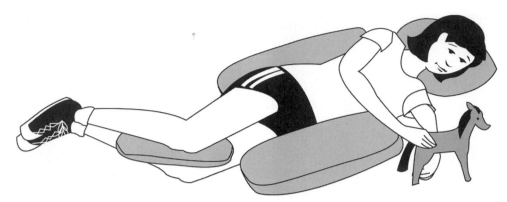

FIGURE 18-7   The side-lying position encourages the child to bring the hands together to play with a toy.

CLINICAL *Pearl*

When placing a child in the side-lying position, remember the following points:

- Alternate side lying to right and left sides.
- Use small towel/blanket rolls or pillows to help the child maintain the side-lying position.
- Provide adequate padded surfaces for shoulders and hips to prevent pressure sores and diminished circulation. Consider placement of towel in between legs to discourage strong lower extremity hip adduction.
- During play and social interaction, make sure that toys and people are presented below the child's eye level to encourage a chin tuck or neck flexion and discourage abnormal patterns of neck extension.

BOX 18-2

Basic Sitting Position

OT practitioners help develop sitting options for children using the following guidelines:

- Hips and knees are flexed to 90 degrees.
- Back rests against chair back.
- The trunk is vertical.
- The body is symmetric.
- The head is aligned with the trunk, at midline, and flexed slightly forward.
- All three back curves (cervical [neck], thoracic [middle], and lumbar [lower]) are present and in good alignment. A small rolled-up towel or a lumbar roll can be used to help maintain the normal curves in the back.
- Both feet are positioned flat on the floor or supported on a raised surface in neutral.
- The tabletop or lapboard is positioned at elbow height. Elbows are flexed at 90 degrees position on armrests, if available.

From Crepeau, E., Cohn, E., & Boyt-Schell, B. (2009). *Willard and Spackman's occupational therapy* (11th ed.). Philadelphia: Lippincott Williams & Wilkins.

Sitting Position

Children must develop sufficient balance between neck and trunk flexors and extensors to be able to sit upright independently. Typically developing children begin to assume the unsupported sitting position around 6 to 7 months of age.[2,7] The sitting position requires the child to maintain postural control of the head, trunk, and extremities against the pull of gravity and requires coactivation of the trunk flexors and extensors. Once children assume a stable sitting posture without having to brace upright using the arms, they can manage weight shifts and move the center of gravity over the base to reach, retrieve, and manipulate objects. This helps refine righting and equilibrium responses. The sitting position provides valuable visual and kinesthetic experiences that advance children's perceptual and cognitive development as well. Many occupations such as feeding, toileting, schoolwork, and play are performed in the sitting position. Therapists frequently evaluate children's sitting posture and provide interventions to facilitate the correct alignment in upright sitting to encourage children participate in chosen occupations (Box 18-2).

Children assume a variety of sitting positions, including long sitting (lower extremity adduction with knee extension), ring sitting (lower extremity abducted, knees flexed to form a circle), tailor sitting (lower extremities abducted and knees flexed and crossed), and side sitting (one lower extremity adducted, one abducted with knees flexed) positions (Figure 18-8). Ring- and tailor-sitting positions offer more stability to children who have weaker trunk muscle tone or poor postural control. The long-sitting position may be difficult for children who have abnormal muscle tone or tightness in the hamstring muscles in the lower extremity. Side sitting requires greater strength and activity from the trunk muscles due to the asymmetric positioning of the lower extremity and weight shift toward

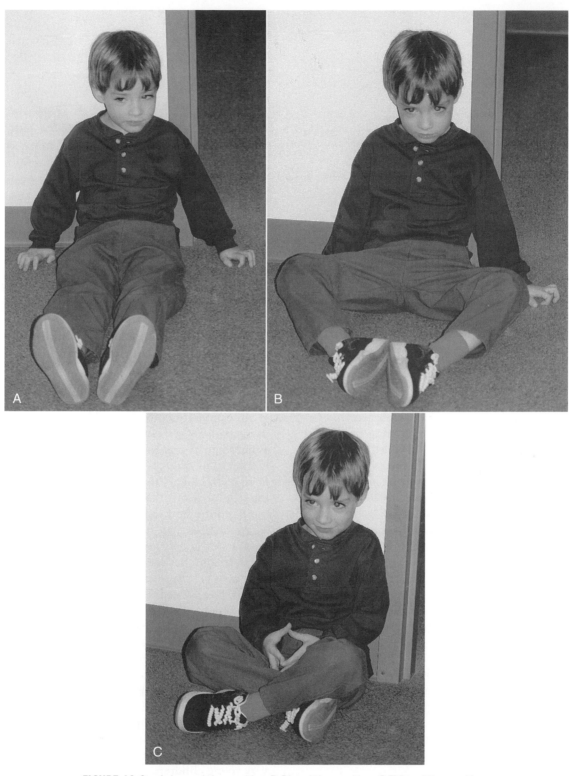

FIGURE 18-8   **A**, Long-sitting position. **B**, Ring-sitting position. **C**, Tailor-sitting position.

one side of the body. W sitting or sitting with the both lower extremities adducted with knees flexed inward such that the legs form a "W" is a stable position that is developmentally appropriate at 10 to 12 months of age, but it is not recommended for children older than 1 year, as it may lead to hip dislocation and continued lower extremity tightness misalignment in the hip and leg muscles (Box 18-3).

Many adapted seats facilitate developmentally appropriate sitting positions and promote participation

BOX 18-3

Sitting Positions

Children with poor trunk stability may favor a W-sitting position because the lower extremities are positioned to provide a wide base of support. W sitting does not require trunk strength or stability and thus makes it easier for children to manipulate objects and play on the floor. However, W sitting may lead to orthopedic problems, including increased risk for hip dislocation, joint deformities, and the aggravation of muscle tightness. W sitting does not allow for rotation, weight shifting, or the opportunity to cross midline. Therefore OT practitioners discourage W sitting by promoting other sitting positions that engage children's postural system and encourage the use of trunk muscles. Alternatives to W sitting include tailor sitting, long sitting, side sitting, or sitting on the OT practitioner's lap, on a bench, or on a ball.

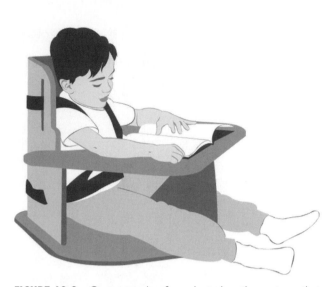

FIGURE 18-9 One example of an adapted seating systems that help inhibit spasticity and compensate for limited postural control.

in activities such as feeding, dressing, playing, and academics. Corner chairs promote scapula protraction (shoulders and arms forward), humeral internal rotation, and trunk stability by providing lateral supports in the seated position (Figure 18-9). Consequently, this type of chair encourages children to bring their hands to the midline within their visual field, which promotes the holding and manipulation of objects (e.g., books, toys, feeding utensils). Many corner chairs have trays that further promote the use of hands in the sitting position. These trays may be positioned in such a way to help children bear weight through the elbows to facilitate hand movements if necessary. Some corner seats provide the option to sit directly on the floor or elevated for to facilitate play at a table. For example, during story time at school, raised corner seats allow for knee flexion in addition to hip flexion in the seated position (e.g., allowing children to sit at table height with peers in the classroom).

Bolster chairs are frequently used for children who demonstrate increased lower extremity muscle tone in the hip adductors and internal rotators. The use of a bolster in between the lower extremities can promote hip abduction and external rotation as children straddle the bolster in the seated position. This allows children to maintain better stability to use their hands for play, academics, or other essential ADLs.

Wheelchairs

Wheelchairs provide the means for children with mobility issues and to actively explore their environment. The OT practitioner, family, and team decide whether a child needs an electric wheelchair or a

standard wheelchair on the basis of many factors. The team makes decisions concerning specialized features of the wheelchair including the type of frame, push handles, rear wheels, front casters, arm rests, leg rests, and wheel locks (Figure 18-10). The appearance of the chair is important to the child, so he or she should participate in selecting the style, fabric, and color. Wheelchairs come in ultralight, light, and heavy-duty weights. The type of seat selected is important for the fit of the chair. Although some children are able to use a solid seat, others may require customized seating cushions, and some may need to use a sling seat. The rear tires may be solid or filled with air (pneumatic). Air-filled tires are easier to push over sandy or rough terrain, but they are not as durable as solid tires. Arm rests can be fixed or removable, full length, desk length, or elevated. Removable armrests make it easier to transfer the child in and out of the wheelchair; full-length armrests provide more stable support for mounting trays or other devices. It is important for the wheelchair to fit the child correctly. The therapist with specialized training in seating and mobility typically conducts the wheelchair evaluation. Some lending programs may allow the use of a temporary wheelchair while waiting for the permanent chair to arrive. OT practitioners may help parents and other caregivers adapt strollers to use as temporary mobility devices for very young children.

MOBILITY

OT practitioners consider the ability of a child to move around his or her environment to learn more about their world. For example, infants roll and crawl to investigate their environments; this provides them with new

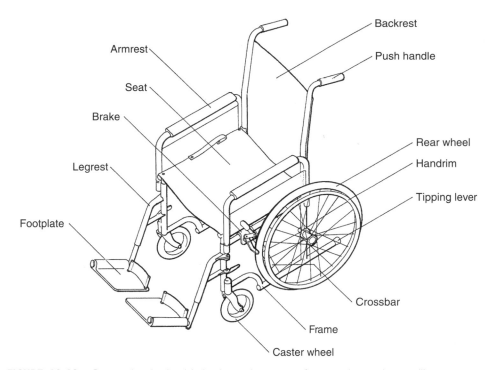

FIGURE 18-10 Conventional wheelchair: the major parts of supporting and propelling structures. (From Ragnarsson, R. T. (1990). Prescription considerations and comparison of conventional and lightweight wheelchairs. *Rehab Res Dev, 2*(Suppl) 8.)

opportunities and experiences to learn and relate to others. OT practitioners may suggest strollers, scooters, adapted tricycles, or other equipment to encourage movements in children (Figure 18-11).

CLINICAL *Pearl*

Some OT practitioners have advanced training in wheelchair seating and mobility. This specialty training offers expertise at sizing and ordering specialized wheelchairs and seating equipment for young children or adolescents. This specialized training may help a practitioner determine the necessary modifications for a child to use a wheelchair at home or in school. For example, a large powered wheelchair cannot be carried up the stairs at a house. Although the chair may fit the child adequately, the parents may require help bringing a specialized power wheelchair into their house or apartment. It may be necessary to build a ramp or to recommend a different type of chair, depending on the child's environment.

Quadruped Position

Once children have sufficient head and trunk control as well as stability at the shoulder and pelvic girdles, they can shift weight from side to side in the prone-on-extended-arms position and will often try to assume the quadruped position to begin to move in their environment. The quadruped position allows children to reach for objects and attempt to move toward motivating toys. OT practitioners frequently work with children on the stabilization and strengthening of the trunk, shoulders, and hips and on equilibrium responses by encouraging children to shift weight while playing in the quadruped position. After learning to assume the quadruped position, children begin to shift weight, often by lifting a hand off the floor to reach for a toy. Initially, this weight shift is brief and may result in a fall. However, after some time and repeated attempts, children are able to reach forward and grasp a toy without falling. Often this allows children to discover that repeating this movement provides momentum, allowing greater freedom to move to rotate in this position. Children enjoy the new movements gained in quadruped as they increase his or her ability to move successfully toward interesting objects. It is through repeated practice that quadruped position quickly becomes a precursor to creeping (forward movement on belly) and crawling (forward movement on hands and knees). This forward movement in quadruped involves dissociation of the hip and shoulder muscles as well as dissociation of movements on the right side of the body from those on the left side. For example, the right hip flexes while the right shoulder extends; meanwhile, the left shoulder flexes while the left hip extends. Rolls, bolsters, and scooter boards can be used to facilitate quadruped position (Figure 18-12).

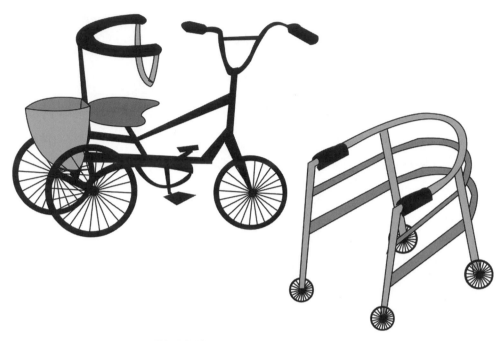

FIGURE 18-11 Types of mobility devices.

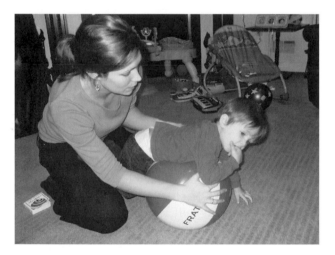

FIGURE 18-12 OT practitioners can use an exercise ball to facilitate the quadruped position.

Half-Kneel/Kneel Position

Children typically assume the half-kneeling or the tall-kneeling position before they attempt to stand. Tall kneeling is an easier position to maintain than half kneeling because it provides a more secure base of support with both lower legs in contact with the support surface. The tall-kneeling position requires less work from the trunk to maintain postural control and equilibrium during weight shifts while playing in this position. Children must develop stronger trunk stability and more mature equilibrium reactions in sitting and tall-kneeling positions before they are able to maintain a half-kneeling position. Gradually, as children gain more motor and balance control, they move from tall kneeling to half kneeling to standing without difficulty.

Because knees are vulnerable to injury, the tall- and half-kneeling positions are typically used during transitions to and from sitting to standing during play activities. OT practitioners help children assume half-kneeling and kneeling positions to do such things as reaching for objects at different surfaces (i.e., low to the ground or at small table). Frequently practitioners help children use external supports to transition (e.g., propping on a wall or perhaps a small table on which they can lean).

Standing Position

The standing position involves full weight bearing through the hips and lower extremities and promotes bone growth, muscle development, and blood circulation. Standing is typically a prerequisite skill for walking and higher-level mobility. Once children gain internal stability in the standing position, they are able to use both hands for play. Children who need positioning assistance to stand may benefit from supine and prone standers. Standers support the body from either the back (supine stander) or the front surface (prone stander) and can be secured in a vertically tilted position. A stander can be reclined if necessary for children who require additional trunk support (i.e., children who are unable to maintain the reclining position on their own). Children with increased trunk muscle extensor tone may benefit from having the stander tilted slightly forward to decrease the muscle tone so that they can maintain the head at

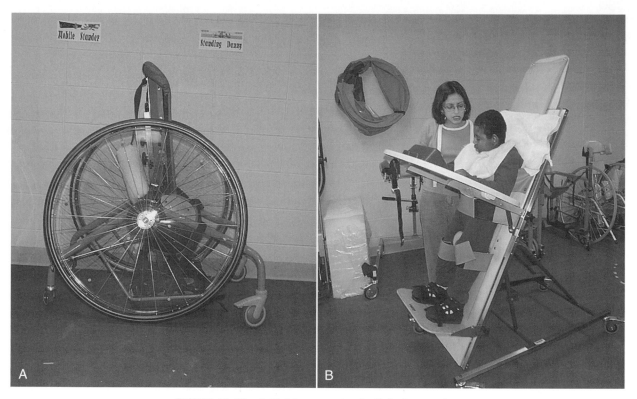

FIGURE 18-13 **A**, Mobile prone stander. **B**, Supine stander.

midline. Freedom standers, standing boxes, and parapodiums provide external support to children who have limited trunk control and stability. These positioning devices allow children to stand upright and use their arms and hands to play, feed, write, or read (Figure 18-13).

> **CLINICAL** *Pearl*
>
> To increase a child's ability to play while positioned in a stander, attach a tray to the front of the stander that allows a child's arms and hands to be placed in front at midline, giving the child the opportunity to explore objects. Positioning two or more children using supine standers close to each other allows for participation in a group activity or game.

THERAPEUTIC POSITIONING

The goal of therapeutic positioning is to provide the necessary support to promote a child's active engagement in occupations, not as a way to improve motor control or strength. Therefore therapeutic positioning provides the external support required to promote function in play, leisure, education, IADLs, and self-care tasks. The goal of therapeutic positioning is to provide children with safe, efficient, and effective postures that enable participation in social, academic, family, and self-care activities.

For example, OT practitioners may provide a corner seat to help a child sit upright during story time at school. When evaluating the usefulness of the seat, the therapist considers that the child will remain in the seat for 15 minutes (the length of story time). The OT practitioner provides a seat with adequate support and one that ensures the child's success. Thus the therapeutic value of the positioning equipment is that it allows the child to participate in story time with his or her peers. (Although the adaptive seat may improve the child's trunk strength and stability over time, the goal of the adaptive chair is to improve engagement in story time at school.)

CASE *Study*

Two-year-old Nathan has a diagnosis of spastic quadriplegic CP. He keeps both his hands fisted, forearms pronated, elbows flexed, and shoulders internally rotated. His hip and knees are flexed and internally rotated and his pelvis is posteriorly tilted keeping his trunk slightly flexed. His feet are plantar flexed and he is unable to sit unsupported, stand or walk. Nathan prefers to play lying prone and he is able to reach for objects with his right arm, but he is slow and inaccurate. After several unsuccessful attempts, he is able to pick up objects placed close to him (within arm's length). The OT goals for Nathan include improving his ability to sit and play with toys, increase skill with self-feeding, and helping him move more efficiently to explore his environment through play.

Nathan has difficulty sitting upright during mealtime; he collapses forward or totally extends back into his posture chair. His mother reports that she typically holds Nathan during mealtime due to these abnormal postures. The therapist provides an adapted insert (corner seat type) for the highchair that helps to position Nathan with his hips flexed forward (anterior tilt) and provides external rotation of his knees and hips and a footrest to stabilize his feet on the base of the chair. The lateral supports provide adequate trunk support.

The OT practitioner adds a pummel secured on the lap tray of the chair, which allows Nathan to hold and stabilize with his left hand, so he can use his right hand to hold the spoon or pick up food. In addition to changes in his positioning at mealtime, the OT practitioner provides Nathan with a small stepstool to sit on when undressing at bedtime. The stool is placed up against a corner of the room, which provides Nathan with external stability as he attempts to doff his socks and pants. The stool has armrests, which Nathan can use to stabilize his left hand and use his right hand more effectively. Sitting on the stool braced against the wall increases his success at dressing tasks as this supports his sitting posture; it also improves the position of his pelvis and reduces his atypical posturing. These positioning devices help Nathan engage in more independent feeding and dressing activities in his home.

OT practitioners use positioning and handling techniques to help children engage to their fullest extent in daily occupations. In addition, OT practitioners use handling techniques to promote improved motor control during the performance of daily tasks and activities. As such, handling involves continual evaluation of children's responses to the practitioner's input (i.e., cues and touching) as it relates to the desired motor movement. This is a dynamic process and therefore requires the practitioner to be aware of how he or she is influencing children's motor and emotional responses. The following section describes handling techniques as described within the framework of neurodevelopmental treatment (NDT). The authors begin with a definition of NDT emphasizing the principles of the theory and conclude with a description of handling techniques, including a case application.

NEURODEVELOPMENTAL TREATMENT
What Is NDT?

Karel and Berta Bobath developed NDT as a technique to help children with functional limitations. "NDT is a problem-solving approach to the examination and treatment of the impairments and functional limitations of individuals with neuropathology, primarily children with cerebral palsy."[3–5,8,9] The goal of NDT is to help children perform skilled movements more efficiently so they can

carry out life skills.[7,9] Therefore, practitioners using NDT must have an understanding of typical movements and how they change across a person's life span. Once practitioners understand typical movements, they can analyze how abnormal muscle tone and abnormal postures interfere with children's movements. OT practitioners can then facilitate normal postures so that children are able to "feel" typical movements. NDT theorists believe that moving in typical patterns improves neural pathways; this makes movements more automatic, which, in turn, helps children perform daily occupations.[9]

NDT Principles

The principles of NDT are based on the theory that movement can be refined through repetition and refinement of successful motor actions. Children can develop improved neural pathways to help them move efficiently and accurately through this repetition and practice.[6–8] OT practitioners use NDT intervention and skilled handling and gentle facilitation at key points of control to help children "feel" normal movement during functional activities. Proximal key points of control include the shoulders, hips, trunk, and pelvis, where the practitioner places his or her hands to guide the children through the movements. Distal key points of control include hands, feet, or head. Through handling and guidance, children are able to repeat and refine movement. New neural pathways may develop over time, resulting in more mature movement patterns and improved quality and accuracy of movements.[3–5,7]

Frequently OT practitioners begin NDT sessions by inhibiting abnormal muscle tone. Inhibitory techniques are used to reduce hypertonicity (increased muscle tone) in children. In the presence of hypotonicity, practitioners use facilitation techniques to increase muscle tone to a more normal level (Table 18-2). Once a child's muscle tone has reached a more normal state, the practitioner facilitates movement, typically through handling during play or goal-directed functional activities. The practitioner follows the child's lead during these activities and helps guide the child through the sequence of typical movement patterns needed to complete the task. The practitioner is careful to allow the child to actively perform as much of the movement as possible on his or her own and provides support only where necessary to allow the child to be successful in the activity.

The following is a summary of NDT principles that guide intervention:[4,7,10]

- The goal of NDT intervention is to improve overall function in daily tasks by increased active use of the trunk and involved extremities.
- Intervention should be individualized and focused on functional outcomes.
  - The OT practitioner may attempt to normalize muscle tone before and during functional movement.

TABLE 18-2

Indicators for Use of Inhibition and Facilitation Techniques

REQUIRED TECHNIQUE	CHILD INDICATORS	STRATEGIES
Inhibition	Hypertonicity Active primitive reflexes Excessive activity and motion Behavioral excitation Excessive sensitivity or reactivity to handling and touch	Sustained pressure to tendon Slow stroking of spine while child is in prone position Rotational movement (trunk and hip rotation) Slow rocking or rolling Heavy joint compression Sustained weight bearing Slow holding movements Wrapping, swaddling Calm music, warm colors, soft noises, dim lights, warm temperatures
Facilitation	Hypotonicity Inactive primitive reflexes, lack of balance reactions Excessive relaxation, semiconscious state Behavioral nonresponsiveness, flat affect Decreased reactivity to handling and touch	Light moving touch Tapping, sweep tapping, alternate tapping to activate contraction Fast vestibular input Heavy joint compression Active weight shifting Quick, variable movements Upbeat music, cool colors, louder noises, bright lights, cool temperatures

- The OT practitioner analyzes musculoskeletal limitations interfering with movement and function.
- The OT practitioner facilitates normal movement patterns, including both passive and active movements that are meaningful to children.
- Treatment emphasizes quality of movement (e.g., accuracy, quickness, adaptability, and fluency) and reproducibility of movement.
- Experience is a driving force for children. New activities build on previous sensorimotor experiences (typical and atypical).
- Target postural control and movement by using key points of control. Proximal points of control (e.g., hips, trunk, pelvis) provide more support to children, whereas distal points of control (e.g., head, hands, feet) require children to perform more of the movement.
- The OT practitioner engages children in "typical" movement and repetition using new movement patterns to develop new neural pathways.
- Children's motivation and active problem solving is considered when developing therapy goals and intervention activities.

Therapeutic Handling

Therapeutic handling is a dynamic process used to help children participate in their daily activities. The benefits of handling include assisting children with learning movements, allowing children to feel functional movements, and facilitating or inhibiting muscle tone that may interfere with movements.[3–5,7,8] Therapeutic handling allows the OT practitioner to feel children's responses to changes in postures and movements and to modify handling as necessary to assist children in successful motor responses (Figure 18-14). Therapeutic handling is used to facilitate normal postural control and movements so that children are able to engage in meaningful and age-appropriate activities.[6] Handling enables the OT practitioner to notice and feel changes in postures and/or movements. Consequently handling is used both in assessment and intervention.[8] OT practitioners following an NDT approach use facilitation and inhibition to correct children's incorrect patterns of movements or positions before they lead to secondary deformities and/or dysfunction.[6]

Children with CP or other neurologic disorders experience muscle tone abnormalities interfering with posture and movement. Abnormal muscle tone affects the children's ability to engage in play, self-care, academics, mobility, and communication. NDT theorists hypothesize that these children experience difficulty "feeling" or "sensing" typical movements and therefore are at risk for developing secondary deformities and/or dysfunctional movement.[1,10] Children with muscle tone abnormalities are frequently unable to correct for changes in posture. They do not feel the changes in movements or may experience a delay in sensing these changes. A delay in the reaction to changes or the absence of sensations, along with abnormal muscle tone, may cause frequent falls, inaccurate movements, or slow clumsy movements.

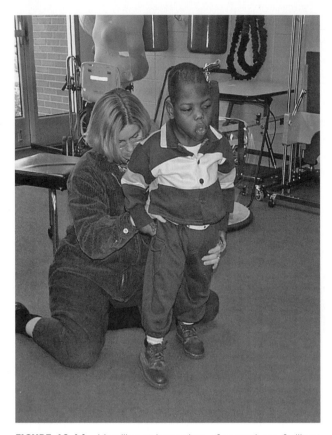

FIGURE 18-14 Handling at key points of control can facilitate movement.

OT practitioners following NDT theory use therapeutic handling at key points of control to help children feel the typical movements. Through practice and repetition of typical movements that occur in meaningful activities, children develop more accurate and efficient movements. They sense typical movements and understand intuitively how it feels to perform movements correctly. Current NDT theory also emphasizes targeting children's motivations and interests for activities during interventions.[7]

Handling Technique

The OT practitioner provides gentle cueing by placing his or her hands on the child at specific key points of control and in a certain manner. The OT practitioner uses hands to provide the child with a directional cue or assist in the weight shift (Figure 18-15). Handling may be used to stimulate a muscle group to contract or relax. The OT practitioner is careful to allow the child time to respond and to gently guide the child's weight shifts. The goal of handling is to improve the child's success and motor control through practice of the movement during the activity and within the actual context of the activity. As the child gains movement control, the practitioner lessens his or her handling or cueing. The goal of NDT is for the child to actively perform the movement.

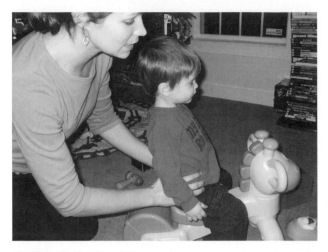

FIGURE 18-15 The OT practitioner uses gentle cueing techniques to facilitate the desired movement.

Practice Application Using NDT

- The OT practitioner evaluates the child's movements by carefully analyzing how the child moves in and out of positions, maintains positions, and responds to changes in the environment. The practitioner examines muscle tone, joint integrity, ROM, and postural control during movements. Furthermore, the practitioner explores the child's motivations for movements and his or her ability to initiate and terminate movements. The quality of movements is also considered.

- As a preparatory method before engaging the child in a therapeutic activity, the OT practitioner may use specific techniques to either inhibit or facilitate muscle tone, depending on the needs of the child. Next, the practitioner helps the child repeat normal patterns of movement while engaging in a functional task. This occurs as the OT practitioner facilitates movements at key points of control and guides the child's movements through therapeutic handling. Repetitive practice of typical movements helps the child develop new neural pathways and eventually the movements become automatic. The OT practitioner uses activities that are meaningful and motivating to the child and the treatment activities should be goal-directed. For example, a treatment session may involve play with siblings or typical peers, which is more reinforcing than solitary play.

- The OT practitioner places his or her hands on the child at either proximal or distal key points of control to help the child maintain postures during functional activities. The OT practitioner facilitates movements by providing the least amount of support needed for the child to be successful. The key to intervention is for the child to correctly perform as much of the movement as possible. The OT practitioner acts as a guide, working to engage the child in more normal movement patterns. OT practitioners are sensitive to the child's movements and are careful to limit extraneous sensory stimulation or cues.

- OT practitioners facilitate a weight shift by gentle cueing in the direction of the desired weight shift through handling. The OT practitioner places his or her hands gently on the child to guide functional movements. For example, when helping a child move from the sitting position to the quadruped position, the OT practitioner may decide to guide the child in completing lateral weight shifts by providing a directional cue to the lateral oblique muscles (flexors) of the trunk (see Figure 18-15).
- When examining a child's movement, the OT practitioner considers that all movements begin with a weight shift. Thus children must be able to initiate a lateral (to the side), cephalo-caudal, caudal-cephalo (head to toe, toe to head) or anterior–posterior weight shift. Children also use righting, equilibrium, and protective extension reactions during movements.

OT practitioners help children assume positions, maintain positions, and transition in and out of positions by facilitating the appropriate weight shift, muscle action (i.e., flexion, extension, rotation), and/or postural reactions (i.e., righting, equilibrium, protective extension). NDT intervention involves continual assessment of how children are moving during functional tasks. The OT practitioner adjusts his or her handling throughout the session according to the child's motor and sensory responses.

CASE *Study*

Applying NDT Interventions

Christina is a 2-year-old who has a diagnosis of right spastic hemiplegic CP. She presents with moderate hypertonicity throughout her right upper and lower extremities. Christina avoids using her right hand during play and holds her right arm in a flexed position; her hand is clenched, with her thumb inside her palm and her wrist flexed. She does not like to bear weight on her right and becomes irritable when touched on her right side. Christina pulls herself up to stand on her left side, leaving her right toe internally rotated and lightly touching the ground. During early therapy sessions, Christina would become upset when the OT practitioner attempted to facilitate a weight shift to the right. Christina loves stuffed animals, especially dogs, and she enjoys music; she will try to dance to all types of music. The OT practitioner at the early learning center observed Christina on the playground and during indoor play activities. Christina plays alongside one other girl, but does not like to be touched (especially on her right side). The OT practitioner decides to use an NDT approach to help Christina use both hands for play and move her body in and out of play positions with ease.

The long-term goals of Christina's occupational therapy are as follows:

- Christina will increase use of her right hand when playing with toys, as measured by her ability to hold a large ball in both hands in 80% of trials.

- Christina will successfully rotate her body to both right and left sides 80% of trials while reaching for a toy in an unsupported sitting position.

To address these goals, the OT practitioner designs an intervention session using a NDT approach and decides to motivate Christina by having her play with stuffed animals during the session. Using facilitatory and inhibitory techniques, the OT practitioner decreases the spasticity in her right upper and lower extremities by gently and playfully stretching them. Next, the OT practitioner facilitates weight bearing to the right, by placing her hands on Christina's hips (as a **key point of control**) and asking Christina to reach for the stuffed animal. Christina begins to get tearful as she senses this weight shift. The OT practitioner quickly praises Christina's efforts and asks her to try to get to the stuffed animal from the other side. Meanwhile the OT practitioner helps Christina open her right hand, by pressing it into her own hand to normalize tone. Christina is able to bear weight leaning on the OT practitioner, and the OT practitioner is able to modify the stretch. As Christina shows signs of fatigue, the OT practitioner changes her position and allows Christina to move to the prone-on-elbows position. In this position, Christina must also bear weight on the right side. The OT practitioner continues to facilitate an open hand posture, by bringing in more stuffed animals. They end the session with a musical game in which Christina stands (supported at the hips) and shows off her latest dance move! The OT practitioner encourages Christina's mother to follow through with these play activities at home.

Current State of Evidence for Using an NDT Approach

NDT intervention is an individual approach to examining and improving movements during the performance of meaningful and functional daily activities, but there continues to be a need for more rigorous clinical studies in order to demonstrate support for wide use in today clinics. A recent systematic review of interventions for children with CP concluded that interventions focused on meaningful goal-directed activity result in better outcomes than a focus on performance components or handling techniques.[8] This systematic review did not support the use of NDT techniques as outlined in current published studies.[8] Of the 15 randomized controlled trials measuring NDT efficacy, 12 (studying 674 children) found no statistically favorable benefits from NDT; these trials were of varying quality (high, moderate, and low), whereas three trials (studying 38 children) showed improvements in body structures and functions such as gait parameters, spirometry, and milestone acquisition. Consequently, OT practitioners selecting to use and NDT should carefully monitor child progress and short-term outcomes to determine benefit. Intervention should always be linked to goal-directed activities that are commonly seen in daily tasks.

SUMMARY

OT practitioners work with children with CP or other neuromuscular conditions whose poor postural control and movement patterns limit their active participation in daily occupations. OT practitioners use their knowledge of positioning and handling techniques to help children succeed in meaningful everyday occupations. Providing external stability through positioning equipment may allow children with CP or other neuromuscular conditions to be successful in a variety of occupations, such as feeding, bathing, play, and academics. OT practitioners using NDT frequently prepare children for movements using sensory techniques to inhibit or facilitate muscle tone to a more normal level. During functional activities, OT practitioners gently guide children by placing their hands at key points of control and facilitating weight shifts and typical movement patterns. While facilitating movements, OT practitioners inhibit abnormal muscle tone and provide supports so that children are able to engage in meaningful activities. Positioning and handling techniques are used to help children engage in social, academic, self-care, and play activities.

References

1. Barthel, K. (2009). A frame of reference for neuro-developmental treatment. In P. Kramer, & J. Hinojosa (Eds.), *Frames of reference for pediatric occupational therapy*. Philadelphia: Lippincott Williams & Wilkins.
2. Bly, L. (1994). *Motor skills acquisition in the first year. An illustrated guide to normal development*. San Antonio, TX: Therapy Skill Builders.
3. Bobath, B. (1967). The very early treatment of cerebral palsy. *Dev Med Child Neurol, 9*, 373–390.
4. Bobath, K. (1980). *A neurophysiological basis for the intervention of cerebral palsy*. London: Heinemann Books.
5. Bobath, B., & Bobath, K. (1984). The neuro-developmental treatment. In D. Scrutton, et al. (Eds.), *Management of the motor disorders of children with cerebral palsy. Clinics in developmental medicine*. Oxford: Spastics International Medical Publications.
6. Case-Smith, J. (2015). Foundations for occupational therapy practice with children. In J. Case-Smith, & J. O'Brien (Eds.), *Occupational therapy for children and adolescents* (7th ed.). St. Louis, MO: Mosby.
7. Howle, J. (2007). *Neuro-developmental treatment approach: theoretical foundations and principles of clinical practice* (3rd ed.). Laguna Beach, CA: NDTA.
8. Novak, I., McIntyre, S., Morgan, C., Campbell, L., Dark, L., Morton, N., et al. (2013). A systematic review of interventions for children with cerebral palsy: state of evidence. *Dev Med Child Neurol, 55*(10), 885–910.
9. Neurodevelopmental Intervention Association. (2008). What is NDT? Available at: http://www.ndta.org.
10. Schoen, S., & Anderson, J. (2009). Neurodevelopment treatment frame of reference. In P. Kramer, & J. Hinojosa (Eds.), *Frames of reference for pediatric occupational therapy*. Philadelphia: Lippincott Williams & Wilkins.
11. Shumway-Cook, A., & Woollacott, M. (2007). *Motor control: translating research into clinical practice*. Philadelphia: Lippincott Williams & Wilkins.

REVIEW *Questions*

1. What are the typical developmental positions seen in early infancy from 1 to 12 months?
2. What are the principles for the proper sitting position?
3. What are some examples of equipment that support positions?
4. What are the principles of NDT?
5. Describe how OT practitioners use positioning and handling during treatment sessions to improve a child's overall functional skills.

SUGGESTED *Activities*

1. Practice moving your body in early developmental positions of prone, supine, side lying, sitting, quadruped, and standing. Consider how you move your center of gravity and manage weight shifts to efficiently move from one position to the next.
2. Practice different facilitation and inhibition techniques on your classmates to improve a child's ability to sit upright with improved back extension.
3. Study the parts of a piece of pediatric equipment (i.e., stander, posture chair, or wheelchair). Practice removing and replacing the detachable pieces and special belt/strapping on the equipment.
4. Using the Internet, research four types of positioning equipment that promote prone positioning, side-lying, sitting, and standing.

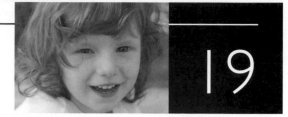

19

Activities of Daily Living and Sleep/Rest

CHAPTER *Objectives*

After studying this chapter, the reader will be able to accomplish the following:

- Describe the progression of activities of daily living (ADLs).
- Describe a collaborative approach to help children develop the ability to engage in ADLs and sleep/rest.
- Develop intervention strategies to improve engagement in ADLs and sleep/rest for children and youth.
- Understand the concept of co-occupation as it relates to designing and implementing intervention for ADLs and sleep/rest.
- Describe remediation, compensatory, and adaptive strategies to help children perform ADLs.
- Identify adaptive equipment and devices that help children perform ADLs.

CHAPTER *Outline*

CASE *Study*

Ten-year-old Ashley and her family were returning home after visiting out-of-town family members during school vacation when her family's car was struck by an oncoming vehicle, ejecting Ashley through the front windshield from the passenger seat. Emergency personnel immediately transported Ashley by ambulance to a local hospital, where she was assessed and transferred via helicopter to a large pediatric acute care hospital. During her hospital stay, Ashley's medical team determined she had sustained a traumatic brain injury (TBI) and an incomplete C6-C7 spinal cord injury (SCI). After multiple diagnostics, surgeries, and daily skilled inpatient rehabilitation, Ashley was discharged to a local pediatric unit within an acute rehabilitation facility.

The occupational therapy (OT) practitioner, with input from the occupational therapy assistant (OTA), evaluates **activities of daily living (ADLs)** and sleep/rest. They begin by conducting an interview with the child and family to determine the child's prior routines, values, and culture.[10]

This chapter addresses ADLs and sleep/rest in children and adolescents. The Occupational Therapy Practice Framework identifies ADLs and sleep/rest as separate occupations. ADLs also may be referred to as personal ADLs (PADLs) and/or basic ADLs (BADLs).[1] ADLs comprise meaningful activities that encompass self-care: bathing and showering, toilet hygiene (e.g., bowel and bladder management), dressing, eating/swallowing, feeding, functional mobility, personal device care, personal hygiene, and sexual activity.[1] The author also describes the occupation of sleep/rest. ADLs and sleep/rest are essential to a person's daily living and well-being.[1,7] This chapter addresses developing the OT intervention plan, implementing therapy, measuring progress, and planning for discharge. Specific intervention strategies and case examples are provided throughout to promote learning.

ADLs AND SLEEP/REST: A COLLABORATIVE APPROACH TO INTERVENTION

Pediatric OT practitioners are faced with a diverse caseload of clients with complex medical and developmental issues. Infants, children, and adolescents may present with multiple diagnoses and symptoms related to conditions that influence their overall level of independence in occupations. OT practitioners view individuals holistically, regardless of age, disease, or disability and therefore individualize the intervention plan to meet the unique needs of each child and his or her family.

Regardless of the setting (e.g., acute care, community, and school), disruption or interference with the process of development not only affects the child but also the family members, caregivers, and friends within the child's

physical and social environments. Client- and family-centered approaches are integral to the OT process, and meaningful activities complement cultural values and beliefs.[1,7] Viewing the child holistically, as an occupational being who has individual habits, roles, and routines is part of the dynamic OT process.[1,10] Client factors support and/or adversely affect performance skills.[1]

OT practitioners working with infants, children, and adolescents facilitate skill acquisition so that children and adolescents can engage in a variety of ADLs. They help children and youth develop healthy sleep and rest routines.[10] Although development typically occurs in a sequential pattern, OT practitioners working with children and adolescents are challenged to think outside the box to determine how internal (e.g., motivation, cognition, emotions, muscle tone) and external (e.g., cultural, physical, environmental) variables influence development. For example, a child diagnosed with a congenital anomaly, acquired disability, or developmental disorder may present with symptoms that interfere with the maturation of functional skills. The child's condition or symptoms may interfere with his or her ability to learn both basic and higher-level skills, which may result in deficits in functional skill development and transfer of learning across multiple contexts.[1,5]

As the OT process unfolds, analysis of occupational performance guides practice. The OT practitioner collaborates with the certified OTA (COTA), the child, and the family. Using a collaborative team approach enhances occupational performance outcomes (e.g., independence in ADLs and sleep/rest). Under the direct supervision of the occupational therapist, the COTA may be responsible for assisting with goal development, selection of intervention approaches, determination of the means of service delivery, and selection of outcome measurements within the intervention planning process, depending on his or her level of service competence. Once the intervention plan is implemented, OT practitioners are responsible for establishing therapeutic rapport, incorporating meaningful activities into treatment, consulting with various professionals, and providing education to the client, family, facility, and community.

Examining sleep and rest can illustrate the importance of collaboration. The practitioner reviews the family's sleep routine with parents to better understand their values, rituals, and home routines. The practitioner collaborates by identifying some factors that may better prepare the child for sleep. A careful observation of the physical environment may reveal areas that may support or hinder the child's sleep. For example, the family may eat sugary desserts, watch television, or play active games before bedtime. For some children this can increase energy levels and disrupt sleep patterns. The practitioner may recommend that the family make adjustments to the routine. Perhaps they can agree to provide warm milk for dessert, have the children read quietly, and quietly talk about the day's events. These calming activities may help the child establish a sleep routine. By collaborating closely with the parents and child, the OT practitioner is able to develop an intervention plan that is meaningful to the child and family.

A DEVELOPMENTAL PERSPECTIVE OF ADLs AND SLEEP/REST

Infants and toddlers rely on others to ensure that their basic needs are met. As they grow older, they begin to engage in self-care tasks such as bathing, feeding, dressing, and bowel and bladder control. They establish sleep/rest routines. They begin to move around the environment (to explore their surroundings). When infants and toddlers are not busy exploring their surroundings or engaged in social interactions, they are typically sleeping or resting. When engaged in occupations, they learn to tolerate sensations, listen to body cues, and use their hands to manipulate objects. Infants born with congenital anomalies or inherited disorders and those born prematurely may experience difficulty tolerating, managing, and learning the skills needed to perform ADLs.[1,4]

Infants, toddlers, and adolescents have many opportunities to engage in ADLs in natural settings and across multiple contexts (e.g., home, day care, community). Peers and siblings often demonstrate how to initiate, sequence, and complete ADL tasks. Parents and teachers play essential roles in teaching children how to engage in ADLs.

Adolescents and teens experience internal variables (e.g., emotions, self-concept, motivation, initiation) and external variables (e.g., peer pressure, social expectations) that influence ADL and sleep/rest performance. Social attention, peer pressure, body image, and sexuality influence occupational performance in activities such as hygiene, dressing, and sexual activity.[1] Chapters 6 to 8 present an overview of the typical sequence of development of occupations.

CO-OCCUPATION

The term *co-occupation* refers to occupations shared by at least two individuals.[12] A naturally occurring co-occupation involves a parent calming his or her child. In this case the child is responding to the parent (social participation), and the parent is engaging in the caregiving role. Infants rely on others (such as caregivers, parents) to provide sensory stimulation, opportunities to develop relationships, and exposure to sensorimotor opportunities for skill acquisition. OT practitioners address deficits in co-occupational performance and consider the complexities of relationships when developing interventions for ADLs and sleep/rest.[9,17]

OT practitioners work with children who come from diverse environments and cultures. Exploration of the environment in early childhood is essential for optimal sensory and motor development. Many children deprived of early sensory experiences (such as those in orphanages) experience long-lasting sensory (such as vision and touch processing) and motor difficulties.[2] Working collaboratively to support the co-occupations of families is helpful to children and may promote the development of ADL skills.

EVALUATION TO INTERVENTION

The OT practitioner completes an occupational profile to better understand a child's strengths and weaknesses and to develop functional goals addressing occupational performance deficits.[1] The occupational profile provides an overall picture of the child's functioning, including contraindications, signs and symptoms, and performance skills. The OT practitioner considers the child's family, culture, and environment during the intervention process.

The guidelines in Box 19-1 may help practitioners design various interventions to address ADLs.

BOX 19-1

Guidelines for Designing Interventions to Address ADL Performance

- Review the occupational profile, including goals and recommendations.
- Ensure all contraindications are taken into consideration during intervention planning and implementation.
- Be comfortable explaining the role of an OTA (in nontechnical terms) to the client and/or the family.
- Use universal precautions during interventions.
- Address the performance deficits and environmental modifications that enable children to be successful in participating in occupations such as ADLs.
- Encourage active client participation and involve caregivers.
- Remember the OT process is dynamic and that alterations to the intervention plan may be indicated over time.
- Consult with the supervising occupational therapist, the client, and the team (including family, caregiver, and staff members) throughout the OT process regarding goals and progress.
- Document progress clearly.
- Report concerns about the intervention process to the supervising occupational therapist.
- Use available professional resources for assistance.
- Collaborate with all team members during discharge planning to ensure that the consistency of care will continue.

INTERVENTION STRATEGIES TO PROMOTE ADLs AND SLEEP/REST
Toilet Hygiene

CASE *Study*

Kara is a 13-year-old girl who was in a motor vehicle accident a month ago. She sustained a fractured right humeral head and now receives outpatient occupational therapy. Because of Kara's current limited upper extremity range of motion (ROM), she requires assistance with toilet hygiene. She is mortified by her need to have someone help her with this personal task and asks the OTA if there is anything that can be done immediately to help her increase her independence to perform the task.

The OTA considers that ROM limitation is temporary due to the fracture. The OTA provides adaptive clothing by suggesting the child wear clothes that do not require she use both hands to fasten or unfasten, and clothes that can be easily removed. The OTA provides Kara with some tips on how to use one hand for toileting hygiene. She decides to carry her own wipes to make sure she can clean herself adequately. By having the wipes in her pocket, she does not have to reach over for the toilet paper. After providing the tips in private, the practitioner asks Kara to go into the bathroom and try them out. The tips help solve the problems that were of concern to Kara, allowing her to feel confident in handling her toileting.

Toilet hygiene involves a full range of activities, including "obtaining and using toileting supplies, managing clothing, maintaining toileting position, transferring to and from toileting position, cleaning body, and caring for menstrual and continence needs (including catheter, colostomy, and suppository management), as well as completing intentional control of bowel movements and urination and, if necessary, using equipment or agents for bladder control."[1,8]

Toilet training can be a challenging process for caregivers. The skilled OT practitioner can assist children and adolescents who have difficulty with toilet hygiene by making this all-important process more manageable. The OT practitioner considers all factors that may interfere with these activities. When "potty training" a child, the practitioner first establishes the family routine and schedules toilet breaks. Children are reinforced for successes in toileting via stickers and/or praise. Before engaging in a toileting program, the practitioner makes sure the child is ready. The first step of any toileting program is for the child to indicate that he or she is wet or soiled. Therefore the practitioner may recommend that the child wear cloth diapers to experience the feeling of being uncomfortable. Starting the program by

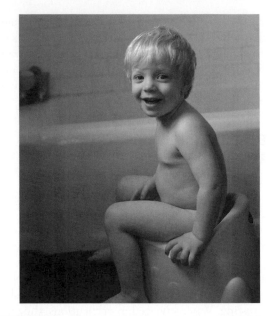

FIGURE 19-1 "Potty training" is a natural part of childhood.

encouraging the child to drink fluids and eat salty foods may help to facilitate necessary urges. At the beginning of any program, parents are encouraged to bring the toddler or child to the toilet often and make the event pleasurable and relaxed (Figure 19-1). Once the child has some successes, the parent can decrease the time on the toilet and begin requiring that the child decide when to go. The gradual decrease in cueing allows the child to become independent. Remaining dry through the night is one of the last components children are able to accomplish. Furthermore, some children have difficulty with sleep and do not wake themselves at night to toilet. The OT practitioner also encourages families to promote the range of toileting hygiene activities as the child is able to gain skill.

A variety of adaptive equipment may be useful for promoting increased independence for toilet hygiene. Grab bars and toilet safety frames provide extra support for transferring onto the toilet. A raised or lowered toilet seat may also be indicated, depending on the specific needs of the child. For some individuals, a bedside commode may be beneficial. A skin inspection mirror can be helpful to individuals who have difficulty cleaning themselves. A variety of toilet tissue aids that allow individuals with limited ROM to clean themselves adequately are also available commercially. Toilet paper holders can be adapted to be maximally accessible.

Bowel and Bladder Management

Bowel and bladder management encompasses both the voluntary control of bowel and bladder movements as well as the use of alternative methods to support bladder control.[1] To optimally manage bowel and bladder functions, which include processes of both volition and intention, an intact neurologic system is essential.[6]

Infants and toddlers begin developing the concept of bowel and bladder functions in addition to processing sensations before developing motor control abilities for the volitional control of their actions. Young children, through either structured or nonstructured programming, have environmental affordances such as education, caregiver assistance, peer-modeling opportunities, and physical setup to support the development of functional skills. During the school-age years, children develop and participate in a consistent routine. Continued adaptations are made in accordance with daily scheduled activities throughout adolescence and the teenage years.

CASE *Study*

Destiny is an 11-year-old girl who attends a private day school for children with complex needs, including behavioral and sensory issues. Destiny's primary medical and educational diagnoses are visual impairment, hearing impairment, and autism. She relies primarily on her tactile, proprioceptive, and vestibular sensory systems for information regarding where she is physically in space as well as in proximity to other persons and objects within her physical environment. In addition to occupational therapy, she receives speech and language therapy and physical therapy services. Destiny also works with a certified orientation and mobility specialist, who teaches those with visual impairment and has advanced training in teaching those with hearing impairments.

Destiny's educational team members are concerned about her new behaviors. This is the third consecutive day of inconsistent behaviors with regard to bowel and bladder management. The para-professional who works with Destiny and her teacher says that Destiny's requests to use the bathroom have been inconsistent with her previous behaviors. Previously, she required only check-ins, but now she requires one-on-one constant supervision because of her tactile-seeking behaviors, including smearing feces on the bathroom walls. The team members also report that her stools are loose and that she has been having multiple "accidents" during the day. They ask the OT practitioner for guidance because Destiny's sensory-seeking behaviors interfere with her safety and hygiene. The OT practitioner contacts her caregiver and learns that over the weekend Destiny experienced difficulty with bowel management due to constipation. Her caregiver reported that Destiny was given an over-the-counter stool softener; misreading of the dosage instructions led to too much of the medication being given and consequently loose stools for the past 3 days. According to the caregiver, this is the first time Destiny has had bowel difficulties since she developed independence in bowel and bladder management. Her pediatrician suggests

stopping the stool softener and encouraging Destiny to drink a lot of water throughout the day.

OT practitioners work with children and adolescents who have difficulties with bowel and bladder management. Common symptoms such as increased urinary frequency, lack of voluntary bowel control, and decreased sensory awareness are associated with multiple diagnoses, especially those associated with injuries to the brain, spinal cord, and/or nerves (e.g., shaken baby syndrome, SCI).[6] Regardless of etiology, bowel and bladder management is an integral occupation requiring remediation and/or compensation.

CLINICAL *Pearl*

When working with children with a diagnosis of SCI at or above the T6 level, monitor for signs and/or symptoms of autonomic dysreflexia (AD). AD occurs when noxious stimulation is unable to reach the brain. Instead, the information (i.e., a full bladder) reaches the spinal cord, which triggers a reflex that results in constriction of blood vessels below the injury leading to increased blood pressure. The brain attempts to send signals to dilate blood vessels, but the information cannot travel past the level of injury. Consequently, blood vessels above the injury dilate but are unable to decrease the overall increase in blood pressure. AD has the potential to result in a heart attack or death. Signs and symptoms include the following:

- Red blotches above the level of injury
- Hypertension
- Nasal congestion
- Chills
- Sweating

If a child or adolescent demonstrates signs or symptoms of AD, the OT practitioner should immediately follow procedures already in place at the facility regarding medical attention. When indicated, the child may benefit from being positioned into the **semi-Fowler's position** to support abdominal relaxation and breathing.[6] The child's head should be elevated (30–45 degrees), and knees should be in either flexion or extension bilaterally. OT intervention addressing bowel and bladder management may help prevent future episodes of AD.[6,14]

CASE *Study*

Ashley, the young girl in the previous case study, who sustained a SCI at the C6-C7 level, lost sensation and volitional control of both bowel and bladder functions. In addition, she has short-term memory loss due to TBI. She is returning to school full time in 1 month. Ashley needs strategies to recall the steps of her bowel and bladder program. Ashley is especially concerned that she will forget the steps for optimal bowel and bladder management and experience embarrassment.

In early infancy and toddlerhood, parent education is essential for learning bowel and bladder management and handling techniques. For children who have experienced acute trauma, discussing self-catheterization or having a caregiver complete tasks for them may cause feelings of embarrassment and frustration. Privacy and dignity are integral aspects of intervention.

Remediation techniques for bowel and bladder management may include therapeutic handling during diaper changes to deal with fluctuating muscle tone, development of an individualized toileting program, and implementation of a behavioral reward program. Compensatory strategies include use of pull-ups or adult diapers, and adult-directed timed schedule. A pediatric client with a hip fracture may benefit from a raised toilet seat to avoid hip flexion. Children and adolescents may need to be trained in catheterization. This training is usually a collaborative effort between the OT practitioner, the nurse, the caregivers, and the child.

Bathing and Showering

Bathing and showering are occupations made up of multiple tasks and sequences, including obtaining and using supplies; soaping, rinsing, and drying body parts; maintaining varied bathing positions; and transferring to and from positions while bathing.[1] Infants and toddlers are at the beginning stages of concept development in that they are just learning the purposes and functions of objects and activities. They have not yet developed meaningfulness to the act of being bathed. For infants and toddlers, bath time provides an opportunity to play and enjoy the sensations while making sense of objects.

Some adolescents view bathing and showering as a meaningful self-care activity that ensures health. Children, adolescents, and teens may have difficulties with bathing and showering for many different reasons (e.g., motor, sensory, cognitive, behavioral, and developmental). The OT practitioner begins with an analysis of the child's strengths and areas for growth (obtained from the occupational profile) to determine the best intervention.[1] The following case studies illustrate intervention strategies for bathing and showering.

CLINICAL *Pearl*

Bath time may be a fun time for those with special needs to work on performance deficits (e.g., ROM, stretching, positioning). For teens, bath or shower time provides the OT practitioner and caregiver(s) the opportunity to work on remediating or compensating for performance skill deficits. Functional skills are developed and generalized over time across varied contexts.[1,18]

CASE *Study*

Molly, a 3-year-old toddler, is referred to occupational therapy following a right proximal humerus fracture with no medical precautions. Areas for growth, identified from the occupational profile, include right upper extremity active ROM and strength, independence in self-care, and endurance during functional play tasks involving right upper extremity use. Her mother is worried about bathing Molly because she is hesitant to hold her and move her right arm.

With children such as Molly who are in need of remediation techniques for orthopedic limitations, the focus is on meeting the client where he or she is currently functioning, facilitating the return to previous functional status, and improving overall independence. Remediation techniques include upper extremity therapeutic exercises (ROM and strengthening) and therapeutic activities to increase active participation and independence. Grading the location of bath supplies on shelves by altering the shelf height or the placement of supplies on the shelves will provide the child with reaching opportunities before entering the bathtub or shower area. Use of warm water creates a therapeutic environment for exercises. OT practitioners may incorporate functional activities. For example, they may have the child reach above shoulder height to retrieve their favorite toys, while physically supporting them in the bathtub as needed. Various-sized water toys, weights, and resistance support the child's intrinsic motivation for play while improving bathing and showering skills. Involving the caregiver in the session helps with carryover or incorporating OT strategies into the child's daily routines.[10] Educating the caregiver on positioning, handling techniques, and overall safety is essential.

Children presenting with neurologic, sensory-perceptual, emotional regulation, and cognitive deficits may have difficulty with aspects of bathing and showering. They may benefit from intervention techniques to improve motor performance to complete ADL activities guided by control or motor learning, neurodevelopmental therapy, sensory integration, or developmental frames of reference. For example, **preparatory activities** for a child with low muscle tone include stimulatory activities such as vibration, whereas calming tasks such as rocking are indicated for children with spasticity.[16] Cold increases muscle tone, whereas neutral warmth relaxes it. These basic concepts are important as the activity demands of bathing and showering call for the ability to retrieve, manipulate, and use various supplies; maintain body position (i.e., standing up against gravity with water resistance or bathing in supine moving within the water); transfer between positions; and wash and dry self.[1]

Remediation may include analyzing activities so that the practitioner can teach small steps via forward or backward chaining (Table 19-1).[14] The OT practitioner

TABLE 19-1

Forward and Backward Chaining Techniques

	DEFINITION	EXAMPLE
Forward chaining	The OT practitioner encourages the child to initiate the first step and complete the process as much as possible before the OT practitioner completes the process. The OT practitioner repeats the steps until the client completes them all.	Child removes clothes, steps into bath, and washes self in tub; caregiver dries child off, dresses child, and empties tub water.
Backward chaining	The OT practitioner assists the child until the last step of the process and then allows the child to perform the last step; the OT practitioner repeats the process allowing the child to complete the next to last step and the last step until the child completes them all.	Caregiver removes child's clothes, washes child in tub, dries child off. Child dresses self and empties tub water.

can facilitate the process by having the child or adolescent initiate the first step of a sequence or complete the last step of a sequence, depending on the chosen intervention approach. The OT practitioner should continue to gradually increase the level of difficulty over time.

CASE *Study*

A 14-year-old adolescent who has been diagnosed with major depression presents with flat affect, decreased socialization skills, and lack of motivation to complete daily grooming tasks before school. On the basis of the information obtained while completing the occupational profile, the COTA plans and implements a sensory inventory to gain more information about the teen's sensory preferences. The adolescent reports a strong preference for warm sensations. The COTA, the teen, and the mother work together to create a strategy to increase the adolescent's motivation and frequency for showering. The collaborative decision to have the adolescent's mother turn on the shower 2 minutes before wake-up time, paired with the verbal cue "Your warm shower is ready," helps the adolescent tolerate the shower three times during the first week. The adolescent's motivation to engage in bathing and showering is facilitated by the intrinsic motivation for experiencing sensations involving warmth and hearing her supportive mother's voice. The adolescent and the mother both report a sense of progress in accomplishing ADLs—an example of successful co-occupational performance.

This example illustrates the importance of collaborating with the child and family to develop a remediation plan. Developing an ADL routine helps reinforce patterns.[10] Combining a positive sensory experience (e.g., warm water) with positive reinforcement from the mother reinforces behaviors and helps establish a routine. In addition to remediation, the OT practitioner may develop

compensatory techniques. For example, children with deficits that interfere with ADL performance may benefit from the following:

- Self-care training using assistive devices or adapted techniques, including long-handled self-care supplies (i.e., sponge), shower chairs, reachers, non-slip tub mats, safety bars, and/or removable shower heads
- Staff supervision and implementation of a visual schedule for an adolescent with cognitive skill deficits residing in a group home setting, which is another possibility for support during occupational participation
- Labeling items in large print and contrasting colors to support pediatric clients with low vision
- Incorporating adaptive techniques such as using a container with one U-shaped side to rest against the client's head for washing hair to eliminate the need to tilt the head backward, which may cause distress
- Ensuring a smooth transition from a bath or shower with a snug towel wrap to help the client handle increased sensitivity to change in temperatures and to provide the sensory supports to maintain an optimal level of arousal
- Educating parents, caregivers, and staff members on the level of supervision needed throughout bathing and showering as necessary
- Rearrangement of a client's bathroom to accommodate a wheelchair and/or shower chair as necessary
- Education on work simplification or energy conservation to support co-occupation and prevent caregiver "burnout," especially when the child's needs are complex and physically taxing for the caregiver

Assistive technology may help children succeed in performing ADLs. Computer-simulated programs for self-care tasks may assist the children in learning the required sequences for bathing and showering before attempting the multistep task in the natural context. Having a concrete visual schedule that includes the day and time for

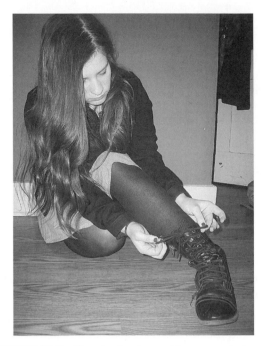

FIGURE 19-2 Dressing involves putting on one's shoes.

bathing and showering is an additional means of cognitive support. (See Chapter 27 regarding assistive technology options.)

Dressing

Dressing involves multiple steps and is influenced by both internal and external variables. It involves selecting clothing and accessories appropriate to time of day, weather, and occasion; obtaining clothing from storage area; dressing and undressing in a sequential fashion; fastening and adjusting clothing and shoes; and applying and removing personal devices, prosthetic devices, or splints. Cognition, perceived self-image, sense of style, and sensory preferences are some potential internal variables that influence the dressing process.

The sequence of dressing includes retrieving clothing items from a storage area and completing dressing/undressing tasks as appropriate. Developmentally, as gross motor movements precede fine motor movements, using fasteners, adjusting clothing and shoes, and the application and/or removal of devices occur after the child is able to complete dressing and undressing tasks.[1] See Figure 19-2 of child putting on shoes. Chapter 7 provides the developmental sequence of the acquisition of undressing/dressing skills.

Infants rely on caregivers to dress/undress them. Toddlers play dress-up and begin to develop basic skills to dress and undress. Figure 19-3 shows children playing dress-up. Children move from play-based dressing activities to dressing in specific attire or uniforms for example, dance and soccer uniforms. The school-aged child moves

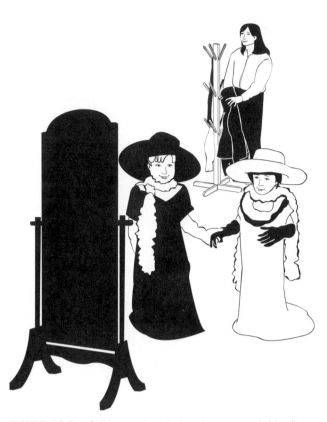

FIGURE 19-3 Children enjoy playing dress-up, and this allows them to practice the skills required, problem solve, and learn. (From O'Brien, J.C., Solomon, J. W. (2013). *Occupational analysis and group process.* St. Louis: Mosby.)

from relying on caregivers to choose clothing to developing an individualized style or preference for certain clothing. Favorite colors, textures, and styles begin to drive a child's intrinsic motivation to independently go through the dressing process. Teens may change clothing preferences in response to peer pressure to look a certain way. The OT practitioner should consider a child's motor and sensory skills, and motivations (e.g., preferences for style) when developing a dressing intervention program.

CASE *Study*

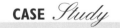

Six-year-old Megan has a diagnosis of status post-left cerebrovascular accident (CVA), with right hemiparesis and right neglect. She has trouble dressing as a result of her difficulty completing the fine motor aspects of dressing. She is able to don and doff large, loose-fitting clothing items with minimal physical assistance and requires moderate verbal cues to use her right upper extremity as an assist during dressing.

Megan presents with right upper extremity spasticity, and her fist remains in full flexion. Despite the cold weather, she comes to the clinic without wearing a jacket. The OT practitioner observes her walking down the hallway. Megan appears comfortable wearing only a sweatshirt and jogging pants; yet, the right side of her waist band is twisted, and the back of her shirt is bunched up at her waist line. She does not verbalize or demonstrate signs of discomfort.

Megan's mother reports that Megan has been having difficulty getting ready for school this week. Reportedly, she is frustrated with even simple dressing tasks such as zipping her jeans and buttoning large buttons. Megan says that she "hates buttoning and zipping" and does not want to work on using her hands, as the right one is "no good anyway." Megan's mother rolls her eyes and says that Megan must learn how to dress herself.

Megan's current short-term goals include fastening four or five large buttons (1-inch in diameter) with minimal physical assistance for accuracy and zipping her jacket with set-up and minimal verbal cues. The OT practitioner decides to work on increasing Megan's motivation to dress herself by discussing her preferences for styles, colors, textures, and clothing. Once they both select an outfit more like that of her teen peers, Megan becomes interested in dressing. She seems more concerned about her appearance and involved in the intervention plan.

Dressing involves a complex sequence of events. OT practitioners apply knowledge of typical development when working with children who are in need of remediation, compensation, and education intervention within this domain (Figures 19-4 through 19-6).[1,15]

Remediation strategies include helping children who exhibit motor and praxis skill deficits through practice with repetition and variation, as described in the section on motor control/motor learning.[15,18] In addition, symptoms related to neurologic conditions, for example, visual neglect, changes in muscle tone, and diminished sensation may require the OT practitioner to incorporate therapeutic handling techniques, including muscle tone facilitation and/or inhibition techniques from the neurodevelopmental treatment (NDT) approach.[16] Conditions resulting in such symptoms as weakness require the OT practitioner to grade the activity demands. For example, a child with fair bilateral upper extremity strength may benefit from therapeutic ROM and strengthening activities. The OT practitioner working with children may have the opportunity to address dressing issues within a natural context, such as when a child changes into a bathing suit for an aquatic therapy sessions. Some children are unable to consistently demonstrate the same abilities across different contexts.[18] Providing OT services within the child's natural environment is ideal, as the task of dressing/undressing has a sense of purpose.

Compensatory strategies that may be beneficial to children include assistive devices and adaptive equipment such as pediatric-sized reachers, button hooks, leg raisers, sock-aids, loops for clothing, shirts and pants without tags, socks without seams, and Velcro fasteners. OT practitioners must be sure that children and their caregivers demonstrate competency in using equipment and devices before recommending them. Children may benefit from visual supports during the dressing process to provide cues regarding initiation, sequencing, and activity completion. OT practitioners should consider the range of motor, cognitive, and emotional performance skills required for dressing. In addition, the consideration of contextual factors (e.g., cultural, temporal) when designing dressing intervention is essential.[1]

A child or adolescent with sensory processing issues may present with difficulties interfering with dressing and benefit from compensatory strategies. (Box 19-2 on p. 366 presents possible strategies.) As praxis is an end product of sensory integration, the ability to develop the idea of how to begin dressing can be a major area of difficulty for some children.[2] For example, some children have difficulty tolerating certain fabrics and types of clothing. Children with sensory processing difficulties may become agitated with clothing that is too snug or has tight waistbands or wrist bands. Some children need to have their new clothes washed before wearing them.

Swallowing/Eating

Swallowing/eating is defined as keeping and manipulating food or fluid in the mouth and swallowing it. Swallowing is moving food from the mouth to the stomach. Feeding, setting up, arranging, and bringing food (or fluid) from the plate or cup to the mouth is referred to as **self-feeding**.[1] Swallowing is a specialized area in OT practice.[1,15] OT practitioners may work on swallowing skills with premature babies in the neonatal intensive care unit setting, or infants and toddlers in a community-based OT program. Swallowing is a complex process that requires intact sensory, motor, and voluntary actions. The OT practitioner typically provides intervention as part of a feeding team. In addition to the infant, child, or adolescent, team members may include the caregiver(s), physician, nurse, speech and language pathologist (SLP), SLP assistant, educator, and para-professionals.

Swallowing involves the oral preparation of food into a bolus, the oral transit phase of moving the bolus from the front of the mouth to the back of the mouth, the pharyngeal phase of swallowing once the bolus passes through the anterior faucial arches, and the esophageal phase of swallow. The OT practitioner can provide interventions to change the voluntary phases of swallow (i.e., oral preparation and transit and activation of the pharyngeal phases) but involuntary peristalsis controls the pharyngeal and esophageal phases of swallowing.

Children who have difficulty swallowing foods and/or liquids are frequently referred for occupational therapy.[15] The role of the OT practitioner may include providing intervention within a feeding group, monitoring a child for signs and symptoms of aspiration during lunch within

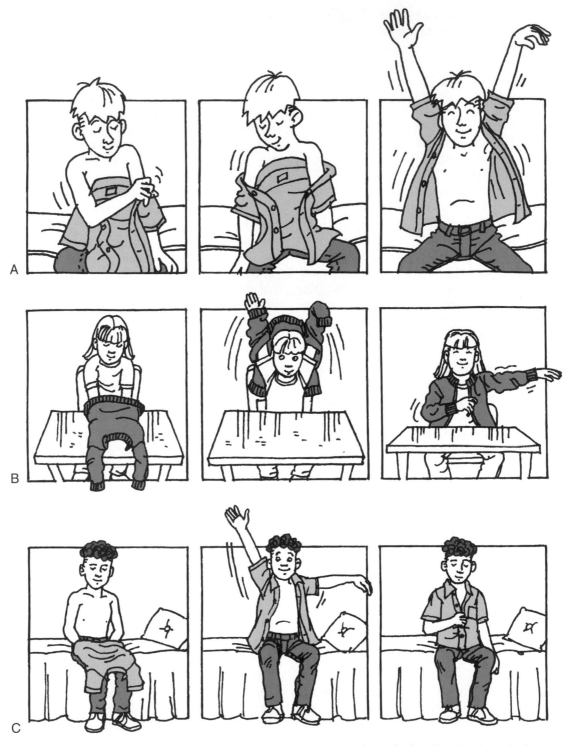

FIGURE 19-4 Adapted methods for putting on a shirt. **A**, Lap and over-the-head hemiplegic method. **B**, Front lap and facing-down method. **C**, Front lap and facing-down hemiplegic method.

the educational setting, and/or providing direct intervention within the acute care setting to a teen recovering from an accident that caused jaw instability. Regardless of the context, intervention planning and implementation of OT services for children who are in need of remediation for swallowing difficulties may include

oral motor/oral sensory programming, NDT muscle tone techniques, jaw rehabilitation (including jaw strengthening programming), and team/or education regarding safe swallowing.[5,15]

OT practitioners may target the child's food preferences, routines, and fine motor abilities to promote

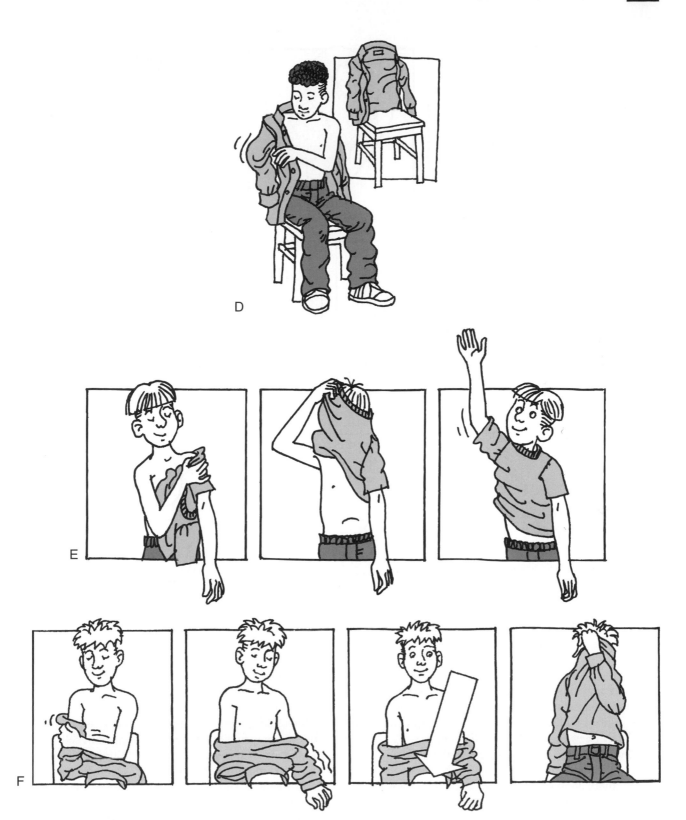

FIGURE 19-4, cont'd D, Chair method. E, Arm-head-arm method. F, Lap-arm-arm-neck method.

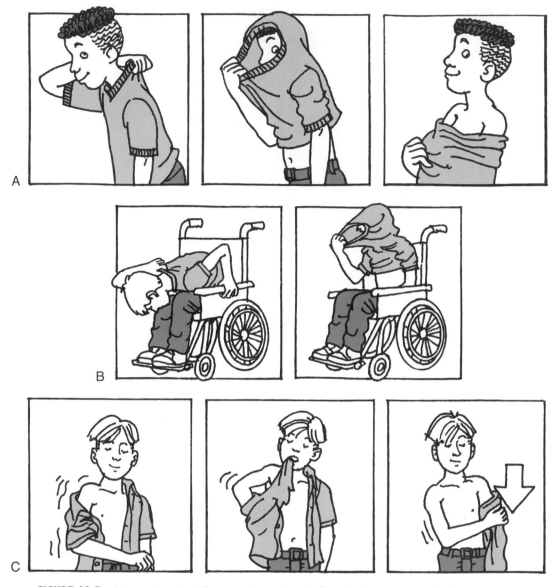

FIGURE 19-5 Adapted methods for removing a shirt. **A,** Over-the-head method. **B,** Duck-the-head-and-sit-up method. **C,** Arms-in-front method.

self-feeding. They may focus on posture and eating behaviors including portion size, hand-to-mouth, manners, and food variety. Intervention may emphasize oral-motor control including tongue, jaw, and lip control to completely chew foods before swallowing.

From a developmental perspective, the suck-swallow-breathe synchrony typically emerges as the first self-regulatory activity during the prenatal period. Infants work on further developing this synchrony, often finding pleasure in drinking from a bottle and/or breast-feeding.[2,3,15] This process provides the infant with the opportunity to bond with caregivers during occupational engagement. The toddler explores foods as well as the self-feeding process via play.

A small play kitchen with a toy refrigerator and a toy oven provide the toddler and young school-aged child with the opportunity to engage in the occupation of self-feeding at both parallel and interactive levels of play. Over time, responsibility for tasks such as setting the dinner table is introduced. Habits and routines may form as the child assumes a role in the process as school-aged children may find meaning in assisting with self-feeding tasks such as set-up and clean-up.[3,10] During adolescence, socialization with peers during self-feeding occurs on a more frequent basis. As the child grows, the contexts change, and transfer of learning is required as self-feeding activity occurs across multiple environments.

As proximal stability precedes distal mobility, swallowing is often correlated with fine motor abilities. An infant may require preparatory activities, including strategies to improve the suck–swallow–breathe synchrony.[2,5] School-aged children may benefit from biomechanical techniques to develop swallowing skills, including therapeutic

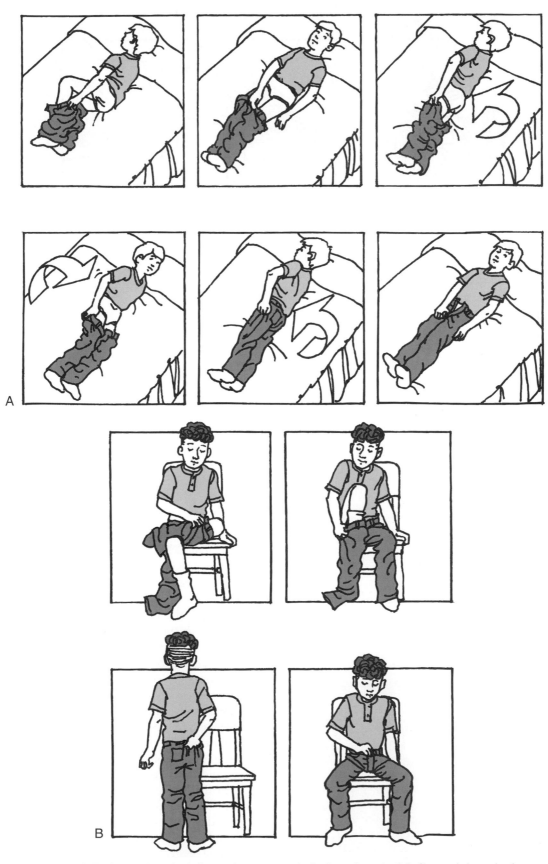

FIGURE 19-6   Adapted methods for putting on pants. **A,** Supine-roll method. **B,** Sit-stand-sit method.

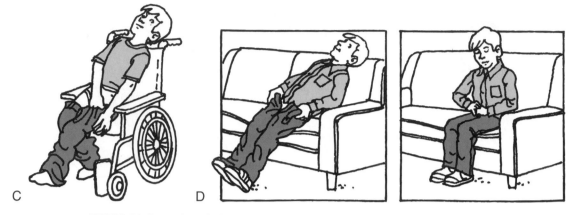

FIGURE 19-6, cont'd **C,** One-side bridge-sitting method. **D,** Bridge-sitting method.

BOX 19-2

*Compensatory Strategies for Children
with Sensory Processing Issues*

- Wash new clothes in familiar detergent before having the child wear them.
- Use detergent with mild or no fragrance.
- Allow the child to pick his or her clothing.
- Be sensitive about the waistbands, wrist bands, and neck region.
- Remove tags completely before the child wears the clothes.
- Some children prefer "gently used" clothes; others want new clothes.
- Not all children will prefer loose clothing; some may prefer tighter-fitting clothing.
- Be aware of each child's individual clothing preferences.
- Ask children to express themselves through colors and styles of clothing.

exercises to increase ROM and strength.[2,7] In addition, reliance on available sensory systems throughout the swallowing process is integral for children and youth.

CLINICAL *Pearl*

Children diagnosed with low vision and/or blindness may require staff and/or caregivers to provide them with information regarding foods and liquids. Ensure that these children receive accurate information and are able to express their likes and dislikes. Do not force a child to eat something that is not a preferred food.

Many school-aged children present with immature swallowing patterns and are in need of remediation. The young child diagnosed with developmental coordination disorder may require practice and repetition with variation, to succeed in carrying his or her milk cartons from the school kitchen to the lunch room, without dropping the tray or losing his or her balance.

CLINICAL *Pearl*

Rothmund-Thomson syndrome (RTS) is a rare genetic disorder characterized by short stature, thumb and/or radial anomalies, juvenile cataracts, gastrointestinal (GI) issues, osteopenia, absent patella(s), alopecia, high risk for bone and skin cancers, and/or poikiloderma (skin rash); 400 cases of RTS have been identified so far in the literature. OT practitioners may work with children with RTS and their families to develop feeding programs that do not cause GI issues. They may help children with RTS complete ADLs by providing assistive technology or teaching children compensatory strategies. OT practitioners may consult with children and families on techniques to promote sleep and rest.

Caregivers provide sensory exploration opportunities to the infant when novel foods and liquids are introduced.[5,16] Toddlers develop feeding preferences, and they may develop fears of new foods.[7] With continued opportunities to explore, try, and develop early swallowing skills, the toddler develops his or her ability to attempt or accept a variety of foods. During the school years and into adolescence, food selection follows a narrower trend, as personal preferences emerge.[3,5] The teenager continues to change preferences based on variables such as peer-group and cultural influences. Nutrition is a major concern in the case of children with eating and swallowing issues. Nurses and caregivers support pediatric clients with severe eating and swallowing issues by administering G- or J-tube feedings or both. In addition, nurses and caregivers provide suctioning for the medically fragile child unable to manage his or her own saliva. Products to thicken liquids such as Thick-it or Simply Thicke, diet adaptations (i.e., puréed consistency for all foods and PediaSure for added nutritional value), change in physical context and/or type of chair for proximal support, and optimal positioning may be indicated to compensate for limited or lack of safe swallowing.

BOX 19-3

Techniques to Promote Swallowing in Children and Adolescents

- Position infants in the semi-reclined position.
- Position toddlers and teens in the upright sitting position, with the neck slightly flexed forward.
- Provide oral-motor stimulation to children who have low oral–motor musculature.
- Vibration, quick stroking (above lip, on cheeks) may improve swallowing.
- For infants with swallowing difficulties, provide jaw control to improve ability to suck on the bottle (by gently holding the fat pads on the cheeks).
- Provide jaw control to help toddlers and adolescents swallow.
- Thicker liquids are easier for most children to control and swallow.
- Do not force children to put anything in their mouths.
- Encourage children to suck on ice pop or something sour.
- Provide a calm setting for the child. Distractions may interfere with swallowing.
- Do not talk to the infant while feeding (this may distract him or her).
- Work slowly with the child. Some children may have a delayed swallow.
- Promote tongue lateralization by encouraging the child to reach both sides of the mouth for food (i.e., place cracker on one side of mouth to encourage tongue movement to side).

BOX 19-4

Strategies to Manage Feeding Problems[19]

- Resolve or control negative medical influences
- Optimize biomechanical alignment
- Improve oral-motor control
- Facilitate positive feeding practices
- Support new skill development

Adapted from VanDahm, K. (Ed.). (2012). *Pediatric feeding disorders: evaluation and treatment.* Framingham, MA: Therapro, Inc.

compensatory pattern of using active wrist extension to promote a tenodesis action, to enable the child to pick up self-feeding materials.[4]

CLINICAL *Pearl*

Children with sustained a neurologic injury at level C6 or above typically have intact active wrist extension. Tenodesis is a typical movement pattern that occurs as a result of the volitional ability to actively extend the wrist against gravity. During active wrist extension, the digits move into a flexion pattern. In contrast, when the child allows his or her wrist to lower (wrist flexion) with the assistance of gravity, the digits typically extend.[11] The tenodesis action can be used to assist with both grasping and release of objects. A wrist–hand orthotic such as a tenodesis orthosis helps facilitate this. OT practitioners should engage children in functional activities that do not require tight digit flexion, as excessive stretching of the flexor tendons may potentially interfere with tenodesis.[11] As a result of having the ability to use the tenodesis action, in addition to appropriate assistive devices and/or adaptive equipment, the child is able to increase his or her overall level of functional independence in ADLs.

Both internal and external factors have the potential to adversely affect a child's ability to swallow safely. Internally, congenital anomalies in the oral cavity, sensory processing issues, and increased muscle tone are examples of common symptoms that interfere with optimal swallowing.[16] OT practitioners may choose to use compensatory strategies with children and adolescents. For example, an 8-year-old diagnosed with Down syndrome might place food at her molars to compensate for decreased tongue coordination and low oral muscle tone. Box 19-3 provides techniques to promote swallowing.

When the OT practitioner chooses to use a compensatory approach, such as altering and/or adapting the task, materials, or the environment, active engagement in swallowing may be supported.[15] Caregivers may engage in the process of swallowing as a co-occupation, setting up self-feeding items close to the child who fatigues easily during reaching tasks. Assistive devices including universal cuffs to hold utensils, self-feeding devices, weighted utensils, and splints (i.e., a tenodesis splint commonly used by a child with status–post C5-C6 SCI) support the

Feeding

Feeding is defined as consuming nutrition by mouth. *Feeding disorder* is a term used to describe behaviors of individuals who have difficulty consuming adequate nutrition by mouth. VanDahm et al. recommend using an integrated intervention approach while providing services for those with feeding disorders.[19] This means having a multidisciplinary team approach to the evaluation and intervention of feeding disorders. Feeding disorders typically involve a combination of several factors that might include medical issues, oral-motor mechanisms, structural misalignment(s), sensory processing issues, behavioral issues, or a combination of all of these factors.[19] Box 19-4 lists strategies to manage feeding problems.

BOX 19-5

Positioning Key Body Parts[19]

- Neck with midline orientation
- Head with midline orientation
- Shoulders level and forward
- Trunk with midline orientation
- Pelvis level (palpate anterior superior iliac crests to determine evenness)
- Hips @ 90 degrees of flexion
- Knees @ 90 degrees of flexion
- Feet neutral and on supported surface

Adapted from VanDahm, K. (Ed.). (2012). *Pediatric feeding disorders: evaluation and treatment.* Framingham, MA: Therapro, Inc.

BOX 19-6

Benefits of Proper Positioning[19]

- Safe swallowing
- Good digestion
- Adequate breathing
- Social participation

Adapted from VanDahm, K. (Ed.). (2012). *Pediatric feeding disorders: evaluation and treatment.* Framingham, MA: Therapro, Inc.

Proper Positioning

Proper positioning is critical to successful feeding experiences. Poor positioning during feeding can lead to difficulties breathing, risk for aspiration, poor caloric intake, regurgitation, and constipation. The OT practitioner should assess postural alignment by observing the position of key body parts. Boxes 19-5 and 19-6 list key body parts and proper alignment guidelines.

CLINICAL *Pearl*

OT practitioners may use rolled hand or dishtowels to provide support that promotes proper body alignment and symmetry.

Transitioning from Breast-feeding or Bottle to Solids

Pediatricians typically recommend introducing cereal and stage 1 baby food between 4 and 6 months of age.[19] Organic and nonorganic problems may make the transition from liquids to solids more difficult. Examples of organic conditions are prematurity, food allergies, and sensory processing issues. Examples of nonorganic conditions are child abuse/neglect, errors in food preparation, and poor feeding techniques. The organic and nonorganic problems may lead to feeding difficulties such as

BOX 19-7

Atypical Oral-Motor Function[19]

- Lip retraction
- Exaggerated tongue protrusion or tongue thrust
- Jaw thrusting with protrusion or retraction
- Lip pursing
- Tongue retraction
- Tonic bite reflex

Adapted from VanDahm, K. (Ed.). (2012). *Pediatric feeding disorders: evaluation and treatment.* Framingham, MA: Therapro, Inc.

food refusal and poor chewing skills. Interventions may include side placement of the food and facilitation of lip/jaw closure. There are eight levels of textures. The first four levels (i.e., smooth puree, mixed smooth and gritty puree, gritty puree, and finely chopped) do not require chewing. The fifth and sixth levels (i.e., finely fork mashed and fork mashed) require vertical chewing, which is an up–down munch pattern. The final two levels (i.e., cut-up whole foods and whole foods) require mature, rotary chewing.[19]

CLINICAL *Pearl*

The recommended sequence of chewing interventions is (a) resistive chewing to encourage coordination among jaw, cheeks, and tongue; (b) chewing food wrapped in mesh or tulle; and (c) chewing whole foods such as cheerios, then crackers, then toast to more difficult-to-handle food items.[19]

Drinking

Drinking is defined as liquid intake by mouth. The continuum of drinking in typical development is breast- or bottle feeding, drinking from a cup with a spout, drinking from an open cup, and drinking from a straw. A typical oral motor function may interfere with successful transition from a nipple to a cup. Box 19-7 presents common oral motor problems that interfere with drinking from a cup. The OT practitioner should identify what is interfering with the child's drinking and provide appropriate interventions. For example, if the child has a poor lip seal on the cup because of an underactive orbicularis oris, the practitioner may facilitate muscle contractions by using quick stretches. If the child is hypersensitive to touch around the mouth, the practitioner may apply pressure to prepare the mouth for the cup.

Weaning from Tube Feeding

Prematurity with a disorganized suck–swallow–breathe triad, a trachea-esophageal fistula, cardiac conditions that lead to fatigue, poor stamina and endurance, and GI issues may lead to a medical decision to insert a feeding tube. The readiness of an infant or child to transition from tube feedings to oral feedings is based on clinical signs, medical stability, resolution of primary medical condition, and the commitment of the family or primary caregiver(s).[19] The Palmer Protocol for Sensory-Based Weaning[12a] is frequently used during the weaning process. First the oral sensitivities are resolved and then oral-motor interventions are provided to improve the function of the structures. The type of food texture introduced depends on the child's tolerance.

CASE *Study*

Jeannie has been Thomas's occupational therapist since he began preschool at age 3. Thomas is now 7 years old and is enrolled in a classroom for students with moderate to severe intellectual disabilities. While he was in preschool, Jeannie and Thomas worked on finger feeding and independently holding and drinking from a sippy cup. Initially, Thomas raked the food into the palms of his left hand and brought his hand to his mouth. He was only able to release the food into his mouth when his hand was in contact with his lips. By the end of his preschool years Thomas independently finger fed himself a variety of finger foods. He used a pincer grasp to pick up his food and released the food into his mouth without touching his hand to his lips. He also held and drank his milk from a sippy cup. By the end of his second year of preschool, Jeannie and the team discussed working with Thomas on spoonfeeding. The team agreed that Thomas was ready to learn to feed himself using a spoon. His individualized educational plan goals and objectives were updated to include independence in spoonfeeding with adaptive devices. Before Thomas began first grade, Jeannie ordered a left-angled built-up toddler spoon and a scoop dish with a suction base/bottom.

During the first several weeks of school, Thomas was fed using the "new" spoon and bowl. He was allowed to explore these devices while waiting for his food to be placed in the bowl. During week 3 of first grade, Jeannie instructed the classroom staff how to provide hand-over-hand assistance to allow Thomas to scoop his food, take the loaded spoon to his mouth, and return the spoon to his plate while chewing before swallowing the food. The classroom staff was also shown how to position the dish to promote scooping against the raised edge. Throughout his meals Thomas had to be monitored closely as he had a tendency to stuff his mouth. Jeannie continued to work with Thomas weekly during lunch to monitor his progress and to update his self-feeding program as he gained skills.

By the end of first grade Thomas was able to scoop his food, take the loaded spoon to his mouth, and bring the spoon back to his plate with physical cuing at his left elbow. He continued to need monitoring so he did not stuff his mouth with food. He was given verbal prompts to chew and was offered opportunities to drink throughout his meals at school. Before summer vacation Thomas's mother met with Jeannie to review his progress with spoonfeeding and suggestions were made for home activities during summer break.

Thomas is now in second grade. He is independent in spoonfeeding, using the adaptive devices. The team has decided to work with Thomas on using a fork as appropriate during meals. Jeannie ordered a small left-angled fork for Thomas. Presently, Thomas uses his adapted spoon independently at school with monitoring of the amount of food in his mouth. He is provided hand-over-hand assistance to stab his food, but he independently takes the adapted fork to his mouth and returns it to his plate. Thomas continues to need a scoop dish during meals.

CLINICAL *Pearl*

When children and youth do not have active forearm supination it is difficult for them to release food into their mouths from a loaded utensil. Angled utensils are a solution to the lack of active range of forearm motion. Angled utensils can be purchased or made. Placing a light-weight utensil in a drawer and applying downward pressure creates an angled utensil.

Developmentally, infants learn to finger feed before learning to use utensils. Self-feeding using utensils involves a sequence of steps: picking up utensil, getting food on the utensil, taking loaded utensil to mouth, releasing food into mouth, and returning empty utensil to plate (see Figure 19-7). Thomas's case exemplifies the use of a developmental frame of reference while providing OT intervention to increase independence in feeding skills.

Functional Mobility

Functional mobility is defined as moving from one position or place to another (during performance of everyday activities), such as in-bed mobility, wheelchair mobility, and transfers (e.g., wheelchair, bed, car, shower, tub, toilet, chair, floor).[1]

A child's functional mobility can be affected in a variety of ways for any number of reasons. Some children have developmental delays that resolve with intensive early intervention services. Other children have mobility impairments and require external support in the form of orthotics or durable medical equipment, such

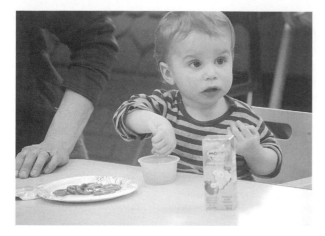

FIGURE 19-7 Self-feeding is an essential activity of daily living. Toddlers learn to hold utensils.

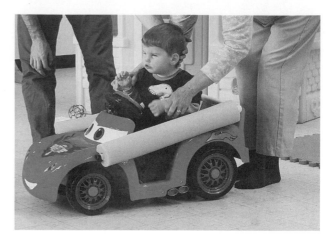

FIGURE 19-8 Toddler plays in adapted car to explore environment.

as a wheelchair, for mobility. In collaboration with the occupational therapist, the COTA determines the most appropriate intervention approach to enable a child to move from place to place to engage in meaningful activities. The child's goals (or desired outcomes), data from the evaluation, and evidence are considered when developing the intervention plan. Intervention approaches include health promotion, remediation and restoration, modification, or prevention.[1]

Health promotion intervention seeks to create and promote activity in the context of daily life.[1] An example of health promotion related to functional mobility is the efforts of pediatricians and early intervention providers to encourage "tummy time" to promote healthy infant motor development.[9] Another example of health promotion encourages children to play outside as a reaction to rising childhood obesity statistics related to sedentary activities.[6]

For some children, the intervention approach for functional mobility may require the OT practitioner to establish, remediate, or restore specific skills.[1] For example, the OT practitioner may work to develop the child's coordination and postural control for mobility. As children grow, there may be a variety of factors that influence skill acquisition. For some children, such as those with neurologic disorders (e.g., cerebral palsy), the use of positioning techniques and orthoses/splints can be used to maintain skills, including those required for functional mobility. Some children may require equipment to modify, compensate for, or adapt to limited movement, such as a brace, pediatric walker, or wheelchair. The needs of the child and the family should be taken into consideration when determining the most appropriate equipment. Infants and toddlers benefit from being able to explore their environments early. Adapting a play toy so the toddler can gain early mobility promotes learning and play (Figure 19-8).

Finally, prevention efforts may be aimed at eliminating potential barriers to occupational performance in the area of functional mobility. A simple prevention effort for a child who is gaining functional mobility but lacks adequate safety awareness includes environmental manipulation in the form of a gate to block off access to stairs or other dangers. Another example of prevention from a therapeutic standpoint is providing education to caregivers of children with neurologic conditions, such as a TBI, about the importance of proper bed and wheelchair positioning; ROM programs, to maintain proper joint alignment for control of abnormal tone and prevention of contractures, should also be provided.[13]

The needs of the child and the family ultimately drive the appropriate interventions for children with impairments that affect functional mobility. The pediatric OT practitioner should identify and build on the strengths of both the child and family. When designing an intervention approach, it is important to consider the various settings and contexts where the child or adolescent is likely to engage in functional mobility.[17]

CASE *Study*

Rosalie was born prematurely at 27 weeks gestation. She qualified for early intervention (EI) services on the basis of her premature birth and other risk factors, including her mother's advanced age and use of narcotics during pregnancy, as well as the family's qualification for a number of state-sponsored welfare services. A reevaluation revealed that Rosalie demonstrates significant developmental delays across all domains (cognitive, self-care, personal and social, fine and gross motor, and receptive and expressive language) and confirms her need for EI services. A developmental specialist is the service coordinator (SC) for the family. Rosalie is still not crawling at 11 months of age. The SC requests OT services to obtain greater expertise regarding gross motor development. After a consultation between the SC and an occupational therapist, it is clear that Rosalie is able to sit with a wide base of support but she cannot maintain trunk control in a facilitated quadruped position. The OT practitioner discovered that Rosalie is not exploring her environment because she is not yet mobile. Providing Rosalie with an adapted toy that serves as a scooter, enables her to move around (lying in prone position and moving her hands and legs) and find toys and objects of interest in the playroom. By showing Rosalie the possibilities, she is now beginning to demonstrate more interest in crawling and moving in the environment. The OT practitioner focuses on postural control each session and provides opportunities to reinforce the mobility Rosalie is beginning to acquire.

Personal Device Care

Personal device care is defined as "using, cleaning, and maintaining personal care items, such as hearing aids, contact lenses, glasses, orthotics, prosthetics, adaptive equipment, glucometers, and contraceptive and sexual devices."[1]

Younger children largely depend on their parents or caregivers to provide personal device care. As children get older, it may be appropriate to take a more active role in the management of their own personal device care. Additionally, managing **personal hygiene and grooming** becomes more important as the child grows older. This process may be difficult for children with disabilities who may not have adequate fine motor coordination. Some children have difficulties with the process skills of temporal organization as well as organization of space and objects, which affect the ability to complete the tasks involved in grooming.[15] OT practitioners may collaborate with nursing to enable children and youth to take care of personal devices as needed.

Personal Hygiene and Grooming

Personal hygiene and grooming is defined as "obtaining and using supplies; removing body hair (e.g., using razor, tweezers, lotion); applying and removing cosmetics; washing, drying, combing, styling, brushing, and trimming hair; caring for nails (hands and feet); caring for skin, ears, eyes, and nose; applying deodorant; cleaning mouth; brushing and flossing teeth; and removing, cleaning, and reinserting dental orthotics and prosthetics."[1] (See Figure 19-9 for child brushing teeth.)

A visual schedule is an approach that may be helpful in remediating such issues within this domain. The COTA may assist with creating a daily schedule to assist with personal hygiene and grooming, as well as personal device care. The visual schedule should be individualized, and the context of the task, as it relates to the client

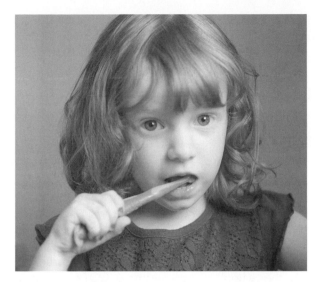

FIGURE 19-9 Brushing one's teeth is considered a task of personal hygiene.

and caregivers, should be taken into consideration. Pictures illustrate the steps in the process and can be posted in a logical place so that the child may utilize the visual aid. Constructing such a schedule often involves trial and error and may need to be amended many times until it works optimally for the child.[15]

A child's or adolescent's satisfaction with his or her own hygiene may often be different from that of the caregiver. It is important to educate the child on the benefits of good hygiene and work with both the child and the caregiver regarding the essential tasks and the frequency of performance.

Some children require modifications due to difficulties in the performance skills of strength and effort. Adaptive equipment may be indicated to promote increased independence for completion of grooming activities. For individuals with limited ability to grasp small handles, a universal cuff can be used to hold a toothbrush, comb, hair brush, or razor.[4,15] Some cuffs can be weighted to provide better control. For difficulties with grip strength, a built-up handle can be useful. Angled or long-handled brushes can be helpful to individuals with limited ROM. Bathroom faucet handles can be adapted to be easier to maneuver. Additional equipment that may assist an individual in completing grooming tasks include the electric toothbrush, floss holder, or water flosser.[15]

CASE *Study*
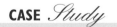

Sixteen-year-old Elliot has Asperger's syndrome. His parents sought OT services because he has difficulty completing his morning and evening hygiene routines in a timely fashion. Elliot worked with an OT practitioner who helped him develop a visual schedule—a number of pictures posted on a single large poster board—that hangs on his bedroom wall. Elliot is having difficulty accessing the visual schedule.

Sexual Activity

CASE *Study*

Damien is a 15-year-old student who lives at a residential school for adolescents with visual impairments. In addition, Damien has a diagnosis of autism. Since entering puberty, he has started to masturbate frequently in public places. This behavior not only makes other students and the staff uncomfortable, but also affects Damien's ability to effectively perform his educational tasks. In collaboration with the school support team, a COTA, under the supervision of an occupational therapist, develops a plan to address Damien's behavior. They begin by introducing the language of labeling "public or not private" and "private" spaces and teaching Damien to understand the difference. Every time he starts to touch himself in a public space, he is brought to his room or to a bathroom and he is taught that masturbation is something people do in a private place. The goal is that once Damien understands the difference, he will ask for private time when he needs it. Once this goal is accomplished, the team slowly has him wait longer and longer. For example, when he asks for private time, the staff member says, "One more (minute, half hour, etc.)." Slowly, Damien is able to increase the time he waits for private time so that the behavior becomes more manageable and appropriate. Damien is better able to attend to his educational occupation.

Sexual activity is defined as "engaging in activities that result in sexual satisfaction and/or meet relational or reproductive needs."[1, p. S19.] Sexual activity becomes an area of increasing importance as children approach adolescence. COTAs may encounter adolescents who may engage in socially inappropriate sexual behaviors, such as masturbating in public, without understanding why it makes others uncomfortable. In some cases, the role of the COTA may be to work with the adolescent to establish and encourage the appropriate context for sexual activity. Creating a plan for appropriate times and places to experience sexual relief can be empowering to the child and help avoid awkward situations.[15]

Sleep/Rest

CASE *Study*

Dora is 25 months old. Her parents have recently moved to a new city for career advancement opportunities. Dora's parents are concerned about her motor development.

She is evaluated by an interdisciplinary EI team. The evaluation results reveal that she has a gross motor delay that qualifies her for OT services through EI.

Dora's parents express concern that she wakes up in the middle of the night and is inconsolable unless she is allowed into her parent's bed. This behavior started shortly after the move when Dora began to wake up crying in the middle of the night. Her parents felt bad about uprooting her and allowed her in their bed to comfort her; however, it has gotten out of control and has now become a nightly occurrence. This has been affecting the entire family's ability to sleep through the night.

After careful evaluation and interview with the parents regarding nighttime rituals, the OT practitioner developed a plan with the parents. The parents' "guilt" regarding the move and anxiety has allowed them to comfort Dora and she enjoys sleeping in their bed. Although some families are comfortable with this, Dora's parents are not able to sleep with her in bed with them and, consequently, they are not getting adequate sleep. Dora is taking an extra long nap in the afternoon. To help the family readjust the bedtime routine, the OT practitioner suggests a gradual decline in the time Dora is allowed in the family bed. Furthermore, the parents will spend 30 minutes "snuggling" with Dora and reading a book before her bedtime, to provide her with the assurance and comfort she enjoys. When Dora awakes at night, the parents will start by only allowing her a short time (to be determined by them) in their bedroom. Dora will go back to her room for the night. Eventually Dora will not be able to go into their bedroom, but be comforted in her own room. The gradual decrease in time that she spends in their bed will help the family sleep patterns.

The OT practitioner considered the family values of having the child sleep in her own room through the night. Some families support a "family bed" and thus, it is important for the OT practitioner to consult based on the family's values.

Sleep/rest is defined as "a period of inactivity in which one may or may not suspend consciousness."[1, p. 520] Sleep is an occupation in its own right, and sleep disturbances have a serious effect on the quality of an entire family's life. Young children may experience sleep disturbances for a variety of reasons (e.g., anxiety, hunger, nutrition, illness, medication, habits). OT practitioners should consult with children and families after carefully evaluating sleep patterns and routines (Figure 19–10). Behavioral interventions may help change inconvenient sleep patterns. OT practitioners understand that knowing the factors contributing to the sleep disruptions is essential when developing a plan. Sensory diets may be helpful in regulating a child's sleep–wake cycle.

OT practitioners should record the time and pattern of sleep of children and their parents. This may reveal a variety of family issues and could indicate health issues of the child. Some medications may interfere with sleep patterns and consultation with a pharmacist may prove

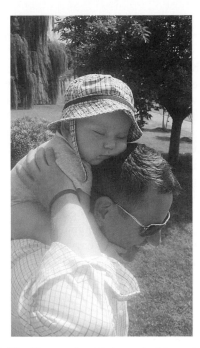

FIGURE 19-10 Sleep and rest is important to optimal occupational performance. Toddlers sleep throughout the day.

useful. Providing young adolescents with strategies to allow them to sleep and cope with anxiety can provide lifelong lessons and promote healthy habits. Sleep is important in coping and performing physical and cognitively and therefore it is essential that OT practitioners design interventions to establish healthy sleep patterns in children and youth.

SUMMARY

ADLs consist of very basic activities in which people engage, such as feeding, dressing, bathing, toileting, hygiene, and sexual activity. Rest and sleep is an occupation that helps the body heal and recover and it is essential for learning. These occupations make up a child and family's routines and when a disruption occurs, it affects not only the child but also the entire family. The OT practitioner plays a key role in enabling children to engage in ADLs and sleep/rest. Through collaboration and individualized intervention planning, OT practitioners provide remediation, compensation, and education strategies to promote engagement in daily living. This chapter provided case examples and descriptions illustrating a variety of ways in which an OT practitioner may facilitate ADL and sleep/rest performance.

References

1. American Occupational Therapy Association. (2014). Occupational therapy practice framework: domain and process (3rd ed.). *Am J Occup Ther, 68*(Suppl. 1), S1–S48.

2. Ayres, A. J. (1972). *Sensory integration and learning disorders.* Los Angeles: Western Psychological Services.

3. Bahr, D. C. (2001). *Oral motor assessment and treatment ages and stages.* Needham Heights, MA: Allyn and Bacon.

4. Desjardins, M., & Basante, J. (2013). Congenital anomalies/amputations/prostherics. In N. Falkenstein, & S. Weiss (Eds.), *Hand and upper extremity rehabilitation* (3rd ed.). St. Petersburg, FL: Exploring Hand Therapy Company.

5. Ernsperger, L., & Stegen-Hanson, T. (2004). *Just take a bite: easy, effective answers to food aversions and eating challenges.* Arlington, TX: Future Horizons.

6. Francis, K. (2007). Physiology and management of bladder and bowel continence following spinal cord injury. *Ostomy Wound Manage, 53,* 12.

7. Boyt-Schell, B., Gillen, G., Scaffa, M., & Cohn, E. (2013). In *Willard and Spackman's occupational therapy* (12th ed.). Philadelphia: Lippincott, Williams & Wilkins.

8. Guide for the Uniform Data Set for Medical Rehabilitation (including the FIM™ instrument), version 5.1. (1997). Buffalo, NY: Uniform Data System for Medical Rehabilitation.

9. Jennings, J. T., Sarbaugh, B. G., & Payne, N. S. (2005). Conveying the message about optimal infant positions. *Phys Occup Ther Pediatr, 25,* 3–17.

10. Kielhofher, G. (2008). Motives, patterns, and performance of occupation: basic concepts. In G. Kielhofner (Ed.). *A model of human occupation: theory and application* (4th ed.). Philadelphia: Lippincott Williams & Wilkins.

11. Lashgari, D., & Yasuda, L. (2006). Orthotics. In H. Pendleton, & W. Schultz-Krohn (Eds.). *Pedretti's occupational therapy practice skills for physical dysfunction* (6th ed.). St Louis: Elsevier.

12. Olsen, J. A. (2004). Mothering co-occupations in caring for infants and young children. In S. A. Esdaile, & J. A. Olson (Eds.). *Mothering occupations.* Philadelphia: FA Davis.

12a. Palmer, M. M. (1998). Weaning from gastrostomy tube feeding: Commentary on oral aversion. *Pediatr Nurs, 23(5),* 475–478.

13. Pearson, L. (1995). *Hands on, TeamRehab Report.* Available at: http://www.wheelchairnet.org/wcn_prodserv/Docs/TeamRehab/RR_95/9504 art2.PDF.

14. Shepherd Center Learning Connections. (2009). *Education model on spinal cord injury: autonomic dysreflexia.* Atlanta, GA: Shepherd Center Inc.

15. Shepherd, J. (2015). Activities of daily living. In J. Case-Smith, & J. O'Brien (Eds.). *Occupational therapy for children and adolescents* (7th ed.). St. Louis, MO: Elsevier.

16. Shoan, S. A., & Anderson, J. (1999). Neurodevelopmental treatment frame of reference. In P. Kramer, & J. Hinojosa (Eds.). *Frames of reference for pediatric occupational therapy* (2nd ed.). Philadelphia: Lippincott Williams & Wilkins.

17. Tieman, B. L., et al. (2004). Gross motor capability and performance of mobility in children with cerebral palsy: a comparison across home, school, and outdoors/community setting. *Phys Ther, 84,* 419–429.

18. Toglia, J. P. (2005). A dynamic interactional approach to cognitive rehabilitation. In N. Katz (Ed.). *Cognition and occupation across the life span: models for intervention in occupational therapy* (2nd ed.). Bethesda, MD: AOTA Press.

19. VanDahm, K. (2012). *Pediatric feeding disorders: evaluation and treatment.* Framington, MA: Therapro.

REVIEW *Questions*

1. What is a collaborative approach to intervention for ADLs and sleep/rest?
2. What activities are considered ADLs?
3. What is meant by co-occupation? Provide some examples of co-occupation.
4. Identify interventions that might be used when working with a child who has difficulties with dressing.
5. How is a compensatory approach used to address ADLs and sleep/rest?
6. What are some remediation activities to address ADLs and sleep/rest?
7. List the five different intervention approaches as outlined in the Occupational Therapy Practice Framework. Provide an example of each approach as used to address ADLs or sleep/rest issues.
8. What is the progression of toileting, dressing, feeding, and bathing?
9. How should the OT practitioner address swallowing issues in children?
10. What is functional mobility?
11. What are some positioning techniques for feeding?
12. What piece of adaptive equipment may be used during hygiene tasks for a client who has difficulty with grasping small objects?

SUGGESTED *Activities*

1. Using catalogs that have assistive technology devices and adaptive equipment for pediatrics, identify a minimum of two items that may be prescribed to promote independence in the following ADLs: bathing and showering, hygiene, bowel and bladder, feeding, dressing, and functional mobility.
2. Observe a variety of children (of different ages) eating and dressing. Discuss their ease and quality of performance as well as the developmental tasks.
3. Observe a child with special needs with regard to feeding and dressing. Discuss the motor performance and developmental tasks involved in this situation. Identify what you can do to make the tasks easier for the child.
4. Develop a list of survey questions regarding the sexual activities of teens. Interview an adolescent with special needs. Discuss overall findings in class.
5. Outline five strategies to improve ADLs. Describe the ADL clearly and examine the steps and motor, cognitive, and sensory requirements. Consider how you would make the tasks easier or more challenging for the child. Describe other factors an OT practitioner would consider before implementing the strategies.
6. Examine the sleep/rest patterns and routines of an infant, toddler, school-aged child, and adolescent. How do they differ? How might an OT practitioner intervene at each stage? What may be interfering with sleep patterns and routines?
7. Describe functional mobility options for toddlers, school-aged children and adolescents. What are the differences and how would these options promote exploration and mobility? Record the cost associated with each option.

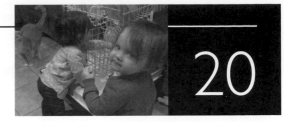

CARYN HUSMAN
BARBARA J. STEVA

Instrumental Activities of Daily Living

20

KEY TERMS

Instrumental activities of
  daily living
Cognitive functioning
Executive functioning
Deficit-specific training
Metacognitive training
Compensation
Social skill training
Task-specific training
Forward chaining
Backward chaining
Scaffolding
Augmentative and
  alternative
  communication
Voice output
  communication aids
Community mobility
Developmental stages of
  mobility
Money management
Fitness
Nutrition
Medication management

CHAPTER *Objectives*

After studying this chapter, the reader will be able to accomplish the following:
- Identify the instrumental activities of daily living (IADLs) and describe how they relate to occupational performance in children and adolescents
- Describe therapeutic activities that an occupational therapy practitioner might use to address difficulties in occupational performance in the IADLs
- Describe adaptations that may be used to improve a child's performance in the IADLs
- Describe intervention strategies that may be used to improve a child's performance in the IADLs

CHAPTER *Outline*

CHAPTER *Outline*—continued

The profession of occupational therapy is defined by its unique focus on "everyday life activities," known clinically as occupations.[5] Occupational therapy (OT) practitioners work to assist adults and children in a wide variety of occupations, thus facilitating opportunities for satisfaction, competence in roles, health, wellness, and quality of life.[5]

Instrumental activities of daily living (IADLs) are defined by the American Occupational Therapy Association (AOTA) as "activities to support daily life within the home and community that often require more complex interactions than those used in ADLs."[5] IADLs comprise an area of occupation that includes activities that are focused on interaction with the environment.[5] More specifically, IADLs involve care of others, care of pets, childrearing, communication management, driving and community mobility, financial management, health management and maintenance, home establishment, meal preparation and cleanup, religious and spiritual activities and expression, safety and emergency maintenance, and shopping. Explanations of these categories, as described by the AOTA Practice Framework are found in Table 20-1.

IADLs are typically multifaceted patterns of occupation. Each occupation can be divided into several tasks, each requiring specific skills. To develop individualized intervention strategies, goals, objectives, and outcomes, the OT practitioner considers the performance skills, performance patterns, and bodily functions; specific task analyses; individual values, roles, and interests; and current barriers to independence for each child. By their very nature, IADLs are optional and may be completed by another person.[5] In particular, IADLs may be optional for children, depending on age, family culture, and culture of the community in which they live. However, performance in IADLs is pivotal for independent living as an adult. Therefore the promotion of skills and independence in this area cannot be understated, especially in the case of children with disabilities as they grow.

This chapter explores the factors and considerations regarding interventions for children and adolescents with cognitive, physical, visual, and communication challenges in the area of IADLs.

COGNITIVE AND EXECUTIVE FUNCTIONING

The OT practitioner assesses the presence and potential impact of any cognitive or physical impairment that could prevent the individual's achievement of independence in a particular skill. Deficits in fine or gross motor skills, strength and endurance, active range of motion (AROM), balance and positioning are assessed, treated and monitored throughout the intervention period.

Due to the complex nature of IADLs, OT practitioners evaluate **cognitive functioning**, particularly **executive functioning**, to develop appropriate goals, objectives, and intervention plans. Children with cognitive impairments often express a decreased awareness of cognitive limitations that could affect realistic goal setting and adjustment to a disability.[51] *Executive functioning* is a term used to describe a set of cognitive abilities located in the frontal cortex of the brain. More specifically, the frontal lobe provides organization and control for all cognitive skills. Cooper-Kahn and Dietzel (2008) described executive functioning as a set of processes that include the following:

- Inhibition: the ability to stop one's actions and thoughts at an appropriate time;
- Shift: the ability to think freely and move from one situation to another to respond appropriately;
- Emotional control: the ability to regulate emotional responses by thinking and responding rationally;
- Initiation: the ability to begin a task, generate ideas, responses, and problem-solving strategies;
- Working memory: the ability to hold information in the mind to use for completing a task;
- Planning/orientation: the ability to manage present and future oriented tasks;
- Organization of materials: the ability to impose order on work, play, and storage spaces; and
- Self-monitoring: the ability to monitor self-performance and measure it against a standard of what is needed and/or expected.[16]

Children with challenges in one or more of these areas may struggle to plan a project, tell a story with details or in sequential order, memorize or recall information, initiate and complete tasks, and retain information while doing another task (recall a phone number while dialing). Although executive functioning is used

TABLE 20-1

Definitions of Instrumental Activities of Daily Living Areas

CATEGORY	DEFINITION
Care of others (including selecting and supervising caregivers)	Arranging, supervising, or providing the care for others
Care of pets	Arranging, supervising, or providing the care for pets and service animals
Childrearing	Providing the care and supervision to support the developmental needs of a child
Communication management	Sending, receiving, and interpreting information using a variety of systems and equipment, including writing tools, telephones (cell phones or smartphones), keyboards, audiovisual recorders, computers or tablets, communication boards, call lights, emergency systems, Braille writers, telecommunication devices for deaf people, augmentative communication systems, and personal digital assistants
Driving and community mobility	Planning and moving around in the community and using public or private transportation, such as driving, walking, bicycling, or accessing and riding in buses, taxi cabs, or other transportation systems
Financial management	Using fiscal resources, including alternative methods of financial transaction and planning, and using finances with long- and short-term goals
Health management and maintenance	Developing, managing, and maintaining routines for health and wellness promotion, such as physical fitness, nutrition, decreased health-risk behaviors, and medication routines
Home establishment and management	Obtaining and maintaining personal and household possessions and environment (e.g., home, yard, garden, appliances, vehicles), including maintaining and repairing personal possessions (e.g., clothing and household items) and knowing how to seek help or whom to contact
Meal preparation and cleanup	Planning, preparing, and serving well-balanced, nutritional meals and cleaning up food and utensils after meals
Religious and spiritual activities and expression	Participating in religion, "an organized system of beliefs, practices, rituals, and symbols designed to facilitate closeness to the sacred or transcendent,"[33] and engaging in activities that allow a sense of connectedness to something larger than oneself
Safety and emergency maintenance	Knowing and performing preventive procedures to maintain a safe environment; recognizing sudden, unexpected hazardous situations; and initiating emergency action to reduce the threat to health and safety; examples include ensuring safety when entering and exiting the home, identifying emergency contact numbers, and replacing items such as batteries in smoke alarms and light bulbs
Shopping	Preparing shopping lists (grocery and other); selecting, purchasing, and transporting items; selecting method of payment; and completing money transactions; included are Internet shopping and related use of electronic devices such as computers, cell phones, and tablets

From American Occupational Therapy Association. (2014). Occupational therapy practice framework: domain and process (3rd ed.). *Am J Occup Ther,* 68(Suppl. 1), 19-20.

continually in daily occupations, it is difficult to evaluate all the aspects that this term encompasses. In addition to formalized test batteries, observation and "hands-on" assessment of task completion are invaluable to the practitioner. Brown, Moore, Hemman, and Yunek found that client reports of independence and actual performance were not always consistent.[9] Real-life experiences were found to be more complex than those portrayed in simulations or in the interview process. The OT practitioner may need to adapt an activity or teach the child to use a compensatory strategy for absent or impaired skills.

Intervention Strategies

Intervention strategies aimed at improving IADL performance for children with impaired cognitive skills can include deficit-specific training, metacognitive training, compensation, social skills training, and task-specific training.

- **Deficit-specific training** involves restoring or improving specific cognitive tasks such as attention, initiation, and problem solving through remedial exercises, grading of tasks, and gradually increasing demands on cognitive performance components.[51]
- **Metacognitive training** works to improve the fundamentals needed to set realistic goals by enhancing self-awareness and skills such as time management, self-control, anticipation, and self-monitoring.
- **Compensation** teaches the child to use alternative methods or strategies to complete a given task. Children can use lists, memory notebooks,

electronic cuing devices, diaries, wall charts, and picture schedules.

- **Social skill training** involves improving interpersonal skills such as nonverbal cues, verbal and nonverbal communication skills, and conflict negotiation skills.
- **Task-specific training**, also referred to as functional skill training, involves systematic training of specific tasks required to complete an activity.

A combination of these techniques may be needed to achieve the most efficient and functional outcomes. Figure 20-1 shows the OT practitioner engaging a child in a craft activity to work on organizing, planning, sequencing, fine motor ability, and problem solving

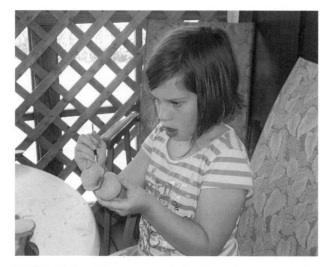

FIGURE 20-1   OT practitioners help children learn to organize, plan, problem solve, and sequence actions to carry out instrumental activities of daily living. Engaging in craft activities is fun for many children and can help them to learn motor and cognitive skills required for instrumental activities of daily living.

required for IADLs. Children enjoy craft activities and this serves as a meaningful activity to develop a variety of skills.

When working with cognitive functioning, the OT practitioner also conducts activity analysis to divide each task into parts and determine specific skill areas the child might be lacking. The OT practitioner may use forward or backward chaining to teach a task. Chaining involves dividing the task into individual steps, teaching each step, and finally putting the steps together. **Forward chaining** involves teaching the task from beginning to end, whereas **backward chaining** involves teaching the task from the last step to the first step. For example, tying shoe laces may be taught using forward chaining, where the child is taught first to tie the initial knot, then to make a loop, wrap the other lace around the loop, push the lace through the hole to make another loop, and finally pull both loops. When using backward chaining, children complete only the last step of pulling the loops to finish the task. Next, they combine the last two steps of pushing the lace through the hole and pulling the loops to complete the task. The OT practitioner continues to add the previous step of the task until the child can completely perform the task.

Figure 20-2 illustrates backward chaining. The OT practitioner in this case gathers all the materials, provides hand-over-hand assistance for scooping, and allows the child to bring the spoon to his mouth and complete self-feeding.

Another way of adapting an activity is to provide faded assistance or grading. This involves providing assistance for all, or a portion, of the activity. As the child improves, assistance is "faded" to encourage the child to perform more of the activity independently. Faded assistance may occur in the form of physical assist or grading

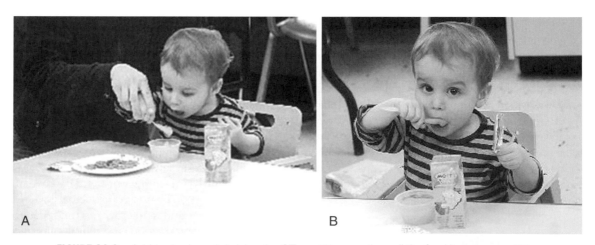

FIGURE 20-2   **A,** Using backward chaining, the OT practitioner gathers all the food items, opens all the containers and prepares the materials. The practitioner uses hand-over-hand assistance to scoop the food. **B,** The child completes the self-feeding task by bringing the spoon to his mouth.

of the activity in the form of adaptations or accommodations to the size of objects, speed, frequency or duration of the activity, height and angle at which the activity is performed, number of steps, complexity, and sensory components of the activity. Verbal and/or physical cues or prompts can be provided to assist the child to recall a specific technique or sequence.

Assistive technology helps children with motor impairments access their living space through environmental control for lights, TV, or other electronic devices. Environmental adaptations such as the positioning of furniture or using positioning or mobility devices can assist children to navigate their environment and complete tasks they may otherwise be unable to complete.

Throughout the assessment and intervention process, the OT practitioner monitors the level of supervision and/or assistance. This includes the ability of the child to perform transfers to and from positions, equipment, and through the environment/community. It is important to collaborate with physical therapy practitioners when assessing the mobility needs of children. The level of assistance a child requires to transfer can change throughout the therapy process as strength, endurance, and cognitive skills improve or decline. The OT practitioner is responsible for educating family and others in how to perform transfers with care taken to ensure proper body mechanics. Types of transfers commonly provided are outlined in Table 20-2. They are required for the child to complete the task safely and successfully. It is important to maintain close communication with family and caregivers of the child to ensure safe follow through of activities outside of the therapy session.

DEVELOPMENTAL CONSIDERATIONS AND TRANSITION

IADLs, particularly home management and meal preparation, are essential for eventual independent living.[18] Typically developing children begin these tasks at age 4 to 6 years, taking on increasing independence from ages 11 to 14. Frequently, children with disabilities begin working on IADL skills later than typically developing children; however, they may need more time with practice to gain mastery. Therefore it is important for children with disabilities to begin engaging in IADLs in the early years. Not only does it help prepare them to transition to adult roles, participation in IADLs in the home also allows the child to socialize with and contribute to their family.[18]

Intervention Strategies

Often, the OT practitioner helps children gain IADL skills most efficiently in the natural setting.[19] The practitioner

TABLE 20-2

Transfers for Safe Movement in the Environment

TYPE OF TRANSFER	
INDEPENDENT	
Assisted	**Close guard**
Minimal assist: Child performs ≥75% of the activity	Child can typically perform the activity without assistance but may require assistance at some point during the transfer
Moderate assist: Child performs ≥50% of the activity	Practitioner is in close proximity to the child, immediately ready to assist
Maximum assist: Child performs <25% of the activity	**Contact guard** Child can perform the activity but has a good likelihood of requiring physical assistance at some point during the transfer Practitioner maintains contact with the child, prepared to provide assistance immediately
	Sliding board Child has enough strength to lift most of the weight off the buttocks and enough sitting balance to move across a surface in a seated position Practitioner maintains close or contact guard position, depending on the ability of the child
DEPENDENT	
One-person lift Two-person lift Mechanical lift	Child is unable to provide meaningful assistance in the transfer Practitioner lifts the child using the appropriate method based on size, weight and environmental conditions in which the transfer is occurring

Pierce, S. L. (2013). Restoring functional and community mobility. In M. V. Radomski & C. A. Trombly (Eds.), *Occupational therapy for physical dysfunction.* Baltimore, MD: Lippincott Williams & Wilkins.

can match the child's specific motor, cognitive, and perceptual abilities to IADL tasks,[43] and provide assistance to the family to determine how to integrate tasks into daily life. The OT practitioner also provides consultation to set realistic goals, challenges, and supports, and to help parents gain skills to help their child as needed. Early facilitation of IADL skill acquisition in the home occurs through play and the parental process of **scaffolding**. OT practitioners target IADLs through scaffolding by engaging children in pretend play and daily household chores. Adults can begin by allowing children to play with the materials used for IADLs and pretend that they are completing the tasks. Next, adults can allow children to do the tasks with them, and then finally allow them to do part of or the entire task independently.[43] Even if adults need to go back and complete some part of the task after the child has finished his or her work, allowing the child to participate in IADLs in their natural setting contributes to skill building and mastery. As children prepare to transition to adulthood, it is important for the OT practitioner to focus on the child's strengths and what he or she is able to do[58] as opposed to his or her deficits. Children with disabilities also must learn to manage and supervise the actions of others so that they can direct their own care.[18] The OT practitioner can facilitate IADLs by giving opportunities for the child to direct the caregiver, and teaching metacognition by asking questions and reflecting on the process of IADLs. Metacognitive and reflective questions include, "What should I do next?" "How did that go?" "Is there anything I should have done differently?" and "How could I do that better?" Building connections in the community is also essential for success.[58]

CASE *Study*

Julie is an 18-year-old high school student. At the age of 16, she was hit by a car while riding her bicycle without a helmet and suffered a traumatic brain injury. Although her residual physical impairments were mild, she continued to be challenged by decreased organization and memory. She received OT services at school, and she and her educational/OT therapy team identified goals that include improved independence in self-organization. Julie has significant difficulty organizing herself at school with respect to homework assignments and class schedules. A memory book/daily planner was provided to assist Julie in organizing activities, although she continued to be forgetful and leave the book in her locker or at home. Julie enjoyed using her cell phone to text and talk with her friends, and was seldom seen without the device. The OT practitioner and Julie worked together to program the phone as a memory aid. Julie learned to access and use the daily planner on the phone, "To Do" lists were set up, and an alarm was programmed to remind Julie of important events. The OT practitioner provided faded assistance in the form of verbal cues, which were then faded to written directions, to help Julie program important events and assignments into the phone. The educational team provided verbal cues to prompt Julie to use the aid during the school day, and the cues were faded as she became more independent. The team also worked with Julie's parents to develop and implement a rewards program for successful use of the cell phone as a memory/organization aid. Each day, whenever Julie used her memory aid independently, she was rewarded with additional computer or video game time

at home, a preferred activity that was typically time limited. Julie's independent organization improved at school and in the community. In time, Julie became more proficient at programming and accessing the aid independently.

COMMUNICATION MANAGEMENT

Communication is an integral part of participation in all daily tasks. Many children receiving OT experience difficulty communicating due to their disabilities or injuries.[22] Communication devices compensate for that difficulty and allow for participation in work, leisure, and social occupations. Communication devices support independence, facilitate greater engagement in learning and progress toward goals, and contribute significantly to occupational performance and quality of life.[56] Furthermore, devices help children with disabilities to socialize, get information, and develop cognitive skills thereby promoting development and decreasing negative behavioral concerns.

Communication devices provide **augmentative and alternative communication** (AAC) to children who are unable to communicate effectively.[47] Children with autism, apraxia, or physical disabilities such as cerebral palsy that prevent the oral structures from being coordinated fluidly for speaking are candidates for a communication device. Children with hearing impairments can use a communication device to communicate with those outside their community without the help of an interpreter. A wide range of communication devices, from low-tech to complex high-tech options, is available. Low-tech communication devices include systems that do not require a form of power for operation, such as an alphabet board, communication board, or book.[22] Mainstream technology including laptops and cell phones can be adapted to provide options for AAC. Other high-tech devices store information and produce auditory communications. High-tech devices are able to store information and produce auditory communications.[21] These devices are also known as speech-generating devices or **voice output communication aids** (VOCAs).

Although communication is classically the realm of the speech and language pathologist, the OT practitioner is an important team member in the selection and training of a communication device. The team considers many different methods, body parts, and sites of control for access of AAC.[22] The OT practitioner assists with the selection of equipment that best fits the child's movement abilities by assessing ROM, motor control, positioning, endurance, visual-perceptual skills, and personal preferences.[22,45,47] The most common and direct method for accessing communication devices requires the use of the upper extremity for operation.[22] If upper extremity movement does not enable the use of a device, children may be able to access AAC through a mouth or head stick, head tracking, eye gaze, and speech recognition technologies.[22] Once the device has been selected, the OT practitioner sets up the child's environment to facilitate ease of use and ergonomic function and works as part of the team to train the child to use the equipment effectively.

Telephones

The telephone and cell phone are the most commonly used communication devices. Children with disabilities can use these devices to ensure safety and security. Cell phone features can be set up to benefit people with motor challenges. One-key dialing, speakerphone, and more rugged phones may be helpful. A common, widely available cell phone adaption is the large number pad. Cell phones can also allow access to text-to-speech applications, and can be adapted with speech-generating technology. Children without the fine motor control necessary to access a cell phone in the typical manner can use eye gaze and scanning switch technology.[22]

Children may require training and repetition for effective use of a cell phone. Picture cards that demonstrate the steps of making a call may be helpful and can be attached to the phone by a key ring. Important phone numbers such as home and emergency numbers should be programmed for one-key dialing or a one-step process. Other phone numbers or the key to the phone's speed dial also can be included on the card attached to the phone. If the child is unable to use the phone to call multiple numbers, the phone can be programmed to call one number only. Families can consult with their cell phone providers for further information.

Low-tech Communication Boards

Low-tech communication boards are simple and inexpensive pieces of equipment for augmenting communication. They are often the first support used to increase a child's ability to communicate. Communication boards may contain pictures of items or activities a child may want or need. In the early stages, the child may use the board to make choices. This is especially effective for children with physical disabilities who are unable to access their environments independently due to motor limitations. Using a communication board, the child is able to indicate with what toys or areas of the room he or she wishes to interact.

More complex communication boards may be suitable for children who lack the motor control to speak and type quickly but have the cognitive ability to communicate and spell. These boards contain frequently used phrases and the letters of the alphabet. The child points to the letters or words with his or her hands, mouth stick, or light pointer to indicate what he or she would like to communicate. Although these systems can be effective, they require an active and participating listener and can be laborious to use. However, they may also be an important first step in facilitating communication and can demonstrate the child's ability to use their cognitive and motor skills to communicate.

Communication boards contain words or hand-drawn, computer-illustrated, or photographic pictures. Several programs that provide a wide range of high-quality illustrations and commonly used pictures are available. Communication boards often come with Velcro so that pictures can be held in place or moved as needed. Picture books organize pictures for communication. Books allow access to a greater number of pictures than communication boards and may be organized by topic for quick and easy location of pictures. Velcro is often placed on the outer cover of the book so that the pictures currently in use can be displayed on the front of the book.

Note: The use of pictures for a communication board should not be confused with the Picture Exchange Communication System, which is explained in greater detail later in this section (Tables 20-3 and 20-4).

Using Pictures to Communicate to the Child

Pictures can also be used as visual supports to assist the OT practitioner in communicating with children.[10] These pictures are called *visual supports* in this text to avoid confusing them with communication boards that children use to communicate their thoughts. When a child uses pictures to function, it is important that the OT practitioner consult with teachers and parents so that the system can be used across various settings.

TABLE 20-3
Common Methods for Using Pictures for Communication During Daily Tasks and Occupational Therapy Sessions

METHOD	DESCRIPTION
Indicating wants and needs	Pictures of daily tasks and items in the environment can allow a child to communicate his or her desired and needed items within those daily tasks, such as what he or she wants to play with, what he or she wants to eat, and to use the bathroom. Eventually a child can be taught to comment when he or she is tired or hungry.
Building words or sentences	Once a person learns to discriminate the pictures, he or she is taught to build sentences, exchange, and point to the pictures on the sentence strip.

Modified from PECS USA: What is PECS? Available at: http://www.pecsusa.com/pecs.php; and Frost, L., & Bondy, A. (2002) *Picture Exchange Communication System training manual,* (2nd ed.). Newark, DE: Pyramid Educational Consultants..

TABLE 20-4

Visual Supports for Participation, Regulation, and Emotional/Behavioral Development

VISUAL SUPPORT	DESCRIPTION
Activity schedule	Pictures may be placed on a strip or page to show the number and order of activities expected. When each activity is completed, the pictures are removed or shifted to another area that indicates the activity is "all done."
First/Then	Two pictures indicate activities that come first and second. This can be an effective motivator if an unfavored activity is followed by a favorite task. For example, use the bathroom and then play a game.
Choice making	Pictures are presented so that a child can choose an activity, toy, or snack. Many or few pictures can be presented, and choices can be made based on therapeutic effect and therapist intentions.
Breakdown of tasks into steps for teaching and independence	Pictures represent the steps of a task. This can increase independence and attention for multistep actions and activities. Examples include grooming sequences, setting the table, or steps for production line work.
Communication of feelings	Pictures of facial expressions can assist children with understanding and identifying their emotions.
Visuals to accompany songs	Pictures that represent verses of songs allow children of all abilities to participate in songs and help explain what the words mean in a concrete manner.
Visuals for support during emotional dysregulation	When children are emotionally dysregulated, they may have difficulty taking in auditory information from others. Pictures may allow people working with them to communicate safe and regulating alternatives to unsafe behavior.
Social stories	Social stories are written about future events that may be difficult for a child to tolerate such as going to a busy store or going trick-or-treating. Pictures are frequently used to make the story easier to understand. These are especially effective for children who have autism spectrum disorders.
Support for visual impairment	Large pictures provide directions for individuals who have difficulty reading small print.

Adapted from Bryan, L. C., & Gast, D. L. (2000). Teaching on-task and on-schedule behaviors to high-functioning children with autism via picture activity schedules. *J Autism Develop Dis, 30*(6), 553–567.

Visual supports are commonly used to communicate expectations, show how many activities are expected, and demonstrate the order of activities.[10] Visual supports can increase on-task behaviors; be used to teach complex topics such as arousal or excitement levels by presenting symbols that young people can understand and relate to; increase self-awareness of emotions and arousal/excitement levels; and be used to augment social stories to ensure children know how to respond and act safely in challenging situations.[10]

OT practitioners consult with a speech and language pathologist on the use of pictures for children (Table 20-5).

CLINICAL *Pearl*

Picture schedules can help structure the therapy session if a child is impulsive or distractible. They can also be useful when a child is avoidant of therapy tasks or has difficulty tolerating nonfavored activities.

Picture Exchange Communication System

The Picture Exchange Communication System (PECS) was created to increase communication for individuals with autism spectrum disorders.[40] PECS has also been found effective for other populations with cognitive, communication, and physical disabilities. The system is put in place by a speech and language pathologist and used under the supervision and guidance of that specialist. Nevertheless, it is important for OT practitioners to have knowledge of the program, which is widely used.

PECS is a systematic method for teaching initiation of communication through the exchange of pictures.[40] Through PECS, a child is taught to use communication to get his or her needs met. The goal is to teach the child to use communication independently. The system is not necessarily a replacement for speech; frequently young children who begin using the program also begin to use vocal language.[40] The OT practitioner continues to use language with a child who uses PECS. However, basic use of the protocol reinforces the work done in speech therapy and improves OT sessions and outcomes (Table 20-6).

TABLE 20-5

Using Pictures or Illustrations During Intervention

TYPES OF PICTURES	PROS	CONS
Photographs	Photographs are necessary for children who do not understand the symbolism of other pictures. They provide an exact communication of objects, people, and places.	Use of photographs requires time and resources, including a compatible digital camera and computer, or actual photographs.
Programs such as Boardmaker®	These programs provide clearly drawn, universally understood symbols for communication. They may be transferred to a variety of settings and are commonly used in school settings.	The program must be purchased and may be expensive. The OT practitioner must learn the computer program for ease of use.
Pictures from the Internet or magazines	Pictures are readily available on the Internet and in magazines.	The quality of the image may vary. Copyright laws must be adhered to.
Hand-drawn pictures	Hand-drawn pictures are readily available and may convey messages for which a specific illustration does not exist.	Quality will vary with drawing skill. Some children may not understand the symbolism of hand-drawn pictures.

TABLE 20-6

Phases of the Picture Exchange Communication System

PHASE	DESCRIPTION
Phase 1	The child is taught to initiate communication by presenting a picture to obtain a desired object such as a toy or a snack. The desired object is provided immediately to reinforce the communication exchange. During this phase only one picture is used, and the child is not asked to determine which picture matches what he or she wants.
Phase 2	The child is taught to initiate communication when others are not readily available and waiting for the picture exchange. To do so, the child is taught to obtain the picture and go to another person to request the object in exchange for the picture. The practitioner begins by standing close by and then moves farther away to make the child persist in the effort to communicate.
Phase 3	The child is taught to distinguish between pictures to get the desired item. Initially, the child distinguishes between two very different pictures such as a snack (a preferred item) and a sock (a nonpreferred or contextually irrelevant item). As the child is successful, more preferred and numerous pictures are presented. These pictures are placed in a binder with loop-and-hook fastener so the student can flip through the pages, find the picture of the desired item, and exchange it.
Phase 4	The child is taught to use a sentence strip. The child places a picture denoting "I want" and the item or activity that he or she wants and exchanges the entire strip with the other person, such as "I want ball."
Phase 5	The child is taught to respond to the question "What do you want?"
Phase 6	The child is taught to make comments about the environment such as "I see" or "I hear."
Continued expansion of vocabulary	The child is taught to use adjectives, verbs, and prepositions to describe the things he or she wants or notices.

Modified from Frost, L., & Bondy, A. (2002). *The Picture Exchange Communication System training manual,* (2nd ed.). Newark, DE: Pyramid Educational Consultants.

High-tech Voice Output Communication Aids

A wide range of high-tech devices and software is available to augment communication for people with disabilities. These include small, handheld devices that contain a few messages; larger devices that are portable, are mountable on wheelchairs, and store large amounts of vocabulary; and complex systems that can be used with computers to export any message the child can type. The handheld and larger portable devices are usually the first high-tech devices used with children, who must learn to use the devices as they are learning to communicate and use vocabulary. It is important that their continued development is taken into account when selecting a Voice Output Communication Aid (VOCA).

VOCAs are the specific hardware that the child accesses for communication. These high-tech communication boards work in the same way as low-tech boards: the child accesses a picture or symbol to communicate with others. However, when the child accesses a picture or symbol on a VOCA, the device releases an audible message so that others can hear it when the child wishes to communicate.

Small devices present a limited number of pictures, sometimes as few as three or five. When activated, the device plays a frequently used sentence or message such as "I want to play" or "I need to go to the bathroom." Some of these devices are able to record specific messages and can therefore be useful for including children who have difficulties with typical occupations of childhood such as giving an oral report or acting in a school play. More complex systems comprise several menus that present words or messages within a theme. The child is able to access many words or messages for each theme. The child first selects a topic from a main menu page and then is able to access a number of words or messages about that theme. For example, the child might access a food theme, in which several choices of favorite foods and snacks are presented. Common themes for young children include foods, bathroom, greetings, weather, songs, and toys. As communication and the use of the device develop, an ever-expanding array of themes may be programmed on complex VOCA. VOCAs can be accessed by a variety of means so that a child can communicate using whichever part of the body he or she is best able to move. If the child has controlled movement of the upper extremity, he or she can access the symbols with fingers on a touch screen. If less volitional movement is available, the child may use a switch to select the appropriate symbol.[30] Switches can be accessed through paddles that are pushed by any part of the body where controlled movement exists. This might be the hand, elbow, or side of the head. Puff-and-sip configurations can be set up for the child who is unable to move any of the limbs in a controlled manner.[30]

OT practitioners play a vital role in teaching children to use switches.[30] First, the OT practitioner provides experiences to help the child learn that the switch causes something to happen. This is most easily achieved with a cause-and-effect toy that moves, lights up, and/or makes sound when the switch it activated. Once the child understands the concept thoroughly, the switch can be used to operate a highly motivating phrase. In the case of some children, this might be "I want a snack" or simply "Hello." Next, the child works with more than one switch to produce more than one communication. In later stages, the OT practitioner works with the child to use the switch to select a picture from the screen of a high-tech VOCA. A common set-up includes a cursor on a screen that moves among various pictures. The child works to press the switch as it lands on a specific picture. In this way, the OT practitioner prepares the child to use technology to select whole words and phrases in a complex communication system.[30]

Other alternative methods for accessing VOCAs include pointers and eye-tracking devices. Pointers may use light-beam or infrared technology to select symbols.[14] Eye-tracking devices follow the movement and gazing of the eyes to select symbols and messages.[8] These adaptations require a significant level of head and eye control as well as high-level cognitive skills.[14]

CASE *Study*

Carl began attending a special purpose preschool program soon after turning 3 years old, when he was diagnosed with autism. He did not use words to communicate at home or in school. When he was strongly motivated to get something, he took an adult's hand to lead him or her to the desired object. In school, Carl rarely displayed interest in free-play activities; he needed direct facilitation from a teacher or an OT practitioner to engage in play activities for short periods. Carl also cried frequently and threw tantrums; at times he was extremely difficult to console. The speech and language practitioner (SLP) introduced the PECS system to the school program. The OT practitioner first worked with the SLP to help Carl learn to use the system. The team used motivating activities and snacks to encourage Carl to use the pictures for communication. The OT practitioner incorporated short activities, cause-and-effect toys, and sensory activities to encourage Carl to participate and communicate during this phase of learning the system. After Carl learned the system, the OT practitioner carried over the use of PECS into other activities such as free play, playground time, and snack. The SLP and the OT practitioner consulted with Carl's teacher and parents to further generalize the use of PECS. Several months later, Carl independently accessed his PECS picture book to request food, toys, and games. He became more engaged and compliant with classroom and therapy activities. He also showed a marked decrease in crying and tantrum episodes across settings. Carl's vocal language, however, did not develop further. Therefore he was evaluated for a VOCA for future use.

Computer Systems for Communication

Computers allow children to communicate via email, blogs, and programs that convert text to audible speech.[8] Many modifications are available so that children can access keyboards and mouse pointers.[8]

Alternative keyboards increase the ease with which a person who has a disability can type.[8] Keyboards may be enlarged or constricted to allow for more success with the keys. The order of the letters also may be customized, so that the most frequently used keys are situated in the home row, or the most important keys clustered in the center for one-finger typing. Keyboards can be designed for use with one or two hands. Furthermore, keyboards can be programmed to produce words or phrases when a combination of keys is pressed. Other adaptations include moisture guards, overlays to increase visual contrast or tactile feedback, and rigid overlays to prevent pressing the wrong buttons.[8]

Computers may be accessed through nontraditional mouse arrangements if the user is unable to effectively use a mouse.[8] A track ball may be helpful for children with limited movement of the upper extremity, but accurate movement at the fingers. The track ball also may be appropriate for the child with full ROM, but who lacks the motor control or stability to move the whole hand or arm to move a standard mouse. Alternatively, a computer screen can be accessed through the use of a switch. Again, a cursor moves between different areas of the screen and the child presses the switch when the cursor pauses on the appropriate area. A child may also use a stick or pointer as a mouse; software is available to interpret head movement as movement of the pointer across the screen.[8] In addition, eye gaze and infrared programs are available for the child with the ability to gaze into a camera in a controlled manner.[8,14] (see Chapter 27 for additional information).

iPad and Tablet Technology

Tablets are common devices in homes, schools, and the community. They are easy to access and do not carry any stigma. Tablet applications have been used to increase social play with children with autism.[35] Tablets are also used for instruction in special education school settings. With the technological advances in communication devices, tablets have also become an increasingly common AAC device that can be accessed by a variety of modes and used for a variety of communications.[22] Tablets can be accessed by tactile means, mouth or head sticks, head or eye gaze, or voice. Tablets can be mounted to a wheelchair for easy independent access. They can be used for digital communication, information storage, and speech generation.

COMMUNITY MOBILITY AND DRIVING

A child's role in regard to **community mobility** changes through the life span and is dependent on the life role and interests of the individual. Progression may involve a car seat/stroller > walking > tricycle/bicycle > school bus > public transportation > driving > dependency on others for transportation and mobility.[48] The clinician should assess client factors to best prepare and modify the human and nonhuman aspects of the environment for access. Human factors may include disability, values, or interests, whereas nonhuman factors involve physical barriers and accessibility.

Developmental Stages of Mobility

The OT practitioner should take into consideration the **developmental stages of mobility** when planning intervention. The infant and toddler typically take on the role of a passenger. The young child begins to explore mobility by creeping and walking. Transportation to and from school on a school bus or on public transportation becomes a focus for the school-aged child. At this time, the child often explores his or her community when riding a bicycle or scooter. As the child grows, increased importance is placed on safety and judgment as the child begins to explore the environment more independently. Crossing the street, reading and understanding street signs and signals, and negotiating curbs and obstacles within the environment become important to independence and safe community mobility. The adolescent and young adult incorporate all of these developed skills as they find independence and autonomy preparing to drive or navigate public transportation.[5] Ultimately, mobility is a necessary life component that leads to better quality of life, fulfillment of roles, access to leisure activities, and engagement in meaningful activities. To provide effective intervention, it is necessary to assess on an ongoing basis the child's strengths and needs in performance areas specific to the mode of mobility that the child is seeking. Visual perception, motor coordination, muscle strength, sensory regulation, and executive functioning affect the successful and independent participation of a child's mobility within the community. Adaptations in the form of mobility devices, supplemental aids, or modifications to the environment may be necessary to attain optimal independence. The child or the caregiver and the OT practitioner work together to develop individualized treatment goals, objectives, and a specific treatment plan to address the child's mobility needs.

Transportation for the Infant, Toddler, and Young Child

The National Highway Traffic Safety Administration (NHTSA) provides clear guidelines for the safe transport of infants, toddlers, and young children.[38] Car seat manufacturers provide detailed weight and age limits specific to each particular seat. Installation methods for car seats vary, and manufacturer instructions should be followed, without exception, when installing the seat in a vehicle. The role of the OT practitioner is to assess the child's physical needs and make recommendations as to the type of seat required. Although no adaptations or modifications should be made that will change the structural integrity of the seat, low-tech modifications, such as towel rolls for head and trunk support, can be made to provide comfort and safety to the child.

The following should be taken into consideration:

- Minimum weight: When assisting a caregiver in selecting a seat for an infant with medical needs, the minimum weight limit needs to be considered, as most commercially available car seats have a minimum weight of 5 pounds. Many premature infants or infants with special needs weigh less than 5 pounds, so customized seats may be required.
- Car bed: A car bed may be required if the infant is unable to tolerate the semi-reclined position.
- Rear-facing–only car seat: These seats are for rear-facing position only. They typically have a carrying handle for portability or as part of a stroller system. A new seat is required when the child reaches the weight limit of 22 to 40 pounds and/or is ready to face forward.[2]
- Convertible and 3-in-1 car seat: A convertible car seat provides a rear-facing position for the infant and converts to a forward-facing seat, when appropriate, as the child grows. The 3-in-1 seat also converts to a booster seat. Many of the convertible or 3-in-1 seats have a higher rear-facing weight limit (40–50 pounds) due to their larger size. The infant remains in the rear-facing position as long as possible to prevent injury in the event of a crash. In the rear-facing position, the seat helps to absorb the force of the crash, whereas a forward-facing seat could cause abdominal or spinal injuries to the small child. A rear-facing seat that accommodates greater weight can be beneficial to children with issues such as small stature, developmental delay, brittle bones, Down syndrome, hydrocephalus, low muscle tone, and poor upper body control.[2]
- Forward-facing seat: A forward-facing seat designed to only face forward is generally used for children at least 1 year of age who have out grown the maximum height and weight limits for the seat. These seats typically use a five-point harness, and, as the child grows, many can be converted into a booster seat when used in conjunction with the vehicle lap-and-shoulder belt.[2]
- Booster seat: Booster seat systems are designed for children who have out grown the height and weight limits of the forward-facing seat with harness. Booster seats elevate the child to a level in which the lap-and-shoulder belts can be properly positioned. The vehicle safety belt should only be used when the child is tall enough for it to cross over the shoulder in the middle of the clavicle and pass over the sternum. The lap belt should sit low and snug across the upper thighs, not the stomach.[2] The shoulder belt should never be placed under the arm or behind the back. This leaves the upper body unprotected and can lead to abdominal or spinal injuries in the event of a crash.[11]

As the child grows and becomes more physically adept, adaptations may be required to prevent the child from releasing the seatbelt or harness. The NHTSA offers a list of the web sites of organizations that provide safety seat inspections to ensure proper installation and use of individual car seats.[38]

- Special car seats and harnesses: Specialized car seats or harnesses can be purchased through certain manufacturers to accommodate more severe physical limitations (Table 20-7).

Lower Anchors and Tethers for Children (LATCH) systems or vehicle seatbelts can be used to anchor a child safety seat in the vehicle with equal safety results. Most passenger vehicles and all car seats manufactured on or after September 1, 2002 are equipped with a LATCH system. The LATCH system consists of metal anchors found in the back seat, in the crack where the back and seat cushions meet. The safety seat attaches directly to these anchors using clips found on the safety seat. An upper tether behind the vehicle seat secures to the upper portion of the safety seat to prevent tipping forward in the event of a crash.[38]

CASE *Study*

Joel is a 5-month-old (2 months adjusted age) boy born prematurely at 27 weeks' gestation weighing 7 pounds. He has been hospitalized since birth due to low birth weight and multiple congenital anomalies. During his hospitalization, Joel tolerated the upright and semi-reclined positions for very brief periods before his oxygen saturation levels decreased to an unhealthy level. A referral was made to the OT practitioner for assistance with positioning to prevent deformity, parent teaching, and discharge planning. The OT practitioner worked with Joel and the family to develop an intervention plan consisting of position changes and activities to build Joel's ability to remain in the upright position. Upon discharge from the hospital, Joel remained in the semi-reclined position for 3 to 5 minutes at a time. The OT practitioner consulted with the family and the medical team to develop a method for Joel's transportation within the community. A car bed was ordered for Joel to provide safe positioning in the back seat of the car. Joel's parents were instructed in positioning. The OT practitioner positioned Joel in the car bed and placed towel rolls at his head, feet, and sides to prevent rolling with the starting and stopping motions of the car. The practitioner also observed the parents position Joel. Joel left the hospital with his parents and continues to receive early intervention services within the home environment to address positioning and developmental skills, as appropriate.

TABLE 20-7

Automobile Safety Seats for Infants and Children

AGE GROUP	TYPES OF SEATS	CONSIDERATIONS
Infant/toddler	Rear-facing only (≤22–40 pounds) Rear-facing convertible seat 3-in-1 seat (40-50 pounds)	Until 2 yr of age OR Child reaches the maximum height or weight allowed by the manufacturer
Preschooler	Convertible seat ("converts" from rear-facing to forward-facing) 3-in-1 seat Forward-facing seats with harness (≤40–80 pounds) Combination seat with harness (≤40–90 pounds) Built-in seat (weight and size limits vary according to vehicle manufacturer) Travel vest (between 20 and 168 pounds and may require a tether)	Any child who has outgrown a rear-facing seat due to weight or height limit
School-aged children	Belt positioning booster seat until the vehicle safety belt fits properly—usually at 4 feet, 9 inches tall and between ages 8 and 12 yr.	Any child whose weight or height is above the manufacturer's limit for their forward-facing seat. A child has outgrown a forward-facing seat when he or she reaches the maximum weight or height limit for the seat, the shoulder is higher than the top harness slots, or the ears are level with the top of the seat. A booster seat should be used until the child can sit all the way back in the vehicle seat with knees bent comfortably over the edge of the seat without sliding forward. The child should be able to maintain this position for the duration of the ride. In addition, vehicle seat belt should fit properly. The vehicle safety belt fits properly when the shoulder belt lies across the middle or the chest and shoulder, not the neck or throat. The lap belt is snug across the upper thighs, not the belly. The seat belt should never be placed under the arm or behind the back as this leaves the upper body unprotected in the event of a crash.
Older children	Shoulder-and-lap belt	All children less than 13 yr should be seated in the back seat.

Data from American Academy of Pediatrics. (2015). *Car seats: information for families for 2015,* https://www.healthychildren.org/English/safety-prevention/on-the-go/Pages/Car-Safety-Seats-Information-for-Families.aspx.

Transportation for the School-Age Child

School buses are designed to use compartmentalization among other features such as size, height, and weight of the vehicle to ensure the safety of its occupants and are not equipped with safety belts. Compartmentalization maintains students in a small padded space between seats with high backs. This prevents the passenger from being thrown forward, over the seat, in the event of a crash.[48] Children with medical or behavioral challenges may require special considerations when using school transportation. Safety seats, seat belts, harnesses, and wheelchair tie-downs may be required to ensure safe transportation.

OT practitioners work with the educational team, including the transporter, to develop a safe plan for transportation and an evacuation plan in the event of an emergency. Since 2002, the American National Standards Institute/Rehabilitation Engineering and Assistive Technology Society of North America (ANSI/RESNA)[3] requires wheelchairs to be dynamically crash tested and mandates specific requirements for wheelchair frames used as seating within a motor vehicle. ANSI WC-20 outlines safety requirements for the seating systems (seat pan, seat back, and attachment hardware) placed into the wheelchair frame after purchase.[4] When securing a wheelchair within any motor vehicle, the chair should be forward facing to prevent injury to the occupant through lateral body shift and/or shearing forces applied to the wheelchair.

When assessing options for school and personal transportation for a child in a wheelchair, all other viable seating options should be exhausted before considering the wheelchair as the seating device for transportation. Children using a wheelchair due to poor endurance or small children using a child safety seat should be transferred out of the wheelchair into a vehicle seat or safety seat for transportation. The OT practitioner provides training to all individuals expected to assist with transfers to ensure proper body mechanics and safe transfers. When not being used as a transportation device, the wheelchair is properly secured within the vehicle to prevent it from becoming a projectile in the event of a sudden stop or crash. If the child cannot be transferred into a vehicle seat due to his or her physical limitations, the wheelchair must be secured using the four-point tie-down system and the three-point occupant restraint system.[46] Shutrump, Manary, and Buning described in detail the requirements of school bus transportation of the student in a wheelchair.[46] Modifications to the school bus are required for proper placement of tie-down systems. The four-point tie-down system consists of four individual anchors (two front and two back) secured to the vehicle floor and then attached to the frame of the wheelchair. Tie-downs are secured to the chair frame as close as possible to the seating surface while remaining below it. Detachable parts of the chair should never be considered for placement of the tie-downs, and straps should form a direct line between the floor and the attachment point, with no wrapping or angling around other chair parts. A shoulder-and-lap belt must be used in addition to any safety belts used for positioning within the chair. The lap belt must fit low and snug across the pelvis, with the lower edge of the safety belt touching the upper thighs. This is typically achieved by threading the lap belt between the armrest and back of the chair. The shoulder portion of the belt must also be snug and positioned over the middle of the clavicle, across the sternum and connect to the lap belt near the hip. Any accessory equipment such as lap trays, backpacks, and communication devices are removed from the wheelchair and secured separately. A power wheelchair must be restrained in this same manner, although it may require an additional set of anchors due to its weight.[46]

Transportation for the Adolescent (Driving)

When the adolescent is ready to attempt driving, the OT clinician evaluates cognitive, visual, physical, and sensory processing abilities that affect this life role. Obtaining a driver's license can affect an adolescent's access to employment, housing, social, educational, and recreational opportunities.[48] The evaluation and care plan for the child considering independent mobility within the community takes into account physical ability, executive functions, visual perception, and visual motor skills,

including coordination and quick use of extremities, ability to cross streets safely, managing social interactions, managing time, handling emergency situations, and caring for self independently. Other skills to consider include map reading, money management, management of emotions/feelings, and regulation of sensory input, as it pertains to tolerating sensory input on a crowded bus, in a traffic jam, and so on.

"Occupational therapists and occupational therapy assistants have the education and training necessary to address driving and community mobility as an IADL."[50] The use of clinical reasoning skills to evaluate and treat the strengths and weaknesses in the areas of performance skills, performance patterns, contexts, and client factors is viewed by the AOTA as a basic role of the OT practitioner. AOTA recommends specialized training for the clinical assessment of vision, cognition, motor performance, reaction time, knowledge of traffic rules, and behind-the-wheel driving skills. Supplementary training and expertise allows the OT practitioner to provide recommendations and assistance in vehicle modifications and driver training. AOTA also requires additional, specialized training for OT professionals who want to work in the area of driver rehabilitation providing direct services to children with health or age-related issues.[5a]

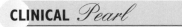

CLINICAL *Pearl*

Many states require licensure as a professional driving instructor before intervention or instruction can be provided to a novice driver or to a driver whose license has expired.

Public Transportation

Adolescents develop independence as they use of public transportation to access peer activities, school, and work. Physical and cognitive limitations can impair successful completion of these activities. The Americans with Disabilities Act of 1990 clearly outlines physical and structural access requirements for all public transit systems.[52] Environmental awareness, directionality, and ability to follow multistep sequences play an important role in achieving independence in this area. The youth is required to combine several skills to complete this task successfully. He or she must purchase tickets using some form of money exchange, choose the appropriate transit system to go to the correct location, and navigate the system safely, including loading and unloading if using a mobility device. Problem solving and multistep sequencing are required to determine what needs to be done during delays or rerouting. Some children may require preteaching on the correct way to purchase tickets and deposit coins/tokens. Anticipation and attention deficits could affect the ability to prepare for the stop and to signal the driver to stop. Intervention may incorporate education on the use of the subway, bus, and road maps. This can be done by setting up a treasure hunt or by simply asking the child to plan a route from one destination to another using a map. It is in the child's best interests to incorporate problem-solving dilemmas into the session. This encourages the child to practice cognitive flexibility and come up with problem-solving strategies. These skills are assessed and applied in the community as much as possible. Simulated environments often do not provide for variables such as increased noise, crowds, delayed schedules, and alternative routing.

Wheelchair Mobility

Mobility for the child with physical challenges must be considered when developing an intervention plan. Brinker and Lewis found typically developing children learn naturally occurring effects and consequences as they interact with their environments through self-initiated mobility such as creeping, walking, and biking.[7] Children limited in self-initiated mobility opportunities because of their physical challenges can demonstrate limited motivation, diminished overall independence, learned helplessness, and diminished cognitive, social, and emotional development. When providing OT intervention to a child with newly acquired limitations, progressive limitations, or limitations that are becoming more difficult as he or she grows, the practitioner may work with the child and/or his or her caregivers to obtain assistive mobility in the form of a wheelchair. Butler found that independent mobility impacted a child's spatial understanding of the environment.[12] A study conducted by Deitz, Swinth, and White found enhanced self-initiated movements and increased attempts for peer interaction after the introduction of a power mobility device.[17] Physical and cognitive impairments that can affect independent mobility, whether power or manual, can include impaired head and eye control, body control, upper body strength, spatial awareness, and motor planning. The child should be assessed and receive instruction in locking and unlocking the brakes; maneuvering the chair through environments with and without obstacles; turning, starting and stopping; and the ability to open or close doors independently. Strength should be assessed for the ability to propel the manual chair over rough, smooth, and angled surfaces as well as up and down hills or ramps. Strength limitations can be addressed in direct therapy sessions through play activities such as throwing weighted beanbags at a target and through weight-bearing activities. The ability to safely maneuver the wheelchair can be addressed in simulated environments using obstacle courses. Before discharging

a child from direct therapy services, these skills should be assessed in the natural environment to ensure that generalization of skills from the simulated tasks to the real-life situation has occurred.

When selecting a wheelchair, the OT practitioner ensures proper fit, allowing for growth adjustments, as most funding sources expect seating systems to accommodate the individual for at least 5 years (see Figure 20-3 for an example of a wheelchair for a young child). Powered mobility versus manual mobility should be evaluated with care. The powered wheelchair is less portable and requires specialized transportation due to its greater weight. It is more costly and requires adequate safety awareness, judgment, and visual perception. Control systems need to be assessed to ensure adequate control and safety. The manual wheelchair is lighter and more portable, is less costly, and can be easily propelled by the user or caregiver. Both chairs can typically accommodate specialized seating systems based on the child's needs. Whichever type of mobility the child uses, he or she should have symmetric hip alignment with hips, knees, and ankles supported at approximately 90 degrees. The seat depth should accommodate the length of the thigh, while allowing 2 to 3 inches of space from the front edge of the seat to the popliteal fossa. The seat width should be approximately 2 inches wider than the widest part of the hip and thighs. The height of the seat back is

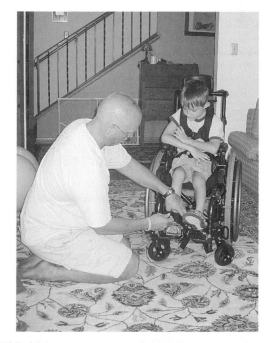

FIGURE 20-3 A well-fitted wheelchair promotes functional mobility so the child may explore the environment and his community. It is important to teach parents how to assure proper positioning. (From Case-Smith, J. & O'Brien, J.(2015). *Occupational therapy for children and adolescents* (7th ed.). St. Louis: Elsevier.)

dependent on the stability and balance of the child, with a higher back required for more stability and support. A low back, preferably below the scapula, is useful for the child with good balance who propels the chair manually. This allows for extension at the shoulders when pushing. Leg rests that are removable are helpful for the child who performs standing transfers. Removable armrests are typically necessary for the child performing sliding transfers and helpful when sitting at a low table. The seat belt and lap tray are also accessories to be considered when selecting a wheelchair.

> ### CLINICAL *Pearl*
>
> When having difficulty seating a child with excessive extensor muscle tone, seating that provides flexion of the hips at an angle slightly more than 90 degrees can inhibit the muscle tone. Placement of the seatbelt on the chair at a 90-degree angle to the thighs can help maintain the position.

> ### CLINICAL *Pearl*
>
> Ensure that children's skin is protected under lap trays, as severe sunburn can occur when using a clear lap tray in direct sunlight.

> ### CLINICAL *Pearl*
>
> Children benefit from early mobility experiences. Adapting scooters can help them experience mobility and investigate their surroundings. Figure 20-4 illustrates a mobility option for younger children and can help them experience movement.

Walkers, Canes, Crutches, and Miscellaneous Mobility Devices

Physical therapy practitioners are responsible for the evaluation, selection, and training in the use of walkers, canes, and other mobility devices. Whereas OT practitioners are involved in facilitating safety in the community and at home while using a mobility device during daily occupations.[41] Figure 20-5 shows the OT practitioner supporting a child's mobility by using a walker to allow the child to engage in play activities. At the same time the physical therapist evaluates the child's ability to use the walker, the fit of the walker, and determining whether any modifications are needed. The anterior or posterior walker provides support to the child and the ability to move the lower extremities, but it requires support. The upper extremities should be

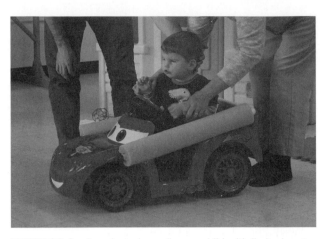

FIGURE 20-4 An adapted car allows a child with limited motor ability to move around the play environment.

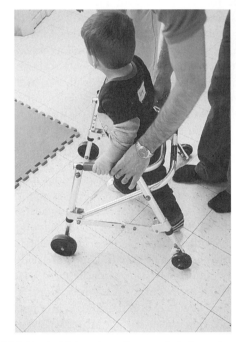

FIGURE 20-5 A child uses a walker to gain independent mobility.

carefully monitored for hyperextension of the thumb and fingers and excessive weight placed on the wrists due to poor lower extremity strength and upright posture. In these cases, a walker with forearm troughs may provide better positioning and support the child. Canes come as straight canes or quad canes. The straight cane has a single end point to provide stability for the child. The quad cane has a single staff with four end points to provide increased stability. Devices such as mobile standers and adapted cycles provide mobility to children with special needs and allow for social interaction within the community setting. Adaptations may be required to provide comfort and optimal positioning and function.

Bicycles, Scooters, Roller Blades

As the child grows, independent mobility becomes more important to his or her autonomy. Bicycling, using a scooter, skateboarding, and skating require advanced development of balance and equilibrium reactions, postural control, and upper and lower extremity coordination. Executive function skills such as attention, initiation, safety awareness, and judgment are considered when evaluating children's mobility and safety. The use of safety equipment such as helmet, elbow pads, and kneepads should be taught before placing a child on a moving object and should be strictly enforced each time the child rides. Judgment and safety awareness are required when crossing a street, riding among pedestrians, and following general riding rules. To ride safely in the community, children and youth must be able to recognize and respond to the meaning of traffic signals and street signs. They also must be able to transfer these skills for a variety of conditions.

Street Safety

Children with disabilities will likely need assistance to learn to navigate their community safely. Repeated exposure and learning opportunities facilitate learning and eventual independence with regard to street safety. The OT practitioner may address street safety during natural learning opportunities and through consultation with parents and teachers.

Street Safety with Young Children

Young children learn about general safety around cars, safety in parking lots, and how to cross the street. OT practitioners encounter natural opportunities to teach children about street safety during school outings, when getting on and off school buses, and when going to and from playgrounds. Although young children are not expected to navigate streets independently, they can learn to play only in safe areas such as driveways and playgrounds, walk on sidewalks and crosswalks, stop when they reach a street, avoid going into the street without an adult, and recognize when it is safe to cross a street. Young children can also be taught to pay attention to crossing guards for assistance.

Street Safety with Older Children

Older children begin to assume independence in maintaining their personal safety when moving through their communities. They learn how to understand traffic signals and road signs and how to navigate city streets. The OT practitioner ensures that they can recognize and understand street signs and traffic signals. Practice in observing street safety rules can be integrated well with community mobility interventions. Additionally, the OT practitioner ensures that children who have intellectual disabilities or communication limitations carry personal identification, which would be vital in case they get lost; this may be attached to a belt or backpack and should include emergency contact information. Furthermore, children who use wheelchairs are encouraged to attach reflective strips to the device and use a strobe light when traveling on the street during dusk or in the dark.

FINANCIAL MANAGEMENT, SHOPPING, AND CARE OF PETS

Children who exhibit impaired use of one or more executive function skills may experience challenges in the areas of financial management, shopping, pet care, and care of others. They frequently have difficulty generalizing skills across environments. They show difficulty sequencing and completing complex tasks associated with each IADL. For example, a child may have difficulty calculating the discounted price while shopping. External aids assist children in accessing and participating in activities independently. For example, a child may carry a calculator or list to remember what to purchase. OT practitioners carefully assess the child's knowledge and skills in each area to determine where to begin the intervention process.

Financial Management

Financial awareness begins in early childhood with imaginary play involving shopping, money exchange, and the awareness that money is required to obtain desired items. In elementary school, children begin to learn to identify names and values of coins and paper currency. Children with learning disabilities or visual-perceptual impairment may have more difficulty distinguishing between items of similar size, for example, a dime and a penny, or a nickel and a quarter. Some children can be taught to distinguish between these items using the texture on the edges of the coins. Coin carriers can also be useful for the child having difficulty distinguishing between coins. Paper currency can be folded differently to distinguish between denominations. These strategies can, however, present difficulties for the child with impaired memory. Children may benefit from a picture book or card with a picture of the bill or coin paired with the value. Children can practice these skills through games, contrived practice, or in a simulated environment such as a school store, where small school items or snacks are sold. In this situation, the children are asked to interact with peers to discuss the prices of items, collect the correct amount of money, sort the bills, and provide change to the customer as necessary. When children are unable to motorically manage coins and bills, a prepaid credit card can allow them to access their funds. The card can be attached to a bag or belt loop with a retractable key ring. This adaptation requires an understanding of money management.

Money management involves understanding amounts of money and accounting for the changes in amounts, budgeting, check writing, depositing and withdrawing money, use of an automatic teller machine, and eventually paying bills. Money management can begin at an early age. Young children can save money for a desired item such as something simple like a snack. As the adolescent seeks employment and earns money, skills for budgeting and using a savings or checking account become more important. Children with disabilities may lack awareness of the cost of items or the ability to plan and sequence these challenging tasks. Children with motor disabilities may need adaptations to successfully manage the fine motor aspects of financial management. OT practitioners can select natural activities to teach the child the value of money. Frequent repetition is important for skill acquisition, and use of a calculator is very helpful.

Next the child learns to budget small amounts of money by anticipating the costs of items and determining how much money they need to complete a task such as buying food for a recipe. Role-playing a restaurant scenario where the child orders the food he or she wants, receives a bill, and pays with paper money and coins is a fun way to work on using money. Roles also can be reversed where the child plays the role of the waiter, tallying the bill, collecting the money, and giving change to the practitioner. Learning to make and follow lists for activities with sequenced steps is an important step toward financial responsibility. As the child masters these early steps he or she can move to budgeting from a bank statement, writing checks, and paying bills. Sample bank statements, blank practice checks, and sample bills are available online. The OT practitioner can work with the child to find the amount due on a bill, write a check for that amount, and determine how much money would be left. Specific physical adaptations include large print, text-to-speech computer adaptations, large checks, and use of templates such as a cardboard check template that exposes the areas of the check that need to be completed. As with all IADLs, skills are practiced in contrived settings and in natural environments for generalization. New skills should always be assessed within the natural environment before discharge from therapy to ensure adequate proficiency.

Shopping

Successful shopping performance skills include the ability to make a list; identify where to purchase the item(s),

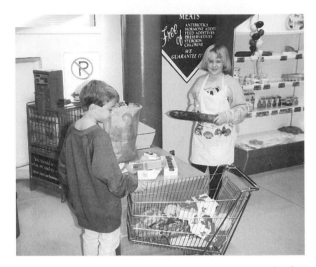

FIGURE 20-6 Children must use many skills to shop for food. (From Case-Smith, J. & O'Brien, J. (2015). *Occupational therapy for children and adolescents* (7th ed.). St. Louis: Elsevier.)

that is, department or grocery store; find and obtain a needed item in the store; calculate the purchase price; maneuver the shopping cart through the store; and complete the currency exchange to purchase the item(s). Figure 20-6 illustrates children engaged in an intervention to develop shopping skills. The child who uses a mobility device may need to call the store to find out about the accessibility and location of elevators. Grocery stores often provide a list of aisle numbers paired with items in the aisle or a map of the store to assist shoppers with disabilities. Shopping lists should be grouped (dairy, bread, soups, frozen items) as much as possible to conserve energy and increase efficiency. Copies of lists with staple items or frequently used items can be prepared, with the child highlighting or circling the currently needed items before each trip. Picture cards assist in identifying specific brands of item. Laminated picture cards can be attached to a ring before shopping and each card removed from the ring as the item is purchased. A calculator can be used to keep track of the cost of items. Children with visual or motor impairments may require a large-keypad calculator for successful use. Simulated environments can be set up in the clinic setting for the child to practice maneuvering a shopping cart through obstacles and finding needed items. The natural setting of the community also affords opportunities to practice communicating and requesting assistance.

Care of Pets

Many children experience great reward and gratification from caring for family pets. Children and adolescents are often expected to assist in the daily care of the family pet. Responsibilities might include feeding, grooming, keeping the environment clean, providing shelter and exercise as needed, and ensuring proper health care

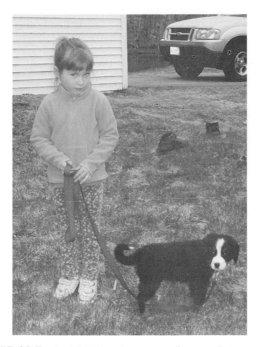

FIGURE 20-7   A child takes her puppy for a walk to care for her pet.

for the pet. Depending on the age of the child, one or more of these activities may be expected (Figure 20-7). Lists and schedules can assist the child with impaired memory skills carry out these responsibilities. Picture lists or schedules can assist the child or adolescent who is unable to read. Adaptations may be required for the child with motor impairment. Larger tools or a cuff for scooping food and cleaning up after the pet may be needed.

HEALTH MANAGEMENT AND MAINTENANCE

Managing one's health is an important IADL. To be healthy, a person must exercise, eat nutritious foods, protect the body, and manage medication regimens. Many children and adolescents do not manage and maintain their health status independently; however, this is an area in which children take an increasingly larger role as they get older. Therefore it is important to address this area continually throughout childhood at the appropriate level for the child.

> **CLINICAL** *Pearl*
>
> Adapted physical education should be recommended when the general gym class does not facilitate a child's participation because it does not meet his or her ability level or provide a safe environment. No student should be deprived of physical education and exposure to physical leisure opportunities.

Exercise

Exercise is a crucial element of health and wellness. Currently, the United States is facing the alarming challenge of increasing numbers of overweight and obese children.[13,15,20] Long-term consequences of obesity include increased risk for diabetes, cardiovascular disease, respiratory disorders, metabolic syndromes, cancers, gallbladder disease, and sleep apnea, as well as lowered self-esteem.[6,15] Furthermore, children with physical disabilities are at an increased risk for obesity.[13,15,20] OT practitioners can take on an important role in the prevention and remediation of obesity in children. (For additional information, see Chapter 15.)

New models of practice have emerged in which OT practitioners can provide structure for **fitness** programs and can work to change the environmental context and perceptions regarding physical activity.[6,15] These programs are especially relevant in school settings. OT practitioners can work creatively to improve access to physical occupations.[15] OT practitioners influence fitness at the community level, for example, by increasing children's participation in active occupations or advocating for an open gym time at the local school.[13]

The OT practitioner can bring a unique and informed perspective to a fitness program.[13,15] The OT philosophy regarding health and wellness can be applied to create programs based on fitness and lifelong participation in healthy physical activities rather than on weight loss. The OT practitioner can play an important role in determining the frequency and duration of physical activity for any individual.[15,20] When focusing on children with disabilities, the OT practitioner can promote activities with just the right challenge, or engage children in activities that will enhance motor skills and ability to participate in social and community occupations.[20] The practitioner also can find motivating ways to promote wellness such as using new technologies like video games.[29] The OT practitioner can provide consultation to teachers and families to include fitness activities in the daily routine of the child. In addition, OT practitioners advocate for children with disabilities to participate in sports or games to their ability, or find resources for adaptive sports.

Additionally, OT practitioners can bring the benefits of exercise to other populations, such as children with mental illness. A review of studies regarding mental health and exercise found that individuals consistently experienced increased quality of life, satisfaction, socialization, and enjoyment from opportunities for exercise.[1] Furthermore, exercise is also considered to be a coping mechanism for people with mental illness.

> **CLINICAL** *Pearl*
>
> Within a school setting, advocacy for healthy choices in the cafeteria and vending machines, and the inclusion of recess and motor breaks positively affects the health and well-being of all students and staff.

Fitness Programs

When developing a fitness program, the OT practitioner first determines the child's current level of physical activity and activity tolerance.[20] Gross motor skills are observed to determine the activities in which the child can participate with little or no assistance. The OT practitioner observes the child's running, jumping, climbing abilities, and ball skills. If these movements are not available or skilled, the OT practitioner determines what parts of the body have the most movements and design activities and games that capitalize on those movements.[20]

Children with significant motor impairments and who lack volitional movement also need special programs for fitness such as passive ROM programs. The OT practitioner can carry out ROM programs and teach the program to the school staff or family members to ensure that the child receives the program each day. When teaching such a program, it is important to provide the information in more than one way and to give informational materials to the learners so that they may review the lessons as needed. For example, ROM is demonstrated, explained verbally, and also explained with words and pictures on an information sheet. The OT practitioner teaches which joints should be moved and how far and in what direction they move. It is important to show the learner where to place the hands, how to watch for signs that the child may be in pain, and when to back off and consult with the practitioner. The OT practitioner can ensure that the teachers and family members are able to safely provide the ROM exercises by asking them to demonstrate their ability before the session ends, and continuing to consult to ensure the exercise is occurring as recommended.

CLINICAL *Pearl*

If a child's ROM decreases, consult your supervisor and/or report this change to the child's doctor. The child may need a splint to provide passive stretch during the day. In extreme cases, casting or surgeries may be necessary.

Adaptive Sports and Activities

People with disabilities may wish to participate in competitive or club sports. The OT practitioner can play a role in identifying potential sports, providing resources and information regarding choices, and assisting with skill development or enhancement for successful participation in such an occupation. The Special Olympics provides competitive options for people with a wide range of abilities. Wheelchair sports as well as sports for those with visual impairments are available in many areas. Other options for children and adolescents of varied abilities include swimming programs, karate, adapted gymnastics, and horseback riding. Physical fitness activities may be accessible via therapeutic recreation programs in the community.

CLINICAL *Pearl*

Children with motor impairments may be better able to learn and participate in ball sports if larger equipment, such as a large ball or bat, is provided.

Nutrition

Nutrition is another area of health maintenance that OT practitioners address during intervention.[13,34] Nutrition information can supplement other OT activities. Nutrition themes can be woven in when working on handwriting, cutting, finger isolation for calculator use, or a variety of other goals. Nutrition information integrates well into activities for financial planning and cooking. Furthermore, the OT practitioner can use games (e.g., board games) to teach the principles of eating well, avoiding an excess of snack foods and sugary drinks, and minding caloric intake. The OT practitioner can work on primary goals such as visual perception and also can heighten knowledge about nutrition through the theme of the game. For example, the OT practitioner may choose to use a healthy food as pictorial theme for matching, sorting, or identifying games.

OT practitioners have affected nutritious eating through novel and creative programs in school systems.[34] In one urban school, occupational therapists advocated for healthier choices at lunch and promoted healthier eating through educational programs regarding food and nutrition.[13] Within school and community settings, OT practitioners advocate for healthy choices in vending machines and snacks.

OT practitioners receive referrals to help picky eaters try new foods. When working with picky eaters, it is important to first consult with an occupational therapist trained in feeding interventions to ensure that no impairments in feeding exist. Once cleared to try a variety of foods, the OT practitioner can encourage pleasurable exposures to new foods. Pushing new foods is not recommended because this can result in a power struggle and decrease the likelihood of the child increasing the food repertoire. Some children may withdraw from foods secondary to sensory processing disorders.[25] If a child gags at the sight or smell of food or withdraws from touching food or certain textures, sensory processing may need to be addressed before success with eating can be achieved. If this is the case, tolerance of smell and tactile experiences may be an appropriate starting point.

When working with picky eaters, practitioners expose them to new foods gradually.[25] The child learns to enjoy mealtimes and experience pleasure through a slow introduction to new foods. New foods can also be introduced through a process known as chaining. First, the OT practitioner needs to determine what specific foods the child eats, as well as the textures, flavors, shapes, and colors of food the child currently enjoys. Next, the practitioner provides exposure to new foods that share some of the characteristics of the familiar foods. For example, if the child enjoys the taste of spaghetti, he or she may be encouraged to try other dishes that have long noodles, are red and white in color, or have a tomato sauce flavor. The child might also try other shapes of pasta, other brands of tomato sauce, or other sauces. The child may also try new tastes by dipping a favorite food in new sauces.[25] Before using food chaining to increase a child's food repertoire, it would be highly beneficial to review the results of a study by Fraker, Fishbein, Cox, and Wilbert[22] (Box 20-1).

A physician is contacted immediately if the child experiences vomiting, retching, choking, spitting up, gagging, ongoing diarrhea, painful swallowing, wheezing, constipation, or lack of appetite during the intervention.[25]

CLINICAL *Pearl*

When working with picky eaters, new foods are best introduced during a planned snack time, rather than during regular meals.

Sexuality

Sexuality is a key aspect of life and plays a vital role in physical and emotional expression. Sexuality becomes an area of concern as children get older. It is especially important to discuss sexuality with adolescents who have

BOX 20-1

Sample Progression to Begin Trying New Foods and Improve Nutritious Eating

- Tolerate new foods in one's space—on the table, on another person's plate, and eventually on the child's plate.
- Touch new foods—this may occur through play, for example, feeding a toy.
- Smell new foods.
- Touch new foods to the cheek or lips.
- Lick new foods.
- Put new foods in the mouth and possibly chew the food with the option of discreetly spitting it out into a napkin.
- Chew and swallow new foods, beginning with one bite or a small bite.

Adapted from Fraker, C., Fishbein, M., Cox, S., & Walbert, L. (2007). *Food chaining: the proven 6-step plan to stop picky eating, solve feeding problems, and expand your child's diet.* Cambridge, MA: Da Capo Press.

cognitive disabilities or difficulty understanding the emotions or intentions of others.[44] Teenage girls and boys with cognitive disabilities may be particularly in need of consultation and coaching with regard to protecting their bodies and developing healthy sexuality.

Some OT practitioners may not feel comfortable discussing sexuality with their clients or other members of the team. However, the importance of this topic as it relates to health and safety cannot be underestimated. This issue can be addressed in several ways.[44] The OT practitioner can advocate for students with disabilities to participate in sexual education in public schools at the appropriate learning level. It may be necessary for the OT practitioner to explain the importance of sex education to teachers, school administrators, or parents and caregivers. Another option for dealing with this issue is direct consultation with the family. This can be achieved through written or oral communication, which might include information materials sent home with the child. Information materials on abstinence, sex education, and safe sex are readily available on the Internet.[44] It is imperative that the OT practitioner obtains consent from an individual's parent or guardian before discussing the topic of sexuality with a minor child.

Medication Management

Children and adolescents require supervision to manage medication regimens. As adolescents mature, they may take more and more responsibility for **medication management.** The OT practitioner should never work alone in teaching medication management. Rather, increasing the child's independence in medication management is a team decision. The parent or caregiver should always be involved in the decision and teaching/learning process. Some parents may want their child to be independent in medication management. The number of children in the family and the educational level of parents may affect the decision. The severity of the disease or disorder and the child's developmental level is considered.[39] Independence in managing medications cannot be taken lightly, as serious consequences may result from missing, duplicating, or misdosing medication.[23] Incorrect medication management can result in functional impairments, hospitalization, or even death.[23] When deciding if a child is ready for increased independence in medication management, the following questions must be asked:

- What would be the consequence if the medication were missed? In other words, how important is each medication dose to the person's health and well-being?[39]
- Does the child willingly take the medication? Does the child take all of the medication when it is presented?

- Can the child tell time? Can the child count correctly?
- Does the child know the names of his or her medications?
- Can the child distinguish between different medications based on size, shape, and other identifiable characteristics?[32]
- Can the child read the label on the medication container to distinguish between different medications?[32]
- Can the child independently open medication containers and manipulate individual pills effectively?
- Does the child have the problem-solving skills to be able to avoid taking too much or too little medication?
- Will the child contact a caregiver or professional for help if confusion or problems arise?[27,39]

Once the team decides to move forward with increasing the child's independence in medication management, the OT practitioner identifies the areas the child needs to work on through the questions just cited. The child may need to work on matching and sorting pills; this can be practiced with small items such as buttons or candy before moving on to pills. Fine motor skills may need to be targeted to promote efficient manipulation of the pills. In this case, grasp and in-hand manipulation are observed and addressed during the intervention.

Effective organization of medications is essential for successful medication management.[23] Intervention techniques include setting up a weekly pillbox and organizing visual reminders such as written cue cards or pictures that display the pill organization accurately that the child can work from.[32] Once the pillbox is set up, the child will need fine motor skills and motor planning to open each segment and pour the pills into the hand.

Once the child can successfully organize the medications, he or she may be ready to begin taking them with more independence. Initially, the child takes the medication independently, but under the supervision of a caregiver. Next, an effective system to remind the child to take the medication is set up.[23] Visual notes and reminders may be helpful. Computer reminders through e-mail and calendar programs may assist computer-savvy individuals.[23] Ongoing success often depends on the generation of routines and habits with regard to taking medications.[27]

Once the child has demonstrated success to this point, the decision to move forward with greater independence can be taken. At first, a telephone call to ensure each dose has been taken is recommended. The amount and type of support a child needs is then individualized. The OT practitioner might consult with caregivers or nurses to assist with determining the level of support that the child requires. Some children may need assistance to set up the weekly pillbox but may be independent enough to take the medication each day. Others may be more independent with medication organization but may need assistance each month to determine which medications need refills. Regardless of the level of independence, it is important that an accurate list of all medications be maintained. It is further recommended that a pill count be regularly conducted to ensure that medications are being taken correctly.[27] Also, additional support should be given whenever a medication regimen changes.[27]

HOME ESTABLISHMENT AND MAINTENANCE

Home management tasks frequently include activities such as cleaning, laundry, and trash disposal, as well as maintenance tasks such as repairs and yard care.[42] For children and adolescents, home management includes occupations that are typically known as chores. The expectations for chore completion vary depending on the family culture and the child's capacity for engagement. Many families of children with disabilities may not require the children to do chores. However, when children participate in doing chores, even simple or adapted ones, they are learning how to complete tasks, role competence, and responsibility. Furthermore, they will likely gain self-efficacy and confidence. Common chores include putting toys and games away, cleaning the bedroom, making the bed, doing laundry, washing kitchen or bathroom surfaces, vacuuming, dusting, and taking out the garbage. Adults with disabilities who experience difficulty with home management tasks have to rely on assistance from others in the community, or they may be unable to live alone.[42] Therefore it is important for children to learn and practice home management tasks as they grow older to prepare them for greater independence as adults.

The OT practitioner consults with parents to suggest home management tasks that are appropriate for the child's abilities, assist with modifications and adaptations to improve success and independence, and provide direct intervention so that the child can learn to do the task as appropriate. OT practitioners also might address home management tasks in the school system as part of a life-skills program or to prepare for transition out of the school system. Young children participate in home management by tidying up toys; they frequently use a "cleanup song" or routine. Clearly marked boxes and shelves also improve performance. Older children begin doing chores at home. It is normally expected that a child will master one or two specific chores independently before completing more complex chores. Such tasks may include taking out the garbage, getting the mail, or washing the kitchen table. As the child shows greater success, independence, and initiative with these tasks, more difficult tasks can be introduced. Positive reinforcements, whether verbal or monetary, increase motivation. Behavioral strategies such as sticker charts or tangible reward systems may be necessary.

Common barriers to independence in home management include cognitive and physical limitations. Methods for assisting children with general difficulties in these areas are described in Boxes 20-2 and 20-3.

MEAL PREPARATION AND CLEANUP

Meal preparation is an important occupation for independence. When learning to prepare meals, children often begin by helping adults with cooking or setting the table (Figure 20-8). As they get older, children may begin to follow simple recipes or prepare simple snacks by themselves (Figure 20-9). Later, adolescents may learn to use the microwave, toaster, toaster oven, range, or oven (Figure 20-10). At each stage, the OT practitioner instructs children in kitchen safety, techniques for safe food handling, and safety with utensils.[26] Depending on needs of the child, the OT practitioner also addresses the use of specific cooking appliances, as well as how to measure ingredients, follow a recipe, clean the workspace, and properly store food.[26] The OT practitioner can modify and adapt tasks, tools, and workspaces to provide interventions that facilitate greater independence with meal preparation. The OT practitioner also can provide educational materials to assist with generalization of skills.[26]

Meal Preparation with Young Children

Young children benefit from assisting with preparation of snacks that do not require cooking and from assisting

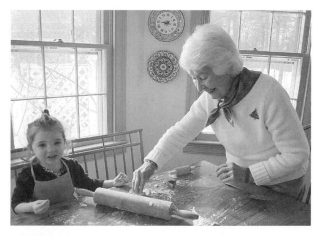

FIGURE 20-8   A toddler helps make cookies with her grandmother.

with obtaining and mixing ingredients for a dish that the adult will cook or bake. These tasks can be integrated into an OT session, school curriculum, or parent activity. Young children might slice bananas with a dull, plastic knife, assemble a fruit salad, sequence the addition of ingredients for trail mix, slice tubes of cookie dough, roll up pieces of deli meat, or stir the ingredients for a cake or mashed potatoes. These activities can be used as creative ways to address many goals such as fine motor,

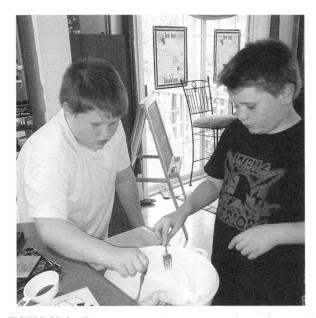

FIGURE 20-9 These two young boys are proud to make a meal "all by themselves."

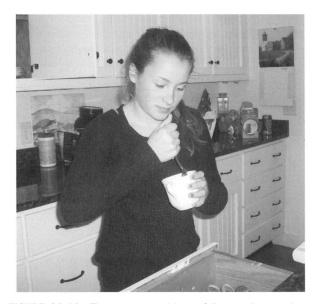

FIGURE 20-10 Teenagers are able to follow recipes and are independent in meal preparation.

sequencing, and prereading goals. They provide a natural venue for discussing healthy eating as well as cultural traditions. They also make excellent group activities. The OT practitioner can find recipe ideas for OT activities in cookbooks for young children.

Meal Preparation with Older Children

Older children may begin participating in snack and meal preparation more independently. The OT practitioner begins with simple snack preparation and observes the child's motor and cognitive skills to determine what

level of cooking suits the therapy sessions best. Older children are likely ready to prepare snacks or lunch foods that require more than one step. Examples include sandwiches, tuna and egg salads, cake mixes, vegetable and fruit salads, and frozen foods that are cooked in the microwave. Older children may begin working on simple cutting and peeling if their fine motor skills are adequate for safe participation. Modifications and adaptations may be required for safety, independence, and success.

Meal Preparation with Adolescents

Adolescents who have achieved the skills necessary to complete the tasks previously noted may begin participating in more complex food preparation. They may work from a recipe and prepare snacks and other foods with multiple steps. Some children may work with printed recipes, whereas others may benefit from recipes that also show the steps in a picture format. They may begin to learn how to use appliances. The OT practitioner observes motor and cognitive skills when selecting the most appropriate appliances. A microwave allows children with physical or visual impairments to cook with greater ease and safety.[31] Microwaves save time, use lighter cookware, decrease fatigue, and are easy to clean.[57] The toaster oven and the crockpot are convenient for children whose physical disabilities may prevent them from using the oven easily.[28] Additionally, these smaller, portable devices will likely be used more often than an oven when the child lives independently.[31] Therefore the OT practitioner may choose to work with these appliances first.

Modifications and Adaptations to Assist with Meal Preparation

> **CLINICAL** *Pearl*
>
> When working with meal preparation, begin with simple snacks that do not require heating. Increase the number of steps or ingredients needed to increase complexity. Move on to microwave preparation before asking the child to use the stovetop or oven.

As children who use wheelchairs get older, kitchen accessibility may become a priority (Table 20-8). The OT practitioner can provide consultation on kitchen modifications to make cooking easier and safer. Using a microwave, crockpot, toaster oven, or cook-top range (burners only) helps avoid more extensive modifications.[28] Wheelchairs need an adequate turning radius in the kitchen, ideally 5 × 5 feet. People using wheelchairs need to get close to the counters, sink, and oven. Counters can be lowered, and adaptive refrigerators,

TABLE 20-8

Cooking Adaptations

ADAPTATION	DESCRIPTION
ADAPTATIONS FOR WORKING WITH ONE HAND	
Utensils with large and ergonomic handles	Provide a larger surface to grasp, hold, and carry the tools
Jar openers	Mount to wall or provide power to open jars and bottles
Electric can openers or those with shelves	Provide power or stability to open cans
Bottle and carton holders	Increase ease of pour for large liquid containers
Stationary bowls	Prevent bowl from slipping while working through suction cups or metal frames
Pot-holding frames	Hold a pot onto a burner to prevent it from moving
Stationary cutting boards	Suction to the work space and hold food stationary with prongs to allow for one-handed cutting
Stationary peelers	Suction to the work space to allow for one-handed peeling
Roller or rocker knives	Allow for one-handed cutting
Stationary scrubbers	Suction to side of sink basin to allow for one-handed dish washing
ADAPTATIONS FOR WORKING WITH LOW VISION	
Contrast-color cutting boards	Improve visibility of food and working materials
Liquid indicators	Indicate when liquid is reaching a certain level
Adjusting level guides for measuring	Provide a tactile method for measuring rather than relying on small printing on liquid measuring cups

Adapted from Infinitec. Infinite potential through assistive technology. Available at: http://www.infinitec.org/live/homemodifications/lowcost alternatives.htm.

sinks, and stovetops that provide space for the cook's knees can be installed. Cabinets and cabinet doors can be removed so the cook can access the workspace while in the wheelchair.[28]

The OT practitioner can train children in mobility in the kitchen. Without modifications to the environment, the child will have to approach the counter or sink sideways in the wheelchair, which is not ideal. To remove items from the refrigerator, the child will have to maneuver the wheelchair sideways to the refrigerator door, open the door, and then move into the space such that the wheelchair keeps the door open and the he or she can reach the items in the refrigerator. Refrigerator contents must be organized in such a way that the child can reach all of the items without stretching unsafely. If the kitchen lacks the space the cook needs, chopping and cold preparation can be done in another location close to the kitchen.[28] The child can use a rolling cart to transport items, or trays can be placed strategically throughout the workspace to ensure safe mobility; cooks who use wheelchairs should never carry hot items on their laps.[28]

CASE *Study*

Robert receives occupational therapy through his school. As part of his transition planning, some goals were set, including that he prepare snacks and simple meals independently. This allows him to eat nutritious foods when home alone and participate in an independent living program after high school. When a certified OTA began working with him, Robert's personal goal was to make macaroni and cheese. The OT practitioner recommended that they start with some other foods so she could observe his skills and ensure that he would be safe using the stovetop. As they worked, the OT practitioner noted that Robert could not maintain his postural control when using both hands despite a chest strap on his chair. Robert needed to support his upper body with one arm when pouring, cutting, stirring, or transporting bowls or pots. Robert and the OT practitioner worked on his positioning to make food preparation most effective and to help him expend his energy more efficiently. He worked at low tables where he could use one arm to support his body while also holding a bowl, rather than working at the higher countertop. They worked on transporting items across the counters with a sliding motion and discussed environmental modifications that would help Robert avoid having to transport bowls, especially hot bowls, over long distances. They also worked on maneuvering Robert's wheelchair to bring him close to the refrigerator and microwave so that he could reach items without compromising his posture. The OT practitioner realized that Robert would not be able to stir or flip an item on the stovetop because he would be unable to support his upper body and stabilize the pot or pan at the same time. Therefore they decided to make microwave macaroni and cheese, and Robert could achieve his goal while ensuring safe cooking practices. The certified OTA also consulted with the physical therapist to determine whether a more supportive system was indicated for increased postural stability.

SAFETY PROCEDURES AND EMERGENCY RESPONSES

Children with disabilities have the same needs and rights with regard to safety and emergency response as do others. In some cases, children with disabilities require a higher level of planning, practice, adaptations, or environmental modifications to ensure their safety. The OT practitioner consults with parents and the staff at schools or day-care centers to ensure the safety of children. Factors to consider include the use of child safety devices, fire safety, safety with strangers, and street safety. Emergency planning must also be given specific attention. Families and schools must plan for expected emergencies, for example, a storm that has been forecast, as well as sudden emergencies. Advance planning is the key to ensuring safety. Refer to the list of resources for specific publications and information on emergency planning.

Child Safety Devices

Some children with disabilities may be more prone to exploring unsafe household substances or lack the judgment to identify unsafe substances. Children with physical disabilities may also require enhanced safety while sleeping in a bed (Table 20-9).

TABLE 20-9

Common Safety Devices

COMMON SAFETY DEVICES	USES
Safety locks and safety latches	Use to close doors, cabinets, and drawers that contain sharp objects, cleaning products, or toxic chemicals
Safety gates	Prevent children from falling down stairs, or entering rooms containing dangerous materials or tools
Door locks and door knob covers	Prevent children from entering some areas at all, such as the area with an unsupervised swimming pool
Electrical outlet covers	Prevent children from touching electrical outlets
Child bed safety rails	Prevent children from falling off the bed

Modified from My Child Safety: Child safety devices. http://www.mychildsafety.net/child-safety-devices.html.

CLINICAL *Pearl*

When recommending safety bed rails, for optimal safety, consider rails that attach at the bottom of the bed rather than at the sides. Older and large-sized children sleeping in full-sized beds may require hospital bed rails.[36]

Fire Safety

Special measures must be taken to ensure the safety of children with disabilities in the event of a fire.[55] They may need to be alerted about the fire and be helped to exit safely. All families should have basic fire escape plans. Government guidelines for a safe fire escape are as follows[24]:

- Install fire alarms on each floor of the home or building.
- Create a fire escape plan with two ways to exit each room.
- Leave immediately if a fire occurs.
- Feel a door before opening; if it is hot do not open it.
- Plan a meeting place outside the house; use a specific location rather than a general "across the street."
- Never go back into the building; wait for the assistance of fire fighters.
- Know the principle of "stop, drop, and roll"; if an individual is unable to do so due to physical disability, he or she should have a small fire extinguisher readily available and be trained in its use.[55]

Recognition of a fire is the first step to a safe escape. Children with visual or hearing impairment will need adapted fire alarms. Devices that vibrate, flash, or flash a strobe light outside the home to alert others ensure that an individual with a disability becomes aware of a fire as soon as possible.[52,53,55]

Escaping a burning building is especially difficult for a child with a physical disability.[55] A plan of escape must be put in place and practiced repeatedly to ensure that all possible obstacles are considered and the extent of assistance that the child will need is fully understood. A family or institution may enlist the assistance of the fire department in developing a safe exit strategy. Additionally, the local fire department can be contacted in advance to provide information about the specific needs of a child with a disability when there is a fire. When formulating an exit plan, ensure that the child's mobility system, such as the wheelchair or walker, can fit through all doors of the escape route. Wheelchair ramps should be installed at emergency exits to ensure easy access for these children. Whenever possible, children with physical disabilities should be housed on the first floor of a building because they will not be able to use an elevator in the event of a fire. New buildings that have only one accessible exit are required to set up a fireproof area equipped with an emergency call system. If such an area exists, the child must be trained in how to get to the area and call for assistance. Schools must have fire escape chairs available when children in powered chairs use the upper floors of school buildings. Families and institutions may also consider making a back-up plan for the eventuality of the child being unable to escape the burning building. In this case fire protection devices, such as sprinkler systems and fireproof partition walls, should be installed. Fireproof blankets and fire extinguishers are also helpful to the individual who needs assistance to evacuate.[55]

Safety with Strangers

All children must be educated about who they can and cannot trust and that they should never go anywhere with a stranger.[37] Children with disabilities may need more intensive and repeated learning opportunities to ensure that they can maintain their safety.

Safety with Strangers for Young Children

Young children learn about dealing with strangers from their parents, preschool, early elementary school, and storybooks. Stranger safety information is easily integrated into the school curriculum and in OT interventions. This issue is commonly addressed through information about the people in the community that children are safe to trust—community helpers such as policemen, firemen, security guards, teachers, and medical workers.[37] OT practitioners can assist children with learning about community helpers through discussions and activities that include coloring, cutting, gluing, or matching pictures of community helpers. OT practitioners also can recommend songs or storybooks to teachers and parents. It is the responsibility of parents and teachers to teach children not to go anywhere with strangers; however, at times, the OT practitioner may see the need to provide guidance to parents about effective methods for communicating this to their children and to teachers about methods for integrating activities to teach this safety lesson into the school curriculum.

Safety with Strangers for Older Children

Older children with disabilities may require repeated learning opportunities and practice with strategies to ensure they understand the rules and methods for keeping themselves safe. Common methods for introducing stranger safety concepts include pictures, movies, and social stories. The OT practitioner can ensure that children know what to do if they are confronted by strangers and provide opportunities for practice through role-play activities. Children can be taught that when a community helper is not present, they can make a loud noise, scream, or yell for assistance. Some children may also carry a whistle or other emergency noisemaker if they are unable make enough noise to get assistance in an emergency.[37]

SUMMARY

This chapter described IADLs, which include communication, community mobility, financial management, shopping, care of pets, health management and maintenance, home establishment and maintenance, meal preparation and cleanup, and safety and emergency procedures. Specifically, the chapter provided thorough descriptions of the IADLs and discussed how OT practitioners help children and adolescents with cognitive, physical, visual, and communication challenges engage in these activities. The chapter provided intervention strategies and discussed the considerations (e.g., family culture, community culture, age, physical setting) that practitioners examine when making clinical decisions. Specific intervention techniques such as forward and backward chaining, compensation, and assistive technology were introduced along with numerous case examples to illustrate sample intervention sessions. OT practitioners play a key role in helping children and adolescents engage in a variety of IADLs, which are important in developing autonomy and life satisfaction.

References

1. Alexandratos, K., et al. (2012). The impact of exercise on the mental health and quality of life of people with severe mental illness: a critical review. *Br J Occup Ther*, 75, 48–60.
2. American Academy of Pediatrics. (2014). *Car seats: information for families for 2014.* Available at http://www.healthychildren.org.
3. American National Standards Institute/Rehabilitation Engineering Research Center on Wheelchair Transportation Safety. (2000). *ANSI/RESNA WC19: wheelchairs used as seats in motor vehicles.* Available at http://www.rercwts.org/rerc_wts2_kt/rerc_wts2_kt_stand/Intro_WC19.html.
4. American National Standards Institute/Rehabilitation Engineering and Assistive Technology Society of North America. (2008). *ANSI/RESNA WC20: Wheelchair Standards/Volume 4: Wheelchairs and Transportation.* Available at http://www.rercwts.pitt.edu/RERC_WTS2_KT/RERC_WTS2_KT_Stand/Standards.html.
5. American Occupational Therapy Association. (2014). Occupational therapy practice framework: domain and process (3rd ed.). *Am J Occup Ther*, 68(Suppl. 1), S1–S48.
5a. American Occupational Therapy Association. (n.d.). The occupational therapy role in driving and community mobility across the lifespan (fact sheet). Available at: http://www.aota.org/About-Occupational-Therapy/Professionals/PA/Facts/Driving-Community-Mobility.aspx.

6. Blanchard, S. A. (2006). AOTA's statement on obesity. *Am J Occup Ther, 60,* 680.

7. Brinker, R. P., & Lewis, M. (1982). Discovering the competent handicapped infant: a process approach to assessment and intervention. *Top Early Child Special Educ, 2,* 1–16.

8. Brodwin, M. G., Cardoso, E., & Tristen, S. (2004). Computer assistive technology for people who have disabilities: computer adaptations and modifications. *J Rehabil, 70,* 28–33.

9. Brown, C., Moore, W. P., Hemman, D., & Yunek, A. (1996). Influence of instrumental activities of daily living assessment method on judgments of independence. *Am J Occup Ther, 50,* 202–206.

10. Bryan, L. C., & Gast, D. L. (2000). Teaching on-task and on-schedule behaviors to high-functioning children with autism via picture activity schedules. *J Autism Dev Disord, 30,* 553–567.

11. Bull, M. J., & Engle, W. A. (2009). Safe transportation of preterm and low birth weight infants at hospital discharge. *Pediatrics, 123,* 1424–1429.

12. Butler, C. (1997). Effects of powered mobility on self-initiated behaviors of very young children with locomotor disability. *Dev Med Child Neurol, 28,* 325–332.

13. Cahill, S. M., & Suarez-Balcazar, Y. (2009). Promoting children's nutrition and fitness in the urban context. *Am J Occup Ther, 63,* 113–116.

14. Chen, S. C., et al. (2004). Infrared-based communication augmentation system for people with multiple disabilities. *Disabil Rehabil, 26,* 1105–1109.

15. Clark, F., Reingold, F. S., & Salles-Jordan, K. (2007). Obesity and occupational therapy. *Am J Occup Ther, 61,* 701–703.

16. Cooper-Kahn, J., & Dietzel, L. (2008). What is executive functioning? Available at http://www.ldonline.org/article/29122/.

17. Deitz, J., Swinth, Y., & White, O. (2002). Powered mobility and preschoolers with complex developmental delays. *Am J Occup Ther, 56,* 86–96.

18. Dunn, L., et al. (2013). Household task participation of children with and without physical disability. *Am J Occup Ther, 67,* e100–e105.

19. Dunst, C. J., et al. (1995). Young children's natural learning environments: contrasting approaches to early childhood intervention indicate differential learning opportunities. *Psych Reports, 96,* 231–234.

20. Dwyer, G., et al. (2009). Promoting children's health and well-being: broadening the therapy perspective. *Phys Occup Ther Pediatr, 29,* 27–43.

21. DynaVox Mayer Johnson. (2014). Available at: http://www.dynavoxtech.com/products/.

22. Fager, S., et al. (2012). Access to augmentative and alternative communication: new technologies and clinical decision making. *J of Ped Rehab Med, 5,* 53–61.

23. Feldman, P. H., et al. (2009). Medication management: evidence brief. *Home Healthc Nurse, 27,* 379–386.

24. Fire Protection Association. Safety tip sheets. Available at http://www.nfpa.org/safety-information/safety-tip-sheets.

25. Fraker, C., et al. (2007). *Food chaining: the proven 6-step plan to stop picky eating, solve feeding problems, and expand your child's diet.* Cambridge, MA: Da Capo Press.

26. Grimm, E. Z., et al. (2009). Meal preparation: comparing treatment approaches to increase acquisition or skills for adults with schizophrenic disorders. *Occup Ther J Res, 29,* 148–153.

27. Haslbeck, J. W., & Schaeffer, D. (2009). Routines in medication management: the perspective of people with chronic conditions. *Chronic Illn, 5,* 184.

28. Infinitec. Infinite potential through assistive technology. Available at http://www.infinitec.org/live/homemodifications/lowcostalternatives.htm.

29. Jacobs, K., et al. (2011). Wii health: a preliminary study of the health and wellness benefits of Wii Fit on university students. *Br J Occup Ther, 74,* 262–268.

30. Jones, J., & Stewart, H. (2004). A description of how three occupational therapists train children in using the scanning access technique. *Austr Occup Ther J, 51,* 155–165.

31. Kondo, T., et al. (1997). The use of microwave ovens by elderly persons with disabilities. *Am J Occup Ther, 51,* 739–747.

32. Kripalani, S., et al. (2007). Development of an illustrated medication schedule as a low-literacy patient education tool. *Patient Educ Couns, 66,* 368–377.

33. Moreira-Almeida, A., & Koenig, H. G. (2006). Retaining the meaning of the words religiousness and spirituality: a commentary on the WHOQOL SRPB group's "A cross cultural study of spirituality, religion and personal beliefs as components of quality of life.". *Soc Sci Med, 63,* 843–845.

34. Munguba, M. C., Valdes, M. T. M., & Da Silva, C. A. B. (2008). The application of an occupational therapy nutrition education programme for children who are obese. *Occup Ther Int, 15,* 56–70.

35. Murdock, L. C., et al. (2013). Use of an iPad play story to increase play dialog of preschoolers with autism spectrum disorders. *J Autism Dev Disorder, 43,* 2174–2189.

36. *My Child Safety: Child safety devices.* (2008). Available at http://www.mychildsafety.net/child-safety-devices.html.

37. *My Child Safety: Stranger danger.* (2008). Available at http://www.mychildsafety.net/stranger-danger.html.

38. National Highway Traffic Safety Administration. (2011). *Simple facts about LATCH.* Available at http://www.nhtsa.gov/Safety/LATCH.

39. Orrell-Valente, J. K., et al. (2008). At what age do children start taking daily asthma medicines on their own? *Pediatrics, 128,* e1186–e1192.

40. PECS USA. What is PECS? Available at http://www.pecsusa.com/pecs.php.

41. Pierce, S. L. (2013). Restoring functional and community mobility. In M. V. Radomski, & C. A. Trombly (Eds.), *Occupational therapy for physical dysfunction.* Baltimore, MD: Lippincott Williams & Wilkins.

42. Powell, J. M., et al. (2007). Gaining insight into patients' perspectives on participation in home management activities after traumatic brain injury. *Am J Occup Ther, 61,* 269–279.

43. Primeau, L. A. (1998). Orchestration of work and play within families. *Am J Occup Ther, 52,* 188–195.

44. Savarimuthu, D., & Bunnell, T. (2003). Sexuality and learning disabilities. *Nurs Stand, 17,* 33–35.

45. Son, S. H., et al. (2006). Comparing two types of augmentative and alternative communication systems for children with autism. *Ped Rehab, 9,* 389–395.

46. Shutrump, S. E., Manary, M., & Buning, M. E. (2008). Transportation for students who use wheelchairs on the school bus. *OT Practice, 13,* 8–12.
47. Sigafoos, J., et al. (2005). Supporting self-determination in AAC interventions by assessing preference for communication devices. *Technol Disabil, 17,* 143–153.
48. Stav, W. (2009). Seatbelts on school buses, not a good idea. *OT Practice, 14,* 18–20.
49. Reference deleted in proofs.
50. Stav, W. B., et al. (2005). Driving and community mobility. *Am J Occup Ther, 59,* 666–670.
51. Toglia, J. (1999). Management of occupational therapy services for persons with cognitive impairments (statement). *Am J Occup Ther, 53,* 605–607.
52. United States Access Board. (1998). *ADA accessibility guidelines for transportation vehicles, September.* Available at http://www.access-board.gov/guidelines-and-standards/transportation.
53. U.S. Fire Administration. Fire safety for people with visual impairments. Available at http://www.usfa.fema.gov/citizens/disability/fswy20.shtm.
54. Reference deleted in proofs.
55. U.S. Fire Administration. Fire safety checklist for people with disabilities. Available at http://www.usfa.fema.gov/citizens/disability/fswy23.shtm.
56. Watson, A. H., et al. (2010). Effect of technology in a public school setting. *Am J Occup Ther, 64,* 18–29.
57. Whiteman, E. (1989). Microwave cookers: their value for people with disabilities. *Br J Occup Ther, 52,* 55–58.
58. Wynn, K., et al. (2006). Creating connections: a community capacity-building project with parents and youth with disabilities in transition to adulthood. *Phys & Occup Ther Ped, 26,* 89–103.

Resource List

ADAPTIVE SPORTS ORGANIZATIONS

Disabled Sports USA: www.dsusa.org
Dwarf Athletic Association of America: www.daaa.org
Great Lakes Adaptive Sports Association: www.glasa.org
Adaptive Sports Center of Crested Butte Colorado: www.adaptivesports.org
International Paralympic Committee: www.paralympic.org
BlazeSports America: www.blazesports.org
National Sports Center for the Disabled: www.nscd.org
National Wheelchair Basketball Association: www.nwba.org
Special Olympics: www.specialolympics.org
United States Association of Blind Athletes: www.usaba.org
USA Deaf Sports Federation: www.usadeafsports.org

DAILY LIVING AIDS COMPANIES

Daily Living Aids for People who are Blind or Visually Impaired: www.annmorris.com
Dynamic Living: www.dynamic-living.com
Independent Living Aids, Inc.: www.independentliving.com
Sammons Preston Roylan: www.sammonspreston.com

REVIEW *Questions*

1. List five IADLs and describe how they relate to occupational performance in children and adolescents.
2. What therapeutic activities might the OT practitioner use to address difficulties in community mobility for a child or adolescent?
3. What are the safety procedures and emergency procedures the OT practitioner may need to address with children and youth?
4. Describe some communication strategies. How would the OT practitioner consult with a speech therapy practitioner? Describe the differences in the two roles.
5. What are some intervention strategies to help a child or adolescent engage in health management and maintenance activities?
6. How might the OT practitioner help a child with physical or cognitive difficulties with home establishment and maintenance?

SUGGESTED *Activities*

1. Choose one IADL in which you currently engage. Describe in detail the tasks involved in this IADL. Describe how your abilities have changed since childhood. Discuss those things that have helped you succeed or have interfered with your ability to perform. How would you help a child perform this IADL?
2. Describe some compensatory strategies to help a child or youth who is visually impaired perform IADLs. What equipment is available? Describe resources in your area.
3. Interview adolescents to better understand their health management and maintenance routines. What issues are they facing regarding sexuality, fitness, and nutrition?

4. Design a meal preparation activity for toddlers, middle school children, and adolescents. Participate in the activity with a child and describe how you had to change your activity to be successful. Examine what you would do differently next time. How did you choose this activity and whom would it benefit?

5. Review the section on community mobility and then explore the options in your neighborhood. Describe the transportation options and consider how a child or adolescent who uses a wheelchair would access such options. Explore how a child would access the typical activities (e.g., school, playground, sports, local places). Present your findings to classmates.

6. Prepare a meal using a variety of cooking adaptations (from class or from local store). Describe how the adaptations changed the task.

7. Visit a speech therapy practitioner and discuss the variety of communication devices. How does the practitioner view the role of the OT practitioner? Communicate with a child who uses a communication device. Discuss this with the speech therapy practitioner and specifically ask about techniques that would help the communication. Provide a summary of your findings to classmates.

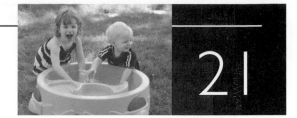

Play and Playfulness

JANE CLIFFORD O'BRIEN
ELIZABETH W. CRAMPSEY

KEY TERMS

Play
Intrinsic motivation
Internal control
Freedom to suspend reality
Pretend play
Playfulness
Framing
Play adaptations
Just-right challenge
Play assessment
Play environment

CHAPTER *Objectives*

After studying this chapter, the reader will be able to accomplish the following:

- Describe the characteristics of play and playfulness and differentiate between the two
- Identify potential barriers to play that children with disabilities may encounter
- Describe ways to facilitate play and playfulness in children who have special needs
- Describe the way that play is used as a tool in occupational therapy sessions to increase skills
- Describe how play is used as a goal of occupational therapy
- Identify occupational therapy observational assessments used to evaluate play and playfulness
- Describe techniques that promote play and playfulness

CHAPTER *Outline*

CASE *Study*

Think about a time in your childhood when you were playing.

- What were you doing?
- Who was with you?
- Were you playing with friends, peers, or siblings?
- Where were you?
- How did you feel?
- What was the expression on your face?
- What did you learn?
- Was playing an important aspect of your day?
- Is your memory a joyful one?

Perhaps you are thinking about a time you and your friends sat on your grandmother's porch and played house. Maybe you were playing school. Perhaps you were on a playground. Recalling these moments brings many happy memories to mind. People remember laughing, making friends, learning and testing skills (such as who could jump the highest), problem solving, and negotiating. These skills are critical to a child's development and provide a foundation for the future.

Children learn motor, social–emotional, language, and cognitive skills through play.[21,27,37] To illustrate this fact, consider a 1-year-old girl playing in the water sprinkler. She must problem solve how to turn on the faucet with the right amount of water. She bends down to feel the cool water in her hands. She is practicing motor planning, squatting, and balancing while receiving the tactile sensation of the water on her hands. As she cups her hands on the sprinkler, she must coordinate her tiny fingers to grasp the nozzle. Cognitively, she pays attention to the water and tries to figure out what happens when she changes her hand position. She is learning the ways in which liquid differs from the solid ground on which she stands. She problem solves to keep the water in her hands and tries to understand the reason it leaks through. Orally, she feels the water on her tongue and swallows the droplets. She sticks her tongue out and gathers the liquid in her mouth, then throat to swallow it. Her 4-year-old brother joins the play activity, and now she must share the sprinkler. This requires flexibility and negotiation, perhaps even the managing of conflict. He laughs and jumps. She watches and smiles and tries to imitate his skills. She is developing social skills. The children repeat the play activities. Watching them, it becomes clear that play requires many skills.

Children learn and refine skills during play.[6] This is demonstrated as children show off feats of strength and agility, problem solve to play a game or perform a motor skill, and work out problems that arise. They communicate to satisfy their needs and decide on rules for the activities by negotiating with group members. Often children spend the entire playtime deciding on the rules of the game or the way the story will unfold. They use their language skills and must become keen observers of nonverbal communication.[9]

Maximizing a child's ability to play interests occupational therapy (OT) practitioners because it is the primary occupation of childhood and critical to the development of skills across all performance areas.[9,24] To appreciate the importance of play, imagine life without it. Life would certainly be lacking without play. Parham and Primeau underscored the importance of play by stating that it may reveal what makes life worth living.[33]

With this appreciation of the importance of play, imagine making a difference in a child's ability to play. Developing a child's play skills comprehensively affects both the child and his or her family. The child is better able to interact with friends, family members, and the environment. Studies show that strong social skill development and play correlate with overall success in life.

OT practitioners work with children to enhance their ability to play and thus can make a difference in their lives.

PLAY

Most adults smile when asked to remember a time when they were playing. They reminisce about childhood memories of favorite toys and activities. They laugh and relate humorous stories such as having mud fights and conducting elaborate neighborhood play events. Adults recall historic events from childhood play such as pretending to be astronauts landing on the moon. They are able to describe the activities, feelings, and skills they gained during play. Most agree that play was, and still is, fun! It provides an opportunity to be carefree. When was the last time you played? When was the last time you were able to be in the moment and stay in the moment to play? When was the last time you pretended? Or laughed with abandon?

Play is generally defined as a pleasurable, self-initiated activity that the child can control.[8] **Intrinsic motivation** is the self-initiation or drive to action for which the reward is the activity itself rather than some external reward.[9] Intrinsic motivation is demonstrated when children repeat activities.[8,9] **Internal control** is the extent to which the child is in control of the actions and to some degree the outcome of an activity.[8,9] Internal control is observed when children spontaneously change the play (e.g., when a 6-year-old boy declares in the middle of a pretend game, "Now I am going to be the good guy"). Intrinsic motivation and internal control are important for the development of problem solving, learning, and socialization skills.

Another element of play is the **freedom to suspend reality**, which is sometimes seen as the ability to participate in make-believe activities, or pretend play (Figure 21-1).[9,40] **Pretend play** develops as children are able to engage in higher cognitive functioning.[37] They begin by role-playing simple everyday actions such as feeding a doll. They are

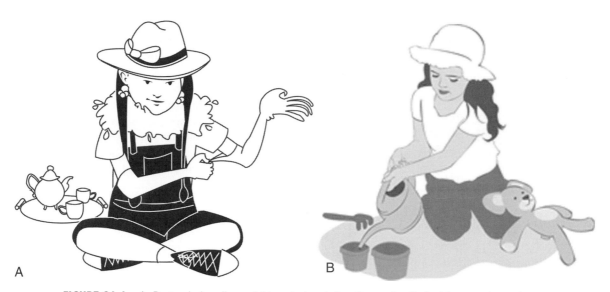

FIGURE 21-1   A, Pretend play allows children to break free from rules. **B,** A girl pretends to plant a garden in her playroom using her toys.

able to engage in elaborate make-believe scenarios as their language and cognitive skills develop.

Freedom to suspend reality also includes teasing, joking, mischief, and bending the rules.[9] Children turn old games into new ones by altering the traditional sequence, changing the rules, creating new situations, and using objects imaginatively during play.

Play is the primary occupation of children and a medium for intervention.[10,21,29,32] Play affords skillful OT practitioners unlimited opportunities to teach, refine, and enable more successful functioning and play. Play allows for the blend of components of reality with imagination allowing an opportunity to learn about social cues and rules while having fun.

CLINICAL *Pearl*

OT practitioners can evaluate the characteristics of play to design interventions. Emphasis is placed on using the child's strengths to improve weak areas. For example, a child who is highly motivated to play but lacks the needed physical skills may be encouraged to perform activities in an alternative way. A child who focuses on the end product (e.g., winning the game) versus the process of play may benefit from participating in play activities that have no end product, such as imaginative play. Turning challenging tasks into play will be more successful than to focus solely on a challenging component for the child or youth.

PLAYFULNESS

Playfulness is defined as one's disposition to play.[9,10] It is a style individuals use to flexibly approach problems and can be regarded as an aspect of a child's personality.[10,11] Playfulness, like play, encompasses intrinsic motivation,

internal control, and freedom to suspend reality, all of which occur on a continuum.[9,11,21]

Children who are engaged in the play process are intrinsically motivated. They show signs of enjoyment and seem to be having fun.[9,11,13] Internal control is evidenced in sharing, playing with others, entering new play situations, initiating play, deciding, modifying activities, and challenging themselves.[9,11,13] Children who use objects creatively or in unconventional ways, tease, and pretend show the element of freedom to suspend reality (Figure 21-2).[10,13]

CASE *Study*

Children lacking playfulness exhibit problems fulfilling their roles as players. For example, 6-year-old Sam has sensory integrative dysfunction. He has difficulty with motor tasks and does not play well with other children. Sam is not spontaneous in activities. He requires time to plan how he will accomplish motor tasks. Sam becomes upset when he does not get his way. He does not like the rules to be changed and has trouble changing pace once he is involved in an activity. Moreover, he does not read the other children's cues and frequently plays too rough. He shows poor body awareness by getting too close to the other children. Sam does not initiate play with his peers. His slow and awkward movements cause him to lag behind. During the OT evaluation, Sam says that he has no friends and no one likes him. His parents are worried that Sam does not have any friends. The goal of his OT sessions is to improve his playfulness so that he can interact with friends in the home, school, and community settings.

The OT practitioner works to develop rapport with Sam and plans fun and playful activities. Sam does not initiate play

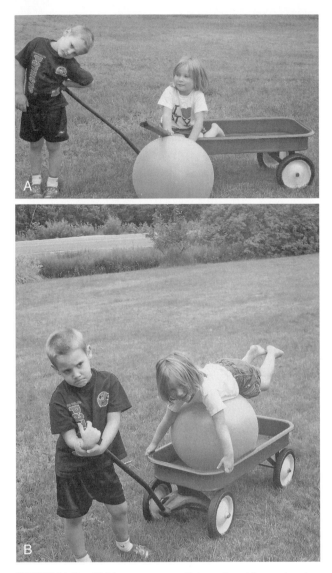

FIGURE 21-2 Children must negotiate and problem solve during play. **A,** A girl and a boy spend time figuring out what to do with the large ball, stick, and wagon. They must negotiate who will pull the wagon. **B,** The boy pulls the wagon while the girl is holding on tight. They challenge their motor skills (e.g., balancing on the large ball). Using objects in unconventional ways (e.g., lying on the ball in the wagon) is part of playfulness.

activities but is cooperative and attempts all of them. The OT practitioner strives to enable him to have fun and be spontaneous during the therapy sessions, hoping that this behavior extends to the home and school settings as well.

During one session, the OT practitioner and Sam engage in a game of Star Wars. Sam, playing Darth Vader, runs after the OT practitioner, saying, "I will get you, Luke." The OT practitioner is thrilled that Sam is initiating play. However, shortly thereafter Sam stops playing, looks at the OT practitioner, and says, "Is it time to go yet?"

Sam exhibits a low level of playfulness. He is not engaged in sustained, intense enjoyment. He focuses on the end product (completing therapy) rather than being

intrinsically motivated to play and be in the moment. Poor internal control is characterized by an inability to enter new play situations, initiate play with peers, share, decide what to do, and challenge himself. Sam is able to engage in pretend play when acting out Star Wars with the OT practitioner but has difficulty reading others' cues, which is evident when he plays too roughly and gets too close to his peers during interactions.

Considering Sam's limitations and the long-term goal of enabling him to play with peers, his OT objectives include the following:

1. Spontaneously initiating a change in activity, at least three times, during a 45-minute supervised play situation.
2. Responding positively (smiling, remain engaged, cooperating with the OT practitioner) when he does not get his way, at least three times during a supervised play situation.
3. Entering a group of peers already playing on the playground and participating in the activity without interrupting the play, at least three times a week.
4. Engaging in a motor challenge during play, at least three times, during a supervised play situation.

Framing situations as play allows children to know what play is so that they may interact accordingly. They are free to pretend, challenge each other, and tease without malice. All of these actions require that children read nonverbal as well as verbal cues. Reading nonverbal cues allows children to realize when they have pushed a boundary too far during play.

CASE *Study*

Scott and Alison are playing in a sandbox, pouring sand on each other. They laugh and watch for cues from each other that say, "This is okay. We are still playing." The game continues, and Alison begins to pour sand on Scott's head. She receives a serious look from Scott. The nonverbal cue says, "Hey, that is a little too close to my eyes. I do not like that." Alison responds with a smile that says, "Oops! I'm sorry," and pours sand on Scott's arm instead. Her nonverbal response says, "Okay, I'll be more careful." This exchange of cues allows the play to continue while they learn to be attentive to each other. They are learning the rules and boundaries of play.

Assessment of a child's playfulness provides information about the way the child processes, problem solves, and manages emotional stress. These skills are important to the child's development and social well-being.

NATURE OF PLAY AND PLAYFULNESS

OT practitioners must understand the nature of play and playfulness to be able to use it effectively as an

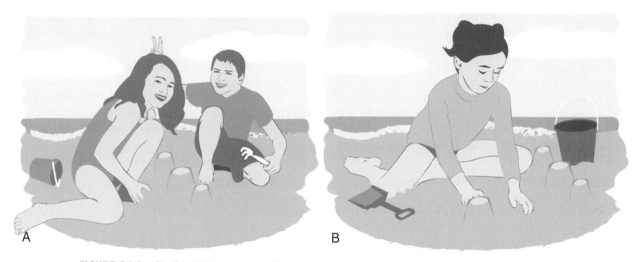

FIGURE 21-3   Playful children may be silly or serious during play. **A,** A boy shows playfulness by his teasing his sister. **B,** The girl is quite serious and concentrates on the task while building a sandcastle.

intervention technique. When children play and are playful, depending on the activity, they may laugh, smile, and be active; they may also be serious, quiet, and totally absorbed in play (Figure 21-3). Play can be frustrating, and it can involve failure. The flexible and spontaneous nature of play and playfulness is demonstrated when children change themes or use toys in unexpected ways.

The process (doing) rather than the product (outcome) provides the primary source of reward in play activities.[9] Children engage in play for its own sake.[10,13] Playful children discover, create, and explore. Therefore no way of playing is right or wrong. Play is a safe outlet for children to challenge themselves and helps them develop skills.

OT practitioners must remember to maintain the nature of play and playfulness during therapy. Children who have special needs may require additional assistance to play.[35] OT practitioners are knowledgeable about the abilities of children who have special needs and are therefore in an ideal position to promote play and playfulness.

PLAY DEVELOPMENT OF CHILDREN WITH DISABILITIES

The normal sequence for the development of play is often delayed in children who have special needs.[27,28] (see Chapter 8 for a discussion of this sequence). This may be the result of limited physical, cognitive, or social–emotional skills.[27,28] For example, a child who is unable to bring the hands to the mouth has trouble exploring the environment. Children who are unable to experience sensations in a typical manner often require intervention to engage in play opportunities, which stimulate their growth and development. If children are not afforded these opportunities, they may exhibit poor play skills.[28,30,35] Changing or modifying the environment (such as modifying the playground for wheelchair

access) helps children who have special needs experience play.[28,30]

Children with special needs may take longer to respond, make less obvious responses, initiate activities less frequently, and be less interactive than other children. They are often passive in their play.[27,28] Children with intellectual deficits exhibit a restricted repertoire of play and language, decreased attention span, and less social interaction during play.[27,28] Children with visual impairments are less interested in reaching out to explore and engage in social exchanges during play.[27] Children with hearing impairments show less symbolic and less organized play.[27]

Children with developmental and physical disabilities commonly experience difficulty playing. They do not have the same play skills as their typically developing peers, and therefore are not exposed to the same play opportunities. These barriers are believed to correlate with deficits in other areas of the child's development such as social and emotional, speech, gross motor, creativity, and problem-solving abilities. Children with disabilities often receive interventions for their diagnosed disabilities and their presenting symptoms; unfortunately, most interventions less often are play-based.[25]

Children with attention-deficit/hyperactivity disorder (ADHD) commonly experience difficulty engaging in cooperative play.[20] They tend to play for shorter periods of time, frequently change their play activity, and have difficulty returning to an activity after an interruption.[15] In structured play settings, children with ADHD often experience trouble transitioning from one activity to another and display more negative play behaviors (such as disrupting and violating established play rules).[20]

Cordier et al. studied children with ADHD to determine how to effectively design a play-based intervention model.[21] They focused on the typical behaviors of children with ADHD, their play environments, and motivating the children. The impulsive and hyperactive behavior in conjunction with poor self-regulation and control may also create deficits in a child's intrinsic control and motivation, a foundational component of play. They suggested that OT practitioners use a client-centered approach to design interventions for children with ADHD focusing on improving their socials skills and reducing tendencies of disruption and domination.[20]

Children with autism spectrum disorders display deficits in communication abilities, social interactions, and range of interests and activities. They can show limited socialization and imagination, which interferes with play. Children with this diagnosis tend to prefer to play alone, and when in groups, they commonly have difficulty detecting and understanding the meaning of verbal and nonverbal social cues displayed by the other children.[39] To successfully promote play, OT practitioners strive to create interventions that are both appealing and motivating to the child.

Children with sensory processing disorder (SPD) and those with developmental coordination disorder (DCD; see Chapters 13 and 25 for explanations of these conditions) may have difficulties with play and playfulness.[14,19] These children may benefit from play-environment adaptations and focus on their ability to play. SPD often interferes with a child's ability to interact with people and objects in his or her environment due to the poorly regulated reaction to multiple inputs (or sensory inputs). Children with DCD experience gross motor delays. Furthermore, once they have mastered tasks, they repeatedly perform the tasks with little variation and show limited flexibility in their movement patterns.[14]

With respect to play, this lack of variability or flexibility causes less interest in play and participation in playgroups. Bundy et al. found that for children with SPD, changing the play setting seems to have more effect on play capabilities than does focusing on remediating praxis (e.g., motor planning).[15] For example, modifying a child's environment to better stimulate interest and inspire confidence may promote expansion of social play skills. Improving social skills and confidence through play may lead to parallel developments in other areas of a child's life and learning experiences.[39]

Children with cerebral palsy (CP) display impaired postural control and functional ambulation, which can be accompanied by emotional and behavioral dysfunction[38] (see Chapter 17). CP affects both physical and cognitive development, including communication skills, and is present throughout an individual's life span. These functional impairments may create significant barriers to a child's development of playfulness. **Play adaptation** refers to modifying the play environment by reducing physical barriers helps increase playfulness in children with CP.[12] Improving communication with parents and peers can also positively influence playfulness with this diagnostic group.[12]

To meet developmental challenges and learn ways to play, children with special needs require assistance.[27,28] OT practitioners must understand typical development and play patterns, and support these children when teaching skills and facilitating play. For example, OT practitioners can increase spontaneity in children by allowing them to discover play materials that have been hidden or placed within reach.[28,35] OT practitioners identify children's strengths and weaknesses, as well as those of the family, to design effective interventions. Capitalizing on strengths increases the success of therapy and facilitates development of advanced play skills.

CLINICAL *Pearl*

Children play in various physical positions. OT practitioners make sure that children with special needs spend time in many positions, such as supine, quadruped, sitting, kneeling, and standing positions. Playtime is not the time to work on positioning. Children should be free to use their arms and hands and feel safe.

INFLUENCE OF ENVIRONMENT ON PLAY

The environment in which play occurs influences children's play. Each child has his or her own unique style of play, which is shaped by age, sex, experiences, family, and environment. Engaging in play depends on a child's feeling of safety, confidence, and interests. Therefore a child's environment may promote or restrict playfulness.[15,39] For example, structuring of school days and the availability of staff members influence play environments and opportunities for children. Currently, many schools have restricted the allotted time for outdoor recesses and have removed equipment from playgrounds. In the past, children commonly played outdoors in wooded areas or cleared fields and mostly did not play with manufactured toys, or have screen time, which promoted social interactions, imaginative play, creativity, and physical activity.[12] Bundy suggested that parental responses to safety concerns have reduced the opportunities for children's play in imaginative and creative ways.[12] For example, parents and teachers promote the "correct way" to go down a slide. Children commonly play on playgrounds—play environments with static play equipment (slides, swings, climbers, etc.) that do not lend themselves to nearly as much imaginative play and creative manipulation.[11,12] For children with physical disabilities, playgrounds can create a barrier to cooperative play with their typically developing peers.

It is important for the OT practitioner to consider a child's environment when assessing play and playfulness. Models such as the Model of Human Occupation and Person–Environment–Occupation examine how the physical or social environment supports or inhibits a child's play.[24] Interventions focusing on changing or modifying environmental factors can be helpful in promoting play skills.

The Importance of Playground and Recess for Children and Youth

Most adults remember playing on a playground at recess as children. What types of things do you remember doing—playing in the sandbox, climbing on a play structure, swinging on swings, spinning on the whirl-a-round, or taking turns on a see-saw? Do you remember playing organized games, such as hopscotch, four-square, kick ball, or tag? Did you play alone, with the same friends, or did you do different things with different peers? How did you feel when on the playground? Chances are you even remember managing some kind of conflict on the playground.

The importance of providing recess to children and youth cannot be minimized. Recess and time on the playground are an essential routine for children. It provides a much needed, most often outside, time for children to get a break. Play aids in the development of social, emotional, physical, and cognitive skills that students need to be successful both in school, as well as in society.[18] Children who participate in play activities learn skills and solve problems needed in adulthood.[1-3] Additionally, there are documented benefits for higher achievement in school and setting a foundation for healthy habits in adulthood. It provides an opportunity to take a break from the rigors of learning, and a chance to recoup energy.[2,3]

The many benefits of physical activity are widely known and accepted, with the Centers for Disease Control and Prevention citing weight control and reduced risk for cardiovascular disease, type 2 diabetes, and some cancers.[16,17] Additionally, physical activity is found to strengthen bones and muscles and increase life expectancy.[17] Research finds that attention to classroom tasks is improved after recess.[22,23] Other benefits of recess and time on the playground include improved mood and an opportunity to practice life skills through play skills. These skills include: cooperation, self-regulation, social participation, turn-taking and sharing, strength and coordination, self-advocacy and self-confidence.[33]

OT practitioners who work in school systems promote participation in all activities and occupations, inclusive of recess. OT practitioners are well positioned to modify activities and environments and support participation.

OT practitioners can promote social participation by identifying opportunities for inclusion and collaboration and by adjusting the playground challenge to the "**just-right challenge**." OT practitioners include students of all abilities and provide opportunities for positive social engagement. Due to the ability of OT practitioners to break down tasks and needs, they can recommend specialized equipment and modifications for accessibility to promote play for children of all ages and abilities.[41,42] Through promotion of proper playground equipment and recess time, OT practitioners create opportunities for children to develop confidence as well as physical, social and emotional skills.[41,42] Through play, caregivers can model and nurture appropriate social behaviors to help children navigate social situations and even help make schools safer for children.[26]

Providing inclusive play spaces for children supports independent and social play in either a supported or free form way. A play space becomes inclusive when it is physically accessible, has activities that are age appropriate and provides a stimulating sensory experience. Kanics described seven primary principles of design when thinking about providing inclusive play spaces.[23] These are included in Box 21-1.

Learning, playing, and growing are largely influenced by children's goals that are accomplished through play and that is how children occupy their free time.[1-3] Play is the primary occupation for children and therefore supports and facilitates the development of physical coordination, emotional maturation, social skills, and social interactions.

RELEVANCE OF PLAY

CASE *Study*

Twelve-month-old Frankie cannot sit up because of hydrocephalus and poor trunk tone. He is nonverbal. He can move his arms but is unable to reach and grasp objects. He occasionally smiles and laughs. His vision is poor. After positioning him properly, the OT practitioner places a mercury switch attached to a flashlight on his arm. When Frankie raises his arm, the flashlight lights up his face. Frankie raises his arm soon after the switch is placed on his arm and smiles when the flashlight lights up his face. He puts his arm down and the light turns off. Frankie laughs and laughs. He repeats this activity numerous times. It is evident that he realizes he is in control of the light. His mother has tears in her eyes. She turns to the OT practitioner and says, "Frankie is playing."

OT changed this family's perception of Frankie by showing them his ability to play, which is both a powerful tool and an important outcome in OT by increasing his social engagement and interaction.

BOX 21-1

Principles of Universal Design

Equitable use	The design is useful and marketable to people with diverse abilities
Flexibility in use	The design accommodates a wide range of individual preferences and abilities
Simple and intuitive use	Use of the design is easy to understand, regardless of the user's experience, knowledge, language skills, or current concentration level
Perceptible information	The design communicates necessary information effectively to the user, regardless of ambient conditions or the user's sensory abilities
Tolerance for error	The design minimizes hazards and the adverse consequences of accidental or unintended actions
Low physical effort	The design can be used effectively and comfortably with a minimum of fatigue
Size and space for approach and use	Appropriate size and space is provided for approach, reach, manipulation and use regardless of the user's body size, posture or mobility

Copyright © 1997 NC State University, The Center for Universal Design. Connell, B.R., Jones, M., Mace, R., Mueller, J., Mullick, A., Ostroff, E., Sanford, J., Steinfeld, M.S., Vanderheiden, G. The Center for Universal Design (1997). *The principles of universal design,* Version 2.0, Raleigh, NC: North Carolina State University.

CLINICAL *Pearl*

Observe the child's movements when deciding where to position a switch. Place the switch where the child can activate it by using movement patterns he or she uses automatically. This promotes play and provides the child with control and immediate success for this cause-and-effect opportunity.

OT practitioners work with families, educators, and other professionals to improve the quality of life for children and their families. Play is vital to a child's development and an important outcome of intervention. OT practitioners who use play may be faced with parents and professionals who do not take them seriously.[8] Engaging parents in discussions from the beginning of the process educates them about the importance of play during therapy sessions. OT practitioners discuss with parents how the session went and the progress made toward the goals. OT practitioners who recognize that parents do not value play as a goal may decide to emphasize the use of play as a tool to increase the child's skills in other areas. Other professionals may take OT practitioners more seriously once they see the progress a child makes in OT. OT practitioners may frequently need to educate parents and other professionals on the purpose of the use of play and its correlation to development, social skills development, engaging in meaningful activities.

To promote play and playfulness, activities recommended for the home should be limited to those that are fun and nonthreatening for the child. The child can engage in activities in which he or she can show off certain abilities to the parents. This is motivating for both the child and the parents. OT practitioners investigate the role of play in children's lives and focus on providing them with a means to play.

Play as a Tool

Play is often used as a tool to increase skill development. Occupational therapy is designed around play activities that will increase skills such as strength, motor planning, problem solving, grasping, and handwriting, which are necessary for the child to function. Using play as a tool to improve a child's ability to function has many advantages. Children typically cooperate and readily engage in play. Most goals can be addressed during a play session because play encompasses a variety of activities.

The characteristics of play (i.e., intrinsic motivation, internal control, and suspension of reality) need to be present when play is used as a tool to improve a child's skills. These characteristics occur within the framework of a play setting. The OT practitioner arranges the environment so that children can choose activities that help meet their goals while having fun. The OT practitioner allows the child to tease, engage in mischief, and face challenges. The practitioner allows the child to participate and engage in the give and take of a social exchange.

CLINICAL *Pearl*

Many household items make novel toys for the clinic and home. Pots and pans can be containers, musical instruments, or even hats. They promote pretend play. Cardboard boxes, grocery bags, and laundry baskets can be used for a variety of play activities. Bring them into the clinic to allow children to explore and be creative with them.

Making therapy sessions fun through play is not always easy. OT practitioners set up an environment to encourage the child to choose activities that foster therapy goals. This is considered the art of therapy.[4,10]

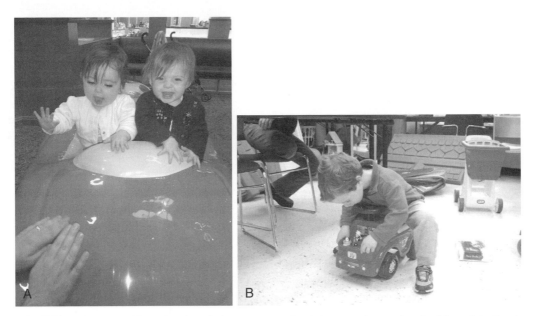

FIGURE 21-4 **A,** Children interact with each other during an occupational therapy play session. Social participation is an important part of play. Setting up the environment to facilitate social interactions helps the children spontaneously interact. **B,** The play environment provides children a chance to explore toys. This child decides to ride the truck (although this is not how the toy is intended to be used; the practitioner allows it to continue to encourage creativity).

The OT practitioner sets up the just-right challenge, which is one that is neither too hard nor too easy.[4,10] The OT practitioner must know the child's strengths and weaknesses to do this effectively. Some children are competitive and enjoy such games. Others fear failure and may be easily intimidated by competitive games. Some children enjoy roughhousing, and others do not. Making a therapy session fun means observing a child's subtle cues and spontaneously adapting the session to maintain a level of excitement and motivation. (Figure 21-4 shows children in a play session that has been set up to encourage play.)

A physically and emotionally safe environment allows the child to feel in control. The OT practitioner designs activities to target specific skills. The child is only aware that the activity is fun. Often the practitioner may need to discreetly change the way the task is performed to get the maximum benefit from the activity. This must be done playfully to keep the flow of the play session going.[21] Sometimes the practice of a skill takes priority over playing.

A critical element of play is for activities to be free from rules. This does not mean that rules are not present in play activities but that they are negotiable. Children may make up new rules and change them during play. OT practitioners provide enough rules for children to feel secure and safe without imposing so many that they do not feel free to play. Both the child and practitioner must have the freedom to change the activity. Therefore, if a child is performing an activity that does not promote therapy goals, the OT practitioner can modify the challenge. This is illustrated in a therapy session challenging the child's balance.

CASE *Study*

David is kneeling on a platform swing and propelling it forward and backward. The practitioner increases the skill level required by saying, "Oh, here come the asteroids," and throwing large balls under the swing. David looks at the OT practitioner, smiles, and says, "Hey, no fair. I didn't know that was coming." The OT practitioner responds, "The asteroids came out of nowhere! Luckily, you are Superman and were able to stay on the spaceship!" The changes are skillfully made so that the session remains playful.

CLINICAL *Pearl*

Children love to swing. Remember that swings are not just for children with sensory integrative dysfunction. Many children benefit from the sensations and movement patterns that accompany swinging.

Children can imagine a therapy session to be a spaceship ride, an Olympic quest, a deep-sea diving expedition, a skiing event, or a leisurely stroll down the alley. Through pretend play the child gains skills in imagination, verbalization, and communication. Equipment can and should be used to promote mastery and allow for novelty. Pretend play allows the OT practitioner to use the same equipment in countless ways that tap into the child's imagination. Teasing, joking, and mischief are parts of play. The child may teasingly throw a soft ball to hit the OT practitioner's head. Children may joke that the OT practitioner cannot perform a skill. Children develop their sense of humor during play.

Play provides an excellent tool for intervention when used correctly because children are highly motivated to participate.[12,27,29]

CASE *Study*

Angie is a 2-year-old girl with hemiplegia on the right side of her body. She lives with her two brothers aged 8 and 9 and her parents. Angie attends day care daily. She receives OT services for 1 hour every week. Her parents report that she does not play well with other children. She grabs their toys, pushes them, and screams as a way of getting her needs met. She does not like to be touched on her right side and does little weight bearing on that side. Angie has a difficult time engaging in play activities. She screams and cries when the OT practitioner touches her on the right arm. She does not initiate play. Angie exhibits decreased active range of motion in her right arm.

The OT practitioner designs an intervention that involves play to increase Angie's use of her right side. (See Chapter 7 for a description of the sequence and development of typical play and useful information for designing this type of intervention.) The OT practitioner considers Angie's age when choosing the play activities. Based on her knowledge of 2-year-old children, the OT practitioner chooses busy and messy play activities. According to Parten, 2-year-olds usually participate in solitary play but do make an effort to interact with other children.[34,36] The OT practitioner notes that 2-year-old children enjoy sensory activities such as playing in sandboxes, water play, and working with Play-Doh. They also enjoy manipulatable toys such as Legos, pop-up toys, and blocks and gross motor toys such as balls, riding toys, and swings.

The child's age and sex, the setting, and the concerns of parents must be considered when writing the goals and objectives of OT. The OT practitioner considers the child's physical capabilities and the factors interfering with her ability to play. Angie has right-sided hypersensitivity. She does not bear weight on the right side. Considering Angie's limitations and the long-term goal that she will use her right hand spontaneously for bimanual activities, Angie's therapy objectives include the following:

1. She will spontaneously reach for objects placed above her head with her right hand, at least five times during a 45-minute therapy session.
2. Using two hands, she will catch a 20-inch ball tossed underhand from 2 feet away, at least three times during a 45-minute session.

3. She will walk on a level surface at least 10 feet while holding on with both hands to a push toy such as a shopping cart.
4. She will use both hands to take apart small objects, such as pop beads, 75% of opportunities without signs of frustration.

Box 21-2 contains sample objectives involving play as a tool for OT intervention.

The OT practitioner designs play activities that incorporate the use of Angie's right side. She plays games rolling a large ball, wheelbarrow racing, and climbing a ladder. She pulls pop beads apart, dresses baby dolls, pours sand and water into containers, and makes confetti out of newspaper. All these activities require Angie to use both arms. The OT practitioner stages the activities in such a way that Angie is successful. The OT practitioner frequently provides Angie with hand-over-hand assistance. She watches for cues from Angie when placing a hand on her arms. The practitioner uses humor and laughter to keep the session playful. Intervention focuses on keeping the atmosphere fun and playful while increasing the functional use of Angie's right arm. The emphasis of the intervention session is to promote bilateral hand skill development. The OT practitioner assists Angie in using her right hand during play.

CLINICAL *Pearl*

Children love little packages. Wrap little items in small boxes and allow the children to unwrap them to improve fine motor skills through play. Have the children wrap up surprises for other children as a fun way to improve hand skills.

Table 21-1 lists toys associated with the development of specific client factors. Angie's case demonstrates the use of play as a tool to improve a child's physical skills. The OT practitioner uses play activities to increase the ability of the child to use her right side.

TABLE 21-1

Toys and Play Activities Designed to Target Selected Client Factors

CLIENT FACTOR	TOYS AND ACTIVITIES
SENSORY FUNCTION (SENSORY AWARENESS AND SENSORY PROCESSING)	
Tactile	Water play, massage, Play-Doh, Koosh balls, glue, beans, sand play, tactile boards, brushing, lotion games, stickers
Proprioceptive	Trampolines, jumping, pulling on ropes, climbing ladders, tug-of-war, pulling a wagon, wheelbarrow walking, pushing
Vestibular	Riding a bike, skateboarding, see-saw, sliding, swinging, Sit and Spin, rocking horse
Visual	Mobiles, toys that move, bright-colored rattles and toys, mirrors
Auditory	Musical toys, bells, rattles, CD players, songs
Gustatory	Food, gum, candy
Olfactory	Smelly markers, Play-Doh, smelly stickers, food
NEUROMUSCULOSKELETAL AND MOVEMENT-RELATED FUNCTIONS	
Strength	Ball games, bike riding, manipulative games, jump rope, Red Rover, London Bridge, swimming, sports
Endurance	Repetitive games, walking, sports, hiking, swimming, bike riding, climbing
Postural control	Trampolines, bike riding, sports, swimming, climbing, walking on uneven terrain
Gross coordination	Outdoor playground equipment, bikes, sports, water, outdoor play
Fine motor	Manipulatives, arts and crafts, small toys, figurines, dolls, dress-up, sewing, coloring, cutting
Oral-motor	Musical instruments, whistles, bubble blowers, pinwheels
MENTAL FUNCTIONS (AFFECTIVE, SELF-MANAGEMENT, COGNITIVE, PERCEPTUAL)	
Affective	
Psychological	Self-esteem board games, art projects, motor challenges
Interpersonal	Pictionary, team games, Twister, new games
Self-expression	Arts and crafts, pottery, clay, dance
Self-management	
Coping skills	Monopoly, life skills game, role playing
Cognitive	
Memory, sequencing	Board games (e.g., Memory, Clue, Monopoly, Candy Land)
Categorization	Card games (e.g., Hearts, Go Fish), sorting, matching games
Spatial operations	Puzzles, models, arts and crafts, Legos, Lincoln Logs
Problem solving	Board games, card games, arts and crafts, puzzles
Perceptual	
Perceptual processing	Puzzles, building blocks, doll houses, farms, building logs, model cars and airplanes, paper dolls, coloring books, mazes, computer games, dress-up, obstacle courses, Simon Says, Follow-the-Leader

Adapted from American Occupational Therapy Association. (2014). Occupational therapy practice framework: domain and process (3rd ed.). *Am J Occup Ther, 68*(Suppl. 1), S1–S48.

Play as a Goal

OT practitioners must be careful to avoid "teaching" play. They model play, cultivate the skills needed for play, and set up the environment to facilitate play. OT practitioners must ensure that play is enjoyable. Increasing the skills required for play is important and beneficial to the child.

OT practitioners must maintain the quality of play.[10,24,36] A child who has the skills needed for play but does not engage in spontaneous and intrinsically motivated activity is at risk. That child may show deficits in play that will carry over to the school, home, and community. Play deficits in childhood may inhibit a child's ability to gain the needed skills for adulthood.[19,36] Therefore, it is important for OT practitioners to target play as a goal of therapy.

The OT practitioner emphasizes the child's approach to activities and the manner in which the child

BOX 21-3

Sample Objectives When Play or Playfulness Is the Intended Outcome of Occupational Therapy Intervention

- Child will initiate one new activity during an adult-supervised play session.
- Child will enter into a play activity (already in progress) without disrupting the group during an adult-supervised play session.
- Child will stay with the same basic play theme for at least 15 minutes during an adult-supervised play session.
- Child will use an object in an unconventional manner spontaneously at least once during an adult-supervised play session.
- Child will share toys with another child (trading toys at least three times) during a 15-minute play session.

plays when play itself is the goal of therapy. For example, when play is viewed as a goal of therapy rather than merely a tool of intervention, the OT practitioner notes the way Angie (see the Case Study on p. 414) engages in play, not just her using her right hand to manipulate a toy. A short-term objective to increase Angie's play might be for her to spontaneously initiate play with a peer at least three times during an adult-supervised play session. Box 21-3 contains sample objectives when play is the goal (intended outcome) of OT intervention.

CASE *Study*

Angie's OT sessions include playmates because she needs assistance playing with others. The OT practitioner designs the environment to encourage Angie to respond to changes and be spontaneous. Angie participates in bilateral activities such as playing with balls, wheelbarrow racing, and ladder climbing. The OT practitioner facilitates a playful attitude in Angie while allowing her to pick the activities and choose the way she will perform them. The OT practitioner facilitates sharing, negotiating, and taking turns, and encourages the child's parents and teachers to facilitate the skills of sharing, negotiating, and taking turns at home and in the school, thus creating many opportunities for Angie to improve her play and playfulness.

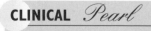

CLINICAL *Pearl*

Invite another child or OT practitioner to keep the play sessions exciting. This is a great way to learn new activities and methods of playing.

CASE *Study*

Angie's second session differs from the first, which targeted the use of her right hand, in that the emphasis is now on both interaction and motor skills as opposed to motor skills alone. The OT practitioner pays close attention to Angie's ability to engage in spontaneous activity, choose a variety of tasks, initiate changes, and read the cues of her peers. The Test of Playfulness (ToP) is used as a framework for the observation, evaluation, and documentation of playfulness.[7] O'Brien and colleagues were able to design play goals after a parental interview and a 30-minute observation of free play using the ToP as a guide.[31]

It is possible to use play as both a tool for therapy and a goal of therapy sessions. In Angie's case, it would be appropriate to work on increasing the use of her right side as well as improving play. This takes skill on the part of the OT practitioner, who must have the trust of the child and read his or her cues very carefully to maintain the child's engagement in play.

ROLE OF THE OCCUPATIONAL THERAPIST AND THE OCCUPATIONAL THERAPY ASSISTANT DURING PLAY ASSESSMENT

The observation of children during play provides OT practitioners with important information. **Play assessment**, in combination with parent, child, and teacher interviews, provides the OT practitioner with necessary information. Bryze supports the contributions of narratives in collecting information on play.[7] These narratives focus on the interviews of parents, caregivers, and children.

OT practitioners use a variety of play assessments when working with children with special needs. Table 21-2 provides descriptions of several play assessments. The occupational therapist is responsible for the evaluation and analysis of information when evaluating play but can delegate portions of the assessment to the occupational therapy assistant (OTA), who can assist in interviewing the teachers and caregivers and observing the children during play. The OT practitioner uses the results of the play assessments to design therapy goals and provide effective intervention. Play assessments provide a foundation for organizing information.

It is not always possible to evaluate children with moderate to severe physical and cognitive disabilities through standardized testing. However, play evaluations may be administered to all children. These evaluations provide the flexibility needed to assess children and give measurable information concerning a child's strengths and weaknesses. For example, the ToP has been found to be reliable in measuring playfulness in children with intellectual disability; the Knox Preschool Play Scale is reliable in measuring play skills in children with multiple disabilities. The Transdisciplinary Play-Based Assessment is designed to be used with all children and includes an

TABLE 21-2

Play Assessments

KNOX PRESCHOOL PLAY SCALE

The Knox Preschool Play Scale (PPS) provides a developmental description of play behavior in four domains[24a]:

1. Space management
2. Materials management
3. Imitation
4. Participation

The PPS is designed for children ages 0 to 6 years. The Knox PPS is easy to administer and score. It requires two 30-minute observations of free play (indoors and outdoors). The revised scale provides age equivalencies to 6 months for children ages 0 to 3 years and yearly for children ages 3 to 5 years.[24a]

TEST OF PLAYFULNESS

The Test of Playfulness (ToP) provides an objective measurement of playfulness.[9,11] Children are observed playing with peers in familiar environments suitable for play for 15 minutes inside and 15 minutes outside. Administration of the scale requires training by viewing videotapes of children playing and scoring them according to ToP guidelines. OT practitioners can use the information to systematically examine playfulness in children to develop intervention plans.[11] It has been found to be an accurate test for assessing typically developing children and those with disabilities.[15]

TRANSDISCIPLINARY PLAY-BASED ASSESSMENT

The Transdisciplinary Play-Based Assessment (TPBA) is a procedure for administering a comprehensive transdisciplinary assessment for children ages 0 to 3 years.[27] The TPBA provides structured guidelines for performing this assessment. OT clinicians can use this procedure to design intervention. The TPBA is an observational assessment that may take as long as 90 minutes to administer. All of the team members participate in the assessment. Information is gained in cognitive, social–emotional, communication and language, and motor skills.[27]

A play history is a semistructured interview designed to obtain information about the child's behavior.[36,40a] The play history is based on the developmental progression of play and examines behaviors in five developmental phases:

1. Sensorimotor
2. Symbolic and simple constructive
3. Dramatic and complex constructive
4. Games
5. Recreational

OT practitioners using this scale must have a firm knowledge of the normal progression of play. The scale provides a framework for gathering information on it.[40a]

CHILDREN'S PLAYFULNESS SCALE

The Children's Playfulness Scale consists of 23 Likert-type format items and uses a 5-point response/scoring system[5a]:

1. Sounds exactly like the child
2. Sounds a lot like the child
3. Sounds somewhat like the child
4. Sounds a little like the child
5. Does not sound at all like the child

Children receive a playfulness score. This scale is efficient and inexpensive and requires no direct observation of the child. Bundy and Clifton, however, questioned the use of this scale for children with disabilities.[14a]

THE CHILD OCCUPATIONAL SELF-ASSESSMENT

The Child Occupational Self-Assessment (COSA) is a self-report evaluation most commonly given to children in school settings but is acceptable in numerous other contexts and in combination with other assesments.[23a,23b] In schools, the COSA is often used to elicit the child's viewpoints and own goals when developing an individualized educational program. Children may complete the COSA as traditionally done, using pencil and paper; to accommodate children with special needs, a card-sort version is available.[23a,23b]

The COSA was developed using foundational components of the Model of Human Occupation, which theorizes that performance is affected by an individual's motivation, habits, physical/cognitive abilities, interests, and environment. The assessment first asks children how they feel about their skills in communication, interaction, motor control, and processing. It then asks children to identify how important that activity is to them. For example, the COSA asks children how well they believe they "keep working on something even when it gets hard." Children then choose from four different options ranging from *I have a big problem doing this* to *I am really good at doing this*.[23a, p. 12] For the same question, children are asked how important that ability is to them, and they may answer again from four choices, ranging from *not really important to me* to *most important of all to me*.[23a,23b]

Continued

TABLE 21-2—cont'd

Play Assessments

TEST OF ENVIRONMENTAL SUPPORTIVENESS

The Test of Environmental Supportiveness (TOES) follows the Person–Environment–Occupation (PEO) model. The TOES is a 17-item assessment administered to children between 15 months and 12 years of age.[15,21a] Children are observed during 15 minutes of free play, as in the ToP, to evaluate what motivates and supports them at play. This assessment can be used to evaluate many different environments, such as day care, home, and the outdoors.[15] Caregivers, playmates, spaces, and objects are four environmental domains that have been found to affect play. The TOES uses a 4-point scaling system to identify the significance of each environmental component in supporting or inhibiting a child's playfulness. The TOES has been found to be a valid and reliable assessment tool that can be used for children with or without disabilities.[15,29a]

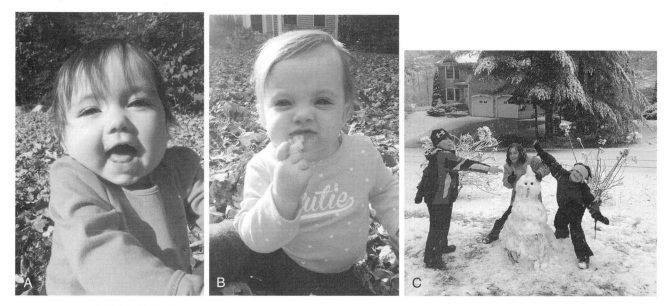

FIGURE 21-5   The environment may afford children with opportunities for playfulness and creativity. **A**, Playing in the leaves is a popular play activity for children. **B**, Toddlers enjoy the sensations and sounds of the fall leaves. **C**, These children are playful and creative as they build a snowman together and enjoy the new snow.

accompanying intervention manual (Transdisciplinary Play-Based Intervention) to assist OT practitioners in intervention planning. The findings obtained from play evaluations are easily translated into measurable goals for therapy sessions that allow clinicians to organize intervention more deliberately, thereby benefiting the children they treat.

TECHNIQUES TO PROMOTE PLAY AND PLAYFULNESS

Fully using play in OT practice is an art and a science. Just as with any intervention, OT practitioners must practice the techniques. The science of using play involves understanding the characteristics, components, and settings that facilitate it. OT practitioners must identify the desired outcome of therapy and evaluate the motor, psychological, and/or social factors interfering with the child's ability to play.

Creating a therapeutic environment involves analyzing a child's skills and determining the way(s) to adapt activities. Knowledge of the development of the motor, cognitive, language, social–emotional, and play skills of children is essential to designing effective interventions. Examination of the environment and knowledge of the child's culture help OT practitioners determine appropriate play activities. Figure 21-5 illustrates how the natural environment facilitates play.

Occupational therapy using play requires the OT practitioner to find the child within him or herself. Playful practitioners practice play and are able to support the child's playful nature. Clinical expertise in the therapeutic use of self is important for understanding the way(s) to evoke play in children and is considered part of the art of therapy. OT practitioners engage in the art of occupational therapy when they connect with the child. Skillful practitioners play effortlessly with children while challenging them to acquire and master new skills. The art of occupational therapy involves weaving clinical judgment, skill, and individual style into successful therapy sessions.

Box 21-4 provides suggestions on how to promote playfulness in occupational therapy sessions.

CLINICAL *Pearl*

Get in touch with your playful side. Spend a day with a child to remember the way it feels to play. Let the child lead you and show you how to play.

Characteristics of Playful Occupational Therapy Practitioners

OT practitioners can cultivate specific characteristics in themselves that promote play (Box 21-5). They must be playful themselves if they wish to treat children effectively and facilitate play and playfulness. Children view a happy, smiling OT practitioner—one who is able to interact joyfully with them—as playful.

It is important for the OT practitioner to establish goals and to structure the intervention setting. However, the OT practitioner must be flexible enough to change the activity based on the child's responses. The OT practitioner needs to be skillful in planning and setting up a playful environment so that the child will choose activities that further the therapeutic goals. This ensures that therapy will be fun for the child. Facilitating play requires that the OT practitioner keep the goals clearly in mind while structuring the environment and adjusting the mode of interaction.[27]

OT practitioners acting as play facilitators pay careful attention to a child's interests, elaborate on his or her verbalizations, and model play behaviors.[27] If an activity is not challenging to a child but he or she is enjoying it, the OT practitioner may decide to continue the activity before increasing the level of the skill required. The child may need to practice the task to gain mastery.[36] Children need to be challenged in all areas of development. OT practitioners need to provide social, cognitive, and motor challenges.

OT practitioners need to be creative to spark children's imaginations during play sessions. A sense of humor is vital; OT practitioners may have to act silly, make mistakes, and even act as a peer to encourage a child to play. From the child's point of view, the OT practitioner may seem to demand that he or she perform tasks that are much harder to them than to the adult. For example, in one intervention session a child asked to play the role of the OT practitioner and then said, "Okay, now stand on your head and clap your hands together behind your back three times. I will time you." This suggests that the degree of challenge the child has experienced during treatment sessions was too much.

BOX 21-4

Suggestions to Promote Playfulness in Occupational Therapy Sessions

I.   Create a playful environment where children can explore, create, problem solve, and participate in social activities.
   - Set up the environment to facilitate playfulness in children and youth.
   - Use curtains or dividers to separate children's and adults' spaces if space is shared in the clinic. Keep the space child-friendly.
   - Change the themes of spaces through paintings or party items (e.g., birds, piñatas, or other decorations).
   - Music adds a playful nature to the space.
   - Include an element of "pretend" in the session.

II. Provide interesting and novel materials that promote creativity and fun.
   - Set up a "tea party" theme by adding a small table, tea set, and pink table cloth.
   - Add the children's favorite toys to the environment. You may ask them to bring one or two to the session.
   - Puppets come in all sizes, so use of them can be easily gradated.
   - Magnetic blocks are easier for children with coordination difficulties.
   - Adaptive toys allow children to hit a switch or pull a lever to activate a toy.
   - Using the finger for painting is easier than using a brush.
   - Sitting in adapted chairs allows children to use their hands better.

III. Develop a safe playful atmosphere that encourages children to be spontaneous and even silly.
   - Change the demands of the task to provide the just-right challenge.
   - Having a limited number of directions for the games makes it easier for children to play them.
   - Change the rules to make children more successful, or bring the target closer.
   - Allow for a variety of positions during play.
   - Remember that eye contact may be overwhelming to some children. In addition, it is not imperative for children to smile to show that they are having fun.
   - Allow the children to make changes to the activity.
   - Use an upbeat and playful tone when speaking to the child.
   - Follow the child's lead.
   - Laugh with the child.
   - Encourage flexible play.

BOX 21-5

Characteristics of Occupational Therapy Practitioners That Promote Play and Playfulness in Children

- Playfulness: Having warm, inviting, and sincere personalities
- Flexibility, creativity, and spontaneity: Ability to change activities and pace based on the needs of the child and to stop activities and create new ones if needed
- Child friendliness: Interacting at the child's level; being familiar with child's terms and current trends. Being familiar with the trendy movies, games, and action heroes is helpful
- Sense of humor: Trying out silly things; laughing at self
- Intuition: Being able to read child's cues (nonverbal and verbal); being aware of signs of boredom, fatigue, or frustration
- Positive reinforcement: Offering sincere praise when child has performed well, has tried very hard, or is in need of support
- Patience: Allowing child to experience some frustration; helping child to work on frustration tolerance through play
- Observational skills: Being able to watch and not intervene at every turn; allowing child to be in control
- Openness: Learning new games and play activities from children; watching children in many settings to keep activities novel
- Fun: Smiling; laughing; playing with children

BOX 21-6

Characteristics of an Optimal Play Environment

- Playful: Provides cheerful, warm, and safe feeling
- Fun and inviting: Is child-friendly; is decorated in such a way that children enjoy being there
- Safe: Keeps children physically and emotionally safe so that they can feel free to explore and play; has mats available
- Novel: Provides various new toys and challenges
- Flexible and creative: Allows children to play in different ways with toys; is arranged to promote a variety of play activities
- Encouraging: Includes adults who facilitate play, are not directive, ensure that the children are safe, assist when needed, and disappear when appropriate
- Creative: Has materials and supplies that promote creativity and not necessarily have an end product; for example, sand, water, clay, and Play-Doh
- Quiet: Allows children some space to be alone if they desire

---

Reading a child's verbal and nonverbal cues provides OT practitioners with information that may help change the play activities. This is important in gaining the trust of the child. Children need to feel that someone is listening to them. Skillful OT practitioners use the child's cues as indicators of stress and emotion. They can assist children in learning to listen to and give cues by nodding and listening to their nonverbal and verbal feedback.

CLINICAL *Pearl*

Provide children with themes for play activities. Ask them to bring in objects from their homes and use them during therapy.

Praising children is highly effective if done properly. They appreciate honest and specific praise. They realize that play can be frustrating and not always successful. OT practitioners need to allow children with special needs to feel frustration and experience failure sometimes.

Playful OT practitioners allow children to make mistakes occasionally. Some of the most playful sessions are those in which the children make mistakes along the way. It is the process that is important.

CASE *Study*

An obstacle course in the clinic is difficult for Jon to climb without falling. He tries numerous times and each time falls into the pillows laughing. He is determined to succeed. He works on this activity until he succeeds in doing it properly. Once he masters the task, he moves on to something new. For Jon, falling into the pillows is almost as fun as staying on the course.

OT practitioners must have a sense of humor. They must take into consideration the setting and the play frame. Therefore, if the child says, "I have a laser gun," during a pretend game, the OT practitioner does not become alarmed. However, a child may be crying out for help during play. OT practitioners should take these opportunities to reach out to the child. Perhaps the most important characteristic of playful practitioners is that they have fun. Children learn the way to play from practitioners who get involved in it. They smile, laugh, and enjoy playing.

Characteristics of the Optimal Play Environment

The optimal **play environment** has specific characteristics (Box 21-6); first and foremost, it is a safe environment.[5]

Children must be safe and feel physically and emotionally safe. The environment should have a variety of age-appropriate toys that the child can choose from.[5,27] These toys need not be expensive; children enjoy playing with ordinary household items and inexpensive readily available items such as boxes, containers, pots and pans.

The OT practitioner should design an environment that promotes novelty, the opportunity for exploration, repetition, and the imitation of competent role models.[21] Novelty makes the session fun and enjoyable, fosters creativity, and creates arousal. An environment that allows for exploration requires arranging toys in such a way that children can look for them, reach them, and investigate the surroundings. Children learn from repetition and should be allowed to do this during play. Repetition is encouraged by the initiation of the same activity with a different theme, goal, or object. For example, the OT practitioner may ask a child to throw a ball at a new target to continue the activity. Being a competent role model requires the OT practitioner to demonstrate playful behavior. Parents and professionals need to give children space to work out play scenarios, and this space must be safe (Box 21-7).

The play space should be arranged to promote a variety of types of play (see Chapter 7).[5] The ways to promote different types of play include the following:

1. Pretend play: Promotes make-believe and may involve using the kitchen table, play food, puppets, and dress-up clothes during play.
2. Constructive play: Designed to allow children to build and create things and involves the use of blocks, Legos, Lincoln Logs, and various other building toys; arts and crafts, paper; crayons, clay, markers, paint, chalk, and scissors; and wind-up toys, beads, and small manipulative toys.
3. Reflective or reading area: A quiet area where children can read and/or write. Items placed in this area may include books, audiotapes, videotapes, paper, and pencils. It can also be a quiet place for a child to simply remove themselves from a busy area or activity to take a breather.
4. Sensorimotor area: An area set up for major motor movements. Toys and equipment present in this area include mats, balls, bikes, swings, balance beams, and trampolines.
5. Exploratory play: Includes multisensory activities such as water, sand, and other tactile play activities.
6. Computer play area: An area that includes a computer with a variety of games.
7. Musical play: Promotes music and involves the use of whistles, rattles, drums, pianos, rhythm games, singing, and tapes.[5]

OT practitioners allow children to express their creativity and spontaneity. Toys have many uses in addition to

---

BOX 21-7

Safety in the Play Environment

- The best safety precaution is to watch all children carefully at all times.
- Plug all electrical outlets with safety caps.
- Ensure that bookshelves are sturdy and will not topple. Anchor shelves to the wall at the top.
- Do not place toys in such a way that they will fall on toddlers' heads when they pull them down.
- Remove all cords to ensure that children do not get caught in them.
- Place mats under all the equipment.
- Pad corners of walls and furniture.
- Know how to perform infant cardiopulmonary resuscitation.
- Be sure that cleaning supplies and medications are out of reach of children.
- Be sure that water tables are closed when not in use.
- Watch for and mop up slippery surfaces.
- Have a first-aid kit available, and frequently review emergency procedures.
- Check out all equipment periodically to ensure that everything is in good working order.
- Clean and disinfect toys and surfaces after each use.
- Follow universal precautions while cleaning up spills.

---

those suggested by the manufacturer. Unless the children are being harmful to others or themselves, allow them to use toys in different ways. Some children may not be aware of the way a toy is typically used. After they have taken some time to explore it, the OT practitioner may demonstrate the expected way without imposing only one method of playing with the toy.

Many children enjoy roughhousing. Children with special needs may also enjoy this. Gentle roughhousing can provide sensory input to them and is often therapeutic and fun. Children of all ages learn through physical contact, and therapy sessions can provide a safe environment for this type of contact. Children may push each other playfully, and adults do not always need to intervene.

CLINICAL *Pearl*

Musical games are fun and playful ways to help a child become more attentive to verbal directions. The child must pay attention to the words of the song or beat of the music to follow along. Some children respond to singing, rhythm or to sing-song instructions.

Playful environments take advantage of themes and are decorated for the occasion. Make sure that the play environment is not too overly stimulating. Use warm colors such as pinks, melons, and yellows.[4] The temperature of the room should be warm, not too hot or cold. Children enjoy being outdoors, so they should be able to play in outdoor settings as well. Children also enjoy places for quiet time and concentration.

The best way to promote play and playfulness in children is to be a playful adult in a playful environment. Arranging the play environment helps OT practitioners become skillful at using the environment therapeutically.

SUMMARY

OT practitioners view play as the major occupation of childhood and believe it is crucial to a child's development. They facilitate the development of play in children with disabilities. Therefore they must understand the characteristics of play if they wish to make significant changes in the play of the children they treat. OT practitioners play an important role in helping parents, teachers, and peers play with children with special needs. The OT practitioners may be able to make simple play adaptations that allow these children to be included with their peers in play.

Play is a fun, spontaneous, internally motivated, and self-directed activity that is free from rigid rules. Playfulness is defined as an individual's disposition to play. OT practitioners typically use play as a tool to improve a child's skills and as a goal for therapy.

OT practitioners expand their use of play by exploring its characteristics and practicing these techniques in the treatment of children. They can have a tremendous impact on the lives of children and their families through fun, creative, enjoyable, and spontaneous activities, allowing children to develop play skills that will carry over to the home, school, and community settings and help prepare the children for adult roles.

References

1. American Occupational Therapy Association. (2011). *Building play skills for healthy children and families.* Available at: http://www.aota.org/Practitioners-Section/Children-and-Youth/Browse/Play/Play-Skills.aspx?FT=.pdf.
2. American Occupational Therapy Association. (2012). *Childhood obesity.* Available at: http://www.aota.org/Practitioners-Section/Children-andYouth/Browse/School/Toolkit/Obesity.aspx?FT=.pdf.
3. American Occupational Therapy Association. (2012). *Recess promotion.* Available at: http://www.aota.org/Practitioners-Section/Children-andYouth/Browse/School/Toolkit/Recess.aspx?FT=.pdf.
4. Ayres, A. J. (1972). *Sensory integration and learning disorders.* Los Angeles, CA: Western Psychological Services.
5. Bantz, D. L., & Siktberg, L. (1993). Teaching families to evaluate age-appropriate toys. *J Pediatr Health Care, 7,* 111.
5a. Barnett, L. A. (1990). Playfulness: Definition, design, and measurement. *Play Culture, 3,* 319.
6. Barnett, L. A. (1998). The adaptive powers of being playful. In M. C. Duncan, G. Chick, & A. Aycock (Eds.), *Play and culture studies* (Vol. 1). Greenwich, CT: Ablex Publishing.
7. Bryze, K. C. (2010). Narrative contributions to the play history. In L. D. Parham, & L. S. Fazio (Eds.), *Play in occupational therapy for children* (2nd ed.). St. Louis, MO: Mosby.
8. Bundy, A. C. (1993). Assessment of play and leisure: delineation of the problem. *Am Occup Ther, 47,* 217.
9. Bundy, A. C. (1997). Play and playfulness: what to look for. In L. D. Parham, & L. S. Fazio (Eds.), *Play in occupational therapy for children.* St. Louis, MO: Mosby.
10. Bundy, A. C. (1991). Play theory and sensory integration. In A. G. Fisher, E. A. Murray, & A. C. Bundy (Eds.), *Sensory integration: theory and practice.* Philadelphia: FA Davis.
11. Bundy, A. C. (2003). *Test of playfulness—4.0.* Sydney, Australia: University of Sydney.
12. Bundy, A. C., et al. (2008). Playful interaction: occupational therapy for all children on the school playground. *Am J Occup Ther, 62,* 522–527.
13. Bundy, A. C., et al. (2001). Reliability and validity of a test of playfulness. *Occup J Res, 21,* 276.
14. Bundy, A. C., et al. (2007). How does sensory processing dysfunction affect play? *Am J Occup Ther, 61,* 201–208.
14a. Bundy, A. C., & Clifton, J. L. (1998). Construct validity of the children's playfulness scale. In M. C. Duncan, G. Chick, & A. Aycock (Eds.), *Play and culture studies* (vol. 1). Greenwich, CT: Ablex Publishing.
15. Bundy, A. C., Waugh, K., & Brentnall, J. (2009). Developing assessments that account for the role of the environment: an example using the Test of Playfulness and Test of Environmental Supportiveness. *OTJR, 29,* 135–143.
16. Center for Disease Control and Prevention. (2012). *Health effects of childhood obesity.* Available at: http://www.cdc.gov/healthyyouth/obesity/facts.html.
17. Center for Disease Control and Prevention. (2012). *Physical activity and health.* Available at: http://www.cdc.gov/physicalactivity/everyone/health/index.html.
18. Clements, R. L. (2000). *Elementary school recess: selected readings, games, and activities for teachers and parents.* Lake Charles, LA: American Press.
19. Clifford, J. M., & Bundy, A. C. (1989). Play preference and play performance in normal boys and boys with sensory integrative dysfunction. *Am J Occup Ther, 9,* 202.
20. Cordier, R., et al. (2009). A model for play-based intervention for children with ADHD. *Austral Occup Ther J, 56,* 332–340.
21. Csikszentmihalyi, M. (1975). *Beyond boredom and anxiety.* San Francisco, CA: Jossey-Bass.
21a. Hamm, E. (2006). Playfulness and the environmental support of play in children with and without developmental disabilities. *OTJR, 26*(3), 88–96.
22. Holmes, R., Pellegrini, A., & Schmidt, S. (2006). The effects of different recess timing regimens on preschoolers' classroom attention. *Early Child Dev Care, 176*(7), 735–743.
23. Kanics, I. (2013). Available at: http://www.aota.org/-/media/Corporate/Files/ConferenceDocs/Conclave/2013SCSchedule/2013%20handouts/HandoutConcurrent16.pdf.

23a. Keller, J., Kafkes, A., & Kielhofner, G. (2005). Psychometric characteristics of the Child Occupational Self Assessment (COSA), part one: An initial examination of psychometric properties. *Scandinavian Journal of Occupational Therapy, 12,* 118–127.

23b. Keller, J., Kafkes, A., Basu, S., Federico, J., & Kielhofner, G. (2005). Child Occupational Self Assessment (COSA) Version 2.1, 2005. MOHO Clearinghouse: University of Illinois at Chicago.

24. Kielhofner, G. (2008). *A model of human occupation* (3rd ed.). Baltimore: Lippincott Williams & Wilkins.

24a. Knox, S. (2010). Development and current use of the Knox preschool play scale. In L. D. Parham, & L. S. Fazio (Eds.), *Play in occupational therapy* (ed 2.). St. Louis: Mosby.

25. Lane, S. J., & Mistrett, S. G. (1996). Play and assistive technology issues for infants and young children with disabilities: a preliminary examination. *Focus Autism Other Dev Disabil, 11,* 96–104.

26. Leigh, I. G. (2013). Preventing bullying: how occupational therapy practitioners can help make schools a safer place for everyone. *OT Practice, 18*(5), 12–16.

27. Linder, T. W. (2000). *Transdisciplinary play based assessment.* Baltimore, MD: Paul H. Brookes.

28. Moran, J. M., & Kalakian, L. H. (1974). *Movement experiences for the mentally retarded or emotionally disturbed child.* Minneapolis: MN Burgess.

29. Morrison, C. D., Bundy, A. C., & Fisher, A. G. (1991). The contribution of motor skills and playfulness to the play performance of pre-schoolers. *Am J Occup Ther, 45,* 687.

29a. Muys, V., Rodger, S., & Bundy, A. C. (2006). Assessment of playfulness in children with autistic disorder: A comparison of the Children's Playfulness Scale and the Test of Playfulness. *OTJR, 26*(4), 159–170.

30. O'Brien, J. C., et al. (1998). The impact of positioning equipment on play skills of physically impaired children. In M. C. Duncan, G. Chick, & A. Aycock (Eds.), *Play and culture studies* (Vol. 1). Greenwich, CT: Ablex Publishing.

31. O'Brien, J. C., et al. (1999). The impact of occupational therapy on a child's playfulness. *Occup Ther Healthcare, 12,* 39.

32. Okimoto, A. M., Bundy, A. C., & Hanzlik, J. (2000). Playfulness in children with and without disability: measurement and intervention. *Am J Occup Ther, 54,* 73.

33. Parham, L. D., & Primeau, L. (2010). Play and occupational therapy. In L. D. Parham, & L. S. Fazio (Eds.), *Play in occupational therapy for children* (2nd ed.). St. Louis, MO: Mosby.

34. Parten, M. (1933). Social play among pre-school children. *J Abnorm Soc Psychol, 28,* 136.

35. Reed, C. N., Dunbar, S. B., & Bundy, A. C. (2000). The effects of an inclusive preschool experience on the playfulness of children with and without autism. *Phys Occup Ther Pediatr, 19,* 73.

36. Reilly, M. (1974). *Play as exploratory learning: studies in curiosity behavior.* Beverly Hills, CA: Sage.

37. Rubin, K., Fein, G. G., & Vandenberg, B. (1983). Play. In P. H. Mussen (Ed.), *Handbook of child psychology* (4th ed.). New York: Wiley.

38. Sipal, R., et al. (2010). Course of behaviour problems of children with cerebral palsy: the role of parental stress and support. *Child Care Health Develop, 36,* 74–84.

39. Skaines, N., Rodger, S., & Bundy, A. C. (2006). Playfulness in children with autistic disorder and their typically developing peers. *Br J Occup Ther, 69,* 505–512.

40. Skard, G., & Bundy, A. C. (2008). The test of playfulness. In L. D. Parham, & L. S. Fazio (Eds.), *Play in occupational therapy for children* (2nd ed.) (pp. 71–94). St. Louis, MO: Mosby.

40a. Takata, N. (1974). Play as a prescription. In M. Reilly (Ed.), *Play as exploratory learning.* Beverly Hills, CA: Sage.

41. Waite, A. (2014). On an even keel: sensory-based strategies for better self-regulation. *OT Practice, 19*(18), 7–10.

42. Waite, A. (2013). Take it outside—occupational therapy's role in making the most of recess. *OT Practice, 18*(5), 7–11.

Recommended Reading

Hamm, E. (2006). Playfulness and the environmental support of play in children with and without developmental disabilities. *OTJR, 26,* 88–96.

Linder, T. (2008). *Transdisciplinary play based assessment* (2nd ed.). Baltimore, MD: Paul H. Brookes.

Muys, V., Rodger, S., & Bundy, A. C. (2006). Assessment of playfulness in children with autistic disorder: a comparison of the Children's Playfulness Scale and the Test of Playfulness. *OTJR, 26,* 159–170.

Parham, L. D., & Fazio, L. S. (2010). *Play in occupational therapy for children* (2nd ed.). St. Louis, MO: Mosby.

REVIEW *Questions*

1. Describe the characteristics of play and playfulness.
2. What is the difference between play and playfulness?
3. How would you facilitate play and playfulness in children with special needs?
4. What characteristics do you possess that would promote play and playfulness in children with special needs?
5. How is play used as a tool in the treatment of children?
6. Describe the way(s) that play can be the goal of therapy.
7. List three play assessments used by OT practitioners. Describe the ways they are administered and the information you gain from them.
8. How can the environment stimulate play and playfulness?

SUGGESTED *Activities*

1. Volunteer to babysit a child with special needs. Play with the child. Reflect on the experience by writing a one-page composition describing the way you felt about the time you spent with the child.

2. Plan and participate in an activity you enjoy with others. Describe the activity, materials needed, and environment. How did you feel during the activity?

3. In a small group, discuss your favorite childhood games and playmates. What types of skills did you learn as a child during play? What feelings do these memories bring to mind?

4. In a small group, role-play the characteristics of OT practitioners that promote playfulness in children.

JEAN WELCH SOLOMON*

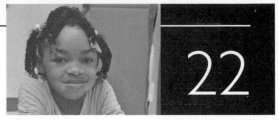

22

Functional Task at School: Handwriting

KEY TERMS

Handwriting
Prewriting strokes
In-hand manipulation
Efficient grasp patterns
Midline crossing
Motor planning
Visual perception
Directionality
Assistive technology

CHAPTER *Objectives*

After studying this chapter, the reader will be able to accomplish the following:

- Identify prewriting strokes, their developmental sequence, and at what age they emerge
- Identify types of efficient grasp patterns used during handwriting
- Explain how handwriting skills affect the ability of children to perform written assignments in the school setting
- Recognize the performance skills required for handwriting
- Describe how visual perception affects handwriting
- Identify the reasons handwriting difficulties occur
- Describe types of handwriting assessments used in pediatrics
- Suggest strategies to improve handwriting or written expression
- Describe assistive technology used as an alternative to handwriting
- Describe individual and group occupational therapy handwriting intervention sessions

CHAPTER *Outline*

*The author would like to acknowledge Monica D. Keen, Diana Bal, Nadine Kuzyk Hanner, Angela Chinners Marsh, and Randi Carlson Neideffer for input to the current edition of this chapter.

425

CHAPTER *Outline*—continued

The most frequent referral for occupational therapists in the school setting is for problems with handwriting.[24] As a result, handwriting intervention programs are often delivered on site at school, either individually or in a small group using an inclusive (integrated classroom) and/or pull-out model of service delivery.[6,7,22] **Handwriting** is one of the functional tasks required of a child in his or her occupation as student. McHale and Cermak reported that as much as 60% of a school day can be spent on fine motor tasks, including handwriting.[24]

Handwriting plays an important role in the educational process. It is associated with the common core standards adopted by the departments of education in most U.S. states.[25] These standards outline the English language art (ELA) and mathematical skills that students are expected to obtain at each grade level throughout their K-12 education. The ELA standards state, among other skills, that a student should be able to demonstrate the ability to write letters and numbers, present ideas in writing, and compose essays. Because handwriting is the most common means a student uses, particularly in elementary grade levels, to demonstrate progress and attainment of skills such as those just mentioned, it is critical to have the ability to produce legible information in an efficient, timely manner. In addition, handwriting is the most common method used by students to take notes and complete tests.[30]

Children use handwriting in noneducational type activities as well. Children often enjoy communicating with family and friends by composing letters, signing their names on holiday cards or on the back of projects for identification. In addition, most children want to feel good about the quality of their work and take pride in what they have accomplished; handwritten work is no exception. Experts claim that illegible handwriting has secondary effects on a child's self-esteem as well as school achievement.[12,23]

Between 10% and 30% of the general elementary school population struggle with handwriting. Many students who receive special education services for a specific learning disorder have difficulty with written expression tasks. The fifth edition of the *Diagnostic and Statistical Manual of Mental Disorders* (DSM-V) categorizes students with specific learning disorders in three core subjects: reading, mathematics, and written expression.[2] For the impairment to be categorized as a written expression–specific learning disorder (previously known as dysgraphia), the student must have errors in spelling, grammar, and punctuation; lack of clarity of ideas; and poor organization of their written work. According to *DSM-V* the combined prevalence for specific learning disorders (reading, mathematics, and written expression) is 5% to 15% across different languages and cultures.[2] Factors that affect the legibility of handwriting include letter formation, horizontal alignment (adhering to margin alignment), size (too large or too small), spacing between letters of words and words, placing of letters and slant.[22,24,28]

Handwriting is one of the tools teachers use to measure a student's academic comprehension. Handwriting allows children to express themselves, learn information, organize their work, and communicate with others. It is vital that occupational therapy (OT) practitioners working in schools address handwriting difficulties to improve students' performances in this functional task or daily occupation.[24,28]

Direct handwriting instruction is not widely provided in the school setting as it is not a requirement in the general

CLINICAL *Pearl*

For many years there have been state education standards defining minimum proficiency required for students in grades K-12 to complete each grade level. With each individual state developing its own criteria there was a lack of uniform expectations. In 2009, development groups comprising state governors, teachers, and other experts created Common Core State Standards. Many states adopted these standards; some states opted out, repealed, or rewrote the standards.[25]

education curriculum in most school districts. Because handwriting is not being taught in the classroom, many students are not learning proper handwriting techniques. Forming letters improperly and inaccurate placement of letters can drastically reduce the legibility and fluidity in the student's writing process. Although it is not part of the general education curriculum, some teachers are still attempting to teach handwriting using formal handwriting programs. There are several widely used handwriting programs from which to choose.[18] These programs offer lesson in both manuscript (print) and cursive handwriting (connected letters). Each is slightly different in appearance and style. Appendix 22-A provides an overview of these programs. Because time is limited, teachers are often unable to consistently monitor the actual day-to-day formation and placement strategies that their students are using while writing. Thus many students are simply drawing the letters without proper formation or directionality (top to bottom). It is challenging to remediate proper letter formation with older children. These poor formation and placement errors become habitual and therefore very difficult to correct.[19]

Howe and colleagues[17] examined the effectiveness of two different approaches: a practiced-based approach based on motor learning theory and a visual perceptual-motor approach based on Beery and colleagues[3] work. For 12 weeks students received OT intervention for the remediation of handwriting deficits. Group A received the intensive practice intervention. Group B received visual-perceptual-motor activities. Table 22-1 provides a review of the two interventions that may be useful when designing handwriting programs. Group A, the students who were given intense opportunities for practice and repetition based on motor learning theory, had significantly greater improvements in handwriting than group B in which the students participated in primarily visual-perceptual-motor activities. The results of this study support using a motor control frame of reference during OT handwriting interventions. (See Chapter 24 regarding motor control/motor learning theory.)[18]

Manuscript writing, which is the most common style used in schools, can be laborious for children. As students get older and continue to experience difficulty

TABLE 22-1

Handwriting Club Group Format

ACTIVITY CATEGORY AND TIME FRAME	INTENSIVE PRACTICE GROUP ACTIVITIES	VISUAL-PERCEPTUAL-MOTOR ACTIVITY GROUP ACTIVITIES
Setup	Sign in on the attendance sheet.	Sign in on the attendance sheet.
Activities designed by therapists using different approaches: 20 min	Answer question of the day in their best handwriting in their journals. Work in handwriting book with a variety of pencils and pencil grips. Select pencils Try on pencil grips Engage in sharing and feedback. When a page is finished, circle the three most legible words. Trade page with another student. Circle the most legible word on each other's pages.	Work on visual perceptual worksheets. Select from a variety of colored pencils or markers of different diameters.
Handwriting activities for both groups: 15 min	Work in commercial handwriting book *Handwriting Without Tears.* Receive instruction (e.g., letter models with arrows, demonstration of letter formation) Text generation: Practice higher-level handwriting skills. Letter writing (e.g., write letters to teachers, classmates, parents or principal on own choice of topic) Recipe contest (e.g., write down favorite snacks and a recipe for how to make them)	Work in commercial handwriting book *Handwriting Without Tears.* Select pencils. Try on pencil grips. Engage in sharing and feedback. When a page is finished, circle the three most legible words. Trade page with another student. Circle the most legible word on each other's pages.
Handwriting game: 10 min	Scattergories, Scutineyes, Mad Libs, or other games that use handwriting on a vertical whiteboard	Scattergories, Scutineyes, Mad Libs, or other games that use handwriting on a vertical whiteboard
Closure	Clean up and go home	Clean up and go home

From Howe, T-H., Roston, K. L., Sheu, C-F., & Hinojosa, J. (2013). Assessing handwriting intervention effectiveness in elementary school students: a two-group controlled study. *Am J Occup Ther, 67,* 26.

with formation of manuscript, many therapists will suggest that students learn cursive handwriting. Because the letters are connected in cursive, it is a more fluid way of writing. Cursive is motorically and perceptually easier for some children due to decreased need to lift the pencil after each letter resulting in less starting and stopping. According to Olsen and Knapton, the end of second grade or the beginning of third is the optimal developmental time to introduce cursive writing.[26] A simplified style of cursive is recommended. The simplified style uses vertical rather than slant letters, such that the letters are similar to those that the students read. Handwriting without Tears *Kick Start Cursive* workbook is a resource to use when introducing cursive handwriting.

> ### CLINICAL *Pearl*
>
> Students in second and third grades frequently show an interest in learning to write their first and last names in cursive.

DEVELOPMENTAL SEQUENCE

Referrals to occupational therapy for handwriting are made based on children not performing at age-appropriate expectations. Teachers notice that the child's handwriting is not as fluent, clear, or legible as his or her classmates. Students are referred to OT practitioners for an assessment of the developmental level at which the child is functioning and the cause(s) for the handwriting difficulties to ensure that appropriate specialized interventions can be designed. Development occurs through the learning, experiencing, and acquisition of the skills. The rate of development and the progression of skills vary in children but usually follow sequential patterns. A discussion of developmental sequence of skill acquisition follows. Select performance skills and client factors that influence the development of foundational handwriting skills are also discussed.

Prewriting

Prewriting strokes are the precursors to forming shapes, letter, and numbers. A child must understand and be able to stroke positional concepts such as *down* (vertical) and *across* (horizontal) before they can put them together to form letters. For example, when providing verbal prompts for stroking the capital letter "L," the student would hear, "Big line down, little line across." The child needs to know what movement down and across mean.

Motor, cognitive, and sensory systems work together for success in prewriting. Children start performing prewriting activities at a very early age. Consider the child putting open hands into the chocolate pudding and rubbing the pudding on the high chair tray in circular motions. Another example is the toddler who takes his or her mom's marker and makes numerous marks on the kitchen wall. As their little hands strengthen, children take crayons and paper and scribble with abandon (Figure 22-1). During this period of prewriting, children hold writing utensils in immature, inefficient grasp patterns (e.g., palmer grasp or digital pronate grasp). As they learn vertical, horizontal, and circular strokes, they start to put them together to make shapes such as squares, rectangles, and crosses. Diagonals require the eyes to cross midline and are the last prewriting strokes to develop. Once the child is able to draw lines that slant left or right they are able to combine the slant lines to form triangles and diamonds. See Box 22-1 for the developmental sequence of acquisition of prewriting strokes.

Efficient Grasping Patterns of a Pencil or Other Writing Tool

Children with handwriting difficulties show a less mature grasp, immature pencil grip, and inconsistent hand preference.[5,20] The most mature grasps are the dynamic tripod and lateral tripod grasps. By definition, in a tripod grasp three fingers are used for holding the writing utensil

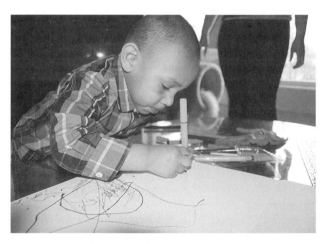

FIGURE 22-1   The child draws a design using a marker.

BOX 22-1

Developmental Sequence of Acquisition of Prewriting Strokes

- 2- to 3-year-olds: vertical and horizontal strokes and then lines
- 3- to 4-year-olds: circles and intersecting strokes and lines
- 4- to 6-year-olds: diagonal lines and the ability to form shapes, i.e. putting the prewriting stokes together into meaningful shapes such as a triangle or square

(Figure 22-2, A). The thumb is bent, the index finger points to the top of the writing utensil, and the writing utensil rests on the side of the middle finger. The last two fingers are curled in the palm and stabilize the hand.[20,29] The lateral quadruped and four-finger grip can be as functional and efficient as the dynamic tripod, lateral tripod, and dynamic quadruped pencil grips in fourth-grade students.[20,29] A quadruped grip (four fingers) is another way children might hold their writing utensils. The thumb is bent, the index and middle finger point to the top of the writing utensil, and the writing utensil rests on the ring finger[20,29] (Figure 22-2, B). Both grasps require that the child be able to dissociate the radial border from the ulnar border of the hand. The web space between the thumb and index finger is closed while writing with a lateral or thumb wrap grasp pattern.

Preschool children have small hands, making it difficult for them to manipulate regular-sized pencils and markers. Some teachers have preschool children use large pencils and/or triangular pencils to promote functional grasps. However, preschool children are encouraged to use short crayons and small pencils for writing/coloring. Crayons are made of colored wax, which provides resistance (strengthening) when coloring. Because of the resistance crayons also provide kinesthetic feedback to the user. Short pencils such as those used for golfing or regular pencils broken in two are perfect for children with small hands. Smaller pencils/crayons help prepare the child's hand for an efficient pencil grip that allows for better control of the pencil.

Knowledge of the progression of grasping patterns is useful to the OT practitioner when evaluating handwriting.[28,29] Cross-thumb (thumb wrap) or static tripod grasps can be fatiguing or painful but offer more stability and power. Tight grasps may limit the variety of movements and make smooth, fluid motions difficult. Writers using tight grasps often press hard on the paper, which results in the formation of dark, sometimes smeared, letters.[28,29]

CLINICAL *Pearl*

Many adults who are successful in active engagement of daily occupations use a variety of pencil grasps with minimum web space and a very tight grasping pattern. Look around and observe the variety of grasping patterns that are used by your classmates or colleagues.

CLINICAL *Pearl*

Recommend a mechanical pencil for the student who has a tight grasp and applies excessive downward pressure onto the pencil. The lead of a mechanical pencil breaks easily, which gives the student immediate visual and tactile feedback if he or she is grasping too tightly or pressing down on the pencil with too much force. Be cognizant of the student's level of frustration if the lead of the mechanical pencil breaks often.

Developmental Stages in Writing Readiness

As children grow and develop, so does their handwriting ability. Table 22-2 provides an outline of the sequence of writing development.[13] The children's ability to manipulate writing/coloring utensils as well as their ability to use their "helper hand" improves. As they become more comfortable with the task of scribbling, coloring, and ultimately writing, their posture during this task changes and matures (Box 22-2).[13] A 2-year-old uses all of his or her fingers to hold a crayon in the palm of the hand. The helping hand is of no use, as the upper extremity is usually retracted at the shoulder, flexed at the elbow, adducted to the side, with slightly bent fingers. This is a position of stability for the child. In addition, the hand performing the scribbling is abducted at the shoulder

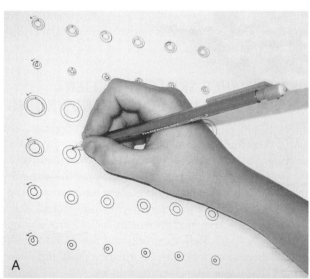

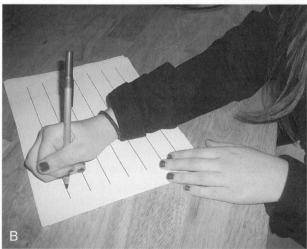

FIGURE 22-2   **A**, Dynamic tripod grasp. **B**, Cross-thumb grasp.

TABLE 22-2

Prewriting Skill Development

ITEM NAME	AGE (MO)
Stirring spoon	12
Scribbling—1 scribble 1-inch long	14
Imitating vertical line 2 inches long	23-24
Imitating horizontal line 2 inches long	27-28
Copying circle—end points within half inch of each other	33-34
Copying cross—intersecting lines within 20 degrees of perpendicular	39-40
Tracing line—deviates <2 times	41-42

Based on Folio, M. R., & Fewell, R. R. (2000). *Peabody Developmental Motor Scales* (2nd ed.). Austin, TX: Pro-Ed.

BOX 22-2

Sequence of the Typical Development of Tool Usage

Children move the whole arm with shoulder movements while holding the utensil in a grasping pattern with the thumb and index finger toward the paper.
- Movement occurs at the forearm, with the shoulder more stable.
- The upper arm and forearm are more stable as movement occurs primarily at the wrist and with the whole hand.
- Movement occurs at the metacarpal joints of all the fingers or with a static tripod grasp.
- Dynamic movement occurs at the thumb and index finger, with the middle finger stabilizing the writing utensil and the ring and little fingers stabilizing and maintaining the wrist angle.

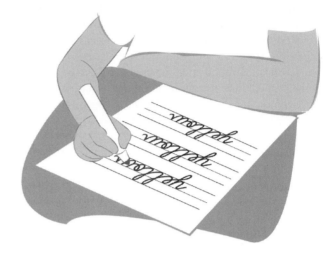

FIGURE 22-3 Students benefit from practicing handwriting. (From O'Brien, J., & Solomon, J. (2012). *Occupational analysis and group process.* St. Louis: Mosby.)

and flexed at the elbow, and the wrist is pronated and does not make contact with the paper at all. The posture of the 3-year-old is more advanced in that the child starts to use the helping hand. The shoulders are still elevated but are not as retracted. All of the fingers may still be used to hold the utensil, and the wrist of the dominant hand continues to be in the air. As the fourth year approaches, the utensil is being held with a more mature grasp. Shoulders are relaxed to a certain extent but continue to be elevated and somewhat retracted for stability. In addition, the child uses the helper hand to hold the paper in a more deliberate fashion. The elbow of the dominant hand is still elevated, and the writing hand still is not making contact with the surface of the table. By the fifth year, a mature grasp has evolved, and the dominant elbow, wrist, and hand all lie comfortably on the surface of the table. See Figure 22-3, which shows the child positioned to write. The shoulders are relaxed, and the child sits confidently at the table for handwriting and coloring activities.

PERFORMANCE SKILLS AND CLIENT FACTORS THAT INFLUENCE HANDWRITING

The American Occupational Therapy Association (AOTA) defines performance skills as motor, process, and communication/interaction skills.[1] Motor skills involve moving and interacting with objects and the environment. Process skills include executive function and cognitive skills. Communication/interactions include skills important in active engagement in social participation. Client factors are body structures and functions of a client. A discussion of select performance skills and client factors that impact handwriting follows.

In-hand Manipulation

In-hand manipulation refers to the precise and skilled finger movements made during fine motor tasks. In-hand manipulation is correlated with handwriting legibility.[21] Figure 22-4 shows a child completing an assessment of in-hand manipulation skills. To perform in-hand manipulation tasks, the child needs to be able to adjust objects within the hand while maintaining the grasp on the object. A general example of this skill is working coins from the palm of the hand to a pincer grasp to deposit the coins into a piggy bank. In-hand manipulation skills during writing are observed when a child rotates the pencil to use the eraser. Another example is manipulating the pencil to write dynamically with a tripod grasp while the ring and little fingers remain still to stabilize the hand.

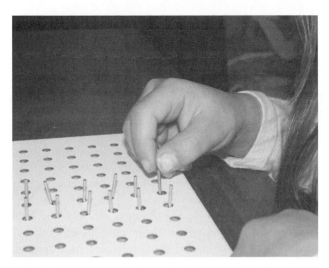

FIGURE 22-4 Manipulating small objects requires fine motor skills and can be used to promote hand dexterity.

In-hand manipulation requires strength, timing, and coordination. Examples of exercises that can strengthen the intrinsic muscles of the hand for improved in-hand manipulation include the following:

- *Translation:* Working items to or from the palm of the hand to or from the tips of the fingers without dropping the items (e.g., moving coins from the palm of the hand to the tips of the thumb and index finger to place coins into the slot of a vending machine).
- *Shift:* Moving objects held with digits proximally or distally (e.g., moving the fingers up or down on the pencil shaft without stabilizing the pencil on an item or surface or "walking" the fingers closer to the tip of a string when stringing beads).
- *Rotation:* Rotating an object using the thumb opposed to the index and long finger (e.g., turning the pencil from lead down to eraser down to erase what has been written).

CLINICAL *Pearl*

Observe how a tool, spoon, or pencil is given to a child. Offering the child the item consistently on one side of the body or to one hand can influence his or her handedness. Frequently, when a right-handed parent sits opposite a child to feed him or her, the child will tend to use the left hand for self-feeding. It is important to present items orienting them to the middle of the child's body.

CLINICAL *Pearl*

Typically the child has established hand preference by age 3. By 3.5 years the child uses a static tripod grasp and has an emerging dynamic tripod grasp by age 4.

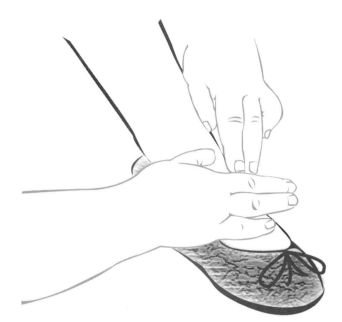

FIGURE 22-5 Child with missing fingers practices tying her shoe.

Active Range of Motion

The OT practitioner evaluates the available active range of motion (AROM) of the trunk, shoulder girdles, elbows, forearms, wrist, and fingers. Contractures or limitations in AROM may interfere with the smooth, coordinated movements required for writing. For example, a student with rheumatoid arthritis may not be able to hold a writing utensil with the tripod grasp. However, when the utensil is placed between the index and long fingers, the child is able to manipulate the writing utensil more comfortably, as this position takes the pressure off of the joints.

Integrity and Structure of Arm, Hand, and Fingers

OT practitioners examine the integrity of the arm, hand, and fingers to determine whether deformities, edema, or open wounds are interfering with writing. Poor integrity of the upper extremity and the hand can cause a lot of pain. This pain may require reduced written assignments and frequent breaks to allow the student to participate fully within the classroom. For example, a student with epidermis bulosa may have blistered, weeping, and peeling skin. In addition, the fingers may be severely contracted. The child may have to hold the writing utensil between the palms of both hands for optimal performance.

OT practitioners examine the child's hand, arm, and fingers to determine whether any structural differences are interfering with the ability to write. Figure 22-5 shows a child who is missing fingers interfering with activities of daily living. For example, some children may be missing digits or have contractures that interfere with writing.

These children may need OT interventions that modify the task.

Posture: Trunk, Shoulder Girdle, Elbow, Wrist, and Finger Stability

When evaluating posture, always start with the trunk. Trunk stability is the very foundation from which the rest of the body gains its stability. Children must call on strong abdominal and lateral muscles to maintain a strong core. Having a strong core enables the child to sustain an upright seating posture during writing. When the child leans or slouches in a chair, it is an indicator that his trunk lacks muscular strength or muscle tone. Interventions to improve posture (such as playing on a ball to improve trunk extension) may help the child write more efficiently (Figure 22-6). When slouching or leaning, the child may compensate by placing the elbows on the writing surface to hold the body up. The child expends so much energy working to maintain an upright position and fatigues quickly, which interferes with coloring or writing. When the child leans on the forearms, the dominant hand cannot be used effectively for writing, and this also impedes the helper hand from stabilizing the paper.

Posture is influenced by the height of the desk and chair. The best sitting position for a child is sitting with the hips and knees at 90 degrees, feet flat on the floor, and the ankles at 90 degrees. The desk should be at a height of two inches above the flexed elbow.[4]

> **CLINICAL** *Pearl*
>
> Alternative seating options in the classroom may promote improved attention to school tasks. Examples include ball chairs, appropriate height stools with back support and oversized pillows at low height tables.

Children must be able to hold the shoulder, elbow, and forearm steady to dynamically use the wrist and fingers for writing. Sometimes children retract their shoulders to keep them steady, which makes it difficult to write effectively. For the most efficient and fluid handwriting the shoulder girdle muscles co-contract keeping the scapula and shoulder joint in a resting, neutral position. The term *elbow stability* refers to the ability of the child to keep the elbow in one position. During handwriting using an **efficient grasp pattern** the forearm is maintained in a neutral position. The term *wrist stability* refers to the child's ability to keep the wrist in one position. Wrist stability is important for the child to perform precise hand skills and to move the fingers more efficiently. The wrist should be straight or slightly extended while writing. Using a vertical surface rather than a horizontal one promotes the development of wrist extension and strengthens the arm and shoulder muscles.[31] For example, try to grasp a hammer with a flexed wrist. The hammer cannot be securely held or controlled because the hand is not in a

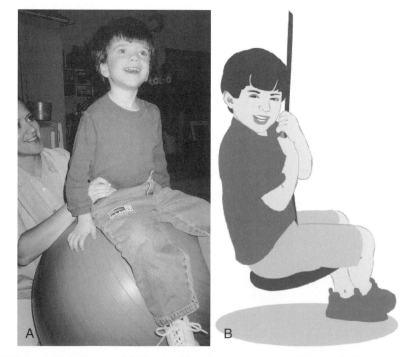

FIGURE 22-6   **A,** Engaging the child by requiring that he remain upright on a ball promotes postural control for sitting necessary for handwriting. **B,** Vestibular stimulation from swinging can promote muscle tone and postural control.

power-grasping pattern. In a slightly extended posture, the wrist stabilizes the hand while using a tool.

The child must be able to hold the nonmoving finger joints steady while writing. OT practitioners examine how much control the child has in keeping the fingers in position. The child who cannot stabilize the joints will have difficulty with fine motor movements. A variety of activities that increase finger strength and finger joint stability are available.

Strength and Endurance

Hand strength and endurance are necessary for performing the complex tasks of writing. The arches of the hand are formed as the intrinsic hand muscles develop. These muscles shape the hand for grasping objects of different sizes, enable skilled movements of the fingers, and control the power and force of prehension. This force is modulated to pick up fragile items, for example, a pencil, or a Styrofoam cup without breaking them. Children with poorly developed hand arches have flat, underdeveloped, weak hands. The lack of hand arching interferes with the strength and coordination. When the arches are well developed, the hand is able to form a bowl in the palm, and distinct creases are seen in the palm. Children with poorly developed arches may compensate by holding the pencil tightly against the palm, showing no web space.

Hand strength that is adequate to hold objects and endurance to repeat motor patterns without fatiguing are important for writing tasks. The process of writing is a continuous one. Therefore promoting optimal muscle strength and endurance for the task is an essential intervention for improving handwriting. Figure 22-7 illustrate activities that promote hand strength and endurance.

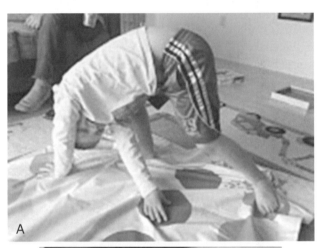

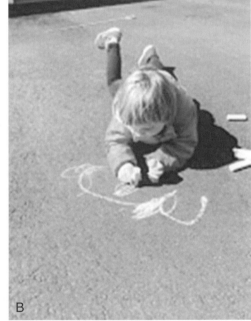

FIGURE 22-7 Children with handwriting difficulties benefit from practice and hand strengthening games. **A,** Twister requires children to lean on their hands, promoting strength. **B,** Drawing with chalk on the ground provides resistance, which promotes hand strength.

Midline Crossing

Melissa, a 5-year-old kindergartner, is right handed. When writing her name, she switches the pencil to the left hand when she gets to the first "s" in her name. She finishes writing her name and then switches the pencil back to her right hand. This is an example of not being able to cross the midline. Another example is using only the right hand to retrieve puzzle pieces on the right and the left hand to retrieve the pieces on the left.

A student should be able to smoothly cross the midline when writing. By definition, **midline crossing** is the ability to continue a motor act (e.g., writing) without switching hands at the point in front of a person's middle. The inability to do so may be an indicator of an immature nervous system. Switching hands at the middle of the paper (hand dominance not established) instead of writing across the paper or moving the paper to the dominant side may indicate difficulty with midline crossing. OT practitioners must determine whether the child is ambidextrous or is unable to cross the midline. A child who is ambidextrous is able to write efficiently with either hand and demonstrate the ability to cross the midline when writing.

Eye-Hand Coordination

The term *eye-hand coordination* (also called *hand-eye coordination*) refers to the control of eye movement coordinated with the control of hand movement, the processing of visual input to guide reaching and grasping, and the use of proprioception of the hands to guide the eyes. Children with poor handwriting skills score lower on eye-hand coordination tasks than those with adequate handwriting skills.[3,23] Examples of poor eye-hand coordination include the inability to pick up an object from a table or the inability to hit a ball with a bat or tennis racket. In terms of handwriting, a student with poor eye-hand coordination has difficulty staying within the lines when coloring or working on a maze (Figure 22-8).

Motor Planning

Children with poor handwriting skills may have deficits in **motor planning** (i.e., figuring out how to move their bodies and then actually doing it) or motor memory (i.e., remembering the motor patterns and being able to repeat them) (Figure 22-9).

Motor planning problems may be due to poor proprioception (poor awareness of muscle and joint position). Children with motor planning difficulties are unable to maneuver around their school environment without bumping into other people or knocking things down.

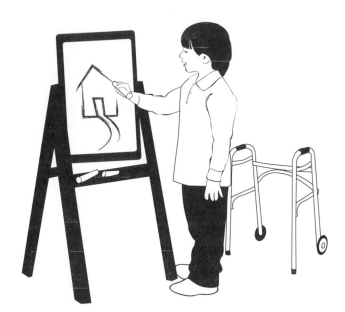

FIGURE 22-8 Using a paintbrush for details requires fine motor coordination. (From O'Brien, J., & Solomon, J. (2012) *Occupational analysis and group process,* St. Louis: Mosby.)

For example, when walking in line and when the line stops, the child unintentionally runs into the back of another student in front or is constantly feeling the walls. Feeling the walls is a means of information for the child about his or her position in space (close to the wall). If the child did not feel the wall, he or she may very well keep bumping into it and sometimes even fall. If even walking down the hall in a smooth, coordinated manner is difficult, then doing a refined task such as moving a pencil over a piece of paper and creating letters could be daunting. Smooth writing requires the ability to motor-plan on a much smaller scale and requires the separation and isolation of finger movements for dynamic grasping patterns.

A well-organized proprioceptive system provides an unconscious awareness of where the body is in space. It helps the child understand the touch and movement that he or she is experiencing. Therefore difficulties with proprioception include not knowing where one's arms or hands are positioned in space with the eyes open or closed, finger identification, and finger isolation. Children with poor proprioceptive abilities do not "feel" the pressure they need to put on the pencil to hold it (so they may squeeze it tightly or hold it too loosely). In this instance they may bear down too hard and write too darkly or not apply enough pressure and write too lightly. These children may need to visually monitor or observe where their hands are positioned on the paper.

The tactile system plays a key role in writing. This important skill requires the ability to feel the pencil and manipulate it without the aid of vision. Some children with handwriting deficits do not feel objects adequately. To fully understand this, try writing while wearing mittens. The lack

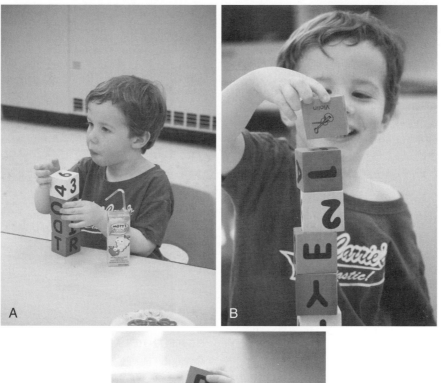

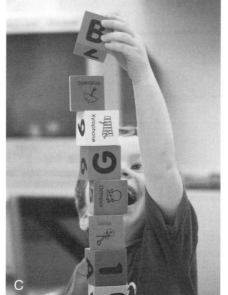

FIGURE 22-9 Precise hand skills and modulation of force are required to grasp a block and carefully build a tower. **A,** The child uses both hands to steady the blocks initially. **B,** The child uses a radial digital grasp to pick up the block. **C,** The child is able to modulate the force with which he releases the block.

of tactile sensation interferes with the ability to manipulate the pencil. To feel the pencil, the child with a poor tactile system may have to hold it more tightly, which interferes with refined movements and results in messy writing.

Visual Perception Skills

Visual perception is not the same as visual acuity. Although a student may *see* a sentence with 20/20 vision,

his or her brain may not *interpret* it accurately. **Visual perception** refers to the way the child makes sense of the visual input. Signs and symptoms of poor visual perceptual skills may include the following:

- May have reversals (*b* for *d*, *p* for *q*) or inversions (*u* for *n*, *w* for *m*)
- Complains that eyes hurt and itch; rubs eyes; complains that print blurs while reading

- Turns the head when reading across the page; holds the sheet of paper at odd angles
- Closes one eye while working; may yawn while reading
- Cannot near and/or far point copy accurately
- Does not recognize an object or word if only part of it is shown
- Misaligns letters; may have messy papers, which can include letters colliding, irregular spacing, letters not on line

CLINICAL *Pearl*

The stimulus item to be copied is in close proximity to the copier's paper and pencil for *near-point* copying.

For example, a student copies problems from a math book onto a piece of paper to perform the calculations. During *far-point* copying the stimulus is a distance from the copier, paper and pencil. Far-point copying is illustrated as the student copies homework assignments from the whiteboard located in the front of the classroom.

Children who have difficulty learning letters or recognizing words will have difficulty understanding the relationships between letters and words. Children need to recognize and perceive the letter forms and understand their differences and similarities before they can write. Figure 22-10 shows an intervention activity to promote visual perceptual skills. Children who do not perform well on visual perception and visual-motor tests typically have poor handwriting skills.

Directionality

The term **directionality** refers to the way print is tracked during reading and writing. Children must know to begin at the top of the page and work toward the bottom and to start on the left-hand side and move to the right. Directionality, or the understanding of which way to go or move the pencil is essential for writing because writing is performed left to right and top to bottom, with some letters placed on the line and some under the line. Forming letters in the correct direction or sequence, orienting them on the page, and starting or stopping letters at the right location are essential for writing.

EVALUATION OF HANDWRITING SKILLS

CASE *Study*

Molly is a first grader at Lincoln Elementary. She sits at a table at the front of the class and loves to participate in most of the classroom activities. She is not able to put

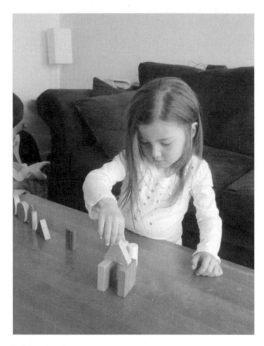

FIGURE 22-10   Building castles with block shapes requires visual-motor and visual perceptual skills.

prewriting strokes together to form most shapes. When encouraged to draw freely, her drawings appear very immature and simplistic. She becomes nervous when it is time to write in her classroom journal and to copy her spelling words from the wipe board (far point copy). She has trouble remembering the letters of the alphabet (working memory), and when called on to identify a letter, she is not always able to provide the correct answer. She struggles with writing letters and numbers. She tends to write large letters and numbers (size issues), so the entire page is covered with very little writing spread all over the paper (margin alignment and placing difficulties). She is able to write her first name, but she starts all of her letters from the bottom of the line (formation errors). Frequently Molly uses multiple strokes to form one letter or number that affects the speed and legibility of her written work.

Handwriting is a multifaceted developmental task. When a student is unable to put prewriting strokes together to form simple shapes, it is quite a challenge, if not impossible, for the student to form a letter. When evaluating a student's handwriting, the OT practitioner looks at myriad components that are needed to successfully perform this task. Visual-motor, perceptual, and fine motor skills are assessed. Considering the child's developmental stage provides insight as to the expectation of where the child's handwriting abilities may fall. In addition, the OT practitioner assesses the child's executive functioning. For example, is the child able to generate ideas for handwriting, remain focused and organized to complete the task in a timely manner, and monitor his or her performance? The OT practitioner analyzes the results of the assessments and observations of the child's skills to determine what components are weak and need to be remediated through individual or small group interventions. Consideration of how the student's sensory processing impacts the child's written expression abilities are assessed.

CLINICAL *Pearl*

Executive function refers to a set of cognitive skills that allows one to plan, organize, sequence, initiate, and stop a task. It allows one to problem solve and maintain focus as well as to monitor and modify behaviors and performance.

Handwriting is an important occupational skill requiring motor, sensory, perceptual, and cognitive abilities.[19,23,27] Formal and informal assessments of the ability to imitate and copy lines and shapes, hold a pencil or tool, and complete perceptual motor tasks help identify the factors for intervention. The OT practitioner is responsible for evaluating all aspects of handwriting, designing intervention and consulting with children, teachers, and parents.[5-7] The goal of occupational therapy in the school is to promote successful participation in the general educational curriculum.[5-7] As such, teachers and parents benefit from recommendations to enhance handwriting skills. Frequently, accommodations allow the student to be successful in written expression tasks at school or home.[5-7]

Assessment

A variety of standardized and nonstandardized assessments are available to determine the client factors interfering with handwriting. Classroom observation is another valuable means to assess handwriting.[7] The following sections describe different types of assessments, classroom observation considerations, and student self-assessments that are used to determine child-specific interventions to improve written expression skills.

Visual Perception and Visual-Motor Assessments

Visual perception is the ability to organize and interpret what is seen. Handwriting requires children to visually perceive the organization of letters and spacing between words. They must also determine the direction of letters (e.g., *b* compared with *d*). Visual perception is required to know where to start writing on the page, sequence the strokes of letters, and space words. When writing, children must recognize that the

sizes of letters do not change the meanings of words. Molly may be experiencing poor visual perception. In this scenario, she is unable to make sense of how letters are formed. Molly may not recognize the differences among *b*, *p*, and *d*.

Visual perceptual tests examine the following skills:

- *Discrimination:* The ability to detect a difference or distinction between one item or picture and another, for example, the ability to identify which picture is not like the others.
- *Visual memory:* The ability to remember a shape or word and recall the information when necessary. With handwriting, children must remember how to form letters, numbers, and shapes. In later school years, this skill is used when remembering how to form the letters to spell words or form multidigit numbers.
- *Form constancy:* The ability to realize and recognize that forms, letters, and numbers are the same or are constant whether they are moved, turned, or changed to a different size. This means that a square is always a square no matter what size or color. An example of visual form constancy relative to handwriting is the child recognizes that the letter J is a "J" whether it is written small or large, darker or lighter.
- *Sequential memory:* The ability to remember a sequence or chain of letters to form a word. With handwriting, children need motor as well as cognitive sequencing. Therefore they need the ability to remember how letters make words and sequence them according to their motor abilities to make those words. For example, when taking a spelling test, the child needs to be able to recall what the word "dog" looks like and remember that it is $d - o - g$ and not $g - d - o$.
- *Figure ground:* The ability to identify the foreground from the background. When looking at pictures, people, or items, it is essential to separate important visual aspects from the background. When writing, children identify written words on lined paper. An example of this is the game of finding hidden objects in a drawing.
- *Visual closure:* The ability to identify a form or object from its incomplete appearance. This enables a child to figure out objects, shapes, and forms by finishing the image mentally, for example, finding a jacket when it is partially covered by others. This ability is required when a letter may not be completely formed.

Visual-motor skills are also known as eye-hand and eye-foot coordination skills. Most assessments used by the OT practitioners evaluate eye-hand skills. Visual-motor assessments examine how well the eyes work with the hands to perform coordinate, precise movements. Box 22-3 presents a list of visual perceptual and visual-motor standardized assessments frequently used by OT practitioners. For a more extensive listing of OT assessments see Appendix 10-A in Chapter 10.

Handwriting Assessments

A variety of handwriting assessments used to evaluate a child's handwriting are commercially available (Box 22-4). Assessments can be standardized or nonstandardized and typically include a clinical observation component. The OT practitioner needs to know the purpose of the evaluation. Do the results need to be standardized? Does the OT practitioner, parent, or teacher want to know where this child's handwriting abilities are in comparison with his or her peers, or is getting an example of the child's handwriting abilities the goal? Is the OT practitioner interested in learning how the child is writing or spacing letters and words? The nature of the evaluation will determine which type of assessment(s) is to be used.

CLINICAL *Pearl*

Another form of nonstandardized assessment can be to compare the work of classmates with the work of the target child. An easy way to do this is to view the work displayed on the wall near the child's classroom. In addition many teachers use a daily writing journal, which the practitioner can use for comparison.

Classroom Observations

Most of a child's handwriting occurs in the classroom. Therefore it makes sense that the student be observed doing this task in this environment. Classroom observations allow OT practitioners to see how children work, how they organize their work/desk surface, and how they use their time. When evaluating a child's handwriting, observation of the child's performance in the classroom is beneficial.

BOX 22-3

Visual Perceptual and Visual-Motor Assessments

VISUAL PERCEPTUAL ASSESSMENTS

- The *Developmental Test of Visual Perception, Second Edition (DTVP-2)* measures visual-motor integration, visual-motor speed, and the components of visual perception such as spatial relations, figure ground, visual closure, position in space, and form constancy.
- The *Motor-Free Visual Perception Test, 3rd edition (MVPT-3;* Colarusso & Hammill) measures nonmotor visual perception in children by testing visual perception without requiring a motor response.
- The *Test of Visual Perceptual Skills, 3rd edition (TVPS-3;* Martin) measures nonmotor visual perception in children by testing visual perception without requiring a motor response.
- The *Jordan Left-Right Reversal Test, 3rd edition (Jordan-3)* measures the ability to recognize reversed images, letters and numbers in isolation and in sequences.

VISUAL-MOTOR ASSESSMENTS

- The *Beery-Buktenica Developmental Test of Visual-Motor Integration, Sixth Edition, (Beery VMI)* measures the ability to integrate visual and motor skills. Visual perception and motor control supplemental tests are available and may be used in addition to the visual-motor integration test to further, and separately, assess perception and fine motor skills.
- The *Test of Visual-Motor Integration–Revised* (Gardner) measures both the reproduction of developmental sequencing of geometric shapes and visual-motor integration.

BOX 22-4

Handwriting Assessments

- The *Children's Handwriting Evaluation Scales* (Stott et al) measures the speed and quality of the child's handwriting skills.
- The *Evaluation Tool of Children's Handwriting (ETCH;* Amundson, 1995) evaluates legibility and speed in six areas of handwriting: (1) alphabet production of lower and uppercase letters from memory, (2) numeral writing of 1-12 from memory, (3) near-point copying, (4) far-point copying, (5) speed, and (6) sentence composition in both manuscript and cursive formation.[15] The ETCH provides legibility scores for the child's age level.
- *The Print Tool* is a nonstandardized assessment from Jan Olsen's Handwriting Without Tears curriculum. "The Print Tool focuses on the eight key components of handwriting: memory, orientation, placement, size, start, sequence, control, and spacing." In addition to being an assessment, The Print Tool also "helps pinpoint the cause of difficulty and provides guidance for a remediation plan specific to the child's needs."
- *The Screener of Handwriting Proficiency* is a free online Handwriting Without Tears tool that assesses writing of numbers and letters generating individual and classroom reports that compare student's handwriting accuracy to same-aged peers using percentiles.

Classroom observation allows the OT practitioner to view the functional task (e.g., handwriting) in the context in which it occurs. Understanding the child's performance within the context of the classroom guides the intervention plan. For example, examination of the *physical context* provides information on such things as classroom space, seating arrangements, the height of the desk, visual stimuli, and environmental supports. Molly may be sitting in a chair that is too high, and the classroom space may not be conducive to writing. In terms of *personal context*, classroom observation may reveal information about Molly's needs. Perhaps she is easily distracted by the noise outside the door or by the decorations on the walls or hanging from the ceiling of the classroom. OT practitioners will want to consider the writing demands of a first-grade classroom as well as Molly's temperament and attitude toward the writing task. From the case study presented earlier, it is apparent that Molly becomes nervous during writing assignments, which provides the OT practitioner a window into her feelings. Temporal context refers to the time of day in which the handwriting task is performed. If handwriting is performed in the afternoon, Molly may very well be tired and restless; however, Molly produces her best work in the morning. Classroom observation may provide insight into how Molly is managing her time as well. Cultural context refers to expectations with regard to the classroom. How organized is the teacher? Are accommodations a natural part of the classroom? Is the classroom too busy for a child who requires a quiet environment for writing? Is the child able to interact easily with his or her peers?

Classroom observations provide valuable information on the factors that may be interfering with function in the classroom. Teachers are able to provide OT practitioners with information about the child's performance in the classroom, classroom expectations, and possible solutions. In addition, the teacher is able to provide the OT practitioner with handwriting samples done by the student at various times of the day.

The Schoodles Pediatric Fine Motor Assessment (PFMA-2) provides a framework for classroom and clinical observations.[14] The PFMA-2 is a performance-based assessment tool that guides therapists' assessment of the observable classroom and underlying skills needed for successful handwriting at school. The PFMA-2 provides a checklist for use during classroom observations. It has a reproducible student workbook to use while assessing the underlying support skills. The PFMA-2 provides age criterion that allows the therapist to compare the student being evaluated to same-aged peers.[14]

> **CLINICAL *Pearl***
>
> Visual or auditory distractions in the classroom may interfere with visual attention to handwriting tasks.

> **CLINICAL *Pearl***
>
> Asking teachers and families what strategies they have used in the past and using those strategies in OT interventions may help children succeed. Matching strategies to the classroom is effective.

Student Self-Assessment of Handwriting

Here's How I Write (HHIW)[8] is a criterion reference assessment with standardized administration procedures. It allows the student to rate his or her perception of his or her handwriting performance. The HHIW has two components: teacher rating and student rating of handwriting. The teacher rating from is completed by the teacher who is primarily responsible for the direct instruction and assessment of written expression school tasks. According to Cermak and Bissell, student self-assessment of handwriting performance is appropriate beginning at grades 2 and 3.[8] HHIW assesses the student's perception and not quality of handwriting. Including children and youth in the assessment, goal setting, and progress monitoring taps into intrinsic factors (such as motivation, self-efficacy and performance standards) and increases academic success.

> **CLINICAL *Pearl***
>
> Make It Legible[21] is a program that uses Willy the Worm self-checklist to assess correct letter formation, proper spacing, use of margins correctly, correct placement and punctuation, proper use of capital letters and correct paragraph indentation. It is available from Therapro (www.therapro.com). Make It Legible is effective in allowing students to assess their work and the work of their peers. It is most appropriate to use with students in grade 2 and above.[21]

> **CLINICAL *Pearl***
>
> Student self-assessment tools are beneficial to track student-specific data.

CONSIDERATIONS FOR HANDWRITING INTERVENTION

OT practitioners evaluate a child's handwriting performance in the classroom. They examine the hand structures and consider health conditions (e.g., physical, psychosocial, or neurologic) that may influence performance, including quality and legibility. The practitioner reviews the context(s) in which handwriting occurs as important to handwriting. For example, a child may experience difficulty performing under stressful test situations. Another child may feel anxious and perform poorly in a crowded classroom. After careful consideration of the multiple factors that influence a child's handwriting performance, the occupational therapist, with input from the occupational therapy assistant develop an intervention plan. The intervention plan provides a clear outline of how the OT practitioner will approach therapy and as such, it helps to identify the targeted activities and focus. This plan is dynamic and flexible, and considers the child's learning style, executive functioning and classroom. As the OT practitioner intervenes, he or she discovers new things about the child and context(s) and adjusts the plan accordingly. As the child progresses, plans and approaches are altered to suit the current situation.

Approaches to Intervention Planning and Implementation

AOTA describes five approaches or strategies that direct intervention planning and implementation[1]:

1. Create or promote
2. Establish or restore
3. Maintain
4. Modify
5. Prevent

Create or promote interventions have a health promotion outcome. Creating an afterschool handwriting program or promoting writing opportunities in the classroom are examples of how an OT practitioner may intervene. Establish or restore interventions have a remediation and/or restoration outcome. OT practitioners may work with a child to gain handwriting skills, hand strength, and coordination (Figure 22-11). The practitioner may help a child who lost handwriting skills after a neurologic injury regain those skills and restore function. Designing and implementing a handwriting group with specially designed instruction in a special education classroom is an example of a remediation strategy. Maintenance interventions support the preservation of occupational performance to meet the client's occupational needs. Practice allows children to maintain and refine skills for occupational performance (Figure 22-12). Revisiting handwriting strategies such as visual or verbal cues allow children to keep their abilities. Interventions using modification involve compensations and/or adaptations to meet the client's occupational needs. Allowing a child to use a tablet for written work, built-up pencil grip, or taping responses

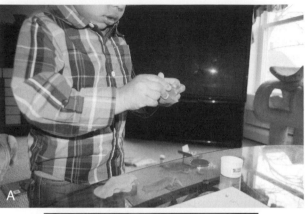

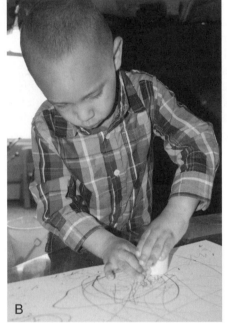

FIGURE 22-11 OT practitioners promote hand strength and endurance for handwriting through play. **A,** This child makes objects with Play-Doh. **B,** He presses the pattern firmly on the Play-Doh.

are examples of classroom adaptations/modifications that allow children to compensate for poor handwriting skills. Preventive approaches are provided to "at-risk" clients to prevent disability having a health promotion outcome. Designing and implementing an afterschool handwriting club for students in the general education classrooms is an example of a strategy that promotes using the proper mechanics of handwriting. OT practitioners use these approaches within the context of universal design for learning.

As mentioned earlier in the chapter, a goal of OT assessment and intervention in an educational setting is to promote participation of all children in the general education curriculum. OT practitioners may apply the principles and strategies of universal design for learning (UDL) to achieve this goal in relation to handwriting. UDL is defined in federal education law as: "research-based

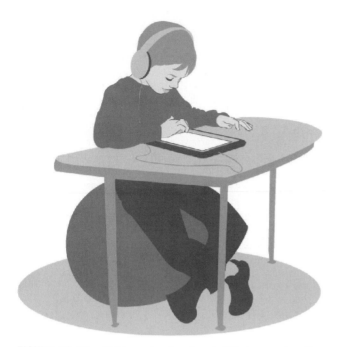

FIGURE 22-12 Children develop hand skills by manipulating objects and practicing movements. (From O'Brien, J., & Solomon, J. (2012) *Occupational analysis and group process*, St. Louis: Mosby.)

framework for designing curriculum—including goals, methods, materials, and assessments—that enables all individuals to gain knowledge, skills, and enthusiasm for learning. UDL provides curricular flexibility (in activities, in the ways information is presented, in the ways students respond or demonstrate knowledge, and in the ways students are engaged) to reduce barriers, provide appropriate supports and challenges, and maintain high achievement standards for all students, including those with disabilities."[16] The OT practitioner may consider learning styles, organization skills, classroom accommodations, compensatory strategies, and environmental structuring when designing OT interventions for handwriting.[16]

Learning Styles

Children learn using various senses and learning styles. Figure 22-13 shows children engaged in a variety of learning styles. Consideration of the child's learning style is helpful in designing interventions and classroom strategies. Some children are tactile or kinesthetic learners, that is, they need to physically feel and act out the task to remember the sequence. These children learn or perform a task better when they are allowed to stand while writing or when given the opportunity to move the body through the act. Using proprioceptive input—such as practicing and feeling the letter formation in the air with or without

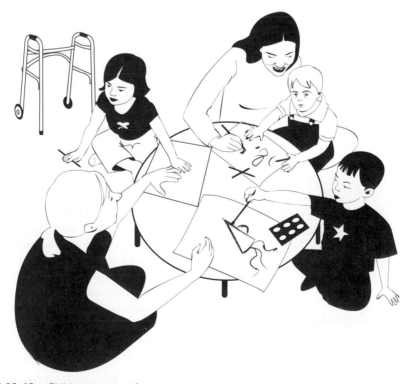

FIGURE 22-13 Children improve fine motor and prewriting skills by seeing, feeling and learning (the practitioner provides verbal cues) regarding letter formation. (From O'Brien, J., & Solomon, J. (2012) *Occupational analysis and group process*, St. Louis: Mosby.)

hand-over-hand assistance for additional tactile sensation of the letter shape—supports their learning. They frequently respond well to physical rewards such as a pat on the back or being sent on errands to the school office.

Children who learn through auditory means write better if they hear or verbalize the letters or words while putting them on paper. These children may talk to themselves while writing, saying the letters and verbally describing the letter formation as they write. Using fun "sayings" for letter formations are also helpful in learning how to stroke a letter. For example, when writing the capital letter "B," the OT practitioner would say, "Big line down. Frog jump up. Now, little curve, and another little curve."

Visual learners rely on visual prompts to replicate shapes, letters, and words. Visual prompts can be something as simple as a dot to remind them where a letter starts or the drawing of a line or box to show where to set/place their letters, or it can be as involved as writing out the letter or word or drawing shapes for the student to trace. Using a variety of bright, neon marker colors is helpful in visually presenting and separating a handwriting task into its components. For example, if you want Buster to trace his name on a line, write his name in neon orange, with a neon green dot to represent the starting point of each letter. However, make the line on which he is to trace his name neon pink. This provides him with all the visual prompts he needs to succeed in the task; yet, it also breaks the activity up into line orientation, starting points for correct letter formation, and visual presentation of his name so that he can remember what the letters look like and how to correctly spell his name. When paired with auditory "sayings" of how to form the letters, Buster gets a sensory-rich explanation of how his name is formed. As Buster becomes more independent in the writing of his first name, the practitioner decreases the amount of visual prompts provided.

CLINICAL *Pearl*

Children have preferred learning styles. For example, visual learners need to see examples, auditory learners need to hear the steps of the process, and kinesthetic learners need to feel and act out the steps of the process.

Executive Function and Organizational Skills

CASE *Study*

Jerome cannot find anything in or on his desk. As a result, he spends too much time looking for papers, folders, or books and misses the lessons. Jerome turns in homework

BOX 22-5

Components of Executive Function

- Inhibition: self-preventing of attending to extraneous stimuli
- Shift: changing tasks or transitioning in the school environment
- Emotional control: maintaining emotions appropriate to the current situation
- Initiation: starting tasks
- Working memory: remembering sequence of current events
- Plan/organize: managing time, assignments and materials to complete tasks
- Organization of materials: keeping desk and book bag organized
- Monitoring: self-awareness of performance

late or loses it in his desk. His papers are often torn and wrinkled. The teacher is sometimes unable to make sense of his writing. When he writes, Jerome does not know where to start on the paper or does not move to the next line, leading to the letters running together or being superimposed. The result of these issues often causes him to receive lower grades.

Having a neat and organized workstation is helpful to all students, especially to those with handwriting difficulties. In addition to having difficulties with organizing their self in preparation for writing (e.g., body position at desk, position of materials on tabletop), they may have difficulties organizing written work on paper. Improper placement and orientation of the letters on the line or improper spacing between words may be seen. Children with poor organizational skills may use letters of varying sizes and wrongly mix uppercase (capital) and lowercase (small) letters in words. Some organizational problems are related to poor visual processing, while others are related to poor motor planning or attention. OT practitioners can help determine the root of the organizational problem. For example, visually figuring out how far apart letters should be placed is a perceptual skill, and moving the fingers to create a letter or form letters counterclockwise requires motor planning. Organization can be taught with frequent reminders and follow-up. Simple systems that the child initiates or helps design are effective. See Box 22-5 for components of executive function. See Box 22-6 for potential intervention strategies to improve executive function and organizational skills.

Classroom Accommodations

OT practitioners may help students and teachers by providing classroom accommodations and strategies

BOX 22-6

Executive Function Intervention Solutions

- Help the child keep desk clean and organized.
- Have the child use folders of different colors for different subjects and cover the textbooks with paper or material of the same color.
- Verbally cue the student; remind the teacher to encourage the student to clear off the writing surface before starting handwriting assignments.
- Make a bag that can be hung on the back of the classroom chair in order to store pencils, scissors, and paper and thus make them readily available.
- Have the child use a planner to record assignments with the teacher checking daily before dismissal.

BOX 22-7

Strategies for the General Education Classroom

- Decrease the amount of written work expected, and reduce redundant written assignments (e.g., completion of 50% of the required work).
- Encourage a buddy system to help with journal keeping or other written assignments. The child can dictate the story to a peer with adequate handwriting, who can write down the story, and the child can then rewrite the story.
- Have the child use a tape recorder so that he or she can dictate a story or tape the teacher's lecture.
- Allow preferential seating and optimal positioning of the student in the classroom. Some children need midline positioning because of decreased visual scanning from one side to the other or one-sided neglect. In addition, auditory learners and easily distracted students frequently need to sit close to the teacher so that they can be more attentive.
- A written list of homework assignments and a checklist of each book or folder that needs to go home can be provided to the child.
- Delegate a packing buddy to help the child pack up at the end of the day to make sure that all of the necessary papers and books are put in the bag.
- Allow the child more time to complete written assignments, or use an outline format for them.
- Grade and emphasize the content of assignments of written expression with a grade for the mechanics of writing.

to encourage success in the classroom. Accommodations or strategies assist with the completion of writing assignments. Children who fatigue easily may not pay attention to or learn from long writing assignments. Writing repetitively may also reinforce inappropriate letter formations. Accommodations that are appropriate for a specific child are included in the accommodation section of the individualized education program (IEP) or as a part of the 504 plan to be followed in the classroom. Box 22-7 lists strategies to assist children in the general education classroom who have handwriting difficulties.

CLINICAL *Pearl*

The primary difference between an IEP and a 504 plan is that students receive special education and related services with an IEP, whereas students do not receive special education or related services with a 504 plan. Different federal laws mandate components of an IEP and 504 plan (see Chapter 4).

Left-Handed Writers

Children who are left-handed may require special accommodations for writing. Writing in a notebook is more difficult for left-handed children because of the placement of the spirals or rings. When writing with the left hand, they find it difficult to see what they have just written because the left hand covers the writing. Left-handed children often place their notebooks angled toward the right and flex the left wrist, which is an awkward posture (Figure 22-14). In the sitting posture, the body is frequently twisted to accommodate the angle of the paper. The left-handed writer tends to push the pencil rather than pull it from left to right. Box 22-8 provides OT interventions for the left-handed student.

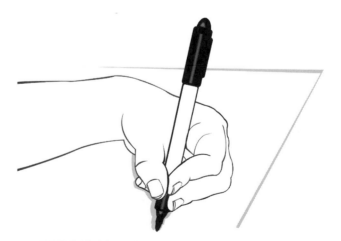

FIGURE 22-14 Left-handed writing is often awkward.

ASSISTIVE TECHNOLOGY FOR SUCCESS IN WRITTEN EXPRESSION

When a student is not successful using handwriting as the primary mode for written expression, the team explores accommodations or modifications that will enhance the

---

BOX 22-8

Interventions for the Left-Handed Student

- Group left-handed children together or at the end of the row so that their hands do not hit the hands of right-handed writers.
- Develop left-to-right directionality. Do exercises on the blackboard to encourage full arm movements, and discourage excessive loops and flourishes in writing.
- Teach vertical writing. Do not insist on a right slant. Left-handed children should be allowed to write with a left-handed slant and with the paper at the midline and angled in the same direction as the forearm.

BOX 22-9

Low-Technology Solutions for Successful Handwriting

- Colored pencils/markers
- Slant boards
- Pencil grips
- Finger positioners (e.g., finger claw)
- Graphic organizers
- Finger spacers/popsicle sticks
- Raised lined or lined colored paper
- Thumb drives for ease of transport across environments and printing of assignments
- Stylus or digital pens
- Weighted pencils
- Mechanical pencils
- Gray box or strips of paper

---

student's occupational performance. The Decoste Writing Profile[9,10] compares the rate of handwriting to the rate of keyboarding. The results of the Decoste Writing Profile guide the team's decision-making process when considering introducing keyboarding as an alternative to handwriting.[9,10] Selected **assistive technology** devices are trialed to determine which is appropriate for the student's success in written expression activities (see Chapter 27 for additional information). The following discussion addresses possible low- and high-technology solutions to increase a child's success with written expression tasks and activities.

CLINICAL *Pearl*

The Decoste Writing Profile is available through Don Johnston (www.donjohnston.com). It is affordable and easy to administer, score, and interpret.[9,10]

Low-Technology Solutions

Low-technology solutions are easy to obtain and use with relative low cost. Box 22-9 provides potential low-technology solutions.

CLINICAL *Pearl*

Low-technology solutions incorporated into general education classrooms support UDL concepts and can facilitate successful writing experiences in the general education classroom. When possible, the OT practitioner should use low- rather than high-technology devices.

High-Technology Solutions

High-technology solutions are not readily available and are more expensive than low-technology solutions. High-technology solutions include:

- Classroom computer workstations
- Laptops
- iPad/apps
- Netbooks
- Portable word processors

Appendix 22-B lists useful Internet resources and iPad apps.

In some circumstances, even after intervention, a student's writing may not be proficient enough to support his or her studies and communication. In such cases, other strategies and compensatory intervention models, such as using a computer (i.e., keyboarding) to support writing are considered.[30] Word processor, netbooks, or iPads are accommodations or supplemental aids that may be used in the classroom with the child who has handwriting difficulties. A student could write out his or her rough draft, or "sloppy copy," and then type the final draft. If the child is using a word processor, it should be presented to the child as early as possible in his or her educational career. The early provision of a word processor does not allow the handwriting difficulties to interfere with written expression skills. The keyboard would improve legibility and reduce spelling errors in written assignments.[15] Most school districts have computer keyboarding skills included in their curriculum; OT practitioners should review what is recommended. Box 22-10 shows a progression of keyboarding development recommended for schools.

Keyboarding requires memorization of where the keys are on the keyboard and how to access the keys and documents. On the one hand, to be a touch typist, timing, rhythm, and bilateral coordination are important. On the other hand, keyboarding does not require spatial organization and directionality, as does handwriting.[27]

Few studies have been conducted on the use and benefits of word processors in comparison with teaching handwriting. Before recommending a word processor or

BOX 22-10

Summation of the Bradley County Grade-Level Technology Expectations

- Kindergarten: Identify all letters, numbers, and other commonly used keys on the keyboard. Know the parts of the computer and how to operate.
- Grade 1: Be familiar with the home keys. Fingers should reach keys, and correct finger positions should be used while typing spelling words. Explore multimedia, use word processing.
- Grade 2: Locate and use symbol keys such as %, ?, Caps Lock, Shift, and Esc. Collect, sort and display data, use drawing tools, use electronic database to locate information.
- Grade 3: Be familiar with punctuation marks, and practice spelling words and fast written expression. At this time, the child should return the hands to the home key promptly after typing. Explore information technologies, build on word processing, awareness of copyright law.

Data from http://www.techcoachcorner2.org. Accessed December 27, 2014.

BOX 22-11

Keyboard Intervention Strategies

- Correct positioning and optimal seating should be provided to the student where the computer is located. Make sure that the screen and keyboard are not too high, the keyboard is aligned at the midline, and the seat is steady.
- Written instructions about how to use the programs should be placed near the computer so that the staff can refer to it if necessary.
- Have the child look across the room periodically to reduce eye strain; also have the child take breaks for stretching exercises.[17]
- Encourage the student to use the right hand on the right side of the computer keyboard and the left hand on the left side. Have the child push the shift key with the little finger and the space bar with the thumb.
- Use a portable word processor or alternative keyboard with enlarged keys to encourage word processor usage in the classroom. Computer keyboards can be altered with Sticky Keys, Filter Keys, or others from the accessibility options of the computer to meet the student's specific needs.

a laptop, the OT practitioner should consider the child's ability to organize his or her work area. Children who are unable to locate their materials may have further difficulty organizing themselves with an additional piece of equipment. A portable word processer may suffice if more than one child uses the computer. A stand-alone computer is beneficial, but computers are frequently located along the wall of the classroom, away from the teacher and classroom peers. Laptops have advantages, but the screen interferes with the visibility of the board or the teacher. Box 22-11 provides keyboard intervention strategies.

CLINICAL *Pearl*

Students will approach keyboarding in a variety of ways. Although the two hands to keyboard method is preferred there are techniques that can be taught to students who have the use of only one hand.

Many of the computer programs used in school computer labs are mouse-driven; that is, the mouse controls most of the action. After the child types his or her name and identification number into the computer, the specific computer lesson comes up. Because many of these programs are mouse-driven, the child is required to move the mouse and click on the correct answer. To do this effectively the child must possess adequate visual and motor skills. The OT practitioner must observe and assess these skills to determine proficiency in using the mouse. The OT practitioner may recommend alternatives to a standard mouse depending on the needs of the child.

The following sample OT intervention session will help the OT assistant (OTA) student to visualize how an actual intervention session might "look" while working with students who have difficulty with written expression activities.

SAMPLE OT INTERVENTION SESSION: "PULL-OUT" GROUP SESSION

- OTA provides services in the therapy room.
- Students are in grade 2 general education and receive special education resource services in subject areas of reading and writing.
- Direct group session outside general education classroom.
- Annual goal: By December 2015, the student will increase correct word sequences from 3 to 15 as measured and documented by the special education teacher.
  - Short-term objective (STO) 1: The student will use correct punctuation at the end of sentences with 90% accuracy as documented by the OT practitioner.
  - STO 2: The student will use correct capitalization at the beginning of sentences with 90% accuracy as documented by the OT practitioner.
  - STO 3: The student will use correct punctuation and capitalization within sentences with 90% accuracy as documented by the OT practitioner.

Sequence of Session

1. Student signs in (first and last name) on large wipe board in designated area: 2 minutes
2. Student "near point" (refers to material located close to student) copies day of the week and date on large wipe board: 2 minutes
3. Student forms the letters of first and last name using thinking putty: 5 minutes
4. Student performs brain gym[11] exercises to promote hand strength demonstrated by certified and licensed OTA (COTA)/L: 3 minutes
5. Student gets assigned handwriting workbook and sharpened pencil: 2 minutes
6. COTA/L provides direct instruction for work sheet(s) to be completed during session: 3 minutes
7. Student completes assigned pages in handwriting workbook: 10 minutes
8. COTA/L provides ongoing feedback per motor control terminology during writing exercises in workbook throughout session and final feedback at the end of the session: 2 minutes
9. Student erases his sign-in information on large wipe board: 1 minute

---

CLINICAL *Pearl*

Brain exercises can be modified (simplified) to promote student success and support handwriting intervention.[11] The exercises can be done in standing or sitting positions. The cross crawl can be changed from contralateral elbow to knee to ipsilateral elbow to knee (www.braingym.com). These activities may promote upper extremity strength for handwriting.

CLINICAL *Pearl*

Students prefer thinking putty to theraputty because of the visual and tactile differences (www.puttyworld.com).

CLINICAL *Pearl*

Special education give writing prompts to measure total words written and correct word sequences. The student(s) is given a topic and 1 minute to think and 3 minutes to write on the given topic. Numeric scores are recorded as a means of documenting progress. Correct word sequences include the correct use of capitalization and punctuation.

SAMPLE OT INTERVENTION SESSION: INCLUSIVE GROUP SESSION

- OTA provides services within first grade general education classroom.
- Four students receive weekly OT intervention and special education resources services in the subject area of ELA.
- OT services provided inside the general education classroom during handwriting block.
- Annual goal: By December 2015 the student will increase total words written from 7 to 19 as measured and documented by the special education teacher.
  - STO 1: The student will use correct spacing between letters, numbers, and words with 90% accuracy in 3-minute writing sample as documented by the OT practitioner.
  - STO 2: The student will use correct placing of letters, numbers, and words with 90% accuracy in 3-minute writing sample as documented by the OT practitioner.
  - STO 3: The student will use correct spacing and placing of letters, numbers, and words with 100% accuracy in 3-minute writing sample as documented by the OT practitioner.

Sequence of Session

1. Yoga poses (stretching) to instrumental, classical music: 3 minutes
2. Pinching, twisting, and popping bubble wrap: 5 minutes
3. Air writing of target letters and words: 4 minutes
4. Brain gym exercises: 3 minutes
5. Handwriting exercises with paper and pencil in handwriting workbook: 10 minutes
6. Self-check work per work booklet instruction and Willy Worm: 3 minutes
7. Brain gym exercises and transition to independent writing in classroom writing journal (sharpen pencil, obtain writing journal, go to assigned desk): 2 minutes
8. OTA monitors assigned students initiation of independent writing in classroom journals: 8 to 10 minutes

---

CLINICAL *Pearl*

Animal walks can be used in lieu of yoga poses. The walks can be static poses without movement being incorporated. Making the sounds of the animal promotes inhalation/exhalation (air exchange).

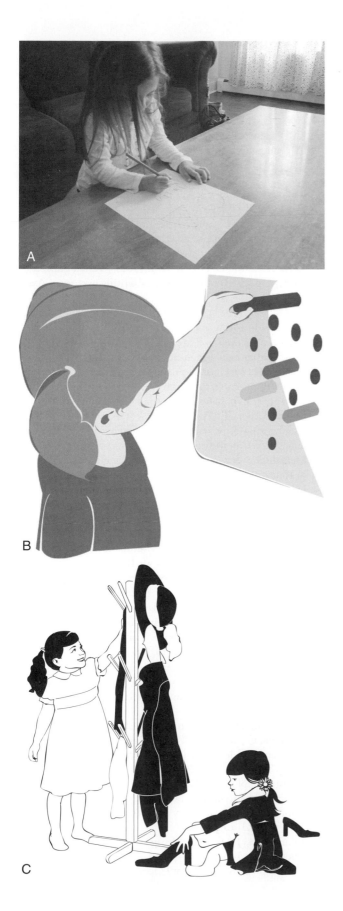

FIGURE 22-15 **A**, Practice copying shapes by "following the dots" can help children gain important motor skills for handwriting. **B**, The OT practitioner designs an activity to practice grasping (pegs and string) and to promote trunk strengthening by requiring the child sit unsupported during the game. **C**, Playing dress-up can help children develop fine motor skills for handwriting. (From O'Brien, J., & Solomon, J. (2012) *Occupational analysis and group process,* St. Louis: Mosby.)

> **CLINICAL *Pearl***
>
> Specially designed CDs with selected music/beats per minute can promote attention to tasks. Some CDs provide background music that may help children focus on intervention or transition throughout the school environment. Advanced Brain Technology (www.advancedbrain.com) sells a variety of music and listening options for children.

OCCUPATIONAL THERAPIST/OTA ROLES IN HANDWRITING ASSESSMENT AND INTERVENTION

The OTA and the occupational therapist work together to assess and provide services to children with handwriting deficits. The occupational therapist is responsible for interpreting assessment results. The OTA may contribute to the evaluation process by completing a handwriting checklist or a standardized assessment to examine the child's skills. The OTA, under the supervision of the occupational therapist, may work directly with the student to promote motor planning, postural stability, visual-motor integration, grasping patterns, and letter formation for writing. The OTA provides handwriting interventions and may lead handwriting groups. Figure 22-15 presents intervention examples. OT practitioners assist children in gaining handwriting skills within the classroom curriculum. The OT practitioner is involved in consultation with caregivers and teachers to provide ideas on remediation and techniques to improve handwriting in the classroom and at home.

SUMMARY

Handwriting is an important area of children's daily occupational performance. OT practitioners analyze the factors that may be interfering with a child's ability to write. The performance skills that may affect handwriting performance include muscle tone, strength, endurance, posture, integrity of structures, visual perception, and sensory processing. In addition to evaluating the underlying factors that may affect handwriting, OT practitioners assess the mechanics of handwriting using specially designed evaluations. Based on the initial data collected and interpreted the occupational therapist in collaboration with the OTA design/implement appropriate interventions to help children succeed in the classroom.

References

1. American Occupational Therapy Association. (2014). Occupational therapy practice framework: domain and process (3rd ed.). *Am J Occup Ther, 68*(Suppl. 1), S1–S48.

2. American Psychiatric Association. (2013). *Diagnostic and statistical manual of mental health disorders, fifth edition* (DSM-V). Arlington, VA: American Psychiatric Association.

3. Beery, K. E., Beery, N. A., & Evans, L. (2004). *My book of letters and numbers*. Minneapolis, MN: NCS Pearson.

4. Benbow, M. (1995). Principles and practices of teaching handwriting. In A. Henderson, & C. Pehoski (Eds.), *Hand function in the child: foundations for remediation*. St. Louis, MO: Mosby.

5. Case-Smith, J. (2002). Effectiveness of school-based occupational therapy intervention on handwriting. *Am J Occup Ther, 56*, 17.

6. Case-Smith, J., Holland, T., & Bishop, B. (2011). Effectiveness of an integrated handwriting program for first-grade students: a pilot study. *Am J Occup Ther, 65*, 670–678.

7. Case-Smith, J., Weaver, L., & Holland, T. (2014). Effects of a classroom-embedded occupational therapist-teacher handwriting program for first-grade students. *Am J Occup Ther, 68*, 690–698.

8. Cermak, S. A., & Bissell, J. (2014). Content and construct validity of Here's How I Write (HHIW): A child's self-assessment and goal setting tool. *Am J Occup Ther, 68*, 296–306.

9. DeCoste, D. (2005). *Assistive technology assessment: developing a written productivity profile*. Volo, IL: Don Johnston, Inc.

10. DeCoste, D. (2014). *DeCoste writing profile*. Volo, IL: Don Johnston, Inc. Available at http://donjohnston.com/decoste-writing-protocol/#.VKGQ2V4CA.

11. Dennison, P. E., & Dennison, G. (1987). *Brain gym*. Ventura, CA: Edu Kinesthetic, Inc.

12. Engel-Yeger, B., Nagauker-Yanuv, L., & Rosenblum, S. (2009). Handwriting performance, self-reports, and perceived self-efficacy among children with dysgraphia. *Am J Occup Ther, 63*, 182–192.

13. Folio, M. R., & Fewell, R. R. (2000). *Peabody Developmental Motor Scales* (2nd ed.). Austin, TX: Pro-Ed.

14. Frank, M., & Wing, A. (2011). *Schoodles Pediatric Fine Motor Assessment: an OT's guide for assessing children ages 3 and up* (3rd ed.). Marshall, MN: Frank and Wing.

15. Handley-More, D., et al. (2003). Facilitating written work using computer word processing and word prediction. *Am J Occup Ther, 57*, 139.

16. Higher Education Opportunity Act. (2008). Pub. L. No. 110-315, 122 Stat. 3078.

17. Howe, T.-H., Roston, K. L., Sheu, C.-F., & Hinojosa, J. (2013). Assessing handwriting intervention effectiveness in elementary school students: A two-group controlled study. *Am J Occup Ther, 67*, 19–27.

18. Hoy, M. M. P., Egan, M. Y., & Feder, K. P. (2011). A systematic review of interventions to improve handwriting. *Can J Occup Ther, 78*, 13–25.

19. Karlsdottir, R., & Stefansson, T. (2002). Problems in developing functional handwriting. *Percept Mot Skills, 94*, 623–662.

20. Koziatek, S. M., & Powell, N. J. (2003). Pencil grips, legibility, and speed of fourth-graders' writing in cursive. *Am J Occup Ther, 57*, 84.

21. Kushmir, G. (2005). Making it legible. Available at http://www.therapro.com/Making-It-Legible-Join-Willy-the-Worm-in-a-Practical-Guide-to-Making-Handwriting-Legible-On-Special-P321042.aspx.

22. Mackay, N., McCluskey, A., & Mayes, R. (2010). The Log Handwriting Program improved children's writing legibility: a pre-test–post-test study. *Am J Occup Ther, 64*, 30–36.

23. Malloy-Miller, T., Polatajko, H., & Anstett, B. (1995). Handwriting error patterns of children with mild motor difficulties. *Can J Occup Ther, 62*, 258–267.

24. McHale, K., & Cermak, S. (1992). Fine motor activities in elementary school: preliminary findings and provisional implications for children with fine motor problems. *Am J Occup Ther, 46*, 898.

25. National Governors Association Center for Best Practices, Council of Chief State School Officers. (2010). *Common core state standards publisher*. Washington D.C.: National Governors Association Center for Best Practices, Council of Chief State School Officers.

26. Olsen, J., & Knapton, H. (2013). *2nd grade printing teacher's guide*. Gaithersburg, MD: Handwriting Without Tears.

27. Preminger, F., Weiss, P., & Weintraub, N. (2004). Predicting occupational performance: handwriting versus keyboarding. *Am J Occup Ther, 58*, 193.

28. Schneck, C. M., & Henderson, A. (1990). Descriptive analysis of the developmental progression of grip position for pencil and crayon in nondysfunctional children. *Am J Occup Ther, 44*, 893.

29. Schwellnus, H., Carnahann, H., Kushki, A., Polatajko, H., Missiuna, C., & Chau, T. (2012). Effect of pencil grasp on the speed and legibility of handwriting in children. *Am J Occup Ther, 66*, 718–726.

30. Weintraub, N., Grill, N. G., & Weiss, P. L. T. (2010). Relationship between handwriting and keyboarding performance among fast and slow adult keyboarders. *Am J Occup Ther, 64*, 123–132.

31. Yakimishyn, J., & Magill-Evans, J. (2002). Comparisons among tools, surface orientation, and pencil grasp for children 23 months of age. *Am J Occup Ther, 56*, 564.

REVIEW *Questions*

1. Name two ways that motor and sensorimotor factors, developmental delays, and visual perception can impede the ability to perform handwriting.
2. How should the wrist and hand be positioned for optimal handwriting performance?
3. How do motor planning difficulties interfere with the child's ability to learn and perform handwriting?
4. Identify two different learning styles, and describe the ways that OT intervention can be adjusted to meet the needs of children with these different learning styles.
5. Outline five different remediation techniques and list the benefits of each strategy.
6. What are the benefits of using a word processor or computer as an accommodation for a child with handwriting difficulties?
7. How should a left-handed student angle the paper, and what other accommodations can be recommended?
8. In what ways does the OTA work with children to improve their handwriting skills?

SUGGESTED *Activities*

1. Observe the variety of pencil grasps that are used. Find out if a tight, nondynamic style of grasp is painful or fatiguing.
2. Try to write with your body in a variety of positions and postures to understand how an awkward posture greatly affects handwriting performance.
3. Use the movement of your shoulder to write instead of the movement of your hand to understand how smooth writing is very dynamic in nature. Evaluate your pencil grasp and writing method.
4. Perform handwriting with the nondominant hand to understand how difficult directionality and letter formation are for some children.
5. Most adults have one learning style that they prefer but are able to use a blend of different styles. Identify what kind of a learner you are.
6. Name the prewriting strokes in their developmental order.
7. In the classroom, what kind of accommodations would be helpful for you to learn?
8. Observe the grasping patterns of people who write with the left hand. How many left-handed writers angle the paper the same way that right-handed writers do rather than angle the paper in the same direction as the forearm?

APPENDIX 22-A

Commercially Available Handwriting Programs

This list provides an overview of some commonly used handwriting programs.

A Reason for Handwriting

A Reason For
700 E. Granite
Siloam Springs, AR 72761
800-447-4332
www.areasonfor.com
This program uses a simplified version of Zaner Bloser's handwriting program and is based on Scripture verses and Christian content. It gives students a practical reason for using their very best handwriting and can be highly motivating.

Callirobics

Laufer
PO Box 6634
Charlottesville, VA 22906
800-769-2891
www.callirobics.com
This program consists of exercises that are repetitive, simple writing patterns done to music. Callirobics can be beneficial to students who are auditory rather than visual learners.

D'Nealian Handwriting

Thurber DN
D'Nealian Handwriting
1 Jacob Way
Reading, MA 01867
www.dnealian.com
This program is developed to ease the transition from manuscript to cursive writing because most of the manuscript letters are the basic forms of the corresponding cursive letters. These letters are formed with one continuous stroke rather than the "ball and stick" method. In addition, many of the letters have a "monkey tail," so the letters are easily converted to cursive formation. The program can be confusing to children who have directionality and orientation difficulties because they do not know in which direction to put the "monkey tail."

First Strokes Multisensory Print Program

The Handwriting Clinic
3314 N Central Expressway, Suite A
Plano, TX 75074
972-412-4119
www.firststrokeshandwriting.com
This program was designed by an occupational therapist and provides a multisensory approach to teaching printing.

Getty-Dubay Handwriting

Continuing Education Press
Portland State University
http://www.cep.pdx.edu/
This program, developed by Barbara Getty and Inga Dubay, is an italicized handwriting program that promotes efficient, simple movements. Exercises to strengthen hand muscles and improve coordination are provided in the book *Write Now: The Comprehensive Guide to Better Handwriting.*

GUIDE-Write Raised-Line Paper

601 SW 13th Terrace, Suite G
Pompano Beach, FL 33069
954-946-5756
www.guide-write.com
GUIDE-write provides products such as raised-line letters and raised-line paper that can be helpful when teaching a student to form letters.

Handwriting Without Tears

Jan Olsen, 1990, 2000
8801 MacArthur Blvd
Cabin John, MD 20818
301-263-2700
www.hwtears.com
This handwriting program uses a developmental approach toward prewriting through cursive writing. The letters are grouped by difficulty in formation of the letter. In addition, the letters are formed with a simple vertical line rather than a slanted line. In this program, there are only two writing lines, a baseline and a center line, which are visually less confusing for children with visual

figure-ground deficits.[10] This program was created by an occupational therapist for her son and is very user-friendly.

Loops and Other Groups

Mary Benbow, 1990, OT Ideas
124 Morris Turnpike
Randolph, NJ 07869
877-768-4332
www.otideas.com
This handwriting curriculum is a kinesthetic program that combines cursive connectors with manuscript letters for a more efficient writing style. The letters are taught in groups that share a common movement pattern. These motor and memory cues are used to help the student visualize and verbalize while experiencing the "feel" of the letters. Mary Benbow is an occupational therapist who provides suggestions for handwriting remediation. Her program is very helpful to students in grades 2 and higher, who have been taught cursive handwriting but have difficulty with letter formation.

Palmer Method

Palmer, A.N. The Palmer Method of Business Writing. The A.N. Palmer Company: New York. 1935.
Embridge, D. (2007). "The Palmer Method: Penmanship and the Tenor of Our Time" in Southwest Review. *Platinum Periodicals, 92,* 327.
This handwriting program has been traditionally used in schools for many years and has been the foundation for handwriting styles. The program begins with the letter "A" and goes through to "Z." It uses a "ball and stick" method, causing the child to lift the pencil as the letters are created. This program is really not used anymore, but teachers tend to teach the "ball and stick" method anyway.

Zaner Bloser Handwriting

2200 W Fifth Ave
Columbus, OH 43215
800-421-3018
www.zaner-bloser.com
This handwriting program is based on the Palmer method but has simplified the material. This program can be easily purchased by schools and has literature and easy-to-use materials to support the handwriting program.

APPENDIX 22-B

Additional Resources

INTERNET RESOURCES

www.handwritingwithouttears.com: handwriting assessments, products, and programs

www.universalpress.com: handwriting assessments, products, and programs

www.southpaw.com: weights for pencils and other sensory intervention products

www.therapro.com: weights for pencils and other sensory intervention products

www.abilitations.com: adapted scissors, pencil grips, weighted pencils, and other supporting products

www.callirobics.com: handwriting program for preschool

www.advancedbraintechnology.com: brain health CDs

www.ablenet.com: assistive technology and training webinars

www.WriterLearning.com: worksheets

www.typingweb.com: timed typing tests and typing programs

www.HaveFunTeaching.com: sentence sequencing, punctuation, capitalization, writing your address worksheets

www.education.com: capitalization/punctuation worksheets

www.worksheetfun.com: cutting/pasting/coloring activities/worksheets

www.k12reader.com: punctuation worksheets

www.scholastic.v Scholastic Story Starters

www.superteacherworksheets.com: picture sequencing, cutting/pasting, punctuation, writing prompts, handwriting worksheets

www.pbis.org/www.pbisworld.com: autism, social stories, behavioral support

www.studenthandouts.com: holiday-themed writing worksheets

APPS FOR MOBILE DEVICES

Visual Memory

- NatureTap (advanced)
- BirdMatching (intermediate)
- Matches! (basic)
- Memory! (basic to intermediate)
- MemoryMatch (basic)
- Veggies (intermediate)

Letter and Number Formation

- LetterToy
- LetterSchool
- Tracing ABC
- ABC Circus
- Letter Quiz
- iWW Lite
- BT Handwriting
- Write ABC & 123
- Trace It

- ABCFunKid Lite
- Cursive

Spelling and Vocabulary Building

- Endless ABC
- Spell Well
- Read Write Spell
- Spell Better

Sentence Building

- Jumbled Sentences 3

Other

- Autism iHelp: opposites
- Autism iHelp: comprehension
- Shiny Party: shapes and sequencing skills
- Jungle Coins: basic coin identification
- Show Me: language comprehension

NADINE K. HANNER
ANGELA CHINNERS MARSH
RANDI CARLSON NEIDEFFER

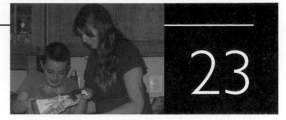

23

Therapeutic Media: Activity with Purpose

CHAPTER *Objectives*

After studying this chapter, the reader will be able to accomplish the following:

- Describe considerations necessary when selecting media for occupational therapy intervention
- Describe the role of the occupational therapy assistant in choosing therapeutic media
- Select developmentally appropriate therapeutic media for different age groups
- Describe the concepts of grading and adapting therapeutic activities based on client factors and activity demands
- Explain the importance of contexts and environment (e.g., cultural, physical, social, personal, temporal, and virtual) when choosing therapeutic media

CHAPTER *Outline*

This chapter serves to introduce the entry-level occupational therapy assistant (OTA) to the definition, background, and application of therapeutic media.

The term **media** (plural of *medium*) is defined as "an intervening substance through which something else is transmitted or carried. An agency by which something is accomplished, conveyed or transferred."[1] **Method** refers to "a means or manner of procedure, especially a regular and systematic way of accomplishing something."[1]

To further clarify these terms in the context of the OT profession, a purposeful activity is chosen to produce desired outcomes for a child and carried out with the use of selected **therapeutic media**. The media and method are chosen for their therapeutic value and individualized for each child's specific needs.

BACKGROUND AND RATIONALE OF THERAPEUTIC MEDIA

In the early days of occupational therapy, arts and crafts were the primary therapeutic activities used by occupational therapists and occupational therapy assistants (OTAs). As social and economic times changed and technology grew, the repertoire of media used in the OT profession expanded and evolved to meet the changing needs of children. Traditional craft activities continue to be used in various practice settings and are of particular value in the treatment of the pediatric population. Children can acquire and practice skills necessary to function in their occupations through the use of crafts as therapeutic media. Furthermore, engagement in crafts is typically an occupation of childhood and thus it lends itself well to occupational therapy intervention. Technology has evolved and many OT practitioners use forms of technology such as tablet computers, electronic games and systems, and applications (apps) as part of the intervention process. This chapter describes the selection and use of traditional and nontraditional therapeutic media as an intervention for children.

SELECTION OF THERAPEUTIC MEDIA

OT practitioners use clinical reasoning skills when choosing therapeutic media for children. Specifically, therapeutic activities are meaningful and motivating while addressing the child's goals. When selecting media, OT practitioners consider the child's interests, therapy goals, **client factors,** performance skills, and performance patterns. They consider the context(s) and activity demands of the activity (refer to the Occupational Therapy Practice Framework 3rd edition for further definition of these terms).[2] Practitioners also evaluate how therapeutic media can be graded or adapted to address the needs of individual children. This chapter provides

an overview of the reasoning necessary to select media for intervention.

Occupation/Interests

OT practitioners use therapeutic media to facilitate and encourage the development of motor, process, and social interaction skills. Matching a child's interests and abilities requires clinical reasoning along with knowledge of the variety of activities available for many age groups. The following questions may help the OT practitioner select meaningful, motivating, and age-appropriate media for children and adolescents:

1. Are the media relevant to the child's age and occupational role (e.g., student, sibling, worker)?
2. Are the media related to the child's current interests and/or hobbies? Can they possibly spark their interest to pursue a new leisure activity (e.g., drawing, computers, photography, needlecraft)?

Goals

Importantly, the OT practitioner selects activities and media to address the child's goals by carefully evaluating the ability of the media and its properties to challenge the child's abilities. The media should naturally challenge the child to repeat motions, thinking, or communication/interaction skills being addressed. The intent of therapeutic activity is to support the child in meeting his or her goals for occupational performance. The OT practitioner considers the following questions when selecting activities (media and methods) for intervention:

1. What specific goals will be addressed?
2. How will the activity (media and method) facilitate the child's goals?
3. Are these media the best choice to facilitate desired outcomes?
4. Is the child interested or motivated to engage in the activity?
5. How will the activity facilitate occupational performance?
6. Can the child relate to the activity?
    7. Is the child familiar with the media being used?
8. Does the media have properties that the child will enjoy?
9. How close does this activity simulate the natural context and actual occupation?

Client Factors

The OTA analyzes activities in terms of client factors to design interventions to meet the child's goals.

Client factors refer to values, beliefs, and spirituality; body functions; and body structures.

Values, Beliefs, and Spirituality

Values are standards and qualities that the child considers worthwhile.[2] Beliefs are those things that the child holds as true and spirituality is defined as the way the child expresses meaning and purpose.[2] OT practitioners working with children should try to understand the child's interests, beliefs, and what they hold as meaningful. Using this knowledge, the practitioner is able to find therapeutic activities that are valued by the child and his or her family.

Body Functions

Body functions include mental and sensory functions; neuromusculoskeletal, muscle, and movement functions; cardiovascular, hematologic, immunologic, and respiratory system functions; voice and speech functions; and skin and related functions.[2] OT practitioners carefully examine each body function to determine how the child or youth may perform. For example, handwriting goals frequently address a body function (e.g., fine motor coordination, visual perceptual processing). Understanding the influence of body function on handwriting helps the practitioner develop intervention plans.

Body Structures

Body structures refer to the anatomic parts of the body.[2] The OT practitioner evaluating handwriting abilities explores the structures of the hand when deciding on intervention strategies. For example, children may have hand deformities requiring compensatory activity or adaptive equipment. The practitioner may have to provide stability to assist a child in writing.

The following questions may be useful in guiding the OT practitioner examine client factors:

1. What does the child enjoy doing? What are his or her interests?
2. What provides the child with a sense of purpose?
3. What body structures (including skin and related structures) are required to complete the activity? What is the child's current body structure status?
4. What physical requirements (i.e., neuromusculoskeletal and movement-related functions, muscle function, movement functions) are needed to complete the activity or use the media (e.g., range of motion [ROM], strength, bilateral integration)?
5. What global or specific mental functions (e.g., level of arousal, motivation, attention, awareness, memory, perception, emotional, experience of self and time) must the child possess to successfully work with the selected media?

6. What sensory functions are required for the child to participate in the activity or with the media (e.g., vision, hearing, vestibular, taste, smell, proprioceptive, pain)?
7. What cardiovascular, hematologic, immunologic, and respiratory system functions are involved?
8. What voice and speech, digestive, metabolic, and endocrine functions are involved?
9. What are the safety issues surrounding the use of the media? Does the child possess the safety awareness to handle the media or participate in the activity without risk (e.g., impulsivity, allergies)?

Performance Skills

Performance skills refer to motor, process, and social interaction actions used during activity.[2] Understanding the complete range of performance skills is necessary when working on handwriting skills. OT practitioners use standardized assessments, clinical observations, and classroom observations to describe performance skill areas that require intervention. For example, handwriting involves motor skills including:

- Aligning paper on desk;
- Stabilizing paper with nondominant hand;
- Gripping pencil in dominant hand;
- Manipulating pencil using tripod grasp;
- Coordinating movement of pencil across paper;
- Calibrating force to press pencil on paper; and
- Using smooth and fluid arm movements for writing (flows).

Process skills refer to how the child interacts with the materials and then problem solves. Process skills include how the child thinks through activities.[2] For example, handwriting involves the following process skills:

- Pacing by maintaining a consistent rate and tempo of writing performance throughout the task;
- Attending to the task;
- Heeding to complete the handwriting task;
- Choosing the pencil to use for the writing sample;
- Using the pencil in its intended way;
- Handling the pencil using a dynamic tripod grasp;
- Inquiring about whether to continue on the next page;
- Initiating by answering the second questions;
- Continuing to write until asked to stop;
- Sequencing letters into words and sentences;
- Terminating the writing upon conclusion; and
- Gathering materials together.

Social interaction skills are addressed frequently in OT intervention. Handwriting may serve as a tool to initiate social interactions (e.g., invitation), continue a friendship (e.g., notes at school), or express oneself.

OT practitioners addressing handwriting may explore the skills required for social interaction. Specifically, handwriting may address social interaction skills in the following ways:

- Approaching or starting an interaction with a peer (e.g., writing an invitation);
- Turning toward a peer when handing him or her a handmade card;
- Making eye contact with peer when passing a note;
- Disclosing opinions and feelings in writing; and
- Using appropriate words of thanks to acknowledge receipt of gift.

Contexts and Environments

Contexts refer to a variety of interrelated conditions that are within and surrounding the child.[2] Contexts includes cultural, personal, temporal, and virtual. The term *environment* refers to the physical and social conditions that surround the child.[2] OT practitioners consider the child's contexts when selecting intervention activities. The OT practitioner may consider the following questions with regard to contextual and environmental influence in activity selection:

1. Is the therapeutic activity consistent with the child's cultural, social, and personal background?
2. What social conditions (e.g., expectations of significant others, relationships with systems such as economic and institutional) surround the activity?
3. What are the personal characteristics of the child, and how will these affect activity selection (e.g., age, sex, socioeconomic status, educational status)?
4. What are the temporal aspects (e.g., stage of life, time of day, time of year, amount of time needed for the activity) of the activity? How will this influence the selection of media?
5. What are the physical characteristics of the activity? In what environment will it take place (e.g., classroom, home, playground)?

Grading and Adapting

OT practitioners may need to change or adjust therapeutic activities to promote success. This is referred to as **grading** an activity. Adapting refers to changing how the activity is performed. The following questions may assist the OT practitioner in grading (changing the degree of difficulty of the activity) activities and adapting (changing how the activity is performed) activities:

1. Can the level of complexity of the activity be increased or decreased according to the child's thought processing level (e.g., decreasing steps or teaching by backward chaining, fading assistance)?
2. Can the media be modified in accordance with the child's physical skills (e.g., less or more resistance, larger or smaller objects)?
3. Can the media be changed to meet the child's sensory function requirements (e.g., placing media on bright background to increase contrast for a child with low vision or using a material with a different texture to accommodate a child's tactile needs)?
4. Are the media versatile enough to be individualized within a group activity?
5. Is adaptive equipment needed or available to enhance the child's performance?
6. Is the child able to work with the media in its intended manner?
7. Do the activity requirements need to be changed (adapted) for success?

Activity and Occupational Demands

Successful intervention planning requires the OT practitioner analyze all aspects of the activity. **Activity and occupational demand** refers to the objects and their properties, space demands, social demands, sequence and timing, required actions and skills, and required underlying body functions and body structures.[2] Analysis of activity demands helps the OT practitioner select appropriate activities and media. The following questions may guide the OT practitioner:

1. Are the tools and equipment necessary to use the media available and in good repair?
2. Are there adequate tools and materials for all of the children?
3. Is there an adequate working surface, open space, and lighting for the activity?
4. What social and communication skills are needed to participate in the activity?
5. What are the steps, sequence, and timing of the activity? Will there be enough time to complete the activity?
6. What skills are required to successfully complete the activity?
7. What body structures are needed to complete the activity?
8. How can the activity be changed for children who have deficits?
9. What are the safety precautions?
10. What is the cost of the activity?
11. Where can the activity take place?
12. Is the adult to child supervision ratio adequate for assistance and safety?

ROLE OF THE OCCUPATIONAL THERAPY ASSISTANT AND THE OCCUPATIONAL THERAPIST IN SELECTING THERAPEUTIC MEDIA

Collaboration refers to "working cooperatively with others to achieve a mutual goal."[3] OTAs deliver OT services under the supervision of and in collaboration with occupational therapists. It is the legal and ethical responsibility of both the occupational therapist and the OTA to ensure that the OTA has the established service competency to choose media that are relevant to the child's occupational goals.

CLINICAL *Pearl*

Service competency ensures that one OT practitioner is able to obtain the same results from a procedure or activity as another. Some ways of establishing service competency are videotaping treatment techniques to be critiqued by an experienced occupational therapist and review of standardized test results to ensure correct administration procedures and accurate scoring. Another method is using competency check-offs for skills such as measuring ROM with the goniometer, manual muscle testing, and safe transfer techniques.

OTAs who do not practice with other therapists nearby (such as those working in some school systems or home health care) can establish **service competency** and expand their skills by seeking an experienced mentor. Pediatric focus groups provide opportunities to collaborate with other OT practitioners and discuss intervention strategies. Furthermore, OTAs may discover new intervention strategies and use of media by attending professional conferences and continuing education. Online resources for media projects and supplies may prove helpful to OT practitioners.

USE OF THERAPEUTIC MEDIA

The OT practitioner uses therapeutic media during the intervention process. The media may be used within the context of a purposeful activity and directly relates to the child's goals. Media may be used as a preparatory activity to address client factors and the underlying skills necessary to achieve the child's goal. Media may be used as a contrived activity, to help a child reach his or her goals. It may also be used as the occupational activity.

CASE *Study*

Seven-year-old Kevin has juvenile rheumatoid arthritis. He is in the second grade. Kevin enjoys art class but has difficulty painting when his joints are inflamed. He also has difficulty holding the paintbrush. The OTA has decided to work on Kevin's goal to improve fine motor skills for academic work by using a painting activity. As a preparatory activity, Kevin and the OTA complete some stretching exercises (both passive and active). The OTA sets up the painting activity that will be conducted in art class later that week. Because Kevin takes longer than the other children to complete his work, the art teacher is pleased that the OTA is able to break down the steps and allow Kevin to get a head start. Furthermore, this allows the OTA to determine what types of adaptations work best for Kevin. She provides Kevin with a paintbrush that has a built-up handle and an easel positioned close to him and at a lower level (so that he does not have to raise his arm as high as the other children). Kevin enjoys painting and is looking forward to finishing his project in art class later in the week.

In this scenario, painting is the goal (fine motor skills to participate in a school activity) and is also the medium (to work on increasing fine motor skills). The OTA is able to help Kevin perform a meaningful activity, which is part of his occupational role as a student. The preparatory activity, in this case, is the stretching and exercising before beginning the painting. The OTA consults with the art teacher and provides the adaptations (built-up paintbrush, and lowered easel height) to ensure Kevin's success. He is invested in the painting and motivated to continue the activity in art class later. The OTA recognizes the importance of using media and activities that are occupation-based and meaningful to the child.

ACTIVITIES

The following section provides examples of how the OTA chooses meaningful and therapeutic activities. Each scenario provides a child's occupational profile, a description of the chosen media and method, suggestions for grading and adapting the activity, and an overview of the required client factors specific to the case. Tables 23-1 through 23-4 provide commonly used therapeutic media for each age group.

Infancy: Birth Through 18 Months

CASE *Study*

Miguel's water play session. Miguel is a 12-month-old boy with a diagnosis of Down syndrome. He receives outpatient OT and physical therapy (PT) services once a week. The goals for occupational therapy include improving Miguel's physical endurance and hand skills for play. During the OT sessions, the OTA works on increasing postural stability for independent sitting as well as improving reaching and grasping skills. This week, the OTA and the physical therapy assistant (PTA) collaborate and plan activities to address Miguel's OT and PT goals in the clinic's pool. The OTA discusses this upcoming session with Miguel's parents who report that he loves to play in the water and that they would like him to develop preswimming skills. Miguel will wear a swimsuit with an attached floatation device for safety while in the pool. To prepare Miguel for the water and increase body awareness, the OTA will rub Miguel's arms, legs, and back with water while naming each body part.

Media/Materials

The media/materials needed are as follows:

- Water
- Kickboard
- Small water toys that require hand skills (e.g., plastic fish, simple squirt toys, etc.)
- Sponge balls of varied resistance
- Beach ball

TABLE 23-1

Examples of Activities for Infancy

ACTIVITY	BRIEF DESCRIPTION OF ACTIVITY OR PRODUCT
Handprint wreath	Arrange cut-out or painted handprints in wreath pattern.
Body awareness dressing/bathing games	Use lotion, soap, powder, and movements while naming body parts during bathing and dressing.
Bubbles	Adult blows bubbles while cuing infant to visually track, reach, and pop.
Multi-texture mat	Can be purchased or home-made for infant to crawl over, walk on, or explore textures.
Cardboard box play	Push/pull infant across floor for vestibular input.
Hand/foot games	Examples are Peek-A-Boo, Patty Cake, and This Little Piggy.
Scooping/Pouring activities	Use various media: water, sand, dirt, rice.
Pots and pan music	Use various-sized pots, pans, plastic bowls, and wooden spoons.
Commercially available developmental toys	Examples are cause-and-effect, sequencing, push/pull toys, stuffed animals, texture books, nesting toys, See and Say, electronic learning systems (such as Leap Pad).

Method

1. The environment was set up with all materials within reach.
2. Miguel should be positioned on the edge of the pool with the PTA providing support at his trunk, as necessary, for safety. The OTA, positioned in front of Miguel, holds up pool toys in various planes to facilitate reaching up, down, and across midline. The OTA carefully monitors Miguel's facial expressions for any

TABLE 23-2

Examples of Activities for Early Childhood

ACTIVITY	BRIEF DESCRIPTION OF ACTIVITY OR PRODUCT
Paper bag puppets	Use paper lunch bags. Cut, glue, or color puppet features onto bag.
Marshmallow people	Use pretzel stick to connect marshmallow body parts.
Birdfeeder	Roll pinecone in peanut butter and birdseed.
Sorting games	Use pincer grasp or tweezers/tongs to pick up small manipulatives for sorting.
Tissue paper collage	Have child crumple up with fingers precut squares of tissue paper and place on glue dots within a defined space.
Parachute	Great group activity! Incorporate with songs. Emphasize up, down, around. Toss items on parachute.
Loop cereal or noodle jewelry	String items on curling ribbon, plastic craft lace, pipe cleaners, etc.
Painting	Examples are finger painting, sponge painting, marble painting, spaghetti painting.
Body movement games	Examples are I'm a Little Teapot, Head and Shoulders, Knees and Toes, and Row, Row, Row Your Boat, obstacle course.
Commercial games/toys	Examples are Don't Spill the Beans, Barrel of Monkeys, Candy Land, Hi Ho Cheerio, Memory, Ants in the Pants, Don't Break the Ice, Mr. Potato Head, Shape Sorter, nesting items, Counting Bears, electronic learning system (such as Leap Pad), tablet computer, and gaming systems.

TABLE 23-3

Examples of Activities for Middle Childhood

ACTIVITY	BRIEF DESCRIPTION OF ACTIVITY OR PRODUCT
Paper chains	Have child cut strips of paper or use precut strips and attach them with various means such as paperclip, staples, glue. Vary colors. Consider cultural differences.
Windsocks	Have child roll construction paper to form cylinder and secure with staples or tape; attach crepe paper streamers along bottom edge; punch holes and thread yarn for hanger; and use markers, stickers, etc., to decorate.
Gingerbread house	Buy a ready-made kit, or provide pint-sized milk carton, graham crackers, stiff icing, and candies to decorate.
Sun catchers	Melt crayon shavings between two pieces of wax paper using iron. Have child make a frame out of popsicle sticks, construction paper, etc.
Paper maché piñata	Provide a thin box. Have child dip tissue or newspaper strips into a flour-and-water mixture (consistency of thin white glue), lay them over box in layers, and allow them to dry completely. Adult slits a hole in the box to fill with candy. Child decorates with paint, stickers, etc.
Body movement games	Examples are Red Light/Green Light, Simon Says, Hopscotch, Animal Walks, and Twister.
Handwriting	Write letters to other children or relatives, letter or word Tic-Tac-Toe, Hangman, handwriting applications.
Commercial games/toys	Examples are Bop It, Hungry Hippo, Connect Four, Tidily Winks, Legos, Mega Links, Uno, Go Fish, Barrel of Monkeys, Pick-up-Sticks, electronic learning devices, tablet computer, and gaming systems.

TABLE 23-4

Examples of Activities for Adolescence

ACTIVITY	BRIEF DESCRIPTION OF ACTIVITY OR PRODUCT
Origami	Fold paper to form 3-D shapes. May use purchased kits or craft book.
Flowerpot découpage	Cut out pictures in magazines, greeting cards, old books. Have child brush découpage glue on back of picture, apply picture to flowerpot, and apply additional découpage glue covering picture and surface completely until entire area is smooth and uniform.
Picture frame	Have child decorate an old picture frame using various media (seashells, puzzle pieces, twigs, gemstones).
T-shirt painting/tie-dye	Provide various fabric paints, stencils, sponges, or brushes to be used on T-shirt. Buy commercial tie-dye kits, or use instructions available in craft books (see references).
Collage	Have child cut out pictures from magazines or catalogs of interest to him or her and glue them onto poster board and add decorative accents as desired (glitter bows, stickers).
CD mobile	Have child decorate and hang promotional or unwanted CDs from fishing line, coat hanger, drift wood, etc.
Rubbings	Have child rub crayons, charcoal pencils, pastels, etc. on thin paper placed over embossed surfaces (building cornerstones, carved wood, coins).
Rubber stamping	Have child create cards, gift tags, and stationary by using commercial rubber stamps and stamp pads.
Scrapbooking	Child can create scrapbook pages using various commercially available items such as stickers/embellishments and by downloading photos from various photo-sharing websites (e.g., Snapfish, Shutterfly).
Commercial games	Examples are Dominoes, Mancala, Pictionary, Jenga, card games, Backgammon, Simon, and Perfection, electronic learning devices, tablet computer, gaming systems, and smart phones.

signs of fear and provides positive feedback while facilitating the "just-right challenge." Once the OTA has ensured Miguel's comfort level, she asks him to kick a large ball positioned in front of him.

3. Once Miguel becomes more comfortable, he is positioned prone on the kickboard in the pool, with the PTA facilitating trunk stability in the prone extension position. Miguel is working on head and trunk control in this position and is encouraged to kick through the water to move forward to reach toys placed in front of him. The OTA holds a sponge ball just below the surface of the water for Miguel to grasp and pull toward him. This movement simulates the dog paddle motion, which is needed for swimming. To improve hand strength, the OTA shows him how to squeeze the water out of the ball to sink a small toy boat.

> ### CLINICAL *Pearl*
>
> Working while in the prone position strengthens cervical, trunk, and scapular musculature. Strengthening these muscle groups will increase overall postural stability and endurance.

Client Factors
Mental Functions
Miguel's level of arousal was sufficient to follow verbal cues provided by the adults, and he was motivated by his enjoyment of water play.

Neuromusculoskeletal and Movement-related Functions, Muscle Functions, and Movement Functions
Miguel reached in various planes with upper and lower extremities, which required stability and mobility of the joints. Although Miguel has low muscle tone, the buoyancy of the water allowed efficient use of his strength and endurance as he moved his arms and legs against the resistance of the water. Miguel needed control of voluntary movement for reaching, grasping, eye-hand coordination, and eye-foot coordination to complete the activity. He also used bilateral integration while reaching across the midline for toys.

Skin and Related Structure Functions
Miguel had skin integrity evidenced by no open wounds or abrasions. This was an important consideration when engaging in water play in a public pool.

Grading and Adapting
Suggestions for grading and adapting the activity are as follows:

- Use a variety of positions and surfaces (e.g., edge of pool for stable surface versus kickboard/raft for unstable surface).

- If a pool is not available, these or similar activities can be carried out using a water table or a bathtub.
- Vary distance and height when presenting objects for reaching and grasping.
- The level of assistance can be increased or decreased according to the child's needs.
- Simulate swimming activities to help prepare children for the occupation of swimming. For example, blowing bubbles, kicking feet, reaching forward, and cupping water are all prerequisite skills for swimming.

The OTA selected water as a motivating medium based on the parent's report of Miguel's enjoyment of water play. Through collaboration, both the OT and PT practitioners were able to safely address Miguel's goals by working in the pool. Furthermore, swimming is an occupation of childhood in which the child and parents were interested.

CASE *Study*

Jessica's handprint/footprint butterfly. Jessica is a 17-month-old child who receives early intervention OT services at her day-care center twice a week. She has a diagnosis of agenesis of the corpus callosum and hypotonia. Jessica's mother would like her to be able to sit independently and tolerate sensory input during bath time. The OTA addresses these aspects of the individualized family service plan (IFSP) by providing controlled sensory input to decrease Jessica's tactile sensitivity and by working to improve trunk stability. The OTA and the preschool teacher collaborate and plan a group activity for Mother's Day that can be adapted to Jessica's needs—a footprint/handprint butterfly (Figure 23-1). As a preparatory activity, the OTA rubs a wet terry washcloth on Jessica's hands and feet using deep pressure while singing a playful song to keep her engaged. During the activity she facilitates transitional movements to various positions to maximize trunk stability and upper extremity weight bearing.

> ### CLINICAL *Pearl*
>
> Many OT practitioners use specific brushing/deep pressure protocols for decreasing tactile sensitivity with the pediatric population. This is a powerful tool and should only be used once training has been completed and service competency established.

Media/Materials
The media/materials needed are as follows:

- Several colors of nontoxic paints in pie tins
- Poster board

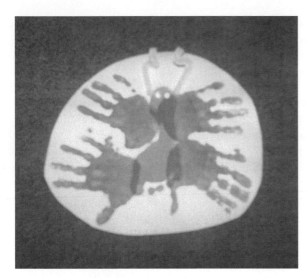

FIGURE 23-1   A butterfly print.

- Soft bristle paintbrush
- Pipe cleaner for antennae (preformed)
- Protective covering for floor
- Glue
- Paper towels

Method

1. The environment should be set up: the floor covered, all materials placed nearby, and the poster board positioned.
2. Sit on the floor behind Jessica to provide supported sitting.
3. While repeating the playful song used during the preparatory activity, brush Jessica's foot with paint and press it on the poster board to form the body of the butterfly. Rotate the paper a half turn, and brush Jessica's hand with paint. Press Jessica's hand onto one side of the body at the top and bottom. Repeat the procedure with the opposite hand to make the other side of the butterfly's body. This forms the wings. Add more paint with the paintbrush, as needed, for detail. Dab Jessica's index finger into the paint, and daub the top of the butterfly's body to form its eyes.
4. After the paint dries, glue on the antennae.

Grading and Adapting

Suggestions for grading and adaptations are as follows:

- Complete in more than one session.
- Provide adapted positioning for external trunk support (e.g., adaptive chair, adult assistance, environmental support).
- Add various media to paint in order to increase tactile input (e.g., sand, uncooked rice, cornmeal).
- Thin paint with water to change tactile input.
- Dip the child's hand into the paint instead of brushing paint onto the palm.

- Apply paint onto the hand with a cotton ball.
- If tactile input is not tolerated, trace the shape of the child's hand, and have child use paintbrush to fill in the shape. Use hand-over-hand assistance as needed.

Client Factors

Client factors addressed and considered for Jessica during this activity are discussed here.

Mental Functions

Jessica needed an appropriate level of arousal to enable her to participate in the activity. She was motivated by the playful way the activity was presented.

Sensory Functions

Proprioception was required for Jessica to sustain various positions such as the upright sitting position and upper extremity weight-bearing position. Jessica's visual functions were stimulated by the bright colors of the paint, and vestibular functions were necessary for her to sustain balance in upright sitting. Her touch functions were sufficient to accept the sensation of the OTA's hand and the texture of the paint.

Neuromusculoskeletal and Movement-related Functions, Muscle Functions, Movement Functions

Although Jessica has low muscle tone, she has sufficient strength and endurance to sustain the upright sitting position and the transitions to various postures with assistance.

Righting reactions were required to reestablish the midline after her painted palm was placed onto the surface of the paper. With minimal assistance, Jessica was able to initiate voluntary movement of her hands and fingers to press her painted palms onto the paper.

The OTA chose the activity based on Jessica's IFSP goals and integrated it into the classroom. Making Mother's Day projects is an important occupation for children of all ages. By considering the demands of the activity, the OTA was able to work on the IFSP goals, namely, trunk stability and decreasing tactile sensitivity, while working in the least restrictive environment. Table 23-1 presents other commonly used therapeutic media for infants.

Early Childhood: 18 Months to 5 Years

CASE *Study*

Pudding painting. Allie is a 36-month-old child with a diagnosis of autism. She receives OT services from a home health agency twice a week. OT interventions focus on improving self-feeding, manipulating objects with hands for play and dressing (fine motor skills), and improving visual-motor skills through imitation of age-appropriate prewriting strokes. Allie demonstrates oral sensitivity.

Allie's mother requested activities that she can do easily with her at home during play. The OTA will model a pudding painting activity that the mother can do with Allie. As a preparatory activity, Allie will squeeze and poke the Play-Doh to prepare her for the tactile input of the pudding as well as to facilitate hand strengthening and digit isolation.

Media/Materials

The media/materials needed are as follows:

- One snack-size pudding cup (choose a flavor and color that the child will like)
- Flat surface such as a cookie sheet or paper plate
- Large pullover shirt that can get messy
- Spoon
- Napkin

Method

The method used comprises the following elements:

1. The environment was set. Because this activity is messy, the work surface was covered and all the materials gathered.
2. Allie donned the pullover shirt with help as needed.
3. Allie opened the pudding cup with assistance as needed. Allie scooped pudding onto the cookie sheet with assistance to sustain grasp or reposition as needed. Allie spread the pudding with her hand.
4. Assisted Allie in establishing index finger isolation, and provided occasional assistance as needed during the activity. Allie imitated prewriting strokes in pudding (i.e., vertical line, horizontal line, circle, and cross) as demonstrated.
5. Once the prewriting activity was over and cleaned up, Allie was given a new pudding cup. With assistance for grasp, she ate the pudding with a spoon as a snack.

Client Factors
Mental Functions
On a global level, Allie was motivated by the new experience of completing prewriting strokes in the pudding. She showed an interest in the new activity. Allie turned when her name was called throughout the activity, showing orientation to person. Specifically, Allie needed sustained attention for 3-minute periods to complete both the visual-motor and self-feeding tasks. Spatial perceptual skills were used throughout the prewriting activity to imitate the strokes.

Sensory Functions
Allie engaged in vestibular functions to sustain dynamic sitting balance while reaching to complete prewriting strokes. Proprioception was necessary to manipulate the pudding, reach, move fingers through the pudding,

and sustain a grasp on the spoon. Touch functions were required as Allie accepted the texture of the pudding both through her fingertips and in her mouth while eating the pudding.

Neuromusculoskeletal and Movement-related Functions, Muscle Functions, Movement Functions
Functional ROM of the upper extremity bones and joints was sufficient to don the pullover shirt. Allie needed control of voluntary movement, specifically eye-hand coordination for both the fine motor and self-care components.

Grading and Adapting
Suggestions for grading and adapting the activity are as follows:

- Use thicker/thinner food textures to change resistance.
- Use items such as pretzel sticks, carrot sticks, marshmallows, or similar items for the child to write with if he or she is tactile defensive.
- Increase/decrease difficulty by having the child imitate, copy, or write from memory.
- Use adaptive equipment such as a scoop bowl or adaptive spoon to increase independence with self-feeding.
- Use nonfood items to practice prewriting and writing skills (e.g. shaving cream, sand, lotion, fingerpaints).
- Vary the working positions (supported sitting, prone on floor, standing, etc.).

After the session is over, the OTA and Allie's mother discussed the process and outcome of the activity. The OTA suggested similar activities using different food items and other prewriting activities so that the mother could participate fully in reaching Allie's goals.

CASE *Study*

Clothespin caterpillar magnets. Four-year-old Carrie attends a child development class in a public elementary school. The class includes children with and without special needs. She receives weekly OT services from the school-based OTA in this setting to support her educational goals in her individualized education program (see Chapter 4). The goals of OT services include addressing difficulty with fine motor, visual perception, and sensory processing (specifically tactile sensitivity). The class thematic unit this week is "Insects." The OTA plans to have the children make clothespin caterpillar magnets. As preparatory activities, Carrie will string large beads onto a pipe cleaner to address fine motor and perceptual skills and search for small plastic items hidden in a rice bowl to decrease tactile sensitivity.

Preparatory activities can be thought of as warm-up techniques to prepare the child for a specific desired action. Activities such as gross motor movements can increase motor planning for tasks such as handwriting. Hand musculature may be developed by upper extremity weight bearing that occurs during activities such as crawling through a tunnel. Similarly, bead stringing can be used to facilitate the pincer grasp needed to hold a pencil for writing.

Media/Materials
Each child will need the following:

- One standard-size wooden clothespin
- Craft glue or wood glue
- Six multicolored pompoms (about half inch)
- One chenille stick (pipe-cleaner) about 4 inches long
- Two small wiggle eyes
- A 2-inch piece of magnet with adhesive backing
- Cotton swabs
- Small dish or paper plate
- Tweezers

Method
1. The environment was set with the table and chair being at the appropriate height and all the materials on the table within reach.
2. The simple color pattern of a completed caterpillar model should be followed.
3. Carrie squeezed glue from the bottle onto a small dish, with assistance as needed.
4. Using a cotton swab to dip into the glue, Carrie spread the glue onto one side of the clothespin. As tolerated, she used her index finger to spread the glue evenly.
5. Following the model for color pattern, Carrie picked out the needed pompoms from a large assortment.
6. She used tweezers to pick up and place pompoms onto glue following the color pattern.
7. Carrie used a cotton swab to apply two drops of glue to the caterpillar's head (first pompom) for the eyes and place two wiggle eyes onto the drops of glue.
8. With assistance, Carrie twisted the pipe cleaner around the side of the clothespin, behind the head of the caterpillar, to form the antenna.
9. Carrie then peeled the adhesive backing from the magnet and placed it onto the back of the clothespins, with assistance as needed.

Client Factors
Mental Functions
Spatial perceptual skills were needed to line pompoms on the clothespin as shown in the model. Interpretation of sensory stimuli (tactile) was required whenever Carrie spread the glue with her fingertips. Choosing pompom color and size required recognition and categorization skills to follow the given pattern of the model.

Sensory Functions
Proprioceptive functions provided feedback necessary for Carrie to sustain adequate pressure when using the tweezers to pick up, move, and place the pompoms without dropping them. Although Carrie's touch functions were hypersensitive, she tolerated a limited amount of input from the glue.

Neuromusculoskeletal and Movement-related Functions, Muscle Functions, Movement Functions
Control of voluntary movement functions were needed during aspects of the activity that required eye-hand coordination to place pompoms matching the given pattern and accuracy in placing the pompoms.

Grading and Adapting
Suggestions for grading and adapting the activity are as follows:

- Use larger/smaller clothespins or tongue depressors.
- Use larger/smaller pompoms.
- When decreased fine motor skills are present, use tongs instead of tweezers.
- Adult uses the glue when the child places pompoms.
- Give more or less assistance depending on child's abilities.
- Instead of twisting the pipe cleaner to make the antenna, the child can glue on a paper antenna.
- Adjust the complexity of the color pattern depending on the child's abilities.
- Adapt the environment. For example, increase or decrease the group size; reduce the amount of materials presented at a time; use a location in the classroom that offers the least visual stimulus.

The OTA conducted this activity in Carrie's least restrictive environment (classroom). By working with the teacher, the OTA was able to design, develop, and implement a therapeutic activity that related both the weekly classroom thematic unit and Carrie's goals. See Table 23-2 for other commonly used therapeutic media for the early childhood age group.

Provide adequate supervision at all times when using small materials to ensure the safety of children. Many children have poor impulse control and safety awareness and may use materials inappropriately.

Middle Childhood: 6 Years Until Onset of Puberty

CASE *Study*

Birthday crown. Six-year-old kindergartener David has a diagnosis of attention-deficit/hyperactivity disorder. He has difficulty completing cutting and handwriting tasks, and the teacher notes that he struggles with puzzles and becomes frustrated easily. David receives school-based OT services once a week to address fine motor and visual perceptual difficulties that interfere with classroom activities. David's teacher has asked the OTA to help David make a "birthday crown" to celebrate his birthday. The OTA agrees to work with David on this activity because it addresses both of David's goal areas and it is a meaningful activity. As a preparatory activity, the OTA has David manipulate firm therapy putty to retrieve beads. The OTA also provides an air-filled cushion for David to sit on during this activity, which may help increase his attention.

Media/Materials

The media/materials needed are as follows:

- Poster board
- Small items for decoration (foam shape stickers, sequins, buttons, etc.)
- Scissors
- Glue
- Cotton swabs
- Stencils (letters and shapes)
- Markers, crayons
- Stapler
- Glitter

Method

1. Set the environment by making sure that the chair and table are an appropriate height and materials are within reach. The amount of visual and auditory stimuli should be reduced the lighting adequate.
2. The OTA drew a crown pattern onto the poster board, and David cut the pattern.
3. The OTA measured David's head, and marked the crown that he would staple later.
4. David decorated the crown (Figure 23-2) by using letter stencils to write his name with correct formation and squeezes glue within the lines of the letters. He worked on his pincer grasp by using a cotton swab to spread the glue and shakes glitter onto the glue. He practiced in-hand manipulation with buttons and sequins that are placed on the crown. David matched and placed foam shapes into predrawn area.
5. David stapled the crown in the previously marked spot, and placed the crown on his head.
6. David cleaned up the area with assistance.

Client Factors
Mental Functions

David was motivated to make the crown for his birthday. He, as most children do, valued the celebration of personal holidays. He was able to modulate his level of arousal to carry the task through to its completion. David was able to sustain attention to complete the multistep task with adaptations (cushion, one-on-one assistance, simple directions). He used perceptual functions to place the stencils neatly in a line, use the correct sequence of letters to write his name, and match and place foam shapes within given areas. He was able to implement problem-solving skills to identify and correct errors in the project. David had to regulate his emotional functions to control his impulsivity. He experienced a positive sense of self by completing and wearing the crown in celebration of his special day.

Neuromusculoskeletal and Movement-related Functions, Muscle Functions, Movement Functions

David's muscle tone and strength allowed him to sustain a grasp on the scissors, hold the pencil correctly, and depress the stapler. Control of voluntary movement for bilateral integration and eye-hand coordination allowed David to stabilize the stencil with the nondominant hand while writing and hold the paper as he cut.

Sensory Functions

Proprioceptive functions were required for David to gradate his movements to use the stapler with appropriate force. These functions also allowed him to move the scissors forward through the paper in a smooth and controlled fashion.

Grading and Adapting

Suggestions for grading and adapting the activity are as follows:

- Provide a model.
- Have the child use tape rather than a stapler if safety is a concern or if strength is poor.
- Have the child use glue sticks, squeeze glue bottle, or use other items to spread glue (paintbrush, cotton ball).
- Give wider/thinner lines to cut.
- Increase or decrease difficulty of crown pattern for cutting.
- Use thicker/thinner paper.
- Use larger/smaller decorative items.

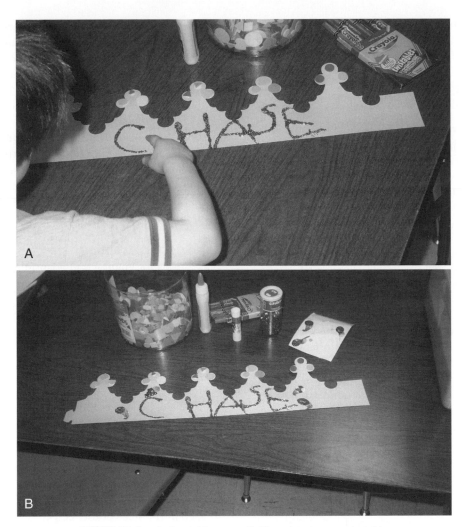

FIGURE 23-2   A, Boy with crown. **B,** Completed crown on table.

- Control the amount of glitter being shaken by partially covering the holes on the top or changing the container that it being used.
- Divide the activity over several intervention sessions depending on the child's attentiveness or needs.

Through collaboration with the teacher a meaningful activity was chosen for the session. The OTA chose preparatory activities that would increase his success in making the birthday crown. The OTA considered David's difficulty attending to tasks and adapted the environment by providing the air-filled cushion.

CLINICAL *Pearl*

Various products are available on the market, such as air-filled cushions and ball chairs, to help children attend to the tasks by providing them with vestibular input controlled by their movements.

CASE *Study*

Crispy rice cereal treats. Casey, a 12-year-old boy with moderate intellectual disability, is a student in a self-contained class at the local middle school. His class often engages in cooking activities to work on their independent living and transitional job training skills. Casey has a short attention span, and the teacher and the OTA have often discussed his inability to carry out multistep tasks to completion. The OTA targets these areas during OT sessions. The class is planning to host a fall luncheon for parents. The students have compiled a shopping list and purchased the ingredients during a community-based outing. The classroom has a full kitchen, and the students will be preparing side dishes for the meal. Casey is making the dessert, a pumpkin-shaped crispy rice cereal treat. After a discussion about the various cultures within the classroom, the teacher and the OTA have decided that it would be most appropriate to make a generic pumpkin motif rather than a jack-o-lantern. The OTA has decided to incorporate the activity within the OT session. She prepares Casey for the activity by carefully reviewing the rules of the session and showing him a sample of the finished product.

Media/Materials

The media/materials needed are as follows:

- 6 cups of crispy rice cereal
- 1 bag of marshmallows
- 2 tablespoons of margarine
- Orange decorative sprinkles
- Spearmint gumdrop leaves
- Pretzel sticks
- Large mixing bowl (microwave-safe)
- Large spoon
- Measuring cups
- Wax paper

Method

1. Set the environment by gathering all the ingredients, and placing the cooking utensils within reach. Have Casey wash and dry his hands.
2. Instruct Casey to open the bag of marshmallows with supervision. Have him empty the contents into the bowl along with the margarine. Have him put the bowl in the microwave for 1 minute; then stir the mixture and microwave it for an additional minute. (Verbal cues may be provided to assist Casey in setting and attending to the microwave timer.)
3. Using potholders, have Casey remove the bowl from the microwave oven.
4. Have Casey measure 6 cups of cereal.
5. He should then pour the cereal into the bowl and mix it thoroughly with the melted marshmallow and margarine mixture using a large spoon.
6. Have Casey wash and dry his hands before handling the food.
7. Demonstrate how to obtain an adequate amount of cereal mixture to form a ball. Have Casey roll the cereal ball in orange sprinkles and place each one on a sheet of wax paper.
8. Have Casey push a pretzel stick into the top and places spearmint candy leaves on each side to make the stem of a pumpkin.
9. Finally, have Casey wash all the items used in warm soapy water; rinse and dry them; and clean the countertops.

Client Factors
Mental Functions

Casey was motivated to complete this activity because his parents were going to be guests.

Casey demonstrated 30 minutes of sustained attention with frequent cueing and verbal directions. He used higher-level cognitive functions to adhere to safety precautions when using scissors and handling hot cooking utensils. Casey had to interpret sensory stimuli visually and use calculation functions to measure the ingredients. He had to plan and execute movements to carry out steps such as pouring ingredients into the measuring containers and emptying them into a bowl. Sequencing skills were needed to follow the recipe and to clean up.

Neuromusculoskeletal and Movement-related Functions, Muscle Functions, Movement Functions

Casey used asymmetric bilateral hand skills to stabilize a mixing bowl while stirring ingredients and forming the rice crispy mixture into a ball. He used symmetric bilateral hand skills to remove the bowl from the microwave oven.

Grading and Adapting

Suggestions for grading and adapting the activity are as follows:

- If tactile sensitivity or defensiveness is a concern, have Casey insert his hands into sandwich bags or food-handling gloves to decrease sensitivity to the texture of the mixture.
- The OTA can complete more of the activity such as touching the mixture.
- Place a nonslip mat under the bowl to increase its stability on the flat surface.
- Adapt the spoon as needed.
- Provide thicker pretzel rods that will not break as easily.
- Provide tongs or tweezers to place items.
- Use visual aids to describe the sequence of activity, such as the steps of the recipe.
- Substitute another dry cereal to change the consistency of the mixture and change the input to Casey's hands.
- Use large visual timers (available from adapted equipment catalogs or educational stores) to provide temporal cues.

The OTA adapted the activity taking into consideration Casey's short attention span by providing verbal cueing and redirection as needed. The OTA coordinated Casey's treatment around the classroom activity so that he could remain in the least restrictive environment and fulfill his role as a student. After discussing the activity with the teacher, the OTA decided to make a pumpkin-shaped dessert for the fall season versus a Halloween jack-o-lantern. Some children in the class did not celebrate Halloween, and thus cultural preferences were respected.

CLINICAL *Pearl*

Many children who have difficulty following verbally issued directions for multistep tasks benefit from visual sequence cards or a visual schedule.

CLINICAL *Pearl*

Before working with food products, ensure that the child has no allergies to items such as wheat or peanuts. Also, consider religious or other dietary restrictions (e.g., gluten-free diets, lactose intolerance).

CASE *Study*

Andre is an 8-year-old boy who has a diagnosis of traumatic brain injury. He presents with hypertonicity of the left upper and lower extremities resulting in decreased ROM, impaired dynamic standing balance, left-side neglect, and impaired executive functions—specifically initiation of activity and sustained attention. In addition, the teacher has reported that Andre avoids tasks involving crossing midline.

The OTA is serving Andre in school. During treatment sessions, she addresses dynamic standing balance, increasing awareness and use of the left upper extremity, and increasing ability to initiate and sustain attention to a task.

Upon the OTA's arrival in the classroom, she finds the teacher leading a small-group activity using the interactive white board. The children participating stand at the white board and use their finger to "drag" the uppercase letters to the corresponding lowercase letter on the board. Although the OTA had a different activity planned for this therapy session, she found the activity that was taking place in the classroom very appropriate for addressing Andre's goals.

Method

1. When it is Andre's turn to participate, he rises from his chair and walks to the whiteboard with close supervision due to impaired gait pattern.
2. The OTA purposefully positions Andre so the information and material he needs to attend to is on his left side. She gives him verbal and tactile cues as needed.
3. The OTA instructs Andre to reach with his left upper extremity to a letter that is at a height that will challenge his dynamic standing balance, ROM of the left upper extremity, and crossing midline.
4. The OTA stands close to Andre to assist him with his reach and in maintaining balance.
5. Andre is instructed to isolate his left index finger to touch the capital letter on the whiteboard and drag it to the matching lowercase letter. When he matches letters successfully, the letters on the whiteboard flash different colors and music is played.
6. The OTA has Andre sit at the front of the group to await his next turn and provides him with verbal cues to assist him in sustaining attention to the activity at hand while the other students take their turn.

Client Factors
Mental Functions

An appropriate level of arousal, impulse control, and sustained attention were needed for Andre to wait his turn while remaining attentive to the activity. Initiation and execution of learned movement patterns were necessary while Andre arose from his seat on the floor, moved toward the white board, and carried out the movements needed for the activity in the correct sequence. Memory and recognition skills were required for Andre to identify and recall which upper- and lowercase letters were correct matches.

Sensory Functions

Andre used his hearing and vision to receive the verbal and visual instructions for the activity as well as information regarding his performance and the performance of others. His vestibular system allowed him to maintain the positions he needed and move without loss of balance. Andre's proprioceptive system allowed him to be aware of the movements of the joints being used at any given time during the activity.

Neuromusculoskeletal and Movement-related Functions, Muscle Functions, Movement Functions

Andre's muscles and joints of the affected upper extremity were challenged as he reached for the letters during the activity. Eye-hand coordination skills as well as crossing of midline were required while touching and dragging the letter across the whiteboard. With close supervision, Andre was able to rise from his seat and walk to the white board despite an impaired gait pattern due to left lower extremity involvement. When given tactile cues, Andre was able to maintain adequate postural alignment while in sitting and standing positions.

Adapting and Grading
Suggestions for grading and adaptations are as follows:

- If index finger isolation is difficult, have Andre use two fingers or his fist to drag the letters.
- A tennis ball can be attached to the end of a dowel rod and Andre can hold the rod and use the tennis ball to drag the letters.
- If Andre has difficulty with shoulder and/or elbow extension to completely reach to the letter, the OTA can provide less or more active assist to facilitate ROM.
- If Andre seems to become fatigued he can sit for a portion of the activity. A therapy ball can be used as alternative seating, with the OTA nearby for safety. This seating will still address balance skills.
- A visual schedule can be created to help clarify the steps of the activity and the OTA can use this to show Andre the steps in preparation since he has difficulty with initiation of tasks.

CLINICAL *Pearl*

Clinicians have access to a wide range of electronic media such as interactive whiteboards, tablet computers, smartphones, and apps that are readily available. With careful consideration of each child's goals, interventions can be planned that are motivating to the child while addressing deficit areas.

Adolescence: Puberty Until Onset of Adulthood

CASE *Study*

Sarah's scrapbooking session. Fourteen-year-old Sarah has a diagnosis of spastic-hemiplegic cerebral palsy. She receives OT services in an outpatient clinic once a week to address difficulties with self-care and leisure due to limited use of her right arm. In a previous session, Sarah and her OTA talked about making a scrapbook containing photographs of Sarah's family's Hanukah celebration. Sarah agreed that she would like to work on such a project. Sarah began the session with preparatory activities to increase sensory awareness and active ROM of her right arm so that she could use it to assist during the scrapbooking activity.

Media/Materials

The media/materials needed are as follows:

- Computer
- Printer
- Photo paper
- Color ink
- Cardstock (culturally appropriate colors and varying thicknesses)
- Scrapbook pages
- Glue
- Adapted cutting equipment
- Stamps and stamp pads
- Hole punch
- String
- Scissors with varied cutting designs
- Stickers, cropping stencils, markers/colored pencils

Method

1. Set the environment by gathering all the materials, adjusting the chair and table to appropriate height to provide support for postural control; position the materials to facilitate reaching and crossing the midline.
2. Have Sarah select and upload photos from her smartphone to the clinic's computer.

3. With the OTA's help, Sarah should print selected photos.
4. Have Sarah crop and organize the pictures onto the desired pages, cut the cardstock to frame pictures with the use of adaptive equipment as needed, stamp phrases or motifs onto background of scrapbook pages, and place stickers on pages.
5. Have Sarah decorate a cover for the book with cardstock, and stickers. She should punch holes with a one-hole punch and secure the book by tying it with string using an adapted one-hand method that she learned from the OTA.
6. Have Sarah clean up the work area with assistance.
7. Have Sarah discuss the family activities shown in the pictures.

CLINICAL *Pearl*

Optimal seating posture for completing fine motor activities is obtained by sitting with hips, knees, and ankles at 90 degrees of flexion. Feet should be flat on the floor or stable surface. The tabletop height should be no more than 2 inches above the bent elbow.

Client Factors
Values, Beliefs, and Spirituality

Sarah was motivated to complete the project because she had positive memories of this important family event that represented her family's values and religious traditions.

Mental Functions

Sarah was aware of person, place, time, self, and others as observed in her description of the events. Thought processes such as recognition were needed to choose the appropriate tools to complete the project. Sarah applied categorization skills as well as perceptual skills to complete tasks such as sorting and placing pictures on the pages, decorating the pages with the stamps, and cutting the borders to frame the pictures. Higher-level cognitive functions such as judgment were used to safely use scissors and cropping tools.

Sensory Functions

Acuity and visual functions were necessary for Sarah to visually locate and distinguish between the materials on the table. Preparatory activities of weight bearing and active and passive ROM helped Sarah retrieve tools and materials with her affected arm.

Neuromusculoskeletal and Movement-related Functions, Muscle Functions, Movement Functions

Sarah needed to sustain postural alignment while working at and crossing midline. ROM was needed for reaching and grasping. The OTA began the session by inhibiting muscle tone (spasticity) in Sarah's right upper extremity to help her use her arm as an assist. Muscle power functions were employed so she could sustain a sufficient grasp on the scissors, hole punch, and stamp. The asymmetric tonic neck reflex was integrated well enough to allow her to turn toward needed materials without abnormal movement patterns impeding the use of her bilateral upper extremities. Eye-hand coordination was required for cropping pictures, arranging photos, and designing the album.

Grading and Adapting

Suggestions for grading and adapting this activity are as follows:

- Vary the thickness of the paper (e.g., thicker paper/ cardstock is easier to hold and gives more sensory feedback during cutting).
- Vary the type of scissors.
- Vary glue (squeeze, stick, etc.)
- Provide adaptive equipment for stabilizing paper.
- Provide a completed scrapbook to use as a model.
- Provide assistance and fade assistance as appropriate.
- Increase/decrease time constraints (e.g., two sessions rather than one).
- Crop pictures via electronic means

The OTA addressed Sarah's goals to increase the functional use of her right arm. She considered areas of occupation as well as personal, cultural, and temporal contexts when choosing the scrapbooking activity. This activity could easily be carried over to the home environment. The OTA adapted the activity to ensure a just-right challenge for the child. (Table 23-3 presents more ideas for activities for middle childhood.)

CASE *Study*

Harry's woodworking project. Harry, an 18-year-old who is moderately intellectually disabled, is getting ready to transition from a self-contained classroom in high school to a sheltered workshop. The interdisciplinary team (school psychologist, job coach, teacher, OTA, speech therapist, Harry's parents, and Harry himself) feels that Harry could complete simple woodworking projects successfully in a supervised workshop setting. The OTA works with Harry weekly for 30 minutes by consulting with his teacher and working toward goals such as improving motor planning to complete multistep activities. The OTA also monitors and provides adapted equipment to help Harry complete fine motor activities more efficiently. Harry's interdisciplinary team agrees he should become familiar with the materials he will be using at the sheltered workshop. The team will examine Harry's adapted equipment needs. The OTA first speaks to personnel involved in the workshop to find out what

equipment is already available. Later, the OTA consults with them regarding Harry's abilities and brings additional equipment that he will be using. Harry decides to make a small wooden jewelry box as an "end-of-the-year" present for his teacher. The OTA requests sequencing cards from the speech therapist to increase Harry's independence in completing the task. Because Harry has a weak grasp, the OTA provides a paintbrush with a built-up handle and a sanding block. The shop environment is safe, conducive to woodworking, and free from distractions. One-on-one assistance is available as needed. The OTA and Harry review the plans of the project and decide that Harry will need two sessions to complete it.

Media/Materials

The media/materials needed are as follows:

- Small wooden box obtained from craft supply store
- Paints and paintbrush (with built-up handle, if necessary)
- Sandpaper and sanding block
- Facemasks to wear during sanding
- Decorations (e.g., faux jewels, shells, colored tiles, stencils)
- Glue
- Cloth
- Picture sequence cards

Method

1. Set up the environment, considering lighting, seating, height of work surface, and positioning of materials. Position Harry to avoid visual and auditory distractions. Protect the work surface with newspaper or drop cloth.
2. The OTA sets up the sequence cards and explains the steps of the activity.
3. Harry dons the mask in preparation for sanding and uses the sanding block to smooth out the small wooden box.
4. Harry cleans all of the surfaces of the wooden box with a soft cloth.
5. Harry applies the paint and lets it dry.
6. Harry chooses decorations and applies them with glue.
7. Harry cleans up the work area.

Client Factors
Mental Functions

Harry sustained attention for 30 minutes to complete the multistep process and safely worked with the materials. His memory was sufficient to remember the procedures, follow the sequence, and use objects for their intended use. Harry relied on perceptual functions to interpret tactile and visual information when sanding and painting the box. Harry smelled the odors of the paint and the freshly sanded wood. He used good judgment and problem-solving skills to determine when and where to sand. Visual cards were useful to Harry. A positive sense of self was reinforced as Harry carried out the process of choosing, constructing, and presenting the project to his teacher.

Neuromusculoskeletal and Movement-related Functions, Muscle Functions, Movement Functions

Harry initiated and sustained sufficient grasp on the surface of the sanding block and the adapted paintbrush despite decreased strength in his hands. Harry showed control of voluntary movement functions when keeping the paint in the correct areas, applying the small objects used to decorate the jewelry box, as well as opening, closing, and manipulating the containers.

Skin and Related Structure Functions

Integrity of the skin was required as protection against sawdust or paint residue getting into open wounds or abrasions.

Grading and Adapting

Suggestions for grading and adapting this activity are as follows:

- Adaptive equipment can be used to increase the child's independence; for example, the paintbrush with a built-up handle. Another example would be a nonslip mat or a jig for stabilizing materials.
- Divide the task into several sessions.
- Use written or pictorial sequencing cards as needed.
- Allow the child to gather, clean, and put away supplies.
- Nonlatex gloves can be worn for skin sensitivities or in the presence of small cuts or abrasions.

The OTA considered Harry's client factors as well as his social and occupational issues when choosing and setting up the activity. Harry felt invested in the project; he was given choices and successfully performed the work with little intervention because of the OTA's careful consideration of activity demands. Table 23-4 presents activities for adolescents.

CLINICAL *Pearl*

Use low-odor paints and finishes in a well-ventilated area. Also, consider any skin allergies that may be present, and take necessary precautions such as using gloves (nonlatex gloves when indicated). When using tools and potentially hazardous materials, ensure that the child has good safety awareness, and provide proper supervision.

SUMMARY

Therapeutic media is an important part of OT intervention. It changes with time and technology and varies according to culture. OT practitioners use media to address child's OT goals. The collaboration between the occupational therapist and the OTA is best served once the OTA has established service competency. Sound clinical reasoning skills are required to choose media that facilitate OT goals and are meaningful to children. Other important considerations include selection of media that are developmentally relevant to children and are graded on the basis of client factors and activity demands. This chapter provided examples of how the OTA uses media to design, develop, and implement intervention activities that present the just-right challenge for each child.

References

1. American heritage dictionary of the English language (4th ed.) (2000). New York: Houghton Mifflin.
2. American Occupational Therapy Association. (2014). Occupational therapy practice framework: domain and process (3rd ed.). *Am J Occup Ther*, 68(Suppl. 1), S1–S48.
3. Punwar, A. J., & Peloquin, S. M. (2000). *Occupational therapy principles and practice* (2nd ed.). Baltimore, MD: Lippincott Williams & Wilkins.

Recommended Reading

Tubbs, C., & Drake, M. (2012). *Crafts and creative media in therapy* (4th ed.). Thorofare, NJ: Slack.

Johnson, C., et al. (1996). *Therapeutic crafts: a practical approach*. Thorofare, NJ: Slack.

Kranowitz, C. (2003). *The out-of-sync child has fun: activities for kids with sensory processing disorder*. New York: Perigee Books.

Kuffner, T. (1999). *The busy books series*. Minnetonka, MN: Meadowbrook Press.

REVIEW *Questions*

1. What should you consider when selecting media?
2. What is the role of the OTA in selecting therapeutic media?
3. Describe why choosing appropriate therapeutic media for different age groups is important.
4. Give some examples of cultural considerations a practitioner makes when selecting therapeutic media.

5. Explain the principle of gradation of therapeutic activities.
6. What purpose do craft activities serve in pediatric OT?
7. Distinguish between preparatory activities and functional activities.

SUGGESTED *Activities*

1. Visit a day-care center or a preschool during a group craft activity. Observe the media used, activity demands, and methods used. Did you notice the staff using any sort of preparatory activities? Considering the results of the activities you observed, do you think preparatory activities would have made a difference in these results? Would the results have been different with OT interventions?
2. Choose a medium and formulate five different activities using the same medium.
3. Consider one of the five activities (chosen from no. 2 above) and adapt/grade it for various client factors (refer to Occupational Therapy Practice Framework, 3rd ed.), age groups, and culture as outlined by this chapter.

4. Plan a craft activity or game considering the following:
   - What materials do you need?
   - How much time will it take to prepare the materials?
   - Can you use the items on hand, or do you have to buy specific items (i.e., playground ball and empty water bottles versus a purchased bowling game)?
   - Which is more cost-effective?

   List the activity demands required to complete your planned craft activity or game for the above question. (Refer to activity demands section of Occupational Therapy Practice Framework, 3rd ed.)
5. Choose a culture other than your own and find a therapeutic media activity related to it. Describe its significance to the culture. Teach classmates how to do the activity.

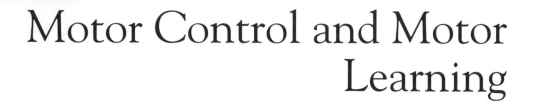

ELIZABETH W. CRAMPSEY
MARY ELIZABETH PATNAUDE

Motor Control and Motor Learning

CHAPTER *Objectives*

After studying this chapter, the reader will be able to accomplish the following:

- Define motor control and motor learning.
- Recognize principles of motor control and motor learning and their application to practice.
- Identify how motor control and motor learning concepts inform interventions.
- Apply concepts of feedback, feedforward, degrees of freedom, coordination and timing, strength/endurance, and muscle tone to intervention strategies.
- Build motor learning and motor control concepts into task-analysis skills for intervention.
- Describe strategies to use motor learning concepts in occupational therapy practice to improve a child's motor control.

CHAPTER *Outline*

To enable a young child to participate in the occupations of childhood, such as play, self-care, school/learning and social interaction, he or she must develop age-appropriate motor skills.[5] Children engage in many activities throughout the course of their days that help them develop and participate in the world around them. Occupational therapy (OT) practitioners provide interventions to children with a variety of conditions to help them acquire motor skills that lead to motor control. These conditions, include, but are not limited to cerebral palsy, developmental coordination disorder, Down syndrome, congenital disorders, and neurologic injury. Children and youth with challenges may have difficulty in their abilities to participate in activities of daily living (ADLs; e.g., feeding, dressing, bathing, playing), instrumental ADLs (IADLs; e.g., care of others, care of pets, meal preparation), rest and sleep, education, and social participation.[3] Having a strong understanding of how to design interventions to help children gain motor function and participate in daily occupations is a paramount skill for OT practitioners. Being able to problem solve creatively, clinically reason, and demonstrate sound decision making will promote best practice when working with children, adolescents, and their families. In this chapter, the OT practitioner will acquire further understanding of these concepts and their role in intervention. The chapter provides clinical examples and strategies to apply motor control and motor learning concepts in intervention.

PRINCIPLES OF MOTOR LEARNING

Motor learning can be defined as the learning and refinement of motor skills over time.[16] This learning takes place as a complex interaction between the child and the environment. It incorporates many factors such as the nature and intensity of the challenge, the cognitive ability of the child, and the contextual demands.[18] To promote the best learning opportunity, finding the "just-right challenge" for the child will be helpful. If the demands are too high, or too low, they will interfere with the child's ability to engage, learn, retain, and adjust appropriately.

Motor learning refers to the intrinsic processes that go hand in hand with children experiencing and participating in meaningful activities that lead to long-lasting changes in motor performance.[8] Motor learning can be incorporated into the teaching–learning process inherent in OT intervention with children and youth. Motor learning refers to the practice of how one teaches movement for success, retention, and engagement in occupational performance.

Motor learning is based on the principles of **neuroplasticity**. Neuroplasticity refers to the ways in which the brain can change by laying down new circuitry and making new neural connections. These changes occur when the brain receives new information or stimuli. An

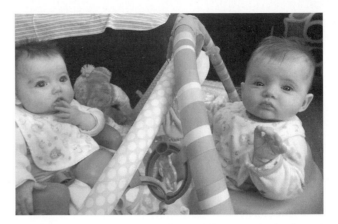

FIGURE 24-1 Swatting at a toy allows infants to gain the control to reach for and manipulate objects.

example of stimuli would be the way a baby's muscles feel when he or she is learning to reach for a toy. A young infant will bat at an object in a seemingly random manner (Figure 24-1). When contact is made with the toy, the brain receives information and begins to lay down the neural circuitry to more accurately reach for it next time. In response to this stimuli, permanent changes are made in the brain. These changes occur easily in the brains of babies and children. This ability of the brain to change, or be "plastic" is very important for learning.[11] Much of the learning that occurs as a result of neuroplasticity requires factors such as **feedback, feedforward,** practice, modeling or demonstration, and transfer of learning. Understanding motor learning concepts provides OT practitioners with sound strategies to use in OT practice to improve a child's motor control. Being well versed in the principles of motor learning will enable the OT practitioner to assist children in motor skill acquisition and control. This enables the OT practitioner to adjust feedback and promote further strategies to aid the child in acquiring motor skills and learning.

Motor learning concepts provide strategies the OT practitioner can use to teach a child to engage in his or her occupations. Specifically, motor learning provides insight into when and how to give feedback; what is the best way to support transfer of learning; how much and what type of practice benefits children. Motor learning research informs the type of activities, practice, and timing of intervention activities. Box 24-1 provides an overview of motor learning principles that may be integrated into OT practice to improve motor control in children in youth.

PRINCIPLES OF MOTOR CONTROL

Motor control refers to the "ability to regulate or direct the mechanisms essential to movement"[16] Motor control research examines the role of the central nervous system (CNS), techniques to quantify movement, and the

BOX 24-1

Motor Learning Principles: Williams*

TRANSFER OF LEARNING
- Skill experiences are presented in logical progression.
- Simple, foundational skills are practiced before more complex skills.
- Skill practice includes "real"-life and simulated settings.
- Skills with similar components are more likely to show transfer effect.
- Practice in natural context with actual objects is most effective.

FEEDBACK
Modeling or Demonstration
- Demonstration is best if it is given to the individual before practicing the skill and in the early stages of skill acquisition.
- Demonstration should be given throughout practice and as frequently as deemed helpful.
- Demonstrations should not be accompanied by verbal commentary because this can reduce attention paid to important aspects of the skill being demonstrated.
- It is important to direct the individual's attention to the critical cues immediately before the skill is demonstrated.
- Allow child time to "figure it out."

Verbal Instructions
- Verbal cues should be brief, to the point and involve one to three words.
- Verbal cues should be limited in terms of numbers of cues given during or after performance.
- Only the major aspect of the skill that is being concentrated on should be cued.
- Verbal cues should be carefully timed so they do not interfere with performance.
- Verbal cues can and should be initially repeated by the performer.
- Verbal cues should emphasize key aspects of movement.

Knowledge of Results and Knowledge of Performance
- A variety of different combinations of both KR and KP typically helps to facilitate learning.
- KP error information may help the performer change important performance characteristics and thus may help facilitate skill acquisition.
- Information about "appropriate" or "correct" aspects of performance helps to motivate the person to continue practicing.
- It is important to balance between feedback that is error-based and that which is based on "appropriate" or "correct" characteristics of the performance.
- KP feedback can also be descriptive or prescriptive; prescriptive KP is more helpful than just descriptive KP in the early or beginning stages of learning.
- KP and KR should be given close in time to but after completion of the task.
- KP and KR should not necessarily be given 100% of the time.

- Learning is enhanced if KP/KR are given at least 50% of the time.
- A frequently used procedure for given KR/KP is to practice a skill several times and then provide the appropriate feedback.

DISTRIBUTION AND VARIABILITY OF SKILL PRACTICE
- Shorter, more frequent practice sessions are preferable to longer, less frequent practice.
- If a skill or task is complex and/or requires a relatively long time to perform or if it requires repetitive movements, relatively short practice trials/sessions with frequent rest periods are preferable.
- If the skill is relatively simple and takes only a brief time to complete, longer practice trials/session with less frequent rest periods are preferable.
- It can enhance skill acquisition to practice several tasks in the same session.
- If several tasks are practiced, divide the time spent on each and either randomly repeat practice on each or use a sequence that aids the overall practice.
- Providing a number of different environmental contexts in which the skill is practiced facilitates learning.
- More practice is not necessarily always better.
- Clinical judgment should be used to recognize when practice is no longer producing changes; at this time a new or different task should be introduced.

WHOLE VERSUS PART PRACTICE
- Whole practice is better when the skill or task to be performed is simple.
- Part practice may be preferable when the skill is more complex.
- If part practice is used, be sure that the parts practiced are "natural units"—that they go together.
- To simplify a task, reduce the nature and/or complexity of the objects to be manipulated. For example, use a balloon for catching instead of a ball.
- To simplify a task, provide assistance to the learner that helps to reduce attention demands. For example, provide trunk support during practice of different eye–hand coordination tasks.
- To simplify a task, provide auditory or rhythmic accompaniment; this may facilitate learning through assisting the learner in getting the appropriate "rhythm" of the movement.

MENTAL PRACTICE
- Mental practice helps to facilitate acquisition of new skills as well as the relearning of old skills.
- Mental practice helps the person prepare to perform a task.
- Mental practice combined with physical practice works best.
- For mental practice to be effective, the individual should have some basic imagery ability.
- Mental practice should be relatively short, not prolonged.

*Adapted from Williams, H. (2011). Motor control: Fine motor skills. In J. Solomon & J. O'Brien (Eds.), *Pediatric Skills for Occupational Therapy Assistants* (3rd ed.). St. Louis: Mosby.

nature, as well as the quality of movement.[12] Motor control addresses posture, mobility, fine motor and gross motor skills and explores motor development throughout the life span. To apply the principles effectively, the OT practitioner must take into account the processing requirements as well as the influence of dysfunction or impairment on movement.[12] For children and youth who exhibit motor challenges, occupational therapists and occupational therapy assistants (OTAs) are in the prime position to integrate their understanding of basic principles of motor control to improve motor functioning related to the child's performance in everyday occupations.

Current motor control theory supports a dynamic systems approach to intervention. Dynamic Systems Theory (DST) suggests that motor control develops and is refined based on an interaction between multiple systems.[16,19] Systems include neurologic, musculoskeletal, psychosocial, environment, and the task or activity requirements. Changing one system will influence others. This approach to intervention suggests that although changing one component may result in improved motor control, OT practitioners will be more effective if they target multiple systems. For OT practitioners this means consideration of the person (skills and abilities, client factors, motivation, goals), task (what type of actions are required), and environment (contexts). Dynamic systems theorists examine multiple factors that influence movement and strategies to improve motor function. Examination of these factors will guide OT practitioners as they develop intervention plans and assess a child's performance.[12] The following principles of motor control guide intervention:

1. **Dynamic Systems Theory** explains the interplay between the neuromuscular system, the environment, cognition, and the intended task.[12] Multiple systems engage and interact with each other, each having their unique role in movement.
2. To fully understand the movement, OT practitioners must acknowledge that change in one system directly affects the others. This ripple effect is critical to understand for successful intervention planning. The goal of motor control intervention is for the child to actively perform under a variety of circumstances.[12]
3. It would not be unusual for one task to involve interactions of many systems such as visual, proprioceptive, kinesthetic, neuromuscular, and tactile systems. This dynamic integration of many systems requires adaptation and subtle changes based on the body's reaction to engagement.
4. To engage in a task, one must first have the intent to move, which is guided by a cognitive process informed by motivation that encourages one to engage in the task.[12]
5. Changes and learning occur due to neuroplasticity.

Three Pillars of Motor Control

Motor control research supports OT concepts of (a) engaging children in meaningful activities that (b) closely mimic occupations of childhood and (c) occur in the natural setting. Figure 24-2 illustrates a child engaging in play with friends in the playroom full of toys. Overall, current motor control theory supports occupation-based, client-centered occupational therapy. Repetition of meaningful activities in the natural context and as one might perform the actual occupation is best for motor learning and motor control. OT practitioners developing motor control intervention adhere to these three pillars of motor control for successful intervention in this area (Figure 24-3).

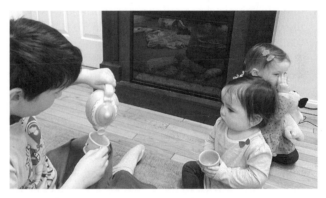

FIGURE 24-2 Activities that mimic the normal occupations of childhood can be very motivating to children and improve motor learning. The infant plays with friends in the busy playroom full of toys.

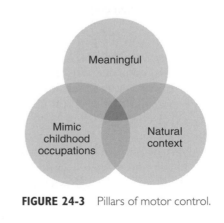

FIGURE 24-3 Pillars of motor control.

1. **Meaningful Activities.** Children engage in activities longer and with better motor control (e.g., reaction time, co-contractions) when the activity is purposeful or meaningful.[7,9,21] OT practitioners value engaging children and youth in purposeful or meaningful activity and current research suggests that the motivation factors produce better quality of movements and stimulate more areas of the brain.[9,10,17] Consequently, targeting intervention to match the child's volition (values, interests, and personal causation) can produce improved outcomes.[9]

   OT practitioners get to know the children they are treating so that they may design interventions that are meaningful to each child. The process of discovering what is meaningful to a child can be very rewarding. To see the eyes of a child light up when discussing his or her favorite toy or where he or she will be celebrating his or her next birthday party can feel magical and really improve the bonding that occurs between the OT practitioner and the child. To understand what is meaningful to a child, OT practitioners may ask the child and/or family members, observe the child interacting with objects, or conduct assessments (e.g., interest checklists, volitional questionnaire). Finding activities that stimulate one's volition is key to occupational therapy practice.

2. **Closely mimic occupations of childhood.** Movement occurs during daily activities and occupations. Children are driven to explore their environment and learn through movements. OT practitioners work with children who experience difficulty moving, which may be due to a variety of factors, including limited desire to move. After determining those activities the child finds meaningful (or interests of which the child is motivated to perform), the OT practitioner develops interventions that closely mimic occupations of childhood. Children are more able to transfer motor skills learned in the actual setting or as close to that as possible. The OT practitioner sets up the environment to mimic natural occupations of childhood, which in many cases is play. This requires the child to perform movements in a variety of ways. Flexibility and adaptability of movement is central to functional movement.

   For example, when working with a child to improve her ability to dress independently, the OT practitioner has pinpointed difficulty with the orientation of clothing. The practitioner sets up the environment to encourage the child to play "dress up" with many different types of clothing, while having the child practice the whole task. The activity can be graded by providing a varying amount of tactile, auditory, and visual cues. Playing dress up is a childhood activity that the child can follow through with at home with her sister. It is a meaningful play activity that will also

help the child develop skills for self-care. OT practitioners who can analyze activities and understand the interplay of the environment, task, and child are able to design intervention activities that facilitate motor learning and motor control.

3. **Occurs in the setting similar to the natural context in which the occupation takes place.** Children learn motor tasks most efficiently, and transfer those tasks into functional activities when they are taught the skills within the context of the whole activity and within the natural context.[4,10,12,20] Although there may be times that a practitioner needs to work with the child to refine a skill, children are most successful if they are taught movement within the context of the occupation being executed. Performing in the natural context provides cues, promotes flexibility of movement, stimulates interest, and targets the child's motivation for performance. It allows for transfer of learning. Therefore OT practitioners should consider the natural context of the activity when designing intervention.

   For example, the child who desperately wants to be successful on the school playground equipment, but struggles with motor control and motor learning will be more motivated to engage in games on the playground. The OT practitioner who provides intervention on the school playground (in the child's natural context) will be able to refine skills and abilities to support success (through remediation or adaptations). These will lead to further practice and engagement from the child. The problem solving and natural planning will inform current and future performance for the child.

CLINICAL *Pearl*

For a child struggling to maintain posture at his or her desk during handwriting tasks, a pull-out method of intervention may not be the most meaningful. However, assessing the child's desk set up for proper height and support, providing appropriate tools and assessing arousal level may facilitate writing in the classroom. A savvy practitioner will be a master of task analysis and adaptation of tasks for the just right challenge.

APPLYING MOTOR LEARNING CONCEPTS TO PRACTICE

Motor learning refers to "how one acquires motor skills and includes type and amount of practice, type and amount of feedback, timing of feedback, type of activities (e.g., bilateral, unilateral, complex, simple), and presentation of tasks for learning."[13] Motor learning concepts can inform OT intervention and are easily integrated into current practice. OT practitioners use these concepts within a meaningful, occupation-based activity within the natural context. Box 24-1 provides an overview of the concepts that can facilitate motor learning. These concepts have evidence to support their use for enhancing motor control. In one study, therapists who used motor learning concepts in practice achieved better intervention outcomes.[17]

Feedback

Feedback informs the learner about his or her progress in acquiring new motor skills. Many forms of feedback exist. Feedback occurs before and after performance (feedforward or feedback) and can be intrinsic (within the child) or extrinsic (provided by an external source). Practitioners provide feedback to children and youth in many different ways (verbal, nonverbal). Feedback can evaluate the performance results (knowledge of results) or aspects of the performance (knowledge of performance). OT practitioners consider the type of feedback, timing of feedback, and motor outcomes when designing intervention. Being mindful of one's feedback can support motor performance.

Feedforward and Feedback

"Feedforward is that intangible abstract representation of sensation that gives us the awareness of what the movement pattern will feel like before we begin to move."[12] Feedforward refers to the adjustments in anticipation of the movement required. For example, a child may position himself or herself to catch a ball by predicting where he or she thinks the ball will go. Client-generated and task-oriented active movements promote engagement and allow the child to register the movement pattern throughout different areas of the CNS. When children are about to engage in a task, they use practice from past experiences as a template. The child receives sensory information regarding a movement. Feedback from a compilation of sensations resulting from the completed movement informs the child about the movement performance. Adjustments based on that performance are made. This experience is stored for the child to pull from for future engagement in the same or similar task.

OT practitioners may help children with feedforward (anticipation) by discussing the movement required. Asking the child to get ready to catch the ball and providing simple cues, such as "are your hands ready?" or "where do you think the ball will go?" can help a child anticipate the movement. Upon completion of the activity, the OT practitioner can encourage feedback by asking the child to reflect on the movement. Both of these activities help facilitate motor control.

Intrinsic Feedback

Intrinsic feedback is the information that children receive following their practice attempt(s). It is based on Adams' theory[2] that sensory feedback occurs in a closed loop and is necessary for the ongoing production of skilled movement. The nervous system processes this sensory feedback by continuously comparing it to previous experiences.[16] The repetition helps to promote neuroplasticity. The child recalls knowledge of how the movement felt and his or her experience of the motor task. For example, as the child crawls through the tunnel, he or she receives intrinsic feedback through weight bearing (Figure 24-4). This feedback then helps the child understand and correct errors or adjustments needed once he or she has acquired motor skill proficiency.

Extrinsic Feedback

Someone other than the child provides extrinsic feedback. It is helpful in identifying errors in the movement, including coordination, timing, sequencing, and motor planning. Extrinsic feedback can help children adjust movements to be more effective. For children with disabilities, OT practitioners may use extrinsic feedback to teach a child a movement. Coaches and physical education teachers use extrinsic feedback to refine skills. Although extrinsic feedback is helpful for learning, OT practitioners consider carefully the timing and degree of extrinsic feedback provided. In the end, the goal of occupational therapy is for the child to problem solve, negotiate, and correct movements as a result of intrinsic feedback. Furthermore, providing too much feedback can interfere with a child's processing. Thus OT practitioners should examine how and when they provide feedback.

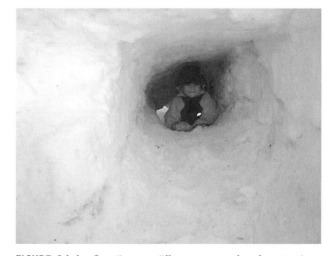

FIGURE 24-4 Crawling on different types of surfaces, such as through a snow tunnel, can increase intrinsic feedback to muscles.

Timing of Feedback

The timing of extrinsic feedback is important to the therapeutic process. Feedback may be provided in various ways, including concurrent, immediate, terminal, and in a delayed manner. Concurrent feedback occurs during the actual movement.[14,15] Immediate feedback occurs just after the movement. Terminal feedback takes place right at the completion of the movement. Delayed feedback occurs after the movement had been completed and a time interval has transpired.

Verbal feedback may be given consistently (after each trial) or sporadically (after some trials).[22] Sporadic feedback after a delay was found to be more beneficial for motor learning than feedback given instantly after movement.[14,15] Delay in feedback across some of the motor trials allows the child to participate in determining what factors play a part in successful or unsuccessful performance.[22] This strategy takes away the dependence on the feedback to learn the skill. OT practitioners should be mindful of when they provide feedback and consider providing a delay in feedback to allow the child to self-reflect, make adjustments if possible. This approach promotes motor learning. However, OT practitioners should consider the stage of learning when determining feedback. Children learning a new motor skills performed significantly better overtime when they received 100% feedback on each trial compared with those children who received less feedback, less frequently.[18]

These findings suggest that children may benefit first from consistent extrinsic feedback when learning a new skill and may use this feedback to self-reflect and develop intrinsic feedback. The goal of OT intervention is to decrease the extrinsic feedback to allow the child to develop intrinsic feedback. OT practitioners may promote intrinsic feedback by providing feedback while a child looks in the mirror as shown in Figure 24-5. Using

simple words for key actions can help the child concentrate on the movement and allow the child to internalize the sensations.

Extrinsic feedback may also be provided by the activity itself. For example, cause-and-effect toys, such as busy boxes or musical toys with a switch that only work when a motor task is successful, provide extrinsic feedback. Another example of extrinsic feedback is working with children on tasks that involve a target as the measure of task completion success. In these cases, the extrinsic feedback is the score of a goal, the sink of a basket, or the connection with a tennis ball. Using this type of extrinsic feedback provides a transition away from the OT practitioner and helps the child rely more on intrinsic feedback.

CASE *Study*

Emily is an 11-month-old with Trisomy 21 (Down syndrome). She demonstrates motor skills at about 8 months. The OT practitioner plans to facilitate both internal and external feedback to promote crawling (i.e., prone on belly, such as commando crawling) then progress her skills toward creeping (i.e., positioned in quadruped). The OT practitioner provides opportunity for Emily to perceive intrinsic feedback while she is developing the prerequisite skills to creep, by providing postural cues and support. The postural cues include positioning the child prone on elbows, or hands while playing on different surfaces (pillows, firm) to allow the child to experience different sensory feedback. The practitioner encourages the child to unweight a hand or adjust a leg to enable her to reach out and manipulate toys or objects placed in the environment. The child is motivated to play with the interesting novel toys. Eventually the child seeks to reach a toy placed higher and the practitioner helps her achieve a quadruped posture (with support). Emily rocks back and forth many times before unweighting an arm and propelling herself forward. By this point, she has experienced weight shifting in a more controlled posture of being prone and prone on elbow. Once Emily has this experience, she will more readily trust her motor skills and try more novel activities.

As the OT practitioner works with Emily, she provides deep pressure to Emily's shoulder and/or hip joints to provide proprioceptive input (intrinsic feedback), which allow her nervous system to more easily perceive the feedback. In addition, handling techniques can be used to facilitate the weight shift. Finally, to facilitate the unweighting of one arm, which is a prerequisite to crawling, the OT practitioner places something motivating and novel in front of Emily. The OT practitioner uses motor control and motor learning concepts by engaging Emily in play (whole task), setting up the play environment, and providing

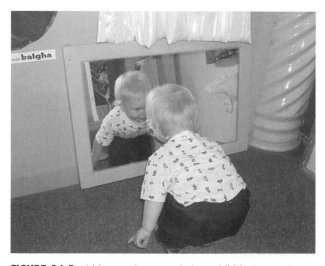

FIGURE 24-5 Using a mirror can help a child incorporate extrinsic feedback into internal feedback.

external feedback (verbal encouragement and short, brief feedback) while stimulating intrinsic feedback for learning. The practitioner considered Emily's personal characteristics (including age) and provided developmentally appropriate activities. The practitioner provided repetitive practice using meaningful activities and shaped (by grading the degree of difficulty) the activities so that Emily was successful. The environment supported Emily's motor skill acquisition by including novelty and safety.

Modeling or Demonstration

OT practitioners frequently use modeling or demonstration to teach children and youth motor skills. Modeling or demonstration involves providing visual information about how to perform a skill or task. This is an effective technique for teaching, especially when the modeling involves demonstration of whole movements. This technique is most effective when presented in the natural context in which the motor task will occur[13] (see Box 24-1). Demonstrations are best if they are provided:

- Before practicing the skill and in the early stages of skill acquisition
- Slowly, without verbal feedback
- After emphasizing critical cues
- Throughout practice and as frequently as deemed helpful

Demonstrations are best if they are given to the child before practicing the skill and in the early stages of skill acquisition. Before demonstrating the skill, the child's attention should be directed toward critical cues. This allows the child to focus on key aspects of the movement. Showing the child the motor actions that are expected can help the child anticipate (feedforward) movements. Young children may observe peers demonstrating movements and imitate them. OT practitioners move deliberately and slowly (not too slowly) to clearly show the child the desired skill. Demonstration should not include verbal feedback as this may reduce attention devoted to the important aspects of the demonstrated skill. OT practitioners provide demonstration throughout practice and as frequently as deemed helpful.

Verbal Instruction

Verbal instructions can be used to teach children and youth motor skills. Typically, practice is preceded or accompanied by verbal instruction or cues. Brief, one to three words of clear, simple key components of the movement positively influence new motor learning.[13] OT practitioners evaluate carefully the key components of movement and focus verbal instructions on those aspects of movement first. Once a child has accomplished the key components, the OT practitioner may provide

additional verbal instruction to refine movement. Providing selected verbal instruction allows the child to focus and be successful. Providing repetitive practice with the same verbal instructions and movement requirements reinforces learning. OT practitioners set up the environment to reinforce key movements.

For example, the practitioner engaged a child in making cookies requiring repetitive hand grasp and strength. The child was engaged in a meaningful occupation that simulated the natural context and provides practice (Figure 24-6). Before the activity, the OT practitioner provided verbal instruction on how to grasp and squeeze the cookie dough. She used simple brief words—"Squeeze 1, 2 (timing) and release." The OT practitioner demonstrated the task using the words and then observed. As the child performed, the practitioner provided feedback after each cookie for the first three. Providing consistent verbal feedback is helpful when one is learning a new skill. The practitioner did not want to continue the extrinsic feedback but rather waited to see if the child self-corrected (intrinsic feedback). The child continued and at one point remarked, "Oops, that cookie is not large enough." The practitioner responded, "What will you do?" and the child answered, "Squeeze harder." The OT practitioner was pleased that the child was able to modify her skills to be successful with the activity. The child looked pleased with her progress and continued.

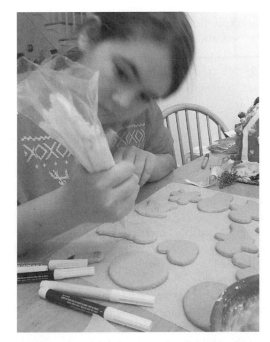

FIGURE 24-6 Occupational therapy practitioners engage children in meaningful activities within the natural context considering the nature of the task, child's abilities, and environment. This child enjoys making cookies, an occupation valued in her family. She is also working on hand strength, endurance, timing, and sequencing.

Paying close attention to the child's nonverbal and verbal feedback helps the practitioner identify the right level of instruction. A skilled practitioner uses many different strategies and is able to individualize strategies for each child. When having a child work on bouncing a ball, the OT practitioner might instruct in the following ways, from simple to more complex:

- Demonstrate using gestures only, no verbal cues.
- Provide minimal verbal cues, such as "Now," "Now," "Now" or "Bounce, bounce, bounce" in time with the activity.
- Grade the verbal instruction to "My turn, your turn."
- Expand further, say "Let's try it again."
- As the child is ready, provide more specific feedback such as, "You are hitting the ball too early (or too late)."
- To help the child refine skills, provide more complex instruction that requires further integration such as "When the ball bounces down, get ready to bounce it back."

OT practitioners use verbal instruction and feedback as praise and to reinforce behavior and performance. However, engaging the child in the process of interpreting his or her success through self-reflection throughout the motor process is a helpful strategy in the child's learning process. Self-reflection promotes problem solving and is internally driven. Consequently, it is best if the child reflects on his or her performance. OT practitioners carefully structure verbal instruction to promote motor learning. They also use verbal feedback to facilitate motor learning by providing children with information regarding their performance and results.

Knowledge of Results

OT practitioners frequently use verbal feedback to provide children with knowledge of their performance. Verbal feedback is most effective when provided immediately following performance. It should be short and meaningful to the child and inform them about their motor success. For example, saying "good job" or "nice one" is not as informative as "you formed your 'b'" or "that one hit the target." **Knowledge of results** (KR) involves information provided from an external source about the outcome, or end result of the performance of a skill or task. KR answers the question: Was the goal achieved? KR is often provided by the therapist during OT intervention.

KR can also be provided as a natural part of the task, if the environment is structured in a way to facilitate the child's awareness. An example of this is bringing a child's attention to his or her performance. This may occur by showing the child the tag on his or her backward pants after a toileting task. Another way to do this is to provide a target with rings on a white board, for the child working on aim, which will let the child know exactly how close (or far away) he or she is from the target. Knowledge of

results is most informative during the retention phase of skill acquisition and learning. Because there are other cues and intrinsic properties and contextual cues to the task, the child can perform without knowledge of results. However, knowledge of results helps with retention as well as transfer of learning.[8, 14]

OT practitioners use knowledge of results to help children retain newly learned motor skills. The knowledge can help a child adjust his or her performance and continue to practice. The following example illustrates how knowledge of results provides reinforcement of skills. During OT intervention a child completes a Lite-Brite task to work on her pincer grasp and visual-motor processing for school. She follows a pattern on the Lite-Brite paper provided. Upon conclusion, she examines the completed paper to see if she pushed the peg hard enough to go through the paper, and to determine whether the pattern followed shows the intended product. This knowledge of results provides extrinsic feedback to support retention of skills. Furthermore, the child is able to evaluate the results, which is desired over the practitioner's evaluation.

Knowledge of Performance

Knowledge of performance (KP) refers to providing information about the nature or characteristic of the movement used to perform the task. The OT practitioner provides information about how the task is performed. KP answers questions, such as: "What did the individual actually do?" or "How did she move to carry out the task?" KP helps children understand how they could adjust or change movements for more accuracy or success. KP provides information to refine movements. For example, the OT practitioner may provide descriptive feedback to the child to help him or her improve performance by stating, "You jumped only a little." The child may take this information and try to jump higher the next time. The practitioner could also state, "You need to jump higher." This prescriptive information indicates what the child must do to improve performance.

OT practitioners provide descriptive and prescriptive knowledge of performance while acknowledging that the child should have an opportunity to reflect on his or her performance errors. It is best if the child is able to change his or her performance of the task through self-reflection.

CLINICAL *Pearl*

When working with children, OT practitioners often feel the need to give a lot of positive feedback, such as "good job" or "yay." However, specific, descriptive feedback enhances the child's ability to learn motor skills. Understanding this may help the practitioner decrease generic feedback such as "good job" and "well done" and increase specific feedback related to KP.

TABLE 24-1

Types of Practice

TYPE OF PRACTICE	DESCRIPTION	STAGE OF LEARNING	OT INTERVENTION EXAMPLE
Blocked	Child practices one skill with short break and returns to that skill. Repetition of the same skill.	Best for refining new motor skill; does not promote transfer of learning; is not as motivating.	Practice picking up 20 crayons and placing in container; rest for 1 minute and repeat.
Distributed	Child practices skill in a variety of ways with short and long breaks. Repetition of different but related skills.	Best to learn new skills; motivating because child engages in variety; promotes transfer of learning.	Engage in art activity to make a fall picture. To make the picture, rip up small pieces of different-colored construction paper (colors of fall leaves), glue them onto the paper, and use crayon to finalize design. (Fine motor skill practice throughout.)
Variable (random)	Best for transfer of learning; child practices actual task in natural context; variety of skills with random rest periods. Repetition of different skills (may or may not be related) and varied practiced.	All stages benefit from this type of practice; best once child has learned basic motor skills (reinforces refinement of skills and transfer).	Child engages in fall-themed activities to work on fine motor skills (make a leaf collage), gross motor skills (trampoline and parachute games), and snack (oral motor skills).

Practice and Repetition

Practice and repetition are frequent strategies OT practitioners use to help children learn and retain motor performance needed for occupational performance. Repetition of motor tasks enhances brain development.[13] The type of practice required varies with stages of learning and tasks. Understanding the types of practice allows OT practitioners to design effective occupational therapy intervention.

There are three categories of practice: blocked, distributed, and variable (Table 24-1). **Blocked practice** refers to repeating the similar movement with short rest breaks, so engagement in the task is much more than the time spent in breaks. The child may practice the same movement component 10 to 20 times. This type of practice is best for fine tuning and refinement of a task, rather than learning a novel or complex task. However, learning parts of a task through blocked practice can be helpful in early learning stages.[22] Because of the nature of this fine tuning or refinement, there will be less transfer of this motor learning using this technique.[13,22] An example of blocked practice includes having a child put pegs in a pegboard or placing coins in a slot, rest briefly and then do the same activity again.

Distributed practice refers to the repetition of different skills that are spread over the course of the intervention session with rest breaks.[22] This practice focuses on broadening the task being practiced. This type of practice is particularly useful in motivating the child to engage and complete an activity and leads to carryover and transfer of learning to other situations. Children will practice a variety of motor skills and, therefore, they receive practice with varied breaks. This type of learning is helpful for children who are learning new tasks. It allows them to learn new skills in a variety of ways that reinforces acquisition of skills.

For example, an OT practitioner using distributed practice to develop a child's fine motor skills for handwriting and play designs an interesting session using a "fall" theme. The session begins with the child tearing small pieces of paper (working on neat pincer grasp), then gluing the pieces on paper (in hand manipulation) and ending with coloring around the picture (tripod grasp). The child gets rest breaks and practices the components for fine motor skills during play in different ways periodically throughout the session. The variety of activities requires the child to adjust his or her motor performance. Distributed practice works best for the learner that is ready to make small changes in real time to complete the task. Distributed practice can be used to teach children parts of the task in the early stages.

Variable practice (also referred to as random practice) incorporates the practicing of many different skills, with periods of rest. This type of practice is helpful for fine tuning of skills, and helpful in the transfer of learning as well. Furthermore, they indicate that better movement quality is attained in whole-task practice and repetition. The child completes a variety of movements with natural breaks.

CLINICAL *Pearl*

During practice of a motor skill, minimal feedback may help older children with retention. More feedback is likely to be most helpful during the practice phase.

CLINICAL *Pearl*

For some children with cognitive abilities (e.g., developmental coordination disorder), discussing strategies of the task, such as handwriting or ball throwing, is helpful for more complex tasks. This may be even better than physical practice. Children may benefit from visualizing motor tasks. For example, the OT practitioner may ask the child to imagine what it would look or feel like to catch the ball in their baseball glove. Talking through movement strategies may benefit some children.

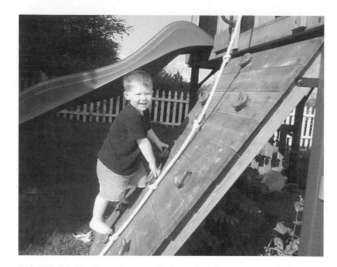

FIGURE 24-7 Learning to climb a climbing structure is fun and prepares the child for play at school.

Transfer of Learning

Transfer of learning refers to applying past learning to new situations, or generalization. Working on this transference requires skillful planning by the OT practitioner. If intervention is not able to occur within the natural context, manipulating environmental factors to closely mimic that natural context will be most helpful. Transfer of learning works best when opportunity is provided for mastery of foundational tasks first. For instance, the practitioner may require the child to master throwing a bean bag to a target first. Then the child incorporates balance skills such as stepping onto a rocker board or uneven surface while throwing. The activity can be further changed to have the child engage in the same activity while swinging to increase the motor demands. The child performs better at the more complex motor skills (balancing while throwing) after successfully performing the initial bean bag throw.

CASE *Study*

Ezekiel is having difficulty climbing on play equipment at school. His school's playground has many different climbing ladders of various inclines (Figure 24-7). Working with Ezekiel in the clinic on climbing clinic ladders to different equipment and creating similar angles and challenges may help him build on this positive clinical experience and so he can transfer those same skills to the playground. Taking this example a step further, the OT practitioner may provide the experience on the actual playground to help problem solve any barriers. Engaging children in the actual activity, which is meaningful, and in the natural context, provides the best motor learning and retention.

APPLICATION OF MOTOR CONTROL CONCEPTS TO PRACTICE

Motor memory includes not only the registration of the influence of the experience, but also the internal feedback from the motor output back into the sensory system. This essentially primes the body to further establish a memory link to that same movement experience. It is after this link is created that the learning occurs. Meaningful repetitive practice where the OT practitioner shapes the movement by requiring more refined or precise movements over time promotes motor memory. OT practitioners frequently target a variety of **motor control** factors through practice and repetition. Using motor learning concepts, practitioners can help children learn movements. Engaging children in meaningful activities that closely mimic occupations of childhood, and that occur in natural contexts, best address motor control.

Meaningful activities are the foundation of OT practice and have been found to increase a child's motor performance. OT practitioners should carefully design meaningful interventions to maximize the child's involvement, volition, and engagement. Children will repeat activities that they find meaningful. OT practitioners use meaningful activities that closely mimic occupations of childhood as both the goal of intervention and the means to achieve the goals. Engaging children in those things (occupations) they want to accomplish seems straightforward. This is the best way to ensure transfer of learning and it helps children learn motor skills. Children and youth who are motivated and desire to engage in activities that are meaningful (such as occupations) will be more successful in performing them. OT practitioners embrace occupation-centered practice and this is essential to motor control.

Engaging a child in meaningful activity in a natural context is the most effective strategy because it allows the child to adapt, problem solve, and respond appropriately and accordingly within the natural context. This in turn reinforces motor control as the interaction is happening in a real environment, rather than a contrived scenario. Performing in the natural context allows for the more likely variables and eventual variation to occur for the child to aid skill acquisition. This reinforces the child's ability to perform activities more naturally, effectively, and automatically in his or her natural context and promotes transfer of learning to a variety of environments. Adjustments made in this natural setting are more meaningful to the child, aiding in skill acquisition. OT practitioners providing intervention to a child within their natural context are urged to allow the child to make mistakes, problem solve, and self-correct to create motor solutions.

Motor control intervention requires the practitioner to examine the person (client factors, performance skills), the task (degree of difficulty), and the environment. A review of selected client factors that may interfere with motor performance is included.

Degrees of Freedom

It may helpful to frame this concept by thinking about the physics of movement. When working with children, considering fulcrum points and lever arms may be helpful during task analysis (see Chapter 11). The addition of strong anatomy foundational concepts will enrich the understanding of limiting degrees of freedom. Joints vary in the amount of movement allowed. This includes the ROM and planes of motion in which it can move. For example, the shoulder girdle can move a full 360 degrees in the sagittal plane. This includes flexion and extension. The shoulder can also move in the frontal and transverse planes, allowing for abduction, adduction, and internal/external rotation. All of these movements refer to the degrees of freedom in which the shoulder can move. All of this mobility may impede a child's ability to control the joint. For fine motor tasks, for example, the child must be able to control the very mobile shoulder joint, as well as the elbow, wrist, and hand joints. To increase control, the degrees of freedom can be limited by holding or stabilizing the joint. For example, to improve upper extremity control needed for writing, the degrees of freedom of the upper extremity can be limited by giving the child a large piece of paper taped to the wall and providing finger paints. The child can hold the distal joints of the hand, wrist, and elbow, while performing a "prewriting" task using primarily the shoulder joint. This activity can be made more challenging by providing a large paintbrush and then smaller paintbrushes and a smaller piece of paper. This example illustrates how the task can be graded seamlessly from easiest to most challenging for the child, from gross activity to seeking more precision and refinement from the child.

Coordination and Timing

Coordination is the activation of specific muscles together.[16] Children and youth with motor impairments often experience challenges with their timing and sequencing of movements.[12] Challenges within the areas of coordination and timing may be a result of a delayed development of the CNS and its ability to efficiently process information.

OT practitioners can address coordination and timing deficits by beginning with gross movements and progressing to more precise movements. OT practitioners can focus coordination intervention by starting with postural control or stability. This may be achieved through intervention or positioning or adaptive equipment. The practitioner provides the child with opportunities to practice coordination by designing activities that require the child to repeat motions and progressively become more accurate. For example, the practitioner may begin by providing a large target area and gradually lessen the target area (to facilitate more precision). The inclusion of music, rhythmic songs, or counting activities into the intervention sessions can promote timing.

Strength and Endurance

Strength refers to the ability to contract a muscle of muscle group against gravity and resistance.[16] Children and youth with motor deficits may experience decreased strength, which negatively affects their ability to engage and perform occupations. In addition to decreased strength, a child with motor difficulties may have poor endurance (i.e., limited ability to sustain muscle contractions over time). OT practitioners can assist children in the development of strength and endurance through the use of meaningful activities.

CLINICAL *Pearl*

Cooking and baking activities can be meaningful tasks for building strength and endurance (Figure 24-8). Kneading bread dough or stirring thick cookie dough can build proximal stability, as well as fine motor muscle strength. In addition, the child can build strength and endurance by carrying ingredients such as bags of flour and sugar, of varying weights. These activities can build meaningful bonds with family and friends, as well.

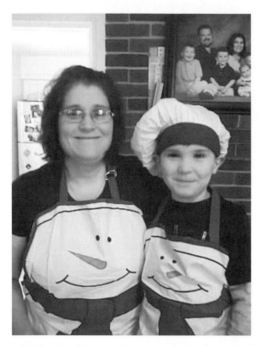

FIGURE 24-8 Cooking can be a very motivating task for children and it lends itself to grading and variability.

Muscle Tone

Muscle tone is the amount of tension in resting muscle or muscle group in response to emotion and gravity.[16] (See Chapter 17 for descriptions of muscle tone fluctuations.) Discrepancies or abnormalities in muscle tone, either hypertonicity or hypotonicity, interfere with motor control. Despite difficulties with muscle tone, OT practitioners focus engagement for children with difficulties in this area on participation in meaningful activities. Rather than focusing on the muscle tone itself, OT practitioners help children engage in the activity. This top-down approach to OT intervention allows children to engage in activity despite abnormal muscle tone. Through engagement in activities, children and youth with muscle tone abnormalities may develop and practice motor skills. Researchers have found evidence to support this approach as shown in studies examining the effectiveness of constraint-induced movement therapy. Children who were encouraged to use their affected hand in repetitive meaningful activity showed improved performance.[1,6,7,21]

SUMMARY

Young children participate in occupations during childhood, such as learning, playing, and socially engaging, that require them to develop and acquire motor skills. OT intervention is provided to enable children to engage in a meaningful way that adds value to their interactions. It is paramount that OT practitioners working with children and youth have a sound understanding of how to design interventions to help children gain motor function and participate in daily occupations. Being able to problem solve creatively, clinically reason, and demonstrate sound decision making promotes best practice when working with children, adolescents, and their families.

Motor learning refers to the learning and refinement of motor skills over time.[16] Participating in and experiencing meaningful activities leads to longer lasting changes in motor performance.[1,4,6–8,17] Motor learning can be incorporated into the teaching–learning process inherent in OT intervention with children and youth. Motor learning helps the child learn from success, retain skills, and engage in occupational performance. The learning that occurs is reinforced by factors such as feedback, feedforward, practice, and transfer of learning. Motor learning is the result of neuroplasticity as the brain develops improved neural synapses or collateral sprouting from practice. OT practitioners use the principles of motor learning to assist children in motor skill acquisition and control.

Motor control refers to the "ability to regulate or direct the mechanisms essential to movement."[16] Motor control refers to the role of the CNS, techniques to quantify movement, and the nature, as well as the quality of movement.[12] OT practitioners evaluate the person (client factors), the task (degree of difficulty), and the environment (context) when considering intervention to improve motor performance. When working to facilitate motor control, OT practitioners develop interventions that are meaningful to the child, closely resemble occupations of childhood and occur within a natural setting.

References

1. Aarts, P. B., Jongerius, P. H., Geerdink, Y. A., et al. (2010). Effectiveness of modified constraint-induced movement therapy in children with unilateral spastic cerebral palsy: a randomized controlled trial. *Neurorehabil Neural Repair*, 24(6), 509–518.
2. Adams, J. A. (1971). A closed loop theory of motor learning. *J Motor Behav*, 3, 111–150.
3. American Occupational Therapy Association. (2014). Occupational therapy practice framework: domain and process (3rd ed). *Am J Occup Ther*, 68(Suppl. 1), S1–S48.
4. Bernie, C., & Rodger, S. (2004). Cognitive strategy use in school-aged children with developmental coordination disorder. *Phys Occup Ther Pediatr*, 24(4), 23–45.
5. Case-Smith, J., Clark, G. J. F., & Schlabach, T. L. (2013). Systematic review of interventions used in occupational therapy to promote motor performance for children ages birth-5 years. *Am J Occup Ther*, 67(4), 413–424.
6. Case-Smith, J., DeLuca, S. C., Stevenson, R., et al. (2012). Multicenter randomized control trial of pediatric constraint-induced movement therapy: 6-month follow-up. *Am J Occup Ther*, 66(1), 15–23.

7. Gordon, A., Schneider, J., Chinnan, A., et al. (2007). Efficacy of a hand-arm bimanual intensive therapy (HABIT) in children with hemiplegic cerebral palsy: a randomized control trial. *Dev Med Child Neurol, 49*, 830–839.

8. Jarus, T., & Ratzon, M. A. (2000). Can you imagine? The effect of mental practice on the acquisition and retention of motor skill as a function of age. *Occup Ther J Res, 20*(3), 163–178.

9. Kielhofner, G. (2008). *Model of human occupation: theory and application* (4th ed.). Philadelphia, PA: F. A. Davis.

10. Mandich, A. D., Polatajko, H. J., Missiuna, C., & Miller, L. T. (2001). Cognitive strategies and motor performance in children with developmental coordination disorders. *Phys Occup Ther Pediatr, 20*, 125–145.

11. Moller, A. R. (2009). *Malleable brain: benefits and harm from plasticity of the brain.* New York: Nova Science Publishers.

12. O'Brien, J., & Lewin, J. (2008). Part 1: translating motor control and motor learning theory into occupational therapy practice for children and youth. *OT Pract, 13*(21), CE1–CE8.

13. O'Brien, J., & Lewin, J. (2009). Part 2: translating motor control and motor learning theory into occupational therapy practice for children and youth. *OT Pract, 14*(1), CE1–CE8.

14. Schmidt, R. A., Lange, C., & Young, D. E. (1990). Optimizing summary knowledge of results for skill learning. *Human Mov Sci, 9*, 325–348.

15. Schmidt, R. A., & Lee, T. D. (2005). In *Motor control and learning: a behavioral emphasis* (4th ed.). Champaign, IL: Human Kinetics.

16. Shumway-Cook, A., & Woollacott, M. (2007). *Motor control: theory and practical applications* (3rd ed.). Baltimore, MD: Lippincott, Williams, & Wilkins.

17. Stueultjens, E. M. J., Dekker, J., Bouter, L. M., et al. (2005). Evidence of the efficacy of occupational therapy in different conditions. An overview of systematic reviews. *Clin Rehabil, 29*, 3–11.

18. Sullivan, K. J., Kantak, S. S., & Burtner, P. A. (2008). Motor learning in children: Feedback effects on skill acquisition. *Phys Ther, 88*, 720–732.

19. Thelen, E. (2000). Motor development a foundation and future of developmental psychology. *Int J Behav Dev, 24*(4), 385–397.

20. Williams, H. (2011). Motor control: fine motor development. In J. Solomon, & J. O'Brien (Eds.), *Pediatric skills for occupational therapy assistants* (3rd ed). St. Louis, MMO: Mosby.

21. Wright, M. G., Hunt, L. P., & Stanley, O. H. (2005). Object/wrist movements during manipulation in children with cerebral palsy. *Ped Rehabil, 8*(4), 263–271.

22. Zwicker, J. G., & Harris, S. R. (2009). A reflection on motor learning theory in pediatric occupational therapy practice. *Can J Occup Ther, 76*(1), 29–37.

REVIEW *Questions*

1. List the principles of motor learning and motor control.
2. Describe the ways in which the principles of motor control and motor learning can be utilized to inform OT practice with children and youth. Specifically address interventions for:
   - Infants
   - Toddlers
   - Preschoolers
   - School-aged children
   - Adolescents
3. List the three pillars of motor control. Discuss ways in which tailoring intervention to the child's age and developmental level relate to these pillars.
4. How does *neuroplasticity* relate to motor learning?
5. Describe how you would integrate at least three motor learning principles (see Box 24-1) into practice.

SUGGESTED *Activities*

1. Observe a child playing on the playground. Describe environmental influences. How does the environment support or hinder the child's movement?
2. Observe a child's movement. Describe the client factors associated with movement. Describe things such as muscle tone, strength, endurance, coordination, balance, quality of movement, timing, and sequencing.
3. Using Box 24-1, identify motor learning and motor control principles used in an OT session (use Evolve site videos).
4. Plan an OT session to target motor skills using motor learning principles. Identify at least four principles to use in the session. Describe how you would integrate them to facilitate motor skills.
5. Plan an OT session to target motor skills by describing how the session uses the three pillars of motor control.
6. Demonstrate the variety of practice, feedback, demonstration, and mental rehearsal techniques used for motor learning.
7. Find new research to describe the effectiveness of motor control techniques. Share findings with classmates.

RICARDO C. CARRASCO
SUSAN A. STALLINGS-SAHLER

25

Sensory Processing/Integration and Occupation

KEY TERMS

Sensory integration
Sensory processing
Sensory integration
  dysfunction
Gravitational insecurity
Sensory processing
  disorder
Sensory modulation
  disorder
Sensory discrimination
  disorder
Sensory-based motor
  disorder
Dyspraxia
Functional support
  capacities
Tactile defensiveness
Sensory seeking
Sensory hypersensitivity
Postural-ocular and
  bilateral integration
  dysfunction
Ideation
Adaptive response
Sensory diet

CHAPTER *Objectives*

After studying this chapter, the reader will be able to accomplish the following:

*   Define the basic principles underlying sensory integration theory, assessment, and treatment
*   Describe sensory-motor, perceptual motor, environmental adaptations, and other approaches used in alleviating sensory processing disorders
*   Articulate the role of the certified occupational therapy assistant in working with children who have sensory processing disorders
*   Describe the taxonomy of sensory processing disorders, including sensory modulation, sensory discrimination, and sensory-based motor disorders
*   Explain how sensory processing disorders affect higher-level cortical processing and development of childhood occupations
*   Describe general principles of occupational therapy screening, observational assessment, and intervention strategies for addressing sensory processing disorders
*   Explain screening, observational assessment, and sensory integration-based intervention strategies for addressing difficulties in sensory modulation
*   Describe screening, assessment, and sensory integration-based intervention strategies for sensory discrimination challenges
*   Articulate general observational assessment and intervention strategies for addressing sensory-based movement disorders of bilateral integration and praxis
*   Identify/describe intervention methods for children who have postural-ocular and bilateral integration dysfunction
*   Identify/describe intervention techniques to work with children who have developmental dyspraxia

CHAPTER *Outline*

Dr. A. Jean Ayres, the originator of **sensory integration** (SI) theory, assessment, and intervention, strongly believed and advocated that the practice of SI by an occupational therapist should take place only at the postgraduate level. SI theory, assessment, and intervention are extremely complex, although the activities appear deceptively easy because they are very playful when effectively implemented by a skilled therapist. However, in settings with close supervision by an appropriately SI-trained and experienced pediatric occupational therapist, the occupational therapy assistant (OTA) can contribute effectively to the intervention program for sensory integration dysfunction.

The term **sensory processing** refers to the means by which the brain receives, detects, and integrates incoming sensory information for use in producing adaptive responses to one's environment.[42-45,50] Children with **sensory integration dysfunction** have a cluster of symptoms that are believed to reflect dysfunction in central nervous system (CNS) processing of sensory input, rather than a primary sensory deficit such as hearing or visual impairment. Dysfunction in sensory processing also does not include the secondary results of a frank CNS birth injury, such as cerebral palsy (CP), or of brain damage caused by stroke or traumatic brain injury. Nor is it used to refer to deficits related to chromosomal or genetic abnormalities such as Down syndrome. This can be confusing to entry-level clinicians because some of these conditions may result in impairments that distort the interpretation of sensations by the brain. For example, a young child with CP may display extreme fear in response to being moved through space, a behavior sometimes termed **gravitational insecurity** when observed in the child with sensory processing dysfunction.[41] However, the origin of the fear response is different. A child with severe spasticity who lacks the movement patterns underlying equilibrium and protective responses has a logical reason to be fearful; the child with sensory processing disorders may react fearfully, even though these self-protective capacities are present in his or her nervous system.

Sensory processing disorder leads to disorganized, maladaptive reactions to and interactions with people and physical aspects of the environment. Such interactions may in turn, produce distorted internal sensory feedback, which reinforces related problems.[5] In many instances, dysfunctional behaviors that perhaps began as sensory overresponsiveness, if not ameliorated, can metamorphose into enduring psychosocial disorders.[45,69]

However, there are several subtypes of sensory processing dysfunction. Although individuals with SI or sensory processing dysfunction share many similarities, they do not all appear the same. Miller and colleagues (2007)[50] developed a helpful visual diagram called the Taxonomy of Sensory Processing Disorders (SPDs). They proposed using the term *SPD* to describe the sensory processing difficulties that impair daily routines or roles. The researchers noted that SPD should be distinguished from the SI Theory and intervention.[50] In collaboration with other occupational therapy (OT) scholars, they have classified SPDs into three categories: **sensory modulation disorders (SMD), sensory discrimination disorders,** and **sensory-based motor disorders.**[50] The categories are further divided into specific subtypes. SMDs and discrimination disorders can be found in one or more sensory systems in any affected individual, namely, vestibular, somatosensory, visual, auditory and olfactory/gustatory. Sensory-based motor disorders include the classically recognized patterns of postural-ocular disorder, bilateral integration/sequencing disorder, and three subtypes of developmental dyspraxia. These are explained in a later section.

Children may have SPDs comorbidly with a primary diagnosis such as autism, learning disability, or attention-deficit disorder; or they may have psychogenic comorbidities related to anxiety, panic, or attachment disorders. A range of levels of severity, from mild to quite severe, exist in SPD. In some children, sensory processing dysfunction may lead to disabling learning problems, causing academic failure.[5] In children with developmental dyspraxia or bilateral coordination challenges, it may be reflected in clumsiness and the struggle of the child to perform everyday occupations that others take for granted. Whereas some children may exhibit impairment in the ability to regulate incoming sensations, others may fail to detect and orient to novel or important sensory information. Together, overresponsivity and underresponsivity to sensory experiences are called SMD.[5,6,9,65,72]

Some types of sensory processing impairment may lead to poor social adaptation; the inability to form close, intimate relationships; and difficulty in expressing and interpreting socioemotional cues.[45] For example, a child with tactile overresponsivity may reject affectionate touch by family members and friends, which may detrimentally affect formation of attachment and friend relationships.[33,59] Difficulties with motor planning may cause awkwardness in skilled movements needed for both structured and unstructured play or may lead the child to be overcontrolling of peer-play situations. They may prefer social fantasy play, which they are better at than social physical play.[63]

Led by the pioneering work of Ayres, together with state and federal legislation supporting inclusive special education, occupational therapists have developed evaluation and treatment strategies for addressing sensory integration dysfunction in the early intervention, preschool, and school-aged populations since the early 1970s. Different strategies may be designed not only for direct treatment with the child, but those that can be implemented in the classroom by teachers, and in the home by family and caregivers. [6,9,31,42,58,65,68,75]

IMPACT OF SENSORY PROCESSING DYSFUNCTION ON INFANT AND EARLY CHILDHOOD OCCUPATION

The early signs of sensory processing problems can be observed even in infancy (Figure 25-1).[66] Parents often report that they have noticed subtle differences—such as lack of cuddling behavior, failure to make eye contact, oversensitivity to sounds or touch, difficulty with the oral-motor demands of suckling, and chewing food—as early as in the perinatal period (Figure 25-2).[46,74] Poor self-regulation of arousal states, irritability, and colic are frequently reported.[1,48,71] In the toddler period, the acquisition of motor, social, and self-care milestones may be delayed. The child may lack normal curiosity about the environment. On the other hand, the child may explore the world in a disorganized or destructive manner, which does not lead to learning and mastery. Figuring out basic whole-body movements, for example, climbing downstairs backward or climbing onto a riding toy, are bewildering and frustrating tasks, which the child may eventually avoid altogether.[64,66]

The preschooler with sensory-based motor planning problems may be unable to organize the body postures and gestures that are appropriate for nonverbal communication, such as the need for affection, to use the toilet, or to request a favorite snack.[63] Typically developing preschoolers can seem almost mesmerized with learning the process of dressing and will attempt the donning and doffing of clothes, shoes, and coats seemingly for hours at a time. However, the child with sensory-based motor planning deficits (called **dyspraxia**) may be dependent on caregivers for assistance and often avoids dressing and

hygiene activities altogether. He or she may handle toys and objects ineptly, constantly damaging or breaking them.

As the child attains school age, the heightened challenges of the elementary grades—sitting at a desk, paying

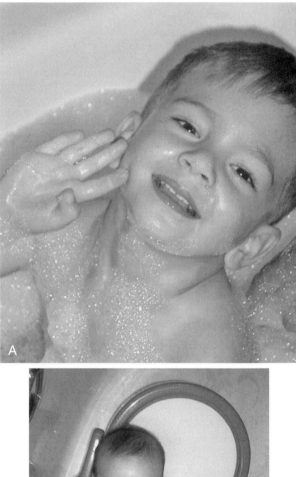

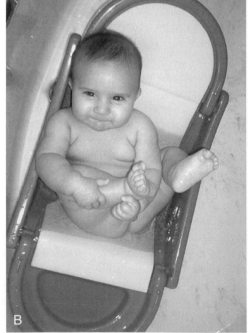

FIGURE 25-1 **A,** Typically developing children enjoy sensory experiences such as bath time. **B,** Typically developing infants enjoy the sensory experience of finding their feet and playing in the bath.

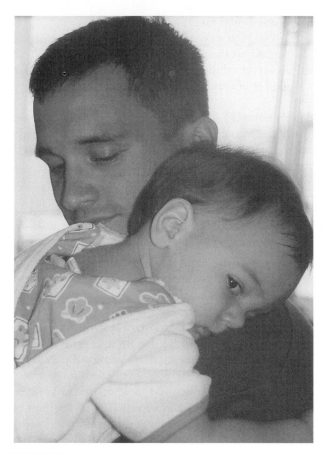

FIGURE 25-2 Whereas typically developing children gain comfort in being held closely by their fathers, those with sensory processing difficulties may find it discomforting.

attention in class, reading, listening, using writing and art tools, and interacting with peers—bring sensory processing dysfunction to light even more. During leisure time, the child may avoid fine manipulative activities or skilled gross motor play, instead preferring more sedentary activities such as watching television, playing electronic games, or looking at books (Figure 25-3). Highly creative and intelligent children may conceal their motor control inadequacies by engaging in verbal make-believe play, which emphasizes imagination and social interaction (with a lot of aimless running around) over toy manipulation and body coordination.

OT practitioners consider observations such as the above behaviors within the context of the child's family system, cultural expectations and norms, and socioeconomic advantages and limitations. As members of a team of professionals, they also use multiple sources of information from co-workers about the child's cognitive, language, and social development because these areas of function have significant effects on the quality of the child's adaptive behavior.[26] A child whose sociocultural and socioeconomic environments do not provide adequate opportunities for movement, exploration, and object play may be at additional risk, and may need

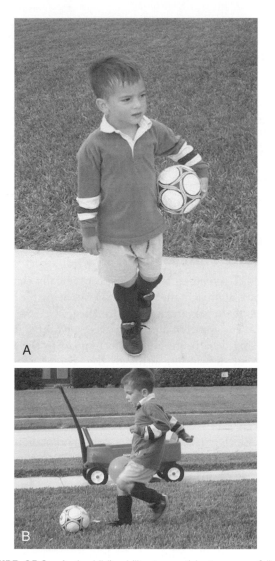

FIGURE 25-3 **A**, A child's ability to participate successfully in leisure/play activities such as soccer requires coordination, motor planning, sequencing, timing, and body awareness. **B**, The child shows adequate coordination, motor planning, sequencing, timing, and body awareness as he kicks the soccer ball in the desired direction.

environmental enrichment to facilitate the emergence of motor planning skills.[75]

WHAT CAUSES SENSORY PROCESSING DISORDERS?

The cause of sensory processing dysfunction remains unknown. However, the pace of neuroscientific investigation has increased greatly in the past decade, leading to support for many of Ayres' original hypotheses about the origins of SPD. First, as stated previously, we know that SPD/SI disorders are not caused by gross "injury" to the brain. In the past, this fact led to the supposition that SI dysfunction was not "real," because no findings could be detected on the imaging techniques available during

Ayres' lifetime. However, the overwhelming, repeated, and consistent standardized test results, together with the advent of advanced psychophysiologic and neuroimaging techniques, are pointing to dysfunction in the lower levels of the brain (as Ayres proposed), and at more "microscopic" levels having to do with synaptic regulation of nerve signals (termed *gating*)[30] through neurotransmitters;[61] or inadequate transmission of neural impulses due to poor integrity of the myelin sheath around nerves in key brain areas for multisensory integration.[57] As these important studies progress, the neurophysiologic basis for sensory processing disorders is gradually being revealed.

SCREENING AND ASSESSMENT OF SENSORY PROCESSING

Initial OT screening and evaluation typically employ a top-down approach, the first tier of focus being the child's daily occupational and role performance.[28,68] However, it may become apparent during this assessment that sensory processing deficits are major contributors to the child's functional difficulties, although the specific nature of the deficits cannot be delineated without further assessment. The OTA may be trained to physically administer a number of sensorimotor screening measures (such as caregiver or teacher questionnaires) and other structured assessments of sensory processing and/or motor performance. However, the interpretation of the results is performed by the occupational therapist, with the OTA providing important insights about the child. The OT practitioner will often collect this type of information on the children referred for OT because sensory processing dysfunction frequently contributes to the occupational performance difficulties for which children are referred, such as poor fine motor/handwriting skills, trouble with self-care tasks, social-emotional problems, or inability to participate in gross motor play activities with peers.

A very important part of the assessment process includes getting initial data from observations of the child by his or her caregivers, teachers, and/or other therapists. If the existence of a sensorimotor processing issue cannot be ascertained, the OTA and his or her supervisor may then decide to administer a standardized screening test. Based on the results of those two sources, an experienced team of OT practitioners may have enough data to formulate an intervention plan. Otherwise, a decision may be made to pursue more comprehensive evaluation of the child's capacities for sensory processing.[19]

A complete sensory processing evaluation typically covers five major areas:

1. Sensory modulation across each sensory system (i.e., tactile, vestibular, visual, auditory, olfactory (smell), and gustatory (taste);
2. Perceptual discrimination ability in most of these areas;

3. Postural-ocular function;
4. Bilateral motor coordination (including organization at and across the midline of the body); and
5. Praxis (the ability to internally visualize and plan skilled or unfamiliar movement actions).[4,15,40]

However, the OT supervisor may elect to focus on fewer areas if the initial OT assessment and SI screening indicate that certain areas are not problematic. The next section illustrates this process with a case study of a typical child referred for occupational therapy assessment.

Observational and History-Taking Assessment

Observation of the child in his or her natural environments is essential because not only can it identify areas in which sensory issues may be present, but it should also demonstrate how those issues affect the child's performance during daily occupational roles and tasks. The main concerns of the child, family, and others usually relate to difficulties with vital age-expected play skills, social activities, capacity for self-regulation, and academic learning that the child must master to grow up successfully. It is to these concerns that attention must be paid, and then, like peeling away the layers of an onion, the "why?" underlying those occupational challenges must be probed.

CASE *Study*

Jason's teacher reports that his letter formation is acceptable, but his handwriting movements are slow and laborious. He presses down so hard that he tears his paper or breaks the pencil lead. He stops frequently to shake or stretch his fingers and complains of pain in his hand. He slouches in his seat, and has trouble sitting in a stable position in his desk. Consequently, Jason fails to complete both classroom and homework written assignments on time, and his grades are suffering. His parents complain that it is a struggle each night at home to get Jason to begin and complete his written homework.

In this case the inability to complete handwritten assignments is the occupational activity that initially brought about the referral. However, assuming that other causes have been ruled out, sensory processing theory and research evidence can be used to analyze the qualitative nature of Jason's handwriting. From this, it can be hypothesized that Jason is receiving insufficient proprioceptive feedback from the joints and muscles in his fingers, so he must bear down harder on his pencil to obtain it, and this assists him in controlling and guiding the pencil. He is further hampered by low muscle tone in his trunk and shoulder girdle,

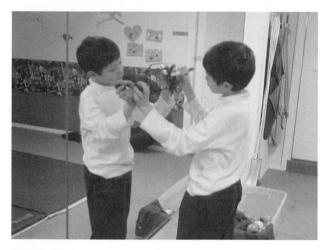

FIGURE 25-4 Children with sensory processing difficulties may experience poor body awareness. Standing while writing may help them become more aware of their bodies and movements. This child writes on a mirror, which also provides visual cues to help him.

which provide inadequate background stability to distal function in the hands, and he must expend extra energy just managing his sitting posture. This attempt to respond adaptively to his impairment slows Jason's progress and creates exceptional fatigue and discomfort in his hand and finger joints, as well as waning attention span. This hypothesis must then be tested by means of a sensory processing evaluation of Jason's somatosensory (tactile-pressure sense) system, as well as his vestibular-proprioceptive system, which is the sensory basis for regulating postural muscle tone. Hence, the reason why we refer to these as "sensory-based motor disorders."

The hypothesis concerning the contribution of sensory processing dysfunction will help shape one or more aspects of the intervention approach, which will probably include activation of Jason's vestibular and proprioceptive systems before seated handwriting activities. Therefore, when relating the SI assessment results to caregivers and other members of the team and in planning a course of intervention, the OT team must bring its interpretation of sensory processing issues full circle to explain concern about the child's occupational performance, which was the original source of the referral. Furthermore, either classroom or direct service interventions to address the underlying sensory processing issues will be recommended (Figure 25-4).

Multiple observation checklists are available for use in sensory processing assessment.[21] Some can be found in pediatric OT textbooks, whereas others are available for purchase from test publishers. Some checklists are informal and based on SI problem behaviors cited in the clinical literature rather than on norms derived from children of various ages. They can be used to gain informative data from teachers as well as caregivers. Such

tools can be helpful if used with the age range intended.[16] Two examples of such tools are the Sensorimotor History Questionnaire and the Teacher Questionnaire of Sensory Behavior (which are available on the accompanying Evolve learning site).[22,24,25]

Formal Assessment Tools

> **CLINICAL** *Pearl*
>
> Informal checklists, as in the examples given in the text above, should never form the entire basis of the conclusions made about a child's sensorimotor functioning.

Formal rating scales are based on knowledge of a child's developmental history and direct observation and are administered by trained professionals who know the child's behaviors, abilities, and preferences well. Such scales are often well researched and standardized on normative groups and fit into the class of SI screening instruments. A summary of them can be found in the literature, and some are described in Table 25-1.[18]

Comprehensive Evaluation of Sensory Processing/Integration

The most comprehensive standardized test battery of SI functioning for children aged 4 years to 8 years, 11 months is the Sensory Integration and Praxis Test (SIPT).[3] These tests include measures of vestibular, proprioceptive, and somatosensory processing; visual perceptual and visuomotor integration; integration between the two sides of the body and brain; and many of the components of the complex set of abilities known as praxis. The praxis tests include measures of postural imitation, motor planning in response to a verbal request, motor sequencing ability, imitation of oral movements, graphic reproduction, and three-dimensional block construction[3,8] (Figure 25-5).

Because of its complexity, only certain licensed rehabilitation professionals with a baccalaureate or graduate degree who have undergone documented rigorous training may administer the SIPT. To become more familiar with the various components of SI evaluation, pediatric OTAs should have a qualified SIPT examiner administer this instrument to them and engage in a reflective discussion of their experiences. This will provide valuable insights about both the process of SI and its assessment.

One of the most challenging aspects of the interpretation of SI and praxis evaluation data is the lack of a concrete one-to-one correspondence between a low score on a particular test and the meaning of that score. Invariably, the SI assessment is about discovering the underlying pattern of sensory disorganization that leads

TABLE 25-1

Summary of Screening or Structured Assessments of Sensory Processing and Sensory-based Motor Dysfunction

NAME OF SCREENING TOOL	STATED PURPOSE	INTENDED AGE RANGE
Test of Sensory Function in Infants[31]	Designed to measure an infant's sensory reactivity and processing to determine the presence and extent of the deficit	4–18 mo
The Infant/Toddler Sensory Profile[35]	By means of the parents' report, measures infant and toddler reactions to everyday sensory events across all modalities	Birth–36 mo
The Sensory Profile[34]	Measures child's responses to sensory experiences as well as perceived movement competence by means of the parents' report	3–10 y
The Short Sensory Profile[49]	A one-page questionnaire with 38 items divided into 7 sections; answers based on a 5-point scale	3–10 y
The Adolescent/Adult Sensory Profile[39]	Self-report; measures responses of teens through mature adults to sensory events in everyday life	11–90 y
The FirstSTEp Screening Test for Evaluating Preschoolers (Parent Checklists)[51]	General screening of major developmental areas, including several creative items of bilateral integration and praxis	2.9 to 6.2 y
The DeGangi-Berk Test of Sensory Integration[32]	A total of 36 items that measure overall sensory integration as well as postural control, bilateral motor integration, and reflex integration	3–5 y
The Miller Assessment for Preschoolers[52]	Broad overview of a child's developmental status; several indices assessing key areas of sensory integration performance	2.9 to 5.8 y
Clinical Observations of Sensory Integration[3] Clinical Observations Based on Sensory Integration Theory[11]	Informal floor assessment primarily assessing a child's postural reactions and oculomotor responses that are included in most neurologic screenings of soft neurologic signs	Various ages; recommended for approx. ages 5–10 y
Bruininks-Oseretsky Test of Motor Proficiency[14]	Both short screening and long evaluation forms included; measures a variety of gross and fine motor skills; includes many items for assessing bilateral coordination	4.6–14.5 y

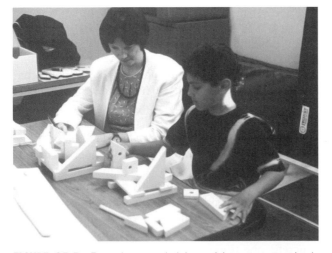

FIGURE 25-5 Formal tests administered by an appropriately trained occupational therapist provide measurable data about various aspects of sensory integration performance. (Photo courtesy of S. Stallings-Sahler.)

to poor performance in one or more functional "end products." In the typically developing child, these end products of well-integrated sensory systems can come in the form of success in functional motor skills such as riding a bicycle or using tools, academic learning skills such as reading and computation, cognitive abilities such as language and abstract thinking, or psychosocial capacities such as emotional attachment and self-esteem. It is the end products of SI that enable children to participate in age-appropriate occupational tasks and roles. However, between sensory organization and these end products there are also intermediate abilities termed *functional support capacities*.[47] **Functional support capacities** represent secondary neurobehavioral, motor, social-emotional, and cognitive proficiencies that are not functional in the occupational sense, but are considered precursors for end products to develop normally. A number of these are measured by the SIPT and other tests and include components such as self-regulatory mechanisms, postural tone, bilateral motor coordination, ability to cross the midline of the body, various subtypes of praxis, cognitive sequencing, and other intermediate-level capacities. Therefore numerous patterns of underlying dysfunction are possible; end product impairments are interpreted according to the way in which the SI and praxis test scores cluster.

CASE *Study*

Two 7-year-old children, Emma and Brian, present with severe handwriting problems along with other fine motor difficulties. However, their SIPT results are distinctly different. Emma's profile displays a low score on copying designs along with many low scores on visual and tactile space perception and low vestibular processing scores, but her scores on the motor accuracy and praxis tests fall within normal limits. By comparison, Brian's SIPT profile also shows a low score on copying designs, with vestibular function, visual, and tactile space perception scores in the normal range. However, his motor accuracy performance is poor, the scores on a number of praxis tests are low, and he has low scores on finger identification, touch localization, and kinesthetic perception.

Both these children had similar end product outcomes (i.e., poor design copying ability), yet their SI and praxis evaluations demonstrated significantly different underlying sensory processing and functional support pathways. Emma's pattern of scores suggests that her poor handwriting and design reproduction skills are probably attributable to impaired visual space perception resulting from poor integration of vestibular, somatosensory, and visual sensory input. On the other hand, disorganized motor planning, which is attributable to the inefficient processing of upper extremity proprioceptive input and a poor body scheme, is the hypothesized source of Brian's impaired handwriting.

Herein lies the difference between a sensory processing evaluation approach and a direct occupation-based assessment model. The former is based on an attempt to measure the underlying neuromotor and sensory mechanisms that support, like the foundation of a building, the function and occupation (in our example, poor handwriting). The latter approach documents and describes the nature of the occupational outcomes. Accordingly, OT interventions based on a top-down teaching strategy to address handwriting issues might look very similar for these two children. However, an SI approach would take the differences in underlying sensorimotor organization into consideration, and the SI treatment program for these two children would look quite different. It should also be noted that these two approaches are not mutually exclusive and probably should be used in tandem, with sensory integration strategies applied first

to prepare the CNS for the direct teaching of the desired occupational skill.

In summary, research using the SIPT as well as Ayres' earlier tests has demonstrated that

1. Various aspects of the components of sensory discrimination, bilateral motor organization, and motor planning tend to group together statistically to form predictable clusters;
2. Developmental trends can be identified in most SI constructs; and
3. Certain sensory systems integrate with one another to give rise to higher-order capacities in behavior and ability.[2,5,7]

With regard to the role of the additional neurobehavioral construct of sensory modulation, although Ayres originally identified the phenomenon of sensory registration disorders, which are now called SMDs, she died before she was able to pursue a more objective method of measurement of these disorders. Fortunately, others have taken up this area of work.[34,35,38,39,53-56,68,73] Research on psychophysiologic measurement has contributed significantly to our understanding in this area.[35,37-39,49,53,55,56,73,74]

SENSORY MODULATION DISORDER

When an OT practitioner hears terms such as **tactile defensiveness,** *gravitational insecurity,* **sensory-seeking,** and **sensory hypersensitivity,** he or she is exposed to some of the clinical language that refers to behaviors representing the class of sensory processing impairments termed *sensory modulation disorder*. Normal sensory modulation is a regulatory process of the CNS that controls the perceived intensity of incoming sensations through the raising or lowering of neuronal thresholds to that sensory input. This is achieved by means of adaptive balancing of inhibition and excitation at many levels of the CNS. Excitation of a neuron tends to lower its threshold to stimulation, thereby allowing more of the sensory input to be experienced in the nervous system. In contrast, if there is more inhibition, the neuronal threshold tends to rise, in effect partially or fully blocking the sensory input from being registered in a person's awareness. Your CNS is regulating sensations in this way as you read this chapter. If it did not, on the one hand, your brain might be so flooded with sensory messages that you would not be able to focus your attention, control your posture, or think about what you are reading. On the other hand, you might have such high sensory thresholds that you over focus, being unable to hear someone calling you from another room, feel a tap on your shoulder, or sense that your body is about to fall out of a chair.

This is only an imaginary taste of what life is like for people with sensory modulation dysfunction. However, some have sensory experiences that are so distorted that everyday sensations are uncomfortable, painful, frightening, or surreal in nature. A woman with agoraphobia and SMD reported to one of the authors that at times she would be walking on a concrete floor in a department store and suddenly feel as if the floor were soft and her feet were going through it, rather than striking the hard surface. At other times, she had trouble falling asleep because she felt as if bugs were crawling on her, or she was unable to get used to the sound of a clock ticking in another room. Children commonly manifest sensory modulation irregularities by their intolerance of such stimuli as clothing, food textures, imposed touch, and household noises (e.g., a phone ringing or an appliance running); or conversely, by not noticing salient stimuli in their environment. Probably the earliest harbinger of SI dysfunction in infancy is unusual overreactivity to touch, taste, or smell. Some forms of gastric reflux in infancy appear to be precipitated not by gastroesophageal abnormalities but by olfactory hypersensitivity, which causes the infant to become nauseous.[67]

Examples of hyper- and hypo-reactivity can be identified as you look through the Sensory History Questionnaire (SHQ) shared previously. Research in which the Sensory Profile and the Adolescent and Adult Sensory Profile were used revealed that children and adults develop behavioral patterns of dealing with their modulation problems, which have been described by Dunn in her model of sensory processing.[12,13,36,38] These patterns tend to divide into four quadrants that are bounded by a continuum of sensory avoidance to sensory seeking, and a continuum of acting in accordance with threshold, to acting to counteract threshold. We all fall within one of these quadrants, but dysfunction lies more at the extreme ends of the continua, where a person's daily life and relationships are more apt to be disrupted by modulatory irregularities. These patterns of sensory modulation are also associated with various types of temperament.[29,70] For more information on this, the reader is referred to the work of Dunn, Miller, Wilbarger, and associates.[35,36,51,56,58,60,65,74,75]

SENSORY-BASED MOVEMENT DISORDER

Sensory-based movement disorder refers to both postural system disorganization due to poor vestibular and proprioceptive processing, and impairments of complex midbrain or cortically controlled internal visualization and motor planning. Children who are found to have sensory integrative problems leading to **postural-ocular and bilateral integration dysfunction** typically manifest poor vestibular-proprioceptive processing, mild hypotonia, a delay in the development of postural and equilibrium reactions, and problems with midline integration. A more motorically involved child will usually exhibit a similar picture of immaturity in postural mechanism development but be compounded by a motor control

condition Ayres and others have termed *developmental dyspraxia*. Of these two conditions, the child with dyspraxia is usually identified more readily because of his or her obvious awkwardness and tendency to have more difficulties with play and acquisition of functional skills.

Postural-Ocular and Bilateral Integration Dysfunction

Of the two broad patterns of sensory-based motor dysfunction, this one is milder in severity. It may be identified by a cluster of several sensory, behavioral, and motor characteristics, including irregularities in sensory modulation; atypical ocular pursuits, convergence, and visual fixation; low duration of postrotary nystagmus; slow or irregular vestibular response to tilt; sluggish postural preferences for inactive positions and sedentary activities; impairments in midline crossing, and delayed establishment of lateral dominance after age 4 (Figure 25-6).[3,48,66]

Other related concerns frequently noted include poor protective, righting, and equilibrium responses during functional movement or clinical assessment; and immature gait patterns such as the use of a wide base, with lateral weight shifting of the lower extremities. To compensate for low extensor muscle tone in the upper body, shoulder girdle positioning may be marked by scapular retraction, scapular elevation, and high-guard arm posturing. (These postural patterns are typical in normal toddler and early preschool development but usually give way to mature

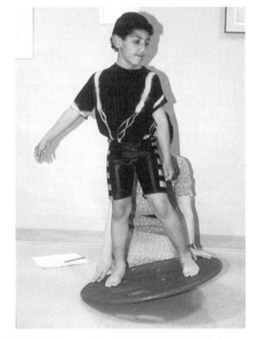

FIGURE 25-6 The quality of this child's equilibrium reactions when tipped on the tilt board provides a window into the integrity of his vestibular-proprioceptive processing. (Photo courtesy of S. Stallings-Sahler.)

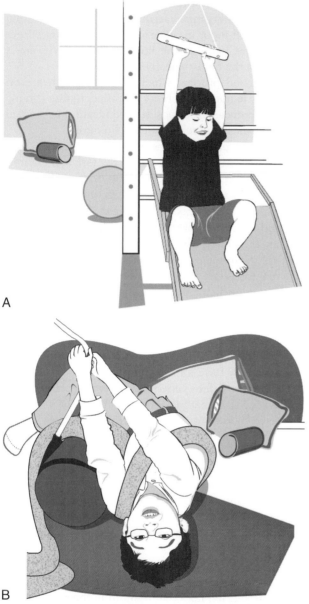

FIGURE 25-7 Children with postural-ocular and bilateral integration dysfunction have difficulty maintaining postures and using both hands together. **A,** The child uses both hands and plans how he is going to lift his legs, hold on, and move down the ramp. This requires processing of postural, vestibular, and proprioceptive information as well as timing and sequencing. **B,** A bolster swing requires postural control and bilateral integration.

postural organization, smooth bilateral-reciprocal movements, and normal lateral dominance during the period between the ages of 4 and 6 years[42,68] [Figure 25-7].)

Assessment of Posture, Ocular Functioning, and Bilateral Integration

Potential problems with postural adaptation can be observed during positions and active movement within the natural environment, as well as the performance of certain items from standardized child development or motor proficiency tests. In infancy, items from tests such as the Bayley Scales of Infant Development-II, the Peabody Developmental Motor Scales-II, and others help OT practitioners understand the child's performance (see Box 25-1 for a list of selected items).[10,43]

For example, the preschooler with low muscle tone and/or difficulties with balance, postural mechanisms, and bilateral coordination, as well as relative symmetry of left/right function may be identified from the items of the Miller Assessment for Pre-Schoolers listed in Box 25-2.[49] Three-year-olds who are at risk for postural and bilateral integration

BOX 25-3

Test Items to Observe Postural Adaptation in 3-Year-Olds

- Airplane
- Diadokokinesis
- Drumming
- Jump and turn
- Monkey task
- Prone on elbows; neck co-contraction
- Rolling-pin activity
- Scooter board co-contraction
- Side-sitting co-contraction
- Upper extremity control
- Wheelbarrow walk

BOX 25-4

Test Items to Observe Postural Adaptation for Postural-Ocular and Bilateral Coordination

- Balance items
- Bilateral coordination items
- Visuomotor control items
- Upper limb speed and dexterity items
- Strength (e.g., observations of postural tone during writing or manipulation tests, play)

deficits will experience difficulty with many items on the DeGangi-Berk Test of Sensory Integration, which are listed in Box 25-3.[32] The Bruininks-Oseretsky Test of Motor Proficiency-II contains many good postural-ocular and bilateral coordination items, which are listed in Box 25-4.[14]

In the child's natural environment or when allowed to explore and play freely in the clinic, postural impairments may be observed in low postural tone, a tendency to move in straight planes rather than using normal weight shifts and trunk rotation imbedded within equilibrium reactions, and difficulty handling changes in surface characteristics, all of which require intact combining of vestibular, proprioceptive and visual processing.[44,62]

Developmental Dyspraxia

Developmental dyspraxia disorder represents the second broad category of sensory-based motor dysfunctions. It is important to realize that children with cognitive impairments will usually have some degree of motor planning difficulty, which is part of the diagnosis of severe developmental delay and is consistent with their development across the board. However, in some cases, sensory processing deficits may also play a role along with the inborn condition. Three major processes are involved in praxis, and impairment in any of them can lead to dyspraxia.

The first and most fundamental process is the ability to register and organize tactile, proprioceptive, vestibular, and visual input in order to assemble accurate internal cognitive maps of the body and the environment with which the body typically interacts.

The second process, which is based on these constructions, requires the ability to conceptualize internal images of purposeful actions, termed **ideation** in the neuropsychological and rehabilitation literature.

The third process is the planning of sequences of movements within the demands of the task and environmental context, including the ability to program anticipatory actions within the next few seconds.

Impairment in praxis ability can occur anywhere within this neurodevelopmental chain of events. On the one hand, children who are most severely impaired lack even that internal visualization of what could be done with many objects. They typically also demonstrate poor registration of (i.e., failure to notice) sensory events. On the other hand, children who have only a planning problem know what could be done, but they cannot program the aspect of "how to do it." These children typically do not have poor registration (sensory hypo-reactivity); in fact, they may have an SMD in the direction of hyper-reactivity or defensiveness. Furthermore, they tend to have poor somatosensory perception of the body for use in motor planning (Figure 25-8). Ayres named the subtypes of developmental dyspraxia based on the hypothesized underlying sensory processing dysfunction associated with each one, in research conducted with the use of the SIPT, building on previous research with the Southern California Sensory Integration Tests.[3,9]

Ayres termed the most common subtype of dyspraxia *somatodyspraxia*. This disorder refers to praxis deficits that result from the inefficient processing of tactile-kinesthetic, proprioceptive, and/or vestibular sensory input within the body. A second type was termed *visuodyspraxia*, which reflects deficits in praxis that result from the poor processing of visuospatial cues, and affects one's ability to program movements in performing a visual construction task such as drawing designs, directing a pen along a line accurately, or building a three-dimensional structure with blocks. In some cases the child may have a combination of these two clusters; this condition is termed *visuo-somatodyspraxia*. A third type is called *dyspraxia on verbal command* and is the result of difficulty translating a verbal command into a motor plan; therefore, it is more language related. For this reason, Ayres proposed that this category of praxis dysfunction is the result of cortical-level left hemisphere dysfunction and is consequently not a true SI disorder, which is by definition subcortical in origin.[2,27,60]

Assessment of Praxis

Praxis difficulties can be observed during many exploratory, play, self-care, school, and physical education

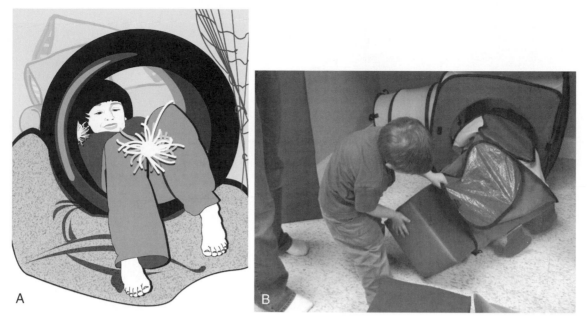

FIGURE 25-8 **A,** A child with developmental dyspraxia may benefit from understanding the concepts of "in and out" while rocking in a barrel. **B,** This child is trying to figure out how to arrange the materials in the tunnel so that he can move through it.

activities. Infants may display problems and frustration with simple adaptive movement responses that challenge their problem-solving abilities within the environment (i.e., "What do I do?"). Some examples might include an inability to figure out how to climb onto a riding toy, how to remove an irritating clothing item on the head, how to imitate simple gestures, or how to lead grownups to do something the child wants done (e.g., opening a door). Children aged 4 to 7 with dyspraxia may struggle to use tools and materials at school properly (e.g., during cutting, pasting, or coloring). They may actively avoid challenging motor planning tasks such as self-dressing, using eating utensils, and playing with manipulative toys; or they may avoid participating in gross motor activities and games requiring praxis ability.[60,66]

Besides the praxis tests of the SIPT, other developmental and motor tests have items that directly test praxis, or the child's quality of execution can be observed. However, as stated earlier, most other tests cannot provide information on underlying sensory processing. In infants, the Bayley Scales of Infant Development-II has the following relevant items:[10]

- Imitates hand movements
- Imitates postures
- Pats toy in imitation

Items on the Miller Assessment for Preschoolers, which are used to observe praxis qualities, include the following:[51]

- Imitation of postures

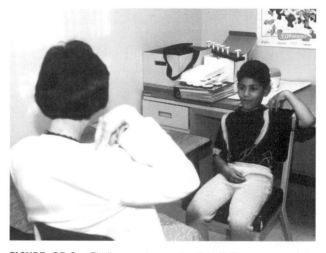

FIGURE 25-9 Challenges to postural imitation are used to assess this aspect of whole-body praxis. (Photo courtesy of S. Stallings-Sahler.)

- Items that require the child to follow the demonstration of the examiner (rapid alternating movements, kneel/stand, walk line, stepping)
- Maze
- Tower and block designs (constructional praxis)
- Block tapping (motor sequencing)
- Puzzle (visuoconstructional praxis)

As Ayres stated, "The child must organize his own brain; the therapist can only provide the milieu conducive in [sic] evoking the drive to do so. Structuring that therapeutic environment demands considerable professional skill"[3] (Figure 25-9).

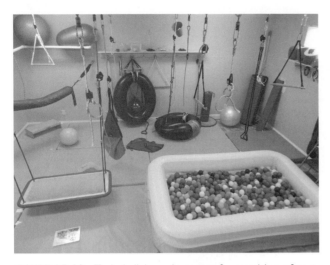

FIGURE 25-10 Typical clinic environment for provision of a variety of sensory integration treatment activities. (Photo courtesy of S. Stallings-Sahler.)

INTERVENTION
General Principles of Sensory Integration Intervention

The central principle of this intervention approach is the provision of controlled sensory input, through activities presented by the therapist, to elicit adaptive responses from the child, thereby bringing about more efficient brain organization (see Figure 25-7).[4] This latter result becomes observable in the increased organization of behavior, movement, and affective expression that is seen in the child. These diverse and multilevel responses are elicited within a rich environment that provides multiple, variable types of sensory experiences with the guidance of a skilled occupational therapist (Figure 25-10). Perhaps the most difficult aspect for new or untrained OT practitioners to comprehend is the absence of an SI "protocol" or "curriculum." (This aspect also needs to be explained carefully to both parents and teachers.) Nor is there a set protocol for treating each of the various types of SI dysfunction, although each type has its unique guiding principles. However, the results of the evaluation should provide the sensorimotor developmental road map that shapes the intervention plan.

SI intervention is centered on the child and guided by the OT practitioner; it is freedom within structure (Figure 25-11). The OT practitioner follows the child's lead but at the same time does not allow the child to run wildly around the treatment space. Nor does the OT practitioner present the child with a predetermined list of "what we are going to do today." How can this be? How do we reconcile these seemingly opposite concepts?

For example, let us begin with the challenge of a child who is running aimlessly around a room or area of a clinic, stopping briefly to look at or touch toys and

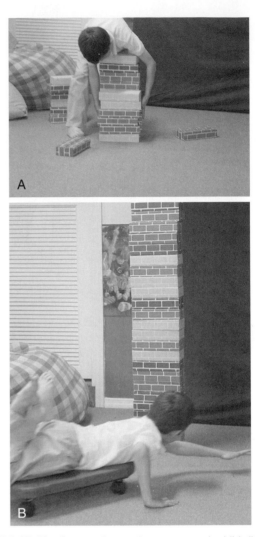

FIGURE 25-11 Sensory integration treatment is child directed and initiated. **A,** This child decides to build a block tower. **B,** The child chooses to knock the blocks down while riding a scooter. This activity provides proprioceptive and vestibular input to the child; it is child directed and fun.

equipment and then charging on to the next room or area. We might ask ourselves, "Is that a 'lead' I should be following?" The answer is yes and no. In this situation, the client is leading his therapist—or at least trying to communicate to him or her. The child is telling the therapist, "I am overstimulated, disorganized, and out of control. I don't know how to modulate and organize all of these novel sensations coming into my nervous system. I need you to help me self-regulate." The OT practitioner must then think critically (and quickly) about how to do this. The questions to consider should be: "What is overstimulating this child? Is the child seeking additional input? What types of sensory input would be calming and organizing to his nervous system? How can I get him to arrest this random running around, and instead channel that poorly directed drive into meaningful exploration and interaction?"

Frequently, the child innately knows what is "hard" for him or her, and will avoid these activities out of anxiety about failure; or lose focus quickly after only superficial engagement. In these cases, child and therapist may collaborate in creating a therapy plan before beginning intervention, where they take turns adding items to the list, with a prior agreement to follow the plan. This strategy provides the child with a sense of control, balanced with risk-taking to attempt the items chosen by the therapist (Figure 25-12).

The treatment of sensory processing disorders appears deceptively easy and playful because the OT practitioner is skilled in directing therapy procedures that are child-directed, active, and result in meaningful **adaptive responses** that promote better brain organization. This ability to "go with the client's flow" derives from the OT practitioner's knowledge of neurobiology; capacity to observe when the child is attempting to make an adaptive response to a challenge; and skill in knowing when to introduce novelty, equipment adjustments, or changes in task difficulty to make the challenges just right. This therapeutic artistry prevents the child from becoming frustrated if the activity is too difficult or bored if the activity is not sufficiently challenging.

CLINICAL *Pearl*

When an appropriately SI-trained and experienced pediatric occupational therapist is available only on a limited basis (or not at all), the certified OTA can contribute effectively to promoting sensory processing with practical intervention strategies.

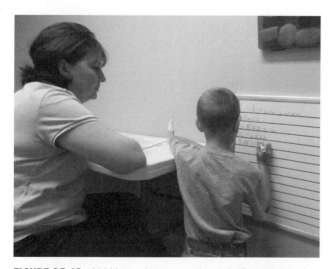

FIGURE 25-12 Writing a therapy session "plan" assists ideation, executive planning, and handwriting skill, while encouraging the child to take risks and share control with the therapist. (Photo courtesy of S. Stallings-Sahler.)

These strategies stand in contrast to the more structured "sensory-motor" or "perceptual-motor" programs often used in adaptive physical education. That type of intervention is typically technique-oriented and repetitive, places emphasis on end-product physical skills, and many times requires a more cognitive orientation on the part of the client. However, if used properly, these specially selected activities may still provide experiences that are rich in helpful sensory input and can be implemented in a variety of settings. Examples of these strategies and intervention activities are shown in Table 25-2 (adapted from Carrasco), as well as the ages and stages of typical development and the corresponding sensory processing levels proposed by Kimball.[20,47]

PROMOTING DIFFERENT LEVELS OF SENSORY PROCESSING AND MOTOR CONTROL
Facilitating Sensory Modulation

Just like intervention for other types of sensory processing disorder, the treatment of sensory modulation dysfunction follows similar guiding principles. Some suggestions are outlined in Box 25-5.[20]

As the child walks into the room, his or her arousal level can be determined by observing behaviors that provide clues about whether he or she is alert, tired, agitated, sleepy, wired, or some other state. This can help the OT practitioner decide whether the planned intervention is appropriate. If the child needs excitation, then it would be appropriate to provide arousing activities that incorporate jumping; fast movements on various swings, rotational or linear. Perhaps vigorous music of the child's choice might be selected, and energy and enthusiasm might be conveyed through the OT practitioner's own voice. Awareness of the child's arousal level tells the OT practitioner where to start, when to adjust, and whether to discontinue a certain activity or type of equipment.

However, if the child seems overaroused (as observed by engaging in random, disorganized, poorly directed activity), the practitioner provides sensory input that will promote healthy inhibition and nervous system organization. This might include rhythmic linear vestibular input on a swing or physioball, while the child engages in an oral-motor activity such as using a "chewie" or blowing bubbles. Generally, activities that promote midline orientation of trunk, upper extremities, oral structures, and eyes are calming and organizing. Sometimes, disorganized behavior can occur during a session and is usually the result of overstimulation and poor monitoring on the part of the OT practitioner. This requires a rebalancing of the child's nervous system by the OT practitioner before the end of the session (Figure 25-13).

If necessary, initial sensory preparation for the session may include methods such as the Wilbarger Protocol

TABLE 25-2

Intervention Strategies to Promote Sensory Processing and Related Developmental and Occupational Information*

LEVEL OF SENSORY PROCESSING	AGE/STAGE	DEVELOPMENTAL TASK	OCCUPATIONAL CHALLENGES	TREATMENT STRATEGIES FOR CLASSIC TREATMENT OF SENSORY PROCESSING DISORDER
Sensory modulation	First 2 y of life	Physiologic homeostasis; self-regulation of arousal and attention Attachment based on self-regulation Primary sensorimotor stage of learning, or learning through sensory input Adaptive reflex behavior to purposeful action Exploratory play	Irritability Poor sleep cycles Intolerance to being held or cuddled or exploring objects and people Poor tolerance to positional changes Frequent startling Slow development but usually within normal limits	Use inhibitory techniques to decrease heightened sensitivity down to levels of functional modulation, with activities rich in one of the following: slow, rhythmical movements; deep proprioceptive input; low-spectrum sounds; dim lighting; minimized environmental sensory input; low-pitched voice and tone. Employ excitatory techniques to alert the central nervous system, such as fast movements; higher and louder pitch of voice; fast, rhythmical sounds or music; light touch; and different textures and consistency of toys and walking surfaces. **Note:** Many individuals with sensory modulation disorder exhibit paradoxical behaviors and responses to treatment. Paradoxical behaviors are manifested when they show hyper-responsiveness to tactile input but hypo-responsiveness to vestibular input; their responses to inhibitory and excitatory strategies may also show such paradoxical behavior, so they respond with excitation when the occupational therapist's intention is for the input to be inhibitory. In such cases, close observation of a pattern of behavior is necessary so that appropriate changes in the strategies can be made as they happen. In such cases, consultation with a supervising occupational therapist trained in sensory integration is warranted.
Continuous sensory modulation	Preschool	Automatic self-regulation Integration of both sides of the body Crossing the midline of the body Development of body scheme Development of gross motor planning Imagination expressed through pretend play	Short attention span Clumsiness Poor articulation Over- or underreaction to slight injury Fear of playground equipment and some walking surfaces (e.g., sand or plush carpet) Very messy and picky eater No awareness of danger and avoidance of novelty Avoidance of peers; a tendency to play with much older or younger children	While conducting activities that promote sensory modulation (i.e., inhibition and facilitation), include those that promote the foundation for the ocular and bilateral integration, balance reactions, and body scheme. Helpful strategies include the use of controlled sensory input that taps the proximal senses (vestibular and somatosensory, especially deep proprioceptive input that includes those of neck proprioceptors and extraocular muscles), which form the foundation for the work of the more distal senses, such as vision and hearing. These strategies should involve the active participation of the child in gross and fine motor activities that require the use of the entire body or parts thereof while moving through space and playing with a variety of objects that he or she can move, manipulate with the fingers, inspect with the eyes, make sounds with, or use some other sense.

TABLE 25-2

Intervention Strategies to Promote Sensory Processing and Related Developmental and Occupational Information—cont'd

LEVEL OF SENSORY PROCESSING	AGE/STAGE	DEVELOPMENTAL TASK	OCCUPATIONAL CHALLENGES	TREATMENT STRATEGIES FOR CLASSIC TREATMENT OF SENSORY PROCESSING DISORDER
Sensory discrimination	Early school age, 5–7 y	Increased skill in differentiating the qualities and characteristics of sensations, such as the intensity, degree, volume, and direction of sensory input Increased fine motor planning Establishment of dominance (lateralization) Flexible social and peer play	Fine motor problems Hyperactivity (often associated with sensory seeking) Impulsiveness Dislike or avoidance of textures in food (lumps), activities (finger painting), and clothing (labels or seams, softness) Difficulty in gross motor activities, with falling or avoidance Accidentally breaks toys or is rough playing with objects or peers	Although system-specific sensory input is useful, a strategy that also provides multisensory input is helpful. The novelty and variety of sensory input provide challenges in differentiating and remembering such qualities as sound, distance, texture, color, movement, and taste but also in categorizing and organizing as well as other challenges. Use activities that promote sensory discrimination during but especially at the end of the treatment session.
Sensory-based movement disorder—postural-ocular and bilateral integration disorder	School age and up (7 y and older) Continued in next age/stage level	Increased abstract thinking Academics More sophisticated tool use Competence in complex skills dependent on previous phases Games with rules and competition	Increased academic problems frequently associated with attention and frustration Poorly or compulsively organized Reversals in writing Continued clumsiness with poor sequencing of tasks Self-esteem problems "Splintered" skills (i.e., lack of generalization ability) Trouble keeping up with peers in activities (especially motor based—slower)	Observe to monitor sensory modulation and behavior regulation that may be expressed as inattention or diminished frustration tolerance and endurance. Provide a balance of movement challenges that incorporate flexional, extensional, and rotational components, preferably during activities that require the child to move the whole body or, when seated at a table or the floor, the arms through space. Infuse the session with experiences that require the crossing of one arm across the midline. Also include activities that require the use of both sides of the body, especially but not only the hands with guidance by the eyes and with one side of the body performing independently or in collaboration with the other.
Sensory-based movement disorder Developmental dyspraxia	Starts with previous level and continues into adolescence and adulthood	Continuation of previous level Concern with physical relationships Team sports Establishing identity Career choice Leisure preferences	Organizational problems (e.g., time management) Trouble finishing homework or tasks started Immature physical skills and social relationships Increased dependence Loses or forgets things May be socially isolated Avoids team sports or chooses heavy contact sports	Observe to monitor sensory modulation. Provide challenges that require active participation in following verbal, written, or other types of directions for task performance and participation such as the construction of two-dimensional end products (e.g., drawings, written work) or three-dimensional constructions (e.g., block towers, obstacle courses). Provide multiple experiences that require the execution of gross, fine, oral, and visuomotor tasks with projected action sequences or those tasks that require planning of movement to hit targets.

*See level-specific treatment guidelines in the following sections.

Adapted from Kimball, J. G. (1993). Sensory integration frame of reference. In P. Kramer & J. Hinojosa (Eds.), *Frames of reference for pediatric occupational therapy*. Baltimore, MD: Lippincott Williams and Wilkins; Carrasco R. C., Sahler S. S. (2005). Sensorimotor history questionnaire—research edition, Winter Park, FL: Fiestajoy Foundation, Inc.

BOX 25-5

Tips for Facilitating Sensory Modulation

- Determine arousal level.
- If necessary, use stimulation protocols.
- Identify the target sensory system(s).
- Monitor cognitive, affective, and physiologic responses to sensory processing demands.
- Compare the consistency of observed behaviors.
- Employ novelty.
- Influence the threshold level.
- Monitor signs of sensory overload or shutdown behaviors.
- Facilitate a balance between seeking and avoiding behaviors and contextual reality.
- Facilitate behavior regulation.
- Prescribe a sensory diet.

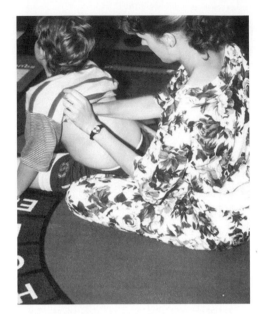

FIGURE 25-14 Therapist promotes the child's initial self-regulation in a treatment session by administering the Wilbarger Protocol, a procedure combining pressure-touch brushing and joint compressions designed by Patricia Wilbarger, M.Ed., OTR/L. (Photo courtesy of S. Stallings-Sahler.)

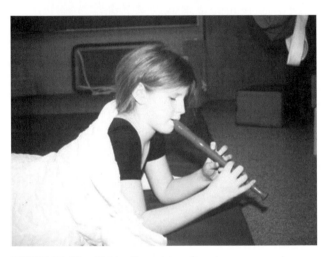

FIGURE 25-13 Child self-regulates after vigorous, arousing vestibular play by engaging in the oral-motor activity of playing a recorder while lying under a weighted blanket. (Photo courtesy of S. Stallings-Sahler.)

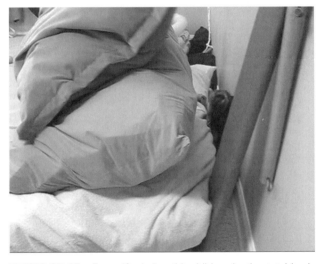

FIGURE 25-15 For self-calming, this child seeks the total body deep pressure provided by a stack of crash pillows. (Photo courtesy of S. Stallings-Sahler.)

if the OT practitioner is correctly trained. If not, the OT practitioner should obtain appropriate training and supervision and emphasize to the family that the protocol needs to be followed consistently at home according to instructions (Figure 25-14). Occupational therapists are increasingly incorporating one of the several auditory integration programs that are now available into their vestibular swing-based intervention. Otherwise, simply being aware of the relative excitatory or calming properties of sound and music, and using them appropriately in a session supports adaptive arousal levels. For example, children often enjoy hearing calming "nature sounds" and receiving total-body deep pressure while lying between two large crash pillows (Figure 25-15).

The focus of sensory processing intervention is aimed toward the organization of multiple sources of sensory input. The focus is also on the lower brain processing of vestibular input integrated with proprioceptive and visual inputs, making it important to identify the target sensory system(s). Ayres proposed that the vestibular system was a major integrator of other senses, and had a significant influence on overall modulation. Pumping a bolster swing to move forward and backward while making postural adjustments in sitting not only provides vestibular input, but also integrates proprioception in the neck, trunk, and eyes. This integration of sensations paves the way for postural integration as well as conjugate eye movements that are necessary for fine and visual-motor activities. However, some behaviors that suggest sensory modulation dysfunction are system specific, such as sensitivity to touch, taste, sights, movement, and smells.

Although movement is a commonly observed end product of efficient sensory processing, the OT practitioner should also monitor cognitive, affective, and physiologic responses to sensory processing demands on an ongoing basis. Sweating, paleness, and other autonomic signs of distress indicate that the sensations being introduced are overwhelming, and the activity should be discontinued. This is always the risk when OT practitioners provide too much passive stimulation to the child without appropriately eliciting adaptive responses that would help the child organize the sensory input.

Cognitive and emotional responses are also helpful windows through which the child indicates whether or not the sensory experience is meaningful. Holding on tightly for comfort when placed on moving therapeutic equipment is an indication that the child is afraid—of the equipment, the rocking, perhaps the OT practitioner, or simply being away from the caregiver. Frustration and anger in the child can be the result of the inability to figure out what has to be done because the task is too difficult; boredom and lethargy can result if the task is too easy.

Behaviors related to hypersensitivity as well as hyposensitivity to sensory input can vary between what is observed at home and in other settings, such as the school or the clinic. These patterns of responsivity can also fluctuate within the same day or from day to day. Ideally, the response would be similar in all settings; so, for example, sensitivity to food textures would be similar at home and in school during snack time. Compare the consistency of observed behaviors; if they are not consistent, consider giving the parents and teachers some tips on how to handle the child who may be manipulative. Sometimes, while observing family dynamics, sleeping and eating patterns may provide information on how to manage SMD. For example, the parents might be able to distinguish between intolerance of certain foods and their child's attempts at controlling the situation or seeking attention, especially if such behaviors are not evident in other contexts such as the school or with grandparents. In these cases, consistency of behavior management together with sensory processing interventions is appropriate.

The introduction of new toys, sounds, smells, and even movement on a swing provides novelty to the interaction and elicits vigilance to new incoming sensations. Employing novelty does not necessarily mean changing the equipment (the toy) or, in the case of a writing activity, the size, shape, and color of the pen or the smell of the ink or the sound that the pen makes with pressure. For some children, too much novelty can be overwhelming,

so it is helpful to introduce novelty in measured ways, embedded in familiar activities to make it more readily acceptable by the child.

Whether the thresholds to sensation are too high or too low, the goal of intervention is to influence and bring them into a range of adaptive homeostasis. Monitor the child's behaviors that suggest the need to raise or lower thresholds, depending on whether he or she withdraws from, seeks, or responds slowly to sensations. Provide activities that provide repetition of similar tasks requiring or producing similar sensations, for example, swinging a ball or throwing it at a target, and sliding down outdoor equipment and ending up in a circle on the sandbox.

While engaging in the above activities, introduce changes in the sequence and other components of the activity to detect signs of sensory overload or shutdown behaviors such as purposeless running around, losing track of the end goal of an activity, a glassy-eyed expression, or simply suddenly becoming quiet, retreating to a corner, or even seemingly falling asleep. Introducing the changes can result in sustained interest and maintained vigilance, thereby influencing attention and purposeful interaction with the environment.

Seeking and avoiding behaviors are often considered "normal" at home but negative in school. Communication with teachers, family members, and OT practitioners is essential, especially when recommending environmental adaptations such as movable seating cushions, wedges, or ball chairs; "fidget" toys; a mini-trampoline in the classroom; or frequent movement breaks for the child. This communication will help facilitate a balance between seeking and avoiding behaviors and contextual reality. Rather than depriving the child of recess as punishment for "disruptive" behaviors, urge teachers to allow the child to go outside to engage in a structured physical activity, such as doing calisthenics or running a lap around the playground (adjusted for age and maturity of the child, of course). This way, the child gets the movement or the vestibular sensory diet he or she needs in order to stay organized for the remainder of the day but still receives a reasonable consequence for the disruptive behavior (Figure 25-16).

The OT practitioner can facilitate behavior regulation by providing different levels of emotional engagement within a session, offering rewards as needed and progressing from immediate to delayed gratification. The OT clinician can provide experiences in detecting not only changes in verbal expression of emotion but also nonverbal communication through body language and facial expressions. This may be through imaginative play experiences or indirectly through role playing with toys or other technology. The OT practitioner can infuse sessions with experiences in detecting changes in feelings about what is going on during the session and the ability to label such feelings.

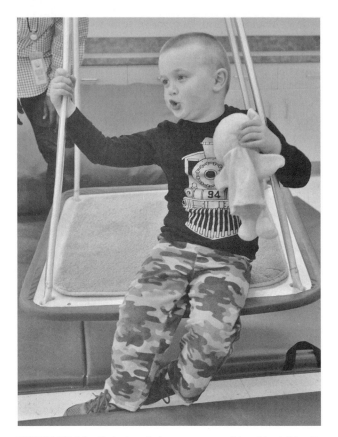

FIGURE 25-16   Swinging during recess provides this child with proprioceptive and vestibular input, integrated with a motor planning challenge, which may help him stay organized when he returns to class.

Tips for Promoting Sensory Discrimination

- Look out for indicators of current or residual modulation disorder.
- Raise modulation level to awareness.
- Identify the sensory "on ramp."
- Infuse activities with controlled novelty.
- Use a variety of materials to infuse novelty.
- Grade complexity of sensory input and adaptive responses.
- Be alert to affective responses.
- Intervene when difficulty comes with diminished visual inspection.
- Keep track of visual dependence, and intervene when its presence or absence is observed.
- Select activities that challenge visual discrimination.
- Provide challenging, age-appropriate, fun activities with intrinsic recognition, matching, and categorization of textures, shapes, sizes, or other characteristics of the object.
- Provide opportunities for auditory localization, sequencing, and figure-ground.
- Challenge localization of sensations.
- Provide opportunities for discrimination abilities.

The OT clinician can prescribe a program of activities that provides sensory experiences on a regular basis (i.e., a **sensory diet**). It may come in the form of a schedule that includes engaging in activities upon awakening in the morning or modulating the nervous system to a more adaptive level when returning home from the day-care center or the school. The sensory diet can include activities designed with and/or provided to the school or family. The activities consider the child's sensory needs on the basis of a comprehensive assessment and diagnosis of SMD but should include a variety of experiences to give the child the opportunity to participate as fully as possible without being threatened by the activities.

Suggestions for Promoting Sensory Discrimination

A summary of suggestions for promoting sensory discrimination for children who have sensory discrimination dysfunction can be found in Box 25-6.

It is important to observe the child for indicators or behaviors that suggest difficulty with sensory modulation or indicate current or residual modulation disorder, such as dyspraxia or postural-ocular and bilateral integration dysfunction. Even when the goals and activities are designed to promote sensory discrimination, it is likely that unresolved or residual SMD will come to the surface; this may be due to several factors, such as the novelty of the activity, stress, the event(s) that happened the previous night or on the way to the clinic, and due to health problems. When this happens, aim for functional modulation and proceed with caution toward your sensory discrimination goal.

Allow the child to be aware of his or her need to seek sensory input (e.g., the reason for the pencil grip, the purpose of the "fidget" toy, the wedge on the chair) as appropriate for age. By raising the modulation level to awareness, the child will hopefully understand and become an active participant in the therapy process.

Although the OT program may be very specific, identify the sensory "on ramp," such as visual versus tactile discrimination goals. The sensory on ramp, or the sensory system that you access to introduce activities, may differ from the goals prescribed by the OT program. For example, the child may be in a vestibular seeking mode when your goal is visual. In this case, activities that provide vestibular input such as running or swinging on the playground may be used as a starting point of the therapy session, but at the same time, visual activities that may in themselves have

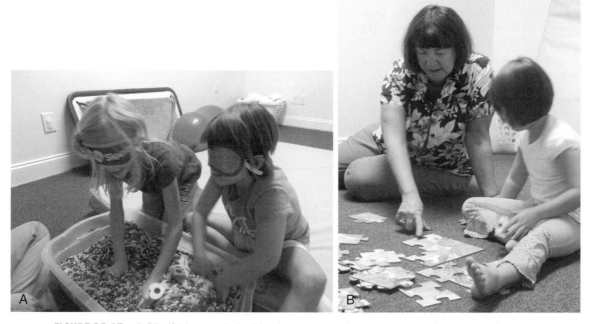

FIGURE 25-17   **A**, Blindfolds to occlude vision increase attention to manual tactile cues used for locating puzzle pieces in a beans-and-rice bath. **B**, The prior task is followed by collaborative assembly of a floor puzzle by these children. Cognitive perceptual tasks are developmentally appropriate at the end of an OT session, after activities to promote sensory integration. (Photos courtesy of S. Stallings-Sahler.)

discrimination components to them may be provided as well (Figure 25-17).

With new sensory input introduced into the sensory experiences, the OT practitioner can promote the detection of new sensations and vigilance for new experiences to come. Infusing activities with controlled novelty is similar to the way in which novelty is effective in managing SMD, only this time it is infused with opportunities to refocus on the variety of the qualities and characteristics of sensations. Additionally, novel activities should be approached with a variety of materials but not at the expense of needed continuation as expressed or observed.

The OT practitioner grades the complexity of sensory input and adaptive responses by matching the child's baseline arousal and processing levels with the sensory components of selected activities and the complexity of the responses expected. As necessary, the demands of the activity should be lowered or raised in relation to the equipment used (e.g., a platform, rather than a bolster or dual-sling swing [Figure 25-18]) or the complexity of the toys used (e.g., limiting the Jenga game pieces to 20 instead of 45).

It is important to observe the child for changes in affect, which serve as indicators of emotional responses to the sensory environment and include reactions to interaction and task demands, and be alert to other affective responses. Observation of the endurance level as well as frustration tolerance, problem solving, and creativity is critical to guiding the intervention session. The OT practitioner

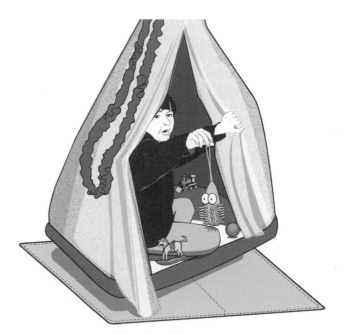

FIGURE 25-18   Swinging on a platform swing provides vestibular and proprioceptive feedback to children. This game requires that the child make adaptive responses in order to pick up tactile toys and place them in a container while moving. The covering over the swing helps calm the child so he is more able to tolerate tactile items. This activity requires timing; sequencing; motor planning; extension through the trunk, shoulder, and elbow; and visual attention.

adjusts the bar as necessary, raising or lowering it for challenges accordingly. It is recommended the reader refer to the BRAINS (Behavior Regulation through Activities for the Integration of Novel Sensations) approach for infusing sensory processing treatment with socioemotional strategies for additional information.[17,23]

When difficulty comes with diminished visual inspection, especially of items that are manipulated, smelled, tasted, or some other sensation, intervention should be provided with reminders, for example, when manipulating zippers, guiding a spoon to the mouth, perceiving when clothing is twisted, finding items such as coins in pockets, or manipulating small objects and tools without vision (e.g., a pencil, spoon, screwdriver). In addition to observing diminished visual inspection, keep track of and intervene when you observe visual dependence, or a lack thereof as in the above situations, or when identifying which body part has been touched when vision is occluded, differentiating smells and tastes without visual cues, or being alert to what certain smells mean, such as burning or gas leaks.

Activities in which letters can be easily reversed or inverted—as in the case of p, b, and q—can be used as selective activities that challenge visual discrimination. Other activities include those that challenge the child to match, recognize, and categorize items according to their qualities such as color, texture, shape, and size and to quickly scan visual images in sequence and those that provide challenges to connect dots, write between lines, play hopscotch, or piece a floor puzzle, all of which demand visual guidance of fine and gross motor movements.

It is recommended that the OT practitioner provide challenging, age-appropriate, fun activities with intrinsic recognition, matching, and categorization of textures, shapes, sizes, and/or other object characteristics, as well as experiences that are rich not only in recognizing symbols and gestures and perceiving depth, distance, the location of borders, boundaries, and spaces between objects but also in differentiating foreground from background images, closure of shapes, and pictures.

Challenge the child to localize sounds, sights, smells, and other sensations by differentiating and remembering similar words and sounds, for example, pat/pack and mitt/meat. Other suggested activities include following instructions with multiple steps and judging the source of a sound, such as turning in the direction of the person calling as well as recognizing the sound of a drum when it competes with the background noise of a toy flute. These activities provide opportunities for auditory localization, sequencing, and figure-ground.

The OT practitioner offers opportunities during and after the session to apply discrimination abilities to ensure their translation into occupations, for example, maintaining balance while taking a shower with the eyes closed or drying the feet with a towel while standing up, maneuvering the body through tight spaces such as in

BOX 25-7

Tips for Remediating Sensory-Based Movement Disorder

- Identify presenting problem(s).
- Promote improved organization of somatosensory body scheme.
- Promote symmetry as well as asymmetry by means of the efficient use of a preferred versus nonpreferred extremity.
- Determine the difficulties and strengths of the practice component(s).
- Infuse the program with constructional activities.
- Infuse the activities with projected action sequences of different types.
- Challenge actions from ideas and images.
- Challenge the ability to learn and smoothly execute new movements.
- Include activities that challenge mouth and tongue movements in coordination with respiration.

an obstacle course, and writing with appropriate pressure on the paper or chalkboard.

Intervention for Sensory-Based Movement Disorders

Many children referred for the treatment of sensory-based movement disorder are also referred for such reasons as fine motor evaluation, writing problems, and delayed development, but rarely for the underlying sensory processing problems. It is therefore important to identify the presenting problem by linking it to the underlying sensory processing deficit through assessment and historical review. By doing so, foundational intervention, sensorimotor treatment, and environmental adaptation can be designed.

For sensory-based movement disorder, promote improved somatosensory body scheme organization with activities such as whole-body playing in a plastic ball bath; rubbing cream/lotion on different parts of the body while discussing each one; brushing oneself with a paintbrush or other type of brush; drawing the silhouette of a body on a long sheet of paper; crawling through a Lycra fabric "tube" while discussing which parts are passing through it; learning to hop-scotch to different patterns on the floor; putting on a new article of clothing; and positioning and adjusting the body on a scooter board, a swing, or even a chair. A summary of remediation for sensory-based movement disorders can be found in Box 25-7 (Figure 25-19).

If the child is hesitant or unable to self-propel a selected swing, the OT practitioner can direct the swing in a direction, speed, or rhythm that would bring about the child's excitation, inhibition, or participation in a purposeful activity as desired. When initial activation of the swing

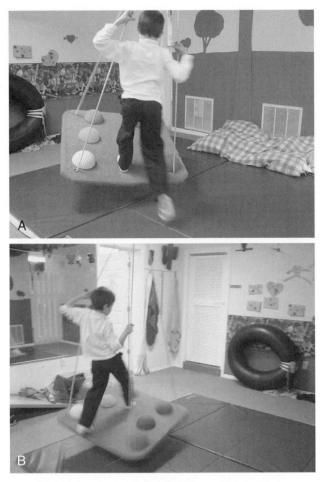

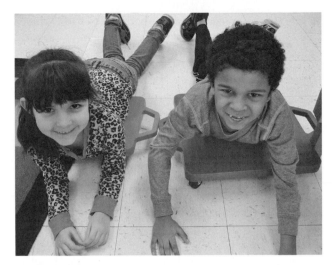

FIGURE 25-20 These children propel themselves on the scooter using bimanual and sometimes bipedal manipulation, which encourages independent and cooperative use of two hands and two feet. This also requires children to effectively sequence and time movements.

FIGURE 25-19 **A,** This child uses the platform swing to challenge his balance and timing. He pretends that he is on a spaceship and must deflect the meteors by hitting them with a "scientific deflector." Children with sensory integration dysfunction may be very creative. OT practitioners can use this creativity to make intervention sessions fun and interesting. **B,** The OT practitioner is able to provide the "just-right" challenge to this activity by controlling the speed of the spaceship (platform swing) and the location of the deflectors (objects to be thrown) and meteors (targets).

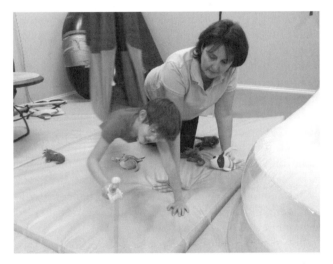

FIGURE 25-21 Prone activities with intermittent linear swinging facilitate this child's vestibular-visual-proprioceptive integration, needed for functional hand use. (Photo courtesy of S. Stallings-Sahler.)

by the OT practitioner is necessary, he or she should nevertheless use clinical procedural reasoning to ask, "How can I facilitate the child's active engagement in this activity?" Sometimes the answer is to sit with, or behind, the child on the swing, assist the child to place and maintain the hands on the ropes or handles, and enable the child to propel the swing with increasing independence.

Tasks that require bimanual manipulation promote symmetry as well as asymmetry by means of the efficient use of a preferred versus nonpreferred extremity. Bimanual or bipedal manipulation encourages the independent as well as cooperative use of two hands or two feet, respectively, such as clapping games, card games, drawing, and sewing (Figure 25-20). Likewise, watch out for overflow movements in the oral area as well as on the opposite side of the body.

Provide challenges to determine the difficulty and/ or strength of the praxis component(s) by asking, "Can you show me a different position to move this swing?" "Can you show me a different way to ride on this scooter board?" or "Can you go through the obstacle course backward?" Such challenges indicate whether the praxis components are cognitive or motor. Include manual motor planning activities, such as making an origami crane, which requires deciding what to do, what sequence to follow, and how to position and move the fingers and paper to accomplish the task (Figure 25-21).

Infuse the program with both two- and three-dimensional constructional activities such as writing, drawing, and block construction, in order to challenge visuopraxis, creativity, and problem solving. Ask the child to creatively determine how to put together objects and materials for play/leisure activities and school/work projects. "Construction" also implies the ability to organize one's belongings and objects in one's environment. "Cleanup time" should be an integral part of the close of every treatment session, as this activity engenders not only organizational ability in the child but also a sense of responsibility and respect for others' belongings that are enjoyed by the child. Challenge 7-year-old clients to design their own obstacle courses during occupational therapy. They may first draw a map of the course on a sheet of paper (two-dimensional construction), then build it (three-dimensional construction), with Socratic questioning and cueing from the OT practitioner. Also, encourage parents to help the child organize his or her own spaces at home, such as the bedroom and/or playroom. Assist the child with developing language and reading/labeling skills and self-organization by having him or her label shelves, drawers, baskets, or room areas with appropriately worded cards or stickers, for example, "Books," "Movies," "Dolls," "Cars and Trucks," "Games," and so on.

Prepare activities with projected action sequences of different types; for example, have the child hit or "latch onto" a target with the force of his or her whole body, with something that is thrown, or have the child draw lines to a target while being aware of cognitive, motor, and affective abilities. Actively engage the child in organizing a series of actions to produce an intentional movement or in figuring out how to do something familiar yet different, such as writing his or her name with the nondominant hand or (more difficult) writing the word "Saskatchewan" spelled backward.

To encourage the development of ideational praxis, design activities that challenge the formulation of actions from ideas and images. Ask the child to perform or translate ideas or images into verbal descriptions, interactions, or products, during play, at school, or at home (e.g., making a kite from a list of materials). Ask the following question: "How would you 'drive' a bolster swing if it were a school bus, spaceship, race car, fishing boat, or some other mode of transportation?" Assist the child to figure out how to play new games or put things together by organizing a series of actions as needed, by asking, "How can we use the equipment to build things like a fort, a spaceship docking station, an igloo, or a Polly Pocket house?" (Figure 25-22).

Fine motor planning can challenge the ability to learn and smoothly execute new movements. Ask the child questions such as: "Can you swing, let go, and land in the big pillow?" "Can you ride your elephant over here and roll over into the hay?" Some activities to challenge fine motor planning include movements required in making

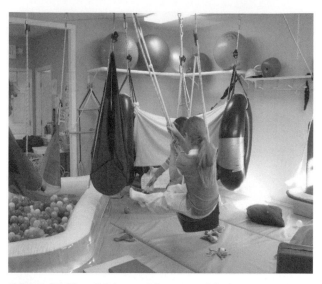

FIGURE 25-22 Children collaborate socially in construction of a "pirate ship" then use play and motor planning skills to move among the different "decks." (Photo courtesy of S. Stallings-Sahler.)

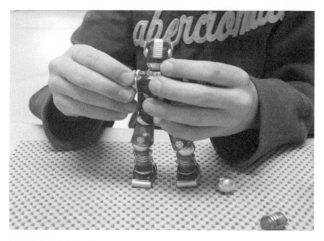

FIGURE 25-23 Fine visual-motor play is enhanced by a foundation of organized sensory processing, laid earlier in the session. (Photo courtesy of S. Stallings-Sahler.)

Mexican "Ojos de Dios" ("God's Eyes"), holiday-themed dream catchers out of colored pipe cleaners; yarn-and-stick projects; origami; simple knots of macramé; or cutting pictures for a scrapbook. Playing with action figures or models also promotes motor process sequencing, constructional praxis, and acceptance of sensory experiences (Figure 25-23).

Include activities that challenge mouth and tongue movements in coordination with respiration, such as those required when eating foods of different textures, sucking sour candy or popsicles, blowing bubbles, blowing cotton balls or ping pong balls across the floor while lying prone on a scooter board, playing wind instruments such as a toy flute, blowing special whistles, and making appropriate facial gestures during interaction.

SUMMARY

This chapter presented a basic review of sensory integration theory, assessment, and intervention strategies. OT practitioners first assess the child's sensory processing abilities and determine the underlying causes for occupational performance deficits. Intervention techniques include following the child's lead and introducing vestibular, proprioceptive, and tactile activities so that the child is challenged to make an adaptive response. The art of occupational therapy includes designing interventions that look like play and in which the child is engaged, whereas the science of occupational therapy involves understanding the neurobehavioral basis of the interventions and outcomes. Explanations of the child's behavioral responses to processing of sensory information to family members and teachers help them understand and help the child participate in daily activities. The chapter provided clinical questionnaires and tips to help OT practitioners design interventions that will be meaningful and fulfilling for the child.

References

1. Als, H. (1986). A synactive model of neonatal behavioral organization: framework for the assessment of neurobehavioral development in the premature infant and for support of infants and parents in the neonatal intensive care environment. *Phys Occup Ther Pediatr, 6,* 3–4.
2. Ayres, A. J. (1989). *Manual: sensory integration and praxis tests.* Los Angeles: Western Psychological Services.
3. Ayres, A. J. (1972). *Integration and learning disorders.* Los Angeles: Western Psychological Services.
4. Ayres, A. J. (1979). *Sensory integration and the child.* Los Angeles: Western Psychological Services.
5. Ayres, A. J. (1974). Sensory integrative processes in neuropsychological learning disability. In A. Henderson, et al. (Eds.), *The development of sensory integrative theory and practice: A collection of the work of A. Jean Ayres.* Dubuque, IA: Kendall/Hunt.
6. Ayres, A. J. (1980). *Southern California Tests of Sensory Integration manual (Rev.).* Los Angeles: Western Psychological Services.
7. Ayres, A. J. (1976). *The effect of sensory integrative theory on learning disabled children: the final report of a research project.* Los Angeles: University of Southern California.
8. Ayres, A. J., Mailloux, Z. K., & Wendler, C. L. W. (1987). Developmental dyspraxia: is it a unitary function? *Occup Ther J Res, 7,* 93–110.
9. Ayres, A. J., & Tickle, L. S. (1980). Hyper-responsivity to touch and vestibular stimuli as a predictor of positive response to sensory integration procedures by autistic children. *Am J Occup Ther, 34,* 375–381.
10. Bayley, N. (1993). *Bayley scales of infant development* (2nd ed.). San Antonio, TX: The Psychological Corporation.
11. Blanche, E. (2002). *Observations based on sensory integration theory.* Torrance, CA: Pediatric Therapy Network.
12. Brown, C., Tollefson, N., Dunn, W., et al. (2001). The adult sensory profile: measuring patterns of sensory processing. *Am J Occup Ther, 55,* 75.
13. Brown, C. (2002). *Adolescent/adult sensory profile.* San Antonio, TX: The Psychological Corporation.
14. Bruininks, R. H. (1978). *Examiner's manual: Bruininks-Oseretsky test of motor proficiency.* Circle Pines, MN: American Guidance Services.
15. Bundy, A. C., Lane, S. J., & Murray, E. A. (2002). *Sensory integration: theory and practice.* Philadelphia: FA Davis.
16. Cammisa, K. M. (1991). Testing difficult children. *Sensory Integration Special Interest Section Newsletter, 14,* 1.
17. Carrasco, R. C. (2003). Building brains with sensory integration. *Adv Occup Ther, 19,* 47.
18. Carrasco, R. C. (1991). Common test instruments. *Sensory Integration Special Interest Section Newsletter, 14,* 3.
19. Carrasco, R. C. (1993). Key components of sensory integration evaluation. *Sensory Integration Special Interest Section Newsletter, 16,* 5.
20. Carrasco, R. C. (2005). *Making sense: classical and practical sensory integration testing and treatment for diverse populations and settings—course manuals.* Marietta, GA: Advanced Rehabilitation Services.
21. Carrasco, R. C. (2001). *Practical information and useful assessments in sensory integration.* Marietta, GA: Advanced Rehabilitation Services.
22. Carrasco, R. C. (1990). Reliability of the Knickerbocker sensorimotor history questionnaire. *Occup Ther J Res, 10,* 280.
23. Carrasco, R. C., et al. (2002). *BRAINS (Behavior Regulation through Activities for the Integration of Novel Sensations): linking sensory integration and emotions with human performance—infusing sensory integration assessment and treatment with socioemotional intervention.* Marietta, GA: Advanced Rehabilitation Services.
24. Carrasco, R. C., & Lee, C. E. (1993). Development of the teacher questionnaire on sensorimotor behavior. *Sensory Integration Special Interest Section Newsletter, 16,* 1.
25. Carrasco, R. C., & Stallings-Sahler, S. S. (2005). *Sensorimotor history questionnaire–research edition.* Winter Park, FL: FiestaJoy Foundation, Inc.
26. Case-Smith, J., & O'Brien, J. (2015). *Occupational therapy for children* (7th ed.). St Louis, MO: Mosby.
27. Cermak, S. A. (1991). Somatodyspraxia. In A. Fisher, E. A. Murray, & A. C. Bundy (Eds.), *Sensory integration: theory and practice.* Philadelphia: FA Davis.
28. Coster, W. J. (1998). Occupation-centered assessment of children. *Am J Occup Ther, 52,* 337.
29. Daniels, D. (2003). *The relationship between sensory processing and temperament in young children.* Unpublished doctoral dissertation, University of Kansas.
30. Davies, P. L., & Gavin, W. J. (2007). Validating the diagnosis of sensory processing disorders using EEG technology. *Am J Occup Ther, 61,* t76–t89.
31. DeGangi, G. A. (1990). *Greenspan SI: test of sensory function in infants.* Los Angeles: Western Psychological Services.
32. DeGangi, G. A., & Berk, R. A. (1983). *DeGangi-Berk test of sensory integration.* Los Angeles: Western Psychological Services.
33. DeGangi, G. A. (2000). *Pediatric disorders of regulation in affect and behavior.* New York: Academic Press.

34. Dunn, W. W. (2014). *Sensory profile 2*. San Antonio, TX: The Psychological Corporation.

35. Dunn, W. W. (2002). *The infant/toddler sensory profile manual*. San Antonio, TX: The Psychological Corporation.

36. Dunn, W. W. (2001). The sensations of everyday life: empirical, theoretical and pragmatic considerations. *Am J Occup Ther, 55*, 608.

37. Dunn, W. W. (1995). *The sensory profile*. San Antonio, TX: The Psychological Corporation.

38. Dunn, W. W. (1999). *The sensory profile: examiner's manual*. San Antonio, TX: The Psychological Corporation.

39. Dunn, W. W., & Brown, C. E. (2003). *The adolescent and adult sensory profile*. San Antonio, TX: The Psychological Corporation.

40. Fisher, A. G., & Bundy, A. C. (1991). The interpretation process. In A. Fisher, E. A. Murray, & A. C. Bundy (Eds.), *Sensory integration: theory and practice*. Philadelphia: FA Davis.

41. Fisher, A. G., & Bundy, A. C. (1991). Vestibular system. In A. Fisher, E. A. Murray, & A. C. Bundy (Eds.), *Sensory integration: theory and practice*. Philadelphia: FA Davis.

42. Fisher, A. G., Murray, E. A., & Bundy, A. C. (1991). *Sensory integration: theory and practice*. Philadelphia: FA Davis.

43. Folio, M. R., & Fewell, R. R. (1984). *Peabody developmental motor scales* (2nd ed.). Chicago: Riverside Publishing Company.

44. Forssberg, H., & Nashner, L. M. (1982). Ontogenetic development of postural control in man: Adaptations to altered support and visual conditions during stance. *J Neurosci, 2*, 545–552.

45. Jacob, R. G., Furman, J. F., Durrant, J. D., & Turner, S. M. (1996). Panic, agoraphobia, and vestibular dysfunction. *Am J Psychiatry, 153*(4), 503–512.

46. Jirgal, D., & Bouma, K. (1989). Sensory integration interview guide for infants. *Sensory Integration Special Interest Section Newsletter, 12*, 5.

47. Kimball, J. G. (1999). Sensory integration frame of reference. In P. Kramer, & J. Hinojosa (Eds.), *Frames of reference for pediatric occupational therapy* (2nd ed.). Baltimore, MD: Lippincott Williams and Wilkins.

48. Mailloux, Z., & Parham, L. D. (2010). Sensory integration. In J. Case-Smith, & J. O'Brien (Eds.), *Occupational therapy for children* (6th ed.). St Louis, MO: Mosby.

49. McIntosh, D. N., Miller, L. J., Shyu, V., & Dunn, W. (1999). Overview of the Short Sensory Profile (SSP). In W. Dunn (Ed.), *The sensory profile: examiner's manual*. San Antonio, TX: The Psychological Corporation.

50. Miller, L. J., Anzalone, M. E., Lane, S. J., Cermak, S. A., & Osten, E. T. (2007). Concept evolution in sensory integration: a proposed nosology for diagnosis. *Am J Occup Ther, 61*(2), 135–140.

51. Miller, L. J. (1993). *Manual: the FirstSTEP screening test for evaluating preschoolers*. San Antonio, TX: The Psychological Corporation.

52. Miller, L. J. (1982). *Manual: the Miller assessment for preschoolers*. San Antonio, TX: The Psychological Corporation.

53. Miller, L. J., & Lane, S. J. (2000). Toward a consensus in terminology in sensory integration and practice: Part I: Taxonomy of neurophysiological processes. *Sensory Integration Special Interest Section Quarterly, 23*, 1.

54. Miller, L. J., Lane, A. E., & James, K. (2002). *Defining the behavioral phenotype of sensory processing dysfunction*. Paper presented at the University of Colorado Health Sciences Center Developmental Psychobiology Research Group 12th Biennial Retreat, "Behavioral phenotypes in developmental disabilities," Estes Park, CO, University of Colorado Health Sciences Center, Developmental Psychobiology Research Group.

55. Miller, L. J., McIntosh, D. N., McGrath, J., et al. (1999). Electrodermal responses to sensory stimuli in individuals with fragile X syndrome: a preliminary report. *Am J Med Genet, 83*, 268.

56. Miller, L. J., Reisman, J., McIntosh, D. N., et al. (2001). An ecological model of sensory modulation: Performance of children with fragile X syndrome, autism, attention deficit/hyperactivity disorder, and sensory modulation dysfunction. In S. S. Roley, E. I. Blanche, & R. C. Schaaf (Eds.), *Understanding the nature of sensory integration with diverse populations*. San Antonio, TX: Therapy Skill Builders.

57. Miller, L. J. & Roid, G. H. (1994). The T.I.M.E. Toddler and Infant Motor Evaluation. San Antonio, TX: The Psychological Corporation.

58. Parham, D. L. (1987). Evaluation of praxis in preschoolers. *Occup Ther Health Care, 4*, 28.

59. Pfeiffer, B., & Kinnealey, M. (2003). Treatment of sensory defensiveness in adults. *Occup Ther Int, 10*(3), 175–184.

60. Reeves, G., & Cermak, S. (2002). Disorders of praxis. In A. C. Bundy, S. Lane, & E. A. Murray (Eds.), *Sensory integration: theory and practice* (2nd ed.). Philadelphia: FA Davis.

61. Schneider, M. L., Moore, C. F., Gajewski, L. L., Larson, J. A., Roberts, A. D., Converse, A. K., et al. (2008). Sensory processing disorder in a primate model: evidence from a longitudinal study of prenatal alcohol and prenatal stress effects. *Child Dev, 79*(1), 100–113.

62. Shumway-Cook, F., & Woolacott, M. (2001). Development of postural control. In F. Shumway-Cook, & M. Woolacott (Eds.), *Motor control: theory and practical application* (2nd ed.) (pp. 192–221).

63. Smyth, M., & Anderson, H. I. (2000). Coping with clumsiness in the school playground: Social and physical play in children with coordination impairments. *Br J Dev Psychology, 18*, 389–413.

64. Stallings-Sahler, S. (2000). Case presentation: child with gastro-esophageal reflux and severe sensory modulation disorder. *Sens Integ Q*, Spring/Summer 2000, pp. 1,6,9,10.

65. Stallings-Sahler, S. (1990). Case report: report of an occupational therapy evaluation of sensory integration and praxis. *Am J Occup Ther, 4*, 650.

66. Stallings-Sahler, S. (1998). Sensory integration assessment and intervention. In J. Case-Smith (Ed.), *Pediatric occupational therapy and early intervention* (2nd ed.). St Louis, MO: Elsevier/Butterworth-Heinemann.

67. Stallings-Sahler, S. (1991). Sensory integration: creating a challenging environment. *Occup Ther Week, 5*(10), 16.

68. Stewart, S. (2004, April). *The relationship between children's intellectual abilities and their socio-emotional presentation in a clinically referred sample*. Paper presented at the Society for Research in Child Development, Atlanta, GA, Society for Research in Child Development.

69. Summers, B. J., Fitch, K. E., & Cougle, J. R. (2014). Visual, tactile, and auditory "not just right" experiences: Associations with obsessive-compulsive symptoms and perfectionism. *Behav Ther, 45,* 678–689.

70. Thomas, A., Chess, S., Birch, H. G., Hertzig, M., & Korn, S. (1968). *Temperament and behavior disorders in children.* New York: New York University Press.

71. Turkewitz, G., & Kenny, P. A. (1985). The role of developmental limitations of sensory input on sensory/perceptual organization. *Dev Behav Pediatr, 6,* 302.

72. Wilbarger, J., & Stackhouse, T. M. (1998). *Sensory modulation: a review of the literature, May 1989.* Available at: http://www.ot-innovations.com/content/view/29/58/.

73. Wilbarger, P. (1984). Planning an adequate sensory diet: application of sensory processing theory during the first year of life. *Zero Three, 5,* 7.

74. Wilbarger, P., & Wilbarger, J. (1991). *Sensory defensiveness in children aged 2-12: an intervention guide for parents and other caregivers.* Denver, CO: Avanti Educational Programs.

75. Williamson, G. G., & Anzalone, M. E. (2001). *Sensory integration and self-regulation in infants and toddlers: Helping very young children interact with their environment.* Washington, DC: Zero to Three National Center for Clinical Infant Programs.

REVIEW *Questions*

1. What is sensory integration?
2. Define and describe sensory modulation disorder.
3. Define developmental dyspraxia, and describe intervention techniques.
4. What are functional support capacities?
5. How does sensory processing affect movement in children?
6. Describe the principles of sensory integration intervention.
7. Identify intervention techniques to work with children who have postural-ocular and bilateral integration dysfunction.

SUGGESTED *Activities*

1. Administer an SI questionnaire to parents of typically developing children. Discuss the results in class.
2. Go to a specialized SI clinic and observe typically developing children playing on equipment. Describe the motor planning and activity levels of the children.
3. Go to a specialized SI clinic and use the equipment for play activities. Note the intensity levels of the experience. How did the activity feel to you?
4. Go through a catalogue, such as that of Southpaw Enterprises, Inc., and develop a list of games and activities for each piece of equipment. Make a notebook containing these activities for future use.
5. Observe an SI session with a child and take notes of examples of how the OT practitioner used the principles of SI treatment (e.g., child initiated, use of suspended equipment, adaptive responses, controlled sensory input).
6. Observe an SI session with a child either in person or by means of videotape. Describe the type of sensory input and the adaptive responses required. How would you modify the activity?

JESSICA M. KRAMER
PATRICIA BOWYER

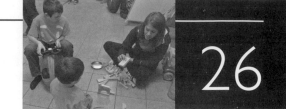

26

Applying the Model of Human Occupation to Pediatric Practice

KEY TERMS

Environment
Volition
Interests
Values
Personal causation
Habituation
Habits
Roles
Performance capacity
Lived body experience
Social groups
Occupational forms/tasks
Environmental impact
Skill
Motor skills
Process skills
Communication/
 interaction skills

CHAPTER *Objectives*

After studying this chapter, the reader will be able to accomplish the following:

- Describe the meaning of the Model of Human Occupation (MOHO) concepts of volition, habituation, performance capacity, the environment, and skill.
- Identify ways to address a client's volition, habituation, performance capacity, environment, and skill in therapy through the use of therapeutic strategies.
- Practice using MOHO concepts to describe and analyze a clinical scenario.
- Become familiar with assessments based on the MOHO that can inform intervention.

CHAPTER *Outline*

Shaun is an 11-year-old boy with cerebral palsy whose handwriting did not improve this year, and who does not try very hard during his biweekly therapy sessions. He continues to fall behind his classmates. Maria is a 2-year-old girl receiving early intervention services after a medically complicated birth. She is just beginning to learn how to dress herself, and giggles with delight after her mother helps her put on her princess costume. Lizzy, a young lady with autism, is beginning vocational training as part of her transition plan, and needs to identify a type of job that will also enable her to be successful given her interests, abilities, and support needs. Sessions with clients, whether infants, children, or adolescents, can either represent a challenge or be an opportunity to make progress toward the achievement of an intervention goal.

Occupational therapy (OT) practitioners have the opportunity to create a therapeutic **environment** that is individualized to each client's preferences and challenges and as a result, more likely to enable young children to reach their occupational therapy goals. So how do you motivate Shaun to practice handwriting so that he does not have to struggle in class? How do you ensure that Maria will learn to successfully perform self-care activities? While working with Lizzy on prevocational skills, what can you do to help identify the employment setting that is most appropriate for her? The Model of Human Occupation (MOHO)[7] is one way to systematically analyze a child's current occupational situation, understand his or her strengths and challenges, and identify the optimal therapeutic environment that will enable him or her to achieve his or her goals.

WHAT IS THE MODEL OF HUMAN OCCUPATION?

MOHO is an occupation-focused, evidence-based, client-centered way of thinking about practice with children and youth. MOHO is concerned with the child's motivation for engaging in occupations, the pattern and organization of occupations, the child's ability to perform occupations, and the influence of the environment on occupations. The main concepts in MOHO are called volition, habituation, performance capacity, and the environment. This chapter defines and explains these concepts. When first learning about these concepts, people may become overwhelmed by all the different definitions. Rather than worrying about memorizing these definitions, it is helpful to keep in mind that the purpose of the concepts is to provide practitioners with a way of systematically thinking about clients and the strengths and challenges they encounter when participating in occupations. As you practice using these concepts to analyze children's occupational participation, it will become easier to remember the different MOHO concepts and their meanings.

MOHO is occupation-focused because the concepts that make it up are focused on understanding the extent to which children are able to participate in the occupations of taking care of oneself, playing, learning, and working. Furthermore, MOHO does not just focus on children's impairments, such as lack of strength or poor visual-motor integration, it also considers what motivates children to participate in occupation, how their participation in different occupations is organized and patterned on a daily basis, and how the environment supports or interferes with participation in occupation.

MOHO is also evidence-based, and the concepts and tools associated with MOHO have undergone almost 30 years of research and development. As of 2015, more than 250 MOHO-related publications of studies, case examples, and theoretical discussions were available to support practice. This research and development has occurred through the collaboration of a network of international researchers and practitioners. Today, MOHO has become the most widely used occupation-focused model in occupational therapy.[4,8,9] This large body of evidence cannot be incorporated into one chapter; the most recent evidence for practice can be easily accessed at the MOHO website: www.moho.uic.edu. The most recent text on MOHO, *Model of Human Occupation: Theory and Application* (4th ed.)[7] also includes a chapter that reviews the evidence supporting the use of MOHO in practice.

Finally, MOHO is client-centered because the concepts are focused on identifying the unique occupational strengths and needs of each client. Although these concepts can be applied to children of any age and with a range of abilities, the understanding gained about each child will be unique and will enable the OT practitioner to individualize OT intervention. MOHO also stresses the importance of incorporating the child's perspective into the therapy process. When working with children and youth, this also includes the family's perspective. Some of the therapeutic strategies introduced in this chapter require the OT practitioner to first obtain the perspective of the child and their family. Observations, informal interviews, and reviewing records and assessments are just some ways of obtaining information about the child and family's perspective.

The remainder of the chapter will introduce MOHO concepts and illustrate how to systematically use those concepts to enhance OT intervention. Readers are urged to practice applying these concepts and remember that MOHO is an occupation-focused, evidence-based, client-centered way of thinking in a systematic way about the clients.

MOHO THERAPEUTIC STRATEGIES

Therapeutic strategies are specific actions that can facilitate client change by influencing the way a child feels,

TABLE 26-1

Therapeutic Strategies and Definitions

THERAPEUTIC STRATEGY	DEFINITION
Advise	Recommend intervention goals and strategies to the child and his or her family.
Coach	Instruct, demonstrate, guide, verbally prompt, and/or physically assist a child while he or she is doing an occupation.
Encourage	Provide emotional support and reassurance to a child during or after an activity.
Give feedback	Share an overall conceptualization of the child's situation or an understanding of the child's ongoing participation in occupations.
Identify	Locate and share a range of personal, procedural, and/or environmental factors that can facilitate a child's occupational participation.
Negotiate	Engage in give and take with the child, his or her parents, and other professionals to achieve a common perspective or agreement about something that the child will or should do in the future.
Physical support	Use physical body to support the completion of an occupational task when a child cannot or will not use his or her motor skills.
Structure	Establish parameters for choice and performance by offering children alternatives, setting limits, and establishing ground rules.
Validate	Convey respect for the child's or parent's experience or perspective.

Adapted from Kielhofner, G. (2008). *Model of Human Occupation: theory and application* (4th ed.). Baltimore, MD: Lippincott, Williams, & Wilkins.

thinks, or does something in the context of therapy. OT practitioners use therapeutic strategies to engage children in therapy and to help create an optimal therapeutic environment. There are nine therapeutic strategies, as shown in Table 26-1. Each therapeutic strategy can be applied in several different ways to address a range of client needs or therapeutic challenges. This chapter demonstrates how OT practitioners use specific therapeutic strategies to address one aspect of the child's volition, habituation, skill, or his or her environment. These examples are provided throughout the chapter in the clinical pearl boxes.

MOHO CONCEPTS: CLIENT FACTORS

Each child brings a unique set of personal factors that influence his or her engagement in occupations. The MOHO concepts that examine these personal, or client, factors are volition, habituation, and performance capacity.

Volition

Volition, or a child's motivation for occupations, is influenced by those activities the child finds most enjoyable (interests), the child's beliefs about what is important (values), and the child's beliefs about his or her ability to effectively perform occupations (personal causation). In combination, these three aspects of volition create a unique pattern of thoughts and feelings that influence how a child anticipates, chooses, experiences, and interprets what he or she does.

Consider Shaun's lack of interest in practicing handwriting. Perhaps Shaun does not find handwriting activities fun, and so is not interested in practicing with his occupational therapy assistant (OTA). It is also possible that Shaun considers it is more important to conserve his energy to perform fine motor tasks other than handwriting, such as eating or using a computer. A final possibility is that Shaun is frustrated with his poor handwriting, and believes that further practice will not improve his handwriting and so he stops trying. By gathering more information, the OT practitioner can determine which of these aspects of volition is influencing Shaun's participation in therapy. The OT practitioner will then be better able to provide an individualized therapeutic environment that is based on Shaun's interests, values, and personal causation.

Interests

Interests are things that a child finds enjoyable and satisfying to do. Usually, children are interested in activities in which they are most likely to be successful and engage without possibility of failure, pain, or difficulty. Therefore interests are inherently motivating; meaning, they are quite likely to encourage a child to engage in a specific activity and a child will usually feel good about him or herself when engaging in a preferred activity. Often, a child may have a pattern of interests that represent a primary interest in one area, such as sports, arts and crafts, or animals. OT practitioners can incorporate a child's interests into therapy activities as one way to facilitate desired change. The following clinical pearl on encouragement provides an example of how a practitioner uses an encouraging strategy to promote interests.

> ### CLINICAL *Pearl*
>
> **Encourage**
>
> The therapeutic strategy of encouraging can be enhanced when it is incorporated along with a child's interests. If a child is unsure, worried, or scared, the impact of encouragement strategies such as verbal assurance ("You can do it") can be strengthened by referring to the child's interests (Figure 26 -1).

For example, Maria's therapist decided to use her interest in dressing up as a princess to encourage her to practice getting dressed. The therapist had Maria decorate a plain shirt with glitter and markers, making it a "princess shirt." The therapist asked Maria to try putting on her shirt so they could pretend to be princesses. However, Maria became frustrated when she was unable to push her arm through the sleeve. The therapist encouraged Maria and drew upon her interest in dressing up by saying, "You can do it, keep trying! I can't wait to play princess with you once you get your princess shirt on!"

Values

Values are those things that a child finds important and meaningful. Values are influenced by a child's culture and context. They result from internalized convictions and are associated with a sense of obligation. These internalized personal convictions define what matters to a child, and may also be a reflection of what matters to other important people in their lives such as a child's family or community. The resulting sense of obligation influences a child's decision to engage in certain occupations over others. Understanding the values a child and his or her family hold can help ensure the OT practitioner provides client-centered therapy. The following clinical pearl provides an example of the importance of using negotiation when values differ.

> ### CLINICAL *Pearl*
>
> **Negotiate**
>
> Sometimes other professionals, parents, and the child differ in the level of importance placed on certain activities, skills, or outcomes. As a result, professionals, parents, and children may not place equal value on the child's therapy goals or for the activities presented during therapy. The therapeutic strategy of negotiation can help practitioners identify intervention activities that are valued by all members of the child's support team, and enable members to reach a compromise that recognizes differences in values.

For example, Shaun's teacher thinks it is important for Shaun to complete handwritten class notes to demonstrate that he is participating in class. However, Shaun's family feels it is more important for Shaun to attend to the teacher and share his ideas during class discussions. Shaun cares most about conserving his energy so that he can complete the full school day. The OT practitioner meets privately with the teacher, Shaun, and his parents to discuss these different values, and negotiates an alternative solution. The teacher will provide Shaun with an outline for each class lecture, and at home each evening, Shaun will add his typed notes to the outline. Shaun will receive class participation points by turning in his typed notes from the previous day and by participating in class discussion. The OT practitioner will stop working on handwriting, and instead help Shaun learn how to type and use voice dictation software. Negotiation allowed the practitioner to identify a solution that recognized the teacher's, Shaun's, and his parents' values regarding learning and class participation.

Personal Causation

Personal causation is a child's sense of competence (sense of capacity) and effectiveness (self-efficacy) for doing different occupations. A child's personal causation is related to his or her awareness of the ability to engage in an occupation. Figure 26-2 illustrates a child's sense of accomplishment from making a unique snow penguin. When a child believes he or she can achieve a desired outcome in an occupation, a sense of self-efficacy is developed. Children's perceptions of their capacity and efficacy guide their activity choices. One child may believe she excels in ball sports and is willing to play all ball-related games,

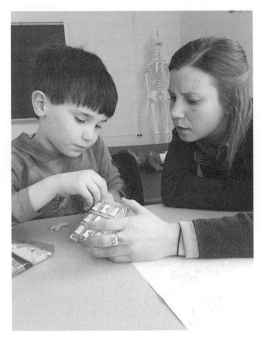

FIGURE 26-1 The OT practitioner provides encouragement to a child who is figuring out what to do next.

another may consider himself "musical" and so he will try to learn how to play a new instrument, whereas another may think she is good at making new friends and therefore is willing to join a new club that meets at the community park. Personal causation is gradually built through continued accomplishments and increases a child's motivation to engage in other occupations. For example, a child who is comfortable walking across the room will be more motivated to explore the environment. A child who enjoys playing games with a brother or sister may feel comfortable initiating interactions with a same-aged peer.

Children and youth do not need to articulate personal causation for OT practitioners to understand how they feel about their capacity and effectiveness. The child who has a good sense of personal causation in an occupation will seek out new challenges, whereas the child who feels a low sense of capacity will avoid new activities (Figure 26-3). For example, a student such as Shaun who is unable write at a high rate of speed may not feel a sense of personal capacity for taking notes in class, and therefore may begin to avoid participation in class. By observing this pattern of behavior, the OT practitioner can determine a child's sense of personal causation.

Volitional Process

The three aspects of volition: interests, values, and personal causation help explain why there are certain activities that are motivating to some children, whereas other children are unmotivated or unwilling to engage in certain occupations. However, how can you change a child's sense of personal causation so that she believes she has the capacity to try a new occupation? How can you help a child identify a new interest? How can you help a child evaluate his values and make choices based on those values? OT practitioners can influence a child's interests, values, or personal causation using the volitional process.

The volitional process is how children experience their participation in occupations. The volitional process includes four steps: anticipation, making choices, experience, and interpretation. A child's interests, values, and personal causation influence each step of this volitional process, as illustrated in Figure 26-4. For example, if a child enjoys movement and swinging, he will most likely anticipate that rocking on a hammock will be enjoyable. As a result, he will be more likely to choose to do the activity of rocking on a hammock in therapy. He is likely to enjoy the experience of rocking in the hammock, and will interpret the activity as enjoyable. Based on this positive interpretation, when encountering this activity in the future the child is more likely to have a positive anticipation of playing in the hammock and choose the activity again.

OT practitioners can try and influence a child's volition by changing the way a child anticipates, chooses, experiences, or interprets an activity. For example, consider Shaun and his poor sense of personal causation regarding handwriting. When Shaun is asked to complete a handwriting activity in therapy, he anticipates that he does not have the ability to successfully complete the activity. The OT practitioner can try and change the way Shaun anticipates this activity by making the activity easier, by making the activity similar to an activity Shaun knows that he is able to complete, or by aligning the activity with one of Shaun's interests. The OT practitioner knows that Shaun enjoys collecting baseball cards, and so the OT practitioner asks Shaun to write a list of his 10 most valuable baseball cards. Making a list is easier than writing full sentences, and Shaun enjoys talking about his baseball card collection. As a result, he has a more positive anticipation of the activity and chooses to complete this activity with the OT practitioner. Although Shaun has some difficulty writing this list, he experiences the activity as more enjoyable because he is thinking about his card collection and sharing his ideas

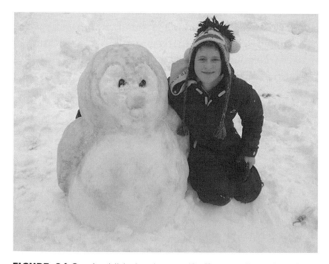

FIGURE 26-2 A child develops self-efficacy when they have achieved a desired outcome. In this case the child feels a sense of pride and accomplishment from making a unique snow penguin.

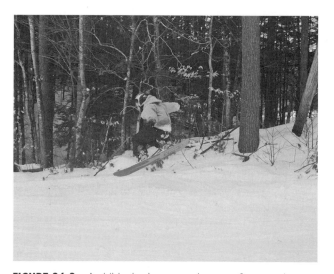

FIGURE 26-3 A child who has a good sense of personal causation will seek out new challenges. Scott tries new "tricks" while snowboarding.

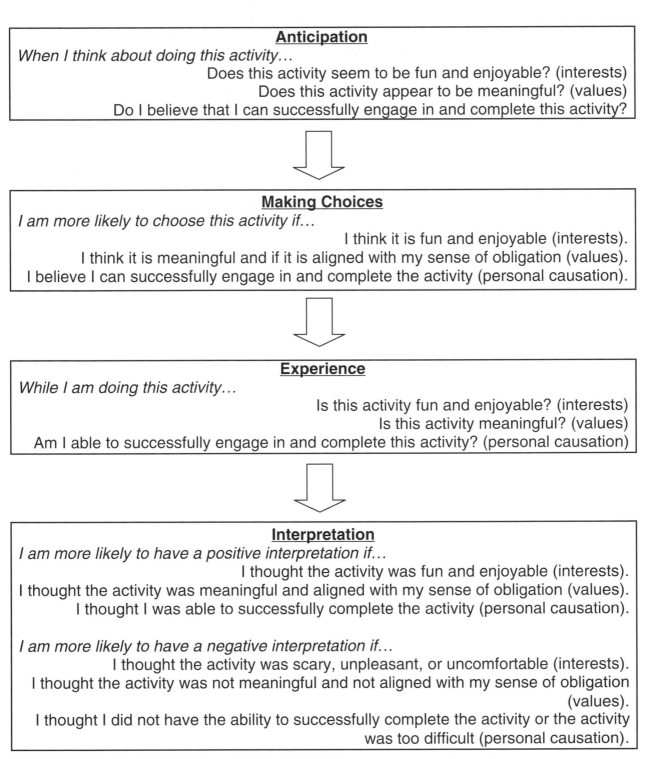

Anticipation

When I think about doing this activity...

Does this activity seem to be fun and enjoyable? (interests)

Does this activity appear to be meaningful? (values)

Do I believe that I can successfully engage in and complete this activity?

Making Choices

I am more likely to choose this activity if...

I think it is fun and enjoyable (interests).

I think it is meaningful and if it is aligned with my sense of obligation (values).

I believe I can successfully engage in and complete the activity (personal causation).

Experience

While I am doing this activity...

Is this activity fun and enjoyable? (interests)

Is this activity meaningful? (values)

Am I able to successfully engage in and complete this activity? (personal causation)

Interpretation

I am more likely to have a positive interpretation if...

I thought the activity was fun and enjoyable (interests).

I thought the activity was meaningful and aligned with my sense of obligation (values).

I thought I was able to successfully complete the activity (personal causation).

I am more likely to have a negative interpretation if...

I thought the activity was scary, unpleasant, or uncomfortable (interests).

I thought the activity was not meaningful and not aligned with my sense of obligation (values).

I thought I did not have the ability to successfully complete the activity or the activity was too difficult (personal causation).

FIGURE 26-4   How a child's interests, values, and personal causation influence the volitional process.

with the OT practitioner. When the list is complete, the practitioner then asks Shaun to type the list into the computer. It takes Shaun a long time to type the list, but he is pleased when he produces a typed list that is easy to read. Although he had some difficulty writing and typing the list, overall, Shaun believes he was able to successfully complete this activity, and interprets his experience as positive.

The OT practitioner believes that the next time this type of activity is introduced; Shaun will be more likely to anticipate a positive experience and therefore will be more willing to engage in therapy activities. By using the steps of the volitional process and thinking about Shaun's interests, values, and personal causation, the OT practitioner can help Shaun reach the desired goal of learning to type.

Habituation

Habituation explains the pattern and organization of a child's participation in different occupations. Habituation is the internalized readiness to engage in consistent patterns of behavior during certain times of day and days of the week, as determined by one's habits and roles. Habits and roles help children organize their lives and make participation in everyday occupations easier.

Habits

When children respond to familiar situations in consistent ways, they are demonstrating a habit. A habit is an acquired tendency to respond automatically to a specific circumstance or environment. **Habits** help children to be efficient and effective when doing familiar, everyday activities. For example, a child who has an organized routine when entering his classroom (hangs up his backpack, then gets out his homework folder and places it in his desk) will be able to quickly put his belongings into the proper place and prepare for the school day. OT practitioners can help children develop new habits or routines to optimize their performance of occupations such as brushing teeth, cleaning their room, or learning a new task at work.

Roles

When a child identifies as a son or daughter, brother or sister, student, soccer player, band member, or worker, he or she is internalizing a role. **Roles** are a set of related actions and attitudes that, in combination, define a culturally and socially familiar status. For example, the role of a student is associated with the actions of attending school, listening to the teacher, participating in classroom activities, playing with classmates, and taking tests. Children are expected to be able to perform the actions associated with their roles, and therapy can be a time for children to learn and practice these role-related actions.

Roles also help children and families define their relationships and actions with others; a child is expected to act differently when interacting with his or her teacher, mother, and best friend. A child who does not identify with any roles will have difficulty interacting with others and participating in activities. In this case, the OT practitioner can use therapy as a time to identify potential roles for a child such as pet owner, class helper, or community volunteer. The following clinical pearl on advising explores the use of this strategy to help children take on and participate in new roles.

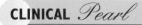

CLINICAL *Pearl*

Advise

OT practitioners can use the therapeutic strategy "advise" to help children take on and participate in new roles.

For example, parents may not expect children to have a role in completing chores around the house because of concerns with accessibility, safety, or task completion. However, learning to complete chores can be an important part of children's development and enables the child to hold a valuable role in the home. The therapist can advise parents of chores that may be appropriate given a child's ability, and identify ways to incorporate that chore into the child's daily routine. For example, a child could take on the chore of "putting away dirty laundry." Laundry baskets could be labeled with different color blocks to help the child sort dirty laundry by color. This type of advice can enable parents to support their child's engagement in new roles.

Performance Capacity

Performance capacity is the third and final MOHO concept addressing personal client factors. Performance capacity is a child's ability to do things as supported by the status of his or her physical and mental components as well as his or her subjective experience of living within his or her body.

OT practitioners can measure the status of physical and mental components, and therefore, this aspect of a child's performance capacity is known as objective. Some examples of physical and mental components that can be measured objectively are strength, intelligence, and proprioception. OT practitioners use other theories to measure, classify, and describe the status of physical and mental components of a child. Therefore MOHO acknowledges the importance of a child's physical and mental components but relies on OT practitioner's use of other frames of reference (biomechanical, sensory integration) to evaluate and explain those components. See the clinical pearl on physical support for an example of how this strategy may be beneficial to practice.

CLINICAL *Pearl*

Physical Support

If a child's physical and mental components make it difficult to complete certain tasks, the OT practitioner can use the therapeutic strategy of providing physical support to help the child successfully complete a task or learn a new skill. This can also help practitioners ensure children's successful experience while doing occupations and can influence the volitional process (Figure 26-5)!

A child's own experience of using and living in his or her body is the subjective aspect of performance capacity, also referred to as the **"lived body" experience**. This aspect is subjective because it is based on the child's unique experience and cannot be measured by another person. However, OT practitioners can try to

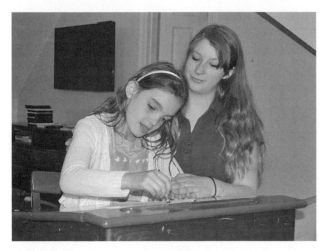

FIGURE 26-5 The OT practitioner provides physical support to help the child stabilize the paper for writing.

gather information to understand a child's subjective experience of using his or her body. For example, a child with sensory integration difficulties and gravitational insecurity may describe the experience of going down a slide as "falling into a black hole." This subjective experience influences a child's sense of capacity and experience of doing occupations as much as the status of their physical and mental components. Awareness of a child's subjective experience helps the OT practitioner to provide a safe and comfortable therapeutic environment. The following clinical pearl on validation provides an example of the importance of validating one's subjective experience.

> ### CLINICAL *Pearl*
>
> #### Validation
> Although there is no formal way to assess or measure a child's subjective experience of using his or her body, the OT practitioner can acknowledge a child's experience using the therapeutic strategy of validation. Practitioners should acknowledge when a child may be scared, unsure, uncomfortable, or in pain when completing therapy activities. For example, a practitioner might say, "I know this is really scary but I won't let you fall" or "If this hurts too much please tell me to stop." The use of this strategy demonstrates respect for the child's lived body experience

MOHO CONCEPTS: ENVIRONMENTAL FACTORS

The MOHO concepts of volition, habituation, and performance capacity address personal client factors that influence participation in occupation. However, MOHO recognizes that the environment also influences children's participation in occupation. The

MOHO concepts that help us think of the environmental factors that directly influence participation are spaces, objects, social groups, and occupational tasks. Additional environmental factors including economic conditions, culture, and political conditions indirectly influence participation and the opportunities available to and demands placed on children. The clinical pearl on structure illustrates how structuring the child's environment may facilitate occupational performance.

Spaces

Spaces are physical places, or contexts that are arranged in ways that influence what children do within those spaces. The unique features or natural or built spaces, such as a grassy hill, a staircase, the current weather, a row of chairs, or the length of a hallway, all influence the extent to which children can participate in different occupations. Other settings influence the types of occupations that take place; a library encourages quiet reading and hunting for books, a playground encourages running and climbing, and a kitchen encourages cooking and eating. OT practitioners can modify and rearrange spaces to ensure accessibility and to encourage a child's participation in specific occupations. One example is rearranging desks so that a child who uses a wheelchair can more easily move about the classroom to obtain materials and interact with classmates.

Objects

Objects are natural or manmade things that children interact and use during occupations. Objects are used in play (blocks), self-care (shoes), mobility (wheelchair), and learning (books). Like spaces, objects also influence the types of occupations children engage in, and the way they perform those occupations. A student such as Shaun can take notes using paper and pencil, or using a computer; the availability of these objects determines how Shaun will take notes in class. OT practitioners may modify existing objects or provide different objects in order to facilitate a child's participation in different occupations. For example, since Maria had a weak grip and difficulty with her fine motor skills, the OT practitioner added a foam handle to her spoon so that Maria could more easily hold her spoon to feed herself. Finally, objects can signify a child's special interests or a role that is important to them. Lizzy takes pride in her role of checking books into the school library, and always carries the clipboard she uses to complete this job. Shaun always carries baseball cards in his backpack, and Maria's room is full of princess toys. OT practitioners can incorporate these objects of interest into therapy sessions to motivate and engage children.

Social Groups

Social groups are collections of people who come together for a variety of formal and informal purposes. Social groups include playgroups, classrooms, worship communities, Internet social networking groups, families, and a neighborhood. In the neighborhood, play with other children may be informally organized by a group of children, but play at school during recess may be formally structured into the daily schedule and may involve specific types of games and activities.

Social groups also influence the types of occupations available to a child and the behaviors those in the social group expect the child to demonstrate. A classroom teacher may expect a child to pay attention, work quietly, and follow classroom rules, whereas a parent may expect the child to play nicely with siblings and eat dinner with the family. OT practitioners can support a child's engagement in occupations by identifying the different social groups a child belongs to, determining the occupations and expectations of each social group, and either modifying those expectations according to the child's ability or helping the child practice those occupations.

Occupational Forms/Tasks

In any culture, there often are common and typical ways of doing specific occupations. Think of playing a game of football, taking a test, or baking a cake; it is likely that each reader thinks of a similar sequence of actions that is required to do these occupations. **Occupational forms/tasks**, are these conventional sequences of actions that are oriented to a specific purpose, and understood by and recognizable to members of a shared culture.[10] For some children, these conventionalized ways of doing occupations are not accessible or possible given their impairments and abilities. OT practitioners can modify the steps in a task or propose an alternative way of doing tasks to enable children's participation in occupations.

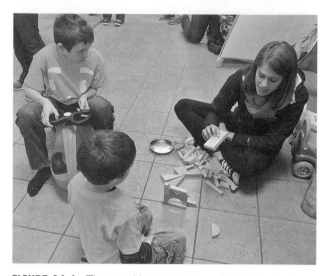

FIGURE 26-6 The practitioner structures this activity by handing the child the blocks so that he is not overwhelmed by all the choices.

THE INTERACTION BETWEEN CLIENT AND ENVIRONMENTAL FACTORS DURING PARTICIPATION

Environmental Impact

Each child is different, therefore, the impact that environmental factors have on a child's participation varies with the uniqueness of each child's impairments and abilities. The extent to which spaces, objects, social groups, and occupational tasks provide opportunities, supports/resources, demands, or constraints on participation is the **environmental impact** for a child. Consider two children with mobility impairments; one child crawls to get around inside of her house, and the other child uses a wheelchair. For the child who crawls, stairs demand the ability to climb, but if that child is able to crawl up stairs, the stairs do not constrain her participation in that environment. However, for the child who uses the wheelchair, if he is unable to meet the environmental demand to climb, the stairs will constrain his participation.

Whether and how a child notices different environmental opportunities, supports and resources, demands, and constraints depends on the child's volition, habituation, and performance capacity. For example, low environmental demands may be boring for one child but calming for another child, and similarly, high environmental demands may engage one child with a variety of interests and strong sense of personal causation yet overwhelm another child with a low sense of efficacy and capacity. OT practitioners should carefully consider how each environment uniquely affects each child's participation in occupations, and attempt to provide spaces, objects, tasks, and social expectations that match the child's abilities and interests and meet their needs. The following clinical pearl on identify provides an example of how a practitioner helps children identify environmental resources.

CLINICAL *Pearl*

Identify

OT practitioners can use the therapeutic strategy to identify, locate, and share a range of environmental factors that provide the appropriate opportunities, supports/resources, and demands. For example, the practitioners working with Lizzy on her prevocational skills determined she enjoyed interacting with people, felt capable of successfully completing three-step repetitive tasks, and was able to organize materials numerically and alphabetically when in a quiet environment. Using this knowledge of Lizzy's interests, personal causation, and skills, the therapist identified that processing simple customer requests and tickets in places such as a snack stand, library, or small movie theater would all be potential employment opportunities that would provide the right balance of opportunities, resources, and demands.

Skill

This chapter already introduced the concept of performance capacity: the child's underlying physical and mental capacities. When a child uses those abilities in the context of a specific environment in order to engage in a task such as dressing, completing a puzzle, or working on homework, we can observe skill. **Skills** are observable, goal-directed actions that the child uses to perform. Skills are influenced by many things: both the environment and the child's personal characteristics. A child's underlying strength may certainly affect the level of skill we observe, but the level of skill a child demonstrates while completing a task is equally influenced by other factors such as the child's level of interest in the task, the objects used to complete the task, and the other people doing the activity with the child. It is important to remember that we cannot "see" performance capacity. However, skills are always actions that we can "see" when a child is working to complete a task or activity. The following clinical pearl on feedback illustrates how giving feedback may help a child gain skill.

CLINICAL *Pearl*

Give Feedback

OT practitioners can give feedback during intervention sessions to help a child understand how he or she is doing with a selected activity. A child can then incorporate the information received and by doing so alter levels of participation. Giving feedback is a valuable way for OT practitioners to help a child have immediate insight into skill performance. A practitioner can provide verbal, physical, or both types of feedback depending on the activity the child is undertaking.

There are three types of skills. **Motor skills** refer to moving one's body or moving objects used to complete tasks. When a child uses her underlying muscle strength and balance to pick a toy off the floor, we observe the motor skill of lifting. **Process skills** refer to the logical sequence of actions, the selection and use of appropriate tools and materials, and the ability to adapt one's performance and actions when encountering problems. When a child decides the steps he will take and the materials needed to complete a homework assignment, we observe the process skills of sequencing and gathering. **Communication and interaction skills** refer to the child's ability to convey intentions and needs and to coordinate social action with other people. When a young adult approaches a teacher to ask a question, we can observe the verbal skills of articulate and speak, and nonverbal skills such as gesture and eye gaze. Coaching is often used to facilitate skill development (see clinical pearl on coaching).

CLINICAL *Pearl*

Coach

When an OT practitioner coaches a child, he or she is providing the child with support to complete a task. For example, a child is working on copper tooling to improve fine motor skills and hand strength as well as tracking and eye–hand coordination. The practitioner notices that the child is missing spots when rubbing the copper to attain the shape of the mold. The OT practitioner "coaches" the child by encouraging him or her to go back over the parts that are not visible from earlier efforts at rubbing the copper with the etching tool. This helps the student to see what needs to be done as well as provide encouragement for him or her to keep working during what may be a period of frustration at not having enough hand strength or fine motor skills.

MOHO-BASED ASSESSMENTS FOR PEDIATRIC PRACTICE CONTEXTS

To systematically consider how factors such as volition, habituation, performance capacity, and the environment impact participation, a range of MOHO-based assessments are available. These assessments help operationalize the MOHO concepts, and can help OT practitioners identify client strengths and needs. OTAs can use these assessments as a way to learn more about the children. They serve as tools to structure interviews and engage in conversations. Therefore practitioners are urged to use the assessments as part of both the evaluation and intervention phases of therapy. Some assessments are designed specifically for children and adolescents; some of these instruments are briefly described here and in Table 26-2. The following summaries explain how OT practitioners may use findings from these assessments to inform intervention.

TABLE 26-2

MOHO-Based Pediatric Assessments

ASSESSMENT	CONSTRUCT ASSESSED	TARGET POPULATION	ADMINISTRATION	ALIGNED AOTA PRACTICE FRAMEWORK DOMAIN
COSA	Youth's perceived competence for and importance of everyday activities at home, school, and the community.	Youth ages 7–17 Able to self-report with support and modifications.	Self-report	Occupational performance Performance skills Performance patterns
PVQ	Children's volition (personal causation, values, and interests) and the effect of the environment on a child's volition.	Children 2–7 Youth who are nonverbal.	Observation	Occupational performance Context and environment Activity and occupational demands
SSI	Fit between the environment, current modifications and accommodations, and a student's unique needs (student–environment fit).	Students who are able to communicate their feelings and contribute to their intervention planning. Originally designed for students with physical disabilities, but applicable to students with other disabilities.	Semi-structured interview	Occupational performance Context and environment Activity and occupational demands
SCOPE	Personal (volition, habitation, and skills) and environmental factors that facilitate and restrict participation in occupations.	Ages birth–21	Range of information gathering techniques (observation, chart review, interviews, etc.)	Occupational performance Performance skills Performance patterns Activity and occupational demands

Other MOHO assessments may also be appropriate for adolescents and young adults. The appropriateness of an assessment for youth should be determined by research demonstrating the use of the instrument with a specific age group, as well as clinical judgment regarding the potential of an assessment to best explain a client's unique circumstances. For more in-depth information on MOHO assessments, readers are encouraged to refer to the *Model of Human Occupation: Theory and Application* text.[7]

Child Occupational Self Assessment[6]

The Child Occupational Self Assessment (COSA)[6] is a client-centered assessment tool and an outcome measure designed to capture youth's perceptions regarding their sense of occupational competence and the importance of everyday activities. The COSA has been used in research with youth aged 7 to 17; however, it may be appropriate for clients as young as 6 or as old as 21. OT practitioners are advised to review the wording of items and rating scales to determine whether the COSA is suitable for

a child. Several formats are available (including paper-and-pencil form with face symbols) and other modifications can be made during administration to make the COSA more engaging and accessible for young people with a range of abilities and needs.

Young people may have perspectives of their performance that are different from adults. When this happens, others may think the self-assessment is inaccurate. However, self-reporting can help young people better self-reflect on their performance. Over time, this self-understanding and self-evaluation can help a young person to be a more effective advocate. Enhancing the COSA self-report with dialogue enriches the information practitioners can gather from the COSA and provides practitioners with the opportunity to demonstrate their value for client-centered practice to pediatric clients.

On the COSA, youth respond to 25 items that ask about everyday activities a young person may do at home, at school, or in the community. The COSA items pertain to different areas of occupations, including self-care, play and leisure, and learning. For each item, the child rates how he or she performs the activity (*big problem* to *really good*) and the importance of the activity (*not important* to *most important of all*). The practitioner looks for "gaps" between youth's competence and importance ratings; activities rated as most important and with the lowest competence ratings may be targeted first during intervention to enhance rapport, build the youth's self-efficacy, and support successful occupational adaptation.

Pediatric Volitional Questionnaire[2]

The Pediatric Volitional Questionnaire (PVQ) is an observational assessment tool that enables the practitioner to better understand the child's personal causation, values, and interests.[2] Items ask about specific behaviors that are easily observed during occupations, and the administrator rates the amount of external support a child requires to demonstrate each behavior. By systematically using several observations in different environments and occupations, the PVQ provides insight into a child's inner motives and provides information about how the environment enhances or attenuates volition. Since the PVQ uses observation, it can be used with young children aged 2 to 7, or may also be appropriate for older children who are not able to express their values, interests, or beliefs regarding their abilities.

Items in the PVQ are grouped into three stages of volitional development: exploration, competency, and achievement. Practitioners can identify whether a child is in the exploration, competency, or achievement phase by identifying where he or she moves from spontaneously demonstrating volitional behaviors to requiring more support. Intervention can then be tailored to the child's current level of volitional development to provide the just-right challenge and encourage volitional growth. For example, children in the exploration stage benefit from a low-risk environment with high levels of support and encouragement. Alternatively, children in the achievement phase have the personal capacity needed to more effectively respond to challenges while engaged in occupation. The PVQ can also be used to document volitional and environmental changes that are outcomes of occupational therapy intervention.

School Setting Interview[5]

The School Setting Interview (SSI) is a semistructured interview designed to assess student–environment fit and identify the need for accommodations for students with disabilities in the school setting.[5] The SSI is to be used collaboratively with the student and is therefore intended for students who are able to communicate their feelings and contribute to their intervention planning (recommended age 10 and older). Although the SSI was originally designed for use with students with physical disabilities, it may be appropriate for students with other disabilities.

The SSI includes 16 items concerning everyday school activities where students with disabilities may need adjustments to be able to participate, such as reading, writing, doing homework, extracurricular activities, and accessing the school building. The student and the practitioner jointly score each item by determining whether any accommodations or changes are needed to maximize participation in each area. The SSI also includes an intervention planning form that records the areas in which changes are required, the specific modifications that need to be made to the physical and social environment, and the specific individuals responsible for executing those changes.

The SSI helps identify gaps between accommodations the student is currently using and what accommodations and assistive technology may be needed to facilitate effective occupational performance in the school context. The SSI also documents when current resources and accommodations support a student's optimal participation; this information can then serve as a guide when planning transitions to new contexts such as a new school or service placement.

Short Child Occupational Profile[3]

The Short Child Occupational Profile (SCOPE) is an occupation-focused assessment that documents how a child's volition, habituation, skills, and the environment facilitate or restrict participation.[3] The SCOPE can be used with children birth to 21 years of age with a range of abilities and diagnoses, and can be used in a range of practice contexts, such as school, home, inpatient and community-practice settings.

Practitioners can gather information to rate the SCOPE in a variety of ways, including observation, interviews, chart review, and by administering other assessments. Practitioners then use this information to rate six subscales: volition, habituation, communication and interaction skills, process skills, motor skills, and environment. Items on the SCOPE are rated based on each child's "individual developmental trajectory"— the capacities a child has the potential to acquire in the future given the child's age, impairment, prior life experiences, and environmental context. This approach enables practitioners to capture each child's strengths as well as challenges using the SCOPE. As a result, items do not require specific behaviors or performance; alternatively, the practitioner uses his or her clinical judgment to determine how each factor uniquely affects each child's participation in occupation. The SCOPE provides criteria statements for each rating to guide practitioners' reasoning.

The results of the SCOPE provide a profile of each child's unique strengths and needs that can be used to guide intervention. For example, high ratings on the volitional subscale suggest that practitioners can harness a child's clearly defined interests or strong sense of efficacy while addressing other needs, such as improving a child's ability to transition between activities or learning new motor skills. The SCOPE also identifies whether the physical or social environment can be modified to better support a child's participation.

MOHO AND THE AOTA PRACTICE FRAMEWORK

The Occupational Therapy Practice Framework[1] is the guiding document of practice for OT practitioners in the United States. Many concepts in MOHO align with the concepts and principles in the framework.

The framework puts forth the two principles that occupations are central to a person's identity and sense of competence, and that the OT process should be driven by collaboration between the practitioner and the child.[1] Using MOHO can help practitioners enact these principles in practice. By considering a child's volition for occupation, practitioners can ensure that intervention focuses on the occupations most important to the child and his or her identity. Attending to a child's habituation—habits and roles—also maintains the focus of evaluation and intervention on participation in occupations meaningful to the individual client. MOHO's attention to the unique effect of each environment on each individual also supports the client-centered approach central to occupational therapy.

OT practitioners can use MOHO concepts to communicate with other practitioners. For example, MOHO's concept of skill is directly aligned with the three skill areas described in the framework: motor, process, and communication/interaction skills.[1] MOHO pediatric assessments are aligned with several domains in the framework. Table 26-2 outlines how each of the MOHO pediatric assessments discussed in this chapter is aligned with specific domains of the framework.

SUMMARY

This chapter examined the concepts of the MOHO as well as reviewed therapeutic strategies for implementing

MOHO. This information provides OT practitioners with a way to explore, understand and address issues that affect a child's abilities. The MOHO helps OT practitioners identify areas in a child's life that are supportive of participation in occupations as well as those that create challenges. MOHO highlights the importance of personal client factors, including volition, habituation, and performance capacity. The MOHO also stresses the importance of different physical and social environmental factors that enhance or impede a child's capacity for participation. Use of the MOHO to methodically and systematically address areas of challenge and to identify strengths of a child supports best practice by focusing on the client. When an OT practitioner uses the MOHO to guide intervention, he or she is using an occupation-focused, evidence-based, and client-centered thought process to guide practice.

References

1. American Occupational Therapy Association. (2014). Occupational therapy practice framework: domain and process (3rd ed.). *Am J Occup Ther*, 68(Suppl 1.), S1–S48.
2. Basu, S., Kafkes, A., Schatz, R., Kiraly, A., & Kielhofner, G. (2008). *The Pediatric Volitional Questionnaire (PVQ), Version 2.1.* Chicago: MOHO Clearinghouse: University of Illinois.
3. Bowyer, P., Kramer, J., Ploszai, A., Ross, M., Schwarz, O., Kielhofner, G., et al. (2008). *The Short Child Occupational Profile (SCOPE). Version 2.2.* Chicago: MOHO Clearinghouse: University of Illinois.
4. Haglund, L., Ekbladh, E., Thorell, L. H., & Hallberg, I. R. (2000). Practice models in Swedish psychiatric occupational therapy. *Scand J Occup Ther, 7*, 107–113.
5. Hemmingsson, H., Egilson, S., Hoffman, O., & Kielhofner, G. (2005). *The School Setting Interview (SSI) Version 3.0.* Chicago: MOHO Clearinghouse: University of Illinois.
6. Keller, J., tenVelden, M., Kafkes, A., Basu, S., Federico, J., & Kielhofner, G. (2005). *Child Occupational Self Assessment. Version 2.1.* Chicago: MOHO Clearinghouse: University of Illinois.
7. Kielhofner, G. (2008). In *Model of Human Occupation: theory and application* (4th ed.). Baltimore, MD: Lippincott, Williams, & Wilkins.
8. Lee, S., Taylor, R., Kielhofner, G., & Fisher, A. (2008). Theory use in practice: a national survey of therapists who use the Model of Human Occupation. *Am J Occup Ther, 62*(1), 106–117.
9. National Board for Certification in Occupational Therapy. (2004). A practice analysis study of entry-level occupational therapist registered and certified occupational therapy assistant practice. *OTJR, 24*(Suppl 1.), S3–S31.
10. Nelson, D. (1988). Occupation: form and performance. *Am J Occup Ther, 42*, 633–641.

REVIEW *Questions*

1. Define the three personal client factors and four environmental factors that influence a child's participation in occupations.
2. Explain the difference between an interest and a value. How can these two concepts be related?

3. Explain the difference between the concepts of performance capacity and skill.
4. In your own words, explain the meaning of environmental impact.

SUGGESTED *Activities*

1. Imagine a clinical challenge you have encountered either through observation or experience. Use the volitional process to think of a way that you could address the child's volition and encourage him or her to engage in the therapeutic activity.
2. Think of one setting such as a bedroom or a classroom and brainstorm all the environment factors within that setting (spaces, objects, social groups, and tasks). Now think of two different clients with two different types of impairments. How does the same setting have a different environmental impact on each child?
3. Think of a child you have worked with in the past, how could you use MOHO to address this child's issue with participation? What conceptual area of MOHO would have helped you develop an intervention to positively affect this child? How would that concept have helped?

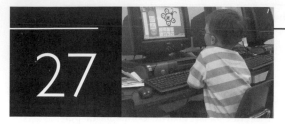

GILSON J. CAPILOUTO
JANE KLEINERT

27

Assistive Technology

CHAPTER *Objectives*

After studying this chapter, the reader will be able to accomplish the following:

- Describe terms, concepts, legislation, and trends in the use of assistive technology in pediatric occupational therapy
- Demonstrate understanding of specific classes of assistive technology available to children with disabilities
- Discuss the role of the occupational therapy assistant as it relates to successful evaluation and implementation of assistive technology services
- Describe best practice strategies required for successful evaluation and implementation of assistive technology services
- Demonstrate understanding of the characteristics of assistive technology and its relative importance in making assistive technology decisions
- Compare and contrast assistive, rehabilitative, educational, and medical technologies
- Provide examples of switch technology and the ways it might be used to assist a child in achieving a goal
- Describe the characteristics of switches and specific considerations when selecting a switch for an individual user
- Describe the ways environmental control units operate and how environmental control unit technology might be used for a child with a disability
- Discuss the role of simple communication technologies for children unable to communicate verbally

CHAPTER *Outline*

Technology continues to influence our lives considerably. We now have a daily dependence on a variety of technologies that include computers, cell phones, and personal digital assistant (PDAs). Each of these technologies has the potential to make our lives a little easier and more comfortable by helping us be more productive and efficient. For people with disabilities, technology is especially important as it can mean the difference between being able to accomplish a task alone and being forced to depend on someone else. In fact, technology has been described as the "great equalizer" for people with disabilities because it provides an important vehicle for maximizing capability.[6,10] The U.S. Congress acknowledged the crucial role of technology in the lives of people with disabilities when, in 1988, it passed Public Law 100-407, titled the Technology-Related Assistance for Individuals with Disabilities Act of 1988.[11] In the preamble to PL 100-407, Congress described four major benefits of assistive technology (AT) for individuals with disabilities:

1. Greater control over their individual lives,
2. Increased participation in their daily lives,
3. More widespread interaction with nondisabled individuals, and
4. The capacity to benefit from opportunities that most people frequently take for granted.

The Tech Act, as it is commonly referred to, allocated a considerable amount of dollars to support the efforts of the states to increase the awareness of the benefits of technology for people with disabilities, funding for the provision of AT devices and AT services, the number of personnel trained to provide such services, and coordination among state agencies and public and private entities to deliver AT devices and AT services.[7]

DEFINITIONS

The formal definition of **assistive technology** (AT), according to the federal government, is as follows: "Any item, piece of equipment, or product system, whether acquired commercially off the shelf, modified, or customized, that is used to increase or improve functional capabilities of individuals with disabilities."* The important thing to remember about this definition is the fact that anything that helps a person be more functional is considered AT. The term *assistive technology* naturally makes one think that AT has to be commercially manufactured and expensive; however, this is not always the case. Also formally defined in the law is the term **assistive technology services,** which includes "any service that directly assists an individual with a disability in the selection, acquisition, or use of an assistive technology device."*

*From Public Law 100-407, January 25, 1988.

The inclusion of a service component is particularly important to occupational therapy (OT) practitioners, and this suggests that those who framed this legislation realized an important truth: equipment alone is not enough; professional services are also required for the evaluation of AT and the training for its use.

Why should we consider the use of AT in the care of individuals with disabilities? A brief look at the World Health Organization's model of disability illustrates the importance of AT, by providing a synthesized view of health from multiple perspectives including individual, biological, and social.[12] Let us say that a child is born without upper extremities (body structures), and so he or she is unable to perform basic activities of daily living (ADLs; activity limitations). If this child is prevented from participating in a local drawing class because of this health condition or activity limitation, then his or her participation has been restricted (participation restriction). AT addresses the health condition aspect of the individual and minimizes activity limitations and participation restrictions by accomplishing multiple objectives. AT might serve to address the environmental factors possibly restricting participation in a desired activity. Such factors might include physical accessibility or attitudes, services, systems, or policies that interfere with the child's options for involvement. Additionally, by identifying and procuring an aid or device that allows the child to meet the goal of drawing, he or she can assume his or her role in society (e.g., a young child who wants to draw) and the health condition is thereby minimized.

> **CLINICAL *Pearl***
> Assistive technology refers to anything that helps a person be more functional in daily life.

> **CLINICAL *Pearl***
> Assistive technology services refer to any service that assists an individual with a disability in selecting, acquiring, and using an assistive aid or device.

ASSISTIVE TECHNOLOGY TEAM

Interdisciplinary teamwork is considered the cornerstone of effective rehabilitation.[2] The need for teamwork is particularly crucial as it relates to the use of AT. The disciplines represented as part of the **assistive technology team** may vary according to the needs of the client and health condition or body functions (Box 27-1). For example, a physical therapist provides important information about gross motor strength and function as well as positioning for function and mobility. The OT practitioner gives valuable input relative to fine motor

Potential Members of the Pediatric Assistive Technology Team

- Child
- Family/caregivers/guardians
- Regular and/or special educator
- Classroom assistants
- Day-care workers
- Physical therapist
- Occupational therapist
- Speech-language pathologist
- Vision specialist
- Audiologist (hearing specialist)
- Physician
- Case worker and/or social worker
- Rehabilitation engineer
- Vendor (assistive technology supplier)

function, participation in ADLs and positioning for access. The speech-language pathologist (SLP) is concerned with overall communication ability as well as specific strengths and abilities related to language comprehension and language expression. The user, and his or her parents, guardians, or caregivers, are always the central members of the team and involved in all aspects of equipment decision making and/or implementation. Additional team members could include a rehabilitation engineer charged with designing or fabricating aids or devices, an equipment vendor who provides medical equipment supplies, or a teacher concerned with using technology to assist a student in meeting his or her educational potential and achieving educational goals. Regardless of which professionals make up an individual team, it is the responsibility of each AT team to work together to decide what technology will be of benefit to an individual user, how it will be used, how equipment will be maintained, and how the impact of the technology will be measured.[4]

CLINICAL *Pearl*

A team approach is necessary for successful AT service delivery.

ROLE OF THE CERTIFIED OCCUPATIONAL THERAPY ASSISTANT

AT services vary depending on the setting and the experience of the individuals comprising the AT team. As such, the role of the certified occupational therapist assistant (COTA) will also vary according to setting and experience. The registered occupational therapist (OTR) and

the COTA are important members of the AT evaluation and service provision team.

At one time or another, the OTR and the COTA may be involved in securing necessary funding for AT, supervising the use of equipment, measuring outcomes related to equipment use, and equipment fabrication and/or adaptation. Additional roles of the COTA include child and family education and instruction in the use of AT as well as education and instruction for other team members such as regular and special educators and classroom assistants.

CHARACTERISTICS OF ASSISTIVE TECHNOLOGY

The term *assistive technology* is used to describe a broad array of assistive aids and devices that include, but are not limited to, aids for daily living, seating and positioning aids, communication aids and devices, environmental control units, aids for persons with visual impairments, and assistive listening devices. As a group, these technologies share common characteristics, which are important to understand in delivering quality AT services (Table 27-1). First, and most important, is a solid understanding of the distinction between "assistive technology" and rehabilitative, educational, or medical technology.[5] The term *assistive technology* should only be used to refer to aids and devices that are used daily to complete a given task. The terms **rehabilitative technology** or **educational technology** should be used when referring to the use of technology as only one aspect of an overall rehabilitation or education program. **Medical technology** refers to the use of technology to support or improve life functions. The following case study illustrates why this distinction is so important.

CASE *Study*

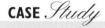

Tyronne has chronic Guillain-Barré syndrome and as a result is unable to use his upper extremities and is nonambulatory. He uses an electric wheelchair for mobility and operates it using a series of switches mounted to his headrest. Because of his upper extremity impairment, Tyronne cannot independently interact with age-appropriate toys. To minimize Tyronne's disability, his OTA has adapted a commercially available, battery-operated toy so that it turns "on" when a switch is activated. The OTA wants Tyronne to use the switch so that he can play independently. To use the switch and adapted toy as AT, the switch would be placed in a location that matched Tyronne's current abilities. This might mean mounting the switch on the headrest of his wheelchair, since his head appears to be his fastest, most energy efficient control site.

Now, let us consider another scenario. Marissa has a developmental disability characterized by gross and fine

TABLE 27-1

Characteristics of Assistive Technology with Definitions and Examples

CHARACTERISTIC	DEFINITION	EXAMPLE
Assistive technology	Technology used daily to improve function	Communication aid
Rehabilitative or educational technology	Technology is only one aspect of rehabilitation or educational program	Software program for teaching ABCs
Medical technology	Technology used to sustain life	Respirator
Low technology	Technology that is easy to obtain and use	Reacher
High technology	Technology that is difficult to obtain and use	Electric feeding machine
Assistive appliance	Aid/device that is beneficial without development of skill	Foot orthotics
Assistive tool	Aid/device that requires development of skill to be useful	Switch-adapted toy

motor delays. Currently, she does not maintain her head in an upright position for any length of time. The OTA is trying to devise activities that encourage Marissa to maintain head control, thereby strengthening the muscles required to develop this skill. The OTA decided that introducing a switch-operated toy may motivate Marissa to maintain an upright head position for increasingly longer periods of time. In this case the strategy may be mounting the switch so that it is activated only when the head is upright. The same technology that was used for Tyronne assistively is now being used for Marissa rehabilitatively.

Recall that the definition of AT emphasizes function, not disability. Because Marissa has to work very hard to activate the toy and this is only one of many activities she is engaged in to increase independent head control, the use of the toy and switch would be considered rehabilitative technology.

CLINICAL *Pearl*

> Assistive technology (AT) targets function, whereas rehabilitative and educational technologies target dysfunction.

You might still be confused as to why this distinction is so important. Consider that in the scenario with Tyronne, the goal is to make technology easy to access. But, in the second scenario, with Marissa, the technology is actually hard to access, because she is being challenged to move in ways that are not easy for her. We would certainly not want an individual to work as hard as Marissa if the goal was daily, independent play. This distinction is important for more practical reasons as well. For example, the use of AT daily (as in the case of Tyronne) or temporarily (as in the case of Marissa) has

a direct effect on considerations of durability, cost, and operational difficulty. If we are going to use a device for the development of a particular skill, we would not want to spend large amounts of money or consider an option that would require a significant amount of lead time to achieve operational competence. Instead, we would limit our options to an aid or device that was relatively inexpensive and easy to learn. This distinction between assistive and rehabilitative or educational technology is also very important for setting technology-related goals as well as gauging our expectations for technology use (i.e., whether we expect AT to be used daily or over a long period of time).

Another characteristic of AT is that it can be categorized as **low technology** or **high technology**.[5] This distinction is somewhat self-explanatory. Low technology is easy to obtain, easy to use, and of relatively low cost. In contrast, high technology is more difficult to obtain, requires greater skill to use, and is frequently more costly. We consider these factors when weighing options for individual users. For example, if we are working with an individual who we know to be "technophobic," then we would probably want to keep our AT options toward the low-technology end. At the same time, we do not want to make AT decisions simply based on the fact that someone enjoys and is comfortable with technology. This author's motto is simple: Never buy a Jaguar when a Volkswagen will do! To be safe, we should always make sure that our decisions about technology are based on the goals and abilities of the child.[7]

The final characteristic of AT that we need to discuss is the distinction between assistive technology tools and assistive technology appliances.[5] The term **assistive appliance** includes any aid or device that provides benefit to the user with little to no training or development of skill. This could include items such as eyeglasses or orthotics. An **assistive tool**, on the other hand, requires the development of skill for it to be of value to the user. Examples of assistive tools include feeding machines, communication aids and devices, and mobility aids. This distinction is especially important when speaking with users and caregivers about their expectations of AT. A good example is the selection of a communication aid or device. Too often, there are misconceptions that if we "just find the right thing," the user will be able to communicate instantaneously. It is important for everyone to be clear about the fact that any communication aid or device is an assistive tool and, as such, requires a certain degree of training before it can be of benefit to the user.

CLINICAL *Pearl*

Assistive appliances such as eyeglasses provide benefit to the user without the development of skill.

CLINICAL *Pearl*

Assistive tools, such as communication technologies, require the development of skill to be of benefit to the user.

ASSISTIVE TECHNOLOGY MYTHS AND REALITIES

In their book on assistive technology, Jan Galvin and Marcia Scherer describe a number of myths and realities with respect to AT, many of which are important to share before moving forward.[7] As already mentioned, AT does not need to be expensive or complicated. A simple pad and pencil can be the perfect communication aid. Moreover, keep in mind that people with the same disability do not necessarily require the same devices. For example, the same wheelchair is not recommended for every person needing one. It is especially important to keep in mind that "assessment," as it relates to AT, is an ongoing process. It is simply not possible to know everything about an individual user in the course of three or even four encounters. Additionally, as users develop and improve their skills as a result of intervention, reassessment of AT needs is warranted. We discuss this further in the section on the assessment process. Lastly, it is important to be open to multiple sources of information when it comes to AT. The field of AT is changing at a remarkably rapid pace, and it is very difficult for any single professional to be familiar with everything that is available. Consequently, consumers, family members, and even vendors can provide valuable input about appropriate technology for individual users.

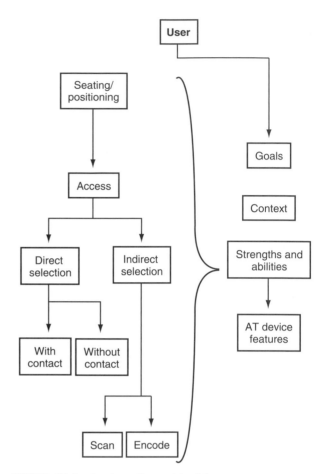

FIGURE 27-1 A schematic model of the assessment process for assistive technology adapted from human factors engineering.

ASSISTIVE TECHNOLOGY ASSESSMENT

Like so many aspects of rehabilitation, AT assessment is a team endeavor. Although COTAs do not conduct evaluations, it is critical to understand the process of evaluation so that the clinical information that is shared with the occupational therapist is valuable in making adjustments to AT goals and intervention procedures for individual users. Numerous approaches to decision making for AT exist. The one discussed here is adapted from a model rooted in the field of human factors engineering.[5] Human factors engineering is a field of study devoted to the interface between man and machines; its application to the field of AT is well suited. As you read this section, it will be helpful to refer to the schematic of the assessment process shown in Figure 27-1.

In rehabilitation, the assessment process is frequently started by administering standardized tests and criteria-referenced measures in an attempt to answer the question, "What can't the individual do?" However, it must be remembered that AT targets function rather than dysfunction, so knowing what an individual cannot do is not very helpful when trying to determine whether technology would be of benefit. Instead, when considering technology, the rehabilitation specialist asks, "What is it the user wants to do?" and/or "What is it the user needs to be able to do?" With these questions as the focus, the AT assessment process begins where it should, with the goals for the user.

When establishing goals for individual users, OT practitioners consider the following:

1. Is this goal rehabilitative or functional?
2. Is this goal shared by the student/user, the family, and other members of the team?
3. Does the goal make sense; is it logical?

You will recall that the distinction between goals that are assistive and those that are rehabilitative affects how equipment is set up (i.e., conserving effort and energy as much as possible [assistive] or as a motor challenge [rehabilitative]) and the type of equipment that is considered (i.e., learning time and cost). Also, when equipment is being considered, intervention goals should be discussed with everyone who has a vested interest in the user because assistive devices frequently require the support of caregivers and other team members for training and maintenance. For example, the OT practitioner, along with the physical therapist, may want to increase a student's exposure to powered mobility as part of a goal focused on independence. However, the student's family is committed to emphasizing the use of a walker and so does not want to consider a power wheelchair. Because the caregivers do not share the goal of powered mobility, it may not be wise to pursue that goal at this time.

Lastly, when establishing goals, it is important to consider whether we are asking the user to do something you and I could/would do. For example, if we have a goal that states the user will attend to an activity for 30 minutes, we have to ask ourselves whether or not we would attend to the same activity for that length of time. Once we have established goals, we can begin to explore whether or not the child's ability to achieve those goals would be enhanced by the use of assistive equipment.

Following the establishment of goals, the next question is, "Where and with whom will the goal(s) be addressed?" This question focuses on the settings for each of the child's goals such as home, school, and/or the community. Each of these has the potential of affecting decisions with regard to devices. For example, one of the user's goals might be to initiate interaction using a communication aid or device. Naturally, we would hope this goal would be addressed across all of the user's physical settings, so one important aspect of any aid or device we will consider would be its portability. The idea of context also includes a social component. For example, will the goal be addressed with familiar or unfamiliar peers, familiar or unfamiliar adults, strangers, or all of the above? Finally, context takes into account the physical contexts of a goal, including temperature (impact of excessive heat or cold), sound (ambient noise), and light (ambient light).

The effect of these factors is fairly obvious. For example, any goal that includes the playground as a setting would need to account for the weather as well as changes in light (natural vs artificial).

The third primary component of assessment involves the specific strengths and abilities of the user. This is where information from specific team members becomes critical. The areas of strength and ability include family, gross motor, fine motor, cognitive, communication, and sensory strengths and abilities. The following case study provides examples in each of these performance skills.

CASE *Study*

Westin is a 9-year-old with cerebral palsy. He is also legally blind. He is believed to have mild intellectual disability. The goal for Westin is functional communication in all settings (home, school, church, community). Currently he uses multiple nonsymbolic forms of communication, including gestures, facial expressions, vocalizations, and simple signs. He has experience using a switch for computer access that includes scanning. The social context for the goal includes familiar peers and non-peers, family, community workers, and strangers. The physical contexts for his goal are inside, outside, school bus, and family van.

Family strengths and abilities include parents who are supportive and involved, insurance coverage for durable medical equipment, and parents who are technology-literate. His gross motor abilities include being able to operate a manual wheelchair with customized seating systems and lap tray for upright support. No plans have been made to alter his system in the next 2 years. With respect to fine motor abilities Westin uses a gross swipe toward objects with fisted hands. Moreover, he uses a head-mounted switch to scan items on a computer screen. Cognitively, he appears to understand much of what is said to him, smiles and laughs when spoken to, makes choices between objects and pictures (groupings of four), and follows two- and three-step commands when they are within his physical capabilities. He uses multiple forms of nonsymbolic communication (vocalizations, facial expressions, body language) as well as simple, adapted manual signs. Information regarding sensory systems indicates his vision is limited to objects and pictures about 4 in. × 4 in., and auditory acuity is within normal limits. Other noteworthy strengths include a good sense of humor, mischievousness, and a friendly and outgoing personality.

This case illustrates a number of key points with respect to assessment. First, note the emphasis on ability. In each domain, we have listed what Westin can do. By taking such an approach, we narrow our equipment options considerably, and with the plethora of equipment available to us, anything we can do to narrow our options is probably good. In the case of communication technologies, we already know we can capitalize on the use of his existing ability to use a head switch for scanning, so we need a device that accepts scanning. In addition, we know he can distinguish as many as four items and can follow three-step directions; this permits us to consider more operationally complex devices.

As various team members gather information, the skills and abilities of the user translate into the necessary features of any aid or device that is considered. For example, if in the course of team conferencing, it is learned that a child has decreased visual acuity, then any aid or device considered needs to include features that account for that, for example, bright colors, tactile features, auditory feedback, and/or magnification options.

Returning to our discussion on assessment, a fundamental aspect is determining how a potential user will interface with an assistive aid or device. This is referred to as **access**. Access is the point of contact between the user and the aid or device that he or she needs to control. For example, you and I "access" the computer via a keyboard and/or mouse. Initially, we work as a team on the identification of a particular "**control site**" or location on the body that can be used to operate a device.[5] Potential sites for controlling aids or devices include hands and fingers, arms, the head, eyes, legs, or feet. Ultimately, the site and movement chosen should represent the fastest, most energy efficient, and most reliable. Following the identification of a control site, the team begins the task of determining the most appropriate form of access for a given user.

One form of access is referred to as **direct selection**. Direct selection is a straightforward method for making a choice or selection.[3,5,7] The keyboard and the mouse are considered direct selection forms of access. For example, when we want to type an "e" we go directly to it and make that selection (by using a finger). Using your hands to operate the joystick on a computer game console is another example of direct selection; when you want to go left, you move the joystick to the left with no intermediate steps involved. Touching a picture to request a drink, using a head pointer or a mouth stick are also considered direct selection techniques.

Each of these examples illustrates direct selection with physical contact. However, for some individuals, physical contact with a control interface is not possible. In such cases, we might consider options that allow for direct selection without physical contact. For example, a person using the eyes to indicate a letter on an alphabet board is using direct selection in the absence of physical contact. A straightforward method of indicating a choice is still used but doing so without physically touching the choice. Another example of direct selection without physical contact would be using a laser pointer to make selections on a display.

As shown in the previous examples, being able to select choices directly is fast and efficient; whether they are letters on a keyboard, directions for a wheelchair, or messages on a communication aid or device. Yet for many individuals with disabilities, direct forms of access are not possible. For these clients, we turn to **indirect selection** access options. Indirect selection requires intermediate steps to make a selection. Now, rather than going directly to the letter on a keyboard, the user might have to scan through the letters of the alphabet via rows and then columns using a switch. To drive a wheelchair, the user might use a switch array corresponding to each direction he or she wants to go (e.g., a switch for "right" and another one for "left"). Alternatively, he or she might use a single switch connected to a directional panel, scanning through the options (i.e., left, right, back, forward). Scanning is one form of indirect selection; another is referred to as encoding.[5] With encoding, the user relies on multiple signals together to specify response. For example, in the case of a person who cannot use his or her hands to operate a wheelchair, a "sip and puff" signal may be used to control the direction of the chair. In this example, varying combinations of signals serve as an encoded language for directional commands such as soft sip, soft puff, forward; and hard sip, soft sip, left. Another example of multiple signal encoding is the Morse code, in which dots and dashes are combined to specify specific letters of the alphabet.

In summary, one important aspect of AT assessment is determining access or how the user will operate or interface with a given device or aid. Two primary forms of access are direct selection, and indirect selection. Direct selection is a straightforward method of indicating a choice or selection. It can be accomplished with or without physical contact. In contrast, indirect selection requires intermediate steps to indicate a response. Indirect selection may be accomplished in one of two ways: scanning or encoding.

Clinically important distinctions exist between direct and indirect selection techniques, and it is important to keep these distinctions in mind. Physically, direct selection is considered more difficult than indirect selection because it requires more refined, controlled movements.[5] However, because all of the elements in the selection set are equally available and do not need to be scanned, direct selection is considered the faster form of device control.[3] Direct selection is also considered less cognitively complex than indirect selection because it is more intuitive.[1] For these reasons, direct selection forms of device control are considered a better option than indirect forms of control. Therefore it is important to thoroughly examine the potential for direct selection forms of access before considering indirect selection techniques.[3,7]

Returning to the model in Figure 27-1, one can see that seating and positioning issues, as well as issues of access, are superimposed on the assessment model aspect of skills and abilities. It is important to keep in mind that muscle tone (e.g., hypertonia and/or hypotonia), the presence of primitive reflexes, skeletal deformities, or movement disorders will all influence access to equipment. Therefore seating and positioning become critical in minimizing the influence of these characteristics on functional device operation. The reader is referred to Chapter 18 for specific information regarding best practice principles of seating and positioning.

ASSISTIVE TECHNOLOGY FOR PEDIATRICS

A number of classes of AT tools should be considered when working with pediatric clients. For the purposes of this chapter, we focus on technology for leisure activities and environmental control and simple communication technologies. Although the focus here is primarily on simple technology solutions, high-technology approaches are also equally important to consider for pediatric populations.

Technology for Leisure Activities

For very young children, "leisure activities" translates to "play." It is important to keep the definition of play in mind because it is easy for us to turn play into therapy. Play is an intrinsic activity engaged in for its own sake, rather than a means of achieving a specific end.[9] Play should be fun, spontaneous, and voluntary. Adapted play refers to the fact that toys are modified to enable children with disabilities to participate and that learning is intentionally incorporated into play activities.[9]

Greenstein suggested that simply observing a child with a particular toy can tell us much about what we need to know before considering adapted toys.[9] First, we should ask ourselves whether a child is playing with a toy because he or she wants to (intrinsic motivation) or because someone else wants him or her to (extrinsic motivation). This is important because research suggests that using rewards to encourage children to engage in an activity will decrease a child's subsequent interest in that activity. It reminds us that children should be playing because they want to. Angelo suggested three possible reasons to explain why children with disabilities do not

engage with toys: (a) they are not interested in the toys (amotivated), (b) frequent failures interacting with toys have reduced their motivation to try (learned helplessness), or (c) they want to play but are physically unable to play with the toys.[9] Adapting toys is helpful to children who are physically unable to play with toys.

The first consideration in adapting play materials for children with disabilities is deciding whether materials simply need to be stabilized.[8] Frequently, children with physical disabilities need a stable surface on which to play so that objects will not move out of their reach. For example, lining a tray with indoor–outdoor carpet and then attaching male Velcro to the base of books, baby dolls, and trucks can serve to hold objects in a stable position and encourage play. A second strategy is to enlarge materials, which serves to enhance visual perception and decrease reliance on fine motor skills.[8] Simple solutions include attaching handles to puzzle pieces and pop-up boxes and placing foam strips around brushes, markers, and utensils to make them easier to hold. Finally, toys can be attached to trays and/or to the children by using elastic bands so that if the toys fall out of reach they can be easily retrieved.

A third strategy is ensuring that all play materials are accessible; as much as possible, children should be able to physically select their own toys and activities.[11] For example, for children in wheelchairs, toys should be attached at chair height on a wall with Velcro or in nets hung from the ceiling. For children physically unable to retrieve their own toys, items should be arranged so that they are easy to select by a gross reach or by pointing. An alternative would be to develop simple picture or object displays that allow children to indicate the toy they want or the game they want to play. For example, attaching actual objects or large photographs to a strip of hard-backed poster board allows children to choose. Choices should be spaced far enough apart to allow children to select a picture of the activity or toy using either a gross upper extremity movement or their eyes (Figure 27-2).

Switch-Activated Toys

Using **switches** to interact with toys and appliances is another form of adapted play. Such adaptations allow children with physical limitations to engage in independent exploration and interaction with the environment. Moreover, using switches with toys can be considered a preliminary activity that serves to develop the skills needed to control a wheelchair or operate a communication device. Switches open and close a circuit, so they operate in the same way as many of the appliances operated on a daily basis, such as televisions, light switches, CD players, and toasters (Figure 27-3).[1] Switches give a person with physical limitations the option to control toys and appliances that he or she otherwise would be physically unable to manage.

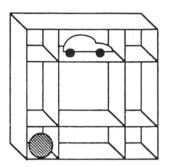

Plexiglass eye gaze object box

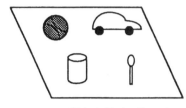

Object Choice Board

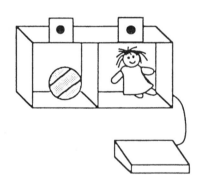

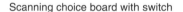

Scanning choice board with switch

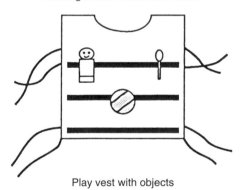

Play vest with objects

FIGURE 27-2 Play activity choice boards. (From Glennen, S., & Church, G. (1992). Adaptive toys and environmental controls. In G. Church & S. Glennen (Eds.), *The handbook of assistive technology.* San Diego, CA: Singular Publishing Group.)

Switches come in all shapes and sizes with varying visual, auditory, and sensory features. When selecting a switch for an individual, consider the following questions:

1. What are the potential control sites for a switch (i.e., head, hand, arm, foot)?

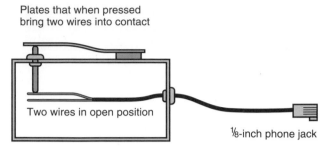

Plates that when pressed bring two wires into contact

Two wires in open position

⅛-inch phone jack

FIGURE 27-3 Anatomy of a switch.

2. What are the functional ranges of motion of potential sites?
3. Does the user have any unique sensory needs that need to be considered?
4. What mounting issues need to be considered?

In fact, just looking at a given switch provides information about its intended user. Keep in mind that manufacturers design switches for very specific reasons—it is not a random process. For instance, OT practitioners ask such questions as, Does the size of the activation surface suggest a person who uses more gross movements or fine movements? Is the switch intended for foot and/or hand activation, cheek/chin activation, or head/thumb activation? Would the physical characteristics of the switch appeal to a child or to an adult? Do the physical characteristics of the switch suggest anything about vision or cognition? What about the strength requirements of the switch? Remember, the task is to match a user's skills and abilities to the features of a switch. The following case scenario provides an example of this process.

CASE *Study*

Twelve-year-old Jayden has a diagnosis of spastic-quadriplegic cerebral palsy. He has also been diagnosed with visual impairment, although the degree of his visual loss is not known. He uses a manual wheelchair for mobility, but is not independent in its use. Although it is difficult to ascertain his precise abilities using standardized tests, his teachers feel that he is responsive to communication and laughs and smiles appropriately when others direct attention to him. He uses multiple nonsymbolic forms of communication, including postural changes associated with excitement and anticipation, swiping at unwanted items with his right upper extremity, and vocalizing to express pleasure and displeasure. His professional team thinks he is a good candidate for an appliance operated by a switch.

Using the Switch Analysis Worksheet shown in Figure 27-4, note the descriptions of each of the pictured switches. Of those presented, which offers features that best match Jayden's described strengths and abilities?

Switch	Picture	Access	Control Site(s)	Sensory Features	Other
1. Lighted Signal Switch ($52.95) **Rapid Assist Technology, Inc.** 614C S Business IH 35 New Braunfels, TX 72130 http://rapidassisttech.com/ 6 1/2"D x 4"H	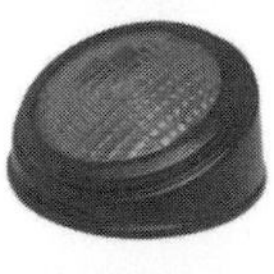	Gross access	Upper extremities; fisted or open hand; foot	Ribbed surface for tactile stimulation; activation feedback; lighted	Angled presentation; suction cup feet
2. Specs Switch ($59.00) **AbleNet, Inc.** 2625 Patton Road Roseville, MN 55113-1308 http://www.ablenetinc.com/ 1 3/8" diameter	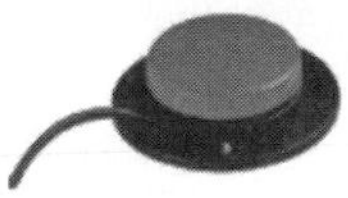	Fine access	Single digit; head; cheek	Activation feedback; bright colors	Various mounting options-velcro strap
3. Pal Pad ($45.00) **Adaptivation, Inc.** 2305-B W. 50th Street Sioux Falls, SD 57105 http://www.adaptivation.com/ index.php 2.5 x 4 x .1 "	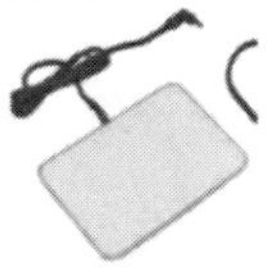	Gross access	Open hand; foot; elbow	Bright color	Completely flat
4. Plate Switch ($50.95) **Enabling Devices** **Toys for Special Children** 50 Broadway Hawthorne, NY 10532 http://enablingdevices.com/ 5" x 8"	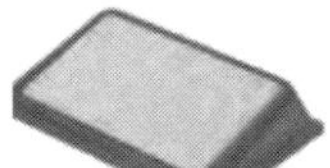	Gross access	Open hand; foot	Activation feedback; bright color	Angled presentation; suction cup feet

FIGURE 27-4 Sample switch analysis worksheet.

If you picked switch 1, congratulations! You are correct. The lighted signal switch offers a relatively large surface area that complements Jayden's gross motor approach to tasks. In addition, it offers sensory features well suited to accommodate his visual impairment, including the fact that it lights up on activation and presents an audible click on activation. Finally, its ribbed surface offers Jayden tactile stimulation as well.

The preceding case reiterates the importance of selecting switches based on individual needs. A worksheet, such as the one provided in Figure 27-4, can help you analyze the options for various clients. If the appropriate switch is not selected, OT practitioners run the risk of drawing conclusions about a student's ability to use a switch that may or may not be incorrect. For example, if switch 2 is the only one available for use, Jayden would most likely be unsuccessful because of its small size and minimal feedback. As a result of his performance with this switch, the team might deduce that he is not capable of using a switch, when, in fact, the switch presented did not accommodate his specific strengths and abilities.

Once a specific switch is selected for trial use, we turn our attention to developing an activity for introducing the switch. The activity should be age appropriate and motivating to the user. It is also important to be precise in the placement of the switch and the appliance or toy, in relation to the user, and to make sure that we repeat that correct placement each time the user engages in switch-activated play. Moreover, trial use of a switch should be carefully monitored before altering the switch or its placement. Users need the opportunity to practice using switches across a variety of activities before changes are considered because switches are considered assistive tools, so some development of skill is required before the switches can be of benefit and before conclusions are made about intervention success or the need for program adjustments.

As stated previously, a number of potential adapted play options are available, depending on the goals for an individual user. Adaptive switches can be used to operate a variety of battery-run or electronic toys and appliances.[8] Switches attach to toys or appliances via cables. More often than not, switches will come with cable attachments. At the end of the cable will be a miniature plug (Figure 27-5, A). Toys or appliances that have already been developed with switches will come equipped with cable receptors in the form of switch interface jacks (see Figure 27-5, B). Alternatively, one can use a battery adapter specifically designed for use with commercially available battery-operated toys and appliances. Battery adapters have a cable receptor with a female phone jack at one end and a copper plate at the other end.

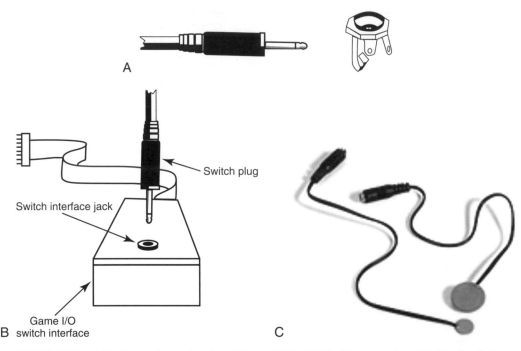

A

Switch plug

Switch interface jack

Game I/O
B switch interface

C

FIGURE 27-5 **A**, Miniature plug: typical sizes ⅛, ¼, and ½ inch. **B**, Switch plug and switch interface jack. **C**, Sample battery adaptor. (**B** from Glennen, S., & Church, G. (1992). Adaptive toys and environmental controls. In G. Church & S. Glennen (Eds.), *The handbook of assistive technology.* San Diego, CA: Singular Publishing Group.)

The copper plate is sized to fit the specific battery type (e.g., AAA, C, D) and is placed between the battery and one of the metal battery contacts, thus interrupting the on/off circuitry (see Figure 27-5, C).[8] Now, when the toy or appliance is placed in the "on" position, it will not operate until the switch is activated. The trick with using both adapted toys and/or battery adapters is that different manufacturers use different-sized cable jacks and receptors, so it is frequently necessary to use adapters to convert between female- and male-type jacks. Resources for battery adapters and cable adapters are included at the end of this chapter.

Finally, it is important to understand the three modes of operation available when using switch technology with individual users. In "momentary" or "continuous" mode, the user must maintain pressure on the switch in order to keep the toy or appliance operating.[1] This is also referred to as the direct mode. Unfortunately, this is not particularly functional. Think about how often you would watch TV or listen to music if you had to continually press the "on" button to do it! Switch-latch timers are devices designed to eliminate this need.[1] To work, the switch is plugged into one part of the switch-latch timer, and the device to be operated is plugged into another part (Figure 27-6). When set in the latched mode, activation of the switch turns the device on, and reactivation of the switch turns the device off. This is a very functional setting for activities such as making milkshakes using a blender or listening to the radio and watching TV. In the timed

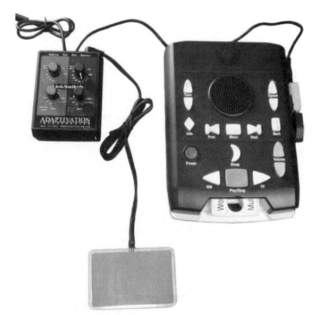

FIGURE 27-6 Switch-latch timer with switch (bottom center) and toy tape recorder (on the right). (From Adaptivation Incorporated: Resources-Handouts: LinkSwitch and Digital Book Player, Sioux Falls, SD, 2014, Adaptivation.)

mode, activation of the switch turns the device on, and it stays on for the amount of time specified; this could be seconds, minutes, or hours. This mode is particularly helpful to determine whether an individual understands that the switch is being used to operate something.

TABLE 27-2

Control Sequence for Environmental Control Systems

INPUT	THROUGHPUT	OUTPUT
Activates system by sending a signal	Receives and transmits signal	Receives signal and gives output
Examples include voice signal, switch activation, and button depression	Examples include radio frequency, ultrasound, and infrared transmission	Examples include lights being turned on or off, volume being turned up or down, CD player being turned on

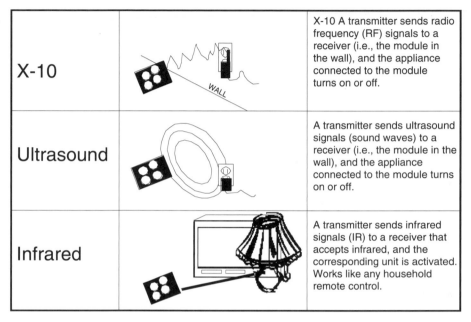

X-10		X-10 A transmitter sends radio frequency (RF) signals to a receiver (i.e., the module in the wall), and the appliance connected to the module turns on or off.
Ultrasound		A transmitter sends ultrasound signals (sound waves) to a receiver (i.e., the module in the wall), and the appliance connected to the module turns on or off.
Infrared		A transmitter sends infrared signals (IR) to a receiver that accepts infrared, and the corresponding unit is activated. Works like any household remote control.

FIGURE 27-7 Three common transmission methods for environmental control units.

For example, using a tape recorder and a switch-latch timer, activation of the switch would result in music being played. When the music stops, the OT practitioner looks for signs that the user understands that the switch and the tape recorder are related somehow. For example, does the user reach for the switch? Does the user reach for the tape recorder? Does the user look at the switch? Does the user look at the tape recorder? These are all signs that the user understands the relationship between the switch and what is being controlled and so can be taught to control devices and toys using switches.

Environmental Controls

Environmental control units (ECUs) are systems that allow an individual to control his or her environment. An ECU consists of an input device, a throughput method, and some form of output (Table 27-2). Three common transmission methods can be used to purposefully manipulate and interact with the environment (Figure 27-7). ECUs offer a motivating option for increasing the functional independence of children with disabilities. ECUs are an important class of AT tools to keep in mind when

considering user goals, as it is an area frequently overshadowed by adapted play technologies and communication technologies. It is important to note that infants as young as 9 months frequently reach for the remote control and proceed to aim it at the television!

Angelo suggested a number of questions be considered when making decisions about ECU options for clients.[1] These questions include asking what the user wants to be able to do, what the user's strengths and abilities are, the context(s) for ECU, and the type of feedback needed by the user. These questions are essentially the same as the ones we used in our assessment model. This model has merit regardless of the class of AT tools under consideration. The following case study illustrates the role of ECU options for pediatric clients with disabilities.

CASE *Study*

Sasha is a 4-year-old with spastic-quadriplegic cerebral palsy. She loves to listen to music and recently received an iPad for her birthday. Sasha's occupational therapist decides to introduce the operation of the iPad with a focus on listening to music because she enjoys that so much. The OT practitioner sets up Sasha's iPad for switch access using directions from imore.com (http://www.imore.com/how-enable-switch-control-motor-accessibility-iphone-or-ipad). By simply going into the settings, and altering the accessibility features, the iPad can operate via switch input and scanning. Moreover, the icons on the opening display can be made larger and the number can be controlled. The occupational therapist decides to have Sasha use the Ablenet's Big Red Twist Switch to access the iPad since she using that switch for access to other items. Using a set-up that includes the switch, the iPad and the APPlicator, Sasha can play her music independently. The APPlicator is a Bluetooth switch interface that has multiple options, including play/pause, skip forward, skip back, and timed play. The OT practitioner decides to introduce the ECU activity using timed play for 15 seconds. This setting will require that Sasha reactivate the switch to continue to play music. Once Sasha gets the idea, the occupational therapist switches over to play/pause mode, giving Sasha complete control. ECU systems for young children are generally straightforward and simple to operate. They offer a level of control that promotes the development of self-determination and empowerment for children with disabilities and so should be incorporated into treatment frequently.

Simple Communication Technologies

Communication technologies (alternative augmentative communications [AAC]) are used in an area of clinical practice that attempts to compensate (either temporarily or permanently) when an individual has difficulty using speech as a primary means of communication. It is important to understand that an AAC device is only one aspect of an individual's communication system, which could also include gestures, facial expressions, body language, and other nonsymbolic forms of communication.

A certified licensed SLP makes decisions about specific aids and devices for individual users. However, it is critical that all team members provide input regarding the specific strengths and abilities of a given user so that the SLP can make an informed decision. Moreover, it goes without saying that all persons involved in the care of an individual using an AAC device would need to understand how the system operates as well as how to interact with an individual using an AAC aid or device.

For the purposes of this chapter, we focus on simple AAC technologies. These are systems that are either manual (i.e., have no electronic components) or simple electronic devices (i.e., use household batteries for operation). Referring back to the assessment model, the SLP looks to various team members to provide input

regarding optimal seating and positioning for access to AAC devices, as well as a user's strengths and abilities relative to direct or indirect selection options and mounting needs. The remaining decisions focus specifically on the language options for AAC. These include how language will be represented (symbol type), what specific words or phrases need to be available to the user (vocabulary selection), what the user will see when they look at the aid or device (display organization), and finally, how messages will be stored and retrieved (message storage and retrieval).

For very young children, simple AAC technologies tend to be activity based. That is, children use specific displays to interact in the context of a specific activity such as snack time, playing with Play-Doh, blowing bubbles, or completing puzzles. Displays tend to include simple line drawings arranged in a row/column format that includes anywhere from 2 to 32 vocabulary items, depending on a child's language ability. Manual displays might involve the use of a vest, eye gaze frame, or single sheet displays depending on individual motor abilities (Figure 27-8).

A number of simple battery-operated AAC systems that take advantage of human-recorded speech to transmit messages are available. The motivation of hearing a spoken message cannot be underestimated in young children for whom speech is difficult. Single-message devices can give children an opportunity to request attention ("Please come here"), request assistance ("Can you help me?"), express a desire ("Please leave me alone"), express recurrence ("Let's do it again!"), or even saying that favorite toddler expression "NO!" Devices designed to present a series of messages (e.g., Step-by-Step

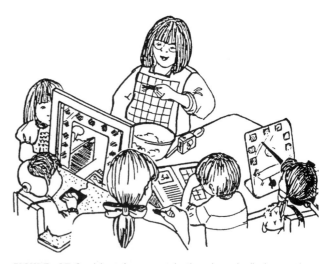

FIGURE 27-8 Manual communication board display options. (From Goosens, C., Crain, S. S., & Elder, P. S. (1994). *Engineering the preschool environment for interactive communication: 18 months to 5 years developmentally* (2nd ed.). Birmingham, AL: Southeast Augmentative Communication Conference Publications, Clinician Series.)

Communicator by Ablenet, Inc.; Sequencer by Adaptivation, Inc.) can provide children with the opportunity to actively participate in story time ("He huffed, and he puffed, and he blew the house down!"), serve as the leader of an activity ("Ready, set, go!"), or tell parents what happened at school that day ("I had pizza for lunch," "We played musical chairs," and "I sat next to Billy on the bus.").

Simple battery-operated devices also come in more complex displays ranging from 2 to 16 possible messages. When using devices with limited messaging capability, SLPs make an effort to program messages that have applicability across a variety of contexts as opposed to those that are limited in use. For example, messages such as "I want a drink" or "I want to eat" are limited in scope. Mealtime and snack time are generally built into one's school day, so the need to request food or drink becomes somewhat moot. More powerful messages such as "my turn," "finished," "more," or "come here" are useful across a variety of activities and will give the child an opportunity to use his or her AAC device multiple times throughout the course of the day.

Visual scene displays (VSDs) are a recent addition to the technology options available to young children. VSD refers to the way messages are stored and retrieved, and although they are created on high-technology devices, they are simple and intuitive to use. Instead of placing graphic symbols in a row/column format, VSDs use contextually rich visual images such as photographs or commercially available images of favorite characters. Such displays provide communication partners with a greater context for interaction and language development. (More information on VSDs can be found at http://leadersproject.org/articles/contemporary-approaches-intervention-visual-scene-displays-vsd.)

Another recent addition to technology options for use with children are apps for mobile devices. The majority of us are familiar with these types of electronic programs given our use of smartphones, tablets, and/or other mobile technologies. Apps are small, self-contained programs that are easy to download and use on a variety of mobile systems. An exciting development in this programming is the easy accessibility of apps for use as AAC programs that can turn readily available mobile devices in to simple AAC systems.

There are multiple apps available for use as one aspect of overall communication. As with other types of AT, several factors must be considered when choosing an app as a potential form of AAC for a given child. All the elements discussed in this chapter regarding child assessment, such as the child's status of motor skills, cognition, and sensory abilities, must be investigated when considering possible apps. Also, the same decisions regarding access (direct vs scanning), language representation systems (e.g., pictures vs photos vs text),

display options, and the most functional way to position the system in relation child must be determined. The characteristics of the app itself must also be assessed to make the best match for the user. Table 27-3 provides a visual display of the possible components that may or may not be available in a given app along with other important factors to consider before selecting a communication app. For example, if voice output is desired, is it offered by the app? Are screen displays premade or can they be customized with personal photos or pictures? Can the app use text rather than pictures only? Does the app allow for scanning with external switches as an access mode? These are all very important issues. If the child cannot use "direct selection" (as described earlier) and must scan using an external switch this may be a problem with many apps. Although Bluetooth technology now allows scanning on an iPad and other such devices, the app itself must also be one that accepts scanning.

Finally, because additional apps become available all the time, cost should be considered (many apps are free or very inexpensive), as well as easy availability to updates and compatibility with other mobile technologies such as an iPad, iPod, iPhone (iOS) or equivalent Android mobile options. An app may appear to be a good match for a given child, but if the family does not have the compatible mobile device, it is not a viable option. Also keep in mind that you want to be able to provide options because the family and the child are the ultimate decisions makers. When looking for apps, always check device compatibility and be sure to read reviews by users before deciding on the options to present a child and his or her family. These reviews are usually included in the description section of the app store you consult.

One last caution when thinking about mobile apps for AAC is the fact that mobile devices are *not* considered dedicated communication systems (i.e., assistive devices used solely for augmentative/alternative communication). Although mobile devices and AAC apps are markedly less expensive than many dedicated AAC instruments, because mobile devices typically serve purposes other than communication, they may not be covered by third-party funding sources.

AAC devices have special cognitive, motor, perceptual, and learning requirements for the people that use them and their communication partners. It is for this reason that successful use of communication technologies involves a coordinated team approach focused on interactive communication and motivating activities. Careful planning and training are required for children to become competent users of AAC systems. Remember, the goal is to reinforce and facilitate any attempt at communication, since what a child has to say is more important than how he or she says it!

TABLE 27-3

Example Decision-Making Chart for Communication Apps

APP NAME	DATE OF ISSUE	OPERATING SYSTEM	PREMADE DISPLAYS	CUSTOMIZABLE DISPLAYS	VOICE OUTPUT
App A	2014	iPad only	Yes	Yes	Yes
App B	2013	Android	Yes	No	Yes
App C	2013	All iOS	Yes	Yes	Yes
App D	2012	All iOS	No	No	Yes

FUNDING FOR ASSISTIVE TECHNOLOGY

Federal legislation provides the foundation for funding for ATs. In other words, lawmakers (senators and legislators) design bills (laws) using input from advocates (in this case, persons with disabilities [PWD], their caregivers, and professionals) that are designed to ensure by law that people have access to the equipment they need.

Before the 1970s, very little legislation addressed the needs PWD. So they and their families relied on private and religious charities, fended for themselves, or just did not have the needed funding. The Rehabilitation Act of 1973 (referred to as Section 504) was the first major piece of legislation for PWD. It established the idea of "reasonable accommodation" (RA) and "least-restrictive environment" (LRE). RA refers to the fact that the needs of PWD must be accommodated so as to not exclude them from the same experiences and opportunities as those of persons without disabilities. RA was written very vaguely and is essentially determined by courts (through law suits). LRE refers to the degree of modifications in a job or academic program that is acceptable. The Rehabilitation Act was patterned after Civil Rights Law. Simply stated, discriminating against individuals because of their disabilities became an act against the law. No person with any disability could be excluded from employment or secondary education solely on the basis of his or her condition. The act mandated that employers and institutes of higher education receiving federal funds accommodate the needs of PWD.

In 1975, Congress enacted a major piece of legislation, also patterned after Civil Rights Law, this time protecting the rights of children with disabilities. The Education for All Handicapped Children Act, P.L. 94-142, later became known as the Individuals with Disabilities Act, or IDEA. In this legislation, handicapped children were acknowledged as people with "certain inalienable rights," which are outlined in Box 27-2.

BOX 27-2

Individuals with Disabilities Act Assistive Technology Mandates for Children with Disabilities

- A free, appropriate education regardless of handicapping condition
- Provision of educational services to the maximum extent appropriate in the least-restrictive environment
- The participation of parents in the educational process
- Due process procedures
- The right to related services (that's us!) to benefit from special education instruction
- The development of an individualized education program—what is going to be done, who is going to do it, where it will be done, when it will be done, and how one will know that it has been completed (functional outcomes)

IDEA, as it pertains to AT, mandated that public schools meet the following criteria:

- Provide evaluation for assistive technology
- Purchase, lease, or provide for acquiring aid or device
- Select, design, fit, customize, adapt, repair, and replace aid or device
- Coordinate and use other services with AT
- Train child and family
- Train professionals

Medicaid is a potential source for funding for AT for PWD younger than age 65 years. However, Medicaid funding for AT is dependent on what categories of service are included in an individual state's plan and how that service is defined by federal and state law or policy (for detailed information about Medicaid and AT see http://209.203.251.64/conf09/Medicaid%20and%20AT.pdf). Private insurance coverage of AT also

TEXT TO SPEECH AND KEYBOARD	ADJUSTABLE LOCATIONS SIZE, VOLUME, VOICES	ACCEPTS SCANNING	REVIEWS	COST
No	No	Yes	Good	$50.
No	No	No	Good	Free
Yes	Yes	Yes	Excellent	$289
Yes	No	No	Good	$ 0.99

depends on individual policies. Often, a specific service such as AT or rehabilitative technology may not be covered by the plan, but a provision for durable medical equipment, which may or may not include the specific AT device or service that OT practitioners want to recommend, may be covered. Historically, private insurers have followed the lead of Medicare/Medicaid in detailing coverage for specific classes of AT tools. Service clubs, foundations, volunteer organizations, and low-interest bank loans should also be considered potential sources of full or supplemental funding for AT. Regardless of the source of funding, AT should be described in terms of the medical benefit to the client, which could include the prevention of secondary disability as well as the impact on quality of life. Specific details regarding expected outcomes and how those will be measured and documented should always be included in a request for funding.

SUMMARY

AT appliances and tools are integral to OT practice. AT fosters functional independence in PWD. The use of AT in pediatrics can motivate children with disabilities early on, and in so doing, it can ward off the negative effect of lack of motivation and learned helplessness. Because the range of AT products and devices is constantly changing, this chapter focused on best practice AT-related principles that will serve the OT practitioner regardless of the specific aid or device in question. Furthermore, because of the dynamic nature of this field, it is imperative that the OT practitioner view his or her role as a member of a team of professionals that always includes family members and consider equipment manufacturers as potential sources of information about the complex and advancing field of AT aids and devices.

References

1. Angelo, J. (1997). *Assistive technology for rehabilitation specialists*. Philadelphia: F.A. Davis.
2. Capilouto, G. (2000). Rehabilitation settings. In S. Kumar (Ed.), *Multidisciplinary approach to rehabilitation*. Boston: Butterworth Heinemann.
3. Church, G., & Glennen, S. (1992). *The handbook of assistive technology*. San Diego, CA: Singular Publishing Group.
4. Clayton, K., & Mathena, C. T. (2000). Assistive technology. In J. Solomon (Ed.), *Pediatric skills for occupational therapy assistants* (1st ed). St. Louis, MO: Mosby.
5. Cook, A., & Hussey, S. (1995). *Assistive technologies: principles and practices*. St. Louis, MO: Mosby.
6. Fallon, M., & Wann, J. (1994). Incorporating computer technology into activity-based thematic units for young children with disabilities. *Infants Young Child*, 6, 4.
7. Galvin, J., & Scherer, M. (Eds.). (1996). *Evaluating, selecting and using appropriate assistive technology*. San Diego, CA: Singular Publishing Group.
8. Glennen, S., & Church, G. (1992). Adaptive toys and environmental controls. In G. Church, & S. Glennen (Eds.), *The handbook of assistive technology*. San Diego, CA: Singular Publishing Group.
9. Greenstein, D. B. (1996). It's child's play. In J. Galvin, & M. Scherer (Eds.), *Evaluating, selecting and using appropriate assistive technology*. San Diego, CA: Singular Publishing Group.
10. Hollingsworth, M. (1992). Computer technologies: a cornerstone for educational and employment equity. *Can J Higher Ed*, 22, 1.
11. Musselwhite, C. (1986). *Adaptive play for special needs children*. San Diego, CA: College-Hill Press.
12. World Health Organization (WHO). (2001). *International classification of functioning, disability, and health*. Geneva: Author.

REVIEW *Questions*

1. What are the types and specific classes of assistive technology?
2. What is the role of the OTA in the evaluation and implementation of AT services?
3. What are the characteristics of AT and its relative importance in making AT decisions?
4. What are the similarities and differences among assistive, rehabilitative, educational, and medical technologies?
5. What are some examples of switch technology?
6. What are specific considerations when selecting a switch for an individual user?
7. What is an environmental control unit, and how does it help a child with disability?
8. What are some simple communication technologies for children unable to communicate?

SUGGESTED *Activities*

1. Examine specific laws that mandate or pay for AT services for children (e.g., Education of All Children Act).
2. Review a variety of switches and develop a notebook describing how they can be used, their cost, and the skills required to use them. Share with classmates.
3. On the Evolve Learning Site, view a video clip of a child who requires AT. Develop a list of possible solutions to allow the child to engage in a variety of occupations.
4. Practice using a variety of AT so you can better understand its use in practice. Visit a vendor fair, assistive technology workshop, or conference that has the newest technology. Present findings to classmates.
5. Develop a resource notebook of communication technologies.
6. Fabricate a variety of educational low technology items that may be helpful in practice (e.g., enlarged print, letters, pictures, matching games). Share with classmates, including source.

Orthoses, Orthotic Fabrication, and Elastic Therapeutic Taping for the Pediatric Population

CHAPTER *Objectives*

After studying this chapter, the reader will be able to accomplish the following:

- Describe key principles, materials, and steps of orthotic fabrication.
- Describe how different types of orthoses can enhance and enable participation of children and adolescents in activities of daily living.
- Understand common pediatric upper extremity conditions, congenital hand differences, and orthotic solutions.
- Define various upper and lower extremity orthoses by name and positioning.
- Describe the role of a certified occupational therapy assistant in orthotic fabrication.
- Describe terms and trends in the use of elastic therapeutic taping to enhance and enable participation of children and adolescents in activities of daily living.
- Provide an overview of application techniques, indications, and contraindications of elastic therapeutic tape.
- Describe the role of a certified occupational therapy assistant in elastic therapeutic taping of children and adolescents.
- Discuss strategies to increase the compliance of children and adolescents with orthoses and elastic therapeutic taping protocols.

CHAPTER *Outline*

Orthoses and/or elastic therapeutic taping may benefit children and adolescents with limited upper and/or lower extremity function by enabling increased participation in activities of daily living (ADLs). Both the occupational therapist (OT) and the occupational therapy assistant (OTA) have important roles in the selection, fabrication, and application of orthoses and elastic therapeutic taping for children and adolescents.

This chapter begins with definitions of the terms *orthoses for immobilization, orthoses for mobilization,* and *elastic therapeutic taping.* The author discusses the general principles and steps involved in the fabrication of orthoses, highlights the characteristics of thermoplastic materials, and offers a general overview of common orthoses for pediatric conditions. Elastic therapeutic taping has been shown to be an effective intervention with different groups of pediatric populations. Goals and application methods of elastic therapeutic taping are also reviewed. Case studies illustrate the principles and concepts for using these techniques with children and adolescents.

DEFINITIONS

Occupational therapists and OTAs often fabricate orthoses to enable children and adolescents to participate actively in their daily routines at home, in school, and in the community.[2] The term **orthosis** is used to describe any support or brace that is placed on a body part. Previously the word *splint* was used and older textbooks may still reflect this term. Orthoses can be fabricated for the upper and/or lower extremity. The purpose of the orthosis varies from individual to individual. An orthosis might support and protect an extremity after injury; provide corrective positioning of a joint with a deformity; assist a weak or injured muscle in active motion; and/or increase functional performance of the extremity (Figure 28-1). For example, an orthosis might immobilize and support an injured and painful wrist during healing or prevent poor elbow positioning during sleep (Figure 28-2). An orthosis might help support a child's wrist in extension to make writing tasks easier, or help a child maintain grasp of a toy. The **wearing protocol** defines the specific **schedule** of orthotic use and must be carefully explained to the child and family members for maximum benefit of the orthosis. The wearing protocol may vary from child to child based on each individual's needs and condition. For example, the wearing protocol of a wrist orthosis following a distal radius fracture may be full time, whereas the wearing protocol of an anti-spasticity orthosis might be 2 hours on and 2 hours off, depending on the severity of the increased tone.[17]

Elastic therapeutic taping, also known as **kinesiologic taping** and/or **kinesio taping,** is an intervention that OT practitioners use to support weak and/or injured muscles or body tissues. Appropriate taping may enable children and adolescents to participate more freely in their daily routines at home, in school and in the community.[13,15,18,19,24–26,28]

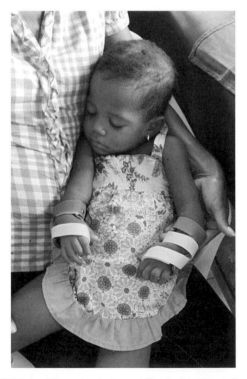

FIGURE 28-1   Bilateral wrist immobilization orthoses for young child with radial club hands. (Printed with permission from CURE Dominican Republic.)

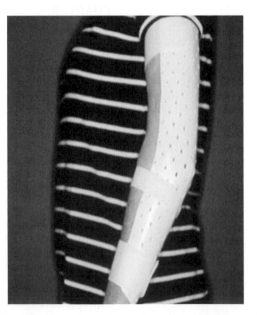

FIGURE 28-2   Posteriorly placed elbow immobilization orthosis (EO). (With permission of Orfit Industries America.)

Basic principles, indications, and contraindications for elastic therapeutic taping for improved muscle control and proprioceptive feedback are detailed.

This chapter covers basic principles and steps of orthotic fabrication and elastic therapeutic taping, and describes common pediatric conditions in which these interventions may be used. The role of the occupational therapy assistant is outlined.

GOALS OF ORTHOTIC FABRICATION

OT practitioners evaluate their pediatric clients to determine whether deficits and/or limitations in performance skills and performance patterns are preventing active participation and engagement in occupations of choice. Adolescents and children engage in schoolwork, play time, sports activities, and family time. Injuries, disease processes, congenital differences, and/or attention disorders may limit this active participation. OT practitioners are skilled at analyzing the pediatric client; his or her occupations, performance skills and patterns; and the child's specific school, home, and community contexts and environments to determine whether an orthosis may be beneficial.[2]

Orthotic fabrication and the use of elastic therapeutic taping are components of the overall treatment plan for any pediatric client. The OT practitioner uses the Occupational Therapy Practice Framework (3rd edition) as a guide to evaluate, identify deficits and limitations, and plan intervention. The framework helps to focus the OT intervention on each individual child within his or her family.[2]

Knowledge of upper extremity anatomy, common pediatric conditions, the disease process, activity analysis, and orthotic fabrication techniques all contribute to the art and science of incorporating orthoses and elastic therapeutic taping into OT interventions.[13,15,17–19,25,26,28]

The main goals of orthotic fabrication are summarized in Box 28-1. The main goals of elastic therapeutic taping are summarized in Box 28-2.

TYPES OF ORTHOSES

Orthoses can immobilize body parts or mobilize body parts and are thus described as either immobilization orthoses or mobilization orthoses. **Immobilization orthoses** can also be called static orthoses. **Mobilization orthoses** can further be divided into **dynamic**, **static progressive**, and **serial static orthoses**.

Dynamic orthoses have components that allow movement. They include elastic elements or coils and springs in the orthotic design. These additions are known as outriggers. Dynamic orthoses may be used to aid in function and/or to improve motion at joints with limitations.

Static progressive orthoses have components that provide a static pull on a stiff joint or on a contracture of the skin to increase passive motion and tissue length. They also have outrigger attachments. Static progressive orthoses are nonfunctional and are used to gain passive motion when joints are stiff and tissue has shortened.

In addition, serial static orthoses may be used to increase passive motion and/or to increase tissue length. However, this orthotic design has no additional components or outriggers and is periodically modified by the OT practitioner to accommodate changes in joint position[17] (Figure 28-3).

Immobilization orthoses can:

- Alleviate pain by supporting injured body parts and allowing them to rest;
- Decrease or prevent contractures by maximizing full joint range of motion (ROM), thus preventing muscle and tendon shortening;
- Provide stability to unstable joints by giving external support to the joint when muscles and ligaments are weakened or strained;
- Improve hygiene or prevent skin breakdown; and
- Protect healing structures.

BOX 28-1

Goals of Orthotic Fabrication

The main goals of orthotic fabrication are as follows:
- Alleviate pain
- Provide support
- Protect healing structures
- Prevent deformity
- Enhance function by assisting weak or paralyzed muscles
- Maintain or correct joint positioning
- Elongate shortened soft tissue structures or contractures

BOX 28-2

Goals of Elastic Therapeutic Taping

- Decrease pain
- Reduce inflammation and edema
- Normalize muscle tone
- Support weak muscles
- Reduce spasms
- Improve range of motion
- Provide muscle reeducation
- Increase circulation

Adapted from Coopee R. (2014). Taping. In M. L. Jacobs & N. Austin (Eds.). *Orthotic Intervention for the Hand and Upper Extremity: Splinting Principles and Process* (2nd ed., pp. 352–372). Baltimore, MD: Wolters Kluwer/Lippincott Williams and Wilkins.

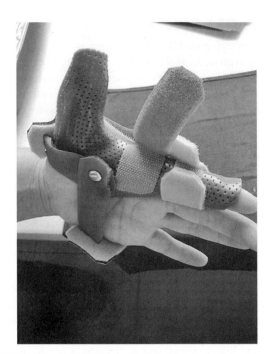

FIGURE 28-3 Serial static orthosis to widen the first web space (hand-finger orthosis [HFO]). (Printed with permission from CURE Dominican Republic.)

An orthosis can hold the hand in proper anatomic alignment, allowing the soft tissues to heal and edema and inflammation to diminish.[6]

Mobilization orthoses can:

- Remodel long-standing dense mature scar tissue;
- Elongate soft-tissue contractures;
- Increase passive joint ROM; and
- Substitute for weak or absent muscle.

CLINICAL *Pearl*

Low-load prolonged stretch (LLPS) refers to a low load of force applied to a stiff joint using an orthosis over a long period. This force is tolerated better and longer than a large load of force applied for a short period. Many mobilization orthoses incorporate the principle of LLPS.

NAMING SYSTEMS

Orthoses have common names used in the clinic that describe either the joints included and/or the positioning of these joints. This naming system is important so that all OT practitioners have a common language when describing the orthoses they provide to their clients.

For example, a **resting-hand orthosis** includes the forearm, wrist, fingers, and thumb and supports the arm in a resting posture. A **short opponens orthosis** immobilizes the thumb in a position of opposition and abduction.

The thumb's interphalangeal joint is left free for pinching activities. But in addition to the common names listed in Table 28-1, OT practitioners need to be familiar with L codes, a method of identifying orthoses for billing purposes. Each L code is associated with a specific orthosis and describes the type of orthosis provided and the upper extremity joints included in the orthosis by letter. (Each upper extremity joint is identified by a letter: S-shoulder, E-elbow, W-wrist, H-hand, and F-finger.) For example, a WHO is a wrist hand orthosis (Figure 28-4).[7] See Box 28-3 for a list of the anatomic names for orthoses.

CLINICAL *Pearl*

Further information on L codes can be found on the following websites:
www.asht.org
http://www.lcodesearch.com/
http://www.medicarenhic.com/viewdoc.aspx?id=2559

PRINCIPLES OF ORTHOTIC FABRICATION

The OT practitioner must be familiar with upper and lower extremity anatomy; the disease process and stages of healing; mechanical principles; and aesthetics in order to provide appropriate orthoses for his or her clients.[6] Several key principles guide the orthotic fabrication process. The required knowledge of orthotic fabrications is summarized in Box 28-4.

Anatomy

The OT practitioner must possess a good working knowledge of anatomy and be familiar with all bony structures, nerve pathways, blood supply, and arches of the involved limb. It is essential to know which bony prominences may be compressed or uncomfortable in the orthosis. The joints and creases provide important landmarks in orthotic fabrication. Orthoses should fully support the intended joint, but not cover the flexion crease of an adjacent joint. Strapping and the edges of the orthosis must not restrict the nerves and the blood supply to the fingers.[3]

Disease Process

After surgery or trauma, the healing limb undergoes what is typically referred to as three stages of healing: inflammatory, fibroplasia, and maturation phases. The appropriate orthosis matches this healing process. During the inflammatory phase, the body part is recovering from the trauma or surgery and is typically swollen and painful. The orthosis provided usually will support and immobilize the healing structures and protect them from sudden movements. During the fibroplasia phase,

TABLE 28-1

Names of Common Upper and Lower Extremity Orthoses

ORTHOSIS	BODY PARTS INCLUDED	POSITIONING/GOALS
Resting hand	Forearm, wrist, fingers, and thumb	Resting posture: wrist in extension, thumb in abduction, MCP joints in flexion and PIP and DIP joints in slight flexion
Short opponens/short thumb spica	Thumb CMC/MP joints	Positions the thumb in functional abduction and opposition
Long opponens/long thumb spica	Wrist and thumb CMC/MP joints	Positions the wrist in functional extension and the thumb in functional abduction and opposition
Dorsal block	Dorsal surface of forearm, wrist, and fingers (and thumb)	Forearm in 0- to 45-degree flexion. MCP joints in maximum flexion, PIP and DIP joints in 0-degree extension
Wrist cock-up	Forearm and wrist joint to end at distal palmar crease	Positions the wrist in function extension
Boutonniere	Finger orthosis includes PIP joint	Positions the PIP joint in maximal extension
Mallet	Finger orthosis includes DIP joint	Positions the DIP joint in slight hyperextension
Radial gutter	Forearm and wrist on radial side	Positions the wrist in neutral deviation, slight extension
Posterior elbow	Posterior side from upper arm and includes entire forearm	Maybe use postsurgery to maintain elbow in flexion
Anterior elbow	Anterior side from upper arm and includes entire forearm	Often used to maintain elbow extension and/or limit elbow flexion
Posterior ankle-foot	Ankle and foot	Controls the amount of dorsiflexion and plantar flexion
Posterior knee	Knee joint	Prevents or reduces knee flexion contracture stabilizes the knee during ambulation rests the knee

CMC/MP, Carpometacarpal/metacarpophalangeal; *DIP,* distal interphalangeal; *PIP,* proximal interphalangeal; *MCP,* metacarpophalangeal.

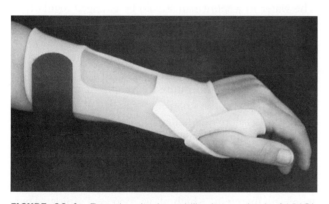

FIGURE 28-4 Dorsal wrist immobilization orthosis (WHO). (With permission of Orfit Industries America.)

BOX 28-3

Anatomic Names for Orthoses

SEWHFO: shoulder elbow wrist hand finger orthosis
SEWHO: shoulder elbow wrist hand orthosis
SEO: shoulder elbow orthosis
EWHFO: elbow wrist hand finger orthosis
EWHO: elbow wrist hand orthosis
WHFO: wrist hand finger orthosis
WHO: wrist hand orthosis
HFO: hand finger orthosis
SO: shoulder orthosis
EO: elbow orthosis
HO: hand orthosis
FO: finger orthosis

Adapted from the American Hand Therapy Society website www.asht.org

the wounds are still healing but the edema is decreasing. The child may begin to move the limb for active exercise and functional activities. The orthosis must continue to support the limb, but may require modifications due to decreased edema and better positioning. The maturation phase implies that the wounds are fairly well healed and the limb and soft tissues and bones are strong enough to support full active motion. Orthoses used in this phase are typically geared toward maximizing active participation in occupations of choice (Figure 28-5) and may be

selected to increase joint ROM and or decrease **contractures** if there are limitations.[9]

Mechanical Principles

Orthoses should firmly support the intended body part and are typically constructed so that they encompass

BOX 28-4

Required Knowledge Base for Orthotic Fabrication

- Knowledge of anatomy: anatomic landmarks, bony structures, nerve and blood supply, joints and creases
- Knowledge of disease process and stages of tissue healing: inflammatory, fibroplasia, and maturation of tissue
- Knowledge of mechanical principles: maximize surface area, support length and circumference of arm, flare material edges away from bones and muscles
- Knowledge of aesthetics and comfort: round all edges of orthosis and strappings, provide appropriate strapping to match size of body part, ensure support and comfort
- Knowledge of thermoplastics: match diagnosis with appropriate material characteristics
- Each orthosis should include three points of contact with the extremity for best distribution of force. The middle force is applied at the joint axis, and the two opposing forces are placed as far away as possible from this point for maximum efficiency in design.

BOX 28-5

Checklist for Enhancing Cosmesis

- Are there any pen marks?
- Are there rough or sharp edges?
- Did you make surface impressions (fingerprints, nail lines, etc.)?
- Is the Velcro adhesive peeling off?
- Did you round the edges of the Velcro loop strap and the corners of the orthosis?
- Did you flair the proximal edges of the orthosis?
- Does the orthosis fit snugly with correct length of straps?

the child. There should be no pen markings on the finished orthosis. The straps should be securely fastened and all Velcro pieces firmly attached. Corners of the straps and the Velcro adhesive should also be rounded so that corners do not peel away over time. See Box 28-5 for a checklist for ensuring aesthetics.

Materials and Equipment Needs

OT practitioners typically fabricate orthoses from low-temperature thermoplastic materials. These materials are activated by immersion in hot water baths known as "splint pans." Some materials can also be activated in ovens. Typical activation temperature ranges from 140°F to 160°F. The water in a splint pan should be changed regularly to avoid buildup of chemical deposits and/or material scraps. There are a wide variety of low temperature thermoplastic materials available on the market and each has different property characteristics.[5] See Box 28-6 regarding the characteristics of low-temperature thermoplastic materials.

In addition to the characteristics described Box 28-6, sheets of thermoplastic materials may have perforations or holes in the splinting material, which allow for ventilation of the skin and make the material lighter in weight. Children or adolescents who live in geographic areas with warmer climates may benefit from the use of these perforated thermoplastic materials, which allow increased airflow. There are many choices of perforation patterns. Catalogues usually feature pictures that demonstrate the different perforation patterns. Always check to make sure the perforation style is suitable for the splint you are making.

The thickness of the material must be taken into consideration as well. Thinner materials such as 1/16-inch and 1/12-inch are better for smaller splints, whereas larger splints may need thicker materials such as 1/8-inch or 3/32-inch. Thinner thermoplastic materials are activated more quickly than thicker materials and cool more quickly as well, meaning they have a shorter working time. Sometimes a thinner material can be used for a large splint by making it circumferential as this type of splint includes

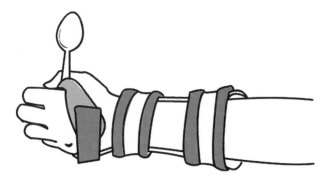

FIGURE 28-5 Wrist extension orthosis with embedded spoon for self- feeding.

two-thirds the length of the forearm and half the circumference of the forearm to evenly distribute the weight of the limb. They offer three points of control or contact with the body part to stabilize the intended joint. The longer the length of the lever arms from the middle point of control ensures a more effective support. Padding placed on bony prominences before orthosis application ensures that structures are protected from pressure. This can be done after orthotic fabrication as well by heating up and bumping out the areas of contact with the bony structures.[4]

Aesthetics

All edges of the orthosis should be carefully trimmed and smoothed so that no rough edges or sharp corners injure

BOX 28-6

Characteristics of Low-Temperature Thermoplastic Materials

Rigidity: The strength of the material. High rigidity is necessary for large splints, specific diagnoses such as spasticity, and splints projecting large forces.

Memory: Ability of the material to return to its original size and shape after being stretched. This is an important concept when frequent remolding of the splint will be necessary, as in serial splinting to increase extension or flexion over time. Memory makes the material more cost-efficient. When working with materials possessing excellent memory, remember to let the splint harden sufficiently before removing or it will lose its shape rapidly.

Conformability or drapability: The way the material conforms to the shape of the hand. Materials with high drapability work best with gentle handling as they conform easily to the arches or bony prominences. Materials with low drapability require firm handling and are recommended for larger splints where this moldability is less important.

Resistance to stretch: The amount of resistance the material gives to being stretched when heated. High resistance means you must work slowly and steadily to stretch the material. Low resistance to stretch means you need to work more quickly and carefully control the material as it stretches.

Coating: A coating may be applied to certain materials to make them easier to work with and less likely to adhere together where no adherence is desired. Coated materials do not bond easily to attachments without having the coating removed. Noncoated materials have very good bonding to themselves and other attachments. Coated materials and noncoated materials each have advantages and disadvantages. The coating can be removed when and if desired.

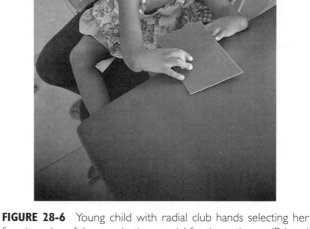

FIGURE 28-6   Young child with radial club hands selecting her favorite color of thermoplastic material for the orthoses. (Printed with permission from CURE Dominican Republic.)

Due to the large number of products available with similar characteristics, it is highly recommended that each OT practitioner requests samples from the distributor or manufacturer to individually test each material and determine its appropriateness for the clinic and specific needs of their pediatric population.

CLINICAL *Pearl*

The following websites provide information on distributors, manufacturers and for general information about low temperature thermoplastic products:
* Chesapeake Medical www.chesapeakemedical.com
* North Coast Medical www.ncmedical.com
* Orfit Industries www.orfit.com
* Patterson Medical www.pattersonmedical.com

Soft Orthoses and Commercially Available Orthoses

Soft orthoses may be purchased commercially or fabricated for children and adolescents who have overly sensitive skin or require minimal support (Figures 28-7 and 28-8). Typically these can be fabricated with Velfoam and/or neoprene, and can also be reinforced with thermoplastic material by dry heating. Soft orthoses are often made as thumb positioning supports for children with cerebral palsy (CP), brachial plexus palsy (Erb's palsy), and/or mild muscle tone.[1,8] Even splints made from Lycra have been shown to be effective.[14]

both the volar and dorsal surfaces and therefore is very stable.

Each specific material has a typical working time, which describes the amount of time from when the material is fully activated to when it is hardened. Novice splint makers may want to choose materials that have longer working times while advanced splinters may be able to work and handle thermoplastic materials that cool and harden quickly.

Thermoplastic materials are now available in a wide variety of colored and patterned options, which may improve compliance with the pediatric population. Make sure the properties of the material are suitable for the specific orthosis needed (Figure 28-6).

See Table 28-2 for a list of low-temperature thermoplastic materials currently available for purchase and a sample of applications.

TABLE 28-2

Currently Available Low-Temperature Thermoplastic Materials

PRODUCT NAME	HANDLING CHARACTERISTICS	APPLICATIONS
Elastic Materials with 100 % memory and elasticity: Aquaplast Aquaplast Watercolors Aquaplast-T Encore Orfit Classic Orfit Colors NS Orfit Natural NS Orfit NS Prism Rebound	Latex-free Translucent or shiny when heated Moderate resistance to stretch Available in ⅛-inch, ¹⁄₁₂-inch, ¹⁄₁₆-inch thicknesses Coated and noncoated Resistant to finger printing Requires no reinforcing Self-bonding	Serial static orthoses Orthoses for spasticity Appropriate for all small finger orthoses, thumb orthoses, resting hand orthoses, wrist and wrist/thumb orthoses and circumferential designs and large orthoses (elbow, knee, long arm, ankle/foot) as well as for ankle-foot orthoses (AFOs) and fracture bracing depending on material thickness
Plastic materials with high drape and conformability: Excel Flexx Rolyan Polyflex II Rolyan Polyform Rolyan Kay Splint Basic	Excellent conformability and drape Minimal memory Moderate rigidity Moderate resistance to fingerprinting Use gravity to assist in orthotic fabrication Available in ⅛-inch, ¹⁄₁₂-inch, ¹⁄₁₆-inch thicknesses	Appropriate for the fabrication of very large to very small orthoses, depending on the thickness of the material Wrist orthoses, wrist/thumb orthoses, hand-based orthoses. All orthoses where excellent support and intimate fit are required
Rubber-based materials: Marque Easy Rolyan San-Splint	Can be worked aggressively without fingerprinting Excellent rigidity without reinforcement Can be softened in a hot air oven as well as in hot water. Heat in oven at 175°F (80°C) for 2–3 min Edges trim easily Latex free	Ideal for medium to large splints Spasticity splints Functional position splints Resting mitt splints Back supports Body jackets Shoe orthotics
Materials with moderate to high resistance to stretch and excellent rigidity: Clinic Colours Ezeform Fiber Form Soft and Stiff Infinity NCM Preferred Omega Black Omega Max Omega Plus Orfibrace Orfit Ease Rolyan Synergy Rolyan Tailor Splint Solaris Spectrum Vanilla	Excellent resistance to markings and fingerprints Materials can withstand firm handling during fabrication Maintains positioning even against high tone and spasticity Maximum resistance to stretch Some have memory and some do not need to test	Appropriate for most types of orthoses, especially large and rigid orthoses, and orthoses for spasticity Long arm orthoses, elbow orthoses, forearm orthoses, wrist orthoses, wrist/thumb orthoses. Excellent for back bracing and ankle supports
Orthoplast II	Excellent drapability, but very rigid material Adheres to self; however, requires solvent for permanent bonding Edges trim and finish well	Ideal for static or dynamic orthoses Finger orthoses Small hand orthoses Wrist orthoses
Orfilight	Extremely lightweight product. Weighs 15%–30% less than other materials. Soft foamy feel with easy to trim edges Moderate memory. Excellent stretch	Finger, toe, and thumb orthoses, hand- and wrist-based orthoses. Lightweight wrist orthoses especially suited for pediatric clients

TABLE 28-2

Currently Available Low-Temperature Thermoplastic Materials—cont'd

PRODUCT NAME	HANDLING CHARACTERISTICS	APPLICATIONS
Silon-LTS	Latex-free product Combines a low-temperature thermoplastic with a therapeutic surface of silicone	Indications for use are burns and hypertrophic scars Use as a prophylaxis after surgery
Orficast Thermoplastic Tape in 1-inch and 2.5-inch rolls	Thermoplastic threads knitted with cotton weave; excellent memory Product offers moldability, conformability and rigidity. No need to make pattern, just cut and wrap Rigidity is increased by the addition of multiple layers	All types of finger orthoses, and hand-based orthoses, and some types of wrist and forearm supports
X-Lite Thermoplastic in rolls of 2-inch and 6-inch	Open-weave design for lightweight applications. Well ventilated Material is self-bonding Rigidity is increased by the addition of multiple layers	Orthoses for positioning and for ADL aids, such as building up tool handles

ADL, Activities of daily living; *AFO,* ankle-foot orthosis

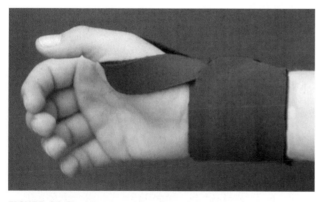

FIGURE 28-7 Neoprene thumb orthosis. (With permission of Orfit Industries America.)

If the child demonstrates contact dermatitis or a prickly heat rash after wearing a neoprene orthosis, he or she may be allergic to the neoprene, and use should be promptly discontinued. Neoprene can also be used as strapping material.[12,22]

CLINICAL *Pearl*

Check the following websites for more information on these commercially available pediatric orthoses:
- Benik Corporation www.Benik.com
- Comfy Splints www.comfysplints.com
- Joe Cool Company www.joecoolco.com
- McKie Splints www.mckiesplints.com
- North Coast Medical www.ncmedical.com
- Patterson Medical www.pattersonmedical.com

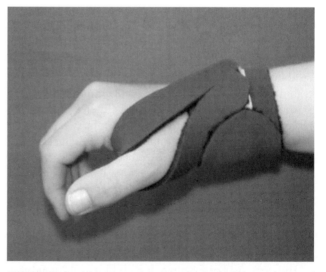

FIGURE 28-8 Neoprene thumb orthosis. (With permission of Orfit Industries America.)

The Evaluation

The OT practitioner may receive the referral for an orthosis from a physician or request a referral after the evaluation. Using the Occupational Therapy Practice Framework as a guide, he or she assesses the child's need for the orthosis.[2] The OTA can contribute to this process. The following areas are evaluated:

1. *Occupations:* Observe the child participating in his or her ADLs. Would the use of an orthosis improve function by allowing the child to be independent in

instrumental ADLs? Or, for example, would it allow the child to stabilize paper for writing tasks? Would the child be able to perform two-handed tasks more efficiently? What ADLs does the child need to perform that might be enhanced with an orthosis, for example, self-dressing or self-feeding?

2. *Client factors:* Assess the child's muscle tone, ROM, strength, contractures. Will an orthosis improve or prevent further loss of any of these components of movement? A thorough evaluation will determine whether ROM is within normal limits. The OT practitioner assesses the child's body structures to determine whether normal or abnormal muscle tone is present. The presence of **spasticity** or increased muscle tone may affect the use of orthoses. For example, an orthosis applied to one area may change the muscle tone and affect the other joints of that extremity. The limb should be assessed for **edema**, or swelling of the limb. Following trauma or surgery, edema is common and should be managed with orthotic use, ice, elevation, and compression. Orthoses made for children with edema may need to be remolded or refitted as the edema decreases over time. Many children and adolescents with special needs develop latex allergies. Some thermoplastic materials or attachments (rubber bands) may contain latex. OT practitioners need to be aware of these potential reactions and use alternative materials.

3. *Performance skills:* Evaluate the child's motor skills and ability to reach, grasp, bear weight on his or her affected limb(s) and stabilize and manipulate objects. What is the child's sensory status? Some children and adolescents are hypersensitive to touch and may not tolerate an orthosis. Nonverbal children may have difficulty indicating they are in pain or discomfort. Careful fabrication of the orthosis, padding around bony prominences, the use of stockinette or a cotton sleeve underneath the thermoplastic material, and careful monitoring help the child with sensory issues tolerate the orthosis. What are the child's processing skills and/or developmental age? The child's age will affect the design and fabrication of the orthosis. For example, if a child is still "mouthing" objects, the orthosis must not contain small pieces or have components that are toxic. Active children may require over-protective orthoses that provide more durability during sports activities. For example, instead of fabricating a hand-based orthosis for a proximal phalanx fracture, a forearm-based orthosis might be prescribed.

4. *Performance patterns:* Assess the child's ability to perform his or her daily routines of getting ready for school in the morning, or getting ready for play dates with friends. How would the use of the orthosis help the child participate in these routines?

5. *Contexts and environments:* Examine the child's environments. Where does the child spend most of his or her time? Is the child able to participate in activities at family activities at home and in school? How would the orthosis help the child participate in school activities with peers? How would the orthosis help the child participate in family activities at home with siblings and parents?

The OT practitioner considers the full domain of occupational therapy (as outlined in the framework[2]) in the evaluation process helps to ensure that the orthoses provided are part of an overall client-centered therapy approach.

The certified OT assistant (COTA) may contribute to the evaluation process and assist in fabricating the orthosis or may fabricate the orthosis, depending on his or her skill level, setting of care, and reimbursement/funding sources. Medicare does not permit OTAs to fabricate orthoses independently.

Steps of Orthotic Fabrication

The steps of orthotic fabrication are outlined in Box 28-7.

BOX 28-7

Steps of Orthotic Fabrication

1. Visualize the orthosis and how it may benefit the child.
2. Draw a pattern of the child's hand on a paper towel.
3. Carefully cut out the pattern and check the fit by placing it on the child's hand.
4. Make adjustments to the pattern as needed.
5. Select the appropriate thermoplastic material. Draw the pattern on thermoplastic material and carefully cut it out inside of the markings.
6. Briefly heat the material to soften enough for cutting.
7. Cut out the orthosis using long and even scissor strokes. Keep the edges smooth.
8. Place the cut orthosis back in the splint pan to fully activate the material.
9. Position the child's extremity in the desired position.
10. Remove the activated orthoses from the hot water and dry briefly on a towel or place flat on the table and pat the towel over the material to remove excess water
11. Check the temperature before placing the orthosis on the child in the desired position.
12. Let fully harden and cool before removing. Trim and round all sharp edges where necessary. Flair the proximal edge by dipping in hot water and pushing it outward slightly with thumb.
13. Add strapping and check for a snug fit on the child.

When fabricating orthoses for young children, especially those with high muscle tone or spasticity, choose a quiet corner or space. Minimize distractions and noise. Play soft music if possible and speak in a calm manner.

Decorate the child's dolls or soft animals to demonstrate the process and make it less frightening (Figure 28-9, A to C).

Secure Strapping Techniques

Young children may not understand the importance of orthotic use and may figure out ways to remove the orthosis if not carefully monitored. Here are some creative strapping solutions to keep orthoses on young patients[22]:

- Place a stockinette sleeve or a tube sock over the orthosis.
- Wrap an Ace bandage or Coban wrap over the orthosis.
- Use buckles or fasteners that require two hands to open.
- Use shoelaces to tie the orthosis closed on the dorsal surface.

- Fit a tubular stockinette or a sleeve from a garment over the orthosis and attach to the child's clothing.
- Use devices typically manufactured for keeping shoelaces tied (Bow Biters). See Figure 28-10, A to D.

Adhere strapping directly to elastic-based thermoplastic materials by scratching away the coating (if present), applying dry heat and firmly pressing the Velcro loop into the thermoplastic material. This ensures that the strap will not get lost. Straps can be removed with pliers if they become wet or dirty.

Children are constantly growing, so there is a need to monitor the orthosis frequently and make adjustments.

OT practitioners carefully evaluate the effectiveness of the orthosis to determine whether it is adequately serving the intended function. See Box 28-8 for key questions to consider when assessing the usefulness of the orthosis.

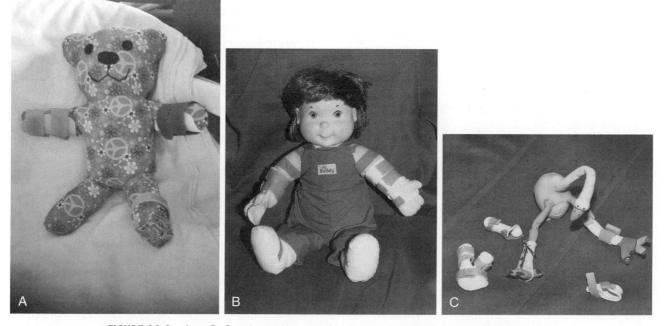

FIGURE 28-9 A to C, Creating orthoses on friends to assist with fear and compliance issues.

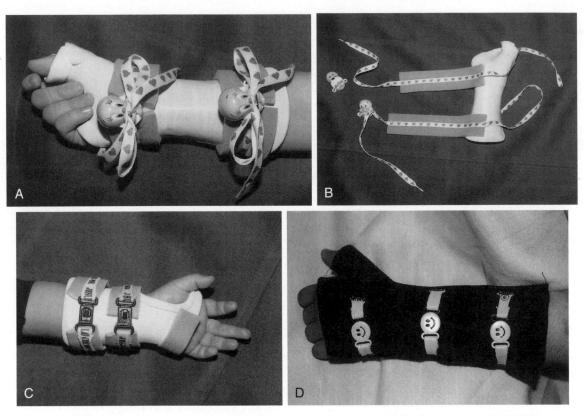

FIGURE 28-10 Creative strapping techniques on wrist thumb immobilization orthoses (WHFO) (**A** and **B**) and wrist orthoses (WHO) (**C** and **D**).

BOX 28-8

The Orthotic Check Out

- Does the orthosis achieve its purpose?
- Does the orthosis maintain the proper position and angles for which it was designed?
- Does the orthosis fit the contours of the palm and/or foot without causing discomfort, redness, irritation?
- Does the orthosis immobilize any joints unnecessarily?
- Is the orthosis long enough to provide proper support?
- Are all edges smooth and all pressure points relieved?
- Can the child or caregiver properly don and doff the orthosis?
- Does the child or caregiver understand the purpose and wearing protocol of the orthosis?
- Is the orthosis cosmetically acceptable to the child

Normal Hand Development

It is critical to appreciate the normal developmental progress of the child's hand to appreciate which activity level suits each child. Orthotic intervention must try to accommodate this development. Normal hand development is outlined in Table 28-3.

Common Pediatric Conditions

Table 28-4 provides a brief description of common pediatric diagnoses and associated orthotic solutions. A review of congenital hand differences and orthotic options are further described in Table 28-5.

The type of orthosis, individual wearing schedule, and rationale for its use will vary among children according to individual needs and the diagnosis.[11,16,23] The following pediatric conditions may require evaluation for an orthotic intervention to enable a child to engage in a variety of occupations.

- Arthrogryposis
- Brachial plexus palsy
- Camptodactaly
- Cerebral palsy (CP)
- Juvenile idiopathic arthritis (JIA)
- Pediatric trigger finger
- Radial club hand
- Syndactaly

Some children and adolescents are born with deformities of the hand or upper extremity, known as congenital hand differences (Figure 28-11). Congenital hand differences can significantly affect normal development. When fabricating orthoses for children with congenital hand differences, the OT practitioner looks

TABLE 28-3

Normal Hand Development

AGE SKILL APPEARS (MO)	UPPER EXTREMITY SKILLS
0–2	Physiologic flexion
2	Grasp reflex
3	Hands together on chest in supine position
4	Grasp reflex diminishing; objects held in both hands at midline; in supine position bears weight on forearm, with more weight on the ulnar than the radial side; pats sides of bottle with hands
5	Two-handed approach to objects, but grasp is unilateral; bilateral transfer; extended-arm weight bearing in prone position; places two hands on bottle, with some forearm supination
6	Weight shifts on extended arms in prone position; sits with a straight back; elbows fully extend when reaching
7	First purposeful release; pulls self to stand
8	Crawls on hands and knees
9	Active forearm supination when reaching
10	Pokes with index finger
12	Uses hands in coordinated manner in which one hand stabilizes and the other manipulates; begins to scribble
15	Releases a pellet with wrist extension and precision

Adapted from Peck-Murray, J. (2014). The pediatric patient. In M. L. Jacobs & N. Austin (Eds.). *Orthotic Intervention for the Hand and Upper Extremity: Splinting Principles and Process* (2nd ed., pp. 585–603). Baltimore, MD: Wolters Kluwer/Lippincott Williams and Wilkins.

TABLE 28-4

Common Pediatric Diagnoses and Orthotic Solutions

DIAGNOSIS	ORTHOTIC SOLUTIONS
Arthrogryposis: Key areas of concern include lack of full joint motion, specifically at the wrists, elbows, and knees/muscle weakness	Immobilization orthoses to prevent deformities and contractures: (wrist flexion and/or extension orthoses, knee and elbow extension and/or flexion orthoses) Mobilization orthoses (serial static) to increase joint range of motion
Brachial plexus palsy/Erb's palsy: Key areas of concern include lack of shoulder external rotation, lack of elbow extension, lack of forearm supination, lack of wrist and thumb motion	Immobilization orthoses to protect and position, prevent deformities and contractures (wrist extension orthoses, elbow extension orthoses, neoprene orthoses) Mobilization orthoses (serial static) to increase joint range of motion
Camptodactaly: Key area of concern is a congenital flexion contracture of the PIP joint of the little finger	Immobilization orthoses to position the little finger in maximum PIP extension
Cerebral palsy/hemiplegia: Involvement on one side of the body. Key areas of concern may include increased tone, shoulder held in internal rotation, forearm pronated, wrist positioned in flexion, as well as a thumb-in-palm deformity. Lower extremity contractures are also a concern	Immobilization orthoses to support and position the extremities, prevent deformities and contractures (wrist, wrist/hand orthoses, neoprene orthoses, thumb abduction orthoses, elbow orthoses), and improve function Mobilization orthoses to increase joint range of motion
Congenital hand differences: Key areas of concern vary depending on specific anomaly and functional ability of individual	Immobilization orthoses to enable function, support and position the extremities, prevent additional deformities and contractures (wrist, wrist/hand orthoses, neoprene orthoses, thumb abduction orthoses, elbow orthoses) Mobilization orthoses to increase joint range of motion

Continued

TABLE 28-4

Common Pediatric Diagnoses and Orthotic Solutions—cont'd

DIAGNOSIS	ORTHOTIC SOLUTIONS
Duchenne's muscular dystrophy: Key areas of concern are soft tissue shortening and contractures	Immobilization orthoses to stabilize weak joints (resting hand orthoses, elbow orthoses, knee orthoses) and prevent deformities and contractures
Juvenile idiopathic arthritis: Key areas of concern include swollen and painful joints	Immobilization orthoses to promote range of motion, provide support and pain relief, prevent deformities and contractures (resting hand and wrist extension orthoses, thumb orthoses, MP joint extension orthoses)
Osteogenesis imperfecta: Key areas of concern include fragile bones and multiple fractures	Immobilization orthoses to protect against frequent fractures, provide increased joint stability (wrist/hand immobilization orthoses)
Quadriplegia: Key areas of concern include muscle tone, positioning to increase function, possible fragile bones over time, and stability for increased motor control	Immobilization orthoses to support and position the extremities, prevent deformities and contractures (wrist, wrist/hand orthoses, neoprene orthoses, thumb abduction orthoses, elbow orthoses), and enable functional activities
Radial club hand: Key areas of concern include radially deviated wrist and often weak thumb or total lack of thumb	Immobilization orthoses to support and position the wrist and fingers (radial gutter type wrist and forearm orthoses, resting hand orthoses, and elbow orthoses) Mobilization orthoses to increase joint range of motion
Rett syndrome: Key areas of concern include muscle atrophy, possible osteopenia with fractures (late stages), and self-abusive behaviors	Immobilization orthoses to protect against self-abusive behaviors (elbow extension orthoses, wrist orthoses)
Syndactaly: Key areas of concern include webbed and contracted fingers	Immobilization orthoses to support and position the fingers (web spacer or finger separators)

Adapted from Peck-Murray, J. (2014). The pediatric patient. In M. L. Jacobs & N. Austin (Eds.). *Orthotic Intervention for the Hand and Upper Extremity: Splinting Principles and Process* (2nd ed., pp. 585–603). Baltimore, MD: Wolters Kluwer/Lippincott Williams and Wilkins.
MCP, Metacarpophalangeal; *PIP,* proximal interphalangeal.

TABLE 28-5

Congenital Hand Differences

SPECIFIC DIAGNOSIS	TYPES	DESCRIPTION	DEVELOPMENTAL ISSUES	ORTHOTIC OPTIONS
Camptodactyly	Infant	Congenital flexion of PIP	Lack of full finger extension	Serial static PIP extension orthosis to extend finger
	Adolescent	Nontraumatic PIP flexion contracture	Lack of full finger extension	Serial static PIP extension orthosis to extend finger
Syndactyly	Simple	Only skin between fingers is involved	Limited finger use	Postoperative orthosis and web space scar management
	Complex	Fusion of fingers through bone and skin	Limited grasp	Postoperative orthosis and web space scar management
Radial ray deficiencies: hypoplastic thumbs	1st degree	Slim thumb	May avoid use of thumb	Soft neoprene orthosis to hold thumb in opposition
	2nd degree	Limited thenar musculature Unstable thumb MP joint Tight web		Soft or rigid orthosis to hold thumb in opposition Postoperative protective orthosis
	3rd degree	Absent thenar muscles Unstable thumb MP joint	Uses scissor grasp between index and middle finger	Rigid orthosis to support thumb Postoperative protective orthosis
	4th degree	Floating thumb	Nonfunctional thumb Uses scissor grasp as above	Postoperative protective orthosis
	5th degree	Absent thumb	Uses scissor grasp as above	Protective orthosis

TABLE 28-5

Congenital Hand Differences—cont'd

SPECIFIC DIAGNOSIS	TYPES	DESCRIPTION	DEVELOPMENTAL ISSUES	ORTHOTIC OPTIONS
Radial ray deficiencies: radial club hands	Type 1	Short radius Hypoplastic thumbs	Normal hand use, except thumbs	Orthosis as needed for thumbs
	Type 2	Hypoplastic radius	Lack of crawling Difficulty weight bearing	Radial- or ulnar-based orthosis Postoperative protective and night orthosis Weight-bearing orthosis
	Type 3	Absent distal radius	Little finger prehension	Radial- or ulnar-based orthosis Postoperative protective and night orthosis
	Type 4	Aplastic radius	Little finger prehension	Radial- or ulnar-based orthosis Postoperative protective and night orthosis
Thumb-in-palm deformity	Type 1	Extensor pollicis brevis and longus deficiencies	Poor prehension, thumb may become contracted in palm	Soft orthosis for day Rigid orthosis for night
	Type 2	Extensor pollicis brevis and longus deficiencies Contractures	Poor prehension, thumb may become contracted in palm	Soft orthosis for day/rigid orthosis for night Postoperative protective orthosis
	Type 3	MP instability	Minimum thumb use	Soft orthosis for day/rigid orthosis for night Postoperative protective orthosis
	Type 4	Miscellaneous deformities	Minimum thumb use	Orthosis as needed
Congenital trigger thumb /fingers		Triggering/crepitus Palpable nodule	May resist use due to pain Limited grasp and release	Orthosis as needed
Arthrogryposis	Distal	Flexed, webbed, and overlapping fingers MP joints in ulnar deviation Adducted thumbs	Limited grasp and release Poor prehension	Serial static and static progressive to increase passive joint range Postoperative

Adapted from Peck-Murray, J. (2014). The pediatric patient. In M. L. Jacobs & N. Austin (Eds.). *Orthotic Intervention for the Hand and Upper Extremity: Splinting Principles and Process* (2nd ed., pp. 585–603). Baltimore, MD: Wolters Kluwer/Lippincott Williams and Wilkins.
MCP, Metacarpophalangeal; *PIP,* proximal interphalangeal

at the child's development and current functioning, determines the purpose of the orthosis, and considers the context in which the child will use the orthosis. The goal of orthoses for children who have congenital hand differences is to improve functional ability for engagement in daily activities. Table 28-5 describes congenital hand differences and associated developmental issues.[10,20,21]

CLINICAL *Pearl*

Give the child a choice in thermoplastic material color or strapping color. Let the child add decorations, such as stickers, jewels, or puppet eyes, to make the orthosis more pleasing and individual.

CLINICAL *Pearl*

Let the child play with a scrap of warm thermoplastic material while the pattern is being made. Make a thermoplastic orthosis for the child's toy figure or stuffed animal.

Strategies to Enhance Compliance with Orthotic Wear

The OT practitioner may fabricate a wonderful orthosis that fits the child or adolescent well and does exactly what the practitioner intends it to do. However, if the child is not motivated to wear the orthosis or dislikes it, the intended goals of the orthotic fabrication will not be met. It is very important to explain the purpose and goals

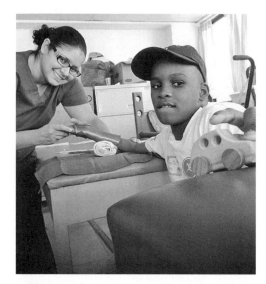

FIGURE 28-11 Eagerly waiting for the thermoplastic material to harden. (Printed with permission from CURE Dominican Republic.)

Name: Timmy Smith	Schedule: 2 Hours ON
Splint: Wrist cock up with ulnar deviation block	2 Hours OFF
	Purpose: Keep hand in a healthy position; stop stiffness and pain

I wear my splint for 2 hours.

Then, I keep it OFF for 2 hours. Then I put it back ON.

My splint helps my arthritis feel better. 😊

My schedule helps me and my OT know when I am wearing my splint.

I stop wearing my splint if I see any red areas or if it hurts.

	SUN.	MON.	TUES.	WED.	THURS.	FRI.	SAT.
8 - 10 am	ON	ON	ON	ON	ON	ON	ON
10 - 12 pm	OFF	OFF	OFF	OFF	OFF	OFF	OFF
12 - 2 pm	ON	ON	ON	ON	ON	ON	ON
2 - 4 pm	OFF	OFF	OFF	OFF	OFF	OFF	OFF
4 - 6 pm	ON	ON	ON	ON	ON	ON	ON
6 - 8 pm	OFF	OFF	OFF	OFF	OFF	OFF	OFF
Bedtime	OFF						

⭐ = YES, I followed my schedule   ✋ = NO, I did not follow the schedule

FIGURE 28-12 Sample orthosis-wearing schedule.

of the orthosis to the child, family members, caregivers, and even school personnel so that they understand its significance and can help with motivating the child to wear the orthosis as outlined (Figure 28-12). If the orthosis enables the child to participate in his or her occupations

of choice, then the wearing protocol is more likely to be followed. It is very important to take the time to explain to the child and family members the importance and goals of the orthosis, and to develop a wearing protocol with them that will be easy to monitor and follow. Younger children may not be capable of understanding the purpose of the orthosis; in these cases the orthosis should be secured in such a way that the child is unable to remove it. Box 28-9 describes strategies to increase compliance with the wearing protocol and secure strapping techniques.

The OT practitioner takes the time to describe the purpose, the wearing schedule, and precautions for wearing the orthosis. OT practitioners use simple language at the child's and family's level of understanding.

Some children and adolescents may see their orthosis as something that makes them "different" from their peers; they may feel as though the orthosis makes them "stand out." These individuals may not want to wear orthoses because of social factors and peer pressure. It is always important to take these concerns into consideration and address them. Allowing the child to select colorful and/or school-colored materials, adding colorful strappings and/or decorating the orthosis are ways that may increase compliance with the wearing protocol and make it something of special value (Figures 28-13 through 28-15).

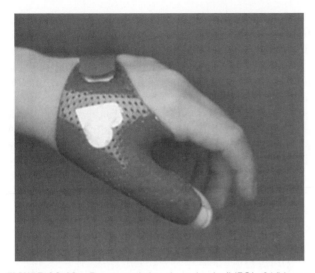

FIGURE 28-13 Decorated thumb orthosis (HFO). (With permission of Orfit Industries America.)

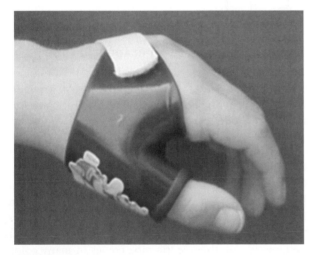

FIGURE 28-14 Decorated thumb orthosis (HFO). (With permission of Orfit Industries America.)

The context and the environment where the child will be wearing the orthosis are also important to consider. If the orthosis is needed during the day at school, make sure the teacher and school professionals are informed so that they can help monitor the wearing schedule. If the child is in a hospital setting, correlate the orthosis wearing protocol with staff shift changes. Include the wearing protocol into the hospital care plan.[21,22]

Constraint-induced movement therapy (CIMT) is an intervention that may include providing an orthosis or cast to immobilize the unimpaired extremity of a child or adolescent with unilateral hemiplegia. This program features intensive repetitive practice of motor tasks, and breaking more complex activities into components of movement for success.[26,27] OT practitioners may be involved in designing a CIMT program for a child and will need to fabricate an appropriate orthosis

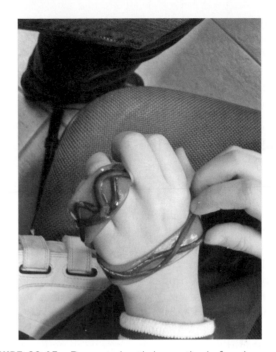

FIGURE 28-15 Decorated anti-claw orthosis for ulnar nerve injury. (With permission of Candida Luzo, hand therapist.)

to effectively block all movement of the unimpaired extremity while engaging the child in active movement patterns involving the hemiplegic arm.

FABRICATION TIPS

Initially, the process or orthotic fabrication may seem very complex and challenging. Each pediatric client has unique needs and challenges. Overtime, the steps of orthotic fabrication become easier to follow and more familiar to the clinician and the method takes less time. Every practitioner develops some tips and strategies along the way to make this process simpler.

The thermoplastic material must be left on the child's arm long enough to harden. This process can be quickened by applying bags of ice chips or wrapping a towel soaked in ice water on the orthosis to cool it more quickly.

SAFETY PRECAUTIONS

It is important to ensure that the tools and equipment needed for orthotic fabrication are off limits to the children or adolescents receiving the orthoses. All scissors and sharp instruments must be kept out of reach. Be careful to prevent hot water from dripping out of the splint pan on to the child, and make sure the splint pan is covered when the orthosis is finished.

Test the temperature of the heated material before placement on the child to ensure that it is not too hot. Do not leave the heat gun on when not in immediate use. Maintain a clean workspace for colleagues and other clients.

With few exceptions, outriggers and orthotic attachments are not recommended for children because these attachments tend to have small pieces that may become detached and consequently are a choking hazard; they could also cause injury to the eyes, ears, and other areas of the body if the child is running and falls on the orthosis.

ELASTIC THERAPEUTIC TAPING

The literature describes three different methods or techniques of applying tape to an individual's body to either facilitate or inhibit movement, provide support, help control edema, and alleviate pain.[13,15,18,19,24–26,28] They are athletic taping, McConnell taping, and elastic therapeutic taping (Kinesio Taping). All taping techniques require advanced training to understand the concepts and practice the techniques without causing harm. Athletic taping is often used to treat sprains, dislocations, and ligament injuries. Athletic tape can be rigid or elastic, but is usually applied in multiple layers to provide a rigid support after an injury.[13] McConnell taping is a method typically used to improve joint alignment, muscle activity, and biomechanics of the body. A sticky under tape is applied first without tension to protect the skin. The heavier tape is applied on top with tension, perpendicular to the muscle fibers (Figure 28-16).

Elastic therapeutic taping is available from many suppliers with a variety of names (Kinseio Tex Tape, Balance Tex Tape, Dynamic Tape, Spider Tech Tape, Rock Tape, Perform Tech Tape) and in a wide range of colors. The original product, known as Kinesio Taping, was first introduced by Dr. Kenzo Kase in the 1970s. Kase developed this intervention to provide pain relief for sports-related injuries. The primary goal of elastic therapeutic taping is to aid the body in self-healing. The use of elastic therapeutic tape is thought to activate the neurologic and circulatory systems by mimicking human kinesiology and normal muscle activity.[13]

Muscles play a primary role in stabilizing body structures, venous circulation throughout the body, lymphatic drainage, and body temperature. Imbalance between muscles and joints may cause movement deficits, pain, and injury. Elastic therapeutic taping is thought to provide additional stability for injured or weak muscles to contract effectively. Studies conducted on children using elastic therapeutic taping methods show positive outcomes. A recent study found that taping the thumbs of children with CP during functional activities reduced the thumb-in-palm deformity.[19] Another study on elastic therapeutic taping of children with CP noted better posture of the head and neck and improved hand function.[24] Researchers also found that the use of elastic therapeutic taping improved upper extremity control and function in a pediatric inpatient rehabilitation population[28] (Figure 28-17).

Before applying any type of tape to a pediatric client, check first regarding possible allergies to the tape or the adhesive. Remove promptly if skin irritations or itchiness occurs.

Application of Elastic Therapeutic Tape

OT practitioners use their knowledge of kinesiology, muscle anatomy, and the fundamentals of OT interventions when applying elastic therapeutic taping to pediatric clients. Children and adolescents who are very active may not be good candidates for taping, since the tape may wear off quickly or fail to stay adhered to the skin. See Box 28-10 for contraindications for taping.

Elastic therapeutic taping has the same weight and thickness as skin. It can be stretched up to 40% more than its length, and is usually made from cotton fibers. The tape has a paper backing that is removed to stretch the tape. Elastic therapeutic tape comes in many colors and patterns and in different widths. After application, it can be worn for several days until the edges start to peel away from the skin.

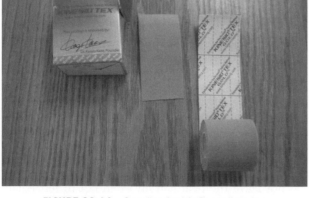

FIGURE 28-16 Supplies for McConnell taping.

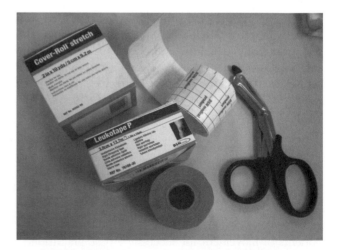

FIGURE 28-17 Supplies for elastic therapeutic taping.

Strategies and techniques for applying elastic therapeutic tape include the following:

- A careful examination of the child's condition to determine whether elastic therapeutic tape may be beneficial. Outline the specific goals of the elastic therapeutic taping with the child and caregivers.
- Advise the child and caregivers about the contraindications to wearing the tape.
- Provide a clear wearing protocol. Be aware that some children may not want to have the tape show. Let children pick their favorite color tape to help with compliance.

BOX 28-10

Contraindications for Use of the Elastic Therapeutic Tape

- Lack of skin integrity: open wounds, infections, scrapes, cuts, burns, newly granulated scars, and cancers or any metastatic diseases
- Poor client compliance
- High activity level of the patient
- Allergies to adhesives
- Application of tape over pain patches such as Lidoderm patches

BOX 28-11

Elastic Therapeutic Taping Techniques

- Apply tape 30 minutes before an activity to allow the skin, muscle, joint, and lymphatic systems ample time to adjust and accommodate the tape and its effects.
- The skin should be dry, free of lotion, and free of excess hair before the tape is applied.
- The tape should be applied in the direction of the movement that is being facilitated or inhibited. For example, when the goal of the tape is to support a weakened muscle, the tape should be placed at the origin of the muscle and end at the insertion of the muscle. To inhibit spasticity in a muscle, the tape should be applied in an insertion-to-origin fashion.
- Once the direction of light pull (e.g., 10%, 20%, etc.) is determined, the center of the tape should be laid over the center of the muscle belly that has to be influenced (i.e., supported, facilitated, or inhibited). After the central portion of the tape is applied to the muscle belly, it should then be pulled proximally to distally.
- Rub the tape gently onto the skin creating a light neutral warmth effect, which will activate the heat-sensitive adhesive property of the tape.
- Blot the tape dry if it has been immersed in water. Rubbing the tape with a towel creates friction and will peel the edges of the tape from the skin.

See Box 28-11 for techniques in application of elastic therapeutic tape.

Treatment of a Tight Muscle to Decrease Spasm

Anchor the tape on the muscle insertion or moveable part of the muscle. Move the limb so that the muscle is on stretch and apply the tape around the lateral and medial borders of the target muscle. End the tape at the origin of the muscle. This application technique is recommended to stabilize joints and relax contracted or overused muscles. It also aids in relaxing the muscles that spasm or muscles that are edematous due to acute injury[13] (Figure 28-18).

Treatment to Support a Weak Muscle

Anchor the elastic therapeutic tape at the site of muscle origin, or the fixed part of the muscle. Move the extremity and the skin so that the muscle and skin are on stretch. Apply the tape on the lateral and medial borders of the target muscle. End the tape at the muscle's insertion. This method might be used for children with CP who have scapular winging due to weak shoulder muscles.[13]

CLINICAL *Pearl*

Advanced training for applying elastic therapeutic tape correctly is recommended.

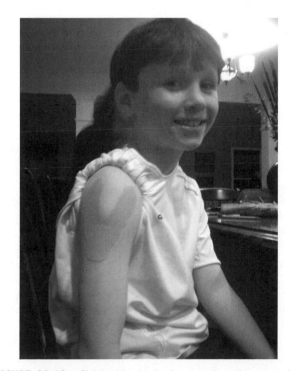

FIGURE 28-18 Child with elastic therapeutic taping over deltoid muscle for support.

Removing the Elastic Therapeutic Tape

- After 6 to 7 days, the tape should be removed by pulling slowly (unlike with an adhesive bandage) in the direction of hair growth.
- Removal should begin with the upper portion of the tape; the tape should be rolled off the skin with the index and middle fingers as if the fingers were walking backward. Lotion, baby oil, canola oil, or medical tape remover may be used over the tape for easy removal.
- The tape can be taken off even while the child is in the shower or swimming pool.
- The tape should stay off for 8 to 24 hours before applying new tape.
- A warm cloth soaked in soapy water should be used to remove any residue. Care should be taken not to scrub abrasively against the skin. The skin should be allowed to breathe and the tape reapplied as needed.

CASE *Studies*

Orthosis to Protect Healing Structures

Sixteen-year-old Kaitlin loves to play soccer. Recently she fell backward on the soccer field and fractured her distal radius, which was immobilized in a cast for 6 weeks. The cast has now been removed, but Kaitlin's wrist is still very painful and her motion is limited. The occupational therapist and the OTA together designed a wrist immobilization orthosis for Kaitlin, protecting her wrist even as she begins an active ROM exercise protocol. Orthoses are often provided after injuries or after a surgical procedure to protect the injured area while complete healing takes place. Kaitlin may remove her orthosis to perform ROM exercises and to perform daily hygiene activities.

Orthosis to Prevent or Correct Deformity

Linda is a 12-year-old girl with sore and swollen wrists due to a recent diagnosis of JIA. Her wrists are beginning to deviate in an ulnar direction, which can lead to the development of contractures, or limitations in movement caused by soft tissue shortening. This abnormal positioning of the wrist joints overtime may lead to permanent deformities and possible joint fusions, which negatively affect function. An immobilization orthosis can protect the affected joints and maintain the normal length of the soft tissue structures, including the ligaments surrounding the wrist joints and the muscles. The orthosis holds the joint in its normal position, provides gentle stress to supporting structures, and promotes the performance of daily occupations.

The occupational therapist evaluated Linda's hand function and painful wrists. The occupational therapist and OTA together designed a wrist immobilization orthosis with ulnar deviation block for Linda. The wrist orthosis held Linda's hand in slight wrist extension while providing a passive stretch to the wrist flexors. The practitioner designed a protocol for orthotic wear of the wrist extension orthosis in 2-hour increments to eliminate joint stiffness.

Orthoses to Improve Hygiene and Prevent Skin Breakdown

Some children require orthoses to protect them from injuring themselves. The OT practitioner must consider safety issues when providing such orthoses and the consequences of wearing the orthosis to the child and to others in his or her environment.

Six-year-old Mark has autism spectrum disorder. He continually picks at his scabs, increasing the risk for infection. The scabs fail to heal and bleed continuously, and they are beginning to scar. The occupational therapist working with Mark decided to provide him with a protective covering for his skin. The COTA, under the supervision of the occupational therapist, fabricated a covering made of stockinette and terry cloth to provide comfort and also cover the existing scabs. However, after several weeks, it became apparent that Mark was able to pick at the scabs after biting through the covering. After collaboration with the occupational therapist, the COTA applied orthotic material over the stockinette so that Mark would be unable to pick at his scabs. Using orthotic devices to prevent a child or adolescent from self-abuse and interfering behaviors may be an adjunctive intervention provided by the OT practitioner.

Orthosis to Enhance Function

Rosa is a 5-year-old girl with CP. She has increased wrist flexor tone and decreased wrist stability, which makes it difficult for her to hold utensils. She is able to sit at a table, but has poor coordination and is continuously dropping her spoon. A wrist immobilization orthosis was fabricated for Rosa to help her hold the spoon (see Figure 28-2). This orthosis provides Rosa with the wrist support she needs to position her wrist in extension, increase hand control and be successful in this important ADL. The OT practitioner uses the principle that external stability may increase mobility. In this case, the orthosis allows Rosa to use her hand and fingers to grasp the spoon. Therefore creating stability around the wrist or elbow with the use of the orthosis may promote improved hand function and allow Rosa to eat independently.

Orthosis to Increase Passive Joint ROM

Jorge is a 15-year-old boy with arthrogryposis. Jorge has developed an elbow flexion contracture of his left arm due to limited active motion of his biceps and triceps muscles. His occupational therapist and OTA decided to try a serial static elbow orthosis to slowly increase passive extension of the stiff elbow joint. If a joint remains in a flexed position

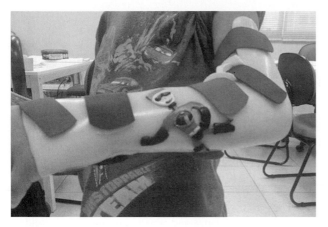

FIGURE 28-19   Decorated elbow orthosis (EO). (With permission of Candida Luzo, hand therapist.)

with limited active movement of the muscles, the risk for bone fusion and permanent deformity increases, which may lead to limited functional use of the hands. Appropriate application of a serial static orthosis to gain passive ROM at a stiff joint will help to stretch and maintain the length of the soft tissue structures. The orthosis applies a continuous LLPS to the muscles and ligaments, holding them in their maximum tolerable end range position. A low-load of force applied over a long period is tolerated better and longer than a large-load of force applied for a short period. Serial static orthosis incorporate the principle of LLPS. The orthosis can be modified on a regular basis to continue progressing the joint to full passive ROM (Figure 28-19).

Initially the elbow extension orthosis held Jorge's elbow in 35 degrees of flexion, but over the course of several weeks, the elbow extension orthosis was periodically remolded to increase the stretch of the stiff elbow into more extension. Jorge wore his elbow extension orthosis in 1- to 2-hour increments throughout the day and was able to achieve nearly full elbow extension, allowing him to participate in more sports activities with his friends.

SUMMARY

The OT practitioner incorporates knowledge of anatomy, physiology, kinesiology, and biomechanics into his or her selection of appropriate interventions to use with the pediatric population. An understanding of the variety of pediatric conditions and fabrication principles help OT practitioners design and fabricate orthoses and apply elastic therapeutic tape. Careful analysis of the many factors influencing the child's occupational performance is necessary when designing an orthosis. OT practitioners work together closely with children and their families to design and fabricate orthoses that meet the individual's goals. Orthoses can be used to promote independent function, prevent deformity, alleviate pain, and improve hygiene. Elastic therapeutic taping can be used as an adjunctive therapy with orthoses to provide support and stability to the extremity to maximize functional participation in daily occupations.

References

1. Abzug, J. M., & Kozin, S. H. (2010). Current concepts: neonatal brachial plexus palsy. *Orthopaedics, 33*(6), 431–437.
2. American Occupational Therapy Association. Occupational Therapy Practice Framework: domain and process (3rd ed.). *Am J Occup Ther,* 68(Suppl 1), S1–S48.
3. Austin, N. M. (2014). Anatomic principles. In M. L. Jacobs, & N. Austin (Eds.), *Orthotic Intervention for the Hand and Upper Extremity: Splinting Principles and Process* (2nd ed.) (pp. 26–46). Baltimore, MD: Wolters Kluwer Lippincott Williams and Wilkins.
4. Austin, G. P., & Jacobs, M. L. (2014). Mechanical principles. In M. L. Jacobs, & N. Austin (Eds.), *Orthotic Intervention for the Hand and Upper Extremity: Splinting Principles and Process* (2nd ed.) (pp. 66–83). Baltimore, MD: Wolters Kluwer/ Lippincott Williams and Wilkins.
5. Austin, N. M. (2014). Equipment and materials. In M. L. Jacobs, & N. Austin (Eds.), *Orthotic Intervention for the Hand and Upper Extremity: Splinting Principles and Process* (2nd ed.) (pp. 84–106). Baltimore, MD: Wolters Kluwer/Lippincott Williams and Wilkins.
6. Austin, N. M. (2014). Fabrication process. In M. L. Jacobs, & N. Austin (Eds.), *Orthotic Intervention for the Hand and Upper Extremity: Splinting Principles and Process* (2nd ed.) (pp. 107–127). Baltimore, MD: Wolters Kluwer/Lippincott Williams and Wilkins.
7. Beresford, M. W. (2011). Juvenile idiopathic arthritis: new insights into classification, measures of outcome, and pharmacotherapy. *Pediatric Drugs, 13*(3), 161–173.
8. Berge, S. R. T., Boonstra, A. M., Dijkstral, P. U., et al. (2011). A systematic evaluation of the effect of thumb opponens splints on hand function in children with unilateral spastic cerebral palsy. *Clin Rehab, 26*(4), 362–371.
9. Bernstein, R. (2014). Tissue healing. In M. L. Jacobs, & N. Austin (Eds.), *Orthotic Intervention for the Hand and Upper Extremity: Splinting Principles and Process* (2nd ed.) (pp. 47–65). Baltimore, MD: Wolters Kluwer/ Lippincott Williams and Wilkins.
10. Bowyer, P., & Cahill, S. M. (2009). *Pediatric Occupational Therapy Handbook: A Guide to Diagnoses and Evidence-Based Interventions.* St. Louis: Mosby.
11. Case-Smith, J. (2006). Hand skill development in the context of infant's play: birth to 2 years. In A. Henderson, & C. Pehoski (Eds.), *Hand Function in the Child; Foundations for Remediation* (2nd ed.) (pp. 118–144). St. Louis: Mosby.
12. Casella, S., & Griffin Scheff, J. (2014). Neoprene orthoses. In M. L. Jacobs, & N. Austin (Eds.), *Orthotic Intervention for the Hand and Upper Extremity: Splinting Principles and Process* (2nd ed.) (pp. 373–390). Baltimore: Wolters Kluwer/ Lippincott Williams and Wilkins.
13. Coopee, R. (2014). Taping. In M. L. Jacobs, & N. Austin (Eds.), *Orthotic Intervention for the Hand and Upper Extremity: Splinting Principles and Process* (2nd ed.) (pp. 352–372). Baltimore, MD: Wolters Kluwer/ Lippincott Williams and Wilkins.

14. Elliott, C. M., Reid, S. L., Alderson, J. A., & Elliott, B. C. (2011). Lycra arm splints in conjunction with goal directed training can improve movement in children with cerebral palsy. *Neurorehabilitation, 21*(1), 47–54.

15. Iosa, M., Morelli, D., Nanni, M. V., et al. (2010). Functional taping: a promising technique for children with cerebral palsy. *Dev Med Child Neurol, 52,* 587–589.

16. Jackman, M., Novak, I., & Lannin, N. Effectiveness of hand splints in children with cerebral palsy: a systematic review with meta-analysis. *Dev Med Child Neurol, 56,* 138–147.

17. Jacobs, M. L., & Coverdale, J. (2014). Concepts of orthotic fundamentals. In M. L. Jacobs, & N. Austin (Eds.), *Orthotic Intervention for the Hand and Upper Extremity: Splinting Principles and Process* (2nd ed.) (pp. 2–25). Baltimore: Wolters Kluwer/ Lippincott Williams and Wilkins.

18. Kara, O. K., Uysal, S. A., Turker, D., et al. (2014). The effects of Kinseio Taping on body functions and activity in unilateral spastic cerebral palsy: a single-blind randomized controlled trial. *Dev Med Child Neurol,* 1–8.

19. Keklicek, H., Uygur, F., & Yakut, Y. (2014). Effects of taping the hand in children with cerebral palsy. *J Hand Ther,* http://dx.doi.org/10.1016/j.jht.2014.09.007.

20. Lutz, C. S., & Kozin, S. H. (2006). Congenital differences in the hand and upper extremity. In S. L. Burke (Ed.), *Hand and Upper Extremity Rehabilitation: A Practical Guide* (3rd ed.) (pp. 659–688). St. Louis: Elsevier Churchill Livingstone.

21. Moran, S. L., & Tomhave, W. (2011). Management of congenital hand anomalies. In T. M. Skirven, A. L. Oster-man, J. F. Fedorczyk, & P. C. Amadio (Eds.), *Rehabilitation of the Hand and Upper Extremity* (6th ed.) (pp. 1631–1646). Philadelphia: Mosby.

22. Peck-Murray, J. (2014). The pediatric patient. In M. L. Jacobs, & N. Austin (Eds.), *Orthotic Intervention for the Hand and Upper Extremity: Splinting Principles and Process* (2nd ed.) (pp. 585–603). Baltimore: Wolters Kluwer/ Lippincott Williams and Wilkins.

23. Sebastin, S. J., & Chung, K. C. (2011). Pathogenesis and management of deformities of the elbow, wrist, and hand in late neonatal brachial plexus palsy. *J Pediatr Rehabil Med, 4,* 119–130.

24. Simsek, T. T., Turkucuoglu, B., Cokal, N., et al. (2011). The effects of Kinesio® taping on sitting posture, functional independence and gross motor function in children with cerebral palsy. *Disabil Rehabil, 33*(21-22), 2058–2063.

25. Souza Neves da Costa, C., Rodrigues, F. S., Leal, F. M., et al. (2013). Pilot study: investigating the effects of Kinesio® Taping on functional activities in children with cerebral palsy. *Dev Neurorehabil, 16*(2), 121–128.

26. Taylor, R. L., O' Brien, L., & Brown, T. (2014). A scoping review of the use of elastic therapeutic tape for neck or upper extremity conditions. *J Hand Ther, 27*(4), 235–246.

27. Wu, W. C., Hung, J. W., Tseng, C., & Huang, Y. C. (2013). Group constraint-induced movement therapy for children with hemiplegic cerebral palsy: a pilot study. *Am J Occup Ther, 67,* 201–208.

28. Yasukawa, A., Patel, P., & Sisung, C. (2006). Pilot study: investigating the effects of Kinesio taping in an acute pediatric rehabilitation setting. *Am J Occup Ther, 60,* 104–1220.

REVIEW *Questions*

1. What are the principles of orthosis fabrication for a child or adolescent?
2. What is the role of the OTA in applying orthoses for children and adolescents?
3. How can the OT practitioner improve the compliance of a child or adolescent in the use of an orthosis?
4. What are the properties of different low temperature thermoplastic materials?
5. How does elastic therapeutic taping benefit children and adolescents?
6. What are the goals of immobilization orthoses?
7. How can the OT practitioner help an adolescent with orthotic wear compliance?
8. What are the different types of mobilization orthoses?

SUGGESTED *Activities*

1. Draw a pattern for a resting hand orthosis and a wrist cock-up orthosis.
2. Locate the bony prominences on the elbow, wrist, and hand and fingers.
3. Demonstrate the functional positions of the wrist and thumb.
4. Create a wearing protocol for a serial static orthosis for a child's stiff wrist.
5. Ask a child or adolescent about his or her preferences regarding an orthosis.
6. Make a compliance checklist for a wearing protocol for Kinesio taping.
7. Create an activity for a child to do while wearing their thumb orthosis for improving function.
8. Use the Cosmesis Check Out to evaluate a completed orthosis and make the necessary modifications.

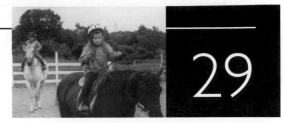

JUDITH CLIFFORD COHN
MASHELLE K. PAINTER

Animal-Assisted Activities and Therapy

CHAPTER *Objectives*

After studying this chapter, the reader will be able to accomplish the following:

- Define and distinguish between animal-assisted therapy and pet-assisted therapy.
- Understand how occupational therapy practitioners use animal- and pet-assisted therapy for the benefit of children and youth.
- Define and distinguish between therapeutic horseback riding and hippotherapy.
- Describe benefits to support use of animal-assisted, pet-assisted therapy, hippotherapy, and therapeutic horseback riding.
- Describe the role of service dogs.
- Identify occupational therapy intervention activities that incorporate the range of therapy options involving animals.

CHAPTER *Outline*

Do you have a pet? If so, take a moment to think about how your pet makes you feel. What is the first pet you remember having? One practitioner had a lightening bug that was kept in a vented jar by the bed. The light from this little bug helped her go to sleep at night. It gave a sense of security.

Animals can reduce social stress, increase motivation, and offer unconditional love (Box 29-1).[10,12] The American Occupational Therapy Association considers care of pets an occupation. Consequently, many occupational therapy (OT) practitioners involve animals in intervention. The trend to involve animals as part of occupational therapy provides a natural motivation for children who may own family pets or are attracted to animals. The focus of this chapter is on animal-assisted activities and animal-assisted therapy. In addition to examples involving small animals (e.g., dogs), the authors discuss involving large animals (e.g., horses) in OT intervention for children and youth. The authors define terms used in practice and provide guidelines for both **pet-assisted therapy** and hippotherapy. The therapeutic benefits of involving animals in practice are presented along with research evidence to support involving animals in a variety of ways in practice. The chapter provides examples of creative ways to incorporate animals into OT intervention.

DEFINITIONS

Originally coined "pet therapy" in the early 1960s, **animal-assisted therapy** and **animal-assisted activities** are rapidly growing fields of study.[15] In 1982, the American Veterinary Medical Association published an official policy statement acknowledging the importance of the human-animal bond to both client and community health.[5] Similarly, organizations such as Pet Partners (formally known as The Delta Society) developed standards around the implementation of animals for therapeutic purposes. Interventions involving the inclusion of animals generally fall into one of two categories: animal-assisted therapy or animal-assisted activities.

When animals work for therapeutic purposes, the activities are known as animal-assisted therapy. Animal-assisted therapy refers to a specific intervention to a select patient that is designed to produce a specific goal.[24] Animal-assisted therapy is a goal-directed intervention directed or delivered by a health/human service professional with specialized expertise, and within the scope of his or her profession. Figure 29-1 shows a practitioner involving a dog to encourage stretching.

Animal-assisted activities refer to events involving animals in which the animal serves as the motivator or facilitates a prescribed movement (e.g., brushing a dog). Animal-assisted activities include the casual "meet-and-greet" activities that involve pets or other animals trained for the purpose of visitation, such as bringing dogs in to a children's cancer ward for comfort.[15] Figure 29-2 shows animal-assisted activity where a dog visits a classroom. Animals included in animal-assisted therapy or activities may be specially trained to work in specific settings and these animals are deemed to have the right temperament to be part of a therapeutic intervention.

Pet-assisted therapy involves working with family pets in a therapeutic environment. These animals are pets trained to work in group settings with a variety of people. As with animal-assisted therapy, pets must have the right temperament to be part of the therapeutic intervention.

Assistant dogs help their guardian with activities such as seeing, walking, hearing, whereas therapy dogs help

---

BOX 29-1

Positive Effects That Animals Have on Humans

- Improve social interaction
- Improve quality of life by increase in self-competence and control over the environment
- Improve cardiovascular health
- Increase in trust
- Acceptance of unconditional love
- Provide structure and purpose
- Improve quality of life through engagement in meaningful occupations (e.g., care of pets)
- Allow child or youth to explore care of pets and interests in animals
- Promote volition (interests, values, belief in self) through interactions with animals

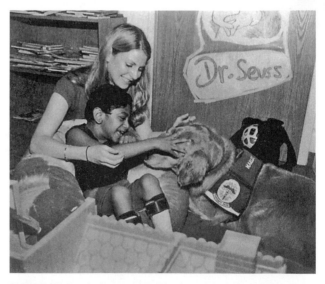

FIGURE 29-1 A dog provides the incentive for a boy to stretch tight muscles. (Photo by Dick Dressel, from Crawford J., & Pomerinke, K. A. (2003). *Therapy pets: the animal-human healing partnership.* Amherst, NY: Prometheus Books.)

in a therapeutic setting. Police, and search and rescue dogs are considered **service dogs**. They have specific roles (e.g., sense the onset of a seizure or retrieve desired item from an inaccessible shelf) for which they must be trained. A service dog is one that assists people with physical or sensory disabilities.[12] Service dogs are legally defined in the Americans with Disabilities Act (ADA).[6] According to ADA, the three types of service dogs are

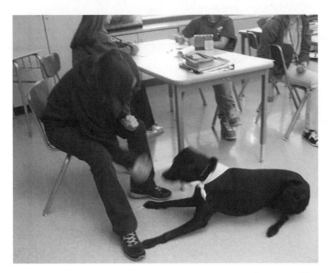

FIGURE 29-2 A pet (Remmy) visits students in a classroom. The session includes reading books about pets and writing a short story, as the dog visits the student.

BOX 29-2

Types of Service Dogs

- A *guide dog* is one that assists a person with a visual impairment or who is blind.
- A *hearing dog* is one that assists a person with a hearing loss or who is deaf.
- A *medical alert dog* is one that assists a person in a medical emergency by detecting specific physiologic changes and locating assistance during medical emergencies.

---

guide dogs, hearing dogs, and medical alert dogs (Box 29-2).[6] A guide dog assists an individual with a visual impairment or who is blind. A hearing dog assists an individual with a hearing loss or who is deaf. A medical alert dog assists an individual in a medical emergency by detecting specific physiologic changes and locating assistance during medical emergencies.[12]

Another way to categorize dogs is as companions or pets, which may include personal as well as institutional pets. A personal pet lives with an individual or family and is a part of that individual's or family's life. An institutional pet resides in a facility or institution such as a skilled nursing facility.

In addition to dogs, horses are frequently used in therapy for children with disabilities to address physical and/or emotional goals. When horses are used as a therapeutic tool, it may be described as either an equine-assisted activity or **equine-assisted therapy. Hippotherapy**, a special form of equine-assisted therapy uses the dynamic three-dimensional movement of the horse to achieve specific therapeutic goals. In the United States, hippotherapy is always provided by an OT practitioner, physical therapist (PT), or speech-language pathologist. **Therapeutic horseback riding** is an equine-assisted activity that primarily focuses on the instruction of riding skills for individuals with disabilities.[14]

OT practitioners may develop animal-assisted activities by incorporating animals into therapy sessions. Because care of pets is an occupation, it is within the OT domain to help children gain necessary abilities to perform tasks associated with pet care.[4] Developing creative interventions by incorporating small or large animals (and/or pets) may benefit children and youth receiving occupational therapy services.

SMALL ANIMALS

Small animals are those that typically weigh less than 40 pounds. Dogs, which are mammals, are one type of small animal. Other types include reptiles such as snakes; amphibians such as frogs; fish; and invertebrates such as hermit crabs and worms (Table 29-1).

TABLE 29-1

Types of Small Animals

CLASSIFICATION	DEFINITION	EXAMPLES
Mammal	Warm blooded with backbone	Dog, cat, rabbit, guinea pig, horse, cow
Reptile	Cold-blooded with horny or scaly skin	Snake
Amphibian	Cold-blooded with smooth skin	Frog, toad, salamander
Fish	Cold-blooded with fins and gills	Goldfish, beta fish
Invertebrate	Cold-blooded without backbone	Worm, snail, hermit crab

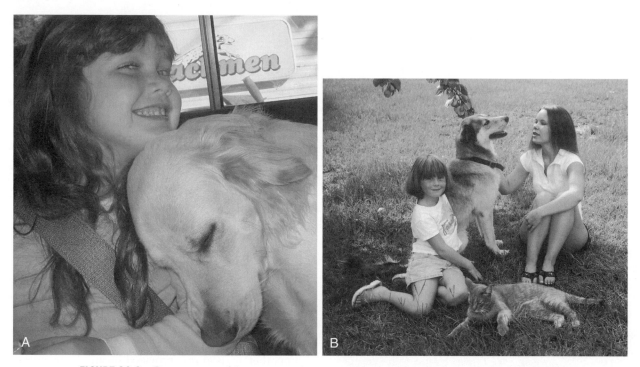

FIGURE 29-3 Dogs are one of the most popular pets and the most frequently used small mammal for animal-assisted services. **A,** A girl cuddles with her pet dog. **B,** Two girls relax in the shade with their pets.

Mammals are animals that have a backbone and are characterized by hair on the skin and mammary glands that produce milk in females. They are warm-blooded animals that maintain a relatively warm body temperature independent of the environmental temperature. Examples of animals that are classified as mammals are dogs, cats, rabbits, and guinea pigs.

Dogs are one of the most popular pets and the most frequently used small mammal for animal-assisted services (Figure 29-3). They offer a large variety of choices. Dogs are small, medium, or large in size and may be purebred or a mix of breeds. Examples of small purebred dogs are dachshunds, Chihuahuas, and cocker spaniels. Large dog breeds include chows, German shepherds, Saint Bernards, Great Pyrenees, and standard poodles. The characteristics of the breed and the individual personality of the dog are both considered when selecting a dog for animal-assisted services or to be a pet. One aspect of a dog's personality is temperament, which refers to the dog's natural or instinctive behavior. When stressed, a dog will respond according to its temperament, and frequently this is characteristic of its breed. For example, chows are known to show an aggressive response under stress.

Training involves teaching a dog to follow commands while being controlled or led by a person. Although dogs can be trained to be obedient, the temperaments of certain breeds may override their training during stressful situations. For example, in crowds of people with much noise and movement, Chows tend to growl and become "snappy."

Reptiles are animals that have a backbone and horny or scaly skin. Reptiles have lungs to breathe. They are cold-blooded animals that do not have a constant body temperature. Legless lizards and turtles are examples of reptiles that intrigue children. A wide range of nonpoisonous snakes may serve as pets or social companions. Reptilian pets tend to require less human attention and care than do other small animals. They require less frequent feeding and handling, which is a consideration in choosing the best animal to be used for animal-assisted services.

Amphibians are cold-blooded animals that have a backbone and smooth skin. All amphibians have gills because at some point in their development, an aquatic environment is required. Amphibians lay eggs to reproduce. Examples of amphibians are frogs, toads, and salamanders. Children and adolescents are usually fascinated by amphibians in their natural environments. Catching, trapping, and releasing frogs or other amphibians in their natural environments require problem solving, timing, sequencing, and precise motor skills (Figure 29-4).

Fish are also cold-blooded animals with backbones, fins for mobility, and gills for breathing. They live in water and require minimum human attention and interaction. Fish that are popular as home and classroom pets include goldfish, beta fish, and kissing fish. Animal-assisted activities involving fish might include increasing occupational performance through caring for them. Fish are not an appropriate choice for animal-assisted therapy, although decorating a fish tank and caring for fish are pleasant activities for children.

Invertebrates are animals that do not have a backbone. Examples of invertebrates are lightening bugs, worms, snails, insects, and hermit crabs (Figure 29-5).

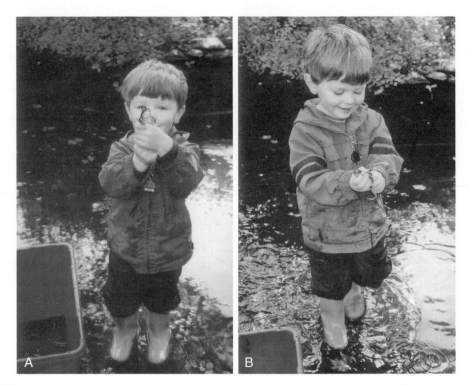

FIGURE 29-4   **A,** A young boy catches and holds onto a frog. **B,** He enjoys feeling the frog in his hands. (Courtesy: Michelle Stone.)

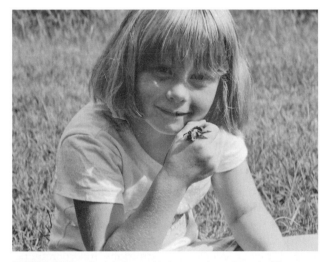

FIGURE 29-5   A girl plays with her pet hermit crab. (Courtesy: Susan Gentry.)

Children who live in rural areas have wonderful opportunities to interact with invertebrates. Hermit crabs and snails are favorites among this class of animal to be kept as pets at home or in a classroom setting.

LARGE ANIMALS

Large animals are those that typically weigh more than 40 pounds. Horses are the most frequently used large animals in animal-assisted services. Other large animals that might be considered for human-animal interactions include farm animals, exotic animals, and marine mammals.

Most farm animals are large and live on a tract of land that is being cultivated for food for human consumption. Examples of large farm animals are horses or mules, pigs, goats, cows, and sheep. Farm animals may have monetary value to the person caring for them. A special relationship of mutual respect is often obvious between the animal and the human caregiver (Figure 29-6).

Exotic animals such as llamas, peacocks, and emus are considered foreign to the United States. Interest in raising exotic animals is growing in many areas of the United States. The potential to incorporate exotic animals into animal-assisted activities and therapy has not been fully explored.

Marine mammals (e.g., dolphins, whales, seals) are warm-blooded animals that live in salty or brackish water. Although they are available for animal-assisted activities (enjoyment or play) on a commercial basis, no known programs incorporating them into animal-assisted therapy exist currently.

CLINICAL *Pearl*

Horses will often lick before they bite another horse or a person. Cows also enjoy licking the salt from human hands. Cows do not have upper teeth and so have no inclination to bite. A horse's tongue is smooth, whereas a cow's tongue is lumpy and coarse.

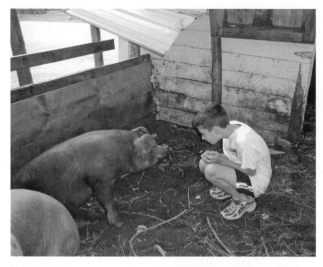

FIGURE 29-6 A young boy feeds his pig and then spends time "playing" together.

BENEFITS OF ANIMAL-ASSISTED THERAPY

Animal-assisted therapy can be used to help children and youth develop psychosocial, social, physical, and educational skills.[10,28,30] The psychosocial benefits of animal-assisted therapy include the following:

- Increase in verbal interactions among group members,
- Increase in attention skills,
- Increase in self-esteem,
- Improvements in depressive symptoms,
- Reduction of anxiety,
- Reduction of loneliness,
- Decrease in behavioral problems, and
- Enhance emotional well-being.[10,13,36]

Children with disabilities benefit from interactions with animals. Children with autism spectrum disorder appear to be more playful and focused when animals are present.[10,21,26] Animals allow OT practitioners to address a variety of therapeutic goals. Therapy animals can help children engage with peers, develop self-esteem, and have fun.[13,36]

Social and motivational benefits include improving willingness to be involved in a group activity, interactions with others and with staff, communication and cooperation, as well as developing empathy and sensitivity.[18,36,37] Children may learn nurturing skills, develop outward focus and interact and open up.[37]

The human-animal bond has been shown to change physical factors including decreasing blood pressure, reducing stress levels, and increasing self-esteem.[37] Children may find it relaxing when an animal is present and this can result in lowered heart rate and blood pressure.[37] Stroking and petting an animal is soothing and calming for children. It may help children feel better and elevate their moods. Children may consider pets to be a part of their family (Figure 29-7).[1] Adamle (2007) discovered

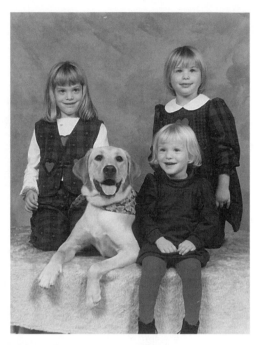

FIGURE 29-7 The human-animal bond is strong and often dogs are considered part of the family.

that a pet therapy program could temporarily fill the absence of previous support systems and be a catalyst for establishing new social relationships.[1]

Pet therapy may help college students suffering from depression.[16] The authors measured depression in 44 students using the Beck Depression Inventory (BDI) before and after intervention (psychotherapy, pet-assisted therapy, or control group that received no therapy). The authors found that BDI scores were significantly lower for those treated with pet-assisted therapy than for those who did not receive this therapy (the control group).[16] Some suggest that pet-assisted therapy can improve a depressed person's self-worth by enabling them to focus on the pet and the environment instead of himself or herself.[29] College students living away from home for the first time often face difficulty. It may be equally as hard for those students to be away from their pets.

To illustrate the breadth of pet-assisted therapy, several higher education institutions incorporate pet therapy activities on campus (i.e., Yale, Ohio State University, Stephens, University of Delaware, Ithaca, Northeastern). The University of Wisconsin, Oshkosh, has a pet-assisted therapy program that is integrated as part of the counseling process. Yale law students can check out a dog, along with their reference materials at the law library as a way to reduce their stress while studying.

Animal-assisted therapy may influence physical factors in children and youth. Specifically, it may improve fine motor skills (brushing, stroking), gross motor skills like balance and coordination (walking the dog), and relaxation (can lower blood pressure). Marcus and Palley (2012) found that dogs lowered pain and stress levels for patients with chronic pain.[25] In the study, patients diagnosed with back pain, fibromyalgia, or unspecified pain and their companions were given the choice to wait in a traditional waiting room or in a room with a therapy dog and its handler. For both rooms, the patients and the companions completed a survey asking what their pain, stress, and energy levels were before they went into the room and when they left the room. For those clients who spent time in the waiting room with the dog, there was a 40% decrease in depression and anxiety scores, 20% in fatigue, and 25% in pain.[25] Dog owners have less heart disease risk due to increased exercise levels, lower blood pressure, lower resting heart rate, lower stress response, and better recovery after a heart attack.[23]

Animal-assisted therapy may provide educational benefits, including an increase in vocabulary and reading fluency, long- and short-term memory, and attitude toward reading.[18,37] The presence of a pet improved the attitude of staff and interactions with patients due to reduced caregiver stress.[18]

PET-ASSISTED THERAPY
Guidelines for Establishing a Pet-Assisted Therapy Program

Practitioners interested in setting up pet-assisted therapy program as part of the OT intervention must follow the guidelines for establishing the program. As an OT practitioner, they must also clearly demonstrate that they are focusing on the child's individualized OT goals. It may be that the OT practitioner works with a person trained in pet-assisted therapy, facilitating therapy goals as the child engages in the activities.

OT practitioners interested in incorporating pet-assisted therapy into intervention begin by understanding the necessary guidelines for establishing a program. A pet-assisted therapy program is conducted in a healthy, safe, and appropriate therapeutic environment for the pet, client, and pet guardian. (Pet guardian refers to the pet's handler or "owner." In professional pet therapy, pets are regarded as family members and therefore not "owned." Thus the term *pet guardian* is preferred.) The following guidelines assure quality pet therapy practice:

1. The pet guardian is a person who is educated in the field of pet-assisted therapy and has adequate insurance. The pet guardian monitors the sessions to determine the length of the treatment based on the current situation and interaction.
2. The therapy pet must be well-mannered and in good health. Additionally, the pet must be current on all shots, seen by a veterinarian on a regular basis, and groomed on a regular basis. The pet practices good obedience skills with the pet guardian on a daily basis. The therapy pet participates in socialization time with

and without other dogs and enjoys recreational activities such as playing fetch with a ball. The pet needs to be happy.
3. Structure of the session:
   - The therapy pet attends sessions with the guardian and is supervised at all times.
   - The therapy pet is given time to adjust to a new situation.
   - The client is given time to build a relationship with the pet and instructed in correct ways to approach a therapy pet and how to treat the pet with respect.

CLINICAL *Pearl*

Cats are the most suitable institutional pets because of their lifestyles (eating and toileting habits, exercise requirements) and independence.

Pet-Assisted Therapy and Occupational Therapy

OT practitioners may set up a pet-assisted therapy program to address physical, social, or emotional goals for children and youth.[22,38] The OT practitioner begins by formulating OT goals and objectives. Next, the OT practitioner determines pet-assisted activities that will best address the child's therapy goals. If the practitioner is certified in pet-assisted therapy, he or she may decide to conduct the sessions. Otherwise, the practitioner may decide to contact a certified pet-assisted therapist to engage the child in a pet-assisted session.

The following steps are essential for setting up a professional pet-assisted therapy program. OT practitioners aware of these steps understand the details involved in this type of programming, which helps assure quality and safety:

- Complete a pet-assisted therapy certification program.
- Contact supervisor or administrator of the setting (e.g., principal).
- Discuss the program ethics, standards, and procedures. Provide copies of the pet's medical record including up-to-date vaccinations, town license, and insurance proof.
- Discuss who will be the pet-assisted therapy liaison.
- Review the evaluation procedure regarding the program.
- Evaluate the suitability of the room and space. (Be sure to determine how to get outside and where the dog can walk, etc.)
- Introduce your pet to the liaison.
- Get photograph releases and permission from parents and guardians for children to participate in the program.
- Dress and act professional at all times; be on time, and be courteous to everyone at the setting.

Although most pet-assisted therapy involves dogs, other pets may serve in these roles (such as rabbits, guinea pigs, cats). Practitioners are encouraged to be creative when designing intervention with animals.

CASE *Study*

OT practitioners may determine that pet-assisted therapy can help children achieve intervention goals. For example, 8-year-old Mark experiences difficulties with functional mobility in the classroom and in making friends. His parents are considering getting him a dog to increase his responsibility at home. The OT practitioner saw Mark become very excited when a dog entered the playground at school. When the practitioner asked Mark, he said he loved dogs and was hoping to get one soon. The OT practitioner contacted a friend who recently completed a pet-assisted therapy course and became certified. Together they planned a 4-week session at school. The OT practitioner received permission from the principal, parents, and teacher. They began the sessions individually with Mark.

The OT practitioner established goals and assisted Mark in the sessions by providing postural support and cuing, and by establishing guidelines for the intervention session. Mark was very excited and enjoyed the sessions. He worked on fine motor skills through brushing, organization by establishing a routine to care for the pet (e.g., get water, take dog for walk, practice simple commands, and provide pet with a snack at end of session), and physical skills through walking and moving to attend to the dog. As he walked the dog, Mark worked on postural control and endurance. The OT practitioner reinforced the activities involved in caring for a pet. The pet facilitator emphasized patience and training and Mark was able to relate to having to practice things longer than some of his classmates. The pet facilitator remarked that all dogs are different and some learn more quickly than others—just like people. He enjoyed having his picture taken with the dog and sharing this with his classmates. Many classmates shared stories about their pets. Mark found it easier to talk with classmates about the pet. Mark looked forward to seeing the dog each week. He was able to demonstrate respect for the animal and his parents eventually bought him his own pet. They felt more confident in his skills.

Session Standards

Each pet-assisted therapy session is unique depending on the needs of the child, the number of children in each group, and the setting. Sessions should not last more than 1 hour and may be shorter if the child and/or pet are tired. Professionals using pet-assisted therapy use their creativity to accomplish the therapeutic goals of the clients. The presence of the pet drives the session. However, the pet is not "performing" but is present. The activity is focused around the pet and the client.

In occupational therapy, the client is the focus of the session and their therapeutic goals drive the session.

Box 29-3 provides sample goals for pet-assisted therapy sessions. Practitioners carefully evaluate how the pet and client will work together to reach the child's goals. To integrate pet therapy with occupational therapy, the practitioner is aware of the pet and how they interact with the child or youth. For example, in the previous case study, Mark walked the dog each week except on 1 week where the dog seemed tired from a busy schedule. On that day Mark practiced commands and wrote a story about caring for dogs. The practitioner does not manipulate the pet, but rather allows the pet and child to interact naturally. It is important to spend time making sure that the child and pet are comfortable and that the child treats the pet with respect. The pet-assisted therapy facilitator makes certain that the pet is safe, secure, and treated kindly. Once the guidelines are in place, the therapy pet is introduced to the client(s) and the session begins.

The OT practitioner recognizes that in pet-assisted therapy the human/pet bond drives the activity. See Box 29-4 and Box 29-5 for sample lesson plans that may be used in occupational therapy. For example, if the client is a child with cognitive challenges the pet's presence may encourage the child to talk about what he or she knows about pets, past pets, or experiences around animals. The child can read to the pet or read stories about the pet and/or engage in activities related to the pet (such as puzzles or pet related games). Figure 29-8 illustrates a variety of books related to the pet. Figure 29-9 shows an adapted puzzle that has been personalized for the children. Personalizing the puzzle by using the pet's photo increases the meaningfulness of the activity and may facilitate more engagement from the child.

CLINICAL *Pearl*

Children love to take home pictures of the animals. These photos preserve the memories and may serve therapeutic purposes. Figure 29-10 is a photo of OT students taken from a session with Remmy.

BOX 29-3

Sample Goals for Pet-Assisted Therapy Sessions

- Child will spontaneously initiate conversation twice with two peers during a 30-minute session.
- To exhibit increased use of right upper extremity for play, child will throw Frisbee 10 times without showing signs of fatigue during a 30-minute play session.
- To show self-efficacy, child will state two things that he or she is proud of after a 30-minute session.
- Given pictorial reminders, child will show success in care of pet by showing that he or she can feed, brush, walk, and care for pet dog for 5 days.
- Child will exhibit improved visual perceptual skills by completing a 6 piece puzzle.

OT practitioners can include the presence of a pet to achieve a variety of physical, psychosocial, or social goals.[34] Throwing a ball to a dog to fetch helps children practice grasping and throwing skills. Using a variety of balls in different sizes can help children gain strength in their hands. Holding, grasping, manipulating, and bilateral hand skills can be practiced. Grooming the pet helps children learn pet responsibility, which is an instrumental activity of daily living (IADL). Timing, holding, grasping, manipulating, and bilateral hands skills can be practiced while playing with the pet. OT practitioners develop many activities with animals and pets that facilitate children's goals.

CLINICAL *Pearl*

Developing pet "playing cards" encourages reading and may serve as a conversation starter (Figure 29-11).

CLINICAL *Pearl*

Creating themed cards can provide novelty to a therapy session and encourage social participation, reading, memory, and attention to details See Figure 29-12 for examples. Everyone enjoys getting a card!

BOX 29-4

Theme: Giving Back to the Community

Group members: Middle school students in service learning class, classroom teacher, pet therapy facilitator, pet (dog named Remmy)

Group goal: Students will identify major issues in society and possible solutions to feel that they can make a difference in their community.

Objective: Students will discuss important societal problems and how pets can help with them. Students will work together to find answers to problems.

Method:
- Hand notecards to students.
- Ask students to think of a serious society problem or issue that is important to them and write it on one side of the card.
- After a few minutes, have the students discuss ways pet therapy can help solve the problems. Write answers on the back of the card.
- Share the problems and solutions with the class.

Conclusion: Pets can help society in a variety of ways and each and every one of us can make a difference.

Samples of students' work: These examples were taken from a middle school service learning class.

PROBLEM	HOW PET THERAPY CAN HELP GIVE BACK TO THE COMMUNITY (STUDENT RESPONSES)
Violence	If someone had a violent problem, pet therapy could help make him or her better.
Bullying	When someone is getting bullied, a dog can be there to make them comfortable.
Discrimination	Not all pit bulls are dangerous. Dogs are reflections of their training. Like people you have to get to know them.
Bullying	It could help the bully with their social problems. They can learn respect and responsibility and they could be nicer.

BOX 29-5

Theme: Be Positive—We All Have to Practice!

Group members: Middle school students in service learning class, classroom teacher, pet therapy facilitator, pet (dog named Remmy)

Group goal: Students will recognize that education and training is necessary for everyone. They will realize that training a dog takes a positive attitude and share that attitude with others.

Objective: Students will learn that everyone responds to positive praise. Students will practice obedience skills with Remmy and realize that training a pet takes time and patience and positive reinforcement.

Method
- Discuss steps to become a certified pet therapy dog.
- Have students practice obedience skills with pet by picking an index card with that skill on it and practicing with Remmy.
- Help students reinforce the skills with treats and praise. Point out how Remmy does so much better with praises and treats.
- Emphasize that dog training requires patience and a positive attitude.
- Explain that just like pets, people respond well to positive praise.
- Assignment: You are to give out a "Dog Treat" card to someone this week who does something nice for you. Write your praise, compliment, or thank you on the back of the "treat" card.
- Next week, report to class how you felt giving away a treat.

Conclusion: Remember service learning is about giving back to your community. Stay positive!

Samples of work: The children were excited to talk about the cards they had given out. One child gave one to his bus driver, another to his mom for making a nice supper, another to her friend who was always there for her, and another to her teacher. They asked for more cards to give out the next week.

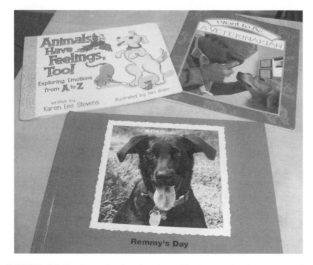

FIGURE 29-8 Developing books with the pet's picture can facilitate reading, attention, and the child's motivation to participate in therapy to reach his or her goals.

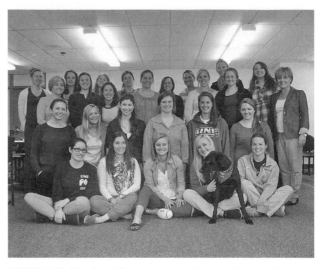

FIGURE 29-10 Providing a photo of the session reminds the children of the experience and may facilitate memories, provide a conversation starter with friends, and encourage social participation. OT students at the University of New England pose for a photo with Remmy after a pet therapy session.

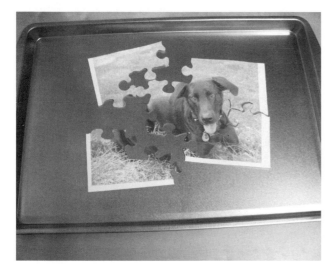

FIGURE 29-9 Puzzles can be created using the pet's picture and adapted for many children. The pieces to this puzzle have magnetic backing so they can be moved easily on the tin sheet.

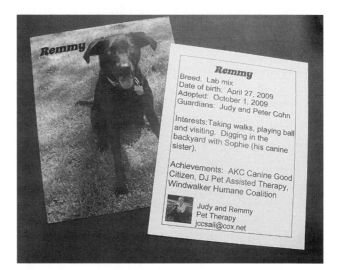

FIGURE 29-11 Pet "playing cards" may help children remember the experience and engage in conversations with others. Practitioners can use the playing cards to encourage attention to details, social participation, language, reading, and memory. The cards can also be used to promote fine motor skills.

EQUINE-ASSISTED THERAPY

Equine-assisted therapy (EAT) is the therapeutic use of horses for treating individuals with disabilities. It is not merely "horseback riding." Published research and anecdotal evidence indicates that using horses for therapy can affect and improve the health and well-being of individuals with a range of physical and emotional limitations in a way that differs from traditional therapies.[2,7,8,17,27,33] Those who choose to work in the EAT field must be trained in both horsemanship skills and have an understanding of disabilities in order to provide a sage and therapeutic experience for the rider. EAT may help children with disabilities enjoy greater

mobility, independence, and function, in addition to receiving the same health and wellness benefits as nondisabled riders.

Hippotherapy vs. Therapeutic Riding

There is often confusion between hippotherapy and therapeutic riding.[3] In some texts, hippotherapy and therapeutic riding are both considered types of EAT and often the current literature will use the terms *equine-assisted therapy* and *therapeutic riding* interchangeably. However, professionals in both the fields of therapeutic riding and hippotherapy are working toward standardizing the terminology so that there is a distinction between the two.[3,33] Box 29-6 provides a comparison of these two terms.[3]

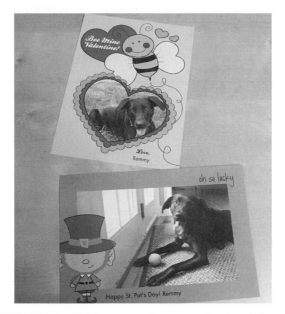

FIGURE 29-12 Children may enjoy personalized cards for special events. These Valentine's and Saint Patrick's Day cards from Remmy provide novelty and fun that helps to stimulate learning.

General Benefits of Equine-Assisted Therapy

Children with disabilities may have absent or impaired walking patterns. The movement of the horse gives kinesthetic and sensory input to the nervous system of the rider, helping to strengthen core muscles, normalize spastic muscle tone, and improve balance and coordination.[2,20,31] One of the main reasons why the horse's movement is so beneficial is because "the motion of the horse transfers movement patterns to the body center (i.e., lumbar spine and pelvic regions), duplicating the patterns man typically executes when walking upright."[8] The horse provides dynamic movement that no other piece of equipment can replicate.[3,9] Another physical benefit of using the horse is the transfer of the horse's body temperature to the rider. Because a horse's temperature is 2 to 3 degrees warmer than a human body's temperature, the extra warmth that is felt by the rider helps to relax and stretch tight muscles, particularly in the legs.[32]

The psychological benefits are sometimes more obvious that the physical benefits. For many riders, being on a horse is a pleasurable experience. It is also a very social activity, with the rider interacting with the instructor, therapists, volunteers, other clients and the horse. Social interaction and "having a good time" are considered equally important components of the therapy session.[32] OT practitioners may find that animal-assisted therapy helps children develop interests,

---

BOX 29-6

Comparison of Hippotherapy and Therapeutic Riding

	HIPPOTHERAPY	THERAPEUTIC RIDING
Definition	Physical, occupational, or speech therapy implemented by a team that includes a licensed, credentialed therapist	Recreational horseback lessons for children with disabilities, completed by a certified therapeutic horseback riding instructor in conjunction with volunteers
Method	The movement of the horse is used as the treatment tool in physical, occupational, and speech therapy.	Recreational horseback riding lessons are adapted to allow the child to ride successfully.
	The horse's movement is essential in meeting therapy goals.	The horse's temperament is essential to learn riding skills.
	The therapist provides direct hands-on intervention at all times.	The riding instructor teaches from center of arena with some hands-on from instructors or volunteers as needed.
	The therapist assesses and modifies therapy based on child's responses.	The riding instructor provides adaptations or suggestions to enable child to ride.
	Reimbursed by medical insurance.	Not covered by insurance.
Goal	To improve neurological functioning in cognition, body movement, organization, and attention levels to improve functioning in daily occupations	To teach the child proper riding position and reining skills; to introduce child to leisure activity.

Data from American Hippotherapy Association (2010): Hippotherapy vs. therapeutic riding: what is the difference? Available at http://windrushfarm.org/downloads/american.pdf.

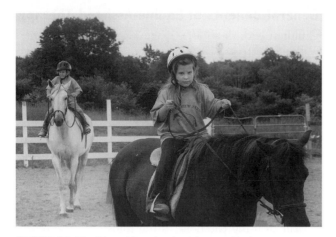

FIGURE 29-13 Two girls enjoy learning to ride horses at summer camp. (Courtesy Cheryl Joyce.)

motivations, belief in their skills (Figure 29-13). For example, Taylor and colleagues found preliminary evidence that with hippotherapy, **volition** (one's interests, self-efficacy, and motivation) may improve in children with autism.[35] The authors used the Pediatric Volitional Questionnaire to measure volition in three children with autism before, during, and after 16 weeks of hippotherapy.[35]

OT practitioners may use EAT to target several cognitive factors needed to engage in occupation:

1. Sequencing: Stopping a horse or hanging rings on a peg can be difficult for child with a physical or neurologic impairment. Dividing the task into individual steps and putting them in the correct order can be helpful in ADLs.
2. Eye-hand coordination: Learning to turn a horse around a cone requires eye-hand coordination.
3. Multitasking: A child must learn to multitask as he or she holds the reins in the correct position while maintaining balance and listening to the instructor's directions.
4. Sensory processing: The child processes sensory input from a variety of sources (tactile, visual, auditory, etc.) while horseback riding.
5. Left-right discrimination: The child discriminates left and right as he or she pulls on the reins to cue the horse to move in a given direction.
6. Spatial orientation: The child learns where the body is in space in relation to other people and objects as he or she maintains body position on the horse.
7. Motor planning: The child must execute motor tasks in the proper sequence and with graded muscle movement, such as holding onto the reins and putting one's feet in the stirrups while moving up and down as the horse moves.[32]

These are examples of some of the tasks emphasized in a therapeutic horseback riding program.

What Makes a Suitable Therapy Horse?

Like other animals that are involved in animal-assisted therapy, not all horses are good candidates as therapy horses. A horse's physical condition, conformation, and temperament are qualities that must be evaluated before inclusion in a therapeutic riding program. Box 29-7 provides some guidelines for selecting a horse for hippotherapy. If the horse is to be considered for hippotherapy specifically, the therapy practitioner should assess the quality of the horse's movement to know whether or not it will produce the right movement and sensation. For example, a horse that does not "track up" (where the hind foot steps into the impression left by the front foot) may produce a stride that is choppy and inhibits the natural movement of the rider's pelvis. This may be fine for a rider with autism who needs more proprioceptive input, but not suitable for a rider with cerebral palsy who needs to be able to relax his or her muscles. A therapy horse must also be sound, which means it does not exhibit any signs of lameness or stiffness in any of its limbs. Horses that have been retired due to arthritis or injury are not appropriate for therapy as it is physically hard work for the horse. In many cases, the horse has to compensate for the lack of balance in a rider, causing the horse's back and legs to become sore. A horse that is not in good physical condition will not last long in a therapeutic riding program. Finally, the ideal therapy horse will have a calm, patient disposition and not be spooked easily.[14] The horse must be able to tolerate being around different types of equipment (wheelchairs, walkers, etc.) and not be bothered by the squealing or accidental kick in the ribs from an excited child. On the other hand, a therapy horse should not be lazy or half asleep on the job. It should be able to readily move forward on command and make upward and downward transitions (changes in speed) easily. The horse should appear to enjoy its work.[32]

Children with a variety of health conditions may benefit from EAT. For example, children with cerebral palsy may benefit from the movement of the horse as it helps to relax their muscles, decrease spasticity, strengthen core balance and stability, and improve head and neck control.[8,9,27] Children who exhibit poor attention span and organization from traumatic brain injury may benefit from hippotherapy as it provides stability, proprioceptive input, and rhythmic movement to help with organization and attention. Research suggests that children with autism spectrum disorder engage in less self-stimulating behaviors, show improved tolerance to sensory experiences, and increased attention after hippotherapy sessions.[26,35] Riding a horse can be a source of pleasure for children with and without disability. It may help them gain self-esteem as they engage in a purposeful activity with peers.[19,30,35]

Some riders may not be suitable for EAT because the risk outweighs the benefit.[2] EAT is not recommended for children under the following circumstances:

1. If the activity on the horse will cause a decrease in the child's function, an increase in pain, or generally aggravate the medical condition.
2. If the interaction is detrimental to the child or the horse.
3. There is always a potential risk for a fall during the activity. Such a fall may cause a greater functional impairment than the child originally had. The possibility of a fall should be given careful consideration.
4. If it is the medical opinion of the physician that EAT would be inappropriate for the child.
5. If the child's own behavior is a contraindication and would prevent a safe treatment session.[31]

INCORPORATING ANIMALS INTO PEDIATRIC OCCUPATIONAL THERAPY PRACTICE

Incorporating animals into the OT process involves several occupations or life activities in which individuals participate (Figure 29-14). Engagement in instrumental ADLs such as care of pets, health management and maintenance, safety procedures, and informal personal education participation might be the outcomes of animal-assisted activities and animal-assisted therapy. The OT practitioner may also decide to use animal-assisted therapy to improve a child's ability to perform certain client factors needed for successful participation in occupations. Children may need to develop problem-solving and fine motor skills or balance to care for pets or interact with an animal. The OT practitioner needs to consider the cultural, physical, temporal, and virtual contexts of the client when incorporating animals into activities and therapy.[4] The activity demands and individual client factors will have an influence on the decision-making

process.[4] The following questions may guide practitioners in decision making concerning animal-assisted therapy:

- Who are your clients?
- Where will the animal-assisted services be provided?
- Are you considering a large animal or a small animal for these services?
- What characteristics are you looking for in the animal?
- What type of human-animal interaction will be involved?
- What are the potential health hazards?
- What pets or other animals are present at the client's home? Does the client have access to them?
- What are the goals of incorporating an animal into the therapy sessions?
- What is the best fit between the animal and the client?

Intervention Planning

Animals can be used in therapy as a modality (i.e., the animal is the tool to improve the skill) or as the goal itself (i.e., caring for the animal is the occupation that the person is trying to master; see Figure 29-14). For either reason, the OT practitioner must carefully analyze the tasks required for client participation in the activity in order to include the animal effectively in therapy sessions. Box 29-8 provides therapeutic outcomes that may be addressed in hippotherapy or EAT. Box 29-9 provides sample goals that may be addressed through hippotherapy or EAT. Once the OT practitioner has established the goals of the therapy session, a decision on the type of animal activity is required, as illustrated by the following case study.

CASE *Study*

George is a 5-year-old boy with limited use of his right arm. He loves animals and has a pet cat that he has been unable to see since his hospitalization. The OT practitioner decides to surprise George in the therapy session and bring in a cat for him to brush using both of his arms and hands. The OT practitioner positions the cat so that George has to reach for and hold it. This is a natural activity for him because it emphasizes his love of animals. The goal of the session is to help George improve motor skills (e.g., the use of his right hand). Therefore, throughout the session, the OT practitioner skillfully adapts the activity in such a way that George has to use his right arm. In this example, brushing the cat is an activity that promotes right arm movement.

Brushing the cat could also be considered the goal of the session (e.g., the occupation itself is the goal) in this

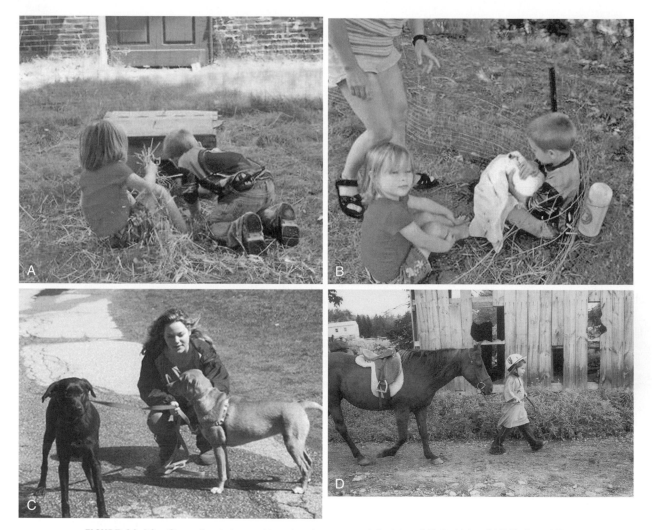

FIGURE 29-14 Care of pets is considered an Instrumental Activity of Daily Living (IADL). **A** and **B,** A boy and a girl care for their bunnies as part of their daily chores. **C,** A girl walks two dogs. **D,** A girl brings a horse back to her stall. (Courtesy Cheryl Joyce.)

scenario because George has a cat at home. Therefore, if one of his chores is to brush his cat, the OT practitioner may want to focus the session on how he will be able to do this despite limited movement in his right arm. In this case the OT practitioner would position the cat in such a way that George would be successful in the task. This would help George adapt and compensate for the limited use of his right arm to be able to effectively fulfill his role as caregiver for the pet.

CASE *Study*

OT practitioners may decide to help children explore their environment through visual, auditory, and tactile means by involving animals in therapy. Exploration helps children develop sensory and problem-solving skills.

Seth, a 2-year-old boy with developmental delays, lived in the inner city. When his OT practitioner proposed using

insects and animals in therapy sessions, Seth's parents smiled and stated that unlike his older brother, Seth never explored a sandbox or the ground. The parents did not realize that because of his delays, he never felt the ground or grass. The OT practitioner planned a session in which sand, worms, ants, and plants would be used. While Seth was playing during this session, his mother pointed out the various objects. The OT practitioner also placed small toys in the sand and allowed Seth to determine whether or not each toy was an animal. Seth smiled and laughed when he picked up a worm and observed its movements. His mother enjoyed teaching her son about the animals and insects and told him stories about her own childhood experiences. This session empowered the mother and reminded her in a subtle way that children at all levels of ability value exploration. Furthermore, Seth was able to experience typical sensations, although they were somewhat different from those of his inner city environment.

Therapeutic Outcomes of Hippotherapy

Improvement in functioning in all areas of occupation by developing the following:
- Muscle tone for improved motor control
- Balance and equilibrium responses
- Gross and fine motor coordination
- Symmetry of motor functions
- Postural control
- Speech and language skills
- Self-efficacy and self-concept
- Body awareness
- Emotional well-being
- Regulation of behavior
- Sense of success

Sample Goals for Hippotherapy

- Child will show ability to engage in the occupations involved in the care and maintenance of horses.
- Child will participate in riding sessions.
- Child will show improved skills and ability in riding horses.
- Child will show improved posture and gait.
- Child will demonstrate grooming and caring for the horse.
- Child will participate in social activities related to horses (e.g., 4-H).
- Child will socialize with others involved in care and maintenance of horses.
- Child will organize and prepare clothing and materials needed to engage in occupations involved in the care and maintenance of horses.
- Child will successfully initiate and complete activities related to horses.
- Child will show adequate problem solving and reactions to experiences related to horses.

Animal-assisted therapy can help children with emotional and/or behavioral difficulties. Animals have a calming effect and are responsive to humans.[11,12,19] Therefore, children can be taught to read the cues of animals, and this new skill may transfer to reading the cues of people in their lives. Caring for animals can be satisfying to children, and teaching animals to perform simple commands to animals can be rewarding. The bond between the child and his or her pet is beneficial, especially in the case of a child who experiences behavioral and/or emotional difficulties. The nurturing nature of animals and the feeling of acceptance created by them help these children. The OT practitioner may need to model the appropriate way to touch an animal and thus help the child bond with the animal. The session may focus on reading the animal's cues, caring for it, or teaching it to do a trick. Through these sessions, the child learns patience, understanding, timing, caring, and perseverance. Caring for animals requires consistency in performance and organization.

Animals may be used as a modality to improve social participation. A child may show his or her pet to friends, meet other children with the same type of pet, or join clubs that discuss the care of animals (e.g., a 4-H club, riding organization, fair). These groups help children learn about and gain interest in their pets and develop a sense of belonging. OT practitioners can help children with special needs participate in these groups by helping them adapt or compensate as needed.

The activities described here are just a few of the many possibilities that animal-assisted therapy offers to children and OT practitioners. Intervention must be centered on the child's and his or her family's needs. OT practitioners should understand the family's culture and attitude toward animals. Many of these activities can be tailored to meet the needs of children with special needs.

SUMMARY

Animal-assisted therapy and animal-assisted activities can be a creative and interesting modality for OT intervention. Many children participate in occupations involving animals, making this a natural fit for occupational therapy. Children of all ages enjoy interactions with animals and occupations that involve them. Understanding the full range of services and training required to provide services under pet-assisted therapy, hippotherapy, therapeutic horseback riding, or EAT allows OT practitioners to make informed decisions regarding intervention options for children and their families.

References

1. Adamle, K. N., Riley, T. A., & Carlson, T. (2007). Evaluating college student interest in pet therapy. *J AM Coll Health, 57*(5), 545–548.
2. American Hippotherapy Association (nd.). Available at: http://www.americanhippotherapyassociation.org/uncategorized/about_aha.
3. American Hippotherapy Association (nd.). Hippotherapy vs. therapeutic riding: what is the difference. Available at: http://windrushfarm.org/downloads/american.pdf.
4. American Occupational Therapy Association. (2014). Occupational therapy practice framework: domain and process (3rd ed.). *Am J Occup Ther, 68*(Suppl. 1), S1–S48.
5. American Veterinary Medical Association official statement. (2014). Human animal bond. Available at: https://www.avma.org/KB/Policies/Pages/The-Human-Animal-Bond.aspx.

6. Americans With Disabilities Act of 1990. (1990), Pub. L. No. 101-336, 104 Stat. 328.

7. Aoki, J., Iwahashi, K., Ishigooka, J., Fukamauchi, F., Numjiri, M., Ohtani, N., et al. (2012). Evaluation of cerebral activity in the prefrontal cortex in mood (affective) disorders during animal-assisted (AAT) by near-infrared spectroscopy (NIRS): a pilot study. *Int J Psychiatry Clin Pract, 16*, 205–213.

8. Benda, W., McGibbon, N. H., & Grant, K. L. (2003). Improvements in muscle symmetry in children with cerebral palsy after equine-assisted therapy (hippotherapy). *J Altern Complement Med, 9*(6), 817–825.

9. Bertoli, D. (1988). Effects of therapeutic horseback riding on posture in children with cerebral palsy. *J Phys Ther, 8*(10), 1505–1512.

10. Blue, G. (1986). The lives of pets in children's lives. *Child Educ*, December. 85–90.

11. Connor, K. (2001). Animal-assisted therapy: an in-depth look. *Dimens Crit Care Nurs, 20*, 20–27.

12. Crawford, J., & Pomerinke, K. A. (2003). *Therapy pets: the animal–human healing partnership.* Amherst, NY: Prometheus Books.

13. Eggiman, J. (2006). Cognitive-behavioral therapy: a case report—animal-assisted therapy. *Topics Adv Pract Nurs (eJournal), 6*(3).

14. Engel, B., & MacKinnon, J. (Eds.). (2007). *Enhancing human occupation through hippotherapy.* Bethesda, MD: AOTA.

15. Fine, A. H. (Ed.). (2006). *Handbook on animal-assisted therapy* (2nd ed.) San Diego: Academic Press.

16. Folse, E. B., Minder, C. C., Aycock, M. J., & Santana, R. T. (1994). Animal-assisted therapy and depression in adult college students. *Anthrozoos, 7*(3) 188–184.

17. Frank, A., McCloskey, S., & Dole, R. L. (2011). Effect of hippotherapy on perceived self-competence and participation in a child with cerebral palsy. *Pediatr Phys Ther, 23*(3), 301–308.

18. Heimlich, K. (2001). Animal-assisted therapy and the severely disabled child: A qualitative study. *J Rehabil, 67*(4), 48–54.

19. Hooker, S. D., Freeman, L. H., & Stewart, P. (2002). Pet therapy research: a historical review. *Holist Nurs Pract, 17*, 17–23.

20. Hulchanski, C. (2008). Horsing around. *Adv Ocuup Ther, 24*, 50.

21. Katcher, A., Friedman, E., Beck, A., & Lynch, J. (1983). Looking, talking, and blood pressure: the physiological consequences of interaction with the living environment. In A. Katcher, & A. Beck (Eds.), *New perspectives on our lives with companion animals.* Philadelphia: University of Pennsylvania Press.

22. Kielhofner, G. (2008). *Model of human occupation: theory and application* (4th ed.). Baltimore, MD: Lippincott, Williams & Wilkins.

23. Marcus, D. A. (2008). *Fit as Fido: follow your dog to better health.* Bloomington, IN: iUniverse, Inc.

24. Marcus, D. A. (2011). *The power of wagging tails: a doctor's guide to dog therapy and healing.* New York: demosHealth.

25. Marcus, D. A., & Palley, G. (2012). Dog therapy in waiting rooms calms and eases pain. 6th World Congress of the World Institute of Pain. Abstract 261. *Pain Med, 13*, 45–57.

26. Martin, F., & Farnum, J. (2002). Animal-assisted therapy for children with pervasive developmental disorders. *West J Nurs Res, 24*(6), 657–670.

27. McGibbon, N. H., Andrade, C. K., Widener, G., & Cintals, H. L. (1998). Effect of an equine movement therapy program on gait, energy expenditure, and motor function in children with spastic cerebral palsy: a pilot study. *Dev Med Child Neurol, 40*, 754–762.

28. National Institute of Health. (September 10–11, 1987). The health benefits of pets. NIH Technology Assess Statement Online, 1987. Available at: http://consensus.nih.gov/1987/1987healthbenefitspetsta003html.htm.

29. Pet Assisted Therapy for Depression (nd.) Available at: http://www.ehow.com/way_5644970_pet_asssisted-therapy-depression.

30. Pitts, J. (2005). Why animal assisted therapy is important for children and youth. *The Exceptional Parent, 35*, 38–39.

31. Professional Association for Therapeutic Horsemanship (PATH). (2014). Available at: http://www.pathintl.org/.

32. Scott, N. (2005). *Special needs, special horses: a guide to the benefits of therapeutic riding.* Denton, TX: University of North Texas Press.

33. Sherer-Silkwood, D. (2003). The difference lies in the perspective. *NARHA Strides, 9*, 14–16.

34. Solomon, J., O'Brien, J., & Cohn, J. (2013). Emerging occupational therapy practice areas. In J. O'Brien, & J. Solomon (Eds.), *Occupational Analysis and Group Process* (pp. 133–142). St. Louis, MO: Elsevier.

35. Taylor, R., Kielhofner, G., Smith, C., Butler, S., Cahill, S., Ciukaj, M., et al. (2009). Volitional change in children with autism: a single case design study of the impact of hippotherapy on motivation. *Occup Ther Mental Health, 25*, 192–200.

36. Watts, K., & Everly, J. S. (May, 2009). Helping children with disabilities through animal-assisted therapy. *The Exceptional Parent*, 34–35.

37. Weston, F. (2010). Using animal assisted therapy with children. *Br J School Nurs, 5*(7), 344–347.

38. Winkle, M. (2003). Dogs in practice: beyond pet therapy. *OT Practice, 8*, 12–17.

Resources

Assistance Dogs International
http://www.adionline.org

American Hippotherapy Association (AHA)
http://www.americanhippotherapyassociation.org/

The Delta Society
www.deltasociety.org
c/o Delta Society, USA
580 Naches Avenue SW, No. 101
Renton, WA 98055–2297

International Association of Human-Animal Interaction Organizations
www.iahaio.org

Professional Association of Therapeutic Horsemanship International (PATH Int'l)
www.pathintl.org

PAWS for Health
www.vcu.edu/paws/benefit.htm

Resources for Games and Activities During Hippotherapy

Adapted Physical Education catalogs
http://www.flaghouse.com

Educational catalogs such as Nasco
http://www.nascofa.com

Freedom Riders
http://www.freedomrider.com

Sportsmark by Signam
http://www.sportsmark.co.uk

REVIEW *Questions*

1. What is an animal-assisted activity?
2. What is animal-assisted therapy?
3. What are the guidelines for establishing a pet-assisted therapy session or hippotherapy session?
4. What are the benefits supported in the research for animal-assisted therapy? Pet-assisted therapy? Equine-assisted therapy?
5. What is the role of the OT practitioner in animal-assisted activity or therapy?
6. What are some occupational therapy intervention activities that may include animals?
7. What are some goals that can be addressed involving animals in OT sessions with children?
8. What contraindications might prevent involving of animals in occupational therapy for a child?

SUGGESTED *Activities*

1. Volunteer at your local Society for the Prevention of Cruelty to Animals (SPCA). Describe the role of caring for the animals. List the steps, tasks, and routine.
2. Volunteer with a therapeutic horseback riding and/or hippotherapy program. Identify the goals for each session and describe the activities designed to address these goals.
3. Develop a list of activities involving pets that could be used in OT practice. Use the framework to analyze client factors and activity demands.
4. Analyze the activities necessary to care for a specific pet. Describe how you might prepare a child to achieve the ability to care for a pet. Consider habits in roles for this occupation.
5. Observe a hippotherapy or pet-assisted therapy program. Conduct an interview with a client and professional to identify benefits of a hippotherapy or pet-assisted therapy program.
6. Develop an OT intervention activity using an animal to achieve specific goals. Describe the goals and steps to the activity. Include materials, time, sequence, client factors and tasks involved. How would you make this activity easier or more challenging if needed.
7. Find a recent research study that examines the benefit of use of animals to intervention. Summarize the findings and report how you would use these findings in OT practice with children and youth.

Glossary

Abduction Moving away from the body; movement away from the midline of the body

Access The point of contact between the user and the aid or device that he or she needs to control

Accommodation Automatic adjustment of the lens of the eye to permit the retina to focus on objects at varying distances; adaptation or special consideration

Achievement stage The late childhood stage (6–11 years of age) in which children successfully accomplish movements and skills. Refers to the refinement of movements and skills

Acknowledgment Providing feedback to individuals, which assures them that they have been "heard"

Acquired condition/Acquired disorder An illness or state of health that is not inherited and interferes with an individual's ability to be functionally independent

Acquired immune deficiency syndrome (AIDS) A severe immunologic disorder caused by the retrovirus HIV (human immunodeficiency virus) that is characterized by increased susceptibility to infections and certain rare cancers; transmitted primarily through body fluids

Active ROM (AROM) Movement at a joint that occurs because of the contraction of skeletal muscle

Activities of daily living (ADLs) Self-maintenance activities such as dressing and feeding; also called basic activities of daily living (BADLs) or personal activities of living (PADLs)

Activity Specified pursuit in which an individual participates

Activity analysis A tool that helps occupational therapy practitioners prioritize, plan, and implement effective treatment; involves identifying every characteristic of a task and examining each client factor, performance component, performance area, and performance context

Activity and occupational demands The objects and their properties, space demands, social demands, sequence and timing, required actions and skills, and required underlying body functions and body structures

Activity configuration The process of selecting specific activities to use during an intervention

Activity demands Those things that are needed to carry out an activity

Activity synthesis Modifying, grading, and/or changing the structure or steps of an activity into a whole; includes adapting, grading, and reconfiguring activities

Acute Extremely severe symptoms or conditions; having a rapid onset and occurring after a short but severe course

Acute medical management Immediate and early management of individuals with a wide variety of medical concerns and conditions

Adaptation Adjustment or change to suit a situation

Adapting activities Modifying or changing a task or using adaptive equipment to make a task easier

Adaptive functioning How able someone is to perform the basic demands of everyday life

Adaptive response The ability of the brain to receive, interpret, and respond effectively to sensory information

Adaptive technology Assistive, adaptive, and rehabilitation devices for people with a disability

Addiction An intense psychological and physiologic craving

Adduction Movement toward the midline of the body

Adjunctive therapy An intervention used to assist with the primary intervention and intervention outcomes

Agonist Prime mover, or the primary muscle, that creates movement at a joint

Agoraphobia Fear of public places and open spaces

Akinesis Absent or reduced control of voluntary muscles

Alignment To move toward a straight line; posturally, to keep body segment bones and joints correctly oriented toward each other, particularly in the proximal areas of the head, neck, trunk, and pelvis

Allergen A substance (such as pollen or mold) that causes an allergic reaction or sneezing, wheezing, itching, or skin rashes because of an abnormally high sensitivity to the substance

Alveolus (plural: alveoli) Terminal sac-like structures of the lungs, which are the sites of gas exchange between the respiratory and circulatory systems

American Sign Language A visual language used predominantly in the United States and in many parts of Canada

Amputation The loss of a body part, often all or part of an arm or leg

Animal-assisted activities Events involving animals in which the animal serves as the motivator or facilitates a prescribed movement (e.g., brushing a dog)

Animal-assisted therapy A goal-directed intervention in which animals are used for therapeutic purposes. It is directed or delivered by a health/human services professional with specialized expertise, and within the scope of his or her profession

Antagonist Opposite of the agonist in action (i.e., lengthens in order to allow shortening of the agonist)

Anatomic position The upright position with the palms facing forward and the arms resting by the sides of the body, legs slightly spread apart, and toes pointing outward

Anterior/ventral Front

Antibody A Y-shaped protein that is secreted into the blood or lymph in response to the presence of an antigen or invading microorganism

Antifat A negative attitude toward persons who are obese or overweight

Antigen Toxins, bacteria, foreign blood cells, or cells from transplanted organs that cause the body to produce antibodies

Anxiety A state of uneasiness, apprehension, uncertainty, and fear resulting from the anticipation of a threatening event or situation

Anxiety disorders When anxious feelings become distressing and interfere with everyday functioning

AOTA Code of Ethics Addresses the ethical concerns of the profession using the seven principles of beneficence, nonmaleficence, autonomy and confidentiality, social justice, procedural justice, veracity, and fidelity to promote and maintain high standards of conduct by all occupational therapy personnel.

Areas of occupation Daily activities in which people engage, including activities of daily living (ADLs), instrumental activities of daily living (IADLs), education, work, play, leisure, and social participation

Arteriole Small artery

Artery Vessel that moves blood away from the heart

Arthrogryposis A congenital disorder marked by generalized stiffness of the joints; often accompanied by nerve and muscle degeneration, resulting in impaired mobility

Articulation Juncture between bones or cartilage

Ascending pathways A nerve pathway that carries sensory information from the body up to the brain

Assistive appliance Any aid or device that provides benefit to the user with little to no training or development of skills. This can include items such as eyeglasses or orthotics

Assistive technology (AT) Low or high technology that allows an individual to acquire or sustain independence

Assistive technology for handwriting Tools and devices that provide assistance to children who struggle with handwriting

Assistive technology device (AT device) A piece of equipment that helps individuals with disabilities to perform occupations or daily activities and is used on a daily basis

Assistive technology service (AT service) Any service that directly assists an individual with disabilities in the selection, acquisition, and/or use of an assistive technology device

Assistive technology team (AT team) A group of professionals who make recommendations and carry out the training of an individual with a disability by using an assistive technology device

Assistive tool Requires the development of skill for it to be of value to the user. Examples include feeding machines, communication aids and devices, and mobility aids

Asymmetric Not symmetric or balanced

Ataxia Abnormal fluctuation of muscle from normal to hypertonic (increased muscle tone); loss of the ability to coordinate muscular movement; loss of the ability to coordinate movements, usually due to fluctuations in muscle tone from normal to abnormally high

Athetosis A type of cerebral palsy characterized by involuntary writhing movements, particularly of the hands and feet; loss of ability to coordinate movement due to the fluctuation of muscle tone from abnormally low to abnormally high; writhing movements

Attention deficit hyperactivity disorder (ADHD) A neurobehavioral disorder characterized by difficulty with attention, hyperactivity, distractibility, and impulsivity

Atom Smallest unit of matter with subatomic parts of electrons, protons, and neutrons. Protons and neutrons are located in the nucleus of an atom. The electrons circle around in the valence(s) that surround the atom's nucleus. The number of electrons in an atom's outermost valence determines how that element bonds with other elements

Augmentative and alternative communication (AAC) Communication tools that help or replace spoken or written words for individuals who have trouble with the production and of comprehension of language

Autism Spectrum Disorder A disorder characterized by severe and complex impairments in reciprocal social interaction and communication skills and the presence of stereotypical behavior, interests, and activities

Autonomic nervous system Involved in maintaining homeostasis by innervating targeted organs throughout the body

Automatic reflex movement Movement that is instinctual, and assists in an individual's development and survival

Backward chaining A way to grade an activity in which an individual learns the last step first; begins with the individual completing the last step after watching the occupational therapy practitioner perform the first few steps and progresses to the individual learning the next to the last step (and so on) until the whole sequence is independently performed

Ball and socket or triaxial joint A freely moving joint such as the hip and shoulder joints; movement occurs in all three cardinal planes

Basal ganglia A group of structures (caudate nucleus, putamen, and globus pallidus) linked to the thalamus in the base of the brain and involved in coordination of movement

Base of support The body structure that carries the weight during static and dynamic balancing

Bathing and showering Typical skills involving soaping, rinsing, and drying the body, which are learned in early childhood

Behavioral change The modification or transformation of behavior

Bilateral motor control Both sides of the body working together during an activity; ability to use both sides of the body in smooth movements simultaneously

Biomechanical frame of reference A framework in which the evaluation and intervention focuses on range of motion, strength, endurance, and preventing contractures and deformities; used primarily with orthopedic disorders

Bipolar disorders Symptoms of major depression alternating with episodes of mania or hypomania characterized by excessive elation and energy, aggressive and disruptive behaviors, low frustration tolerance, and impulsive behavior

Bladder and bowel management Encompass both the voluntary control of the bowel and bladder movements as well as the use of alternative methods to support bladder control

Blocked practice Repeating similar movement with short rest breaks, so engagement in the task is much more than the time spent in breaks

Blood pressure The pressure that the circulating blood puts on the walls of the vessels

Body awareness Internal sense of body structures and their relationships to each other

Body image An attitude toward one's own body

Body mass index (BMI) Measurement based on one's height and weight and calculated on (weight/[height]$^2 \times 703$)

Bolus Solids and semisolids that have been chewed (masticated) and mixed with saliva before being swallowed

Bone Dense, semirigid, porous, calcified connective tissue that forms the major portion of the skeletal system in the human body and other vertebrates

Bone density Thickness of bone

Brain plasticity Lifelong ability of the brain to reorganize neural pathways

Brainstem The portion of the brain that is continuous with the spinal cord and comprises the medulla oblongata, pons, midbrain, and parts of the hypothalamus, functioning in the control of reflexes and such essential internal mechanisms as respiration and heartbeat

Burn An injury to body tissue caused by thermal, electrical, chemical, or radioactive agents

Capacity Ability to perform

Capillary A thin-lined blood vessel that connects arterial blood supply with venous blood supply; exchange of nutrients and waste products occurs in the capillary beds

Carbon An abundant, nonmetallic element that is found in inorganic and organic compounds; highly reactive in binding with other elements because of the number of electrons in its outer valence or shell

Carbon dioxide (CO$_2$) A compound that consists of one atom of carbon and two atoms of oxygen that is necessary for photosynthesis in plants and is a waste product of cellular respiration in animals

Cardiac disorders Conditions that involve the heart and/or blood vessels

Care of others The physical upkeep and nurturing of other human beings

Cardiovascular system/circulatory system Organ system consisting of the heart, blood vessels, and blood that functions in the transport and exchange of nutrients and waste products throughout the body

Cartilage Tough, elastic, fibrous connective tissue found in various parts of the body

Cellular respiration Process that takes place in the mitochondria of cells, during which chemical reactions result in the production of adenosine triphosphate (ATP), which is the source of energy for other chemical reactions

Centennial vision Recognizes occupational therapy as a science-driven and evidence-based profession that continues to meet the occupational needs of clients, communities, and populations

Center of gravity The midpoint or center of the weight of a body or object (in standing adult, this is midpelvic region)

Central nervous system (CNS) Brain and spinal cord

Central vision "Center of gaze"; straight-ahead vision

Cerebellum A large portion of the brain, serving to coordinate voluntary movements, posture, and balance in humans, being in back of and beneath the cerebrum and consisting of two lateral lobes and a central lobe

Cerebral cortex   The furrowed outer layer of gray matter in the cerebrum of the brain, associated with the higher brain functions, such as voluntary movement, coordination of sensory information, learning and memory, and the expression of individuality

Cerebral palsy (CP)   A motor function disorder caused by a permanent, nonprogressive brain defect or lesion; characterized by a disruption in the volitional control of posture and movement; produces atypical muscle tone and unusual ways of moving

Cerebrum   The anterior and largest part of the brain, consisting of two halves or hemispheres and serving to control voluntary movements and coordinate mental actions

Cerebrovascular accident (CVA or stroke)   Condition that involves the disruption of blood flow to the brain, which may result from a blockage or rupture of an artery resulting in partial or total loss of motor and sensory control on one side of the body

Characteristics of low temperature thermoplastic materials   Can be softened in hot water and placed directly on the skin. They are most appropriate for upper limb injuries

Child- and family-focused activity analyses   Analysis of the intervention and identification of the strengths and weaknesses of the child and family

Child-directed   The child takes the lead or initiates the movement, activity, or goals

Chromosome   A threadlike, linear strand of deoxyribonucleic acid (DNA) and its associated proteins that carry genes and pass along genetic information

Circumduction   Combination of flexion, abduction, extension, and adduction in such a way that the distal aspect of the extremity moves in a circle

Clients   Persons, groups, and populations within a community being classified as a group

Client-centered   An approach to treatment whereby the occupational therapy practitioner includes the client in every part of the evaluation and intervention programs, including the decision about the plan of action

Client factors   Components of activities required that affect performance and are specific to each client

Closed fracture   Broken bone does not penetrate the skin

Coactivation   Secondary to reciprocal innervations that means that two or more muscles are sent a message from the nervous system to become active or to contract/relax simultaneously

Co-contraction   Contraction of both the agonist and the antagonist to provide stability at a joint

Cognition   The mental processes of the construction, acquisition, and use of knowledge, as well as perception, memory, and the use of symbolism and language

Cognitive–behavioral therapy   Examines the relationship between thoughts, feelings, and behaviors

Cognitive functioning   An intellectual process by which one becomes aware of, perceives, or comprehends ideas. It involves all aspects of perception, thinking, reasoning, and remembering

Cognitive memory   Recall of thought

Cognitive sequencing   Mentally perceiving the steps of an activity

Collaboration   Working cooperatively with others to achieve a mutual goal

Common Core State Standards (CCSS)   Educational expected outcomes applicable to all students receiving public education.

Common names of orthoses   Arch supports, shoe inserts, orthotics

Comorbidities   Two or more existing medical or health conditions

Communication technologies   Used in an area of clinical practice that attempts to compensate (either temporarily or permanently) when an individual has difficulty using speech as a primary means of communication

Communication/interaction skill   A performance skill involving language and psychosocial skills

Community   A "person's natural environment, that is, where the person works, plays and performs other daily activities"; "an area with geographic and often political boundaries demarcated as a district, county, metropolitan area, city, township, or neighborhood … a place where members have a sense of identity and belonging, shared values, norms, communication, and helping patterns"; locality in which a group lives and participates in daily occupations

Community-based home care   Meets the needs of people who prefer to receive long-term care services and support in their home or community, rather than in an institutional setting

Community-based practice   A practice with a public health perspective that focuses on health promotion and education; a practice within a community

Community-built practice   Skilled services are delivered by health practitioners through a collaborative and interactive model with clients

Community mobility   Mobility in the community or outside the home

Compensatory movement patterns   Patterns of movement used because of reduced control of voluntary muscle

Competency stage   The toddler or middle childhood stage (2–6 years of age), in which children learn basic motor and performance skills

Compliance   Cooperation with recommended regimen, e.g., wearing an orthosis or changing positions

Compound Consisting of two or more substances or elements

Constraint-induced movement therapy (CIMT) An intervention that may include providing an orthosis or cast to immobilize the unimpaired extremity of a child or adolescent with unilateral hemiplegia

Consultation The act or process of providing advice or information

Consultative Providing advice or recommendations

Context Conditions, including physical, personal, temporal, social, cultural, and virtual conditions, surrounding the client that influence performance

Contraction Movement of the myofibrils (actin and myosin) in such a way that shortening of the muscle or increased tension in the muscle occurs

Contracture Soft tissue tightness that interferes with movement at a joint or joints; a limitation in movement caused by soft tissue shortening that may result in a "stiff" or fused joint

Control site Location on the body that can be used to operate a device

Contusion An injury that does not disrupt the integrity of the skin and is characterized by swelling, discoloration, and pain

Co-occupations Refers to occupations shared by at least two individuals

Cortical blindness The total or partial loss of vision caused by damage to the brain's occipital cortex

Cranial nerves Twelve pairs of nerves that come directly from the brain

Cri-du-chat syndrome A rare genetic condition caused by the absence of part of chromosome 5; also known as *cat's cry syndrome* because it is recognized at birth by the presence of a kitten-like cry

Crush wound A break in the external surface of the bone caused by severe force applied against tissues

Cultural competence The ability to effectively interact with people from different cultural and socioeconomic backgrounds

Cultural considerations Thoughtful consideration of the client's customs, beliefs, and expectations, which may be part of the larger society to which the individual belongs

Decubitus ulcer A pressure sore caused by lying in the same position; *decubitus* means "to lie down"; sores that result from pressure on the skin over a bony prominence or as the result of continuous pressure on any area

Deformity Bony fixation of a joint

Deltoid tuberosity Bony landmark on the proximal, lateral aspect of the humerus, which is the location of insertions for anterior, middle, and posterior muscles

Demyelinization Destruction of the myelin sheaths that surround nerve fibers

Deoxyribonucleic acid (DNA) A nucleic acid that carries genetic information and is made of nucleotides and repeating sugar-phosphate groups

Descending pathways A nerve pathway that carries motor information from the brain down to the body

Development The act or process of growth and/or maturation

Developmental coordination disorder (DCD) Disorder characterized by motor coordination that is markedly below the chronologic age and intellectual ability and significantly interferes with activities of daily living

Developmental disorder A mental and/or physical disability that arises before adulthood and lasts throughout one's life

Developmental dyspraxia Neurologic disorder of motor coordination manifested by difficulty thinking out, planning out, and executing planned movements; difficulty with motor planning that is the result of sensory processing problems

Developmental frame of reference A framework in which intervention is provided at the level at which the child is currently functioning and requires that the occupational therapy clinician provide a slightly advanced challenge

Developmental milestones Skills that are common at different stages in development

Developmental stages of mobility The progression and sequence of moving from rolling to move, crawling (on belly), creeping (on all fours), walking, to running. This sequence occurs in a sequential pattern, although the rate may vary

Diaphragm Dome-shaped muscle that separates the thorax from the abdomen and functions during inhalation/exhalation

Digestion Mechanical and chemical processing of food

Digestive system Organ system consisting of the digestive tract and associated body structures that function in the mechanical and chemical breakdown of what is eaten into nutrients that the body can use at the cellular level

Diplegia The distribution of affected muscles in individuals with cerebral palsy, in which the musculature of the lower extremities is more affected than that of the upper extremities

Direct selection A straightforward method for making a choice or selection. Using your hands to operate the joystick on a computer game console is an example of direct selection

Dislocation Displacement of the normal relationship of bones at a joint

Distributed practice Repetition of different skills that are spread over the course of the intervention session with rest breaks

Disruptive behavior disorder   A mental disorder characterized by socially disruptive behavior that is typically more distressing to others than to the individual with the disorder

Distal   Farther away from the body

Domain   A sphere of knowledge, influence, or activity

Down syndrome   A genetic disorder caused by the presence of an extra chromosome 21, which results in mental and motor delays in dressing and undressing—putting on (donning) and taking off (doffing) one's clothes—which are essential, basic self-care skills learned in infancy and early childhood

Dressing   Involves multiple steps that are influenced by both internal and external variables. It involves selecting clothing and accessories appropriate to time of day, weather, and occasion; obtaining clothing from storage area; dressing and undressing in a sequential fashion; fastening and adjusting clothing and shoes; and applying and removing personal devices, prosthetic devices or splints

Duchenne muscular dystrophy   The most common form of muscular dystrophy; characterized by pseudohypertrophy of muscles, especially the calf muscles; seen in males only

Due process   Parents' ability to take legal action against a school if their child's educational rights are violated; derived from the words *due*—owed or owing as a natural or moral right—and *process*—to proceed against by law

Dynamic balance (dynamic equilibrioception)   Ability to move through the environment without falling over

Dynamic systems theory   Explains the interplay between the neuromuscular system, the environment, cognition, and the intended task. Multiple systems engage and interact with each other, each having their unique role in movement

Dynamic orthosis   An orthosis that allows movement in desired joint(s); a splint that assists an individual with movements

Dyskinesias   Abnormal movements, most obvious when a child initiates a movement in one extremity, that lead to atypical and unintentional movement of other muscle groups of the body

Dysphagia   Difficulty with swallowing

Dyspraxia   Difficulty with motor planning

Dystonia   Neurologic movement disorder, in which sustained muscle contractions result in twisting and/or repetitive movements and abnormal postures

Early intervention programs   Promote the function and engagement of infants and toddlers and their families in everyday routines by addressing areas of occupation

Eating   The ability to keep food and fluids in the mouth, move them around inside the mouth, and swallow them

Eating disorder   A mental disorder characterized by a disturbance in eating behavior

Ecologic model   A model that studies the relationship between humans and their physical and social environments

Edema   Swelling or increased fluid secondary to an inflammatory response

Education   The process of receiving instruction and facilitating learning

Educational activities   Tasks that promote learning, especially in academic areas such as reading, writing, and math

Educational technology   The use of technology as only one aspect of an overall rehabilitation or education program; for example, a software program for teaching ABCs

Efficacy   Capacity for beneficial change

Efficient grasp patterns   The forearm is maintained in a neutral position and the wrist straight or slightly extended on a vertical or horizontal surface

Elastic therapeutic taping/kinesiological taping/kinesio taping   An intervention using special tape that occupational therapy practitioners use to support weak and/or injured muscles or body tissues

Element   Substance composed of atoms; each element on the periodic chart has a consistent number of protons equal to the number of electrons

Elimination disorders   Conditions that involve the voluntary or involuntary repeated voiding of urine or feces in inappropriate places

Endocrine system   Organ system comprising the endocrine glands located throughout the body that controls body functions through the secretion of hormones

Endometrium   Inner lining of the uterus that is shed during menstruation

Endurance   Activity tolerance; capacity to perform exercises or activities over time

Environment   The physical and social features of the specific context in which a child or adolescent engages in occupations

Environmental control unit (ECU)   A system that allows an individual with limited motor control to operate electrical devices such as telephones, room lights, and televisions

Environmental impact   The extent to which physical or social aspects of an environment provide a specific child or adolescent with opportunities, supports, demands, or constraints

Environmentally induced disorder   An atypical condition that results from an environmental toxin (such as lead)

Equifinality   The inability to predict how a given situation or event in the present will develop in the future

Equilibrium reactions/equilibrium responses Automatic, reflexive, compensatory movements of body parts that restore and maintain the center of gravity over the base of support when either the center of gravity or the supporting surface is displaced; complex postural reactions that involve righting reactions with rotation and diagonal patterns and are essential for volitional movement and mobility; responses that begin at 6 months and persist throughout one's life

Equine-assisted therapy/activities Activities in which horses are used as a therapeutic tool. Frequently used in therapy for children with disabilities to address physical and/or emotional goals

Esotropia Type of strabismus in which one or both eyes turn inward

Eukaryotic cell A cell that has a membrane-bound nucleus that contains genetic information

Evaluation The process of using formal and informal measures to quantify an individual's performance in areas of occupation

Evidenced-based practice Practice based on review and critique of research and proof of efficacy

Exceptional educational need (EEN) The determination that a disability or handicapping condition exists and interferes with the child's or adolescent's ability to participate in an educational program

Executive functioning A set of cognitive abilities located in the frontal cortex of the brain. It includes inhibition, shift, emotional control, initiation, working memory, planning and orientation, organization of materials, and self-monitoring

Exotropia Type of strabismus in which one or both eyes turn outward

Exploration stage The infancy or early childhood stage (0–2 years of age), in which the child seeks out stimuli; the child is just beginning to move and perform skills

Extension Straightening a joint increasing the angle

Fading assistance A method of grading an activity by gradually reducing the level of assistance given until the individual performs the activity independently

Facilitation/excitation Planned, graded physical guidance techniques used to improve movement coordination by increasing inadequate muscle tone, altering sensory responsiveness, and/or altering behavioral states (e.g., hands-on facilitation techniques that are targeted at key postural points such as the shoulders, trunk, and hips)

Feed backward Reflective movements in response to stimuli (e.g., throwing ball at a target and reflecting on where it hit)

Feed forward Anticipatory movement to prepare for a motor response (e.g., deciding where to run to catch a ball)

Feeding The process of bringing food and fluids to the mouth from containers such as plates, bowls, and cups

Feeding and eating disorders Eating disorders that include anorexia nervosa, bulimia nervosa, binge eating, and body dysmorphic disorder

Fetal alcohol syndrome A disorder that occurs as a result of excessive alcohol consumption by the mother during pregnancy; includes birth defects such as cardiac, cranial, facial, and neural abnormalities, with associated delays in physical and mental growth

Fine motor skill The ability to use the small muscles of the body, especially those of the hands, to perform tasks

Fitness The condition of being physically fit and healthy to enable one to fulfill a particular role or task

Fixation Contraction of muscle(s) to create stability at a joint; may be normal or abnormal

Flexion Bending a joint decreasing the angle

Forward chaining A way to grade an activity in which an individual learns each step from the beginning; begins with the individual starting the sequence and ends with the occupational therapy practitioner finishing what the individual has not yet learned

Fracture A break, rupture, or crack in bone or cartilage

Fragile X syndrome A disorder characterized by a nearly broken X chromosome; the signs and symptoms may include an elongated face, prominent jaw and forehead, hypermobile or lax joints, flat feet, and intellectual disability

Frame of reference Framework that helps the occupational therapy practitioner to identify problems, evaluate, develop intervention, and measure outcomes

Framing Posing situations as certain occupations (e.g., play) so the client understands and acts accordingly

Free, appropriate public education (FAPE) Free public education that is mandated for all children, adolescents, and young adults with disabilities and who are between 3 and 21 years of age

Freedom to suspend reality The ability to participate in "make-believe" or activities in which the participants pretend; the ability to create new play situations and interact with materials, space, and people in ways that are fluid, flexible, and not bound to the constraints of real life

Functional mobility Moving from one position or place to another during performance of everyday activities, such as in-bed mobility, wheelchair mobility, and transfers

Functional support capacities Represent secondary neurobehavioral, motor, social-emotional, and/or cognitive proficiencies that are not functional in the occupational sense but are considered prerequisites for the end products to develop normally

Fussy baby syndrome   Condition in which the infant is easily upset and given to bouts of ill temper; associated with infants who have sensory regulatory disorders

Gastroesophageal reflux disease (GERD)/gastric reflux   Condition in which the acid chyme from the stomach is regurgitated into the esophagus

Gene   A hereditary unit with a specific sequence of DNA that occupies a specific space on a chromosome and determines a specific characteristic of an individual

General sensory disorganization   Disorders in which sensory systems are providing inaccurate information; may be associated with impairments in the tactile, vestibular, and/or auditory systems; also associated with infants who are characterized as "fussy babies"

Genetic conditions   Disorders that occur as a result of abnormal or absent genes

Guillain-Barré syndrome   A syndrome that is characterized by the demyelinization of the peripheral nerves, which causes temporary paresis or paralysis

Glenohumeral joint   The articulation between the head of the humerus and the glenoid fossa of the scapula

Global mental functions   Refers to consciousness, orientation, sleep, temperament and personality, and energy and drive

Gradation   A systematic progression of activities

Grading activities   Changing one or more aspects of a task (usually by increasing or decreasing demands) to make it easier or harder to perform; modifying activities

Gravitational insecurity   Extreme fear or anxiety that one will fall when the feet are not in contact with a supporting surface

Gross motor skills   Activities that require the use of the larger body muscles (e.g., shoulders, hips, and knees)

Growth   Development; increase in size

Habits   Acquired tendencies to respond and perform in consistent ways in familiar or common environments or situations

Habituation   The internal readiness a child or an adolescent has to demonstrate a consistent pattern of behavior guided by habits and roles; this readiness is associated with specific temporal, physical, or social environments

Hair   Filament mostly made of protein that grows from follicles located in the dermis

Half-kneeling   A resting position supported by the knee of one leg and the foot of the other leg with the thighs and trunk somewhat upright

Handling   Methods of providing specific sensory input to individuals with atypical muscle tone, posture, and movement; touching and manipulating with the hands

Handwriting   Used in both educational and noneducational activities, measures a student's academic comprehension, and allows children to express themselves, learn information, organize their work, and communicate with others

Health (World Health Organization [1948])   "Health is a state of complete physical, mental and social well-being and not merely the absence of disease or infirmity"; condition of optimal well-being of an organism

Health promotion   Create and promote healthy activity in the context of daily life

Hearing impairment   A disorder in the auditory system that may be a sensorineural or conductive disorder; relationships exist among hearing impairments and the vestibular system, balance, and chronic otitis

Heart rate (pulse)   Beats of the heart per minute

Hematology units   Hospital setting that specializes in treatment of blood disorders

Hemiplegia   The distribution of affected muscles in individuals with cerebral palsy, in which only the musculature on one side of the body is affected

High technology   Technology that is expensive and not readily available, such as computers, environmental control units, and powered wheelchairs

Hippotherapy   A special form of equine-assisted therapy that uses the dynamic three-dimensional movement of the horse to achieve specific therapeutic goals

Home care   Care that takes place in the client's residence

Home health company   An agency that contracts with nurses and occupational therapy and other practitioners to provide home-based services

Home management activities   Tasks that are necessary to obtain and maintain personal and household possessions

Homeostasis   Tendency of maintaining a relatively stable internal environment

Horizontal abduction   Moving the body part in the horizontal or transverse plane such that the distal aspect of the extremity moves *away* from the midline of the body

Horizontal adduction   Moving the body part in the horizontal or transverse plane such that the distal aspect of the extremity moves *toward* the midline of the body

Hydrogen   The lightest and most abundant element in the universe; one of the most abundant elements found in living matter

Hypersensitive   Increased sensitivity or awareness

Hypertonicity   Abnormally increased muscle tone associated with atypical postural alignment and decreased range of motion at joints; also known as *high tone* or *spasticity*

Hypertropia   Type of strabismus in which there is a permanent upward deviation of one eye

Hyposensitive   Decreased sensitivity or sensory awareness

Hypotonicity   Abnormally decreased muscle tone associated with atypical postural alignment and excessive range of motion at joints; also known as *low tone* or *flaccidity*

Hypotropia   Type of strabismus in which a permanent downward deviation of one eye is present

Hypoxia ischemia   Lack of oxygen caused by lack of blood supply

Ideation   The ability to conceptualize internal representations of purposeful actions

Ideational praxis   A higher-level cognitive function; a component of praxis (a process that includes developing a concept or idea, planning, and executing a motor action)

Identity   The individual and contextual factors that constitute self-perception

Immobilization   Fixing a position of a joint to prevent movement at that joint

Immobilization orthoses   Orthoses that provides stability to unstable joints by giving external support when muscles and ligaments are weakened or strained and decreases or prevents contractures by maximizing full joint range of motion

Immune system   Not a distinct organ system, but rather a coordination of the interaction of many of the organ systems in response to inflammation or infection; activated by the presence of potentially pathogenic organisms or substances

Inclusion   Models that are based on the premise that children with special needs should be educated in a regular classroom (instead of a self-contained classroom), with support personnel or services provided in that classroom (instead of pull-out services)

Inclusion model   Models in which children with disabilities are able to spend time in general education classrooms

Incontinence   Inability to control bowel and/or bladder

Individualized education program (IEP)   The written educational plan developed by a team, which includes the student's strengths and weaknesses as well as annual goals and short-term objectives

Individualized education program team   The team of parents, teachers, special educators, occupational therapy clinicians, and others, that determines a student's need for services

Individual family service plan (IFSP)   The written intervention plan that is developed by the IFSP team and has as its focus family priorities and resources

Individuals with Disabilities Act (IDEA)   Encourages occupational therapy practitioners to work with children in their classroom environments and provide support to the regular education teachers (integration); it also encourages schools to allow students with disabilities to meet the same educational standards as their peers

Inferior/caudal   Toward the feet or tail

Inflammatory response   A localized protective reaction in response to irritation, injury, or infection, which is characterized by redness, pain, swelling, and sometimes reduced movement or function; an immune system response

In-hand manipulation   Moving objects within the hand

In-home services   Occupational therapy services provided within a client's home

Inhibition   Planned, graded physical guidance techniques used to reduce excessive muscle tone, calm overly excited behavioral states, and decrease sensory hypersensitivity; suppression

Innervation   The distribution of nerve supply

Insertion of a muscle   The opposite end of a muscle relative to the origin that moves during a muscle contraction

Instrumental activities of daily living (IADLs)   The complex activities of daily living that are needed to function independently in the home, at school, and in the community

Integumentary system   Organ system consisting of the skin and associated structures and functions as the first line of defense against potential invading microbes

Intellectual disability   Below-average cognitive functioning that causes developmental delays and impairments in multiple areas of occupation, including social participation, education, ADL and IADL skills, and play/leisure

Intelligence quotient (IQ)   A ratio of tested mental age to chronologic age that is usually expressed as a quotient (i.e., the result of dividing one number by another) and multiplied by 100; determined by using a standardized test that measures an individual's ability to form concepts, solve problems, acquire information, reason, and learn

Interactive model   A model in which the service provider and the recipient of the services act upon each other in such a way that the services provided meet the needs of the recipient

Interest   What a child or adolescent finds enjoyable or satisfying

Internal control   The extent to which individuals are in charge of their own actions and the outcome of an activity

Intervention   Actions taken to improve a situation or condition

Intervention plan   A detailed description of the goals, methods, and expected outcomes of therapy

Intrinsic motivation   A prompt to action that comes from within the individual; drive to action that is rewarded by doing the activity itself, rather than deriving some external reward from it

Involuntary   Under smooth muscle or cardiac muscle control

Joint   Articulation between two or more bones at which movement may occur

Joint protection techniques   Ways of protecting the joints, compensating for decreased ROM during exacerbations, and completing activities with less stress on the joints

Just right challenge   Activities that are not too difficult or easy for the client to complete.

Juvenile rheumatoid arthritis   A chronic disorder that begins in childhood and is characterized by stiffness and inflammation of the joints, weakness, loss of mobility, and deformity

Key points of control   The body structures used during handling to promote active movement

Kinesio taping   Taping of joints and muscles to provide support and stability without affecting circulation of movement or range of motion

Kinesthesia   Sense that detects weight and movement in muscles, tendons, and joints

Kneeling   A resting position supported by the knees with the thighs and trunk somewhat upright

Knowledge of performance   Provides information about the nature or characteristic of the movement used to perform the task

Knowledge of results   Involves information provided from an external source about the outcome, or end result of the performance of a skill or task

Kyphoscoliosis   A condition in which both kyphosis and scoliosis of the vertebral column are present

Kyphosis   An exaggerated rounding of the back

Larynx   "Voice box"; a cartilaginous organ of the respiratory system located between the pharynx and the trachea that houses the vocal cords

Lateral   Farther away from the midline of the body

Lateral or external rotation   Moving a body part away from midline; only possible in triaxial joints or the hip and shoulder joints; during this rotation, the head of the femur or the head of the humerus moves out of the articulating fossa

Lateral weight shift   Transferring the body's weight away from the midline or laterally

Learned helplessness   Condition in which one has learned to behave as if helpless or unable to perform activities/occupations

Least restrictive environment (LRE)   A classroom setting with minimum limitations; associated with the premise that children with disabilities have the right to be with nondisabled children

Legitimate tools   Instruments that are in accordance with the established and accepted standards of a profession or discipline

Leisure   Freedom from the demands of work; engaging in a nonobligatory activity that is intrinsically motivating during free time

Leisure activities   Activities that are not associated with time-consuming duties and responsibilities

Leukemia   A group of pediatric health conditions involving various acute and chronic tumor disorders of the bone marrow

Level of arousal   The amount of alertness and attention needed for an activity; must be at the optimum level for learning to take place

Levels of supervision   The amount of oversight required for the occupational therapy practitioner to perform duties

Life cycle   The events that typically occur during one's life

Ligament   Sheet or band of tough fibrous tissue that connects muscle to bone or supports an organ

Linguistic skills   Language abilities

Living matter   Organic matter (matter containing carbon)

Lobes and hemispheres   The brain is divided into right and left hemispheres and the frontal, temporal, parietal, and occipital lobes

Long-term care   Care that is provided in a residential facility when a family or primary caregiver is unable to meet an individual's medical needs; includes the goals of providing appropriate medical care and therapeutic intervention

Low load prolonged stretch   A low load of force applied to a stiff joint using an orthosis over a long period that is better tolerated than a large load

Low technology   Technology that is inexpensive, easy to obtain, and simple to produce

Lymph   Watery fluid found in lymph vessels and nodes

Lymph nodes   Small bodies located on the lymphatic vessels that filter bacteria and other foreign materials from the lymph fluid

Lymphatic system   Organ system consisting of lymphatic vessels and associated structures that functions in transport and exchange as well as responding to an immune response

Matter   Anything that takes up space and has mass or weight

Media   An intervening substance through which something else is transmitted or carried on; an agency by which something is accomplished, conveyed, or transferred

Medial or internal rotation   Moving a body part toward the midline or medially; only occurs in the hip and shoulder joints during which the head of the femur or the head of the humerus turns inward

Medial   Closer to the midline of the body

Medical/surgical units   A specialized unit providing 24-hour medical attention to various diagnoses or conditions

Medical technology   The use of technology to support or improve life functions (e.g., a respirator)

Medication management   Strategies to enhance and integrate medication adherence into patients' daily routines

Memory   The ability to store, retain, and retrieve information

Metabolism   Sum of all chemical reactions that occur in an organism

Method   A means or manner of procedure, especially a regular and systematic way of accomplishing something

Midline crossing   The ability of a body part (e.g., hand or foot) to spontaneously move over to the other side of the body to work there

Mild intellectual disability   A category of intellectual disability in which an individual has a below-average IQ (ranging from 55–69) and typically requires intermittent support; generally allows the individual to master academic skills ranging from grades 3 to 7, although more slowly than other students

Misalignment   Misplacement

Mobilization orthoses   Orthoses that allows body movement. This can further be divided into dynamic, static progressive, and serial static orthoses

Model of Human Occupation (MOHO)   Framework developed by Dr. Gary Kielhofner that views human occupation as a dynamic concept consisting of volition, habituation, and performance capacity and influenced by the environment

Model of practice   Framework that helps occupational therapy practitioners organize their thinking

Moderate intellectual disability   A category of intellectual disability in which an individual has a below-average IQ (ranging from 40–54) and typically requires some level of support as an adult; generally allows the individual to master academic skills at grade 2 level, although significantly more slowly than other students.

Molecule   Smallest part of a substance that retains the chemical and physical properties of the substance and is composed of two or more atoms

Monoplegia   One extremity involvement

Mood disorder   A mental disorder characterized by a disturbance in mood

Morphogenetic principle   The theory that systems tend to evolve and adapt to the larger environment

Morphostatic principle   The theory that systems tend to maintain the status quo (i.e., stay the same)

Motor control   Ability to move smoothly and efficiently

Motor control frame of reference   Follows a task-oriented approach that encourages the repetition of desired movements in a variety of settings and circumstances

Motor disorders   Characterized by deficits in the acquisition and execution of coordinated movements

Motor learning   The techniques used to teach someone how to move

Motor memory   Recall of action patterns within body structures such as muscles and joints

Motor neuron   Also known as *effector neuron*, as it causes a motor response at the effector site

Motor planning   The ability to formulate and carry out a skilled motor act from beginning to end

Motor skill   A performance skill involving objects; includes gross and fine motor skills

Multidisciplinary   Relating to multiple fields of study involved in the care of clients; suggests that although the various disciplines are working in collaboration, they are also working in parallel, with each distinct discipline being accountable and responsible for its tasks and functions regarding client care

Muscle tone   The degree of tension in muscle fibers when a muscle is at rest; the degree of elasticity and contractility in the muscle tissue; the resting state of a muscle in response to gravity and emotion

Muscular system   Organ system consisting of skeletal, smooth, and cardiac muscles that functions in the movement of the body or materials through the body by the contraction and relaxation of muscles; additional functions include maintenance of posture and heat production

Nails   Horn-like envelopes, made of the protein *keratin*, which engulf the distal aspect of the phalanges of the digits of the fingers and toes known as *fingernails* and *toenails*

Natural environment   Usual or ordinary environment

Negotiation   Process of making decisions and resolving disputes

Neonatal intensive care unit (NICU)   A specialized unit that addresses the acute or extremely severe symptoms or conditions of infants so that they can be physiologically stable

Neurobiology   Biology that focuses on the nervous system

Neurodevelopmental disorders   Impairments of the growth and development of the central nervous system

Neurodevelopmental treatment (NDT)   A therapeutic approach used when working with clients who have neurologic disorders and difficulty controlling movements, which interferes with function; occupational therapy clinicians providing NDT need to have advanced training; techniques include direct handling techniques to increase a client's independence

Neuroembryology   The study of the formation and development of the brain and nervous system in the embryo

Neurologic conditions   Congenital or acquired disorders such as spina bifida and Erb's palsy, which affect the central or peripheral nervous system

Neurologic rehabilitation Restoration intervention that focuses on treating neurologic impairment(s)

Neuron Smallest unit of the nervous system that consists of a cell body, dendrites (which carry impulses *to* the cell body) and axons (which carry impulses *away* from the cell body) with myelin sheaths that increase the rate of impulse propagation

Neuroplasticity The ways in which the brain can change by laying down new circuitry and making new neural connections after receiving new information or stimuli

Nervous system Organ system consisting of the brain, spinal cord, and peripheral nerves that regulates the responses to internal and external stimuli; functions in communication within and without and controlling the response to stimuli

Nitrogen A nonmetallic element that is found in all proteins; one of the most abundant elements found in living matter

No Child Left Behind Established in 2001 to increase the standards for teaching and improve the results of student learning; supports the use of scientifically based practices by occupational therapy professionals working in the educational setting

Nonnormative life-cycle events The unanticipated events of life, such as the frequent hospitalization of a young child or premature death of a child or parent

Nonprogressive Not getting worse

Normal Occurring naturally; not deviating from the standard

Normative life-cycle events The usual and expected events of life, such as birth, starting school, and adolescence

Nutrition The science that interprets the interaction of nutrients and other substances in food in relation to maintenance, growth, reproduction, health and disease

Nystagmus Unintentional jittering of one or both eyes

Obesity Excessive body weight caused by an accumulation of adipose tissue or fat

Obligation Social, legal, or moral requirement

Obsessive-compulsive and related disorders Recurring, disruptive, intrusive thoughts that cause anxiety and compulsive, ritualistic, repetitive patterns of behavior that reduce the anxiety

Occupation An activity that has unique meaning and purpose for a person

Occupational forms/tasks Conventionalized sequences of action that are coherent, oriented to a purpose, sustained in collective knowledge, culturally recognizable, and named

Occupational identity Combination of interests, values, and abilities in the pursuit of a realistic choice of a job or a career path

Occupational therapy intervention process model (OTIPM) A model for occupational therapy evaluation and intervention in which a client-centered, top-down, occupation-based approach is used

Occupational Therapy Practice Framework Manuscript developed to assist occupational therapy practitioners in defining the process and domains of occupational therapy

Oncology units Hospital settings that specialize in cancer treatment

Open fracture Involves an open wound, where complications are more common

Optimize Maximize

Oral defensiveness Aversion to harmless oral sensations

Oral hygiene Typical skills that are learned in early childhood, such as brushing the teeth

Oral–motor development Maturation of the oral–motor structures

Origin of a muscle Part of the muscle that attaches to bone or muscle and is stationary during a muscle contraction

Organ Aggregate of several different types of tissues to perform a particular function

Organ system Aggregate of organs that perform specific function(s)

Orthopedic condition A disorder that involves the skeletal system and associated muscles (i.e., joints and ligaments)

Orthosis Refers to an orthotic device; a term used interchangeably with splint; a bracing system designed to control, correct, and/or compensate for bony deformities or muscle imbalance; an external orthopedic appliance

Orthotics A specialty within the medical field concerned with the design, manufacture, and application of orthoses

Outpatient services Care that is provided to a client that does not involve an overnight stay

Oxygen A nonmetallic element that is necessary for cellular respiration; one of the most abundant elements found in living matter

Paraplegia Paralysis or loss of motor and sensory control in both legs

Parent and child support groups Groups that address important issues to both the parent and the child to help maximize the child's participation in daily activities.

Partial-thickness burns Second-degree burns that involve the epidermis and portions of the dermis

Passive ROM (PROM) Movement that occurs at a joint secondary to an outside force

Pathologic fracture Broken bone caused by a disease or health condition

Pediatric acute rehabilitation programs A specialty service that may be found in a children's hospital or rehabilitation hospital. Acute rehabilitation programs are directed by a pediatric physiatrist and provide occupational therapy, speech therapy (ST), and physical therapy (PT) services five to six times a week for 3 hours per day

Pediatric intensive care unit (PICU) A specialized unit that addresses the critical medical needs of the infant, child, or adolescent from birth to 21 years

Pediatric medical care system A group of individuals (professional, paraprofessional, and nonprofessional) who form a complex and unified whole dedicated to caring for children who have health disorders

Perception Process of understanding sensory information

Perceptual coping strategies Defining events, situations, and crises in ways that promote adaptation

Performance capacity The ability of a child or adolescent to do things provided by the status of his or her underlying objective physical and mental components; also influenced by the child's or adolescent's subjective experience

Performance skills The observable elements of action, including motor skills, process skills, and communication/interaction skills

Periods of development Specific developmental stages categorized by age, including infancy, early childhood, middle childhood, adolescence, and adulthood

Peripheral nervous system (PNS) All nerves located outside the brain and spinal cord that connect the central nervous system to body structures such as limbs and internal organs; peripheral nerves, spinal nerves, cranial nerves, and nerves associated with the autonomic nervous system

Peripheral vision "Side vision"; the ability to see objects outside of the line of vision or center of gaze

Peristalsis Involuntary movement of food through the digestive tract

Personal causation A child's or an adolescent's sense of capacity and efficacy for occupations

Personal device care Using, cleaning, and maintaining personal care items

Personal hygiene and grooming skills Typical skills such as face washing, hand washing, and hair care that are learned in early childhood

Pervasive developmental disorder (PDD) A collection of disorders marked by delays in communication and social development; difficulties understanding language relating to events, objects, and/or people; atypical play skills and transitions; and repetitive movements or maladaptive behavior patterns; a group of pediatric health conditions affecting a variety of body functions and structures with a wide range of severity

Pet-assisted therapy Involves working with family pets in a therapeutic environment. The pets are trained to work in group settings with a variety of people

Pharynx Muscular organ that connects the mouth to the esophagus; movement of the bolus in pharynx occurs secondary to peristalsis

Phosphorus A nonmetallic and highly reactive element found in phosphates; most abundant salt found in living matter

Phosphate An inorganic chemical that is a salt

Physiologic flexion Total body flexion of a neonate primarily due to the position in utero

Pica behavior Craving and eating inedible items such as plaster and dirt

Play Any spontaneous or organized activity that provides enjoyment, entertainment, amusement, and/or diversion; an experience that involves intrinsic motivation, with emphasis on the process rather than product and internal rather than external control; a make-believe experience that takes place in a safe, nonthreatening environment

Play adaptations Changes in materials or activities to promote successful play for children who have disabilities

Play and leisure Intrinsically motivated occupations that provide enjoyment and entertainment or activities that are not committed to obligatory occupations

Play assessment Observations of children during play by the occupational therapy practitioner

Play environment The setting in which the occupational therapy practitioner assesses children at play; consists of child-friendly toys and materials

Play goals Outcomes of play during the occupational therapy process

Playfulness Abstract noun derived from the adjective *playful;* a behavioral or personality trait characterized by flexibility, manifest joy, and spontaneity

Positioning Specific ways of placing an individual to maintain postural alignment, provide postural stability, facilitate normal patterns of movement, and increase interaction with the environment; can include the use of adaptive equipment; placing the body in a position usually with the aid of equipment to maintain the position

Posterior/dorsal Back

Postural (skeletal) alignment Mechanically efficient position or alignment of joints of the neck and trunk

Postural mechanism A term used to encompass muscle tone, postural tone, equilibrium, and righting responses, as well as protective extension reactions

Postural-ocular and bilateral integration dysfunction Sensory-based motor dysfunction characterized by a cluster of several sensory, behavioral, and motor characteristics

Posture and positioning   The way in which the body is positioned when one is sitting or standing

Postural stability   Equilibrium in the neck and trunk that provides a base of support in such a way that controlled mobility of the arms and legs is possible; the ability to maintain equilibrium and balance or return to the original position after displacement from that position

Postural tone   Underlying contraction of skeletal muscles that allows the body structures to maintain their position in space

Prader-Willi syndrome   A genetic health disorder that involves chromosome 15; characterized by varying degrees of intellectual disability, overeating habits, and self-mutilating behavior

Praxis   The ability to conceptualize, organize, and execute nonhabitual, novel motor tasks; motor planning

Praxis and developmental dyspraxia   Dyspraxia is a disorder characterized by an impairment in the ability to plan and carry out sensory and motor tasks, which is known as poor praxis

Prematurity   Being born before full term; a baby born after less than 37 weeks' gestation from the mother's last menstrual day (per the World Health Organization [WHO])

Preparatory activities   Methods and tasks that are used during a treatment session to target specific skills or client factors in preparation for engagement in occupations

Prescriptive   The role of the occupational therapist in working with a child in a directive manner, providing the family and the child with a plan

Pretend play   Play that involves symbolic games, imagination, and suspension of reality

Pressure sore   An ulceration caused by the death of cells due to lack of blood supply

Prevocational skills   Abilities that are needed for a vocational or work setting

Prewriting strokes   Precursors to forming shapes, letter, and numbers

Primitive reflexes   A group of movement patterns that begin emerging at birth and continue until approximately 4 to 6 months of age; reflexes that are controlled primarily by the lower brain centers; reflexes that enable the body to respond to influences such as head or body position mechanically and automatically with a change in muscle tone; reflexes that provide the developing infant with numerous consistent posture and movement patterns for early interaction with the environment

Principles of development   The guidelines and general progression of growth and performance skill attainment

Process skill   A performance attribute involving cognition

Profound intellectual disability   A category of intellectual disability in which an individual has a below-average IQ (25 or lower) and requires pervasive support throughout life and extensive assistance with ADLs; physical disorders generally accompany cognitive limitations

Pronation   In an erect (sitting or standing) position turning the palm down to face the floor

Prone   Positioned on stomach

Proprioception   A sensory system having receptors in the muscles, joints, and other internal tissues that provide internal awareness about the positions of body parts

Proprioceptive feedback   Muscle–joint input that provides information regarding position in space and/or in relation to objects

Prosthesis   A device designed to replace a missing part of the body or to make a part of the body work better

Protective extension reactions   Postural responses that are used to stop a fall or prevent injury when equilibrium reactions cannot do so; responses that involve straightening of the arms and/or legs toward a supporting surface

Proximal   Closer to the body

Psychogenic   Originating in the mind or in emotions

Psychosocial development   Theory that identifies the psychological and social stages through which a healthy developing human passes from infancy to late adulthood (e.g., Erik Erickson's 8 stages of psychosocial development)

Psychosocial occupational therapy   The area of clinical practice that provides services to children and adolescents with mental health problems

Psychosocial skills   Performance components that refer to an individual's ability to interact in society and process emotions; include psychological, social, and self-management skills

Public health approaches   Approaches with a focus on health promotion and prevention in populations

Quadriplegia (tetraplegia)   The distribution of affected muscles in individuals with cerebral palsy, in which the musculature of all four extremities is affected; may also affect the musculature of the neck and facial areas

Radial deviation   Moving the wrist radially or toward the thumb

Range of motion (ROM)   The amount of movement available at a specified joint; measured with a goniometer by occupational therapy practitioners

Readiness skills   Those abilities in the performance components and areas that are necessary for engaging in activities related to education, home management, care of others, and vocation

Reading the child in context   A moment-to-moment observation and analysis of a child's relationship to the social and physical environments and the child's responses to the therapeutic process; a tool that helps occupational therapy practitioners plan and implement treatment

Reciprocal innervation The distribution of nerve supply to antagonistic muscles, which allows one muscle to be excited and contract while the other muscle is inhibited, thus relaxing the muscle(s); excitation of the agonist with inhibition of the antagonist thus allowing movement at a joint

Referral A request for a screening or evaluation to determine whether one would benefit from occupational therapy services

Rehabilitation Services provided to an individual experiencing challenges in areas of physical function or limitations in participation in daily activities. Interventions enable to achievement and maintenance of daily functioning

Rehabilitative technology Use of technology as only one aspect of rehabilitation or educational program

Related services Required services provided by schools that include transportation, physical therapy, occupational therapy, speech therapy (ST), assistive technology services, psychological services, school health services, social work services, and parent counseling and training

Relaxation Lengthening of a muscle; loosening up

Reproductive system Organ system of female and male reproductive organs that function in sexual reproduction

Resources Support in the form of time, money, friends, and family; supplies, equipment, and personnel that provide support

Respiratory distress syndrome (RDS) A disease in newborns (especially premature neonates) characterized by difficulty breathing, cyanosis, and formation of a glossy membrane over the alveoli of the lungs

Respiratory rate Number of breaths per minute

Respiratory system (pulmonary system) Organ system consisting of the lungs and associated structures that functions in gas exchange with the environment

Righting reactions Responses that maintain the alignment of body parts; postural reactions that occur in response to a change in the position of the head and body in space; reactions that bring the head and trunk back into an upright position in space; involve extension, flexion, abduction, adduction, and lateral flexion; begin to emerge between 6 and 9 months of age and persist throughout life

Robotics Engineering science and technology of robots, including the design and manufacturing of robots

Roles A socially or personally defined status that is associated with actions or attitudes

Role delineation The clear separation of responsibilities between the registered occupational therapist and the certified occupational therapy assistant

Rote learning The acquisition of behaviors that become routine, though not always fully understood or carried out with sincerity; learning that usually occurs through memorization and repetition

Routines Provide sequence and structure to daily life

RUMBA criteria Method of writing and evaluating goals; RUMBA stands for *r*elevant, *u*nderstandable, *m*easurable, *b*ehavioral, and *a*chievable (attainable)

Scapular elevation Upward movement of the scapula

Scapular depression Downward movement of the scapula

Scapular protraction Movement of the scapula *away* from the midline of the body

Scapular retraction Movement of the scapula *toward* the midline of the body

Scapular winging A condition in which the vertebral borders of the scapulae move away from the thoracic wall, especially during weight-bearing through the arm as result of muscle weakness

Schizophrenia spectrum A serious chronic condition that is difficult to diagnose and has a significant genetic predisposition. It can present with symptoms of severely disturbed behavior similar to autism

Scholarship Form of leadership that enables practitioners to expand their knowledge base and to maintain competence

Scoliosis A sideways curvature of the spine

Screening An informal or formal measure that determines an individual's need for occupational therapy evaluation and intervention

Sebaceous glands Microscopic exocrine glands found in the dermis of the skin that secrete sebum to lubricate the skin and hair

Sedentary activities Activities with no physical activity

Seizure A condition in which an individual has sudden convulsions, as in individuals with epilepsy

Self-concept The total person that the child or adolescent envisions himself or herself to be

Self-efficacy The individual's perception of his or her own capabilities

Self-esteem Pride in oneself; self-respect

Self-feeding Feeding, setting up, arranging, and bringing food from the plate or cup to the mouth

Self-regulation Ability to calm self

Semi-Fowler's position Client's head elevated 30 to 45 degrees and knees either in flexion or extension bilaterally

Sensorimotor frame of reference An intervention approach that focuses on using sensory input to change muscle tone or movement patterns; used with children and adolescents who have disorders of the central nervous system

Sensory diet A carefully designed activity plan for sensory input a person needs to stay focused and organized

Sensory discrimination   Ability to discern and assign meaning to specific sensory stimuli

Sensory input   The basic sensations of touch, sound, and movement that influence the parts of the central nervous system that govern and produce skilled, automatic movements

Sensory integration (SI)   The organization of sensory input to produce an adaptive response; a theoretical process and treatment approach; addresses the processing of sensory information from the environment; includes discriminating, integrating, and modulating sensory information in order to produce meaningful, adaptive responses; occupational therapy clinicians may have advanced training and certification in *Ayres Sensory Integration*® *(ASI)* through Western Psychological Services and the University of Southern California

Sensory integration frame of reference   An approach to intervention developed by A.J. Ayres that utilizes suspended equipment and child-directed activity to facilitate adaptive responses and thereby improve central nervous system processing

Sensory modulation   Interpreting and filtering sensory information

Sensory modulation disorder   Impairment in the ability to regulate incoming sensations or failure to detect and orient to novel or important sensory information

Sensory neuron   Also known as *affector neuron*; sends sensory information to be processed by the central nervous system

Sensory processing   The means by which the brain receives, detects, and integrates incoming sensory information for use in producing adaptive responses to one's environment

Sensory system conditions   Diseases, impairments, or deficits in visual, auditory, vestibular, gustatory/olfactory, or tactile functioning

Service competency   The process ensuring that two individual occupational therapy practitioners will obtain equivalent results (i.e., replication) when administering a specific assessment or providing intervention

Service dogs   Dogs that assists people with physical or sensory disabilities. They have specific roles (e.g., sense the onset of a seizure or retrieve desired item from an inaccessible shelf) for which they must be trained

Severe intellectual disability   A category of intellectual disability in which an individual has a below-average IQ (ranging from 25–39) and typically requires extensive support throughout life; generally, individuals may be able to learn basic self-care skills, although they are unable to live independently as adults

Sexual activity   Engaging in activities that result in sexual satisfaction and/or meet relational or reproductive needs

Shaken baby syndrome   A cluster of impairments resulting from an infant being jerked violently back and forth. A severe type of head injury; occurs when an infant and/or child is shaken violently resulting in the brain hitting against the skull. Symptoms include lethargy, tremors, vomiting, coma, and/or death, depending on the extent of the damage

Side-lying   Position referring to lying on one's side

Sitting   A resting position supported by the buttocks and thighs with the trunk somewhat upright

Skeletal system   Organ system consisting of bones, cartilage, and joints that protects and supports internal organs and other body structures; works with the muscular system to create movement at joints

Skill   Observable, goal-directed action that a person uses or demonstrates when performing a task

Skin   Largest organ in the human body; first line of defense for the immune system to guard against potentially harmful invading microbes

Skin integrity   Condition of the skin

Skin irritation   Painful reaction of the skin to chemical or mechanical forces

Sleep/rest   A period of inactivity in which one may or may not suspend consciousness

Sleep-wake disorders   Conditions in which an individual has poor quality, timing, and amount of sleep

SOAP note   A method of documentation that contains the following subject areas: subjective (thoughts, feelings, and verbalizations), objective (session goal and what occurred), assessment (summary of objectives), and plan (future objectives and session goals)

Social groups   Collections of people who come together for formal and/or informal purposes and who influence the things a child or adolescent does when interacting within those social groups

Social interaction skills   Occupational performance skills observed during an ongoing stream of social exchange

Social participation   Associated with the organized patterns of behavior that are expected of a child interacting with others within a given social system, such as the family, peers, or community

Social skills   Skills that promote effectively living and interacting within a community

Soft tissue injury   Damage to muscles, nerves, skin, and/or connective tissue

Somatodyspraxia   Inadequate processing of tactile, proprioceptive, and kinesthetic information that causes difficulty in motor planning

Somatosensory system   Sensory system that processes tactile, proprioceptive, and kinesthetic information

Spasticity A state of increased tone in a muscle with associated exaggerated deep tendon reflex; increased muscle tone; hypertonicity; often occurs when a stretch reflex is activated in a muscle

Specially designed instruction An instruction that has been modified or adapted to meet the specific learning needs of a student with a disability

Specialty clinics Clinics that focus on specifics aspects of care. Examples include hand therapy, spina bifida clinics, cystic fibrosis clinic, etc.

Specific learning disorders Difficulty learning key academic skills during the developmental period

Specific mental functions Factors that refer to attention, memory, perception, thought, higher-level cognition, language, calculation, sequencing complex movements, psychomotor capacity, emotion, and experience of self and time

Spina bifida Split spine (a common disorder seen by the occupational therapy practitioner); comprises three types: occulta, meningocele, and myelomeningocele; common to treat children with myelomeningocele-type spina bifida because of its associated sensory and motor deficits

Spinal cord The bundle of nerve fibers and associated tissue that is enclosed in the spine and connects nearly all parts of the body to the brain, with which it forms the central nervous system

Splint A device that immobilizes, restrains, or supports a part of the body

Splinter skill A specific, often complex task mastered by a child who lacks the underlying developmental capabilities to perform it; usually attained through compensatory methods and practice rather than by remediating the underlying developmental components

Spontaneity Acting without effort or premeditation; driven by internal forces

Sprain A traumatic injury to the tendons, muscle, or ligaments around a joint and characterized by pain, swelling, and discoloration

Standing A resting position supported by the feet with the legs, thighs, and trunk somewhat upright

Static balance (static equilibrioception) Ability to maintain a posture or position without falling over

Static orthosis An orthosis that prevents movement in a desired joint

Stereognosis The ability to identify objects through touch

Stereotypical attitudes Ideas and judgments held about a person based on appearance or other factors

Strabismus "Crossed eyes"; condition in which the eyes do not line up when focusing

Strength Ability of a muscle or muscle group to move against gravity and additional resistance; power

Subacute Condition between acute and chronic

Subluxation An incomplete or partial dislocation of a bone below the joint

Substance abuse A pattern of behavior in which the use of substances has adverse consequences

Substance dependence A pattern of behavior in which substances continue to be used despite serious cognitive, behavioral, and physiologic symptoms

Substance-related disorder A mental disorder resulting from the inappropriate use of drugs, medications, or toxins

Suck–swallow–breathe (s-s-b) synchrony A skill used continuously throughout life that allows an individual to breathe while simultaneously and unconsciously sucking in and swallowing food, drink, and saliva; its disruption can interfere profoundly with development

Superior/cephalad Toward the head

Supination Turning the palm up toward the ceiling

Supine Position referring to being on one's back

Switch A device used to break or open an electric circuit; an item that connects, disconnects, or diverts an electric current; used with children who have disabilities in order to promote successful interaction with computers, battery-operated toys, and powered mobility systems

Symmetric Balanced or evenly distributed, such as weight through the trunk and hips when sitting in chair

Symmetry Alignment of the body in such a way that the head is in the midline position, the trunk is straight, and the weight is distributed equally on both sides of the body

Tactile defensiveness Aversion to touch

Task-focused activity analysis Identifies the physical, social, and mental factors involved in a specific task

Team collaboration Working together and sharing knowledge to obtain a common goal

Teratogen Anything that causes the development of abnormal structures in an embryo and results in a severely deformed fetus

Thalamus Dual-lobed mass of gray matter buried under the cerebral cortex within the brain that is a structure of the limbic system and is involved in sensory perception and regulation of motor functions

Therapeutic horseback riding An equine-assisted activity that primarily focuses on the instruction of riding skills for individuals with disabilities

Therapeutic media Activities that are meaningful and motivating to clients and address their goals

Therapeutic relationship Trusting connection and rapport established between practitioner and client through collaboration, communication, therapist empathy and mutual respect.

Therapeutic use of self The occupational therapy practitioner's "planned use of his or her personality, insights, perceptions, and judgments as part of the therapeutic process" (Punwar & Peloquin, 2000, p. 285) and conscious use of self in therapy as "the use of oneself in such a way that one becomes an effective tool in the evaluation and intervention process" (Mosey); the art of using oneself to successfully promote engagement in chosen daily activities

Tic disorder A mental disorder characterized by tics or involuntary muscle contractions

Tissue Aggregate of cells to perform a particular function

Top-down teaching Teaching that begins with the whole and works down to the individual components

Touch Information received via skin receptors; includes light touch, deep pressure touch, pain, and temperature

Toilet hygiene Typical skills that are learned in early childhood such as clothing management, maintaining toileting position, transferring to and from toileting, and cleaning the body

Tongue thrust A movement in which the tongue extends outside the lips, interferes with swallowing, and causes food to be pushed outside the mouth; often seen in individuals with cerebral palsy or Down syndrome

Top-down approach Focuses on occupations as the means and ends and emphasizing client-centered care

Trachea "Wind pipe"; a cartilaginous tube that connects the larynx to the bronchi of the lungs through which oxygen and carbon dioxide flow

Transdisciplinary "Across" disciplines; this approach involves a variety of professionals who work closely with children and may, in fact, share roles. Team members may work on goals of another profession

Transition plan Plan for change, refers to going to another stage, such as moving from middle to high school or high school to independent living

Transitional movement Movement from one position to another

Trauma Any stressor-related disorders characterized by traumatic or stressful events that result in anxiety-based and/or fear based behaviors that interfere with an individual's active and successful engagement in daily occupations

Traumatic brain injury (TBI) Condition in which there is serious injury to the brain that causes neurologic impairment; a result of acute trauma to the brain; multiple symptoms are associated with the diagnosis of TBI, which vary widely from mild to severe; mild symptoms include loss of consciousness, headache, and blurred vision; moderate or severe TBI symptoms include similar symptoms, in addition to vomiting or nausea, pupil dilation, seizures, slurred speech, weakness or numbness in the extremities, and agitation

Typical Exhibiting qualities, traits, or characteristics that identify a group; not deviating from the standard or norm

Ulnar deviation Moving the wrist ulnarly or toward the little finger

Unilateral Involving one side of the body or one arm/leg

Universal precautions Use of protective barriers such as gloves, gowns, aprons, masks, and/or protective eyewear to decrease risk for exposure to diseases and/or infections

Urinary system Organ system consisting of the kidneys and associated body structures that function to filter nutrients and waste products from blood and other fluids that circulate throughout the body; additional functions include resorption of nutrients and elimination of waste products

Validation Process of establishing evidence

Value Things that a child or adolescent finds important and meaningful

Variable practice Incorporates the practicing of many different skills, with periods of rest. This type of practice is helpful for fine tuning of skills, and helpful in the transfer of learning

Vasculature The arrangement or the distribution of blood vessels in an organ or body part

Vein Vessel that moves blood to the heart

Venule Small vein

Vertebral column Part of the axial skeletal system that comprises vertebrae and functions to protect the spinal cord and to support the body

Vestibular input Linear and/or rotational movement information received in the inner ear

Visuodyspraxia Visual constructive and praxis deficits

Visuomotor integration Ability to coordinate movements through vision

Visuomotor skills Coordination of the eyes with the hands or other body parts in such a way that the eyes guide precisely controlled movements; also referred to as visuomotor integration skills and eye–hand skills or eye–foot skills

Visual accommodation The ability of the eyes to change optical power to maintain focus on an object

Vision impairment A condition of decreased visual acuity or impaired processing of visual input

Visual perception The ability to interpret and use what is being or has been seen

Vocational activities Work-related activities that typically have a monetary incentive or salary; abilities/skills needed for an occupation, trade, or profession

Voice output communication aids (VOCAs) Electronic devices used to supplement or replace speech or writing for individuals with severe speech impairments, enabling them to verbally communicate their needs

Volition   A child's or adolescent's pattern of thoughts and feelings about himself or herself that occur as he or she anticipates, chooses, experiences, and interprets his or her engagement in occupations

Voluntary   Under skeletal muscle control

Wearing protocol or schedule   The specific schedule of orthotic use that varies from child to child and is based on each individual's needs and conditions. It must be carefully explained to the child and family members for maximum benefit of the orthosis

Weight shift   Transferring of body weight from one structure to another

Whole skills   Occupations or activities that can be done automatically (i.e., without thinking)

Wilbarger protocol   Intervention regimen designed to reduce sensory hypersensitivity

Work   An area of occupation that includes employment and volunteer activities

Work simplification/energy conservation techniques   Analyzing and dividing tasks to a simple level to conserve energy; use of large versus small muscle groups

World Health Organization (WHO)   Specialized agency within the United Nations that acts as the coordinating authority on international public health

Bibliography

Ayres, J. (1972). *Sensory integration and learning disorders.* Los Angeles, CA: Western Psychological Services.

Ayres, J. (1985). *Developmental dyspraxia and adult-onset apraxia.* Torrance, CA: Sensory Integration International.

Cornelia de Lange syndrome: United States National Library of medicine: http://ghr.nlm.nih.gov/condition□cornelia-delangesyndrome.

Kielhofner, G. (2008). *Model of Human Occupation: theory and application* (4th ed.). Philadelphia: FA Davis.

May-Benson, T.A., & Cermak S. A. (2007). Development of an assessment for ideational praxis. *Am J Occup Ther, 61,*148–153.

McKinley, W., Silver, T., Santos, K., Pai, A. (2008). Functional outcomes per level of spinal cord injury. http://emedicine.medscape.com/article/322604-overview.

National Institute of Neurological Disorders and Stroke. (2015). *NINDS Pervasive Developmental Disorders Information Page* (adapted from the National Institutes of Neurological Disorders and Stroke, National Institutes of Health). http://www.ninds.nih.gov/disorders/pdd/pdd.htm.

National Institute of Neurological Disorders and Stroke. (2002). *Traumatic brain injury: hope through research.* NIH Publication No. 02-2478. Washington, DC, NIH.

Preamble to the Constitution of the World Health Organization as adopted by the International Health Conference, New York, 19-22 June, 1946; signed on 22 July 1946 by the representatives of 61 States (Official Records of the World Health Organization, no. 2, p. 100) and entered into force on 7 April 1948.

Rothmund-Thomson syndrome (RTS). http://ghr.nlm.nih.gov/condition-rothmundthomson-syndrome.

Stroke. http://www.nlm.nih.gov/medlineplus/ency/article/000726.htm. Accessed 06.10.10.

The American Heritage® Dictionary of the English Language (4th ed.). http://dictionary.reference.com/browse/

"What is NDT?" www.ndta.org/whatisndt.php. Accessed 06.10.10.

INDEX

Note: Page numbers followed by "b", "f" and "t" indicate boxes, figures, and tables, respectively.